SCIENTIFIC FOUNDATIONS
OF
OBSTETRICS AND GYNAECOLOGY

Scientific Foundations of Obstetrics and Gynaecology

Edited by

ELLIOT E. PHILIPP

M.A., M.B., B.Ch. (Cantab.), F.R.C.S. (England), F.R.C.O.G.

*Consultant Obstetrician and Gynaecologist, Royal Northern Hospital
and City of London Maternity Hospital, London.*

JOSEPHINE BARNES

M.A., D.M. (Oxon), F.R.C.P. (London), F.R.C.S. (England), F.R.C.O.G.

*Consultant Obstetrician and Gynaecologist, Charing Cross Hospital
and Elizabeth Garrett Anderson Hospital.*

and

MICHAEL NEWTON

M.A., M.B., B.Ch. (Cantab), M.D. (Pennsylvania), F.A.C.S., F.A.C.O.G.

*Clinical Professor, Department of Obstetrics and Gynecology. Pritzker School of Medicine, University of Chicago.
Attending staff, Chicago Lying-in Hospital. Director, The American College of Obstetricians and Gynecologists.*

LONDON

WILLIAM HEINEMANN MEDICAL BOOKS LTD

First Published 1970

Reprinted 1971

S.B.N. 433 25100 X

Printed in Great Britain at the Pitman Press, Bath

PREFACE

The object of this book is to compile and integrate the basic scientific information on which the clinical practice of Obstetrics and Gynaecology depends.

It is an international volume with contributors from many countries and many disciplines ranging from cell biology to statistics. The authors were chosen as recognised authorities in their particular fields; or because the work they had done would soon make them so.

In our briefing to our contributors we asked that each chapter "should contain the background material necessary for understanding current advances and should include recent and pertinent information in the field. Its emphasis should be on the basic scientific data, but it should be related to current practice in obstetrics and gynaecology".

On the whole the writers have kept to their brief, and we the editors have not substantially altered the material sent to us. Nor have we altered the English phrasing, except in the case of one or two authors whose native language is not English. Thus American authors have freely used their own terminology, phrasing and spelling, and other authors whichever style they chose for themselves. We have accepted this divergence in style and language feeling that any changes we could have made towards greater uniformity would unwisely have destroyed the individuality in the writing.

We did not dictate very rigidly the length any chapter should be; on occasions we have cut here and there and on other occasions have asked the authors to expand their work. As a result we have noticed that the approach to basic sciences differs markedly depending on whether the writer works primarily in the laboratory or is primarily a clinician.

For us this unevenness adds to the interest and we hope it will do so for our readers. Some re-duplication has deliberately been permitted to demonstrate differences in approach and to allow extra emphasis on important findings and implications.

Our gratitude to our contributors, our publishers and our secretaries and especially to Mrs. Mary Burd who has not only been a secretary but the perfect intermediary between "all interested parties" is here most sincerely expressed.

We should also like to express gratitude to all those authorities who have so generously permitted reproduction of their published work and illustrations. We have acknowledged this whenever we knew the source and if inadvertently any single source is omitted, this has occurred in spite of the greatest care to see that all sources are correct and that none have been left out.

We hope that the intention of our publishers that a bridge shall have been built between the work of the laboratory and the work of the clinician in Obstetrics and Gynaecology has been fulfilled.

THE EDITORS

SPECIAL ACKNOWLEDGEMENT
Section III, Chapter 8

We record our indebtedness to the many obstetricians and pathologists who have helped us. It is not possible to thank them all by name here. We wish to thank Dr. G. A. K. Missen who presented us with the 14-day embryos. Prof. J. S. Baxter very generously placed at our disposal the 'Gar' embryo, and Prof. T. B. Johnston gave us permission to examine the H.R.I. embryo; to both we are very grateful. It would, however, be remiss not to single out Mr. H. Arthure, Miss Josephine Barnes, Miss Gladys H. Dodds, Miss A. Dickins, Dr. D. Haler, Mr. B. Eton, Mr. O. Lloyd, Miss Janet Bottomley, Dr. Alice Townsley, Mr. Bentall, Dr. A. Gresham and Dr. J. Rack who have, often at great personal inconvenience, made so many specimens available to us.

We also must thank Messrs. A. Campbell, J. W. Cash, J. F. Crane, J. A. F. Fozzard, M.A., F.R.P.S., K. Iles, G. Oakes, E. J. Park, F.I.S.T., K. W. Thurley and R. H. Watts, and Mrs. Elizabeth Green and Mrs. Janet Parker.

W. J. HAMILTON
J. D. BOYD

This book is dedicated to the memory of
WILLIAM CHARLES WALLACE NIXON

CONTENTS

SECTION I

GENERAL

SECTION II

FEMALE GENITAL TRACT

SECTION III

OVUM AND FOETUS

SECTION IV

BLOOD AND THE CARDIOVASCULAR SYSTEM

SECTION IX

THE CENTRAL NERVOUS SYSTEM

SECTION X

ENDOCRINOLOGY

LIST OF CONTRIBUTORS

E. C. AMOROSO, C.B.E., M.D., F.R.C.O.G., F.R.C.S., F.R.C.P., F.R.S.
Emeritus Professor of Physiology, Agricultural Research Council, Institute of Animal Physiology, Babraham, Cambridge.

HEINZ BARTELS, M.D. (Tubingen)
Professor of Physiology, Medizinische Hochschule, Hanover.

GEOFFREY M. BERLYNE, M.D., F.R.C.P.
Director of Nephrological Unit, Central Negev Hospital, Beersheba, Israel; Professor of Medicine, Wayne State University School of Medicine, Detroit, U.S.A.; Reader in Medicine, University of Manchester.

J. S. BIGGS, M.B., B.S., M.R.C.O.G.
Senior Lecturer in Obstetrics and Gynaecology, University of Brisbane; Formerly Lecturer in Obstetrics and Gynaecology, University of Aberdeen.

W. D. BILLINGTON, M.A., B.Sc., PH.D.
Research Officer, Department of Zoology, University of Oxford; Lecturer in Zoology, Merton College, Oxford.

C. E. BLANK, M.B., PH.D.
Reader in Medical Genetics, Sheffield University; Consultant in Human Genetics, United Sheffield Hospitals.

G. L. BOURNE, F.R.C.S., F.R.C.O.G.
Consultant Obstetrician and Gynaecologist, St. Bartholomew's Hospital, London.

H. BOUTOURLINE YOUNG, M.D., M.R.C.P.
Research Associate in Human Growth and Development, Harvard University, Assistant Professor of Paediatrics, Yale University.

DAVID BOWSHER, M.A., M.D., Ph.D.
Director, Laboratory of Neurobiology, Department of Anatomy, University of Liverpool; Honorary Clinical Assistant, Regional Neurosurgical Unit, Walton Hospital, Liverpool.

J. D. BOYD, M.A., M.D., D.Sc., F.R.C.O.G.
Late Professor of Anatomy, in the University of Cambridge; Late fellow of Clare College, Cambridge. Formerly Professor of Anatomy, in the University of London at The London Hospital Medical School.

W. BRUMFITT, M.D., Ph.D., M.R.C.P., F.C.Path.
Consultant Clinical Pathologist, Edgware General Hospital, Middlesex; Senior Lecturer in Bacteriology, Wright-Fleming Institute, St. Mary's Hospital, and Honorary Consultant Bacteriologist, St. Mary's Hospital, London.

H. J. CAMPBELL, B.Sc., Ph.D.
Senior Lecturer, Institute of Psychiatry (Department Physiology), London.

R. W. CARRELL, M.B., Ch.B., B.Sc. Hons. (N.Z.), Ph.D. (Cantab.)
Senior Registrar in Clinical Biochemistry, Addenbrookes Hospital, Cambridge 1965–1967; Chemical Pathologist, Christchurch Hospital. New Zealand.

C. O. CARTER, D.M., F.R.C.P.
Director, Medical Research Council Clinical Genetic Unit, London; Honorary Consultant in Genetics, The Hospital for Sick Children, London.

ROMA N. CHAMBERLAIN, M.B.Ch.B., D.C.H., D.R.C.O.G., C.P.H.
Former Principal Medical Officer, Ministry of Health. Lecturer in Paediatrics at St. Mary's Hospital Medical School, London; Co-Director of the British Births Survey 1970 of the National Birthday Trust and Royal College of Obstetricians and Gynaecologists.

T. E. CLEGHORN, M.D., B.Sc., M.R.C.P., F.C.Path.
Director, North London Blood Transfusion Centre, Edgware.

A. P. CONDIE, M.B., Ch.B., M.R.C.O.G.
Consultant Obstetrician and Gynaecologist, Edgware General Hospital, Edgware, Middlesex.

T. A. CONNORS, Ph.D.
Senior Lecturer, Department of Pharmacology, Institute of Cancer Research, Royal Cancer Hospital.

A. T. COWIE, M.R.C.V.S., Ph.D., D.Sc.

A. CARLETON CROOKE, M.A., M.D., F.R.C.P.
Consultant Endocrinologist, United Birmingham Hospitals; Director, Department of Clinical Endocrinology, The Women's Hospital, Birmingham; Honorary Reader in Medicine, Birmingham University.

JOHN A. DAVIS
Professor of Child Health and Paediatrics, University of Manchester.

C. J. DEWHURST, M.B., F.R.C.S., F.R.C.O.G.
Professor of Obstetrics and Gynaecology, Institute of Obstetrics and Gynaecology, Queen Charlotte's Hospital and Chelsea Hospital for Women, London.

S. J. FOLLEY, Ph.D., D.Sc., F.R.S.
Research Professor, in the University of Reading and Head of the Physiology Department, National Institute for Research in Dairying.

L. L. FRANCHI, B.Sc., Ph.D. (Nott.).
Senior Lecturer in Microanatomy, Anatomy Department, The Medical School, University of Birmingham.

HAYAMI FUJIMORI, M.D., Ph.D.
President of the Ninth Annual Meeting of the Japanese Society of Nuclear Medicine; Honorary member of the Japanese Society of Obstetrics and Gynaecology; Formerly Professor and Chairman, The Department of Obstetrics and Gynaecology, Osaka City University Medical School, Osaka, Japan. Consultant, the Shiseikai Kansai Hospital (The Alumni Hospital of Tokyo Women's Medical College).

R. L. GADD, M.D. (Manc.), F.R.C.S. (Ed.), F.R.C.O.G.
Clinical Lecturer, Department of Obstetrics and Gynaecology, University of Manchester; Consultant Obstetrician and Gynaecologist, St. Mary's Hospital, United Manchester Hospitals.

CARL AXEL GEMZELL, M.D., Ph.D.
Professor and Chairman, Department of Obstetrics and Gynaecology, University Hospital, Uppsala, Sweden.

JEAN GINSBURG, M.A., D.M. (Oxon).
Consultant Physician, Endocrine Unit, Royal Free Hospital; Senior Lecturer in Endocrinology, Royal Free Hospital Medical School, London.

C. GOPALAN, M.D., Ph.D., F.R.C.P.E.
Director, Nutrition Research Laboratories, Hyderabad, India.

W. J. HAMILTON, M.D., D.Sc., F.R.C.S., F.R.C.O.G., F.R.S.E.
Professor of Anatomy in the University of London at Charing Cross Hospital Medical College, sometime Regius Professor of Anatomy in the University of Glasgow, formerly Professor of Anatomy in the University of London at the Medical College of St. Bartholomew's Hospital.

C. W. H. HAVARD, M.A., D.M., M.R.C.P.
Consultant Physician, Royal Northern Hospital, Royal Free Group of Hospitals and Saint Mark's Hospital, London.

SHEILA G. HAWORTH, M.B., B.S., M.R.C.P.
Fellow in Fetal Physiology and Neonatology, Columbia University, New York.

B. M. HIBBARD, M.D. (London), Ph.D. (Liverpool), F.R.C.O.G.
Senior Lecturer in Obstetrics and Gynaecology, University of Liverpool; Honorary Consultant Obstetrician and Gynaecologist, United Liverpool Hospitals and Liverpool Regional Hospital Board.

ELIZABETH D. HIBBARD, M.D. (Aberdeen), D.Obst.R.C.O.G.
Lecturer in Obstetrics and Gynaecology, University of Liverpool.

ARTHUR HOLLMAN, M.D. (Lond.), F.R.C.P.
Consultant Cardiologist, University College Hospital, London.

DAVID HULL, B.Sc., M.R.C.P., D.C.H., D.Obst. R.C.O.G.
Consultant Physician, Hospital for Sick Children, Great Ormond Street, London.

ROSALINDE HURLEY, LL.B., M.D., M.C.Path.
Consultant Bacteriologist, Queen Charlotte's Maternity Hospital, London; Lecturer, The Institute of Obstetrics and Gynaecology, University of London.

A. G. I. INGELMAN-SUNDBERG, M.D.
Professor of Obstetrics and Gynaecology, Royal Caroline Institute; Chairman of the University Department of Obstetrics and Gynaecology, Sabbatsberg Hospital, Stockholm; Scientific Consultant, Swedish National Board of Health and Welfare; Scientific Consultant, Medical Board of Swedish National Defence.

S. LEON ISRAEL, A.B., M.D.
Professor of Obstetrics and Gynaecology, School of Medicine, University of Pennsylvania; Director, Department of Obstetrics and Gynaecology, Pennsylvania Hospital.

L. STANLEY JAMES, M.D.
Professor of Paediatrics, Columbia Presbyterian Medical Center, Columbia University, New York.

M. F. JAYLE
Professeur de Biochimie, Faculté de Médecine de Paris.

B. E. JUEL-JENSEN, M.A., B.M. (Oxon), Cand.med. (Copenhagen).
Consultant Physician, Radcliffe Infirmary, Oxford; Clinical Lecturer in Medicine, University of Oxford.

W. LANGREDER, Professor, Dr. Med. et res nat., University of Mainz, Hohenlimburg Hospital.

R. J. B. KING, B.Sc., M.Sc., Ph.D.
Head of Hormone Biochemistry Department, Imperial Cancer Research Fund, London.

A. I. KLOPPER, B.Sc., Ph.D., M.D., F.R.C.O.G.
Reader in Obstetrics and Gynaecology, University of Aberdeen.

KERMIT E. KRANTZ, B.S., B.M., M.S. (Anatomy), M.D.
Professor and Chairman, Department of Gynaecology and Obstetrics, University of Kansas Medical Center, Professor of Anatomy, University of Kansas Medical Center, National Civilian Consultant Gynaecology and Obstetrics, Surgeon General, U.S. Air Force.

G. C. LIGGINS, M.B., B.S., F.R.C.S. (Ed.), F.R.C.O.G.
Senior Lecturer, School of Obstetrics and Gynaecology, University of Auckland, New Zealand.

MARY G. MCGEOWN, M.D., Ph.D., F.R.C.P.E.
Consultant Nephrologist Physician in Charge, Renal Unit, Belfast City Hospital; Honorary Lecturer in Nephrology, Queen's University of Belfast.

IAN MACGILLIVRAY, M.D., Ch.B., F.R.C.O.G.
Regius Professor of Obstetrics and Gynaecology, University of Aberdeen; Formerly Professor of Obstetrics and Gynaecology in London University at St. Mary's Hospital Medical School.

PAMELA J. MALPOIX-HIGGINS, Ph.D.
Research Assistant, Faculté des Sciences, University Libre de Bruxelles, Belgium.

T. MANN, C.B.E., M.D., Sc.D., Ph.D., F.R.S.
Professor of Physiology of Reproduction in the University of Cambridge; Director of the A.R.C. Unit of Reproductive Physiology and Biochemistry, Cambridge.

E. MARLEY, M.A., M.D., D.Sc., F.R.C.P., D.P.M.
Reader in Pharmacology, Institute of Psychiatry, University of London; Honorary Physician, The Bethlem Royal and Maudsley Hospitals.

A. STUART MASON, M.D. (Cantab.), F.R.C.P. (Lond.).
Consultant Endocrinologist, The London Hospital and Oldchurch Hospital, Romford, Essex; Honorary Consultant, Endocrine Department, New End Hospital, Hampstead.

LUIGI MASTROIANNI, Jr., M.D.
Professor and Chairman of Obstetrics and Gynaecology, School of Medicine, University of Pennsylvannia.

J. CHASSAR MOIR, C.B.E., Hon.LLD., M.M.S.A. (Hon. Caus.), M.A., M.D., F.R.C. (Edin.), F.R.C.O.G.
Emeritus Professor, Obstetrics and Gynaecology, University of Oxford.

N. B. MYANT, D.M., M.R.C.P.
Director, Medical Research Council Lipid Metabolism Unit, Hammersmith Hospital, London.

P. W. NATHAN, M.D., F.R.C.P.
External Scientific Staff, Medical Research Council, The National Hospital for Nervous Diseases, London.

L. C. PAYNE, B.Sc., Ph.D. (Cantab.), F.B.C.S.
Formerly Director, Medical Automation Experiment Unit, University College Hospital, London; Medical Computing Consultant.

E. E. PHILIPP, M.A., M.B., B.Ch., F.R.C.S., F.R.C.O.G.
Consultant Obstetrician and Gynaecologist, Royal Northern Hospital and City of London Maternity Hospital, London.

SIR GEORGE WHITE PICKERING, M.D., F.R.C.P., F.R.S.
Master of Pembroke College, Oxford; Emeritus Regius Professor of Medicine, University of Oxford.

D. G. PORTER, M.Sc., Ph.D., B.Vet.Med., M.R.C.V.S.
Lecturer in Physiology, Department of Physiology, Royal Veterinary College, London.

MAY REED, B.Sc., Ph.D.
Member of Medical Research Council's Scientific Staff at the National Institute for Medical Research (1958–1961), Member of Medical Research Council's Neuro-endocrinology Unit in Department of Human Anatomy at Oxford.

PHILIP RHODES, M.A., M.B., F.R.C.S., F.R.C.O.G.
Professor of Obstetrics and Gynaecology, in the University of London at St. Thomas's Hospital Medical School.

C. R. RIZZA, M.D. (St. And.), M.R.C.P. (Ed.).
Consultant Physician, Oxford Haemophilia Centre; Clinical Lecturer in Haematology, University of Oxford.

JOSEPH J. ROVINSKY, M.D., F.A.C.S., F.A.C.O.G.
Associate Professor of Obstetrics and Gynecology, The Mount Sinai School of Medicine; Attending Obstetrician and Gynecologist, The Mount Sinai Hospital, New York; Chief Obstetrician and Gynecologist, City Hospital Center at Elmhurst, New York.

J. W. SCOPES, M.B., Ph.D., M.R.C.P.
Senior Lecturer, Institute of Child Health, London University; Honorary Consultant Children's Physician, Hammersmith Hospital.

D. M. SERR, M.D.
Associate Professor of Obstetrics and Gynaecology, University of Tel-Aviv Medical School. Director, Department of Obstetrics and Gynaecology, Tel-Hashomer Government Hospital, Israel.

SHEILA SHERLOCK, M.D., F.R.C.P. (Lond.), F.R.C.P. (Edin.), F.A.C.P. (Hon.).
Professor of Medicine in University of London at the Royal Free Hospital School of Medicine; Consultant Physician, Royal Free Hospital.

LANDRUM B. SHETTLES, B.A., M.A., Ph.D., M.D., D.Sc., F.A.C.S., F.A.C.O.G.
Diplomate of American Board of Obstetricians and Gynecologists, Diplomate of Pan American Medical Association In Obstetrics and Gynecology. Assistant Professor in Clinical Obstetrics and Gynecology, College of Physicians and Surgeons, Columbia University, and Assistant attending Obstetrician and Gynecologist, Columbia-Presbyterian Medical Center, New York.

L. STEINGOLD, M.B., Ch.B., F.R.C.Path.
Consultant Pathologist, St. Andrew's Hospital, London and Poplar Hospital, London.

C. N. SMYTH, D.M., B.Sc. (Eng.), F.I.E.E., F.Inst.P.
Formerly Senior Lecturer and Nuffield Research Assistant to the Obstetric Unit. Senior Lecturer in Experimental Surgery, University College Hospital Medical School. Consultant in Clinical Measurements, University College Hospital, London.

C. C. SPICER, M.R.C.S., Dip. Bact., Dip.Roy.Stat.Soc.
Senior Epidemiologist, Public Health Laboratory Service; Statistician, Imperial Cancer Research Fund; Chief Medical Statistician, General Register Office; Director, Medical Research Council, Computer Unit, London.

J. D. STEPHENSON, B.Sc., Ph.D.
Research Worker, Institute of Psychiatry, University of London.

G. W. THEOBALD, M.A., M.D. (Cantab.), M.R.C.P. (Lond.), F.R.C.S.E., F.R.C.O.G., L.M. (Rotunda).
Honorary Research Fellow, University College Hospital, Obstetric Hospital, London; Late Consultant Obstetrician and Gynaecologist, St. Luke's Maternity Hospital, Bradford; Formerly Professor of Obstetrics and Gynaecology, Bangkok; Ex-Assistant Master, The Rotunda Hospital, Dublin.

H. G. TUCHMANN-DUPLESSIS, M.D., Ph.D.
Professor, Faculté de Médicine, Paris; Biologiste, Hopitaux de Paris; Directeur, L'Ecole des Hautes Etudes.

J. W. URSCHEL, B.A., M.Sc., M.D., Ph.D., C.R.C.P.(C.).
Research Assistant, Department of Physiology, Institute of Psychiatry, London. Department of Psychiatry, University of Alberta, Canada.

S. WAY, F.R.C.O.G.
Lecturer in Gynaecological Oncology, University of Newcastle upon Tyne; Surgeon, Gynaecological Research Department, Queen Elizabeth Hospital, Gateshead on Tyne.

C. P. WENDELL-SMITH, M.B., B.S., Ph.D. (Lond.), D.Obst., R.C.O.G., M.A.C.E.
Professor of Anatomy in the University of Tasmania; Honorary Anatomist to the Royal Hobart Hospital, Hobart, Tasmania.

M. E. WHISSON, M.B., B.S.
Senior Lecturer, Department of Pharmacology, Institute of Cancer Research, London.

LEIF WIDE, M.D.
Assistant Professor of Clinical Chemistry, University Hospital, Uppsala, Sweden.

SIR BRIAN WINDEYER, F.R.C.P., F.R.C.S., F.F.R.
Vice Chancellor of the University of London; Professor of Radiology (Therapeutic), University of London; Director, Meyerstein Institute of Radiotherapy, The Middlesex Hospital, London.

SECTION I

GENERAL

1. THE CELL

P. MALPOIX-HIGGINS

INTRODUCTION

The schematic picture given in Figure 1 illustrates the important structures involved in the vital functions of the living cell: reproduction, nutrition, locomotion, energy production. Briefly, the genetic material in the nucleus transmits hereditary characters at cell division (mitosis and meiosis) and also controls, in the interphase cell, most

exchanges, in which nucleus and cytoplasm influence one another, and where nucleocytoplasmic exchanges and diverse other metabolic phenomena vary from one cell to another, at different stages in the life of the cell itself, and in that of the organism of which it is part.

Since Schleiden, the botanist, and Schwann, the zoologist, first put forward their theory of "cell-doctrine" in

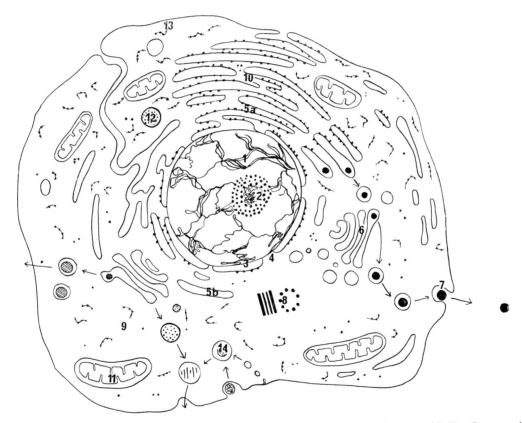

Fig. 1. Diagram of a typical cell based on ultrastructural studies and present experimental data (courtesy of P. Van Gansen and H. Bruge).
1. The nucleus, 2. The nucleolus; granular and fibrillar regions are visible, 3. Nuclear membrane, 4. Nuclear pore, 5. Endoplasmic reticulum:
5a: rough endoplasmic reticulum, 5b: smooth endoplasmic reticulum, 6. Golgi body, 7. Elimination of polysaccharides, 8. Centrioles: one
in longitudinal section, the other in cross section, 9. Free ribosomes and polysomes, 10. Ribosomes attached to membranes, 11. Mitochondria,
12. Lysosome, 13. Cell membrane, 14. Phagosome.

of the major synthetic processes. In the cytoplasm, the mitochondria are responsible for energy production, whereas the ribosomes and polysomes, both free and associated with the endoplasmic reticulum, are the main sites of protein synthesis. Apart from such fundamental facts, it is difficult to generalize. The cell must indeed be thought of as a dynamic unit of life, in constant movement, undergoing continuous intracellular and extracellular

1939, our knowledge of living cells has greatly increased. Original techniques and ideas have created a new and rapidly evolving science: "Molecular Biology", itself an interesting meeting place for many scientific disciplines. With the electron microscope, ultrastructure can now be visualized in minute, molecular detail.

Phase contrast microscopy has been successfully combined with microcinematography for the study of cells cultivated *in vitro*. Interference microscopy permits the measurement of the dry mass of parts of the cell, and provides a valuable reference unit for other cytochemical measurements.

The ultraviolet microscope permits the estimation of the nucleic acid content of the cell, and its use in conjunction with other techniques has furnished a great deal of interesting data. For instance, high resolution, rapid scanning, spectrophotometric techniques have recently been developed which enable the distribution of DNA (deoxyribonucleic acid) along the chromosomes to be determined with a resolution of $0.3\,\mu$. Cytological findings are being confirmed and completed by biochemical work, and vice versa. Radioisotopes and a multitude of techniques for their measurement have increased our knowledge of cell metabolism. The concepts which once required an ingenious flash of understanding, like the initial perception, in the early forties, by Brachet and Caspersson working independently, of the importance of the relationship between ribonucleic acid and protein synthesis, are now being subjected to minute analysis and being confirmed by elaborate techniques.

1. The Molecular Basis of Cell Function

Knowledge of nucleic acid structure and its relation to function have enabled extensive interpretation of living processes in terms of macromolecular structure.

Bacteriophage and bacteria have served the initial experimental study of many of the problems of cell metabolism, because of their low level of complexity. Thus, the demonstration by Hershey and Chase (1953) that bacteriophage DNA carries the viral genetic information from parent to progeny was an early important step toward the understanding of fundamental biological processes: growth and inheritance.

Given the basic chemical structure of DNA (shown in Figure 2a), X-ray diffraction studies and molecular model building enabled Watson and Crick (1953a, and b) to postulate that the DNA molecule in fact consists of two polynucleotide chains joined together by hydrogen bonds between base pairs: wherever the nucleotide base adenine (A) occurs in one chain, thymine (T) occurs in the other; similarly, guanine (G) always pairs with cytosine (C).

Biological Functions of the DNA Molecule

Two fundamental biological processes are performed by the DNA molecule:

(1) *reproduction*, which involves the accurate *replication* of the DNA molecule itself and its segregation between daughter cells;

(2) *growth and differentiation*, which involves the *transmission* of the genetic message contained in DNA to *complementary RNA molecules* which code for *specific proteins*.

Replication of DNA

In order for DNA to replicate, the 2 polynucleotide chains which are wound helically around a common axis, have to come apart, so that each can act as a "template" on which a new complementary chain can be laid down.

Meselson and Stahl (1958) were the first to demonstrate experimentally that each molecule of DNA in the coli bacterium is composed of *equal parts* of newly synthesized DNA and DNA present in the previous generation (this is called semi-conservative replication). (Fig. 3.)

A further important step was the isolation by Lehman, Bessman, Simms and Kornberg (1958) of an enzyme called DNA polymerase, able to synthesize in the test tube chains complementary in base sequence to small segments of DNA offered as templates, given the presence of the required precursors. Since then it has become possible to "visualize" the duplication of the DNA molecule by autoradiography (Cairns, 1963). Escherischia coli was used for this technique: its genome is composed of only one DNA molecule, the duplication of which occupies virtually the entire cycle of cell division. This single chromosome is circular, while replicating. It duplicates by forming a fork, and from this single fast moving locus, two new daughter limbs are formed, each containing one strand of new material and one strand of old.

Recent experiments have revealed that DNA polymerase makes few, if any, errors in replicating DNA in the test tube (Goulian, Kornberg and Sinsheimer, 1967). A "polynucleotide-joining" enzyme, which catalyses the covalent joining of two opposite ends of DNA chains, has been isolated and purified. Its addition to an *in vitro* system for DNA replication, enables such accurate replication of one of the strands of viral DNA that a duplex circular viral DNA genome identical to the one produced *in vivo*, is obtained (made up of the template (+) strand and the newly synthesized (−) strand). The *biological activity* of the molecule so obtained is a major proof of accurate replication; other physical and chemical criteria make the evidence complete. Such techniques should be applicable to the duplex circular genomes of other viruses and to DNA molecules of comparable structure from cellular organelles like mitochondria, and may open up a new field of *in vitro* genetics, (by insertion of base and nucleotide analogs into living genomes). However, in higher organisms the genome is composed of not one, but many DNA molecules, grouped together in chromosomes that contain not only DNA, but also proteins and other macromolecules.

The analysis and *in vitro* synthesis of such DNA (which has not been shown to be circular) is therefore a much more complex problem. Moreover, according to a recent publication (Couch and Hanawalt, 1967) the DNA polymerase system which functions so successfully *in vitro* may only correspond to a "repair" mechanism. As we have mentioned, only *one* of the strands of the ϕX-viral DNA is synthesized in the test tube, whereas the *simultaneous* synthesis of the two strands, as required for the complete synthesis of a DNA duplex at a single locus, may require yet another enzyme.

The Genetic Code

The exact sequence of the four bases: A, G, T and C attached to the backbone of repeating groups of phosphate and a five carbon sugar, represents the DNA code, composed of triplets of nucleotides, for protein synthesis.

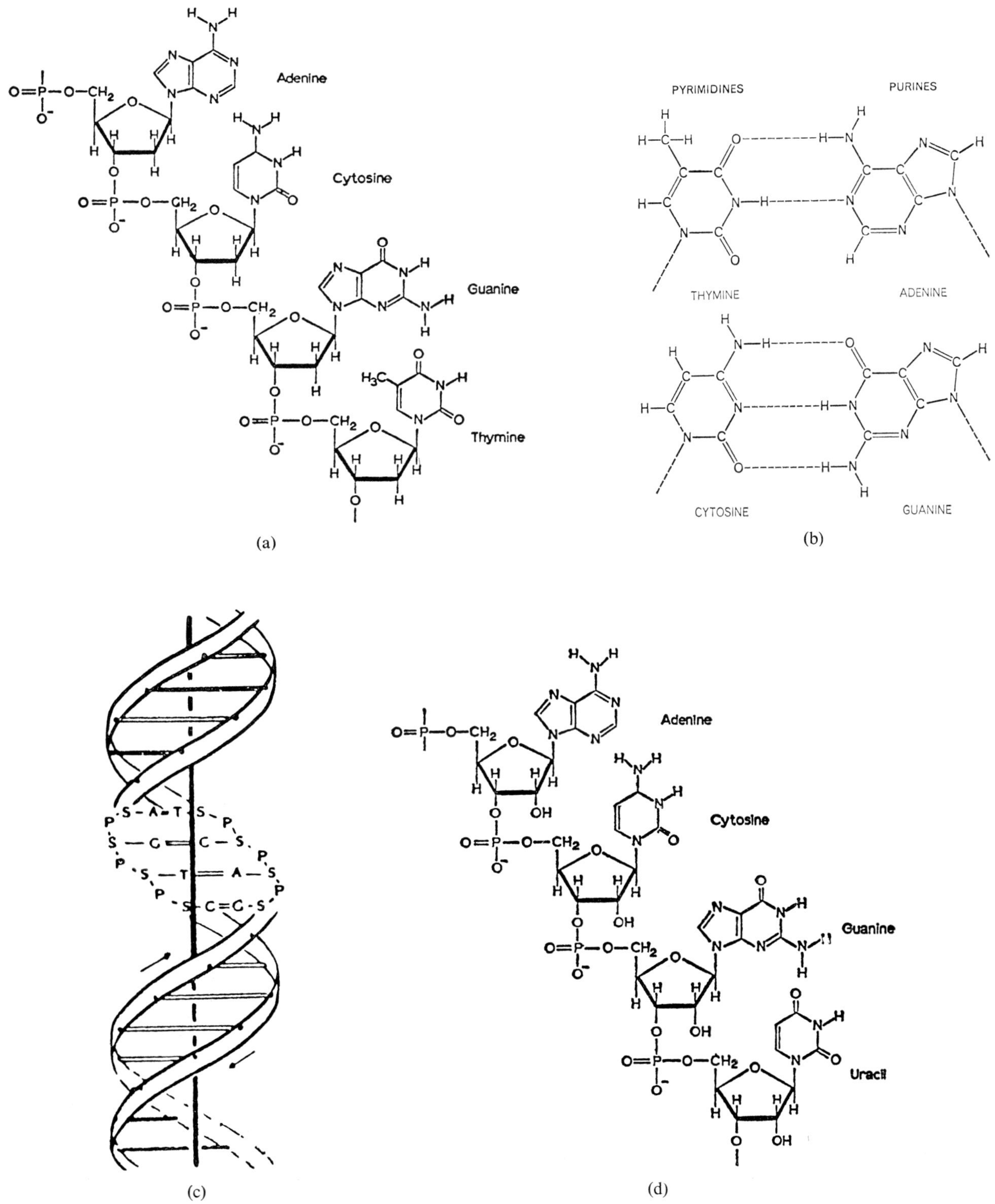

(a)

(b)

(c)

(d)

FIG. 2. (a) Diagram of the DNA molecule. (b) Diagram of the pairing of the four bases in DNA. Cytosine is linked to guanine, and thymine to adenine, by hydrogen bonds. (c) Diagram of the DNA double helix. Alternating sugar (S) and phosphate (P) groups form the backbone. One of the four bases (A, G, T or C) is attached to each sugar. Hydrogen bonds link the bases. (d) Chemical structure of RNA resembles that of DNA, except that it contains a ribose instead of a deoxyribose sugar, and in place of the base thymine, uracil (U) is found.

Before the coded message can be *translated* during the assembly of amino acids into proteins, it is first of all *transferred* to another type of nucleic acid: ribonucleic acid (RNA). The structure of the latter, also given in Figure 2d, is very similar to that of DNA; it differs in containing a ribose instead of a deoxyribose sugar, and in containing uracil (U) instead of thymine as the fourth base of its code, which is therefore made up of A, C, G and U. Ribonucleic acids (RNAs) which carry this coded message from the DNA to the site of protein synthesis, are called messenger RNAs (mRNAs).

The nucleic acid message and the corresponding polypeptide chain are known to be colinear, in that units (codons) composed of triplets of nucleotides in the nucleic acid chain correspond to units (amino acid residues) in the polypeptide chain. (See Sec. IV Chap 4. Eds.)

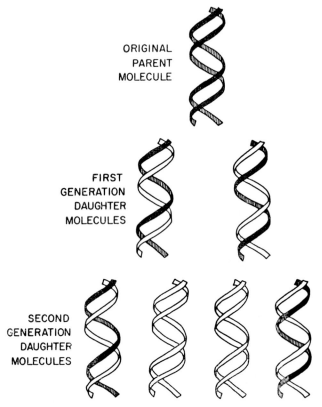

FIG. 3. Model of semi-conservative replication of DNA (after Meselsohn and Stahl, 1958).

RNA Synthesis and its Regulation

RNA is synthesized on a single strand of DNA by a process called *transcription* which, like DNA replication, therefore requires the separation of the 2 DNA strands of the duplex.

The way in which the transcription process is initiated or cut off, has been the object of an elaborate theory proposed by Jacob and Monod (1961) and which has been shown to be applicable to slight changes in their surrounding milieu by the synthesis of specific proteins. In such organisms, small molecules can trigger off the synthesis of

messenger RNAs for whole chains of enzymes by acting on a controlling "operator" site on DNA, which itself influences the DNA sequences (cistrons) coding for a group of enzymes. (Fig. 4).

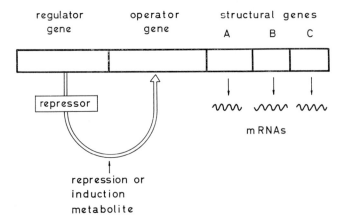

FIG. 4. Double genetic control of enzyme synthesis in bacteria (after Jacob and Monod, 1961). The molecular organization of proteins is determined by *structural* genes. The activity of the structural genes is controlled by two determinants called *regulator* and *operator* genes, *Repressors* which can either be activated (repression) by specific metabolites or inactivated (induction), act as intermediaries between regulator and operator genes. Several structural genes may respond to a single operator site: grouped operator and structural genes form, together, the *operon*.

Protein Synthesis

Protein synthesis occurs on the surface of ribosomes. These small particles are made up of two sub-units, each containing both RNA and proteins (structural proteins and enzymes). Ribosomes have specific surfaces that bind mRNA and amino-acids attached to the "adaptor" molecule: tRNA. The ribosomes are thus the site of encounter of previously activated amino acids, brought to them by specific transfer RNA, of messenger RNA, and of enzymes involved in the formation of the peptide linkage.

The process of polypeptide assembly on ribosomes is shown schematically in Figure 5: it is the fundamental step in protein synthesis on polysomes, and is called *translation*.

2. The Complexity of Eukaryotes

Many of the fundamental molecular mechanisms related to nucleic acid and protein synthesis in biological systems, have been elucidated in the simplest of living organisms: viruses and bacteria, whose genome is usually composed of only one long DNA molecule. Basic functions in the cells of higher organisms are similar.

The genetic code based on triplets of bases in nucleic acids is universal. But control mechanisms and regulatory processes are certainly *not identical* in prokaryotes and eukaryotes. Indeed, in the interphase nucleus of the latter, the genetic material of the cell is separated from the cytoplasm by a nuclear envelope; the size and complexity of the genome itself, and its macromolecular support in the chromosomes, is quite different. The process of transcription most often takes place in the nucleus, while that of translation (assembly of polypeptides on ribosomes) occurs in the cytoplasm. But this is not always so, as we

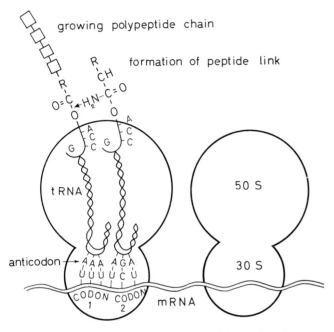

FIG. 5. *Messenger RNA* brings the coded instructions for the assembly of amino acids to form protein molecules A triplet of bases, the *codon*, in mRNA, specifies each amino acid. Activated amino acids are brought to the ribosomal site by a transfer RNA carrying a complementary triplet, the *anticodon*, which is the site recognizing the codon. On the larger subunit (50S) of the ribosome, there is a specific site for accepting transfer RNA. A specific site for mRNA exists on the smaller ribosomal unit (30S). The ribosomes move along the messenger RNA while the code is being read, and in this way, by stepwise addition of amino-acids, the polypeptide chain is built up.

shall see in looking more closely at the cell and its organelles. It is therefore useful to construct a simple schema illustrating present knowledge on the subject of control mechanisms in higher organisms (Fig. 6); this diagram excludes the "operon" concept of Jacob and Monod, since experimental evidence of its existence in eukaryotes has not yet been found.

The rich complexity of the situation, and the idea of cell science as a rapidly evolving subject, will be easier to grasp if we simultaneously select several interesting and original aspects of present day cell research to illustrate the fundamental picture. For instance, present studies on the *distribution of DNA* are revealing *the presence of some of this genetic material outside the nucleus, in or associated* with certain *cytoplasmic organelles. Long lived messenger RNAs* represent, moreover, a cytoplasmic reserve of genetic information and therefore render the cytoplasm independent of nuclear control, as far as protein synthesis is concerned, for periods of time which vary with the length

of life of the messengers. This is why an important aspect of cell studies is that of *nucleocytoplasmic relations* and the extent to which nuclear control of cytoplasmic events is reciprocated by cytoplasmic control of nuclear metabolism. A closely related paradox concerns *oogenesis, embryogenesis and cell differentiation.*

The changing patterns of nucleic acid metabolism throughout the life cycle of higher organisms, beginning with the oocyte, is a fundamental aspect. All the somatic cells of multicellular animals seem to contain an identical quota of DNA in their chromosomes. Yet during morphogenesis, they develop slowly into quite different cells and

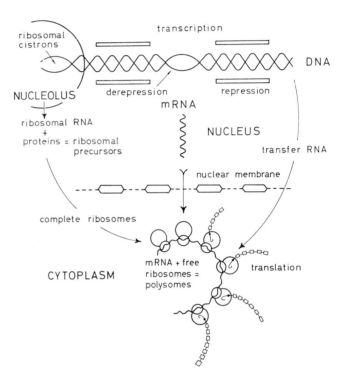

FIG. 6. Diagram of present knowledge of regulatory mechanisms in higher organisms. Several types of RNA are transcribed on the DNA of the genome: —messenger RNA (mRNA); —transfer RNA (tRNA); —ribosomal RNA (ribRNA), and, probably, other unidentified RNAs, or RNAs whose role is not yet known. RNA transcription requires the separation of the two strands of DNA at a given genetic locus, since RNA synthesis takes place on a single strand of DNA. Factors responsible for the repression and derepression of specific gene loci have not yet been identified in higher organisms. Association of DNA with histones may non-specifically repress the majority of the genome. Histone stabilize the double-stranded inactive form of DNA (Frenster 1965, 1966, 1967), whereas other polyanionic substances like acidic proteins, complementary RNA, hormones, stabilize the active form in which the two strands are separated.

tissues, with varying patterns of metabolism. The epigenetic mechanisms for specific and stable somatic selection have yet to be completely explained.

An interesting picture emerges when we examine the structure and function of the cell in relation to these problems.

I. THE STRUCTURE AND FUNCTION OF THE CELL AND ITS ORGANELLES

A. THE NUCLEUS

1. Chromosomes and Chromatin

(a) Chemical Composition and Ultrastructure of the Chromosomes

The presence of DNA in the nucleus was revealed as early as 1924 by the specific Feulgen reaction. Double helix molecules form the basic linear element of the chromosomes (the chromonema) (Fig. 7). Whether the

microscope. Their morphology has been most readily studied in the metaphase or anaphase of mitotic division, when the chromosomes are condensed throughout their length. A recently developed technique involving the spreading of mitotic or meiotic chromosomes on an air-water interphase renders their examination by electron microscopy much more easy (Kleinschmidt, Lang, Plescher, Hellman, Haas, Zahn, Hagedorn, 1961; Wolffe and Hewitt, 1966): the chromosomes are thus seen to be multistranded at all stages of prophase, but to lose this apparent multistrandedness at metaphase, when the chromosome fibres become more tightly coiled. An

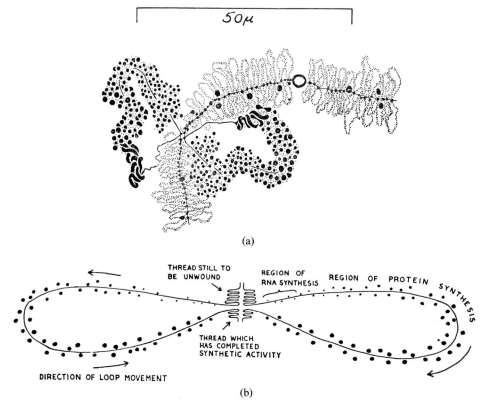

(a)

(b)

FIG. 7. Schema showing structure of lampbrush chromosomes (after Gall and Callen, 1962). Courtesy National Academy of Science. (a) part of chromosome XII from an oocyte of the newt *triturus cristatus*. Normal loop pairs and giant granular loops are shown. (b) model of loop function proposed by Gall and Callan.

DNA of the large chromosomes of higher organisms occurs in uninterrupted strands, or whether the discontinuity observed after ^{3}H–thymidine labelling implies discontinuity of the DNA, is not yet clear (Plaut and Nash, 1964; Freese and Freese, 1963). A single eukaryote chromosome certainly contains many molecules of DNA grouped in units of indeterminate length, called microfibrils.

Initially, electron microscopy of thin sectioned material supplied only limited information concerning the fine structural organization of the chromosomes, in part because of their complexity, in part because of the difficulty of interpreting their 3 dimensional structure on the basis of the 2 dimensional picture obtained with the electron

attempt to analyse the chemical composition and molecular organization of the microfibrils of interphase nuclei on an ultrastructural level, by combining such surface spreading techniques with various enzymatic and other extraction procedures, has led Bastia and Swaminathan (1966) to suggest that the 500, 250 and 100 Å microfibrils observed in many electron microscope preparations represent different orders of coiling of a basic 40 to 50 Å microfibril. Uncoiling of microfibrils can be brought about by treatment with 1 molar ammonium acetate and trypsin, suggesting that Zubay's 1964 model (Fig. 8) implicating histones in the supercoiling of DNA is correct.

DNA is indeed always associated in the chromatin with other molecules, notably basic and acidic proteins, RNA and phospholipids. In this connection, it is interesting to remember that a double DNA helix is about 20 Å thick, whereas the mitotic chromosome of a mammalian cell is

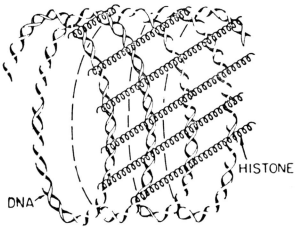

FIG. 8. Model of histone/DNA association (after Zubay, 1964). Courtesy Holden Day, San Francisco, U.S.A. The superhelix of DNA is shown in the form of a double spiral, and the α helix of the histones forms bridges between different parts of the DNA.

1 μ thick (i.e.: 10,000 Å) and 2 to 10 μ long. The table below gives examples of chromosome composition, as determined on isolated metaphase chromosomes by biochemical methods (Cantor and Hearst, 1966; Maio and Schildkraut, 1967).

TABLE

CHROMOSOME COMPOSITION

Type of Cells	Percentage composition of Chromosomes		
	DNA	RNA	TOTAL PROTEINS
HeLa	16	12	72
L-2 ascites tumor	13·5	13·8	68·3

Cytochemical tests (Alfert and Geschwind, 1953) also clearly show the presence of proteins in the chromatin: the histones were the first to be recognized, hence the name "nucleohistone" given to the substance of the chromosomes. Numerous studies have attempted to define their structural or regulatory function with respect to the DNA of the genome. Basic proteins (histones) may be important in ensuring the structural organization of the chromosomes (Bastia et al., 1966; Zubay, 1964); they may also "depress" genomic function, though the similarity in composition of histones from different tissues does not encourage the hypothesis of a specific role, as initially attributed to them by Stedman and Stedman (1950) (cf. Busch, 1965; Bonner and Ts'O, 1964). The acidic proteins of the chromatin may act more specifically on gene activity (Wang, 1967; Paul and Gilmour, 1968).

A new technique involving discrete fluorescent labelling and sensitive ultramicrospectrophotometric determination of the patterns of distribution of DNA (Caspersson, Farber, Foley, Kudynowsky, Modest, Simonsson, Wach

and Zech, 1968) may soon provide further insight into the functional structure of metaphase and interphase chromosomes.

(b) Euchromatin and Heterochromatin

The apparent chromatin network of the interphase cell viewed under the light microscope is really an artefact produced by the contraction of the chromatin and the removal of the nuclear sap by a process of fixation. Yet differential staining reactions for light microscopy revealed long ago that chromatin is made up of two parts: *euchromatin* and *heterochromatin*.

Under the electron microscope, too, this distinction is clear: euchromatin stains less readily than heterochromatin with heavy metals after osmium fixation. Nuclei having abundant euchromatin are generally more active metabolically (in RNA synthesis) than those containing coarse masses of intensely staining heterochromatin. The inactive nucleus of the orthochromatic erythroblast is extensively heterochromatized, for example. On the contrary, the nucleus of the basophilic erythroblast active in RNA and protein synthesis, is much less intensely stained (Fawcett, 1966). Biochemical studies on isolated fractions of euchromatin and heterochromatin have also revealed certain physical and chemical differences: the former seems to contain a slightly higher proportion of acidic molecules (phosphoproteins, ribonucleic acids, for example) whereas the DNA of the latter seems to be more highly condensed, perhaps because it is maintained in a repressed, condensed state by closer association with histones (Stedman and Stedman, 1950; Frenster, 1963). To summarize, heterochromatin does not possess major functional genes, is late replicating, and shows a reduced rate of transcription.

(c) The DNA Content of the Chromosomes

When total amounts of DNA per nucleus or per chromosome are determined, cells of higher organisms are generally found to contain more DNA per haploid chromosome than can be accounted for by their most probable number of genes. In Drosophila giant chromosomes, many cytogenetic observations suggest that one gene is probably located in one band or chromomere, and the amount of DNA in each unit seems to be higher than would be expected (Beermann, 1965). DNA "redundancy" (gene amplification) has also been demonstrated by biochemical techniques involving DNA–DNA dissociation and reassociation (Kohne, 1967). Kohne attributes a special role in evolution to redundant DNA. Callan (1967) explains redundancy by the assumption that each chromomere consists of an initial "master" gene and a number of tandemly linked "slave" genes. Redundancy of the "nucleolar-organizer" region in the supernumerary nucleoli of oocytes will be described further on.

Analyses using ultracentrifugation in caesium chloride gradients in different animal species, notably mammals, has revealed the presence, besides the major DNA component, of given buoyant density, of a second DNA component sedimenting differently (Bond, Flamm, Burr and Bond, 1966). In the mouse, for instance, it corresponds to 10 per cent of the nuclear DNA, and is randomly distributed throughout the nuclear genome in arrays of about 60,000 base pairs. These "multiple" genes are all identical, and one wonders how such sequences are protected against mutational shifts. The function of such so called "satellite" DNA is still unknown.

(d) Chromosome Replication and Cell Division

The method of replication of the DNA of the chromosomes is fundamentally similar to that already described, that is "semi-conservative" replication following separation of the 2 strands of the duplex (Taylor, Woods and Hughes, 1957; Prescott and Bender, 1963; Simon, 1961; Walen, 1965).

Whereas chromosome replication may take only a few seconds in bacteria and occupy practically the whole of the cell cycle, in higher organisms it may last several hours or days, and only occurs during a finite period, the "S" period, corresponding roughly to 40 per cent of the cell cycle. (Fig. 9.)

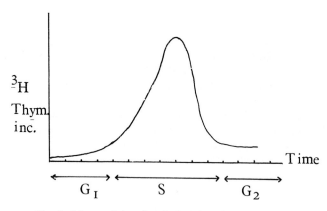

FIG. 9. Schema of the cell cycle, based on the incorporation of thymidine —³H. DNA is only synthesized during the "S" phase, in relation to mitosis.

The several phases of the cell cycle are usually defined in a simplified manner, as follows:

(1) MITOSIS, with its classical phases;

(2) INTERPHASE, the non-dividing phase, itself subdivided into three periods in relation to the replication of the DNA of the chromatin:

(a) G1: post-mitotic, involving the synthesis of proteins and RNA, but not of DNA;

(b) S: the period during which DNA replication occurs; many of the proteins of the chromatin are synthesized at the same time as the DNA.

(c) G2: a post-synthetic period during which the cell prepares for a new mitosis.

The actual situation is much more complex than this schema would suggest. The total protein content of most cells increases continuously throughout the cell cycle, but the pattern of synthesis of individual proteins varies considerably. Some authors have also described the synthesis of small quantities of DNA during G1.

There is a group of cells in higher organisms which ordinarily do not divide but can do so after an appropriate

stimulus (e.g. regenerating liver, or rat kidney cells stimulated by a single injection of folic acid). Such quiescent cells that can be induced to divide have an additional phase, the latent phase, called G_0.

A combination of pulse labelling and DNA autoradiography suggests that the long fibres of which the chromosomal DNA is composed are made up of many tandemly joined sections in each of which DNA is replicated at a fork-like growing point (Hubermann and Riggs, 1968). In Chinese Hamster cells most of these sections are probably less than 30 μ long, and the rate of replication per growing point is 2·5 μ per minute or less. Replication of DNA in these mammalian cells seems to proceed in opposite directions at adjacent growing points which initiate replication simultaneously.

Reproducible asynchrony of DNA synthesis has been found to be characteristic, and the sequence of synthesis of the DNA of different chromomeres appears to be very specific (Plaut, Nash and Fanning, 1966). The presence of *early* and *late* replicating DNA has been shown by autoradiography and by other techniques (Ficq and Pavan, 1961; Lima de Faria, 1959; Hsu, Schmid and Stubblefield, 1964; Mueller and Kajiwara, 1966; Govosto, Pegorano, Maserga and Rovera, 1968) (cf. Plates Ia and Ib). In the main, the early replicating complexes correspond to euchromatin, the late replicating DNA to heterochromatin. Quantitative evaluation of synthetic activity in single chromosomes and their segments has been established (Gilbert, 1962; German, 1964), and one of the first illustrations of asynchrony was the discovery of the female X chromosome, replicating at a very late stage and thus easily differentiated from the other chromosomes. The existence of metabolically labile DNA at certain stages of the cell cycle has also been recorded (Gavosto, 1967; Sampson, Katoh, Hotta and Stern, 1963; Ficq et al., 1961; Pelc, 1962, 1963; Lima de Faria, 1962): the synthesis of DNA outside the normal cycle of DNA replication in relation to mitosis suggests a special metabolic function for these macromolecular fractions.

Chromosome replication involves the formation by replication or synthesis of all the molecular species which give the chromosome form, regulate its metabolic activity and enable it to function during the cell cycle. Some protein synthesis precedes DNA synthesis (during the G1 period), while many of the important proteins (like histones) of the chromosomes, seem to be mainly synthesized during the same S period of the cell cycle as DNA (Prescott and Bender, 1963; Bloch and Godman, 1955; Busch/Hnilica, Taylor, Mavioglu, 1963; Umana, Updike, Randall and Dounce, 1964). However, nuclear protein synthesis usually continues during the G2 period, after DNA replication has finished.

The importance of chromosomal proteins, which may regulate DNA replication (Lehnart, 1964) or RNA synthesis (Frenster, 1965), has resulted in numerous studies of their rate of synthesis in relation to nucleic acid synthesis. There is some indication that the rates of synthesis of histones and acidic nuclear proteins vary under different conditions of growth (Hnilica and Kappler, 1965) and that different fractions play specific roles in the regulation of nucleic acid synthesis (Bonner, Dahmus, Fambrough, Huang, Marushige and Tuan, 1968).

(e) Synthesis of Messenger RNAs

Apart from the replication of DNA, which occupies only a limited part of the cell cycle, a most important function of the chromatin is that of RNA synthesis, i.e.

vitro, that special 'messenger' RNAs having a different base composition from ribosomal RNA, are synthesized at a different rate from the latter. They are not necessarily short-lived, as they are in bacteria. Moreover, since no mRNA has been shown to be capable of coding for a specific cell protein *in vitro*, we cannot assume that these special kinds of RNA are necessarily mRNAs (see review

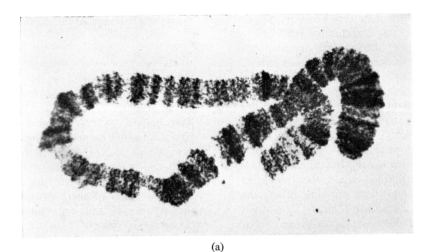

(a)

(b)

PLATE Ia and Ib. Polytene chromosomes isolated from Dipteran salivary glands, labelled with (a) ³H-thymidine, (b) ³H-uridine, and submitted to autoradiography (courtesy of A.FICQ). Labelling with precursors of RNA and of DNA clearly shows the localization of specially active bands, or chromomeres, and asynchronous labelling.

the transcription process. As we shall see further on, the greater part of the cell's RNA is ribosomal RNA, which is synthesized on a small part of the DNA of the chromatin, itself called the nucleolar organizer, and associated with the nucleolus. On the other hand, messenger RNAs which carry precise information for the synthesis of specific proteins are synthesized on active DNA segments in the euchromatin. The way in which these segments are selected for transcription remains an enigma. It has been shown very clearly by autoradiography, biochemical analysis of nuclear RNA, and of RNA synthesized on chromatin *in*

of this question by Chantrenne, Burney and Marbaix, 1967).

A distinction must also be made between RNAs which are synthesized *and broken down in* the nucleus, and which probably play a regulatory role, and the informational mRNA molecules which leave the nucleus in a form not yet accurately defined, to join the ribosomes in the cytoplasm (Harris, 1964; Scherrer, Marcaud, Zajdela and Gros, 1966; Spirin, 1966; Hadjilov, 1967).

What is clear from both autoradiography and biochemistry, is that in any differentiated cell, only certain segments of the DNA genome are transcribed: the others are in a repressed state, and never function to synthesize RNA. Some segments function for short periods of the cell cycle or life cycle of the organism, then cease to function. The study of these phenomena is a vast field of research in itself.

2. The Nucleolus

Cells engaged in active protein synthesis contain two or more *nucleoli*, which vary in size and number from cell to cell. The nucleoli disappear during cell division and reform in the new daughter nuclei under the influence of special regions of the chromosomes called "nucleolus organizer" regions. With electron microscopy, the nucleolus can be seen to be made up of two zones, one granular (granules 150 to 200 Å in diameter), the other fibrillar (fibrils about 50 Å in diameter). Radioautography combined with electron microscopy (Plate IIA) has shown that RNA synthesized in intranucleolar (but chromosomal) DNA, is first found in the fibrillar region, then moves to the granular region to associate with proteins, during the initial process of ribosome formation (Granboulan, 1964; Geuskens, 1966; Perry, 1962). As far as is known at present, the formation of functional ribosomes is not completed in the nucleolus. Analysis of this phenomenon, using centrifugation in sucrose gradients, has shown that ribosomal components sedimenting at 45 S are probably formed first, and only break up afterwards to smaller components (28 S–35 S and 16–18 S). They are thought to migrate in this form through the nuclear membrane into the cytoplasm, where they give rise to "complete" ribosomes, formed of two sub-units (50 S and 30 S), one of which associates with messenger RNA to form the rosette or bead-like polysomes active in protein synthesis, the other larger unit being more particularly associated with the growing polypeptide chains (Fig. 5) (Benedetti, Bont, Bloemendael, 1966). Hybridization experiments, which demonstrate the affinity of complementary nucleotide sequences in DNA and RNA by allowing them to associate together under special experimental conditions, have shown that only a small proportion of the genome (about 0·3 per cent of the DNA), is required to control the biosynthesis of ribosomal RNA, the same genomic site being able to function repeatedly at a given speed (Yankofsky and Spiegelman, 1962; Ritossa and Spiegelman, 1965). In this way, 0·3 per cent of the genome controls the synthesis of 80 per cent of the RNA of the cell (i.e. the ribosomal RNA). We thus have proof of the direct control of the formation of cytoplasmic ribosomal RNA, which is long lived and very stable, on a specific locus of DNA in the nucleolus. This DNA has actually been detected by electron microscopy, and its nature has been checked by treatment of the nucleolus with DNase, which removes it entirely (Van Gansen, 1968, Plate IIB). Some authors suggest that its synthesis is not synchronous with, but independent of, the synthesis of the rest of the DNA of the nucleus (Frayssinet, Lafargue and Simard, 1968). In some cells, at special periods, unusually rapid synthesis of ribosomal RNA requires reduplication of the appropriate DNA segments: this phenomenon is referred to as "gene amplification". Supernumerary nucleoli in amphibian oocytes contain, for instance, an extra quantity of special segments of DNA responsible for ribosomal RNA synthesis (Dawid, 1966; Miller, 1964, 1966; Porkouska, MacGregor and Birnstiel, 1968).

Attempts to characterize endoreplication of ribosomal cistrons (segments of DNA responsible for ribRNA synthesis) in somatic cells have so far proved unsuccessful, however (Ritossa, Atwood, Lindsley, Spiegelman, 1966).

3. Nuclear Enzymes

The nucleus of course contains the enzymes required for the duplication and synthesis of at least the major part of its own constituents (Georgiev, 1967; Patel, Hawk and Wang, 1967): for instance, DNA and RNA polymerase have been shown to be present in the chromatin. The basic and acidic proteins of the chromosomes are generally assumed to be synthesized in the nucleus by a mechanism similar to that operating for cytoplasmic protein synthesis; however, a few reports are begining to suggest that some, at least, of these proteins may be synthesized in the cytoplasm and only later move into the nucleus (Das, 1967; Bloch, 1964; Goldstein and Plaut, 1967; Borun, Scharff and Robbins, 1967). On the other hand, it is not impossible that certain specific protein fractions are synthesized in the nucleus by a mechanism which differs fundamentally from that occurring in the cytoplasm for the greater proportion of the cell's proteins (Freedman, Honig and Rabinovitz, 1966; Malpoix and Zampetti, 1968).

Glycolytic enzymes and those connected with nucleotide metabolism also occur in large quantities in the nucleus, as well as smaller amounts of hydrolytic enzymes. Many of the essential respiratory enzymes seem to be lacking, so that the nucleus probably depends mainly on the cytoplasm for its supply of energy. However, some of the cytochromes have recently been shown to be present in calf thymus nuclei.

B. THE CYTOPLASM

The cellular matrix in which cytoplasmic organelles and ergastoplasm occur, and which is bounded on one side by the nuclear envelope, and on the other by the plasma membrane, is called the hyaloplasm. Free ribosomes and polysomes, various droplets like lipid droplets, and inclusions like the glycogen granules, can be seen in it, as well as filamentous structures and microtubules. It of course contains various types of mRNA, tRNA, sugars, nucleosides, nucleotides, soluble proteins (among which are many enzymes) and structural proteins.

Cytoplasmic Organelles

(a) Mitochondria

Mitochondria, viewed under the electron microscope, are seen to have a fairly complex structure (Plate IIIa and c). Each is bounded by a double membrane: an external, smooth boundary, and an inner much folded structure forming incomplete transverse septa within the mitochondrion (the cristae mitochondriales). The internal,

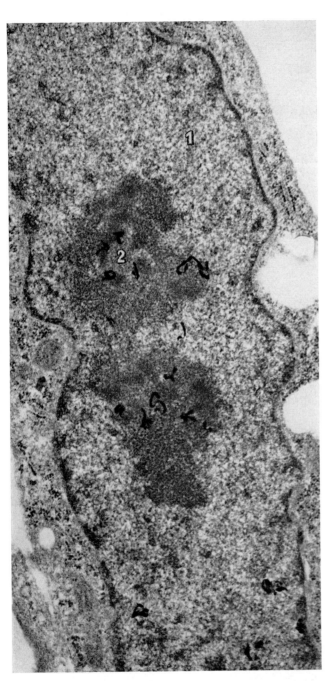

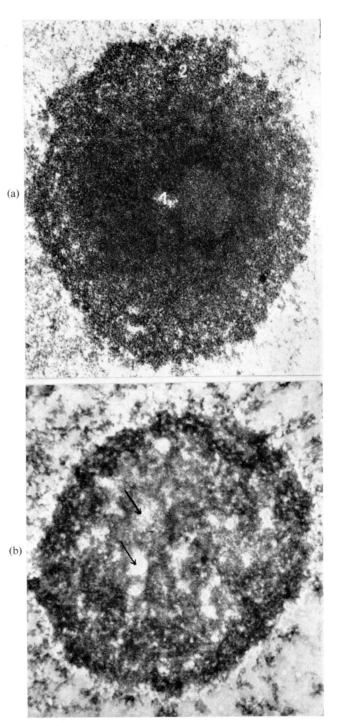

(a)

(b)

PLATE IIA. The nucleus (1) and the nucleolus (2) of a monkey kidney cell in culture, examined by electron microscopy after incorporation of ^{3}H-uridine for 5 minutes ($\times$ 30,000). Radioactivity appears in the *fibrillar* region of the nucleolus first (courtesy of M. Geuskens).

PLATE IIB. Nucleolus of Xenopus laevis egg. (a) normal nucleolus in which fibrillar (1) and granular (2) regions are clearly visible. (b) after treatment with deoxyribonuclease: visible removal of DNA. (courtesy of P. Van Gansen).

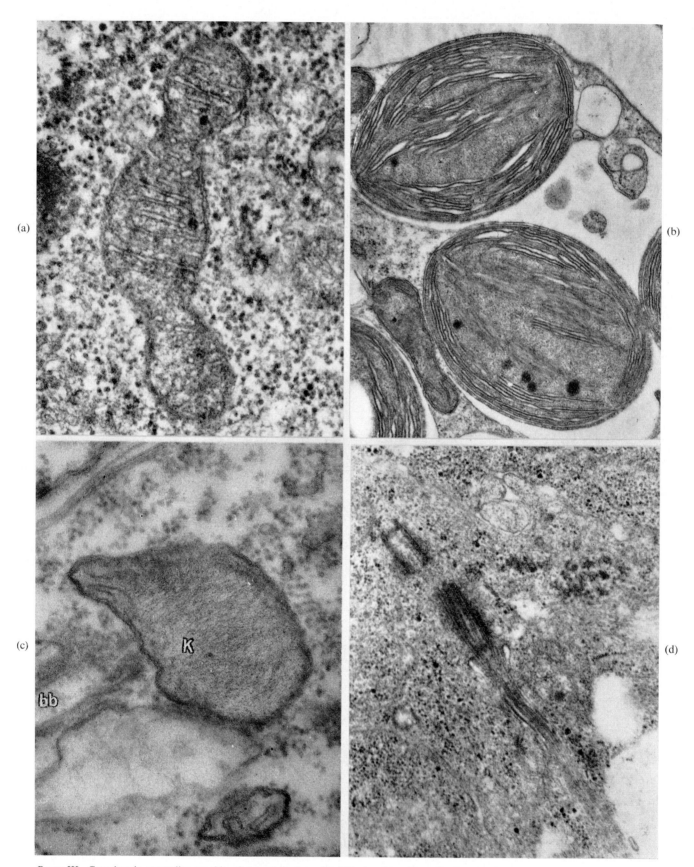

PLATE III. Cytoplasmic organelles capable of autoreplication: (a) Mitochondria of a cell of a gastrula stage embryo of the amphibian *xenopus laevis* (×6000) (courtesy of P. Van Gansen). (b) Chloroplast of the green alga: *Acetabularia mediterrania* (×20,000) (courtesy of M. Boloukhere). (c) Kinetoplaste (K) of the flagellate *Crithidia luciliae*. The material is fixed according to Ryter and Kellenberger. The section shows the double membrane, a few cristae of the associated mitochondrion and the closely packed DNA fibrils. The kinetoplast is always found near the *basal body* (bb) of the flagellum. (d) Two centrioles of an interphase cell of a chick embryo, neurula stage (×40,000). The centriole is cut longitudinally. Fine microtubules are also visible (courtesy of P. Messier).

homogeneous matrix consists of proteins and lipids, and contains randomly scattered "dense" granules 300 to 500 Å in diameter. The membrane may well contain contractile proteins, for the mitochondria undergo frequent changes in shape and volume, moving sinuously throughout the cytoplasm. 25 per cent of the proteins of the mitochondrial membranes are enzymes of the respiratory chains, the cytochromes linked to the Krebs cycle. Energy released by oxidative phosphorylation in mitochondria is transferred to adenosine diphosphate and made available in the form of adenosine triphosphate. The mitochondria are indeed the energy generating sources of the cell.

Mitochondrial DNA

The fact that they contain stable, self-replicating DNA, usually differing in base composition from nuclear DNA, has only recently been discovered (Nass, 1963; Dawid, 1966, 1968; Steinert, 1960, 1967); mitochondrial DNA from various sources has been found to be circular (Sinclair and Stevens, 1966; Hudson and Vinograd, 1967; Nass, 1966, 1967). Mitochondrial ribosomes have also been isolated and found to possess ribosomal RNA differing in sedimentation constant and base composition from cytoplasmic ribosomal RNA (Kuntzell and Noll, 1967). Labelling of mitochondrial proteins in vivo and in vitro has shown these organelles to be capable of independent protein synthesis (Howell, Loeb and Tomkins, 1964; Rifkind, 1967). However, microsomes labelled in vitro can transfer labelled material into both the soluble and insoluble proteins of the mitochondria during a reaction that requires ATP and, probably, GTP (Kadenbach, 1967).

It therefore seems likely that while the mitochondrion contains the genetic information required for the synthesis of some of the mitochondrial components, others may be synthesized elsewhere in the cell. It is interesting, in this connection, to note that "cytoplasmic mutations" affecting mitochondrial DNA have been found to be responsible for the transmission of biochemical and biological characteristics (Mounoulan, Jacob and Slonimsky, 1966, 1967). Such phenomena raise interesting problems concerning the relationship between cytoplasmic factors and nuclear DNA.

The evolutionary origin of the mitochondrion is unknown; some authors think they have evolved from microorganisms that originally parasitized the cytoplasm of the large host cell. Such endosymbionts would, according to this hypothesis, have become non-pathological and finally, an integral part of the host cell. It must be said that mitochondria resemble prokaryotic microorganisms in size, mode of duplication, in the possession of circular DNA molecules, and in ribosomal size.

(b) Plant chloroplasts (Plate IIIb), organelles responsible for photosynthesis, also possess a high degree of autonomy, and their DNA has physical characteristics which distinguish it from nuclear DNA (Green, Heilporn, Limbosch, Bouloukhère and Brachet, 1967). Beautiful electron micrographs showing the conformation of DNA in chloroplasts have recently been achieved by Woodcock and Fernandez-Moran (1968). Chloroplast DNA can replicate (Heilporn-

Pohl and Brachet, 1966) and chloroplasts can multiply (Shephard, 1965), in the absence of the nucleus. Chloroplast DNA moreover codes for chloroplast ribosomal RNA (Sager and Hamilton, 1967), and comparative sedimentation studies have shown the latter to be the smallest ribosomes (together with the 66 S ribosomes of the photosynthetic bacteria), yet examined (Kuntzell et al., 1967). Protein synthesis in chloroplasts has also been shown to be subject to regulatory agents which do not affect cellular protein synthesis, (Brawerman and Eisenstadt, 1967).

The fact that both chloroplast and mitochondrial ribosomes can be distinguished from other cytoplasmic ribosomes, suggests that certain features of ribosomal structure and function may confer specificity, in relation to protein synthesis, to these particles. Comparative sedimentation studies certainly indicate an apparent increase in cytoplasmic ribosomal size accompanying evolution to higher forms and a possible phylogenetic relationship affecting the ribosomes of prokaryotes and eukaryotes (Reisner, Rowe and Macindoe, 1968; Kuntzell and Noll, 1967).

(c) Centrioles (Plate IIId). The centrioles are also endowed with genetic continuity and can replicate in anucleate fragments (sea urchin eggs: Harvey). Situated at opposite poles of the spindle apparatus during mitosis, they are known to contain RNA and protein, and to consist of a hollow cylinder 300 to 500 μ in diameter, the walls of which contain 9 tubules. Centriole replication occurs by orthogonal budding from a parent centriole (Gall, 1961), and, using synchronized HeLa cells, has been shown to occur in synchrony with nuclear DNA synthesis and mitosis, beginning at or near the initiation of DNA synthesis and being completed by G2 (Robbins, Jentzsch and Micali, 1968). These self-replicating organelles probably contain DNA too, although this has not been demonstrated: if they do, such DNA might code for at least some of the proteins of the spindle apparatus and control the formation of microtubules (cf. basal bodies). Electron microscope examination (Robbins et al., 1968) shows physical continuity between pericentriolar vesicles and newly forming spindle tubules.

(d) The basal bodies, (Plate IIIc), **found at the base of all cilia and flagella,** are similar in structure to the centrioles. In certain cells, their functions seem to be interchangeable: as the sperm cell matures, for instance, a centriole gives rise to a flagellum and becomes a true basal body. The distinction which exists seems to be one of function, rather than of structure; the similarity may imply some homology between the structure of the microtubules (Porter, 1966) of the spindle apparatus and that of the microtubules found in flagellae, and produced in relation to the basal bodies. Stephens (1968) notes that the outer fibres of sea urchin sperm flagella, which resemble most other microtubules reported in the literature, are composed of 40 Å globular subunits arranged longitudinally. Their protein nature has been confirmed and found similar to muscle actin, plasmodial actin and the proteins of the mitotic apparatus.

The basal bodies contain DNA, as has been shown by

fluorescence microscopy and deoxyribonuclease sensitive incorporation of tritiated thymidine (Randall and Disbry, 1965; Sonneborn and Plaut, 1967); it therefore seems likely that this DNA codes for the proteins of the cilia.

Morphologically, typical cilia consist of a complex fibrous axoneme embedded in a matrix and enclosed by a membrane. The axoneme itself contains a bundle of nine outer fibres, and two central fibres that run continuously along its length; these fibres are mostly of protein nature (as seen above) and also contain a high percentage of ATPase activity in relation to the energy required for ciliary movement (Gibbons, 1965).

increased quantities of hydrolases, like cathepsin, which are actively synthesized to that end. Such enzymes also intervene when the corpus luteum of the ovary degenerates.

Paradoxically, hydrolytic enzymes might, at some stages, stimulate protein synthesis. Monroy (1965) has found that ribosomes from unfertilized sea urchin eggs synthesize very little protein, as compared with fertilized eggs, but brief exposure to proteases *stimulates* protein synthesis *in vitro* by these otherwise inactive ribosomes.

Lysosomes take part in specialized types of autolysis (as mentioned above, in the case of the corpus luteum), and in intracellular digestion. Foreign particles (bacteria,

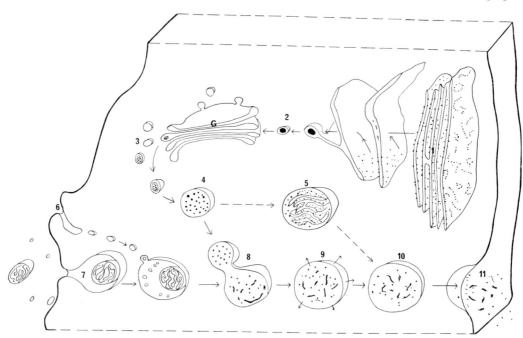

FIG. 10. Illustration of the relationship between lysosomes, endoplasmic reticulum, Golgi body, and digestive vacuoles (courtesy of P. Van Gansen and H. Bruge). 1. Endoplasmic reticulum. 2. Proteins secreted in the endoplasmic reticulum are transferred to the Golgi apparatus (G). 3. Prolysosomes. 4. Complete lysosome containing enzymes. 5. Autophagic vacuole. 6. Pinocytosis. 7. Phagocytosis. 8. Junction of lysosome and phagosome permits digestion of phagocytized or pinocytized material. 9. Digestive vacuole. 10. Residual body. 11. Excretion.

It would be interesting to study the biogenesis of cilia, growing from basal bodies, in a system responding to hormone, like that described by Brenner, 1967: ciliogenesis during the menstrual cycle of the Rhesus monkey oviduct.

(e) Lysosomes. The biogenesis of the cytoplasmic particles called lysosomes is little known: they are probably produced by the ergastoplasm via the Golgi saccules and vesicles (Fig. 10). They are membrane bound particles so heterogeneous in their fine structure that no particle seen in an electron micrograph can be identified with certainty as a lysosome on the basis of morphological criteria alone. First identified by De Duve, Gianetto, Appelmans and Wattiaux (1953), they have been found to contain a number of hydrolytic enzymes (acid hydrolases, acid phosphatases, ribonucleases, deoxyribonucleases). After the death of the cell, the liberation of these digestive enzymes leads to necrosis. These enzymes may also play an essential role at certain stages: during the metamorphosis of the frog, the degeneration of the tail requires

for instance, in the case of leucocytes) are ingested by a process known as endocytosis or phagocytosis. The cell membrane folds inwards to form a pocket enclosing the particles in "phagosomes". Lysosomes become attached to phagosomes and discharge enzymes into them, forming secondary lysosomes in which the foreign particles are digested. Indigestible material remains segregated within "residual bodies" which may remain in the cell for a long time, or may fuse with the cell wall and so discharge their contents (Fig. 10).

(f) Endoplasmic reticulum (Plate IVa). This is the name given to the polymorphous network of membrane systems forming partially continuous trabeculae or cisternae throughout the cytoplasmic matrix of many cells. It is continuous with the nuclear envelope and with the external membrane of the cell. Its origin is not clear; authors have concluded differently that it derives from the nuclear membrane, the nucleus, the Golgi apparatus, the mitochondria, and the plasma membrane. Its basic protein-lipid structure is similar to that of the other cell membranes, like the nuclear envelope, but its composition as to structural proteins and enzymes may vary from cell to cell and even from one region of the cell to another. It contains, for instance, nucleoside diphosphatases, glucose-6-phosphatase, acid phosphatase; it is one of the sites of concentration, with the Golgi apparatus, of substances secreted by the cell, and is also involved in intracellular transport.

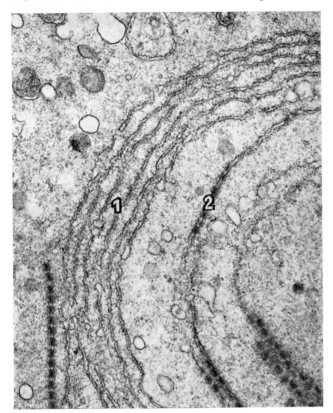

PLATE IVa. Light nucleate fragment of sea urchin egg (Arbacia): ergastoplasm (endoplasmic reticulum) (1) and annulate lamellae (2), (×20,000; courtesy of M. Geuskens). Ribosomes are seen in association with the membranes of the endoplasmic reticulum, and free in the cytoplasm. Annulate lamellae, resembling the nuclear membrane in structure, are found in oocytes and in cancerous cells.

Present data suggests that the membranes of the endoplasmic reticulum also contain a special type of RNA, perhaps mRNA, which is so firmly attached to the membrane that even detergents (deoxycholate) or chelating agents (ethylenediaminetetracetate) are unable to separate it from them (Pitot, 1965; Shapot and Pitot, 1966; Rodionova and Shapot, 1966). Cytochemical evidence of this fact has recently been given by the demonstration, using electron microscopy, that it is possible to remove membrane RNA by treatment with ribonuclease (Bal, Krupal and Cousineau, 1967).

Ribosomes and polysomes attached to the outer surface of many of the cisternae form "*rough endoplasmic reticulum*". The polysomes on rough endoplasmic reticulum probably synthesize both membrane and secretory proteins, whereas *smooth membranes* (which lack associated ribosomes) seem to have specific functions like that of synthesizing drug metabolizing enzymes (liver), steroid hormones (testicle and adrenals), carotenoids (retina), and glycogen (liver). The ribosomes and polysomes seem to be attached to the membrane by the nascent protein they are synthesizing (Sabatini, Tashiro and Palade, 1966; Chefurka and Hayashi, 1966). The degree of attachment of polysomes to membranes also seems to depend on the nature and metabolic state of the tissues; they are much more firmly attached in healthy liver than in hepatoma, and this difference is paralleled by the capacity of the former to modify its enzyme activity in function of metabolic requirements, capacity which is partially or entirely lost in cases of hepatoma. Shapot and coworkers (1965, 1966) have suggested that this fact, taken in conjunction with the presence of mRNA in the membrane itself, may mean that cytoplasmic membranes stabilize certain kinds of mRNA, some of which may be able to control discontinuous protein synthesis independently of permanent, genetic, DNA control. Bal and coworkers suggest that this mRNA might well account for membrane bound synthesis of various enzymes and structural proteins of membranes. Interestingly enough, Attardi and Attardi (1967) have described a membrane associated RNA of *cytoplasmic* origin in HeLa cells. Here again a structural basis seems to exist which may confer long-term "independence" to the cytoplasm, *vis-à-vis* the nucleus, although this property may be of a restricted character, and still controllable by nuclear genes.

A lot can be learned about the ergastoplasm by studying its appearance during embryogenesis, or by following its biogenesis in cells which respond to certain inductive substances by the proliferation of the endoplasmic reticulum. For instance, the administration of phenobarbital to rats induces simultaneously, in the parenchymatous cells of the liver, the synthesis of certain "drug metabolizing" enzymes, and the augmentation of the number of ribosomes and polysomes attached to them (Kato and Gelboin, 1965; Orrenius and Ericson, 1966). Some of the latter only remain attached to the membrane during its formation, then detach from it, so that rough ergastoplasm gives rise to smooth ergastoplasm. Recent experimental data (Dallner, Siekevitz and Palade, 1966) have confirmed that the structural proteins and enzymes of the membranes are synthesized on the polysomes of the rough ergastoplasm and thence transferred to the smooth walled cisternae.

The secretory proteins of the cell are probably synthesized by the ergastoplasm: some may be transferred to the external milieu via the cisternae; some (catalases, peroxidases) may be stored in "dense bodies"; others reach the lysosomes via the Golgi bodies (Fig. 10).

(g) **The Golgi bodies** (Plate IVb). The Golgi bodies are continuous with the endoplasmic reticulum and may well represent a collection centre for cytoplasmic secretions (Novikoff, 1961; Fawcett, 1966). They are less polymorph than the endoplasmic reticulum itself, being composed of piles of saccules dispersed in the hyaloplasm. Each stack corresponds to a dictyosome. Small concave discs 1–3 μ in diameter, are visible. The Golgi apparatus is rich in phospholipids, phosphatases, and proteins. The vesicles often contain secretions which may either stay in the cytoplasm, or be thrown out, e.g. formation of the acrosome of spermatozoids from the vesicles of the Golgi apparatus, or the formation of the skeletal membrane of vegetative cells, which is polysaccharide in nature (pectin). The frequent presence of acid phosphatase and the nature of certain cavities of the Golgi apparatus clearly suggest that lysosomes take their origin there. Novikoff (1961) has

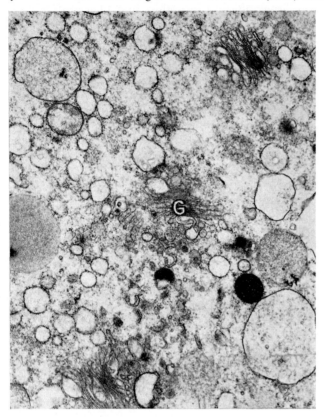

PLATE IVb. Light nucleate fragment of a sea urchin egg (Arbacia). *golgi apparatus* (G) (×17,000) (courtesy of M. Geuskens).

proposed that the Golgi body may represent the site of origin of the ergastoplasm; the intimate relation between endoplasmic reticulum, the other cell membranes, and the Golgi apparatus, suggests a common origin for them all (GERL complex of Novikoff).

To conclude this brief account of nuclear and cytoplasmic structure, let us stress the fact that although the DNA of the nucleus has been shown to code for the synthesis of messenger, ribosomal and transfer RNAs which are required for the synthesis of the majority of the specific proteins of the cell, cytoplasmic DNA may well exert independent genetic control on the synthesis of some of the proteins of the cytoplasm. The fact that certain cell organelles (centrosomes, chloroplasts) are able to replicate autonomously, adds to the interest of this enigma. Proliferation phenomena in certain cells, like that of the biogenesis of endoplasmic reticulum in the absence of nuclear replication, are equally interesting. Cytoplasmic inheritance may interfere much more with nuclear inheritance than was once thought. A new evaluation of such

theories as that of Morgan, who suggested long ago that heterogeneity of the cytoplasm is an important factor influencing nuclear differentiation in developing embryos, is also required. A large excess of cytoplasmic DNA has for instance been found in some oocytes (amphibian and sea urchin eggs); some of it is mitochondrial, but a great deal is bound to the yolk platelets and may represent a precursor of nuclear DNA to be used up during the frequent mitoses of the cleavage period. Eggs are known to receive a certain amount of ready made information of purely *maternal* origin (Spirin, 1966; Nemer, 1968). A great deal has yet to be learned before we can fully understand the way in which each somatic or germinal cell attains a certain stability of expression of interdependent nucleocytoplasmic factors.

II. NUCLEOCYTOPLASMIC INTERACTIONS

A. THE NUCLEAR ENVELOPE

The nuclear envelope (Plate Va) seems to be reconstituted in the telophase of cell division by the coalescence of vesicular elements of the ergastoplasm, and is therefore regarded as a derivative of this cytoplasmic organelle, or as a special part of it which, for some functional reason, is intimately associated with the interphase chromosomes (Fawcett, 1966). Its outermost membrane (75 Å) thick is continuous with the ergastoplasm and bears on its cytoplasmic surface ribosomes and polysomes. A perinuclear space 400 to 700 Å wide, which seems to be continuous with the cavities of the endoplasmic reticulum (Watson, 1955; Marinos, 1960), separates it from the inner nuclear membrane. Whereas cell organization is considerably modified at cell division by the disappearance of the nucleoli and the mingling of cell sap and cytoplasm, in the interphase cell, nucleocytoplasmic exchanges through the nuclear envelope seem to be strictly controlled, and the small nuclear annuli 300 to 500 Å in diameter are probably not freely communicating fenestrations, but sites of regulated transfer of materials (Warren, 1966). Even ion exchange is subject to strict control; the concentration of certain ions in the nucleus may indeed have some importance in relation to hormone action and derepression of genomic sites (Kroeger, 1966). Yet large molecules like RNase, albumins and globulins have been shown to enter the cell nucleus, and to traverse the nuclear membrane (Brachet, 1958, 1959; Coons, Leduc and Kaplan, 1951).

B. THE INFLUENCE OF THE NUCLEUS ON THE CYTOPLASM

The synthesis of every type of RNA in the nucleus, under genetic control, is of course the basis of nuclear control over cytoplasmic events. The segregation of the chromosomes during mitosis and meiosis therefore decides to a large extent the genetic constitution of the daughter cells. The factors determining repression and derepression of specific gene loci, and which are perhaps in part localized in the chromatin, in turn control the development of specific cell types, synthesizing specific proteins.

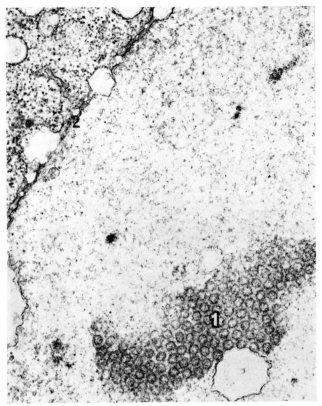

PLATE Va. Nuclear membrane of a cell of a mussel (Myrilus) egg, cleavage stage (1) in tangential section, (2) in transverse section ×13,000 (courtesy of M. Geuskens).

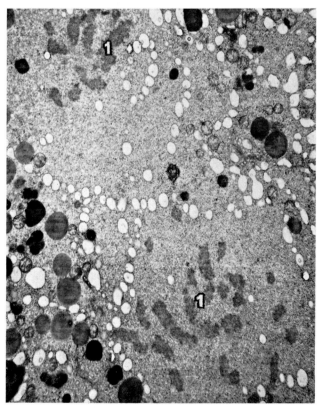

PLATE Vb. Mitosis (anaphase) in a mussel (Mytilus) egg, early cleavage stage (×4500): 1: chromosomes.

C. THE INFLUENCE OF THE CYTOPLASM ON THE NUCLEUS

Nucleocytoplasmic exchange is not a "one way" phenomenon. Recently, Goldstein and Plaut (1967) have provided evidence that, in amoeba, certain proteins shuttle back and forth between nucleus and cytoplasm. Cytoplasmic synthesis of some of the nuclear proteins has been convincingly demonstrated by these and other authors.

Moreover, it is now well established that the cytoplasm can regulate the metabolism of the cell nucleus and induce, or arrest, the synthesis of DNA. The effect of recipient cytoplasm is seen when the nucleus of a G2 phase Amœba is transferred to the cytoplasm of an S-phase (DNA synthesizing) cell: the inactive nucleus begins to synthesize DNA (Prescott and Goldstein, 1967). Adult nuclei injected into frog egg cytoplasm swell up and begin to synthesize DNA, although unable to do so before being separated from their original cytoplasm (Graham, Arms and Gurdon, 1966; Gurdon, 1967). Radioautography has revealed that cytoplasmic proteins entering the nucleus are responsible for this induction of DNA synthesis. Such proteins normally appear as a result of pituitary hormone action on mature oocytes, and their appearance involves both DNA and RNA synthesis (Dettlaff, 1965; Brachet, 1967c). Of course, transplantation experiments can only be performed with certain types of cells, and the proportion of transplanted nuclei entering mitosis decreases the later the developmental stage from which they are taken. Di Berardino and King (1967), who have very long experience of nuclear transfer experiments, think that irreversible changes render most adult, differentiated nuclei incapable of total rejuvenation. On the contrary, the work of Harris (1967) supports the idea that adult nuclei have not permanently lost their genetic totipotentiality, since when inactive red cell nuclei are introduced into HeLa cell cytoplasm, by a special procedure based on treatment with inactivated Sendhi virus, RNA and DNA synthesis recommences in the former.

D. LONG-LIVED MESSENGER RNAs

Not a minor complicating factor in the study of nucleocytoplasmic interdependence, is the ubiquitous existence in the cytoplasm of the cells of higher organisms, of messenger RNAs transcribed in the nucleus, but so long-lived as to confer lasting autonomy to the cytoplasm. Enucleate cytoplasm can in fact survive and develop for a considerable, though variable, period in the absence of the nucleus. This is particularly well exemplified in the case of Amoeba and also of the alga Acetabularia, useful because of the ease with which it can be enucleated, and which has provided a good deal of information on the degree to which the cytoplasm can survive in the absence of the nucleus and, notably, on the duration of life of the messenger RNAs able to retain for weeks, in the cytoplasm, the genetic message imparted to them by the DNA of the nucleus (Brachet, 1960, 1966b, 1967b).

E. CHANGING PATTERNS OF NUCLEOCYTOPLASMIC EXCHANGE

The nature of nucleocytoplasmic exchanges however, certainly varies, according to the age and specific characteristics of a given cell. In embryonic amphibian cells (Van Gansen, 1966), the nuclear membrane is highly convoluted: long, finger-like prolongations of the nucleus penetrate into the cytoplasm. Nuclear "blebs" seeming to involve membrane and nuclear matrix probably facilitate the movement of certain substances from nucleus to cytoplasm (Toro and Olah, 1966). Granular or rodlike RNase digestible material has been shown, by electron microscopy, to be able to migrate through the pores into the cytoplasm; it seems to derive from the chromosomes and might well be messenger RNA bound to protein (Stevens and Swift, 1966; Kessel, 1966).

A great deal of interesting data on changing nucleocytoplasmic relations throughout embryonic development has been published by Brachet (1944, 1957, 1960, 1967a, b, c). The role of the nucleus is relatively reduced at certain stages of development: eggs can cleave in the absence of the nucleus. But when cell differentiation begins at gastrulation, nuclear activity is required to control the synthesis of new messenger RNAs. Lethal hybrids between different species of amphibian and sea-urchin eggs have provided interesting evidence of this critical difference between early cleavage and later stages of development (subsequent to gastrulation), as far as nuclear function and control are concerned. In developing eggs of interspecific frog hybrids (Hennen, 1967), it has been shown that cytoplasmic factors can modify chromosomal function, inducing gross changes in chromosome number and karyotype. Denis (cf. Brachet, 1967d) has shown that lethality in such hybrids results from an inbalance between paternal and maternal DNA replication and mRNA transcription: the replication of paternal DNA is slowed down, whereas its transcription is accelerated tenfold.

Levitan (1967) has also recently reported a maternal factor of cytoplasmic origin, in Drosophila, capable of breaking paternal chromosomes.

The diversity of the relationship between nucleus and cytoplasm according to the type of cell and the stage in its life cycle, brings us to the final chapter in this brief review, that of cell specialization.

III. CELL DIFFERENTIATION

The basic scheme: DNA makes RNA, RNA makes proteins, and the fundamental picture of the cell as we have described it, make up a simplified picture. When we look at the fertilized egg which, in its unique structure, contains all the information required for the development of a specific multicellular organism, we realize that a great deal of detailed analysis is required before we can understand how the basic mechanisms are selectively applied in developing embryos and in differentiated adult cells.

Oogenesis

The mechanism controlling the differentiation of the oocytes themselves is not understood, nor is the period of migration and multiplication which, in mammals, precedes the arrival of the germ cells in the cœlomic epithelium from their site of origin in the endoblast (Pasteels, 1964; Chretien, 1966). One may wonder what distinguishes the differentiation of the germinal epithelium from that of the other, somatic, tissues. Nuclear transfer experiments (Briggs and King, 1952) showing that a somatic nucleus can replace the nucleus of a fertilized egg and give rise to a complete individual, would suggest that similar mechanisms govern both types of differentiation. Perhaps one of the essential differences resides in the biological controls leading to meiosis?

After an initial period of multiplication, during which the primordial germ cells give rise to numerous oogonia, a certain number of the latter begin the initial phases of meiosis: leptotene, zygotene, pachytene, and arrest in diplotene (the dictyate stage). In mammals, all these phases occur in the *foetal* ovary. The injection of labelled thymidine to pregnant mice and to newborn female mice (Borum, 1966) has shown that oocyte nuclei are only labelled if injections are given *before* birth; the mammalian oocyte thus receives its initial quotient of genetic information very early. During the long, waiting dictyate stage, DNA content remains constant at the tetraploid level: homologous chromosomes are already paired, in preparation for the following maturation division: they remain paired in the germinal vesicle from the birth of the female until adulthood. During that time, both nucleus and cytoplasm of the oocyte increase in volume. In amphibians, it has been shown that both RNA and protein synthesis are taking place (Ficq, 1955; Gall and Callan, 1962).

Electron microscope study of a mature mammalian ovum, still in the dictyate stage (Sotelo and Porter, 1959) shows a large cell surrounded by the zona pellucida, in which microvilli from the surface of the oocyte, and macrovilli from the follicular cells, probably facilitate transfer of material from the follicle cells to the oocyte. In the large "germinal vesicle" (nucleus of the dictyate oocyte) the chromosomes are not visible as such, but exist in a dispersed state. A single large nucleolus, which may attain 6μ in diameter, is visible. The nuclear membrane is double, with typical "pores". In the cytoplasm, we observe: free ribosomes, spheroidal mitochondria, smooth vesicles representing early endoplasmic reticulum (there is no "rough" ergastoplasm), Golgi elements, and peculiar "multivesicular bodies" consisting of vesicles up to 0.6μ in size with small vesicles inside them; these structures are analagous to lysosomes. The cytoplasmic organelles (multivesicular bodies, mitochondria, smooth vesicles) tend to accumulate in perinuclear and cortical regions (Fig. 11).

This is the structure which, after maturation division and fertilization, is going to develop and differentiate into a new, adult individual. In view of the fact that mitochondria contain DNA and that ribosomes seem to show some kind of phylogenetic evolution (Kuntzell, *et al.*, 1967; Reisner *et al.*, 1968), one may wonder what is the relationship between the origin of the egg mitochondria and the multiplication of nuclear DNA, and to what extent

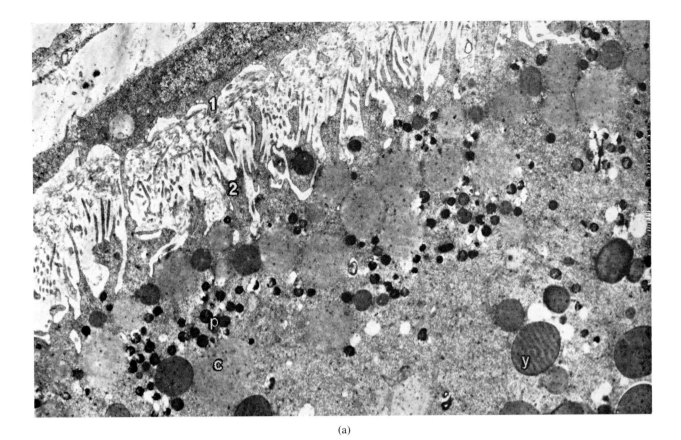

(a)

(b)

PLATE VI. (a) Follicular cell and border of an oocyte of the amphibian *xenopus laevis* ×6000 (courtesy of C. Thomas). Prolongations (macrovilli) from follicle cells (1) penetrate the oocyte. They are met in the intermediary zone by microvilli from the oocyte (2). This intermediary zone contains collagen and mucopolysaccharides. In the oocyte (p) pigment, (c) cortical granules, (y) yolk platelets. (b) Villosities in the peripheral region of an amphibian oocyte *Xenopus laevis* (detail from B) (×40,000) (courtesy of C. Thomas). (1) microvilli, (2) granules: ribosomes and glycogen, (3) fibrillar material, (4) cortical granules, (5) pigment granules.

egg ribosomes (still unattached to the ergastoplasmic membranes), may differ from some of those present in adult, differentiated tissues. The early biogenesis of smooth vesicles also requires to be elucidated. Another

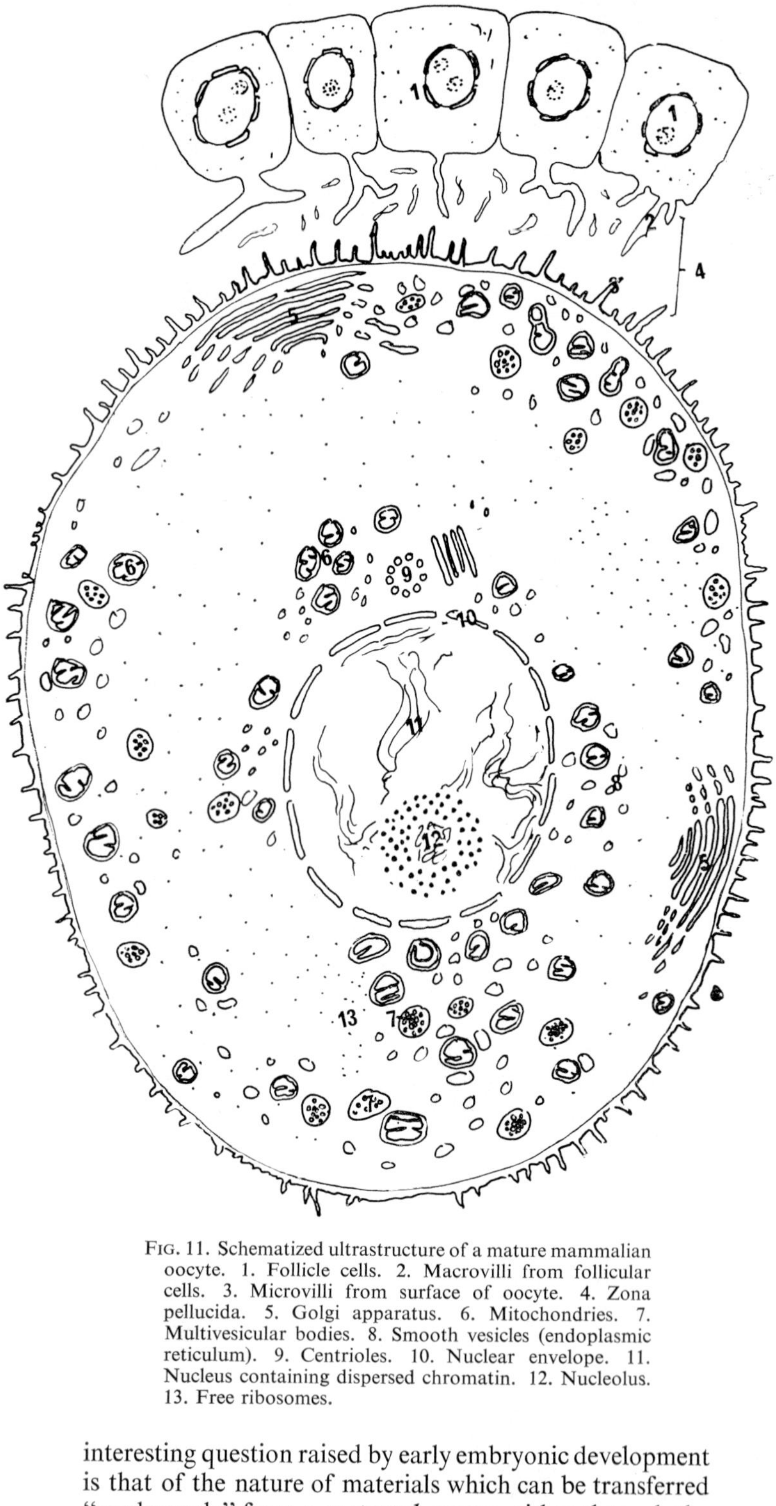

FIG. 11. Schematized ultrastructure of a mature mammalian oocyte. 1. Follicle cells. 2. Macrovilli from follicular cells. 3. Microvilli from surface of oocyte. 4. Zona pellucida. 5. Golgi apparatus. 6. Mitochondries. 7. Multivesicular bodies. 8. Smooth vesicles (endoplasmic reticulum). 9. Centrioles. 10. Nuclear envelope. 11. Nucleus containing dispersed chromatin. 12. Nucleolus. 13. Free ribosomes.

interesting question raised by early embryonic development is that of the nature of materials which can be transferred "ready made" from a maternal source, either through the follicle cells or, in a direct way, in the shape of cytoplasmic organelles in the ooplasm. In some, perhaps special, cases, DNA has been shown to move out of the nurse cells

and enter the egg cytoplasm by phagocytosis (Artemia: Fautrez-Firlefijn, 1951).

Much more is known about early macromolecular syntheses in amphibian and sea-urchin eggs (Brachet, 1967c, e, f; Nemer, 1967) than in mammalian eggs: in the swollen dictyate nucleus numerous nucleoli appear, each containing one or more nucleolar "rings" of DNA which represent a high degree of amplification of the ribosomal cistrons. In fact, most of the RNA synthesized in the nucleus during that stage is ribosomal RNA. Messenger RNA is synthesized in small quantities (equivalent to about 2 per cent of total RNA synthesis), and also transfer RNA (Slater and Spiegelman, 1966; Davidson, Crippa, Kramer and Mirsky, 1966). During amphibian oogenesis, cytoplasmic DNA is also synthesized: it includes not only mitochondrial DNA (Dawid, 1965, 1966), but also DNA associated with yolk platelets (Brachet, 1967c). The latter is probably characteristic of eggs containing a high yolk reserve, and is therefore likely to be almost or entirely absent in mammalian eggs.

Maturation and Fertilization

In mammals, a pituitary (F.S.H.) hormone stimulates maturation in the adult female: the oocyte nucleus resumes meiosis and initiates changes in the follicle which lead to ovulation. At diakinesis, chiasmata are formed and the crossing over of genetic material produces various recombinations; the chromosomes, each composed of paired chromatids, arrange themselves on the spindle. Anaphase follows, the chromosomes travel apart, moving towards opposite centrosomes and at telophase two new daughter nuclei are formed. One belongs to the secondary oocyte, the other to the first polar body. The second meiotic division follows immediately. The chromosome number is now reduced by half, such that the final pronucleus has a *haploid* number of chromosomes. Ovulation in most mammals occurs during metaphase II, and sperm entry is required to stimulate the completion of the second meiotic division and the emission of the second polar body.

The fine structure of the human ovum in the pronuclear stage has been studied by Zamboni, Bell and Bach (1966): in the cytoplasm, the multiplication of the mitochondria, the increase in the number of smooth vesicles of the endoplasmic reticulum and of multivesicular bodies, as well as the number of Golgi elements, indicate the increasing complexity of the cytoplasm. Annulate lamellæ, which can be regarded as nuclear adjuncts formed as an elaboration of the nuclear envelope, appear at this stage.

Simultaneously with the clumping of the chromosomes in the late telophase of the second maturation division, a number of nucleoli appear; they become more prominent and numerous as the pronucleus enlarges (Fig. 12). After coalescence of this initial group of nucleoli, a secondary set appears, and this in *both* pronuclei. Some of these seem to blend with the nucleoplasm, some with the cytoplasm just before the fusion of the two pronuclei. The first segmentation division, followed by the reappearance of nuclei, is accompanied by a renewed formation of nucleoli, and the same sequence of events is repeated. Biochemical studies of these phenomena have not been carried out, but it seems logical to suppose that the numerous nucleoli each contain nucleolar organizer regions which totalize considerable amplification of the ribosomal cistrons of the genome. DNA synthesis begins both in egg and sperm pronuclei 3 to 6 hours after activation in rabbit eggs (Szollosi, 1967), so that the zygote nucleus contains four times as much DNA as the spermatozoon before the first cleavage.

It should be remembered that maturation division involves the mixing of the nuclear sap with the cytoplasm, after years of separation. It can be produced experimentally in amphibian eggs, using pituitary hormones,

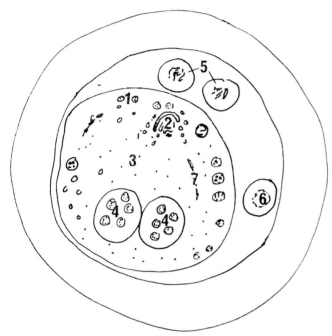

FIG. 12. Schema of Human Ovum in the Pronuclear State. 1. Mitochondria. 2. Golgi. 3. Cytoplasm containing free ribosomes. 4. Pronuclei containing numerous nucleoles. 5. First polar bodies. 6. Second polar body. 7. Annulate lamellae.

and has produced interesting experimental results (Brachet, 1965a; Van Gansen and Schram, 1968; Dettlaff, 1964). For instance, DNA containing particles move into the cytoplasm, accumulate in the cortical cytoplasm, then disappear. RNA and protein synthesis are known to occur during maturation. After fertilization, the cytoplasm of the oocyte, in many species, seems to be organized into special regions which will play a specific role in the future development of the fertilized egg (cf. the polar lobe of molluscs, the grey crescent of amphibians, the early symmetrical organization of mammalian eggs). The potential differences between the various regions of the egg probably depend largely upon the distribution of cytoplasmic materials (macromolecules and organelles). The influence of the cytoplasm upon nuclear metabolism cannot be overstressed.

With the reestablishment of the diploid number of chromosomes, and in the presence of the essential cytoplasmic factors, the long process of embryonic development begins, impossible to describe in all its complexity

in a few short paragraphs. Suffice it to remember that cleavage is a phase of rapid cell multiplication, with no externally visible cell differentiation, dominated by the rapid synthesis of DNA required for mitosis. In amphibians, it involves no ribosomal RNA synthesis, and only slight synthesis of heterogeneous (probably messenger and transfer) RNAs. Segregation of cytoplasmic material still continues in such a way as to map out different regions, of greater or lesser importance in the control of morphogenetic events.

Changing Patterns of Genetic Expression in Early Embryonic Development

The synthesis of mRNAs of different lifetime and nature characterizes different embryonic stages, as observed by a number of authors using the molecular hybridization technique (Denis, 1966; Whiteley, McCarthy and Whiteley, 1966; Glisin, Glisin and Doty, 1966). Denis has shown, for instance, that in amphibian embryos, as development progresses, the variety of messenger RNA molecules in the embryo increases. Early embryos may, like the sea urchin egg, contain "pre-existing" mRNA molecules and polyribosomes of maternal origin, as well as an early formed supply of new and different mRNA molecules synthesized during the initial cleavage stages. During long "waiting periods", certain forms of mRNA are "masked" and inactive (Monroy, 1965; Spirin, 1966). Sea urchin eggs at the 4 blastomere stage, for example, seem to contain three different kinds of structures, all of which contain messenger RNA: (1) informasomes: newly synthesized mRNA-protein complexes; (2) light polyribosomes, and (3) heavy polyribosomes (containing preformed mRNA of maternal origin), which can be distinguished from one another by their rate of sedimentation in sucrose gradients.

It has been shown that mRNA synthesis is activated at a crucial stage in development; in amphibian eggs, at the very beginning of gastrulation, mRNA synthesis increases a hundredfold. Different gene loci come into action at different stages of morphogenesis: some DNA sites are only active in early embryos (gastrulae and neurulae), others in later stages; these *early* and *late* functioning loci could be called "transient" genes; other genomic sites are active both in embryonic and adult organisms (Denis, 1966). The existence of gradients in RNA content and synthesis has also been established (Brachet, 1944, 1960; Bachvarova, Davidson, Allfrey and Mirsky, 1966).

Later Stages of Differentiation

During the early stages of embryonic life (gastrulation), the layers of cells which will form the mesodermal, endodermal and epidermal tissue, are segregated. The next step involves the final stabilization of the synthetic pattern of the differentiated cell: tissue specific proteins are synthesized for the first time. A number of different embryonic systems (lens differentiation, blood cell differentiation) are being investigated to discover the essential steps in the differentiation of a given tissue.

Gene Derepression

Molecular hybridization (Brachet, 1967d) has so far been unable to distinguish between the DNA extracted from the different organs of a given species or between the DNA obtained from embryo or adult amphibians. Yet this same technique distinguishes clearly between DNA from different species. It is not impossible that small differences exist, undetectable by present techniques. But if the genome of different organs and tissues is identical, as is generally thought to be the case, its differential expression at somatic level has to be explained in terms of changes at transcription and translation level.

Using isolated chromatin, isolated DNA, or systems in which DNA and chromatin proteins are reassociated, it has been found that a number of inhibitors of RNA synthesis, like histones and polylysine, stabilize the inactive double stranded helical form of DNA. On the other hand, substances which stabilize the active single stranded loop form of DNA (hormones like testosterone, estradiol, RNA polymerase, complementary RNA, acidic proteins) are found *in vitro* to stimulate DNA template function (Frenster, 1965, 1966a, b, c, d; Bonner *et al.*, 1968). Using a combination of two new *in vitro* techniques, that of hybridization and that of test tube verification of the priming activity of isolated DNA, or DNA combined with different protein fractions of chromatin, Paul and Gilmour (1965a, 1966b, 1967) have come to the tentative conclusion that basic proteins (histones) repress inactive genetic sites in a non-specific manner, whereas a specific polyanionic fraction (containing protein and/or RNA) might select the activity of certain sequences of DNA which, in turn, code for the mRNAs specific for distinct cell proteins.

The polytene chromosomes of dipterans have been shown to respond to histones or hormones injected *in vivo* by decreased or increased RNA synthesis respectively, and this in certain bands (Clever, 1967; Desai, 1967). Histones injected into the blastocele of amphibian embryos (Brachet, 1964) inhibit new syntheses of RNA which normally commence at gastrulation. Added histones have also been found to inhibit morphogenesis in early chick embryos (Malpoix and Emelinckx, 1967). Analysis of preparations of chromatin from various embryonic and adult tissues of the chicken, has shown that whereas the ratio histone/DNA remains fairly stable throughout development, acidic protein/DNA ratios change (Dingman and Sporn, 1964). Other authors have shown differences in turnover of acidic proteins in tissues in differing metabolic states (normal and tumoral tissues, for example: Hnilica *et al.*, 1965).

Several hormones stimulate the synthesis of RNA in specific target organs (for instance: estradiol in the uterus: Talwar, Segal, Evans and Davidson, 1964) and it has been suggested that they act as derepressors by interacting with histones (Sluyser, 1967). Mueller (1967) has detected both nuclear and cytoplasmic protein receptors for estrogen in the uterus, the response of which involves acceleration of both protein and RNA synthesis. Erythropoietin, a glycoprotein hormone, has clearly been shown to stimulate haematopoiesis in embryonic mouse liver at a stage when this organ is becoming an effective haematopoietic organ (Cole and Paul, 1965). But hormone action may involve several different steps, and the initial effect may not be at gene level (Korner, 1966).

A great deal of evidence certainly points to the necessity for change in the association between certain specific protein fractions and the DNA of the chromatin, in order for RNA synthesis to take place (cf. Fig. 6). This change in state, leading to strand separation in preparation for the transcription process, may represent only one aspect of gene activation.

Many interpretations of experimental results have led different authors to invoke regulatory mechanisms resembling those which have been described for bacteria (Jacob *et al.*, 1961) in higher organisms (cf. Granick and Levere, 1964). However, no conclusive evidence has yet been brought of the existence of regulator, operator and structural genes functioning exactly as in bacteria, in higher organisms. We are therefore far from being able to explain the process of tissue differentiation in detail.

"Differentiation" of DNA?

Recent studies of the priming ability of DNA from various organs of the Axolotl (Chapronier-Rickenberg and Justus, 1966) have shown that even when 90·6 per cent of the protein present in the chromatin has been removed, the priming ability of the DNA of different tissues varies. The authors conclude that such variations must either be due to a very small quantity of protein (less than 1 per cent) or to another mechanism, perhaps even to structural changes in the DNA itself, or to such changes as the methylation of DNA during maturation. This latter hypothesis rejoins that of Scarano, Iaccarino, Grippo and Parisi (1967), who consider that methylation of DNA may be a vital factor in the process of differentiation. Cytochemical and biochemical results obtained in our laboratory also tend to prove the existence of differences (in relation to acid hydrolysis) in the DNA of different tissues (Brachet, Guermant and Hulin, 1968); but these differences may be due to changes in the association between DNA and the proteins of the chromatin. Experimental findings concerning the rate of hybridization of DNA with DNA have revealed (Kohne, 1967) a high degree of redundancy of DNA sequences in the genome of eukaryotes (unlike in prokaryotes); this high redundancy level may be responsible for the *apparent* similitude of the DNA of all somatic cells, as studied by present techniques.

Technical improvements in the extraction and characterization of DNA are rapidly teaching us more about different types of DNA, both in the nucleus and in the cytoplasm. As we have seen, certain "satellite" DNAs can be distinguished from the major part of the genome by measurement of their buoyant density in CsCl gradient ultracentrifugation. Using this technique, Rosenkranz and Lipsky (1965) have found a gradual shift in the values of buoyant density of DNAs isolated at various stages of embryonic development of the American sea-urchin.

The functional significance of such differences at gene level has still to be explained, and until the fine structure of all the DNA of each of the chromosomes has been fully analysed, it is impossible to exclude *a priori* the intervention of changes in state or structure of DNA in relation to somatic differentiation. The ageing of cells may also imply radical changes after a certain lapse of time.

Specificity or Non-specificity of Ribosomes?

The discovery of messenger RNA led rapidly to the assumption that ribosomal specificity was not a logical necessity, and therefore, that all ribosomes were likely to be identical. It has only recently been discovered that chloroplast and mitochondrial ribosomes differ from the other cytoplasmic ribosomes. It would therefore be a mistake to exclude, *a priori*, the possibility that fine differences in structure and composition may intervene in deciding whether a given population of ribosomes is able to interpret a given code message for a specific protein. Slight differences in ribosomal structure might equally well determine further distinctions between different cytoplasmic regions of the egg. The early, rapid, production of numerous ribosomes by supernumerary nucleoli may have significance in relation to this problem.

Perhaps this brief account will serve to introduce the cell and its many remaining mysteries. The amazingly accurate techniques now at our disposition and the gradual accumulation of careful and detailed analyses of biological systems should lead to an even deeper understanding of fundamental biological mechanisms. Time, and new research approaches can only hasten our discoveries. The reproductive system is itself a fascinating subject for analysis at ultrastructural and molecular level, and present day research in this direction holds great promise, both on a scientific, and a human, level.

REFERENCES

Alfert, M. and Geschwind, I. (1953), "A Selective Staining Method for Proteins of the Cell Nucleus," *Proc. Nat. Acad. Sci.*, (*N.Y.*), **39**, 991.

Attardi, B. and Attardi, G. (1967), "A Membrane Associated RNA of Cytoplasmic Origin in HeLa Cells." *Proc. Nat. Acad. Sci.* (*N.Y.*), **58**, 1051.

Bachvarova, R., Davidson, E. H. (1966), "Nuclear Activation at the Onset of Amphibian Gastrulation," *J. Exp. Zool.*, **163**, 285.

Bal, A. L., Krupal, P., Cousineau, G. L. (1967), "Localization of RNA in the Membrane Systems of Developing Embryos of Sea Urchins," *J. Cell Biol.*, **35**, 8A.

Bastia, D. and Swaminathan, M. S. (1967), "Ultrastructure of Interphase Chromosomes," *Exp. Cell Res.*, **48**, 18.

Beerman, W. (1965), "Operative Gliederung der Chromosomen" *Naturwissenschaften*, **52**, 365.

Benedetti, E. L., Bont, W. S., Bloemendaal, H. (1966), "Structural Aspects of Polyribosomes and Endoplasmic Reticulum Fragments Isolated from Rat Liver," *Nature*, **210**, 1157.

Bloch, D. P. and Godman, G. C. (1955), "A Microphotometric Study of the Synthesis of Deoxyribonucleic Acids and Nuclear Histones." *J. Biophys. Biochem. Cytology*, **1**, 17.

Bloch, D. P. (1964), "Genetic Implications of Histone Differentiation." in *The Nucleohistones*, Ed. J. Bonner and Ts'O (Holden Day Inc.).

Bond, H. E., Flamm, W. G., Burr, L. E. and Bond, S. B. (1967), "Mouse Satellite DNA. Further Studies on its Biological and Physical Characteristics and its Intracellular Localization," *J. Mole. Biol.*, **27**, 289.

Bonner, J., Dahmus, M. E., Fambrough, D., Huang, R. C., Marushige, K. and Tan, D. Y. H. (1968), "The Biology of Isolated Chromatin," *Science*, **159**, 47.

Bonner, T. and Ts'O, O. (1964), *The Nucleohistones*, ed. Holden Day, San Francisco, London, Amsterdam.

Borum, K. (1966), "Oogenesis in the Mouse," *Exp. Cell Res.*, **45**, 39.

Borun, T. W. Scharff, M. D. and Robbins, E. (1967), "Rapidly Labelled Polyribosome Associated RNA having the Properties of Histone Messenger," *Proc. nat. Acad. Sci.*, **58**, 1977.

Brachet, J. (1944), "Synthesis and Localization and Physiological Role of the Nucleic Acids," in *Chemical Embryology*. New York: Interscience.

Brachet, J. (1957), *Biochemical Cytology*. New York: Academic Press.

Brachet, J. (1958), "The Action of Ribonuclease on the Enzymatic Activities of Living Cells," in *Proceedings of the International Symposium on Enzyme Chemistry, Tokyo*.

Brachet, J. (1959), "Nouvelles observations sur les effets de la ribonuclease *in vivo* sur les œufs de batraciens," *Acta Embryologica et Morphologiæ Experimentalis*, **2**, 107.

Brachet, J. (1960), "Chemical Embryology of Vertebrate Eggs: Biochemical Interactions between the Nucleus and the Cytoplasm during Morphogenesis and the Biochemistry of Differentiation," in *The Biochemistry of Development*. London: Pergamon Press.

Brachet, J. (1965a), "Emission of Feulgen Positive Particles during the *in vitro* Maturation of Toad Oocytes," *Nature*, **208**, 596.

Brachet, J. (1965b), "Acetabularia," *Endeavour*, **24**, 155.

Brachet, J. (1966a), "L'enigme des acides désoxyribonucléiques cytoplasmiques," *Scientia*, **101**, 1.

Brachet, J. (1966b), "Regulatory Mechanisms of Protein Synthesis in the Absence of the Nucleus," *Biochim. Biophys. Acta*, Symposium Lunteren, p. 330.

Brachet, J. (1967a), "Exchange of Macromolecules between Nucleus and Cytoplasm," *Protoplasma*, LXIII, p. 86.

Brachet, J. (1967b), I. "Le role du noyau cellulaire et des acides nucléiques dans la morphogénèse"; II. "Morphogénèse et synthèse des protéines en l'absence du noyau cellulaire," in *L'Embryologie Experimentale a la Biologie Moleculaire*, E. Wolff. Dunod, ed., Paris.

Brachet, J. (1967c), "Biochemical Changes during Fertilization and Early Embryonic Development," *Ciba Foundation Symposium on Cell Differentiation*, p. 39.

Brachet, J. (1967d), "Les techniques d'hybridisation moléculaire et le concept des RNA messagers," *Bull. Acad. Belg. Cl. Sci.*, **4**, 288.

Brachet, J. (1967e), "Protein Synthesis in the Absence of the Nucleus," *Nature*, **213**, 650.

Brachet, J. (1967f), "Synthesis of Macromolecules and Maturation of Starfish Oocytes," *Nature*, **216**, 1314.

Brachet, J., Hulin, N. and Guermant, J. (1968), "Acid Lability of Deoxyribonucleic Acids and Cell Differentiation," *Exp. Cell Res.*, **51**, 509.

Brawerman, G. and Eisenstadt, J. M. (1967), "The Nucleic Acids Associated with the Chloroplasts of Euglena Gracilis and their Role in Protein Synthesis," in *Le Chloroplaste, croissance et vieillissement*, by C. Sironval. Masson et Cie, ed., Paris.

Brenner, R. (1967), "Ciliogenesis during the Menstrual Cycle in Rhesus Monkey Oviduct," *J. Cell Biol.*, **35**, 16A.

Briggs, R. and King, T. J. (1952), "Transplantation of Living Nuclei from Blastula Cells into Enucleated Frog Eggs," *Proc. nat. Acad. Sci.*, **38**, 455.

Busch, H. (1965), *Histones and other Nuclear Proteins*. New York, London: Academic Press.

Busch, H., Steele, W. J., Hnilica, L. S., Taylor, C. W. and Mavioglu, H. (1963), "Biochemistry of Histones and the Cell Cycle," *J. cell. comp. Physiol.*, **62**, Supplement 1, 95.

Cairns, H. J. F. (1963), "The Bacterial Chromosome and its Manner of Replication as seen by Autoradiography," *J. Molecular Biolog.* **6**, 208.

Callan, H. G. (1967), "The Organization of Genetic Units in Chromosomes," *J. cell Sci.*, **2**, 1.

Cantor, K. P. and Hearst, J. E. (1966), "Isolation and Partial Characterization of Metaphase Chromosomes of a Mouse Ascites Tumor," *Proc. nat. Acad. Sci.*, **55**, 642.

Caspersson, T., Farber, S., Foley, G. E., Kudynowski, J., Modest, E. J., Simonsson, E., Wach, U. and Zech, L. (1968), "Chemical Differentiation along Metaphase Chromosomes," *Exp. Cell Res.*, **49**, 219.

Chantrenne, H., Burney, A. and Marbaix, G. (1967), "The Search for the Messenger RNA of Hæmoglobin," *Progress in Nucleic Acid Research*, **7**, 173.

Chapronier-Rickenberg, D. M. and Justus, J. T. (1966), "The Ability of DNA from Various Organs to Prime RNA Synthesis *in vitro*," *Biochem. Biophys. Acta*, **129**, 326.

Chargaff, E. (1950), "Chemical Specificity of Nucleic Acids and Mechanisms for their Enzymic Degradation," *Experientia*, **6**, 201.

Chefurka, W. and Hayashi, Y. (1966), "The Effect of Trypsin on Rough Endoplasmic Membranes," *Biochemical and Biophysical Research Communications*, **24**, 633.

Chretien, F. C. (1966), "A Study of the Origin, Migration and Multiplication of the Germ Cells of the Rabbit Embryo," *J. Embryology and Experimental Morphology*, **16**, 591.

Clever, U. (1967), "Control of Chromosome Puffing" in *The Control of Nuclear Activity*, p. 161, ed. L. Goldstein, Prentice Hall Int., London.

Cole, R. and Paul, J. (1966), "The Effects of Erythropoietin on Hæm Synthesis in Mouse Yolk Sac and Cultured Fœtal Liver Cells," *J. Embryology and Experimental Morphology*, **15**, 245.

Coons, A. H., Leduc, E. H. and Kaplan, M. H. (1951), "Localization of Antigen in Tissue Cells" (6th paper in the series: "The Fate of Injected Foreign Proteins in the Mouse"), *J. Exp. Med.*, **93**, 173.

Couch, J. and Hanawalt, P. C. (1967), "DNA Repair Replication in Temperature Sensitive DNA Synthesis Deficient Bacteria," *Biochemical and Biophysical Research Communications*, **29**, 779.

Dallner, G., Siekevitz, P., Palade, G. E. (1966), "Biogenesis of Endoplasmic Reticulum Membranes," *J. Cell Biol.*, **30**, 31A.

Das, N. K. and Alfert, M. (1967), "Cytochemical Studies on the Concurrent Synthesis of DNA and Histone in Primary Spermatocytes of Urechis Campo," *J. Cell Biol.*, **35**, 31A.

Davidson, E., Crippa, M., Kramer, F. and Mirsky, A. E. (1966), "Genomic Function during the Lampbrush Chromosome Stage of Amphibian Oögenesis," *Proc. nat. Acad. Sci.*, **56**, 856.

Dawid, I. B. and Wolstenholme, D. R. (1968), "Ultracentrifuge and Electron Microscope Studies on the Structure of Mitochondrial DNA," *J. Molecular Biology*, **28**, 233.

Dawid, I. B. (1965), "Deoxyribonucleic Acid in Amphibian Eggs, *J. Molecular Biology*, **12**, 581.

Dawid, I. B. (1966), "Evidence for the Mitochondrial Origin of Frog Egg Cytoplasmic DNA," *Proc. nat. Acad. Sci.*, **56**, 269.

De Duve, C., Gianetto, R., Appelmans, F. and Wattiaux, R. (1953), "Enzymic Content of a Mitochondrial Fraction," *Nature*, **172**, 1143.

Denis, H. (1966), "Gene Expression in Amphibian Development," *J. Molecular Biology*, **22**, 269.

Dettlaff, I. A. (1966), "Action of Actinomycin and Puromycin upon Frog Oocyte Metabolism," *J. Embryology and Experimental Morphology*, **16**, 183.

Desai, L. and Tencer, R. (1968), "Effects of histones and polysine on the synthetic activity of the giant chromosomes of salivary glands of dipteran larvae," *Exp. Cell. Res.*, **52**, 185.

Di Berardino, M. A. and King, T. J. (1967), "Development and Cellular Differentiation of Neural and Nuclear Transplants of Known Karyotype," *Developmental Biology*, **15**, 102.

Dingman, C. W. and Sporn, M. B. (1964), "Studies on Chromatin," *J. biol. Chem.*, **239**, 3483.

Fautrez-Firlefijn, N. (1951), "Etude cytochimique des acides nucléiques au cours de la gamétogénèse et des premiers stades du développement embryonnaire chez Artemia salina," *Arch. Biol.*, **62**, 391.

Fawcett, D. W. (1966), *An Atlas of Fine Structure. The Cell, its Organelles and Inclusions*. Philadelphia and London: ed. W. B. Saunders, Inc.

Ficq, A. (1955), "Le métabolisme de l'oogénèse étudié par autoradiographie," *Arch. Biol.*, **62**, 391.

Ficq, A. and Pavan, C. (1961), "Métabolisme des acides nucléiques et des protéines dans les chromosomes géants," *Pathologie et Biologie*, **9**, 756.

Frayssinet, C., Lafargue, C. and Simard, R. (1968), "Incorporation de thymidine tritiée dans le DNA de foie de rat," *Exp. Cell Res.*, **49**, 40.

Freedman, M., Honig, G., Rabinowitz, M. (1966), "Control of Nuclear Histone Synthesis in the Chicken Reticulocytes," *Symposium International sur le Noyau Cellulaire*, 9–12 May, Rijswick.

Freese, E. B. and Freese, E. (1963), "The Rate of DNA Strand Separation," *Biochemistry*, **2**, 707.

Frenster, J. (1965a), "Nuclear Polyanions as Derepressors of Synthesis of RNA," *Nature*, **206**, 680.

Frenster, J. (1965b), "A model of Specific Derepression within Interphase Chromatin," *Nature*, **206**, 1269.

Frenster, J. (1965c), "Localized Strand Separation within DNA during Selective Transcription," *Nature*, **208**, 894.

Frenster, J. (1965d), "Correlation of the Binding to DNA Loops or to DNA Helices with the Effect on RNA Synthesis," *Nature*, **208**, 1093.

Frenster, J., Allfrey, H. and Mirsky, A. E. (1963), "Repressed and Active Chromatin Isolated from Interphase Lymphocytes," *Proc. nat. Acad Sci.*, **50**, 1026.

Gall, J. G. and Callan, H. G. (1962), "H³ Uridine Incorporation in Lampbrush Chromosomes," *Proc. nat. Acad. Sci.*, **48**, 562.

Gavosto, F. (1967), "Autoradiography Studies in Normal and Leukemic Human Chromosomes," *Progress in Nucleic Acid and Molecular Biology*, **7**, 1.

Gavosto, F., Pegoraro, L. and Masera, P. and Rovera, G. (1968), "Late DNA Replication Pattern in Human Hæmopoietic Cells. A Comparative Investigation using a High Resolution Quantitative Autoradiography," *Exp. Cell Res.*, **49**, 340.

Georgiev, G. P. (1967), "The Nature and Biosynthesis of Nuclear RNAs," *Progress in Nucleic Acid Research and Molecular Biology*, **6**, 259.

German, L. (1964), "Identification and Characterization of Human Chromosomes by DNA Replication Sequence," in *Cytogenetics in Tissue Culture*, ed. R. J. Harris, **3**, 191. New York: Academic Press.

Geuskens, M., Bernard, W. (1966), "Cytochimie ultrastructurale du nucléole," *Exp. Cell Res.*, **44**, 579.

Gibbons, I. R. (1965), "Chemical Dissection of Cilia," *Arch. Biol. (Liège)*, **76**, p. 317 (Symposium Vésale, Bruxelles, 19–24 Octobre 1964).

Gilbert, C. W. (1962), "Time Sequence of Human Chromosome Duplication," *Nature*, **195**, 869.

Glisin, V. R., Glisin, M. and Doty, P. (1966), "The Nature of Messenger RNA in the Early Stages of Sea Urchin Development," *Proc. nat. Acad. Sci.*, **56**, 285.

Goldstein, L. and Plaut, M. (1967), "Protein Interactions between Nucleus and Cytoplasm," in *The Control of Nuclear Activity*, ed. L. Goldstein, Prentice Hall, International Inc.

Goldstein, L. and Prescott, D. (1967), "Nucleocytoplasmic Interactions in the Control of Nuclear Reproduction and Other Cell Cycle Stages," in *The Control of Nuclear Activity*, ed. L. Goldstein, Prentice Hall, International Inc.

Goulian, M., Kornberg, A., Sinsheimer, R. L. (1967), "Enzymatic Synthesis of DNA: XXIV Synthesis of Infectious Phage ϕX174 DNA," *Proc. nat. Acad. Sci.*, **58**, 2321.

Graham, C. F., Arms, K. and Gurdon, J. B. (1966), "The Induction of DNA Synthesis by Frog Egg Cytoplasm," *Developmental Biology*, **14**, 349.

Granboulan, N. and Granboulan, P. (1964), "Cytochimie ultrastructurale du nucléole," *Exp. Cell Res.*, **34**, 71.

Granick, S. and Levere, R. D. (1964), "Heme Synthesis in Erythroid Cells." *Progress in Hematology*, IV, Grune and Stratton, U.S.A.

Green, B., Heilporn, S., Limbosch, L., Boloukhere, M. and Brachet, J. (1967), "The Cytoplasmic DNAs of Acetabularia Mediterranea," *Proc. nat. Acad. Sci.*, **58**, 1351.

Gurdon, J. B. (1967), "On the Origin and Persistance of a Cytoplasmic State inducing Nuclear DNA Synthesis in Frog Eggs," *Proc. nat. Acad. Sci.*, **58**, 545.

Hadjilov, A. A. (1967), "Ribonucleic Acids and Information Transfer in Animal Cells," *Progress in Nucleic Acid Research and Molecular Biology*, **7**, 196.

Harris, H. (1964), "Transfer of Radioactivity from Nuclear to Cytoplasmic RNA," *Nature*, **202**, 249.

Harris, H. (1967), "Artificial Heterokaryons of Animal Cells from Different Species," *J. Cell Sci.*, **1**, 30.

Heilporn-Pohl, V. and Brachet, J. (1966), "Net DNA Synthesis in Anucleate Fragments of Acetabularia Mediterranea," *Biochim. Biophys. Acta*, **119**, 429.

Hershey, A. D. and Chase, M. (1953), "Independent Functions of Viral Protein and Nucleic Acid in Growth of Bacteriophage," *J. gen. Physiol.*, **36**, 39.

Hnilica, L. S. and Kappler, H. A. (1965), "Biosynthesis of Histones and Acidic Nuclear Proteins under Different Conditions of Growth," *Science*, **150**, 141.

Hnilica, L. S. (1967), "Proteins of the Cell Nucleus," *Progress in Nucleic Acid Research and Molecular Biology*, **7**, 25.

Howell, R. R., Loeb, J. N. and Tomkins, G. M. (1964), "Characterization of Ribosomal Aggregates Isolated from Liver," *Proc. nat. Acad. Sci.*, **52**, 1241.

Hsu, T. C., Schmid, W. and Stubblefield, E. (1964), "DNA Replication Sequences in Higher Organisms," in *The Role of Chromosomes in Development*, M. Locke, ed., pp. 83–112. New York: Academic Press.

Hubermann, J. H. and Riggs, A. D. (1968), "On the Mechanism of DNA Replication in Mammalian Chromosomes," *J. Molecular Biology*, **32**, 327.

Hudson, B. and Vinograd, J. (1967), "Catenated Circular DNA Molecules in HeLa Cell Mitochondria," *Nature*, **216**, 647.

Jacob, F. and Monod, J. (1961), "Genetic Regulatory Mechanisms in the Synthesis of Proteins," *J. Molecular Biology*, **3**, 318.

Kadenbach, B. (1967), "Synthesis of Mitochondrial Proteins. Demonstration of a Transfer of Proteins from Microsomes into Mitochondria," *Biochim. Biophys. Acta*, **134**, 430.

Kato, R., Loeb, L., Gelboin, H. (1965), "Increased Sensitivity of Microsomes from Phenobarbital Treated Rats to Synthesize Messenger RNA," *Nature*, **205**, 668.

Kessel, R. G. (1966), "An Electron Microscope Study of Nucleocytoplasmic Exchange in Oocytes of Ciona Intestinalis," *J. Ultrastructural Research*, **15**, 1.

Kohne, D. W. (1967), DNA Replication. VIIth International Embryological Conference, Interlaken, 4–8 September.

Kroeger, H. (1966), "Potentialdifferenz und Puff Muster," *Exp. Cell Res.*, **1**, 64.

Kuntzell, H. and Noll, H. (1967), "Mitochondrial and Cytoplasmic Polysomes from Neurospora Crassa," *Nature*, **215**, 1340.

Kleinschmidt, A. K., Lang, D., Plescher, R. C., Hellman, W., Haas, J., Zahn, R. K. and Hagedorn, A. Z. (1961), *Naturforsch.*, **16b**, 730.

Lehman, I. R., Bessman, M. J., Simms, E. S. and Kornberg, A. (1958), "Enzymatic Synthesis of Deoxyribonucleic Acid," *J. Biol. Chem.*, **233**, 163 and 171.

Lehnart, S. M. (1964), "The Inhibition of DNA Synthesis in Nuclear Protein," *Biochim. Biophys. Acta*, **80**, 338.

Levitan, M. (1967), "A Maternal Factor which Breaks Paternal Chromosomes," *J. Cell Biol.*, **35**, 196.

Lima De Faria, A. (1959), "Differential uptake of Tritiated Thymidine in Hetero and Euchromatin in Melanopus and Secale," *J. Biophys. Biochem. Cytology*, **6**, 457.

Lima De Faria, A. (1962), "Metabolic DNA in Tipula Oleracea," *Chromosoma*, **13**, 47.

Maio, J. J. and Schildkraut, C. L. (1967), "Isolated Mammalian Chromosomes," *J. Molecular Biology*, **24**, 29.

Malpoix, P. and Emelinckx, A. (1967), "Effects of Histones on Morphogenesis and Differentiation in Chick Embryos," *J. Embryology and Experimental Morphology*, **18**, 143.

Malpoix, P. and Zampetti-Bosseleer, F. (1968), "Inhibition différentielle par l'actinomycine et la puromycine de la synthèse des protéines nucléaires et cytoplasmiques," *Arch. Int. Physiol. Biochim.*, **76**, 382.

Marinos, N. G. (1960), "The Nuclear Envelope of Plant Cells," *J. Ultrastructural Research*, **3**, 328.

Meselson, M. and Stahl, F. W. (1958), "The Replication of DNA in Escherischia coli," *Proc. nat. Acad. Sci.*, **44**, 671.

Miller, O. L. (1964), "Extrachromosomal Nucleolar DNA in Amphibian Oocytes," *J. Cell Biol.*, **23**, 60A.

Monroy, A., Maggio, R. and Rinaldi, A. M. (1965), "Experimentally Induced Activation of the Ribosomes of the Unfertilized Sea Urchin Egg," *Proc. nat. Acad. Sci.*, **54**, 107.

Mounoulan, J. C., Jacob, H and Slonimsky, P. P. (1966), "Mitochondrial DNA from Yeast 'Petite' Mutants: Specific Changes of Buoyant Density Correspond to Different Cytoplasmic Mutations," *Biochemical and Biophysical Research Communications*, **24**, 218.

Mounoulan, J. C., Jacob, H. and Slonimsky, P. P. (1967), "Molecular Nature of Hereditary Cytoplasmic Factors Controlling Gene Expression in Mitochondria," in *The Control of Nuclear Activity*, p. 413.

Mueller, G. C. and Kajiwara, K. (1966), "Late Replicating DNA," *Biochim. biophys. Acta*, **114**, 108.

Nass, M. (1966), "The Circularity of Mitochondrial DNA," *Proc. nat. Acad. Sci.*, **56**, 1215.

Nass, M. (1967), "The Circularity and Other Properties of Mitochondrial DNA of Animal Cells," in *Organizational Biosynthesis*, ed. H. Vogel, O. Lampen, V. Brysen. New York and London: Academic Press.

Nass, M. and Nass, S. J. (1963), "Intramitochondrial Fibres with DNA Characteristics," *J. Cell Biol.*, **19**, 593.

Nemer, M. (1967), "Transfer of Genetic Information during Embryogenesis," *Progress in Nucleic Acid Research and Molecular Biology*, **7**, 243. New York and London: Academic Press.

Novikoff, A. B. (1961), "Lysosomes and Related Particles," in *The Cell*, II, ed. Brachet, J. and Mirsky, A. New York and London: Academic Press.

Orrenius, S. and Ericsson, J. L. E. (1966), "Enzyme Membrane Relationships in Phenobarbital Induction of Synthesis of Drug Metabolizing Enzyme Systems and Proliferation of Endoplasmic Membranes," *J. Cell Biol.*, **28**, 181.

Paul, J. and Gilmour, R. S. (1966a), "Template Activity of DNA is Restricted in Chromatin," *J. Molecular Biology*, **16**, 242.

Paul, J. and Gilmour, R. S. (1966b), "Restriction of Deoxyribonucleic Acid Template Activity in Chromatin is Organ Specific," *Nature*, **210**, 992.

Paul, J. and Gilmour, R. S. (1968), "Organ Specific Restriction of Transcription in Mammalian Chromatin," *J. Molecular Biology*, **34**, 305–316.

Paul, J. (1967), "Masking of Genes in Cytodifferentiation and Carcinogenesis," in *Ciba Foundation Symposium on Cell Differentiation*, p. 196. London: J. and A. Churchill.

Pasteels, J. (1964), "La lignée germinale chez les reptiles et ches les mammifères," in *L'Origine de la Lignee Germinale*, ed. E. Wolff. Paris: Hermann.

Patel, G., Hawk, O. R. and Wang, T. H. (1967), "Partial Purification of a DNA Polymerase from the Non-histone Chromatin Proteins of Rat Liver," *Nature*, **215**, 1488.

Pavan, C. (1965), "Chromosomal Differentiation," *National Cancer Institute Monograph*, no. 18.

Pelc, S. R. (1962), "Incorporation of Tritiated Thymidine in Various Organs of the Mouse," *Nature*, **193**, 793.

Perry, R. P. (1962), "The Cellular Sites of Synthesis of Ribosomal and 4 S RNA," *Proc. nat. Acad. Sci.*, **48**, 2179.

Pitot, H. C. (1965), *Perspectives in Biology and Medicine VII* 1964–1965, p. 50.

Plaut, W., Nash, D., Fanning, T. (1966), "Localized DNA Synthesis in Polytene Chromosomes and its Implications," in *The Role of Chromosomes in Development*, ed. M. Locke, p. 113. New York: Academic Press.

Porter, K. R. (1961), "The Ground Substance. Observations from the Electron Microscope," in *The Cell*, II, p. 621, ed. J. Brachet and A. Mirsky. New York: Academic Press.

Porter, K. R. (1966), "Cytoplasmic Microtubules and Their Functions," *Ciba Foundation Symposium on the Principles of Biomolecular Organization*. London: J. and A. Churchill.

Porkouska, E., Macgregor, H. C., Birnstiel, M. L. (1968), "Gene Amplification in the Oocyte Nucleus of Mutant and Wild Type Xenopus Lævis," *Nature*, **217**, 649.

Prescott, D. M. and Bender (1963), "RNA and Protein Replacement in the Nucleus during Growth and Cell Division and the Conservation of Components in the Chromosomes," in *Cell Growth and*

Cell Division, ed. R. J. C. Harris, p. 111. New York: Academic Press.

Prescott, D. M. and Goldstein, L. (1967), "Nuclear–Cytoplasmic Interaction in DNA Synthesis," *Science*, **155**, 469.

Randall, J. and Disbrey, C. (1965), "Evidence for the Presence of DNA at Basal Body Sites in Tetrahymena Pyriformis," *Proc. roy. Soc.*, B, **162**, 473.

Reisner, A. H., Rowe, J. and MacIndoe, H. M. (1968), "Structural Studies on the Ribosomes of Paramecium. Evidence for a Primitive Animal Ribosome," *J. Molecular Biology*, **32**, 587.

Ritossa, F., Atwood, K., Lindsley and Spiegelman, S. (1966), "On the Chromosomal Distribution of DNA Complementary to Ribosomal and Soluble RNA," *National Cancer Institute Monograph* **23**, 449.

Ritossa, F. and Spiegelman, S. (1965), "Localization of DNA Complementary to Ribosomal RNA in the Nucleolus Organizer Region of Drosophila Melanogaster," *Proc. nat. Acad. Sci.*, **53**, 737.

Robbins, E., Jentzsch, G. and Micali, A. (1968), "The Centriole Cycle in Synchronized HeLa Cells," *J. Cell Biol.*, **36**, 329.

Rodionova, N. P. and Shapot, V. S. (1966), "Ribonucleic Acids of the Endoplasmic Reticulum of Animal Cells," *Biochim. biophys. Acta*, **129**, 206.

Rosenkranz, H. S. and Lipsky, D. (1965), "A Preliminary Survey of the Properties of DNA during Embryonic Development," *Biological Bulletin*, **129**, 413.

Sabatini, D. D., Tashiro, Y. and Palade, G. E. (1966), "On the attachment of Ribosomes to Microsomal Membranes," *J. Molecular Biology*, **19**, 503.

Sagar, R. and Hamilton, M. G. (1967), "Cytoplasmic and Chloroplast Ribosomes of Chlamydomonas," *Science*, **157**, 709.

Sampson, M., Katoh, A., Hotta, Y. and Stern, H. (1963), "Metabolically Labile DNA," *Proc. nat. Acad. Sci.*, **50**, 459.

Scarano, E., Iaccarino, M., Grippo, P. and Parisi, E. (1967), "The Heterogeneity of Thymine Methyl Group Origin in DNA Pyrimidine in Developing Sea Urchin Embryos," *Proc. nat. Acad. Sci.*, **57**, 1394.

Scherrer, K., Marcaud, L., Zajdela, F., Breckenridge, B., Gros, F. (1966), "Etude des RNA nucléaires et cytoplasmiques à marquage rapide dans les cellules érythropoïétiques aviaires différenciées," *Bull. Soc. Chim. Biol.*, **10**.

Shapot, V. and Pitot, H. C. (1966), "Isolation and Fractionation of Ribonucleic Acids from the Smooth Endoplasmic Reticulum of the Rat Liver," *Biochim. Biophys. Acta*, **119**, 37.

Shephard, D. C. (1965), "Chloroplast Multiplication and Growth in the Unicellular Alga. Acetabularia Mediterranea," *Exp. Cell Res.*, **37**, 93.

Simon, E. H. (1961), "Transfer of DNA from Parent to Progeny in a Tissue Culture Line of Human Carcinoma of the Cervix (strain HeLa)," *J. Molecular Biology*, **3**, 101.

Sinclair, J. H. and Stevens, B. J. (1966), "Circular DNA Filaments from Mouse Mitochondria," *Proc. nat. Acad. Sci.*, **56**, 508.

Slater, P. W. and Spiegelman, S. (1966), "An Estimation of Genetic Messages in the Unfertilized Echinoid Egg," *Proc. nat. Acad. Sci.*, **56**, 165.

Sluyser, M. (1967), "Interaction between Hormones, Histones and Deoxyribonucleic Acid," in *Regulation of Nucleic Acid and Protein Biosynthesis*, ed. Konigsberger and Bosch, Netherlands. Amsterdam: Elsevier Publishing Company.

Sonneborn, J. S. and Plaut, W. (1967), "Evidence for the Presence of DNA in the Pellicle of Paramecium," *J. Cell Science*, **2**, 225.

Sotelo, J. R. and Porter, K. R. (1959), "An Electron Microscope Study of the Rat Ovum," *J. Biophys. Biochem. Cytology*, **5**, 327.

Spirin, A. S. (1966), "On Masked Forms of Messenger RNA in Early Embryogenesis and in Other Differentiating Systems," *Current Topics in Developmental Biology*, ed. A. Monroy, A. Moscena. New York and London: Academic Press.

Stedman, E. and Stedman, E. (1950), "Cell Specificity of Histones," *Nature*, **166**, 780.

Steinert, M. (1960), "Mitochondria Associated with a Desoxyribonucleic Acid Synthesizing Body in Trypanosoma Mega," *J. Biophys. Biochem. Cytology*, **8**, 542.

Steinert, M. and Van Assel, (1967), "Réplications coordonnées des acides désoxyribonucléiques nucléaires et mitochondriales chez Crithidia luciliæ," *Arch. int. Physiol.*, **75**, 370.

Stephens, R. E. (1968), "On the Structural Proteins of Flagellar Outer Fibres," *J. Molecular Biology*, **32**, 277.

Stevens, B. J. and Swift, H. (1966), RNA Transport from Nucleus to Cytoplasm in Chironomus Salivary Glands," *J. cell. Biol.*, **31**, 55.

Szollosi, D. (1967), "Time and Duration of DNA Synthesis in Rabbit Eggs after Sperm Penetration," *Anat. Rec.*, **154**, 209.

Talwar, G. P., Segal, S. J., Evans, A. and Davidson, O. W. (1964), "The Binding of Estradiol in the Uterus. A Mechanism for Derepression of RNA Synthesis," *Proc. nat. Acad. Sci.*, **52**, 1059.

Taylor, J. H., Woods, P. S., Hughes, W. L. (1957), "The Organization and Duplication of Chromosomes as Revealed by Autoradiography Studies using Tritium Labelled Thymidine," *Proc. nat. Acad. Sci.*, **43**, 122.

Toro, I. and Olah, I. (1966), "Nuclear Blebs in the Cells of the Guinea Pig Thymus," *Nature*, **212**, 315.

Umana, R., Updike, S., Randall, J. and Dounce, A. V. (1964), "Histone Metabolism," in *The Nucleohistones*, p. 200, ed. Bonner and Ts'O. San Francisco, California: Holden Day.

Van Gansen, P. and Schram, A. (1968), "Ultrastructure et cytochimie ultrastructurale de la vésicule germinative et du cytoplasme périnucléaire de l'oocyte mûr de Xenopus lævis," *Journal of Embryology and Experimental Morphology* in press.

Walen, K. H. (1965), "Spatial Relationships in the Replication of Chromosomal DNA," *Genetics*, **51**, 915.

Wang, T. Y. (1967), "The Isolation, Properties and Possible Function of Chromatin Acidic Proteins," *J. biol. Chem.*, **242**, 1220.

Warren, K. B. (1966), *Intracellular Transport*. New York and London: Academic Press.

Watson, M. L. (1955), "The Nuclear Envelope. Its Structure and Relation to Cytoplasmic Membranes," *J. Biophys. Biochem. Cytology*, **1**, 257.

Watson, J. D. and Crick, F. H. C. (1953a), "Molecular Structure of Nucleic Acids," *Nature*, **171**, 737.

Watson, J. D. and Crick, F. H. C. (1953b), "Genetic Implications of the Structure of DNA," *Nature*, **171**, 964.

Whiteley, A. H., McCarthy, B. J. and Whiteley, H. R. (1966), "Changing Populations of Messenger RNA during Sea Urchin Development," *Proc. nat. Acad. Sci.*, **55**, 519.

Wolffe, S. L. and Hewitt, G. M. "Strandedness of Chromosomes," *J. Cell Biol.*, **31**, 31.

Woodcock, C. L. F. and Fernandez-Moran, (1968), "Electron Microscopy of DNA Conformations in Spinach Chloroplasts," *J. Molecular Biology*, **31**, 627.

Yankofsky, S. A. and Spiegelman, S. (1962), "The Identification of the Ribosomal RNA Cistron by Sequence Complementarity," *Proc. nat. Acad. Sci.*, **48**, 1069.

Zamboni, L., Mishell, D. R., Bell, J. H. and Baca, M. (1966), "The Structure of the Human Ovum in the Pronuclear Stage," *J. Cell Biol.*, **30**, 579.

Zubay, G. (1964), "Nucleohistone Structure and Function," in *The Nucleohistones*, ed. Bonner and Ts'O. San Francisco: Holden Day.

2. BIOCHEMICAL ASPECTS OF TUMOURS OF THE FEMALE REPRODUCTIVE TRACT

R. J. B. KING

Despite the availability of tissue from the reproductive tract of women, very little is known about the metabolic processes occurring in tissues such as normal human endometrium, let alone tumours derived from these tissues. The pioneering work of people such as Mueller and Gorski (Gorski, 1968) on the effect of oestrogens on protein and nucleic acid synthesis in the rodent uterus has yet to be translated into studies of the human reproductive tract.

The mechanism of carcinogenesis in any of the human tissues or organs is virtually unknown, although a great deal of work has been performed on experimental animals. Since the technique of placing hydrocarbon coated threads in the cervix or uterus of rodents was introduced, an increasing number of studies are being made on tumour induction in these organs but, to date, these have largely been confined to studies on the effect of hydrocarbons and hormones on tumour induction and on the histological structure of the tumours (Baba and Von Haam, 1967).

Because of the paucity of information on the induction and properties of tumours of the reproductive tract, this chapter will first deal with the current ideas on the mechanism of carcinogenesis in organs such as liver and skin and then see how applicable these ideas are to the tissues of the reproductive tract, especially with regard to the influence of hormones on these tissues.

Mechanisms of Carcinogenesis

Of the generalized theories of carcinogenesis that have been proposed, the two-stage hypothesis (Berenblum, 1964) is especially useful in considering the role of hormones in neoplasia. In its simplest form, this states that there is an initiating and promoting stage of carcinogenesis, the former being very rapid when compared with promotion. Chemicals are known that are purely initiators (urethane), promoters (croton oil) or mixtures of the two (certain hydrocarbons), but the role of hormones as either initiators or promoters has not been well studied. Numerous cases can be cited to show that steroidal hormones are involved in the production of various tumours but, in most cases, it is not known if the steroids are affecting initiation or promotion. The possible exceptions to this are the cases where the initiator and promoter seem to be the same compound as in the production of renal tumours in hamsters by oestrogen. Even here the possibility that, for example, oestradiol is the initiator whilst one of its metabolites is a promoter has not been tested. As far as human tumours are concerned, the evidence is even more ephemeral. There is no conclusive proof that steroidal hormones are initiators although they can certainly influence the growth of human tumours.

Two examples of the complexity of the situation are, first, the demonstration in skin carcinogenesis, that corti-costeroid deficiency augments promotion but has no effect on initiation. Considerations such as this might explain the paradoxical results that, depending on conditions, ovariectomy can either increase or have no effect on production of cervical tumours in mice by hydrocarbons (see later). Secondly, with hydrocarbon-induced tumours of the uterus, oestrogens appear to act as promoters in mice and rabbits but not in rats (Baba and Von Haam, 1967).

In the simplest case initiation can be thought of as an hereditary change in a cell while promotion represents the conversion of this cell into a recognizable tumour. It is tempting to think that promoters act by causing hyperplasia, thus allowing the cancer cell to exert itself but this view is too simple because, although all promoting agents cause hyperplasia, all agents causing hyperplasia are not promoters (Walpole, 1959). What do initiation and promotion mean in molecular terms? This is best considered in relation to current theories on metabolic control mechanisms (Heidelberger, 1964). Briefly, these theories imply that the availability of the genetic information encoded in the DNA is controlled by repressor molecules (proteins?) which can be either activated or inactivated by relatively small molecules. There is no concensus of opinion as to whether the initial reaction in carcinogenesis is directly or indirectly on the DNA or by an effect on a non-nuclear component. A direct chemical interaction between carcinogen and DNA is suggested by the work of Brookes and Lawley (1964), whilst an indirect effect on DNA is embodied in the lysosomal theory of carcinogenesis put forward by Allison (1968). Heidelberger (1964) favours the non-nuclear mechanism as far as skin carcinogenesis by hydrocarbons is concerned. It is very probable that different carcinogens act at different cellular loci. No evidence is available as to the site of the initial reaction in cells of the reproductive tract although in the hamster kidney, which develops tumours after prolonged oestrogen treatment, very little oestradiol gets into the nucleus, which would tend to favour a non-nuclear carcinogenic effect of oestradiol on this tissue.

In contrast to this, a reasonable amount of information is now available about the growth promoting activity of oestrogens, especially that of oestradiol. The initial reaction is the binding of oestradiol to a protein which eventually results in increased nuclear and cytoplasmic RNA synthesis. This in turn provides the templates for increased cytoplasmic protein formation. One of the oestradiol-binding proteins is in the nucleus but a cytoplasmic oestradiol-binding protein has also been demonstrated in the uterus (Gorski, 1968). It is not known if this represents a mechanism for transporting oestradiol into the nucleus or if it is the first stage of a non-nuclear action of oestradiol. Whilst very little is known about the biochemical effects of oestrogens on tumours of the reproductive tract, it is noteworthy that human endometrial carcinomas can take up oestradiol, some of which is in the nucleus and also that oophorectomy decreases RNA synthesis in the transplantable rat uterine Guérin T8 carcinoma. These fragmentary results indicate that the mechanism whereby oestrogens affect normal tissues will provide a good basis for experimentation on tumours.

Biochemical Changes in Tumours Relative to the Tissue of Origin

The difference in aerobic and anaerobic glycolysis of tumours reported 45 years ago by Warburg has stimulated an awe-inspiring volume of work on metabolic properties of tumours and, in view of this, it is surprising that agreement has not yet been reached as to whether this change in metabolism is an essential part of carcinogenesis. This aspect will not be discussed further.

From the myriad reports of differences between normal and neoplastic tissues it is difficult to get a general picture of what changes have occurred, but Pitot and co-workers (Pitot and Cho, 1965) have now presented evidence that one of the fundamental biochemical faults in the cancer cell is a partial loss of the mechanism that regulates enzyme synthesis. This is an adaptation of the deletion theory of carcinogenesis. The net result of this is that altered amounts of certain enzymes are produced and that the enzyme synthesizing system has an altered response to enzyme inducers such as hormones. The actual enzymes that are altered will depend on the tissue being studied.

These metabolic changes may simply affect the cancer cell itself or, as in the case of ovarian tumours, have very pronounced systematic effects remote from the tissue of origin.

Application of these Results to Tumours of the Reproductive Tract

The author feels that the ideas outlined above can be applied advantageously to the study of tumours of the reproductive tract but, due to the small amount of information available on this subject, a great deal of conjecture must be introduced. Only tumours of the endometrium, cervix and ovary will be discussed.

Endometrium

If one accepts the view that, in women, there is a progression from normal endometrium → cystic hyperplasia → adenomatous hyperplasia → carcinoma *in situ*, it is reasonable to think that as oestrogen is involved in the early stages of this progression, it is also concerned in the other stages. Available evidence supports this view (McKay, 1965). The positive correlation between the occurrence of adenocarcinoma and oestrogen-secreting ovarian tumours on the one hand and with prolonged oestrogen therapy (up to 2 years) on the other hand has been questioned on statistical grounds. Similarly, it has been suggested that the association of adenocarcinoma with cortical stromal hyperplasia of the ovary is due to the production of oestrogen by these cells but direct evidence for this is lacking. On the other hand, the positive correlation of

cancer of the endometrium with a failure to ovulate for one reason or another is well documented. The anovulatory conditions include primary or secondary amenorrhea, irregular bleeding, infertility or the menopause. It is not clear if this relationship indicates an effect of anovulatory conditions on the initiation or promotion of the tumour or both. As the peak incidence of this type of tumour occurs 10 years after the menopause, it suggests that the effect of this type of anovulation must occur relatively early in the life of the tumour. The preliminary results of the beneficial effects of long term administration of contraceptive progestogens also points to an hormonal influence on the genesis of the tumour.

It is not clear if the effect of anovulation is due to prolonged oestrogen stimulation in the absence of progesterone, to prolonged absence of progesterone or whether the occurrence of regular menstruation results in the loss of potential cancer cells. The first possibility would necessitate a direct effect of progestogen in inhibiting either tumour induction or growth whilst the latter would be due to a secondary effect of the progestogen. The beneficial effects of progestogen treatment on endometrial carcinoma show quite clearly that these steroids can act directly on at least some of these tumours although the pituitary may also be involved.

Metabolic characteristics of endometrial carcinomas. In premenopausal patients, the histological appearance of the carcinoma often resembles that of the adjacent normal tissue which shows that the tumour is, in certain cases, influenced by endogenous hormone levels. The influence of progesterone in changing normal, regenerative endometrium to the secretory type suggested a possible treatment of the carcinomas with progestational agents. This would divert the cellular activities from proliferation to secretion and thus limit the growth of the tumour. This approach has now been well documented for cases of inoperable endometrial carcinoma (Kistner, Griffiths and Craig, 1965). Steroids that have been shown to be beneficial include progesterone, 17α-hydroxyprogesterone, 17α-acetoxy 6α-methylprogesterone, 6α-methyl 17α-propynyl testosterone and 3β, 17β-diacetoxy 17α-ethenyl 19-nor-testosterone. The results so far indicate that only about 30 per cent of the patients get objective remission after this type of treatment.

It is clear that endometrial carcinoma can be categorized as a hormone associated tumour and has some of the characteristics of this type of neoplasm. Thus both hormone (progestogen) responsive and unresponsive conditions have been described and the former type tend to grow more slowly. There is evidence that in other responsive and unresponsive tumours (rat and human breast, hamster kidney, mouse lymphosarcoma) there is a loss of ability of the unresponsive tumour to bind the effector hormone (King, 1968) and it is tempting to speculate that a similar situation may exist in the endometrium. It should, however, be pointed out that no convincing evidence has yet been presented to show that progesterone is specifically bound in the uterus of experimental animals or humans. One could also ask the question as to whether a lack of progestogen effect on the unresponsive tumour is really due to a loss of response to progestogen or to a process of cell division that is not dependent on oestrogen and therefore cannot be diverted to a secretory condition by progesterone.

The histochemical evidence provided by Thiery and Willighagen (1967) shows that enzymes such as leucine aminopeptidase, adenosine triphosphatase and non-specific esterase are altered in the tumour and that there is some correlation of the degree of morphological differentiation and the enzyme content of the tumour such that the more anaplastic the tumour, the lower the level of enzymes measured. Also of interest in this study was the observation that treatment of patients with progestational agents altered the enzyme content of most of the tumours but the morphological and histochemical changes did not always coincide. This again highlights the question, what does one mean by the term "hormone responsive" tumour? In this case, if one uses the enzymic data, the majority of the tumours are responsive whereas the clinical and pathological data indicate that only about 30 per cent of the tumours can be defined in this way.

Cervix

Prolonged oestrogen treatment of mice gives a low yield of tumours of the cervix but the most efficient method of tumour induction is by implantation of an hydrocarbon impregnated thread. With this technique, the response to hormonal manipulation is dependent on the dose of hydrocarbon. Thus, Murphy (1961) obtained no significant effect with ovariectomy or stilboestrol on tumour production by prolonged methylcholanthrene treatment; when treatment was reduced to four weeks, the simultaneous administration of stilboestrol decreased the latent period and gave a seven fold increase in the number of tumours. Pregnancy did not affect the yield of tumours. Other reports (Islam and Zaman, 1965) indicate that ovariectomy can increase the yield of tumours. The reason for this difference is unknown but could be due to different effects of hormone manipulation on initiation as compared to promotion (see earlier). The aetiology of human cervical tumours is unknown although the earlier mean age of occurrence, the effect of parity and sexual habits suggest that different factors are operative here than in the endometrium.

Where enzyme differences such as glucose-6-phosphate and 6-phosphogluconate dehydrogenase have been detected in human cervico-vaginal tumours it would appear that, as the tumour becomes more anaplastic, the greater the enzyme difference becomes relative to the normal tissue. This is in agreement with the observation that, with hydrocarbon induced carcinoma of the portiovaginalis of the mouse, as the tumour becomes progressively more anaplastic (by repeated transplantation) the glucose-6-phosphate and 6-phosphogluconate dehydrogenase rise (see Thiery and Willighagen, 1965).

The increased levels of 6-phosphogluconate dehydrogenase in human cervical tumours has led to the development of a test for this tumour by measurement of this enzyme in vaginal fluid. Unfortunately, this is less specific than had been originally suggested, for it gives a high proportion (about 30 per cent) of false positive results caused by other inflammatory conditions and also, possibly by low oestrogen excretion.

Other metabolic differences between normal and neoplastic human cervix include glucose, lactate and amino-acid utilization and enzymes of the tricarboxylic acid cycle.

Ovary

Like so many other tissues, the ovary is susceptible to carcinogenic hydrocarbons such as dimethylbenzanthracene. The experiments that have been carried out so far provide a good illustration of how rapid initiation can be relative to promotion. In the experiments described by Jull, Streeter and Sutherland (1966) ovaries removed from mice 24 hours after a single oral dose of dimethylbenzanthracene and then transplanted into untreated mice produced an incidence of 30–40 per cent granulosa cell tumours 4–10 months later. The initiating process took a few hours whereas the promotion stage took several months. Surprisingly, when normal ovaries were cultured for 48 hours *in vitro* with dimethylbenzanthracene and then transplanted into untreated mice, no tumours appeared. It is possible that hormones are also required but neither the *in vivo* or *in vitro* results were affected by testosterone, progesterone or corticosterone. Paradoxically, deoxycorticosterone abolished the effect of dimethylbenzanthracene when given *in vivo* but helped produce tumours in the *in vitro* studies.

The metabolic characteristics of ovarian tumours are governed by the cell of origin. In experimental animals, most of the tumours are of the granulosa cell type whilst a number of types have been described in humans (Morris and Scully, 1958). Granulosa cell tumours produce predominantly oestrogenic effects although cases are not uncommon that exhibit no clinical or pathological evidence of endocrine function. Rare cases of virilism have also been reported. In contrast to this, the Sertoli–Leydig cell tumours usually produce virilization although occasional apparently non-functioning tumours have been reported.

These findings indicate that, in most cases, the neoplastic ovarian tissue retains at least part of its steroidogenic activity although it is not known if the pathway of steroid biosynthesis is the same in the normal and neoplastic tissue (Griffiths, Grant and Symington, 1964).

Also of interest are the reports of hormone secretion associated with metastatic tumours in the ovary where the primary tumour was of a non-endocrine tissue. This effect has been described as being due to a stimulation of the ovarian stroma by the tumour mass. Oestrogenic, androgenic and progestational effects have been reported from such tumours (Scott, Lumsden and Levell, 1967).

REFERENCES

Allison, A. C. (1968), "Lysosomes and the Response of Cells to Toxic Materials," in *Scientific Basis of Med., Annual Rev.*, Chapter II.

Baba, N. and Von Haam, E. (1967), "Experimental Carcinoma of the Endometrium," *Progr. exp. Tumor Res.*, **9**, 192.

Berenblum, I. (1964), "The Two-stage Mechanism of Carcinogenesis as an Analytical Tool," in *Cellular Control Mechanisms and Cancer*, p. 259. Edited by Emmelot, P. and Mühlbock, O. Amsterdam: Elsevier Publishing Co.

Brookes, P. and Lawley, P. D. (1964), "Reaction of some Mutagenic and Carcinogenic Compounds with Nucleic Acids," *J. Cell and Comp. Physiol.*, **64**, 111.

Gorski, J. (1968), in *Recent Progress in Hormone Research*, **24**, in press.

Griffiths, K., Grant, J. K. and Symington, T. (1964), "Steroid Biosynthesis *in vitro* by Granulosa-theca Cell Tumour Tissue," *J. Endocr.*, **30**, 247.

Heidelberger, C. (1964), "Studies on the Molecular Mechanism of Hydrocarbon Carcinogenesis," *J. Cell and Comp. Physiol.*, **64**, 129.

Islam, K. M. N. and Zaman, H. (1965), "Effect of Ovariectomy on 20-methylcholanthrene Induced Dysplasia of the Mouse Uterine Cervix," *Acta Cytol. (Balt.)*, **9**, 446.

Jull, J. W., Streeter, D. J. and Sutherland, L. (1966), "The Mechanism of Induction of Ovarian Tumours in the Mouse by 7, 12-dimethyl benz (α) anthracene," *J. Natl. Cancer Inst.*, **37**, 409.

King, R. J. B. (1968), "An Hypothesis of Hormone Dependence and Independence of Mammary Tumours," in *Factors influencing the Prognosis of Breast Cancer*. Edinburgh: Livingston & Co.

Kistner, R. W., Griffiths, C. T. and Craig, J. M. (1965), "Use of Progestational Agents in the Management of Endometrial Cancer," *Cancer*, **18**, 1563.

Morris, J. McL. and Scully, R. E. (1958), *Endocrine Pathology of the Ovary*. New York: C. V. Mosby & Co.

Murphy, E. (1961), "Carcinogenesis of the Uterine Cervix in Mice: Effect of Stilbestrol after limited Application of Methylcholanthrene," *J. Natl. Cancer Inst.*, **27**, 611.

Pitot, H. C. and Cho, Y. S. (1965), "Control Mechanisms in the Normal and Neoplastic Cell," *Progr. exp. Tumor Res.*, **7**, 158.

Scott, J. S., Lumsden, C. E. and Levell, M. G. (1967), "Ovarian Endocrine activity in Association with Hormonally Inactive Neoplasia," *Amer. J. Obstet. Gynec.*, **97**, 161.

Thiery, M. and Willighagen, R. G. J. (1965), "Enzymes and Malignancy," *Lancet* ii, 244.

Thiery, M. and Willighagen, R. G. J. (1967), "Enzyme Histochemistry of Adenocarcinoma of the Endometrium including Hormone-induced Changes," *Amer. J. Obstet. Gynec.*, **99**, 173.

Walpole, A. L. (1959), "Initiation and Promotion in Carcinogenesis," in *Ciba Foundation Symposium on "Carcinogenesis,"* p. 41.

3. CHROMOSOME ABNORMALITY AND CYTOGENETIC ANALYSIS IN OBSTETRIC AND GYNAECOLOGICAL PRACTICE

C. E. BLANK

Introduction

Developmental processes are initiated and controlled by the interaction of inherited predisposition and environment. The units of heredity, the genes, are carried on the chromosomes, which consist of deoxyribonucleic acid (DNA) and protein. Man normally has 46 chromosomes; 22 pairs of autosomes and a pair of sex chromosomes, XX in the female and XY in the male. Duplication or deficiency of chromosomal material may cause genetic imbalance severe enough to prevent normal development, or indeed be incompatable with life.

Chromosome abnormality, in particular sex chromosome abnormality, is an important cause of primary amenorrhoea, male infertility and other developmental anomaly of sex. At least one in six patients who come to the attention of the gynaecologist because of failure to menstruate spontaneously have a sex chromosome abnormality or a male sex chromosome complement. Amenorrhoea is permanent in both these groups of patients. About 10 per cent of male patients attending infertility clinics have a demonstrable sex chromosome abnormality; a further 10 per cent have an abnormality of their autosome chromosome complement. About one in four miscarriages are produced by chromosome abnormality of the foetus.

Identification of the sex chromosome complement, or sex chromatin state, can be a particularly useful aid to diagnosis and prognosis in primary amenorrhoea, male infertility and where external genitalia are ambiguous.

Chromosome analysis may be carried out on the leucocytes of blood, the fibroblasts of the dermis and other connective tissues, the cells of the bone marrow and, rarely, cells undergoing meiosis in the gonad. A chromosome analysis is possible within four days of obtaining a specimen for blood culture.

Chromosome Complement

Although human chromosomes differ in length and shape, Fig. 1, it is not possible at present to recognize with confidence 23 individual pairs of chromosomes. In practice between 10 and 12 groups of chromosomes can be distinguished, Fig. 2. Chromosome abnormality is presumed where the number of chromosomes in a group is different from the normal or where the morphology of a particular chromosome is different from the normal. The important groups to consider with regard to sex chromosome abnormality are the 6–12 + X group and the Y + 21–22 group.

Late Replicating X Chromosome

It is a particularly fortunate circumstance that one X chromosome in the female undergoes DNA replication out of phase with the rest of the chromosome complement. This late replicating chromosome can be studied (Fig. 3) using autoradiographic techniques. Autoradiography is a useful aid to the identification of extra or abnormal chromosome material. A structurally abnormal X chromosome is always the X chromosome which replicates late. Where more than two X chromosomes are present, the additional X chromosomes also replicate late.

Sex Chromatin

A valuable ancillary to chromosome analysis in the investigation of developmental anomalies of sex is the determination of the sex chromatin state. A convenient tissue to study for sex chromatin is the buccal mucosa,

Fig. 4. The sex chromatin body (Barr body) is a single X chromosome in a tightly coiled (heteropyknotic) form. In a normal male a Barr body is never seen; in a normal female between 20 and 50 per cent of nuclei show a single Barr body, the actual count depending to some extent on the staining technique and method of counting.

Individuals with a single Barr body in a proportion of buccal smear nuclei have two X chromosomes; individuals with two, three or four Barr bodies in a proportion of nuclei have three, four or five X chromosomes respectively.

however, technically easier to make a satisfactory blood smear preparation.

Gonadal Differentiation

It is the presence of a Y chromosome that determines the development of embryonic testes. Even where two, three or four X chromosomes are present a single Y chromosome is sufficient to determine that the bipotential gonad shall become a testis; albeit with poorly differentiated and subfunctional tissue. On the other hand the

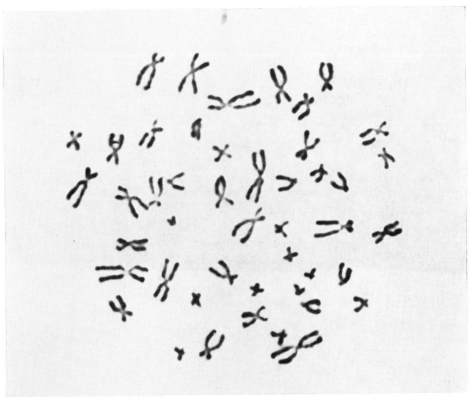

FIG. 1. Human white blood cell in metaphase of mitosis; a stage in cell division particularly suitable for chromosome analysis.

If sex chromatin is absent then only one X chromosome is present. A large, or small, Barr body may indicate an abnormality of an X chromosome. If the proportion of cells showing a Barr body is outside normal limits, or the distribution of cells containing Barr bodies is uneven, a sex chromosome abnormality may be suspected, e.g., a low sex chromatin count sometimes indicates that the patient is a mixture of cell types with respect to sex chromosome complement (sex chromosome mosaicism).

A second type of sex chromatin body is the drumstick, observed in polymorphonuclear leucocytes. In a normal female an excess of six drumsticks per 500 polymorphonuclear leucocytes are observed. A normal male has very few. Like the Barr body the drumstick is a heteropyknotic X chromosome. Drumsticks are not easy to score, even by the expert, and not as much information is to be obtained by examination of a blood smear for sex chromatin as examination of buccal smear. It is,

presence of two complete X chromosomes, without a Y chromosome, is necessary for the completion of ovarian development. The development of internal and external genitalia is secondary to the type and degree of differentiation of the gonad.

Disturbance of the normal XX or XY pattern will influence the development of the embryonic gonad. An apparent exception to this rule is the XXX female, who is fertile and appears to have normal ovarian tissue.

While a normal XX or XY sex chromosome constitution is essential for the differentiation of normal ovarian or testicular tissue, factors other than sex chromosome makeup may also influence the development of the gonad and/or genitalia.

Lyon Hypothesis

X chromosome activity in the mammalian female is quantitatively similar to that in the male, despite the fact

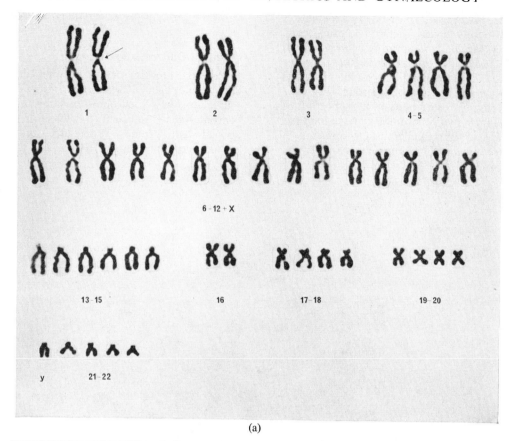

(a)

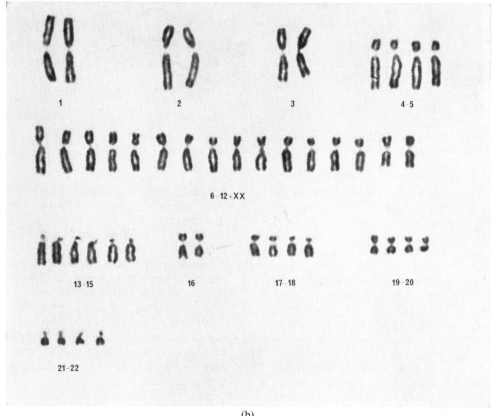

(b)

FIG. 2. Chromosomes arranged into groups according to length of chromosome and position of centromere. (a) Male karyotype and (b) Female karyotype. Arrow indicates centromere.

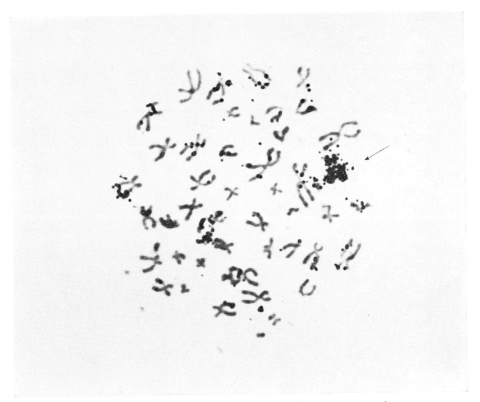

FIG. 3. Autoradiograph. Late replicating X chromosome arrowed.

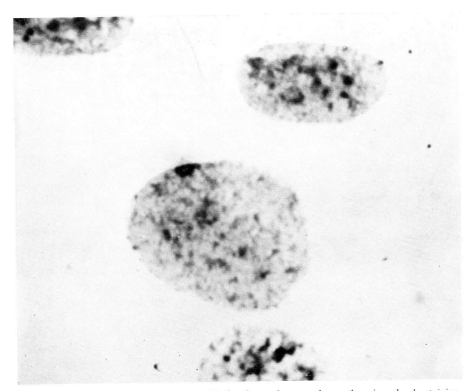

FIG. 4. Sex chromatin in buccal mucosa. Under the nuclear membrane there is a deeply staining body about 1 μ in diameter.

that the female has two X chromosomes and the male only one. At an early state of embryonic development one of the two X chromosomes in cells of the XX embryo is randomly inactivated (Lyon hypothesis). This has the effect of compensating for the double dose of gene products that would otherwise result. Thus the female is a functional mosaic; one cell population expressing the genes of the paternal X and the other those of the maternal X. However, not all of this inactivated chromosome is non-functional for it is apparent that segments of both

one chromosome less. Loss of a chromosome may also occur as a result of anaphase lag, where a chromosome is simply not included in either daughter nucleus. Non-disjunction or anaphase lag may occur at first or second stage of meiosis; non-disjunction at both stages would give rise to zygotes with two, three or four chromosomes extra, e.g. XXXXY.

The commonest structural abnormality observed in developmental anomaly of sex is "isochromosome" X; where the abnormal X chromosome consists of two long

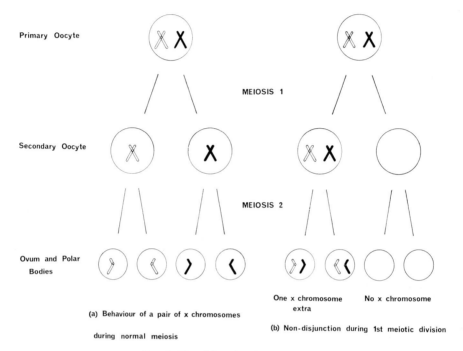

Primary Oocyte

MEIOSIS 1

Secondary Oocyte

MEIOSIS 2

Ovum and Polar Bodies

One x chromosome extra   No x chromosome

(a) Behaviour of a pair of x chromosomes during normal meiosis

(b) Non-disjunction during 1st meiotic division

FIG. 5. Non-disjunction during meiosis.

X chromosomes are necessary for normal gonadal development and indeed for normal growth.

Gene inactivation, late labelling and heteropyknosis are concommitant phenomena in that it is always the heteropyknotic (sex chromatin forming) X chromosome which is late labelling and genetically inactive.

Origin of Sex Chromosome Abnormality

Sex chromosome abnormality may conveniently be divided into three main types: (i) error in the number of chromosomes present; (ii) structural abnormality; and (iii) mosaicism. Each of these three types is observed as a cause of developmental anomalies of sex.

Error in the number of sex chromosomes present, either an extra chromosome, or chromosomes, or an absent chromosome usually arises as a result of misdivision in parental gametogenesis. Non-disjunction (Fig. 5), refers to the failure of homologous chromosomes to enter different daughter nuclei and results in the formation of a cell with one chromosome extra and a cell with one chromosome less. At fertilization this will result in the formation of a zygote with one chromosome extra or

arms rather than a long arm and a short arm. This abnormality can be referred to an error in division during gametogenesis.

The presence of two or more chromosomally distinct cell lines in the same individual is called chromosome mosaicism. This situation arises following non-disjunction or anaphase lag, (Fig. 6), during early embryogenesis. The original zygote may have a normal or abnormal chromosome complement.

Parents of patients with an XXY sex chromosome complement or an XXX sex chromosome complement are, on the average, older than parents in the general population. This increase in parental age is mainly due to the greater age of the mother. It would then appear that non-disjunction leading to the formation of a gamete with an extra X chromosome is more frequent in older women than in younger women and is probably more frequent during oogenesis than during spermatogenesis. On the other hand there is some evidence that the fathers of patients with an isochromosome X are older than is usual. This state can then more often be assigned to misdivision during spermatogenesis.

Chromosome Abnormality in Developmental Anomaly of Sex

While an analysis of sex chromosome complement has aided considerably our understanding of the origin and pathogenesis of developmental anomaly of sex and helped delineate and characterize specific syndromes, there is still a great deal of controversy with respect to the definition and designation of particular clinical syndromes. It is not the purpose of this article to contribute to this

into sex chromatin negative and sex chromatin positive varieties on the buccal smear findings.

Almost all cases of sex chromatin negative Turner's syndrome have a particular chromosome abnormality (Fig. 7), only one sex chromosome, an X, is present. XO/XY mosaicism may occasionally be observed.

Examples of sex chromatin positive Turner's syndrome may be shown to have an abnormal X chromosome, the most common of which is an isochromosome X (Fig. 8),

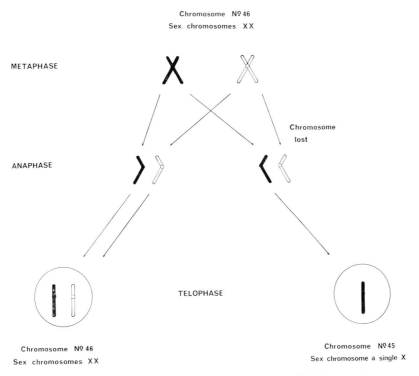

FIG. 6. Anaphase lag at first cleavage division, producing XX/XO mosaicism.

fascinating discussion. Further reading is suggested in the Bibliography.

Among the syndromes usually or sometimes due to sex chromosome abnormality are Turner's syndrome, Klinefelter's syndrome, Hermaphroditism and Pseudo-hermaphroditism. Phenotypic sex is at variance with chromosomal sex in Testicular Feminization and sometimes in Pure Gonadal Dysgenesis.

Turner's Syndrome (synonyms: ovarian agenesis, gonadal dysgenesis)

Primary amenorrhoea, dwarfism and absent secondary sex characteristics usually bring the young person to the attention of the gynaecologist at the expected time of puberty. They have infertile female external genitalia with an under-developed vagina and uterus and undifferentiated "streak" gonads without ovarian follicles. Other stigmata of Turner's syndrome include: webbing of the neck, a "shield" chest, cubitus valgus and co-arctation of the aorta. Urinary gonadotrophins may be greatly increased.

It is convenient to divide cases of Turner's syndrome

or to be a mixture of cell types. A common sex chromosome mosaicism is XO/XX; where parts of the body have an XO chromosome complement and parts have a normal chromosome complement. Other, more complicated, mosaics have been described, in each case one cell line contains only one complete X chromosome. A few patients with streak gonads and some of the somatic stigmata of Turner's syndrome, have an apparently normal chromosome complement. In these patients it is usually debatable whether the clinical features are sufficient to justify the label "Turner's" syndrome.

In some sex chromatin positive patients with clinical features of Turner's syndrome, or with features reminiscent of Turner's syndrome, absence of a part of one X chromosome is apparent. Where dwarfism is a clinical feature the deletion usually involves the short arm of the X.

Pure Gonadal Dysgenesis

Patients who fit this diagnosis have primary amenorrhoea and fail to develop secondary sex characteristics at puberty but do not have the somatic stigmata of Turner's syndrome. Gonadal tissue is undifferentiated. They are usually shown

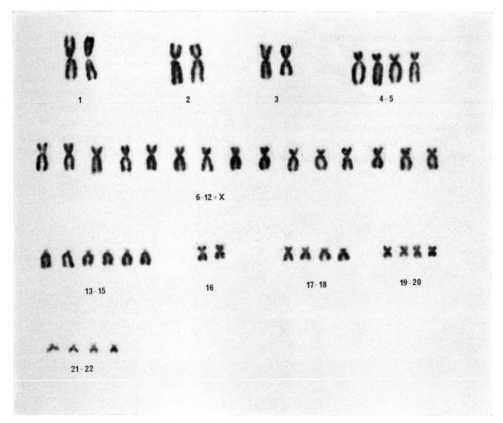

FIG. 7. Karyotype in sex chromatin negative Turner's syndrome. Chromosome number 45; only 15 chromosomes in 6—12+X group, and no Y chromosome. Presumptive XO.

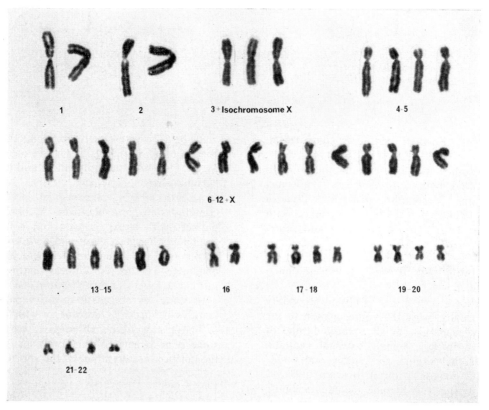

FIG. 8. A karyotype frequently seen in sex chromatin positive Turner's syndrome. Chromosome number 46; one chromosome missing from 6—12+X group and one extra in group 3. This individual has one normal X chromosome and one abnormal X chromosome (which looks like a No. 3 chromosome). Only one short arm of X is present.

to have either an XX or an XY sex chromosome complement without obvious chromosome abnormality.

Klinefelter's Syndrome

Klinefelter's syndrome is an important cause of infertility. It occurs in about one in ten azoospermic males and in about one in a hundred hypospermic males. The external genitalia are unmistakably male but at puberty the testes remain small. Facial and axillary hair are sparse. Pubic hair may be of female distribution. Bodily

Klinefelter's syndrome from the sex chromatin positive (True) Klinefelter's syndrome, most cases may be distinguished on testicular histology.

Hermaphroditism

Hermaphrodites have differentiated ovarian tissue, with ovarian follicles and differentiated testicular tissue.

Most hermaphrodites are sex chromatin positive and usually have an apparently normal female chromosome complement. Two mechanisms which may account for

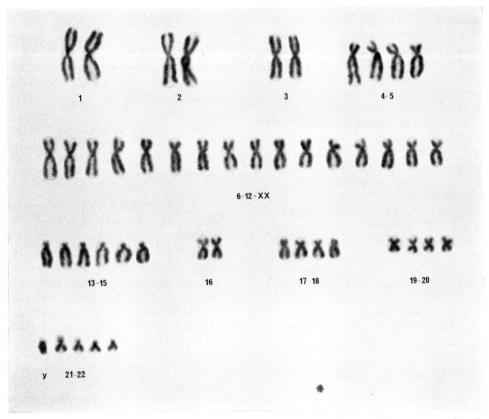

FIG. 9. Karyotype usually seen in sex chromatin positive Klinefelter's syndrome. Chromosome number 47; 16 chromosomes in 6—12+X group and a Y chromosome.

configuration may be eunachoid and there may occasionally be mammary development. Mental subnormality is sometimes a feature. After puberty, urinary gonadotrophins may be greatly increased and the testes show hyalinization of the seminiferous tubules, absent germ cells and Leydig cell hyperplasia.

All sex chromatin positive cases of Klinefelter's syndrome (sometimes called "True" Klinefelter's syndrome) have a demonstrable chromosome abnormality, (Fig. 9), with a cell line containing at least two X chromosomes and a Y chromosome.

Sex chromatin negative patients with clinical features of Klinefelter's syndrome ("False" Klinefelter's syndrome) usually have an apparently normal male chromosome complement.

Although it is sometimes difficult on clinical examination alone to distinguish sex chromatin negative (False)

the development of testicular tissue in the absence of a Y chromosome are outlined below. Sometimes, however, sex chromosome mosaicism may be demonstrated. Where sex chromosome mosaicism is observed, one cell line has a Y chromosome and is presumably responsible for the development of differentiated testicular tissue, and the other cell line lacks a Y chromosome but usually has two X chromosomes, and is presumably responsible for development of differentiated ovarian tissue. Sex chromosome mosaicism may be observed in less than one fifth of sex chromatin positive hermaphrodites.

The origin of two types of differential gonadal tissue in the same individual is a focal point in understanding normal gonadal differentiation. It is then worth mentioning two possible mechanisms which may account for gonadal development in hermaphrodites not the result of XX/XY, or similar, mosaicism. It is theoretically possible, but difficult to demonstrate, that part of a Y chromosome may be transferred to an X chromosome (translocated). If the translocated fragment on this compound chromosome is inactivated when the X chromosome to which it is attached is inactivated (See Lyon hypothesis) but active when this X is active, then the individual will be a mosaic, with respect to sex chromosome activity, of XX/XXY type. This type of mosaicism would be expected to produce a mixture of gonadal tissue; the XX functional cell line being responsible for the development of ovarian tissue, the XXY functional cell line being responsible for the development of testicular tissue. It is interesting to note that, in individuals where this mechanism operates, testicular tissue would never be more developed than that observed in Klinefelter's syndrome. An alternative view, which may be labelled the "Balance Hypothesis", is that chance embryonic events can dominate gonadal differentiation where ovary or testis determiners are of very nearly equal strength. For this to occur it is necessary to postulate either: (i) that both ovary and testis determiners are normally present in the chromosome set of the normal female and, by chance, may occur in nearly equal potency; or (ii) that testis determiners are occasionally transferred from the Y chromosome to other chromosomes (translocation or unequal crossing over).

Sex chromatin negative hermaphrodites are very rare. An apparently normal XY chromosome makeup was described in those analysed for chromosome complement. It is perhaps worthy of note that mosaicism may easily be overlooked, especially if only one tissue, e.g., blood, is analysed for chromosome complement. XO/XY mosaics with some features of hermaphroditism have been described. Usually, however, differentiated ovarian tissue is absent from these patients and they are more properly designated male pseudohermaphrodites.

Female Pseudohermaphroditism

Patients in this group are sex chromatin positive with a normal female chromosome complement. They usually suffer from the adrenogenital syndrome or from transplacental masculinization of a female foetus. In either event the masculinization affects the external genitalia only. Internally they are normal females with bilateral differentiated ovarian tissue, a normal uterus and normal fallopian tubes.

Male Pseudohermaphroditism

These are males whose testes fail fully to masculinize the external genitalia in foetal life. Differentiated gonadal tissue is testicular, but may be intra abdominal or inguinal and unilateral or bilateral. Most male pseudohermaphrodites have an apparently normal XY chromosome complement. Examples of XO/XY mosaicism may, however, enter into this clinical category.

In the extreme variety of this condition the external genitalia and mammary development are normal female but the vagina is short and the uterus absent. Patients with this "Testicular Feminizing" syndrome develop as females except for sex hair and menstruation. This variety of male pseudohermaphroditism is the result of gene mutation and has a familial incidence.

XO/XY Mosaicism

XO/XY mosaicism has been described in: (i) Examples of gonadal dysgenesis, where the gonads are undifferentiated streaks of fibrous tissue; (ii) Examples of male pseudohermaphroditism, where differentiated gonadal tissue is testicular; and (iii) Patients in whom there is some histological support for a diagnosis of hermaphroditism. Differences in gonadal pathology observed in XO/XY mosaicism are probably a consequence of varying distribution of the two cell types in the developing gonads.

Other Sex Chromosome Abnormality

An extra X chromosome may be associated with mental subnormality in the absence of overt developmental anomaly of sex. Triple X females (XXX) only rarely develop primary or secondary amenorrhoea. There seems to be a rough correlation with the number of extra X chromosomes and the degree of mental subnormality present.

Chromosome Analysis where Developmental Anomaly of Sex is Considered

Where developmental anomaly of sex is suspected an appreciation of the sex chromatin state and/or chromosome complement can give an indication of the nature and differentiation of the gonads present or suggest the need for further investigation. It need hardly be emphasized that chromosome analysis is no substitute for gonadal biopsy. Specimens for sex chromatin and chromosome analysis (blood culture) are easily obtained with little inconvenience to the patient.

Where a condition known to be caused by specific chromosome abnormality is suspected the finding of the specific chromosome abnormality is virtually diagnostic of the condition. Although an apparently normal chromosome complement does not necessarily refute the suspected diagnosis, it does make this diagnosis less likely. While some patients with clinical features compatible with a diagnosis of Turner's syndrome or Klinefelter's syndrome, but with an apparently normal chromosome complement, may have an undetected chromosome abnormality, e.g., mosaicism, it is probable that in most the clinical features have an origin other than that of chromosome abnormality.

Turner's syndrome

Where primary amenorrhœa, sexual infantilism, short stature and other physical stigmata of Turner's syndrome are present the experienced practitioner has little difficulty in making a diagnosis, even in the absence of direct evidence of streak gonads. A sex chromatin negative state indicates an XO chromosome complement. A sex chromatin positive state indicates an abnormal X chromosome (usually an isochromosome) or XO/XX mosaicism. Chromosome analysis is usually of academic interest only.

There are, however, many examples of primary amenorrhoea and sexual infantilism where the clinical features, although suggestive, are insufficient to make a confident diagnosis of Turner's syndrome or "streak gonads." In these patients, Table 1, sex chromatin and chromosome analysis is a very useful indicator of the nature and state of differentiation of the gonads and may emphasize the need for laparotomy or peritonoscopy. The patients may be sex chromatin negative or sex chromatin positive. The sex chromatin negative variety usually have a simple XO chromosome complement. Sometimes, however,

individuals ascertained before puberty, will have a relatively normal puberty. One sex chromatin negative XO adult with the somatic stigmata of Turner's syndrome bore a child. This must, however, be very rare. Speculating as to the gonadal development of XO/XX mosaics ascertained before puberty, without evidence of gonadal pathology, must be exceedingly hazardous.

Pure Gonadal Dysgenesis

Sexual infantilism and primary amenorrhoea may, of course, occur in patients without the somatic stigmata of

TABLE 1

SEX CHROMATIN AND CHROMOSOME COMPLEMENT OF 50 CONSECUTIVE PATIENTS REFERRED TO THE CENTRE FOR HUMAN GENETICS, SHEFFIELD, FOR CHROMOSOME ANALYSIS BECAUSE OF FAILURE TO MENSTRUATE SPONTANEOUSLY

Fifty-four per cent had either a sex chromosome abnormality or an XY chromosome complement. Where short stature is a feature, 75 per cent had an abnormality of the sex chromosome complement. These patients cannot be regarded as typical of those referred to a gynaecological clinic.

Additional Clinical Features	Sex Chromatin State	No.	Sex Chromosome Complement	No.
Sexual infantilism. Short stature (less than 5ft.) and other somatic stigmata of Turner's syndrome	Negative	6	XO¹	6
	Positive	1	XO/X Isochromosome X¹	1
Short stature. Other somatic stigmata of Turner's syndrome not prominent	Negative	8	XO¹	7
			XO/XY²	1
	Positive	9	XO/X Isochromosome X¹	1
			XO/XXX³	2
			XX⁴	6
Normal stature. Somatic stigmata of Turner's syndrome not prominent	Negative	6	XO¹	2
			XY⁵	4
	Positive	8	XX⁴	8
Clinical details not recorded	Negative	2	XO¹	1
			XY⁵	1
	Positive	10	XO/XX³	1
			XX⁴	9

1. Streak gonads presumed.
2. Left gonad a streak; right gonad a poorly differentiated testis.
3. Streak gonads or poorly differentiated gonads presumed.
4. If differentiated gonadal tissue present it is presumed to be ovarian.
5. If differentiated gonadal tissue present it is presumed to be testicular

XO/XY mosaicism may be observed. The sex chromatin positive patients usually have an abnormal X chromosome, e.g., an isochromosome or XO/XX mosaicism. An XO/XY mosaic may have a poorly developed intra-abdominal testis and an XO/XX mosaic may have differentiated ovarian tissue.

The somatic stigmata of Turner's syndrome can occur without sexual infantilism and gonadal dysgenesis (Ullrich's syndrome). The condition is not usually associated with chromosome abnormality. In a prepubertal female it is important to distinguish this state from incipient Turner's syndrome. The finding of a sex chromosome complement characteristic of Turner's syndrome would infer gonadal dysgenesis and failure to develop secondary sex characteristics at puberty and make sterility very probable. It is, however, important to emphasize that ovarian tissue, containing follicles and ova, has been observed in XO individuals in infancy and early childhood. The possibility exists that some XO

Turner's syndrome. Some of these patients, difficult to put in any particular clinical category (apart from Testicular Feminization, see below), have an abnormality of the sex chromosomes, e.g., XO/XX mosaicism or a deleted X chromosome. Most, however, have an apparently normal chromosome complement, although the chromosome sex may be at variance with the phenotypic sex. In these patients the finding of an apparently normal XX or XY sex chromosome complement indicates that if differentiated gonadal tissue is present, it is ovarian or testicular respectively.

Testicular Feminization

Testicular feminization is not associated with chromosome abnormality; although chromosomal sex (XY) is at variance with phenotypic sex. This diagnosis is usually made on clinical examination alone. A negative sex chromatin state and/or the demonstration of an XY chromosome complement is sound confirmatory evidence.

The gonads are, of course, testes and may be intra-abdominal.

Klinefelter's Syndrome and Male Sterility

The finding of an XXY chromosome complement, or its equivalent (e.g., XXXY), in a male investigated for infertility indicates severely impaired or absent spermatogenesis and is usually diagnostic of Klinefelter's syndrome.

XXY/XY mosaics may come to the attention of the clinician for reasons other than investigation of infertility, e.g., the investigation of mental subnormality. Some of these patients do not have physical features of Klinefelter's syndrome and have testes capable of normal function. An assessment of fertility must depend on more direct investigation, in particular examination of ejaculate.

While the majority of boys diagnosed as sex chromatin positive XXY males before puberty will develop the physical features of Klinefelter's syndrome and be sterile, a small proportion will not. Some of these will be undetected XXY/XY mosaics.

Recent research indicates that abnormality of chromosomes other than the sex chromosomes may also be a cause of subfertility. Assessment of the probability, and likely products, of fertilization in such patients is, at present, very difficult.

Ambiguous External Genitalia

Although ambiguous external genitalia may first come to the attention of the medical practitioner at puberty, e.g., with mammary development in an apparent male, most patients with ambiguous external genitalia are recognizable at birth. Indecision is usually as to whether the person is an underdeveloped male or a masculinized female.

Most commonly the child is a masculinized female with normal internal genitalia, masculinization occurring either as a manifestation of the adrenogenital syndrome or as a result of hormone therapy given to the mother in early pregnancy. In these cases the infant will be sex chromatin positive. If the child is sex chromatin negative then it is likely that he is an under-masculinized male.

Hermaphroditism must be suspected if the external genitalia are ambiguous, one gonad is in the scrotum or inguinal canal and the patient sex chromatin positive; the finding of an XY/XX or similar (see above) mosaicism would make this diagnosis virtually certain.

Although a simple sex chromatin analysis is sufficient to indicate the nature of the gonads in most cases of doubtful sex, and may quickly exclude the adrenogenital syndrome, a full chromosome analysis may occasionally give useful additional information.

Recurrence Risk of Conditions due to Chromosome Abnormality

Where chromosome abnormality is the cause of developmental abnormality of sex it is usually the result of an isolated event occurring in the gonad of one or other parent or of misdivision during the early embryogenesis of the patient. The parents have normal chromosome complements. The risk of a second occurrence in a subsequent pregnancy is low. The patients are themselves infertile.

About one quarter of early abortions are of chromosomal origin. These abnormalities are usually due to isolated events occurring in chromosomally normal parents and are unlikely to recur.

Certain, well recognized, types of congenital abnormality are due to autosomal abnormality The great majority of these are isolated occurrences in chromosomally normal parents. However, where chromosome abnormality is present in a parent the risk of recurrence in each succeeding pregnancy is usually greater than one in 10.

(This Chapter could be read in conjunction with the chapters by C. J. Dewhurst (Sec. III Chap. 6.) and C. O. Carter (Sec. XII Chap. 4.). Eds.)

BIBLIOGRAPHY

General

Bartalos, M. and Baramki, T. A. (1967), *Medical Cytogenetics*. Baltimore: The Williams and Williams Co.

Hamerton, J. L. (editor) (1962), *Chromosomes in Medicine*. Heinemann.

Overzier, C. (editor) (1963), *Intersexuality*. London: Academic Press.

Miller, Orlander J. (1964), "The Sex Chromosome Anomalies," *Amer. J. obstet. gynec.*, **90**, 1078.

Specific

Lyon, M. E. (1966), "Sex Chromatin and Gene Action in the X-chromosome of Mammals," in *The Sex Chromatin*, pp. 370–386, editor, Moore, K. L. Philadelphia: W. B. Saunders Co.

Ferguson-Smith, M. A. (1965), "Karyotype-phenotype Correlations in Gonadal Dysgenesis," *J. Med. Gen.*, **2**, 142.

Ferguson-Smith, M. A. (1963), "Chromosome Studies in Klinefelter's Syndrome," *Pro. Roy. Soc. Med.*, **56**, 577.

Jones, H. W., Jr., Ferguson-Smith, M. A. and Heller, R. H. (1965), "Pathologic and Cytogenetic Findings in True Hermaphroditism: Report of Six Cases and Review of Twenty-three Cases from the Literature," *Obstet. gynec.*, **25**, 435.

Ferguson-Smith, M. A. (1966), "X–Y Chromosomal Interchange in the Etiology of True Hermaphroditism and of XX Klinefelter's Syndrome in Intersexuality," *Lancet*, **2**, 475.

Ford, C. E. (1963), "The Cytogenetics of Human Intersexuality," in *Intersexuality*, editor C. Overzier. London: Academic Press.

McIlree, Maureen E., Price, W. H., Court Brown, W. M., Tulloch, W. Selby, Newsame, J. E. and Maclean, N. (1966), "Chromosome Studies on Testicular Cells from Fifty Subfertile Men," *Lancet*, **2**, 69.

4. SEMEN

T. MANN

Mammalian semen, as ejaculated, is a suspension of spermatozoa in seminal plasma. The spermatozoa originate in the testes, and are stored in the epididymides. At ejaculation, they come in contact with seminal plasma which consists of the secretions produced by the epididymides, vasa deferentia, ampullae, vesiculae seminales, prostate gland, Cowper's glands (bulbo-urethral glands) and Littré's glands (urethral glands). Because the composition of the ejaculate depends on the relative proportion of spermatozoa and the various accessory secretions, samples of semen obtained from different species or from different individuals, even if belonging to the same species, can show marked variations.

General Characteristics of Semen and the Assessment of Semen "Quality"

Normal fresh semen has the appearance of a creamy, slightly greyish or yellowish fluid. In most mammals it is ejaculated in a liquid or semi-liquid form. In some species (dog, bull, ram), it remains liquid, but in others it forms either a gel, as in the boar, or a firm coagulum, as in the mouse, rat, and guinea-pig.

Human semen, when freshly ejaculated, appears gel-like or "clotted" but within about 20 minutes it liquefies spontaneously and until that happens, sperm motility is negligible. That is why microscopic evaluation of sperm motility in a human ejaculate can only be done when liquefaction has been completed. The coagulation-liquefaction process, characteristic of human semen, is thought to involve several enzymic reactions. The first of these is the action of a clotting enzyme of prostatic origin on a fibrinogen-like protein secreted in the seminal vesicles; the result is the formation of a fibrin-like clot. In the next reaction, called fibrinolysis, fibrin is broken down to smaller fragments by another enzyme of prostatic origin, which is plasmin-like in character. The third stage involves further proteolysis of the lysed fibrin, and leads to the formation of peptides, as well as amino-acids. These amino-acids too, can undergo further enzymic changes, due to the presence in semen of certain deaminases and aminotransferases (transaminases). That is why the protein content of a human semen ejaculate does not remain constant but undergoes rapid change, a factor which must be taken into account in the quantitative analysis of seminal proteins, peptides, and amino-acids.

The volume of a normal human ejaculate varies from 2 to 6 ml., and averages about 3·5 ml. Each ejaculate contains between 50 and 150 million spermatozoa per ml, but, provided that motility and morphology are good, even much lower sperm concentrations down to 20 million/ml., are still compatible with fertility. However, sperm counts below 20 million/ml. must be regarded as a sign of oligospermia. In addition to the variations normally encountered in volume, sperm concentration, and motility, there is also much variability in sperm morphology, that is the percentage of abnormal sperm cells with defects in the head, middle-piece and tail, or "immature" in character. Useful reviews of that subject are found in the monographs of Williams (1965) and Amelar (1966) as well as articles by MacLeod (1964), Hartman, Schoenfeld and Copeland (1964) and Freund (1966).

It is important to bear in mind that various extraneous factors can influence sperm concentration, motility and morphology in different ways. An interesting example is the effect which the frequency of ejaculation has on various aspects of so-called semen quality. As MacLeod and Gold (1951, 1952) have shown, in normal men a prolonged period of continence (up to 10 days) is generally associated with a rise in the ejaculate volume and sperm concentration, accompanied by a decrease in the percentage of active, that is motile, spermatozoa. However, this does not apply to oligospermic men, because in these cases continence may lead either to a small increase of sperm concentration, or to a decrease. Conversely, an excessively high frequency of ejaculation, even in normal men, tends to diminish the number of spermatozoa available for ejaculation. According to Freund (1963) the extra-gonadal sperm reserve, that is the total reserve of spermatozoa in the ampullæ, vasa deferentia and the epididymides, can be depleted in normal men by an average of 2·4 emissions per day during a depletion period of 10 days. Just like spermatozoa, the "replacement" of seminal plasma is also a time-dependent process. It takes more than a day to replenish the reserve of secretory fluid in the human seminal vesicles, as shown by the fact that if two ejaculates are collected from the same individual within 24 hrs, the second one usually contains less of a characteristic vesicular constituent such as fructose. In the bull, on the other hand, where the seminal vesicles can store a large volume of secretory fluid, the so-called exhaustion test brings about a depletion of spermatozoa much more rapidly than a deficiency of seminal plasma. This is illustrated by one of our own experiments (Mann, 1948) in which eight ejaculates were collected from a bull within 1 hour. As a result of these multiple collections the concentration of spermatozoa fell from 1,664,000 sperm/μl. in the first, to 98,000 sperm/μl. in the last ejaculate. In contrast, the concentration of fructose which in the bull, as in man, comes from the seminal vesicles, only decreased from 760 mg./100 ml. in the first, to 690 mg./100 ml., in the last ejaculate.

To assess the "quality" of semen correctly, it is also necessary to take into account the fact that in many species, including man, the different portions or "fractions" of the ejaculate are not identical in make-up, but follow one another in a definite order of sequence. This has been demonstrated repeatedly by the use of the so-called split ejaculate method which depends on the collection of separate fractions of the same ejaculate. Human semen can thus be subdivided into at least three fractions, referred to respectively as pre-sperm, sperm-rich and post-sperm. Normally ejaculation is initiated by the secretion of the Cowper's gland, with the prostatic secretion and spermatozoa following next, and the seminal vesicle secretion appearing last. According to Lundquist (1949) the prostatic secretion contributes from 13 per cent to 33 per cent, and the seminal vesicle secretion from 46 per cent to 80 per cent, of the entire ejaculate. Under special circumstances, however, due perhaps to disturbances in the nervous mechanism which controls the normal ejaculatory process, the normal sequence of ejaculation can be seriously upset. In our own studies we came across disturbances of that kind when examining split ejaculates from certain apparently infertile thoroughbred stallions. A reversal of the usual pattern of ejaculation has also been noted in men (Amelar and Hotchkiss, 1965).

When evaluating the "quality" of semen it is also worth remembering that the motility and the fertilizing ability of the spermatozoa can, under certain rather special circumstances, become dissociated from each other. Normally, good sperm motility is so closely correlated with fertilizing capacity that in the practice of semen appraisal measurement of motility is used as a reliable criterion of sperm "quality". Because, however, motility is associated with the sperm flagellum, that is, the midpiece-tail part of the spermatozoon, whilst the fertilizing ability is located in a different region of the sperm cell, namely in the sperm head, these two sperm "qualities" can be separated; as for example, in the semen of certain infertile bulls which produce ejaculates composed entirely of "decapitated" spermatozoa, that is, sperm-heads completely detached from (fully motile) tails. Another example of a similar nature is provided by the well-known fact that semen which has been exposed to a large dose of X-rays, usually shows normal or near normal motility, but its fertilizing ability is either *nil* or pathologically altered.

As yet, the best criterion of the fertilizing capacity of spermatozoa is their actual ability to fertilize an ovum under conditions *in vivo*. This is assessed on the basis of the so-called conception rate, that is the number of successful pregnancies expressed as percentage of the total number of inseminated females. For the time being, assessment by "conception rate" continues to be the main method of evaluating fertility, at any rate in veterinary practice (Maule, 1962; Cole and Cupps, 1968). It would of course, be much simpler and less tedious to be able to assess "male fertility" by means of a fertilization test *in vitro*. On an experimental level this has already been achieved, but because the quantitative aspects of the *in vitro* fertilization method have not as yet, been worked out in detail, the procedure for the time being, is not ripe for use in clinical practice.

Motility, on the other hand, can be assessed quickly and reliably by various methods, including direct microscopic observation, cinematographic recording of sperm velocity, scanning with a television camera, photoelectric devices, and measurements of electrical impedance change frequency. In addition, quick and dependable methods are now available for assessing the ratio between live or motile, and dead or immotile, spermatozoa. The most frequently used method of this kind is the determination of the incidence of dead spermatozoa by "live-dead differential staining". Certain stains, as for example, eosin, are readily taken up by dead, but not live, spermatozoa. Another means of assessing sperm motility under conditions *in vitro* is the so-called "cervical mucus penetration test", in which a drop of semen is placed on a microscope slide close to a drop of cervical mucus, and the penetration of spermatozoa into the mucus is followed microscopically (Harvey, 1954; Tampion and Gibbons, 1963).

Structural and Chemical Characteristics of Spermatozoa

The total length of a human spermatozoon is about 0·05 mm., but of that length only about 1/10 is due to the sperm-head, and the remainder is made up by the flagellum. The spermatozoa of large domestic animals, such as bull, boar and ram, are approximately the same size. A diagrammatic representation of a mammalian spermatozoon is given in Fig. 1.

The human sperm-head has the shape of an oval flattened body, about 4·6 μ long, 2·6 μ wide, and 1·5 μ thick. It is taken up largely by the sperm nucleus which is filled with closely packed chromatin consisting of deoxyribonucleoprotein. The anterior part of the nucleus is covered by the acrosome, a cap-like structure made up of lipoglycoprotein material; in the acrosome are located various enzymes, including hyaluronidase and protease.

The sperm flagellum, which connects with the sperm-head in the so-called neck, is essentially composed of two parts: the middle-piece, which is about the length of the sperm-head, and the tail. The tail can be further subdivided into the principal-piece and the end-piece. Along the whole length of the middle-piece and tail run centrally a number of contractile protein fibrils which together form the so-called axial filament complex. In the middle-piece where the axial filament complex is best developed, its structure is made up of nine coarse fibres which together compose the "outer cylinder", and nine much finer fibres, each of them double-barrelled, which together compose the "inner cylinder". In addition, right in the centre of the axial filament system are located two more fine fibres, which are referred to as the "central pair".

In the middle-piece, but not in the tail, the entire axial filament complex is surrounded by mitochondria, arranged in the shape of the so-called mitochondrial-sheath. In that sheath, chemically distinguished by a high content of aldehydogenic phospholipids, are located a number of enzymes associated with the metabolic activity of spermatozoa, including the entire cytochrome system and numerous dehydrogenases. In the tail, the axial filament complex is covered on the outside by a spiral fibrous structure known as the tail-sheath. This sheath however, terminates a little distance short of end of the tail, thus exposing the terminal portion of the axial filament system or the so-called end-piece. The sperm-tail also contains some enzymes, notably adenosinetriphosphatase which, by its action on adenosinetriphosphate, provides probably directly, the energy required for sperm motility. Detailed information on the ultrastructure of the human spermatozoon is to be found in a paper by Ånberg (1957).

The Composition and Function of Seminal Plasma

The seminal plasma, that is the fluid composed of the various secretions of the male accessory organs, provides the vehicle in which the spermatozoa are ejaculated. In its physical and chemical properties the seminal plasma differs in many ways from other body fluids. One of its characteristic features is the presence of a wide range of highly active enzymes, including those mentioned before, which are responsible for the phenomenon of semen coagulation and liquefaction. Among the seminal plasma enzymes are several very active phosphatases,

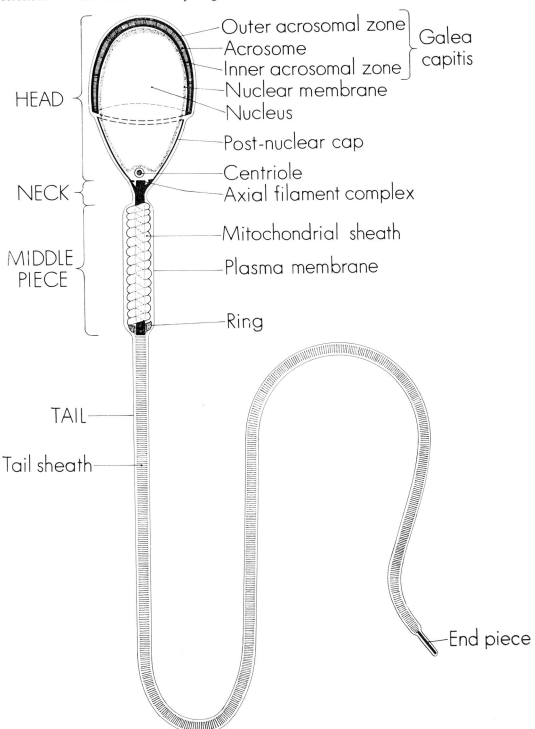

FIG. 1. Diagrammatic representation of a spermatozoon from: T. Mann, "The biochemistry of semen and of the male reproductive tract," Methuen: London.

including the acid phosphatase, which in man originates chiefly from the prostate gland. The activity of the acid phosphatase is so characteristic of human seminal plasma, that it is used in forensic medicine as a sensitive criterion for the detection of seminal stains (Kind, 1964). At least two other normal constituents of the human seminal plasma, namely choline ("Florence test") and spermine ("Barberio test") have also been used in the past for a similar purpose. These two substances belong to a large group of nitrogenous bases which abound in the seminal plasma. The oldest known is undoubtedly spermine, as the characteristic shape of the spermine phosphate crystals has been noted already by Leeuwenhoek, who mentions this specifically in his letter to the Royal Society of London, dated November, 1677.

In many mammals, including man, the seminal plasma contains fructose as the main sugar (Mann, 1946). In man, seminal fructose is derived mostly from the seminal vesicles, and to a lesser extent from the ampullae. The concentration of fructose in the human ejaculate is of the order of 100–500 mg./100 ml. The determination of fructose, which is based on the use of a simple colour reaction with resorcinol, requires no more than 0·1 ml. semen. It provides not only a quantitative measure of the seminal vesicle contribution to the make-up of the human ejaculate, but can serve as a useful diagnostic means for the detection of an occlusion of the ejaculatory ducts (the small ducts through which the spermatozoa and vesicular secretion jointly enter the urethral canal). Fructose-free azoospermic ejaculates have also been encountered in men with aplasia of vasa deferentia (Marberger, Marberger, Mann and Lutwak–Mann, 1961; Amelar and Hotchkiss, 1963).

The human prostate secretes apart from the acid phosphatase a number of highly characteristic substances, among them several proteins and mucoproteins, best distinguishable by immunological, electrophoretic and chromatographic methods (Soanes, Shulman, Mamrod, Barnes and Gonder, 1963; Mann and Rottenberg, 1966; Mischler and Reinecke, 1966). Moreover, the human prostate secretes a large amount of citric acid, of which the human ejaculate may contain as much as 1 g./100 ml. Just as fructose can serve as a reliable criterion of seminal vesicle activity, citric acid provides a similarly sensitive indicator of prostatic function.

Determinations of seminal fructose and citric acid can also serve as indicators of the androgenic status of the male. A low level of fructose in semen is sometimes associated with certain forms of hypogonadism, which is not unexpected if one recalls the fact that both the growth and secretory activity of the seminal vesicles closely depend upon the availability and stimulatory influence of testosterone (Mann, 1967). Another property of fructose in semen is its role as substrate for the metabolism of spermatozoa. Human spermatozoa differ from those of e.g. ram or bull, by showing a relatively low capacity to respire, but their anaerobic metabolism is similarly high. Approximately 2 mg. of fructose are utilized by 10^9 spermatozoa during 1 hour incubation at $37°$.

One more group of seminal plasma constituents deserves special mention, namely the so-called prostaglandins. These substances are unsaturated twenty-carbon fatty-acids, characterized by the presence of a cyclopentanone ring, and endowed with blood-pressure lowering and smooth-muscle stimulating properties. Nearly twenty prostaglandins have so far been isolated, several of them from human semen (Bergström, Ryhage, Samuelsson and Sjövall, 1962). The rapid development in this field is best surveyed in the voluminous prostaglandin bibliography recently published by Pike (1967). Prostaglandins appear to account for all, or most, of the strong smooth-muscle stimulating activity which human seminal plasma exerts on the uterus under *in vitro* conditions.

Sperm "Maturation", "Capacitation", and Survival in the Reproductive Tract

At the time when they leave the testis and the epididymis, the spermatozoa are neither motile nor fertile. They acquire both these properties during the passage in the epididymis. The process of sperm "ripening" or "maturation", does not, however, end in the male tract. In several mammalian species spermatozoa freshly deposited in the female, are incapable of fertilizing the ovum, although they are motile, until they have remained in the reproductive tract of the female for long enough to undergo the so-called "capacitation" process, usually of several hours duration. The fascinating subject of "sperm capacitation" has been extensively reviewed in a recent symposium (Duncan, Ericsson and Zimbelman, 1967).

Apart from "capacitation", numerous other factors influence the survival of mammalian spermatozoa in the female tract. Those of particular importance are listed by Noyes and Thibault (1962) as follows: anatomy and physiology of the female reproductive tract; sperm concentration and motility; rate of sperm passage, and in particular, the number of spermatozoa reaching the uterus and oviducts; the time during which the spermatozoa remain there; the hormonal state of the female at the time of semen deposition; the dilution of spermatozoa by the secretory fluids produced in the female reproductive tract; and the response of the female tract itself to the presence of spermatozoa, of which sperm phagocytosis forms only one but not the least important aspect. All these and probably other as yet undiscovered factors, contribute to the success of fertilization of an ovum by a spermatozoon.

The time which elapses between the moment of sperm deposition and the moment of fertilization is of course, of singular importance. Sperm motility as such is, no doubt, an important factor in this respect. But even immotile spermatozoa, when deposited in the cervix, have been shown, in the cow at any rate, to be capable of reaching the oviducts quickly, a fact from which it must be deduced that spermatozoa do not depend solely upon their own motility, but traverse the uterus also passively by concomitant contractions of the female reproductive tract.

The Ratio between Male and Female-producing Spermatozoa

Assuming that 50 per cent of the spermatozoa leaving the testes, carry the female-producing X-chromosome in their haploid nucleus, while the remaining 50 per cent are endowed instead with the male-producing Y-chromosome, and assuming further, that both X- and Y-carrying spermatozoa reach the site of fertilization in equal numbers, one would expect on fertilization a primary sex ratio of 1:1. Much effort has been directed, particularly in recent years, towards altering that ratio by artificial means, and thus influencing the sex ratio. Counter-streaming centrifugation (Lindahl, 1958), electrophoresis (Gordon, 1957) and differential sedimentation (Bhattacharya, Bangham, Cro, Keynes and Rowson, 1966; Schilling, 1966; Bedford and Bibeau, 1967) were the main methods used in attempts to separate male- and female-determining spermatozoa from ejaculated semen. Occasionally success has been reported, but much more work is needed before the problem of controlling the sex-ratio can be considered as satisfactorily and reproducibly solved.

REFERENCES

Amelar, R. D. (1966), *Infertility in men. Diagnosis and treatment.* Philadelphia: F. A. Davis Co.

Amelar, R. D. and Hotchkiss, R. L. (1963), "Congenital Aplasia of the Epididymides and Vasa Deferentia: Effects on Semen," *Fertility and Sterility*, 14, 44.

Amelar, R. D. and Hotchkiss, R. L. (1965), "The Split Ejaculate. Its use in the management of male infertility," *Fertil. and Steril.*, 16, 46.

Ånberg, A. (1957), "The Ultrastructure of the Human Spermatozoon. *Acta. obstet. Gynec. scand.*, 36, Supplement, 2.

Bedford, J. M. and Bibeau, A.-M. (1967), "Failure of Sperm Sedimentation to influence the Sex Ratio of Rabbits," *Journal of Reproduction and Fertility*, 14, 167.

Bergström, S., Ryhage, R., Samuelsson, B. and Sjövall, J., "The Structure of Prostaglandins E, F_1 and F_2," *Acta chem. scand.*, 16, 501.

Bhattacharya, B. C., Bangham, A. D., Cro, R. J., Keynes, R. D. and Rowson, L. E. A. (1966), "An Attempt to Predetermine the Sex of Calves by Artificial Insemination with Spermatozoa separated by Sedimentation," *Nature*, 211, 863.

Cole, H. H. and Cupps, P. T. (1968), *Reproduction in Domestic Animals*, 2nd edition. New York and London: Academic Press.

Duncan, G. W., Ericsson, R. J. and Zimbelman, R. G. (ed.) (1967), "Capacitation of Spermatozoa and Endocrine Control of Spermatogenesis," *Journal of Reproduction and Fertility*, Supplement No. 2.

Freund, M. (1963), "Effect of Frequency of Emission on Semen Output and an Estimate of Daily Sperm Production in Man," *Journal of Reproduction and Fertility*, 6, 269.

Freund, M. (1966), "Standards for the Rating of Human Sperm Morphology," *International Journal of Fertility*, 11, 97.

Gordon, M. J. (1957), "Control of Sex Ratio in Rabbits by Electrophoresis of Spermatozoa," *Proc. nat. Acad. Sci. (Wash.)*, 43, 913.

Hartman, C. G., Schoenfeld, C. and Copeland, E. (1964), "Individualism in the Semen Picture of Infertile Men," *Fertil. and Steril.*, 15, 231.

Harvey, C. (1954), "An Experimental Study of the Penetration of Human Cervical Mucus by Spermatozoa *in vitro*," *J. Obstet. Gynæc. Brit. Emp.*, 61, 480.

Kind, S. E. (1964), "The Acid Phosphatase Test," *Methods of Forensic Science*, (Curry, A. S., ed.), 2, 267.

Leeuwenhoek, A. van (1677), "Observationes D. Anthonii Lewenhoeck, de Natis e semine genitali Animalculis." Letter dated November, 1677, and published in 1678, in *Philosophical Transactions of the Royal Society*, 12, 1040.

Lindahl, P. E. (1958), "Separation of Bull Spermatozoa carrying X- and Y-chromosomes by Counterstreaming Centrifugation," *Nature*, 181, 784.

Lundquist, F. (1949), "Aspects of the Biochemistry of Human Semen," *Acta physiol. scand.*, Supplement 66.

MacLeod, J. (1964), "Human Seminal Cytology as a Sensitive Indicator of the Germinal Epithelium," *International Journal of Fertility*, 9, 281.

MacLeod, J. and Gold, R. Z. (1951), "The Male Factor in Fertility and Infertility. IV. Sperm morphology in fertile and infertile marriage," *Fertil. and Steril.*, 2, 394.

MacLeod, J. and Gold, R. Z. (1952), "The Male Factor in Fertility and Infertility. V. Effect of continence on semen quality," *Fertil. and Steril.*, 3, 297.

Mann, T. (1946), "Metabolism of Semen. 3. Fructose as a normal constituent of seminal plasma. Site of formation and function of fructose in semen," *Biochem. J.*, 40, 481.

Mann, T. (1948), "Fructose Content and Fructolysis in Semen. Practical application in the evaluation of semen quality," *J. agric. Sci.*, 38, 323.

Mann, T. (1964), *The Biochemistry of Semen and of the Male Reproductive Tract*. London: Methuen.

Mann, T. (1967), "Appraisal of Endocrine Testicular Activity by Chemical Analysis of Semen and Male Accessory Secretions," *Ciba Foundation Colloquia on Endocrinology*, 16, 233. London: J. and A. Churchill.

Mann, T. and Rottenberg, D. A. (1966), "The Carbohydrate of Human Semen," *J. Endocr.*, 34, 257.

Marberger, H., Marberger, E., Mann, T. and Lutwak-Mann, C. (1962), "Citric Acid in Human Prostatic Secretion and Metastasizing Cancer of Prostate Gland," *Brit. med. J.*, i, 835.

Maule, J. P. (ed.) (1962), *The Semen of Animals and Artificial Insemination*. Farnham Royal, Bucks: Commonwealth Agricultural Bureaux.

Mischler, T. W. and Reineke, E. P. (1966), "Some Electrophoretic and Immunological Properties of Human Semen," *Journal of Reproduction and Fertility*, 12, 125.

Noyes, R. W. and Thibault, C. (1962), "Endocrine Factors in the Survival of Spermatozoa in the Female Reproductive Tract," *Fertil. and Steril.*, 13, 346.

Pike, J. E. (1967), *The Prostaglandins*. Research Laboratories, the Upjohn Company, Kalamazoo, Michigan.

Soanes, W. A., Shulman, S., Mamrod, L., Barnes, G. W. and Gonder, M. J. (1963), "Electrophoretic Analysis of Prostatic Fluid," *Investigative Urology*, 1, 269.

Schilling, E. (1966), "Experiments in Sedimentation and Centrifugation of Bull Spermatozoa and the Sex Ratio of Born Calves," *Journal of Reproduction and Fertility*, 11, 469.

Tampion, D. and Gibbons, R. A. (1963), "Swimming Rate of Bull Spermatozoa in Various Media and the Effect of Dilution," *Journal of Reproduction and Fertility*, 5, 259.

Williams, W. W. (1965), *Sterility*, 2nd edition. Published by the author. Springfield, Massachusetts.

SECTION II

FEMALE GENITAL TRACT

1. THE ANATOMY AND PHYSIOLOGY OF THE VULVA AND VAGINA AND THE ANATOMY OF THE URETHRA AND BLADDER

KERMIT E. KRANTZ

Vulva

The vulva is comprised of the external genital organs of the female, including the mons pubis, labia majora, labia minora, clitoris and the glandular structures which open into the vestibulum vaginae. The size, shape, and coloration of the various structures comprising the vulva as well as the hair distribution vary between racial groups as well as between individuals. The normal pubic hair in the female is distributed in an inverted triangle with the base centred over the mons pubis. However, in approximately 25 per cent of women, extension of hair upward along the linea alba is not abnormal. The type of hair, in part, is dependent upon the pigment structure of the individual. It varies from heavy, coarse, crinkly hair in the negro to sparse, fairly fine, lanugo type hair seen in the Oriental. The length and size of the various structures of the vulva are influenced by the pelvic architecture, in addition to its influence as to the position of the external genitalia in the perineal area. The external genitalia in the female have their exact counterparts in the male. Reference to each of these will be made in the description of the gross and microscopic anatomy.

Labia Majora

The labia majora are comprised of two rounded mounds of tissue originating in the mons pubis and terminating in the perineum forming the lateral boundaries of the vulva. They are approximately seven to nine cm. in length and two to four cm. in width varying in size depending upon the height, weight, race, age, parity and pelvic architecture of the individual. Ontogenetically, these permanent folds of skin are homologous to the scrotum of the male. Hair is distributed over their surfaces extending superiorly in the area of the mons pubis from one side to the other. The lateral surfaces are adjacent to the medial surface of the thigh with the formation of a deep groove when the legs are together. The medial surfaces of the labia majora may oppose each other directly or are often separated by protrusion of the labia minora. The cleft that is formed by this opposition anteriorly is termed the anterior commissure. Posteriorly, it is less clearly defined and termed the posterior commissure. The middle portion of the cleft between the two labia has been termed the rima pudendi. Hair distribution over the mons pubis and labia majora may vary from individual to individual. The greater amount of hair is seen anteriorly becoming less posteriorly to absence on the medial surfaces.

The microscopic structure of the labia majora and its superficial layers reveals the following: cross section through the skin shows hair follicles penetrating through the skin which has poor rete peg and papilla development. The epithelium is stratified squamous in type similar to that seen in other areas of the body. Underlying the skin is a thin poorly developed muscle layer called the tunica dartos labialis whose fibres for the most part course at right angles to the wrinkles of the surface forming a criss-cross pattern. Deep through the dartos layer is a thin layer of fascia best recognizable in the old or the young because of the large amount of adipose and areolar tissue present. This tissue is rich in elastic fibres. Numerous sweat glands are found in the labia majora, the greater number being present on the medial aspect. In the deeper substance of the labia majora are longitudinal bands of muscle which are contiguous and continuous with the ligamentum teres uteri (round ligament) as it emerges from the inguinal canal. Occasionally a persistent processus vaginalis (Canal of Nuck) can be seen in the upper region of the labia. In most women it has been impossible to differentiate the presence of the cremaster muscle beyond its area of origin.

Microscopic nerve endings (Table 1) are of seven distinct types. The first of the modalities of touch is the presence of the Meissner corpuscles. These corpuscles are normally situated in the connective tissue of the papilla of the normal skin. They contain both myelinated and unmyelinated fibres which branch and terminate among flattened cells. These terminal cells appear to be modified connective tissue cells which act as receptor endings. They vary in size and number depending on location, age, and degree of development of the individual. Their prime purpose is that of tactile differentiation. The second modality are Merkel tactile discs, present in great abundance. A Merkel tactile disc is considered to be a modification of the Meissner corpuscle and may be the terminal endings that penetrate the epithelium, each becoming attached to a modified squamous cell. A translucent area surrounds each cell in the area of attachment. The nerve fibre itself terminates in a small disc-like arrangement in great numbers. There is evidence that the modified squamous cell to which the nerve ending is attached is sloughed periodically, requiring regeneration of the nerve. The inability of these to be sloughed at the proper time or changes in the superficial layers of the skin as in estrogen deprivation results in thinning of the layer of condensation or zonal cornification and the stratum corneum of the superficial layer reducing the threshold for stimulation . . . hence the symptom of pruritus. The third modality are peritrichial endings, similar to those seen elsewhere in the body. The nerve endings are arranged in a basket-like arrangement with the free nerve endings terminating between the cells at the root of the follicle. They are primarily myelinated in origin.

The second major modality are pressure endings. Pacinian type corpuscles vary in number from person to person. They are situated in aggregates within the fat of

arousal and orgasm during pelvic engorgement is no doubt significant. Pain fibres, the free nerve endings in the skin, arise from both myelinated and unmyelinated fibres. The myelin sheath is lost prior to the element's entry into the epithelium. The fibres, after the stratum germinativum, continue their branching to terminate as very fine endings approximately ·1 μ in diameter with a small bead at the tip which frequently appears to end within an epithelial cell. In addition, many of the free nerve endings will terminate between the muscle cells and in the walls of the

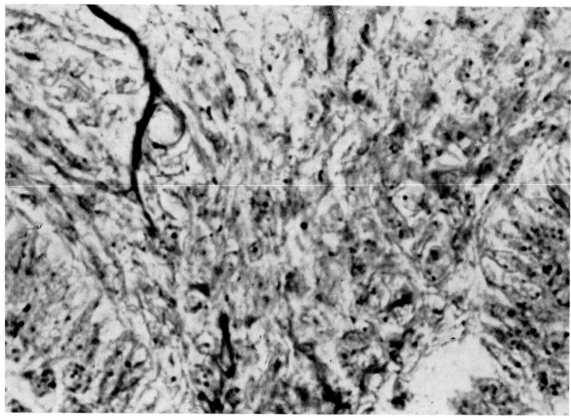

FIG. 1. Section through terminal endings of a Meissner corpuscle in the skin of the labium minus (×950).

the labia majora. The Pacinian type Vater-Pacini corpuscle modulates the sensation of deep tension pressure. They are the only type of nerve endings that can be seen macroscopically, often with the naked eye. A single large myelinated fibre connects with a central pore and acts as a cylinder in the centre of the corpuscle. Surrounding this core are concentric layers of modified connective tissue cells distended with fluid. The nuclei of the lamellæ can be distinctly seen as they protrude into the fluid spaces. A distinct capsule surrounds the entire corpuscle. When cut in cross section, the corpuscles frequently appear like transected onions. Smaller forms of the same corpuscle are frequently called the corpuscles of Herbst. The corpuscles are unevenly distributed throughout the labia majora, often in aggregates together as well as frequently within nerve bundles within the labia majora adjacent to the artery and vein and nerve bundles. The role these corpuscles within nerve bundles may play in sexual

blood vessels. These fibres are unmyelinated. The distribution of the free nerve endings is uniform over the entire surface of the labia majora. Other special type nerve endings such as Ruffini corpuscles and Dogiel-Krause corpuscles are seen. The Ruffini corpuscle lies deep in the subcutaneous connective tissue of the skin. It is composed of a loose arborization of nerve fibres. These fibres terminate in flattened plates in an area containing a nucleated granular substance. Whether these corpuscles send endings further on into the skin as some workers presume or are connected with Dogiel-Krause bulbs as others think is not entirely clear. Their exact role is unknown, though many investigators feel that they perceive temperature while others feel they are pressure endings of sexual perception in the genital area. The corpuscles of Dogiel-Krause and Golgi-Mazzoni and the genital corpuscles of Krause vary tremendously in size and shape. Often they appear like degenerated Pacini corpuscles except that there is an extensive arborization within the corpuscle. This extensive arborization is connected to a myelinated fibre which may terminate in an end bulb, or as some workers believe, in a Ruffini corpuscle or as free endings within the skin. The matrix of a corpuscle is granular, with connective tissue nuclei being visible. The corpuscle may be oval, round, or varied in shape. Investigators feel that this group of endings acts as cold receptors while, in the genital region, they are receptors of sexual stimuli, or perhaps a combination of both. The distribution of these nerve endings varies. Heavy concentration of Ruffini corpuscles is seen throughout the labia majora with a smaller number of Dogiel-Krause corpuscles present in comparison to other areas of the external genitalia. No one has reported a complete absence of this type of nerve ending. Their exact role in sexual stimulus has not yet been totally ascertained.

with the inferior hemorrhoidal pattern. In addition, on each side the posterior labial veins connect with the external pudendal vein terminating into the great saphenous vein (saphena magna) just prior to its entrance (saphenous opening) in the fossa ovalis. This extensive plexus not infrequently shows itself by the presence of extensive varicosities during pregnancy and in cases of pelvic lesions causing obstruction of the large veins.

The lymphatics of the labia majora are extensive with two systems being utilized: one which lies superficially (under the skin) and the other deeper within the subcutaneous tissues of the labia majora. From the upper two-thirds of the left and right labia majora superficial lymphatics pass toward the symphysis and there turn laterally to join the medial superficial inguinal nodes. These nodes drain into the superficial subinguinal nodes overlying the saphenous fossa. The drainage is into and

TABLE 1

QUANTITATIVE DISTRIBUTION OF FREE NERVE ENDINGS IN SELECTED REGIONS OF THE FEMALE GENITALIA

	Touch			Pressure	Pain	Other types	
	Meissner corpuscles	Merkel tactile discs	Peritrichial endings	Pacinian corpuscles	Free nerve endings	Ruffini corpuscles	Dogiel–Krause corpuscles
Mons veneris	++++	++++	++++	+++	+++	++++	++
Labia majora	+++	++++	+++	+++	+++	+++	++
Clitoris	+	+	0	++++	+++	+++	+++
Labia minora	++	++	0	++	++	++	+++
Hymenal ring	0	+	0	0	+++	0	0
Vagina	0	0	0	0	+ Occasionally	0	0

The arterial supply into the labia majora comes from the internal and external pudendals with extensive anastomoses. Within the labia majora is a circular arterial pattern originating inferiorly from a branch of the perineal artery; in the anterior lateral aspect, from the external pudendal artery; and superiorly a small artery from the ligamentum teres uteri. The inferior branch from the perineal artery which originates from the internal pudendal as it emerges from Alcock's Canal forms the base of the rete with the external pudendal arteries. These arise from the medial side of the femoral and occasionally from the profunda arteries just beneath the femoral ring and course medially over the pectineus and adductor muscles to which they supply branches. Penetrating the fascia lata adjacent to the fossa ovalis to pass over the round ligament with a branch to the clitoris, they terminate in a circular rete within the labium majus. Surgical intervention within this area as well as traumatic lesions to the labia majora will often involve this arterial pattern.

The venous drainage is extensive in the form of a plexus with greater anastomoses than are seen with the arteries. The veins, in addition, have communication with the dorsal vein of the clitoris, the veins of the labia minora, and the perineal veins, as well as communications

through the femoral ring (fossa ovalis) to the nodes of Rösenmueller or Cloquet (deep subinguinal nodes) to connect with the external iliac chain. The superficial subinguinal nodes in their situation over the femoral trigone also accept the superficial drainage from the lower extremity as well as drainage from the gluteal region. This may include afferent lymphatics from the perineum. In the region of the symphysis pubis the lymphatics anastomose in a plexus between the right and left side. Therefore, any lesion involving the labia majora allows direct involvement of the lymphatic structures of the contralateral inguinal areas. The lower pole of the labium majus has superficial and deep drainage, shared with the perineal area. It will in part drain through afferent lymphatics to superficial subinguinal nodes; from the posterior medial aspects of the labia majora it may join the lymphatic plexus surrounding the rectum.

The innervation of the external genitalia has been studied by many investigators. It is from the lumbar and sacral plexus. The iliohypogastric nerve originates from T-12 and L-1, and traverses laterally to the iliac crest between the transversus and internal oblique muscles, at which point it divides into two branches: (1) the anterior hypogastric nerve which descends anteriorly through the skin over the symphysis to supply the superior portion of the labia majora as well as the mons pubis, and (2) the posterior iliac—to the gluteal area.

The ilioinguinal nerve originates from L-1 and follows a course slightly inferior to the ilio-hypogastric nerve, with which it may frequently anastomose branching into many small fibres which will terminate in the upper medial aspect of the labum majus.

The genito-femoral nerve (L-1 to L-2) emerges from the anterior surface of the psoas muscle to run obliquely

Labia Minora

The labia minora are two folds of skin that lie within the rima pudendi and measure approximately 5 cm. in length and 5 mm. to 1 cm. in thickness. The width varies according to age and parity, measuring 2 to 3 cm. at its narrowest diameter to 5 or 6 cm. at its widest with multiple corrugations over the surface. They begin at the base of the clitoris where the fusion of the labia is continuous with the prepuce of the clitoris, extending posteriorly and medially to the labia majora at the posterior commissure.

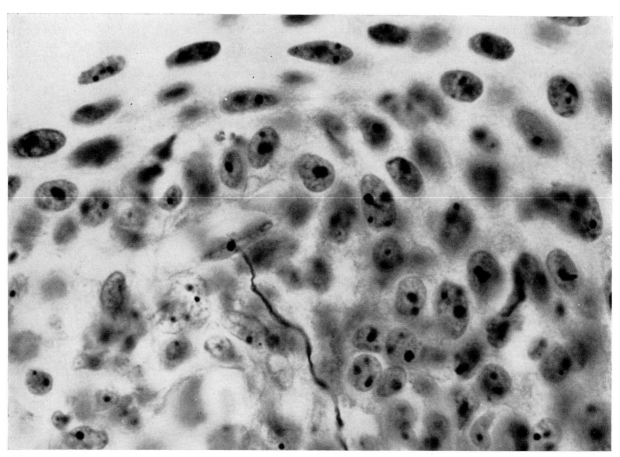

Fig. 2. A tactile disk of Merkel in the epithelium of the labia minora. Note the single unmyelinated fiber terminating in a small knoblike swelling attached to a meniscus of a modified epithelial cell (×950).

downward over its surface to branch in the deeper substance of the labium majus to supply the dartos muscle and that vestige of the cremaster present within the labium majus. Its lumboinguinal branch continues downward onto the upper part of the thigh.

From the sacral plexus the posterior femoral cutaneous nerve, originating from the posterior divisions of S-1 and S-2 and the anterior divisions of S-2 and 3, divides into several rami which in part are called the perineal branches. These supply the medial aspect of the thigh and labia majora. These branches of the posterior femoral cutaneous nerve are from the sacral plexus. The pudendal nerve, composed primarily of S-2, 3, and 4 often with a fascicle of S-1, sends a small number of fibres to the medial aspect of the labia majora.

On their medial aspects, superiorly beneath the clitoris, they unite to form the frenulum of the clitoris adjacent to the urethra and vagina to terminate along the hymen on the right and left sides of the fossa navicularis ending posteriorly in the frenulum of the labia pudendi just superior to the posterior commissure. A deep cleft is formed on the lateral surface between the labium majus and the labium minus. The skin on the labia minora is smooth and pigmented. The colour and distension of the organ will vary depending on the level of sexual excitement and the pigmentation of the individual.

Microscopic examination reveals poor rete pegs and papillae development in the stratified squamous epithelium. The subcutaneous tissue is richly supplied with nerve bundles and blood vessels. The labia minora are characterized by the absence of adipose tissue for most of the length. They contain no hair follicles. The sebaceous glands are found predominantly on the lateral surfaces while sweat glands are evident on both medial and lateral surfaces. The sweat glands appear for the most part to be similar in structure to those seen elsewhere in the body. They are homologous to the urethral glands of Littré of the cavernous portion of the male urethra, and are termed the lesser vestibular glands of the female. Smooth muscle fibres, continuation of the dartos, are found within the

than in the labia majora. There is a rich supply of Ruffini-type corpuscles but an even greater supply of Dogiel-Krause corpuscles in the labia minora.

The main source of arterial supply occurs from anastomoses from the superficial perineal artery, branching from the dorsal artery of the clitoris, and from the medial aspect of the rete of the labia majora. Similarly, the venous pattern and plexus is extensive. The venous drainage is to the medial vessels of the perineal and vaginal veins; directly to the veins of the labia majora; to the

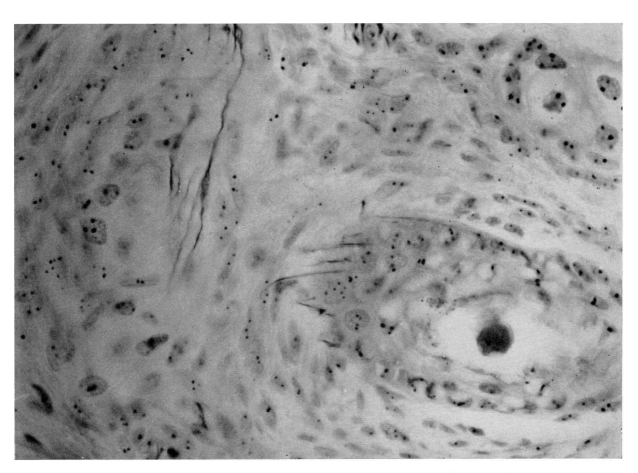

FIG. 3. A cross-section of a hair follicle in the labium majus demonstrating adjacent unmyelinated fibers. The thin unmyelinated elements terminating between the epithelial cells of the outer root sheath are peritrichial endings (×500).

labia minora. They are arranged in a pattern at right angles to the surface grooves, giving the labia the appearance of containing rugae.

The innervation of the labia minora varies. In some individuals, there is a paucity of specialized nerve endings, while in others, they are found to be located in the superior portion. In still others, the nerve endings are distributed evenly throughout the labia. There are approximately a third the number of Meissner corpuscles and Merkel tactile discs found in the labia majora. There is a total absence of peritrichial endings because of the absence of hair follicles. Fewer or the same number of Pacinian corpuscles exist as in the labia majora. Free nerve endings (modulating pain) are less numerous in the labia minora

inferior hemorrhoidals posteriorly; and to the clitora veins superiorly.

The lymphatics medially may join those of the lower third of the vagina superiorly and the labia majora laterally, and go to the superficial subinguinal nodes and to the deep subinguinal nodes. In the mid-line, the lymphatic drainage goes with that of the clitoris—communicating with that of the labia majora to drain to the opposite side.

The innervation of the labia minora originates in part from fibres that supply the labia majora as well as branches from the pudendal nerve as it emerges from Alcock's Canal. These branches may come from the perineal nerve. The labia minora and the vestibule area are homologous to the cavernous portion of the urethra of the male. The short membranous portion, approximately one-half centimetre of the male urethra, is homologous to the middle portion of the vestibule of the female.

The Clitoris

The clitoris is the homologue of the dorsal part of the penis and is an erectile organ consisting of two small erectile cavernous bodies terminating in a rudimentary glans clitoridis. The erectile body, the corpus clitoridis consists of its two crura clitoridis and the glans clitoridis composed of erectile tissue and contains an integument, hood-like in shape, termed the prepuce. On its ventral surface there is a frenulum clitoridis, the superior medial junction of the labia minora. The skin covering the clitoris superiorly and including the prepuce is stratified squamous epithelium richly supplied with sebaceous and sweat glands. Rete pegs and papillae are prominent. In the glans itself there is an absence of glands as well as rete pegs and papillae.

The blood supply to the clitoris is from the dorsal

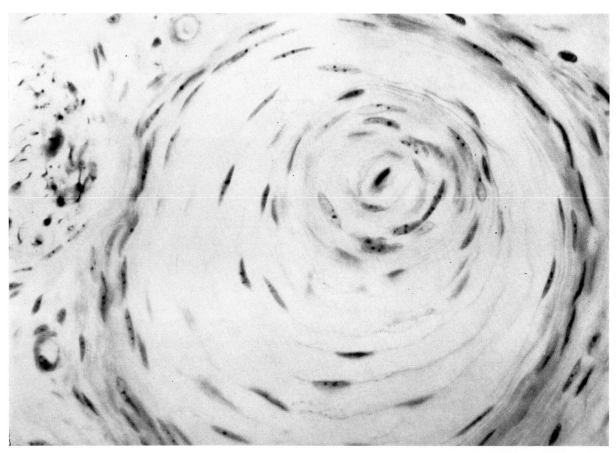

Fig. 4. Cross-section through a Pacini corpuscle within a nerve bundle in the region of the clitoris. Note the presence of adjacent bundles of myelinated and unmyelinated fibers as well as the central filament of the corpuscle (× 500).

with its overlying skin and prepuce, appearing similar (though smaller) to its homologue, the glans penis. It extends from the arch of the symphysis pubis upward and outward being captivated in its position by the anterior portion of the vulva. The cavernous tissue, homologous to the corpus spongiosum urethrae of the male, is not found in the female in the clitoris; however, its corresponding type of tissue exists in the vascular pattern of the labia minora. At the lower border of the pubic arch, a small fibrous band that is triangular in shape extends on to the clitoris (suspensory ligament) to hold it in place and to separate the two crura, which at this point turn in and downward, then laterally close to the inferior rami of the pubic symphysis. The crura lie inferior to the ischiocavernous muscles and bodies. The glans is attached superiorly at the fused termination of the crura. It is

artery of the clitoris, the terminal branch of the internal pudendal artery, which is the terminal division of the posterior division of the internal iliac (hypogastric) artery. As it enters the clitoris, it divides into two branches —the deep and dorsal arteries. Just prior to entering the clitoris itself, a small branch passes posteriorward to supply the area of the external urethral meatus.

The venous drainage of the clitoris begins in a rich plexus around the corona of the glans running along the anterior surface to join the deep vein and continuing downward to join the pudendal plexus from the labia minora, majora and perineum, to form the pudendal vein.

The innervation of the clitoris is through the terminal branch of the pudendal nerve, from the sacral plexus, as previously discussed. It lies on the lateral side of the dorsal artery and terminates in branches within the glans,

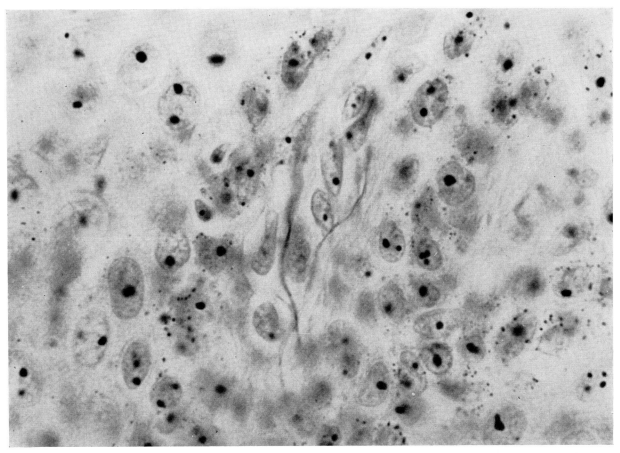

FIG. 5. Microscopic section through the labium minus demonstrating a nerve branching in the stratum germinativum prior to termination as free nerve endings (×950).

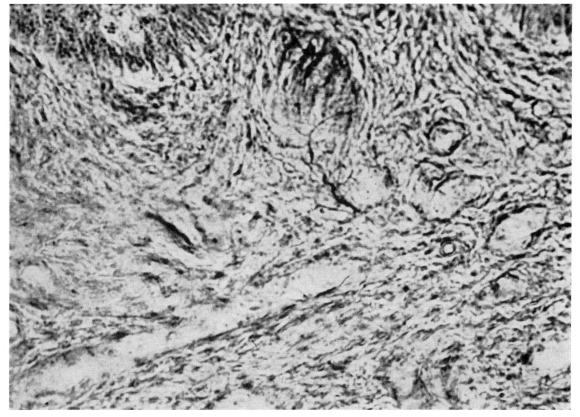

FIG. 6. Ruffini corpuscle lying in the tunica propria of the skin (×250).

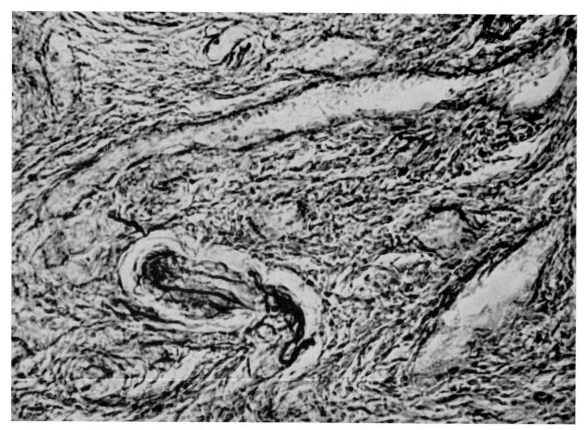

Fig. 7. A Dogiel-Krause corpuscle cut in longitudinal section (× 160).

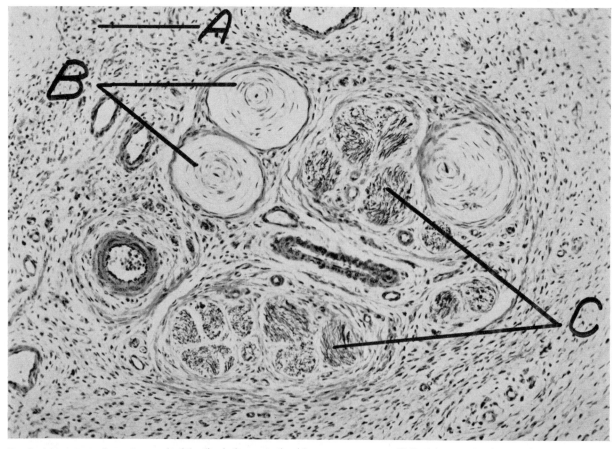

Fig. 8. A low-power photomicrograph of the clitoris demonstrating (*a*) corpus cavernosum, (*b*) Pacini corpuscles, (*c*) nerve bundles. Note the vascularity of the nerve trunk and the presence of Pacini corpuscles within the epineurium (× 160).

corona and prepuce. The nerve endings seen in the clitoris vary from patient to patient from a total absence within the glans of the clitoris to a rich supply primarily located within the prepuce. The modalities of touch, Meissner and Merkel tactile discs, are less in number than in the labia minora. Peritrichial endings are absent. Pacinian corpuscles in all sizes are seen in great abundance, their distribution following no set pattern. A fair abundance of free nerve endings (pain) is present. Ruffini and Dogiel-Krause corpuscles follow the distribution previously described. They may be abundant, or scarce, in the clitoris. In the latter case, they will be found in greater numbers either in the prepuce or in the labia minora. There may be a total absence in the clitoris itself. This becomes clinically significant when one considers the great emphasis that has been placed upon the clitoris in sexual satisfaction in the female.

The lymphatic drainage of the clitoris is primarily that of the labia minora, the right and left side having access to contra-lateral nodes in the superficial inguinal chain. In addition, through its extensive network, there is added access downward and posteriorly to the external urethral meatus toward the anterior portion of the vestibule.

Vestibule

The area of the vestibule is that area bordered by the labia minora laterally, posteriorly by the frenulum labiorum pudendi or posterior commissure, and anteriorly by the urethra and the clitoris. Inferiorly, it is bordered by the hymenal ring. The opening of the vagina or junction of the vestibule with the vagina is limited by a membrane stretching from the posterior and lateral sides to the inferior surface of the external urethral orifice, termed the hymen. Its shape and openings vary, and depend on age, parity, and sexual experience. The form of the opening may be infantile, annular, semilunar, cribriform, septate, vertical; and it may even be imperforate. In the case of the parous and post-coital individual, the tags of the hymenal integument are termed carunculæ myrtiformes. The external urethral orifice which is approximately two to three centimetres posterior to the clitoris on a slightly elevated and irregular surface with depressed areas on its lateral sides may appear to be stellate or crescentic in shape. It is characterized by many small mucosal folds around its opening. On its lateral sides and directly upon its surface are the orifices of the para- and peri-urethral glands (Ducts of Skene, Aztruc). At approximately 5 and 7 o'clock, just external to the hymenal ring, are two small papular elevations which represent the orifices of the ducts of the glandulæ vestibulares majores or larger vestibular glands (Bartholin) of the female. The fossa navicularis is the area that exists between the frenulum labiorum pudendi and the hymenal ring. The skin surrounding the vestibule is stratified squamous in type with a paucity of rete pegs and papillae.

The blood supply is an extensive capillary plexus which has anastomoses with the superficial transverse perineal artery. A branch comes directly from the pudendal anastomosis with the inferior hemorrhoidal artery in the region of the fossa navicularis; the blood supply of the urethra anteriorly, a branch of the dorsal artery of the clitoris and the azygos artery of the anterior vaginal wall also contribute. The venous drainage is similarly extensive in network involving the same areas described for the arterial pattern.

The lymphatic drainage has a distinct pattern. The anterior portion, including that of the external urethral meatus, drains upward and outward with that of the labia minora and the clitoris. The part next to the urethral meatus may join that of the anterior urethra, which empties into the vestibular plexus to terminate in the superficial inguinal nodes, superficial subinguinal nodes, and the deep subinguinal nodes and into the external iliac chain. The area of the fossa navicularis and the hymen may join the lymphatics of the posterior vaginal wall intertwining with the intercalated lymph nodes along the rectum which follow the inferior hemorrhoidal arteries. This becomes significant when malignancy involves this area. Drainage, therefore, occurs through the pudendal as well as the hemorrhoidal chain and through the vestibular plexus onto the inguinal region.

The innervation of the vestibular area is primarily from the sacral plexus through the perineal nerve. The absence of the usual modalities of touch is noted. Meissner corpuscles and peritrichial endings are absent, the latter because of the absence of hair follicles. A small number of Merkel tactile discs are present. Pacinian corpuscles appear to be lacking. An abundance of free nerve endings (pain) is present especially in the vestibular portion of the hymenal ring. Ruffini and Dogiel-Krause corpuscles are conspicuous by their absence.

Larger Vestibular glands

The glandulae vestibulares majores (larger vestibular glands or Bartholin glands) are situated as previously described, with a duct measuring approximately 5 mm. in size. The gland itself lies just inferior and lateral to the bulbocavernosus muscle. The gland is tubular and alveolar in character with a thin capsule and connective tissue septa dividing it into lobules where occassional smooth muscle fibres are found. The epithelium is cuboidal to columnar, pale in colour, with the cytoplasm containing mucigen droplets and colloid spherules with acidophilic inclusions. The epithelium of the duct is simple in type, and its orifice may be that of the vestibule, i.e. stratified squamous. The secretion is a clear, viscid, glairy, and stringy mucoid substance—pH alkaline. Secretion is active during sexual activity. However, after the thirtieth year of life, the glands undergo involution, shrink in size, and become atrophic. The arterial supply to the greater vestibular gland comes from a small branch on the bulbocavernosus muscle, penetrating deep into its substance. Venous drainage is with that of the bulbocavernosus body. The lymphatics drain directly into those of the vestibular plexus, having access to the posterior vaginal wall along the inferior hemorrhoidal channels. They also drain via the perineum into the inguinal area. Most of this minor drainage is along the pudendal vessels in Alcock's canal. This, in part, explains the difficulty in dealing with malignancy involving this gland. The greater vestibular gland

(Bartholin) is homologous to the bulbourethral gland, Cowper's gland, Deverney's glands, Tiedmann's glands, or Bartholin glands of the male. The innervation of the greater vestibular gland is from a small branch of the perineal nerve which penetrates directly into its substance.

Musculature

The muscles of the external genitalia and cavernous bodies are homologous to those of the male though less well developed. The *bulbocavernosus muscle* and deeper bulbus vestibuli or cavernous tissue arise in the midline, from the posterior part of the central tendon of the perineum where each opposes the fibres from the opposite side. Each ascends around the vagina enveloping the bulbus vestibuli, the cavernous tissue (the corpus cavernosus bodies of the male) to terminate in three heads: the fibrous tissue dorsal to the clitoris; the tunica fibrosa of the corpus cavernosa, overlying the crura of the clitoris; and thirdly, decussating fibres which join those of the ischiocavernosus to form the striated sphincter of the urethra at the junction of the middle and lower thirds of the urethra. The blood supply is from the perineal arterial branch of the internal pudendal artery as it arises at the anterior part of the ischiorectal fossa. Deep to the Colles fascia and crossing between the ischiocavernosus and bulbocavernosus muscles, it sends one or two branches directly into the bulbocavernosus muscle and vestibular body continuing anteriorly to terminate in the dorsal artery of the clitoris. The venous drainage is with the pudendal plexus. In addition, posteriorly, it is in part with the inferior hemorrhoidal veins and laterally with the perineal vein, a branch of the internal pudendal vein. The lymphatics run primarily with those of the vestibular plexus with drainage inferiorly toward the intercalated nodes of the rectum, and anteriorly and laterally with the labia minora and majora to the superficial inguinal nodes. Contralateral drainage in the upper portion of the muscle and body is evident.

The *ischiocavernosus muscle* and its attendant cavernous tissue arises from the ischial tuberosity and inferior ramus of the ischium, enveloping the crus of its cavernous tissue in a thin layer of muscle ascending to and over the medial and inferior surfaces of the symphysis pubis to terminate in the anterior surface of the symphysis pubis at the base of the clitoris, and to send decussating fibres to the region of the upper and middle thirds of the urethra to form the greater part of the voluntary sphincter of the urethra. Its blood supply is through perforating branches from the perineal artery as it ascends between the bulbocavernosus and ischiocavernosus muscles to terminate as the dorsal artery of the clitoris. The innervation is from an ischiocavernosus branch of the perineal division of the pudendal nerve.

The *transversus perinei superficialis* muscle of the perineum arises from the inferior ramus of the ischium as well as from the ischial tuberosity. These fibres extend across the perineum and are inserted into the central tendon of the perineum meeting those from the opposite side. Frequently, muscle fibres from the bulbocavernosus, the puborectalis, the superficial transverse perinei, and

occasionally the external anal sphincter will interdigitate. The blood supply is from a perforating branch from the perineal division of the internal pudendal artery. The nerve supply is from the perineal division of the pudendal nerve. In the cavernous substances of both the bulbocavernosus and ischiocavernosus muscles, Pacinian corpuscles and Dogiel-Krause corpuscles are present.

It should be noted that the area termed as the inferior layer of the urogenital diaphragm is a potential space depending upon the size and development of the musculature in the area, the parity of the female, and pelvic architecture. It contains loose areolar connective tissue with fat interspersed. The bulbocavernosus muscles with the support of the superficial transverse perinei muscles and the puborectalis muscles act at a point of fixation on each side for the support of the vulva and external genitalia as well as for the vagina.

Vagina

The term vagina, named by Colombo, means sheath. The vagina serves as the intermediary or connecting organ between the external genitalia and the uterus. In the adult, it varies in length from 7 to 10 cm.; the posterior wall being approximately 1·5 to 2 cm. longer. One of its more notable topographical landmarks are the rugæ vaginales, folds of the vagina, that pass medially upward and posteriorly on either side toward the midline connecting to a longitudinal ridge in the midline known as the column rugarum. In the area of the urethra this ridge becomes more prominent and is termed the urethral carina. In the region of the origin of the urethral carina, a deep lateral groove and fold are present. This, in conjunction with a similar fold less prominent in the posterior vaginal wall at the upper level of the levator ani, is known as the "fold of Shaw."

The anterior vaginal wall terminates in a circular fissure around the cervix uteri where the cervix projects into the vagina. The groove or space thus formed between the cervix and the anterior vaginal wall is termed the fornix. The vaginal opening is partially covered by the hymen. The transverse section of the undistended vagina varies from stellate, just within the hymenal ring, to H shape, under the urethra and the middle third, to a crescent shape, just below the cervix. In older women where atrophy has occurred, the organ may be crescent shaped in its entirety.

The vagina of the nulliparous reclining woman assumes a downward direction of 55° to the vertical in its lower two-fifths, 10° in the second two-fifths, and approximately 55° in the upper fifth. The overall angle is 30°. These changes of direction cause the vagina to take the shape of an S or italic letter *f* curve as it descends into the pelvis. The long axis of the vagina forms an angle of 90° with that of the normal anteverted uterus. The cervix uteri, therefore, is situated opposite to the posterior vaginal wall. Anteriorly, the vagina is intimately related with the urinary bladder and the urethra throughout its length. The inferior surface of the bladder lies adjacent to the anterior surface of the vagina along its entirety. The urethra, in the upper third of its length, assumes a similar relationship. The lower two-thirds of the urethra enters into a close anatomical relationship with the anterior vaginal wall, thus involving the anterior portion of the lower third of the vagina. In the region of the upper third of the urethra at its junction with the bladder, heavy bands of tissue pass on the anterolateral walls of the vagina adjacent to the levator ani muscles (puborectalis) with similar fibres from the urethra and vesical neck to traverse on to the rami of the pubic symphysis—the *puboprostatic ligaments* of the female. The presence of a thick connective tissue layer interposed between the vagina and the bladder and the upper third of the urethra has been termed "pubocervical fascia" and "musculofascial sheet". Some have felt this layer was most probably synonymous with the puboprostatic ligaments. Most recent studies have substantiated the absence of a fascia; instead the presence of a loose areolar connective tissue adventitia of the vagina is found, having no supporting capacity. The ureters may be observed on either side in the region of the upper third of the vagina as they enter the muscularis of the bladder. They course in an oblique direction along the anterolateral margin of the vesicovaginal junction, and actually exist as distinct entities between the bladder and the anterior vaginal wall. Posteriorly, the upper fourth of the vagina is related to the rectouterine space, the cul-de-sac, (pouch of Douglas), which is covered with peritoneum. The middle half of the vagina is in close relationship to the rectum, only the adventitia of both organs being interposed. Behind the lower fourth of the vagina, the anal canal has begun and the two organs are separated by the sphincters of the anus and rectum, as well as the interposing perineal body containing the origin of the bulbocavernosus and insertion of the superficial transverse perineal muscles. In the region of the hymen, the vagina is covered on its lateral aspects by the bulbocavernosus muscles and bodies. The fact that this muscle invests the vestibular bulbs or cavernous bodies is the reason it long has been termed the sphincter vaginae.

The blood supply of the vagina is unique, being rich in order to maintain its various segments during the descent of the head during labour. Superiorly, the blood supply originates from the uterine artery which gives off a descending branch, the cervicovaginal artery. This corresponds to the inferior vesical artery of the male. On either side it sends a branch to the cervix to form the coronary artery of the cervix circumventing the cervix by anastomosing anteriorly and posteriorly. The anterior anastomosis forms the azygos artery of the anterior vaginal wall which descends in the midline downward within the adventitia of the vaginal musculature; the posterior artery has approximately five lateral branches on either side until it terminates in an anastomosis in the region of the external urethral meatus with the descending (urethral) branch from the dorsal artery of the clitoris. The lateral vaginal arteries or continuation of the inferior vesical arteries continue on the anterolateral walls of the vagina. These vessels divide similarly, sending branches anteriorly toward the midline and posteriorly on the lateral sides to anastomose with the azygos artery on the anterior vaginal wall and with the hemorrhoidals on the posterior vaginal

wall. Not infrequently terminal branches of the internal iliacs, known as arteriovaginalis, similarly may supply this region. When this occurs, the inferior vesical artery supplies the middle half of the vagina. The lower half of the vagina is supplied by ascending branches of the middle hemorrhoidal arteries. The latter divide to send rami to the anterior, as well as posterior, walls of the vagina. The various rami of the arteries supplying the vagina (both right and left sides) meet in the midline on the anterior, as well as posterior surfaces, to form the anterior and posterior azygos arteries of the vagina. These similarly terminate with a final anastomosis between the urethral branch of the dorsal artery of the clitoris which originates from the perineal branch of the internal pudendal artery anteriorly, and, with hemorrhoidals at the level of the rectal sphincter posteriorly. The posterior vaginal wall, therefore, gets part of its blood supply from the middle and inferior hemorrhoidal vessels.

The venous drainage of the vagina is through a series of plexuses: in the lower portion of the vagina the drainage is along the urethra on to the perineum and into the dorsal vein of the clitoris, as well as into the middle hemorrhoidal venous plexus. The greater part of this drainage is perineal in direction (internal pudendal plexus), terminating in the internal pudendal vein. This vein may be single or paired, and communicates directly with the hypogastric veins of its side. The upper vaginal venous plexus joins the uterine and cervical veins to drain directly into the hypogastric veins.

The lymphatics of the vagina are closely related to those of the adjoining organs. They begin with an easily demonstrable mucosal plexus and drain into a deeper muscular network. The collecting trunks form a definite pattern. The muscular plexus forms an irregular network on the anterior and posterior surfaces of the vagina with anastomoses between both sides. This multitude of small lymphatics coalesce into larger channels, usually two to four in number.

There is some disagreement as to the direction of flow along the lateral walls of the vagina. The trunks may drain in three distinct directions: superior, middle, and inferior. The superior group of lymphatics join those of the cervix, while the middle group of collecting vessels course along the vaginal arteries toward their origin. The superior group of lymphatics follow the cervical vessels to the uterine artery, where they pass the ureter both superiorly and inferiorly accompanying the uterine artery, to terminate in the medial chain of the external iliac nodes. It has been observed that some of these lymphatics may enter the node of the obturator foramen. The middle group, which drains the greater part of the vagina, terminates in a hypogastric node at the origin of the vaginal artery. It is not infrequent to observe small nodes along their course. There are in addition intercalated lymph nodes in the rectovaginal septum. They are primarily responsible for the drainage of the rectum and part of the posterior vaginal wall. The distinctly separate lymphatic drainage of the posterior vaginal wall from that of the anterior vaginal wall may in part explain the late involvement of the posterior vaginal wall in carcinoma of the cervix. On the other hand, involvement of the posterior vaginal wall with carcinoma of the rectum becomes possible. The third, or inferior group of lymphatics, supplies the area around the hymen. These vessels form frequent anastomoses between right and left sides and course in two distinct directions. In part they curve upwards to anastomose with the middle group of the vagina to terminate in the respective pelvic nodes, while the remaining channels enter the vulva to drain into their respective group of inguinal nodes with contralateral accessibility.

The anastomoses of the vaginal lymphatics are many. Superiorly, they join readily with those of the uterus and cervix and, in the middle and inferior areas, with the vulva, urethra, and rectum. The vagino–urethro–vesical lymphatic relationship has been one of conjecture. There is little doubt that there is a distinct separation between the vesical and vaginal drainage. This separation is not clear, however, in the region of the lower two-thirds of the urethra. Because of the intimate relationship of the urethra with the anterior vaginal wall the urethra joins, at least for its most part, the vaginal lymphatics (inferior group) to drain onto the vulva. There is no doubt that connections do occur between the posterior vaginal wall and the rectum in the lower third of the vagina. The drainage, however, is not maximal along this route, which follows that of the rectal stalk. The pararectal nodes for the most part are distinctly different from those of the previously described paravaginal chain. There has been considerable conjecture concerning the flow of the lymph into the vagina from the vulva and possible retrograde flow from the hymenal area. The evidence at the present time leads one to conclude that this does occur, but not by preference. The uterovaginal nodes of Sappey (hypogastric nodes of the vaginal arteries at the junction of vaginal arteries, ureter, and uterine arteries), as well as the nodes in the base of broad ligament and the uterovaginal wall, may be considered intercalated nodes and are inconstant in number and position.

The gross innervation of the vagina has been studied, for the most part, with that of the uterus. The pelvic autonomic system originates with the superior hypogastric plexus. The middle hypogastric plexus passes into the pelvis to the immediate left of the midline. At the level of the first sacral vertebra the plexus divides into branches going to the right and left sides of the pelvis. These branches form the beginning of the inferior hypogastric plexus. The inferior hypogastric plexus is therefore a divided continuation of the middle hypogastric plexus, the superior hypogastric plexus, the presacral nerve, or the uterinus magnus. This group of nerves descends into the pelvis in a position posterior to the common iliac artery and anterior to the sacral plexus, curves laterally and finally enters the sacrouterine folds or ligament. The medial segment of the primary division of the sacral nerves S-2, 3 and 4 with some question of fibres from S-1 and occasionally from S-5 send their fibres (nervi erigentes) into the pelvic plexus within the sacrouterine folds. Therefore, the plexus appears to contain both sympathetic (inferior hypogastric plexus) and parasympathetic (nervi erigentes) components. Within the base of the broad ligament an

extension of this plexus contains many ganglia. The ureter occupies a position superficial to the ganglia. The plexus is supplied by the middle vesical artery.

No specific pattern of the supply to each adjacent organ has been described. The greater number of nerves appears to enter the uterus in the region of the isthmus, whereas a lesser number of fibres descends along the lateral aspects of the vagina. These fibres are both pre- and postganglionic. This pattern is similar to that of the arteries that supply the vagina. In addition to sending rami to the vagina, the vesical branches, in part, go directly to the bladder together with its blood supply. Small ganglia may be noted between the bladder and the vagina in the loose areolar connective tissue separating the two organs. Ganglia may be noted along the lateral vaginal wall adjacent to the vaginal arteries, as well as along the sides of the rectum in the rectovaginal junction.

The supports of the vagina have been discussed at length by many anatomists and surgeons. Because of its position as the connecting organ between the external genitalia and the uterus, its supports have an intimate relationship with the urethra, bladder, and rectum. In the introital area, specifically the isthmus, the vagina is supported by the bulbocavernosus muscle. Just beyond the bulbocavernosus muscle, at approximately the junction of the lower and middle third of the vagina, the levator ani muscles may be palpated with ease. This is the second most significant point of support for the vagina. The vagina abuts directly against the levator ani muscle (puborectalis) at this point and anteriorly to the pubic symphysis through the puboprostatic ligaments. From this point into the pelvis to the cardinal ligaments there is no lateral support for the vagina. The bladder, anteriorly, does not give the vagina any support whatsoever, resting upon it only as an adjacent organ. Posteriorly the rectum lies in apposition to the vagina but with little to no support other than what can be obtained from the junction of the rectum and the posterior vaginal wall on the lateral sides. This allows the superior portion (upper third of the vagina) to be relatively easily distendable, which has been reported a natural phenomenon occurring during sexual excitement. Large bands of tissue radiate out toward the lateral walls in the region of the isthmus of the cervix (junction of the vagina with the uterus). These bands of tissue have been termed variously: ligaments of Mackenrodt, or cardinal ligaments. Their postero-medial aspects have been called the uterosacral ligaments, the medial aspect of the base of the broad ligament. The cardinal ligaments, originating at the junction of the isthmus of the uterine cervix with the corpus of the uterus, course outward in a fanlike pattern toward the lateral pelvic walls, being perforated by the vessels and nerve elements as they descend in the pelvis. A natural defect exists within the cardinal ligaments at the point the ureter passes over the uterine artery. A large number of ganglia exist at this site (the plexus of Frankenhäuser). The support of the vagina may be summarized to be from three sources: the ligaments of Mackenrodt or cardinal ligaments, in its uppermost portion; the puborectalis muscle of the levator group, with the puboprostatic ligaments at the junction of the middle and lower third; and, bulbocavernosus muscle and body in the region of the vestibule.

The microscopic anatomy of the mucosa of the vagina is unique in its structure and in its response to the various hormones. The epithelium is a thick (·15 to ·2 mm.) uncornified stratified squamous type of epithelium lacking any glands. The transition of squamous epithelium into the simple columnar epithelium of the endocervix is not abrupt, (2–9 mm.), forming what is commonly termed the transitional zone. The epithelium of the vagina consists of three main layers: a basilar layer composed of oval cells with prominent nuclei; an intermediate layer of larger, flatter cells with nuclei; and, an inconstant zone of cornification with superficial cornified cells containing pyknotic nuclei that demonstrate the greatest response to hormonal stimulation.

The cyclic response of the epithelium to estrogen stimulation was first reported in the guinea pig by Stockard and Papanicolaou and in the human by Dierks. Since that time much work has been done to further demonstrate the cyclic and hormonal variations in the vaginal epithelium. Electron microscopy has demonstrated that the epithelial cells are connected syncytially with each other through bridges of protoplasm. No definite cell limits are observed in these areas. Bizzozero's nodules were observed in the protoplasmic bridges. Spaces under the protoplasmic bridges connect with each other to terminate finally in the lumen of the vagina. Densifications are seen in the epithelial cells; but, no keratinization is noticeable. The cytoplasm of the epithelial cells contains two types of fibrils, the coarser of which, tonofibrils, run from cell to cell, thus forming an integrated system in the epithelium.

The lamina propria is relatively thicker than usual. It contains a fairly thick network of collagenous fibres with an interlacing network of elastic fibres. Papillae indent the epithelium through its length, but are more prominently seen on the posterior wall. They are more apparent in the nulliparous individual and may play a significant role in aiding the epithelium to stretch during parturition. A rich blood and lymphatic supply are seen within the lamina propria and again in the submucosa. Through the latter layer are found the larger blood vessels, the lymphatics, and the few nerves that supply the epithelium. The lymphatics may form small aggregates, intercalated nodes, similar to the Peyer's patches of the bowel. These aggregates have also been observed in the adventitia surrounding the organ, where occasionally they may be recognized on gross examination.

The arteries in the vagina are tortuous in their course and appear somewhat spiral in nature, whereas the veins are of a more sinusoidal in pattern. The looseness of the submucosa and its somewhat different vascular pattern may be a natural development with that of the epithelial rugae, to allow the great distension of the vagina necessary for parturition. Any rigidity of the lamina propria would not be to the advantage of the distension needed in parturition. This allows a more direct access of any infectious or malignant process to the deeper lymphatics and blood supply.

The muscle pattern of the vagina is continuous with the muscle of the uterus. The outer layer of muscle in the uterus runs in a longitudinal fashion and at the region of the isthmus passes outward and into the base of the broad ligament to form the superior surface of the cardinal ligaments or the ligaments of Mackenrodt. The outer layer of smooth muscle of the vagina, longitudinal in direction, forms a similar pattern composing the inferior surface of the cardinal ligament. An inter-digitation of the fibres within the cardinal ligament occurs. The ratio of muscle to connective tissue varies, although usually it is 1 to 3. The longitudinal muscle fibres continue along the length of the vagina to the region of the hymen where they gradually disappear in the connective tissue of the vestibule. On the anterior vaginal wall (lower third) the longitudinal muscle fibres are found to be more displaced by the urethra than diminished in number. The inner muscle layer of the vagina is developed more poorly, forming a spiral-like course appearing in microscopic sections as somewhat circular in pattern. Where the urethra traverses the anterior vaginal wall, the circular fibres circumvent and include the urethra. Striated fibres from the bulbocavernosus and ischiocavernosus muscles may be seen as they ascend from the lateral sides and surround the urethra to form the striated voluntary sphincter. Fascia surrounds the vagina and the presence of pubocervical fascia has been much disputed since first proposed by Bonney as a "musculo-fascial plane." Although there are investigators who still believe that such fascia exists, the greatest evidence at the present time supports its absence. This can be readily confirmed in microscopic sections. An inner sparse longitudinal muscle layer is inconstant and poorly developed but does exist with the fibres terminating in the region of the isthmus of the cervix, turning inward and descending into the cervix proper.

Microscopically the innervation of the vagina demonstrates the presence of fine nerve endings (free in type) to the blood vessels in the lamina propria. Connections exist between the ganglia seen in the adventitia of the vagina and the muscularis: some of the fine fibres penetrate to the mucosa to terminate as free nerve endings. No demonstrable relationship has been shown between the nerve fibres in the vagina and responses of the mucosa to hormonal stimulation. Vater-Pacinian-type corpuscles have been observed in the adventitia surrounding the vagina, but none within the organ itself. Microscopic ganglia are apparent in the adventitia surrounding the vagina and along the lateral walls adjacent to the blood vessels. Fibres have been traced, both pre- and post-ganglionic, from the inferior hypogastric plexus and the nervi erigentes to the ganglia. In the upper third of the vagina, the ganglia are frequently situated between the bladder and the vagina with the ganglian cells being both pseudo-unipolar and multipolar in type. Unmyelinated fibres from, and passing through, the ganglia have been observed to supply the muscularis and blood vessels; an occasional fibre penetrates to the mucosa and terminates in the free endings in the basal layer. The mucosa of the vagina is for the most part without innervation. The nerves along the sides of the vagina appear to be in a wavy pattern similar to that seen in the broad ligament adjacent to the uterus. This wave effect may be a protective device for the nerves during the distension of the vagina during parturition. Nerve bundles from the nervi erigente and along the sides of the rectum, containing an artery and a vein, will often have within the fascicle a Vater-Pacinian-type corpuscle which would allow transmission of pressure brought through the endings during any period of vaso-dilation or vascular engorgement in the region.

PHYSIOLOGY OF THE VULVA AND THE VAGINA

The physiology of the vulva and the vagina is intimately concerned with the act of reproduction. The first is its response during sexual stimulation. The vulval response to sexual stimulation begins primarily with vascular engorgement in the area of the mons pubis accompanied by perspiration from the sweat glands. The labia majora, depending upon the parity of the woman, play a specific role. They appear, according to the studies of Masters and Johnson, to thin and flatten out against the perineum with a slight elevation upward and outward away from the introitus completing the change at the time the plateau level of sexual tension is achieved. Under prolonged sexual excitement the labia majora may become markedly engorged with venous blood and have been noted to become edematous: resolution follows orgasm. However, it has been noted the labial vessel congestion may persist for a period of two to three hours during detumescence.

Under sexual excitement the labia minora expand to two to three times their normal size in diameter. The tumescence of the labia minora at the peak of the excitement phase results in a definitive colour change of pink to bright red in colour. This colour change may involve the prepuce of the clitoris. This change has been termed by Masters as the "sex-skin" change. The degree of this response is in part dependent upon the parity of the individual, being less in the multiparous than in the nulliparous. Masters notes that no woman ever has been observed to attain an orgasmic release without first displaying the specific "sex-skin" or labia minora colour changes. The colour change returns fairly rapidly toward normal following orgasm.

Under sexual stimulation some secretion may come from the lesser vestibular glands. The greater vestibular glands (Bartholin's glands) respond to sexual stimulation by secretory activity; secretion is mucoid, small in amount and deposited into the fossa navicularis That amount secreted in the excitement phase appears to play an insignificant role in coitus. The Bartholin gland near the age of 30 begins to show a progressively diminishing function.

The clitoris during sexual excitement demonstrates a definitive pattern. The prepuce reacts with tumescence with the labia minora. The clitoris itself, specifically the glans, demonstrates vasocongestion to the point of tumescence. However, erection as seen in the male does not occur. The tumescence of the glans when developed persists as long as any significant degree of sexual excitement is present.

During sexual excitement specific changes occur within the vagina. Accordingly Masters and Johnson describe a copious transudate occurring in the vagina with tumescence in the bulbocavernosus and ischiocavernosus bodies, forming the orgasmic platform during the plateau phase, increasing during orgasm. The upper two-thirds of the vagina for the most part dilates with a full vaginal expansion and a lengthening of the posterior fornix during resolution. The vagina at that time is no longer distended.

During the excitement phase, the vascular engorgement within the pelvis would also involve the nerve bundles. As previously stated, the Pacinian type corpuscles within the nerve bundles, susceptible to the vascular changes, may play an active role in tripping the orgasmic phase of sexual excitement.

The vulva and vagina during pregnancy, labour and delivery play more a passive than active role. During the progressive months of gestation, the increased employment of the collateral circulation of the vagina and the vulva progressively adapts the organ to the needs of parturition. Softening of the introital area is evident as a result of the high progesterone levels and vascularity. Hypertrophy of the vaginal muscles, similar to that of the uterus, and concomittant hypertrophy of the vaginal mucosa also occurs. From the onset of labour to the culmination in parturition, the rhythmic contractions of the uterus resulting in dilatation of the cervix also occur actively in the musculature of the vagina. Early in labour the vagina appears to be long with the cervix difficult to palpate due to the vaginal depth and lack of accessibility. As labour progresses and dilatation of the cervix occurs the vagina shortens. The rugae accommodate the distension of the vagina as the presenting part moves downward toward the levator support. The bladder is displaced upward and anteriorly to the symphysis and therefore out of the pelvis. The rectum in its position posteriorly is compressed into the hollow of the sacrum with any of its contents being expressed ahead of the presenting part. Descent of the presenting part, specifically in cephalic presentation, with dilatation of the vagina and descent onto the levator support is relatively painless. Dilatation of the levator ani muscles and emergence of the head upon the vulva results in a maximum amount of dilatation in a relatively fixed region of the vagina. The act of parturition requires displacement of the transverse perinei and the bulbocavernosus muscles downward and laterally. The external anal sphincter is depressed downward just ahead of the presenting part. The lower two-thirds of the urethra intimately involved with the anterior vaginal wall is unable to be displaced upward with the bladder; therefore, it is lengthened and protrudes ahead of the presenting part. During parturition the relatively fixed region of the hymenal ring must dilate. A midline perineotomy (incision or guided lacerations) is most effective to minimize trauma to vital supports of the vulva, bulbocavernosus, and transverse perinei muscles. The over-distension of the vagina due to the presenting part and body of the infant forms a temporary sacculation. If it occurs too rapidly or dilatation is beyond the resilience of the vagina, rupture of the vaginal musculature may occur. This is often demonstrated by a cuneiform groove on the anterior wall and a tongue-like protrusion on the posterior wall of the vagina. Therefore return of the vagina and vulva to the non-pregnant state is dependent upon the tonus of the muscle, degree of distension of the vagina during parturition and the resolution to the nonpregnant state.

Urethra and Bladder

The urethra of the human female varies from 2·5 cm. in the child to 8·0 cm. in length in the adult; averaging 5·25 cm. The urethra assumes an angle of approximately 16 degrees from the external to the internal meatus as measured against a horizontal line of reference—the anterior vaginal wall. The lower two-thirds of the urethra is inseparable and an integral part of the anterior vaginal wall.

The arterial supply of the urethra is divided into segments. The upper third of the urethra receives its arterial supply through anastomoses from the vessels of the bladder. The middle and lower third receive direct branches from the vaginal artery on either side on the anterolateral aspect of the vagina as well as from the azygos artery in the midline. Because the urethra and the vagina in this region are inseparable, their blood supply is communal in nature. The venous drainage of the upper third of the urethra is with that of the bladder through the inferior, middle, and superior vesical veins; and inferiorly, through the clitoral venous plexus. The innervation of the urethra is from the hypogastric plexus in conjunction with that of the bladder and anterior vaginal wall by ganglia in juxtaposition to the base of the bladder.

The anterior urethral lymph flow is into the vestibular plexus with connecting channels to the superficial inguinal nodes. The posterior urethra has three directions of flow: (1) the anterior superior portion lymphatics course into the posterior bladder wall and hence to the external iliac chain; (2) the anterolateral and lateral regions drain into the lateral bladder wall where the channels may course to the internal group of the external iliac chain, to the hypogastrics, or even into the obturator group; and (3) the posterior aspect courses either into the posterior surface of the bladder and thus into the uterine channels or into the vessels of the anterior portion of the urethra. The lymphatic drainage of the dome of the bladder is separated into that of the right and left side, in addition to being separate from the base of the bladder.

Decussating fibres from the bulbocavernosus and ischiocavernosus muscles surround the middle third of the urethra to form the voluntary (striated) sphincter of the urethra. Just superior to this sphincter, the urethra passes between the puborectalis muscles of the levator ani group.

Adjacent to the vagina and levator ani and on the lateral sides of the urethra in the middle and upper third arise bands of connective tissue traversing anterolaterally onto the pubic ramus of each side. These, because of their similarity to like structures in the male, are termed the puboprostatic ligaments of the female.

The entire urethra of the female is homologous to the prostatic portion of the urethra in the male. No specific layers of bladder musculature nor evidence of an internal sphincter is demonstrable.

The bladder on its lateral, superior and posterior surfaces is covered by a thin layer of areolar connective tissue. Blood supply to the bladder is in part derived from the obliterated hypogastric arteries. The superior vesical artery, in most instances, divides into three branches; the two superior ones supply the bladder dome, while the inferior branch (middle vesical artery) enters the bladder tissue on its posterolateral surface to supply the region of the trigone. Frequently, branches of the inferior vesical artery course into the base of the bladder. Veins form no specific pattern; instead, they form a large plexus which frequently anastomoses with the hypogastric vein and its main tributaries. On its superior and lateral surfaces, this venous plexus is termed the plexus of Santorini (pampiniform).

Lymphatic drainage of the bladder is through two main routes: (1) the anterior bladder wall channels which course along the obliterated hypogastric artery to the nodes of the posterior abdominal group; and (2) the vessels of the posterior bladder wall which either drain into the channels of the anterior bladder wall or follow the course of the superior vesical artery to the posterior abdominal nodes. Anastomoses are common between lymphatics of the cervix and those of the base of the bladder.

The nerves, abundant, inconstant in number, and arising from the hypogastric and pelvic plexuses, do not accompany the blood vessels to the bladder.

Because the mucous membrane of the urethra forms many longitudinal folds, the shape of its lumen varies from stellate to crescentric. The epithelial lining may vary. In the region of the external urethral meatus, the epithelium is stratified squamous in type, changing to pseudo-stratified until, nearing the vesical neck, transitional epithelium becomes apparent. The bladder itself is lined by transitional epithelium. Small aggregates of lymphocytes may be noted in the longitudinal folds of the urethral mucosa.

The glands surrounding the urethra form no specific pattern. They are dispersed among the longitudinal muscle fibres of the urethra being most prominent in the lower third, though they frequently extend along the entire course of the urethra to the vesical neck. The glands, simple tubular in type, are lined by a simple columnar epithelium. Secretion can be noted within the lumina of many of the glands. The glands form the pattern of the paraperi-urethral glands as described by Huffman. These have previously been called the ducts of Skene or Aztruc.

The ducts of the glands are simple and enter directly into the urethra except in the lower third where they frequently traverse parallel to the urethra for several millimetres to open directly to the outside (Skene's ducts). Their number is not constant. The ducts, in most instances, are lined by simple columnar epithelium, with pseudo-stratified epithelium frequently being present in the duct near its junction with the urethra.

The smooth muscle of the urethra is in two patterns, longitudinal and circumferential. The longitudinal fibres originate in the region of the external urethral meatus and lie adjacent to the lumen. They increase numerically along the course of the urethra toward the bladder. In the region of the vesical neck the bundles of the longitudinal muscle fibres intermingle with the circular smooth muscle of the urethra, both to merge into the muscle bundles making up the musculature of the bladder. The circular smooth muscle begins in the lower third of the urethra. The fibres are sparse in number, surround the entire urethra and are intimate with the smooth circular muscle of the vagina which lies superior and inferior to them. The urethral muscle is in a spiral pattern outside the longitudinal muscle bundles. They increase in number along the lower and middle thirds of the urethra. In the upper third of the urethra and in the vesical neck, the circular fibres form into bundles to intermingle with the bundles of the longitudinal muscle to form the muscle bundles which constitute the musculature of the bladder. Besides the circumferential smooth muscle of the vagina in the lower half of the urethra at the junction of the middle and lower third of the urethra there are decussating fibres from the bulbocavernosus and ischiocavernosus muscle that enter from the lateral sides to surround the urethra and form a distinct bundle (sphincter). This is the voluntary or striated muscle sphincter of the urethra. The smooth circular and longitudinal muscle of the urethra is continuous as well as contiguous with the smooth muscle of the bladder. The number of layers of muscle in the bladder are, therefore, a result of the interlacing of these urethral layers—the thickness of the layer being dependent upon *the degree of* distension of the organ. At the junction of the middle and upper third of the urethra on the anterolateral aspects of the vagina and urethra abutting against the levator ani muscles are the heavy bands of connective tissue coursing obliquely and anteriorly to the pubic rami (the puboprostatic ligaments).

The microscopic innervation of the urethra and bladder consists of small bundles of nerves containing both myelinated and unmyelinated fibres, originating in part from the parasympathetic ganglia along the lateral margin of the urethra and vagina, perforating the urethrovaginal septum. Several myelinated nerve fibres can be noted to enter the striated sphincter of the urethra. These are found to originate from a branch of the perineal nerve. Some free nerve endings (of the pain type) are present in the urethra and bladder. The epithelial lining of the bladder is transitional in type. No glands are present within the bladder. The muscle is entirely smooth in type. Between the bladder and the anterior vaginal wall is a thin layer of areolar connective tissue containing nerves and small blood vessels. The arteries and veins as they enter the bladder substance form capillary plexuses that are extensive adjacent to the mucosa of the bladder. Anastomoses between the vascular supply of the bladder and the urethra are easily demonstrable. Numerous parasympathetic ganglia are found in the loose investing connective tissue of the bladder. The cells within these ganglia are uni and bipolar in type. Both myelinated and unmyelinated elements are seen to enter and leave the ganglia, thus demonstrating pre and post ganglionic elements as well as visceral afferents No specialized nerve endings can be observed in the bladder wall.

REFERENCES

Allen, E. and Doisy, E. A. (1923), "An Ovarian Hormone: Preliminary Report on its Localization, Extraction and Partial Purification, and Action in Test Animals," *J. Amer. Med. Assc.*, **81**, 819–821.

Aronson, H. (1866), *Beiträge zur Kenntnis der centralen und peripheren Nervenendigungen*. Berlin, Germany: O. Dreyer.

Ayre, J. E. (1944), "Cyclic Ovarian Changes in Artificial Vaginal Mucosa," *Amer. J. Obstet. Gynec.*, **48**, 690–695.

Bahr, G. F. and Moberger, G. (1956), "Beitrag zur Kenntnis der Feinstruktur des Vaginal-epithels des Menschen," *Z. Geburtsh. Gynäk.*, **146**, 33–42.

Ballantyne, J. W., and Williams, J. D. (1891), "The Histology and Pathology of the Fallopian Tubes," *Brit. Med. J.*, **1**, 107, 168.

Beneventi, F. A. and Marshall, V. F. (1956), "Some Studies of Urinary Incontinence in Men," *J. Urol.*, **75**, 273–284.

Bense, W. (1868), "Ueber Nervenendigungen in den Geschlechtsorganen," *Z. rat. Med.*, **33**, 1.

Bodian, D. (1936), "A New Method for Staining Nerve Fibres and Nerve Endings in Mounted Paraffin Sections," *Anat. Rec.*, **65**, 89.

Bonney, V. (1923), "Diurnal Incontinence of Urine in Women," *J. Obstet. Gynaec. Brit. Emp.*, **30**, 358–365.

Briesky, A. (1887), "Diseases of the Vagina," in *Cyclopedia of Obstetrics and Gynecology*, **10**, 216–219. New York, N.Y: Woods.

Bröse, P. (1910), "Ueber die Sensibilität der Inneren Genitalorgane," *Gynäk.*, **34**, 1532.

Bruhns, C. (1898), "Über die Lymphgefässe der weiblichen Genitalien, nebst einigen Bemerkungen über die Topographie der Leistendrüsen," *Arch. Anat. Ent.*, 57–80.

Baumm, E. (1921), *Grundriss zum Studium der Geburtshülfe*. 9th ed. **3**, 516. Wiesbaden, Germany: Bergmann.

Calmann, A. (1898), "Sensibilitätsprüfungen am weiblichen Genitale nach forensischen Gesichtspunkten," *Arch. Gynäk.*, **55**, 454.

Carrad, H. (1884), "Beitrag zur Anatomie und Pathologie der kleinen Labien," *Z. Geburtsh. Gynäk.*, **10**, 62.

Cateula, J. (1930), "Nouvelle Note sur les Lymphatiques du Vagin," *Ann. Anat. path. et Anat. Normale med. chir.*, **7**, 903–904.

Celegran, G. T. (1899), *Hernia cul-de-sac*. Paris, France: Thesis.

Chrischtschonowitz (1871), *Beitrag zur Kenntnis der feinen Nerven in der Vaginalschleimhaut*. Vienna, Austria.

Cohnstein, I. (1881), "Zur innervation der Gebärmutter," *Arch Gynäk.* **18**, 384.

Colombo, Matteo Realdo (Colombus, Matthaeus Realdus) (1559), *De re anatomica*. Libri XV. Venetiis, ex typog. N. Beuilacquoe.

Coujard, R. (1951), "Quelques considérations sue le système nerveux autonome uterovaginal," *Gynéc. et obstét.*, **50**, 270–296.

Cowperthwaite, A. C. (1888), *A Textbook of Gynecology Designed for the Student and General Practitioner*," 5–7. Chicago, Ill: Gross and Delbridge.

Cruveilhier, J. (1844), *The Anatomy of the Human Body*. First Am. from the last Paris ed. Edited by G. S. Pattison. New York, N.Y.: Harper.

Curtis, A. H. (1946), *Textbook of Gynecology*. 5th ed. p. 33. Philadelphia, Pa.: Saunders.

Dahl, W. (1915–1916), "Die Innervation der wieblichen Genitalien," *Z. Geburtsh. Gynäk.*, **78**, 539–601.

Danesino, V. (1951), "Prime indagini conil metodo al cloruro d'oro del Ruffini sul plesso nervoso utero-vaginale nei feti umani," *Arch. ostet. e ginec.*, **56**, 51.

Danesino, V. (1951), "Particolarità strutturali delle espansioni nervose nei genitali esterni di mammiferi (nota preventiva)," *Arch. ostet. e ginec.*, **56**, 158.

Davenport, H. A. and Kline, C. L. (1938), "Staining paraffin sections with protargal; experiments with Bodian's method; use of n-propyl and n-butyl alcohol in Hofker's fixative," *Stain. Tech.*, **13**, 147.

Davis, C. H., Ed. (1935), *Gynecology and Obstetrics*. **1**, 13. Chap. 1, "Anatomy of the Female Pelvis," by E. J. Carey. Hagerstown, Md.: W. F. Pryor.

Deter, R. L., Caldwell, G. T. and Folsom, A. I. (1946), "Clinical and Pathological Study of the Posterior Female Urethra. *J. Urol.*, **55**, 651–662.

Dickinson, R. L. (1949), *Human Sex Anatomy*. 2nd ed. Chap. 4, 34–39. Baltimore, Md.: Williams and Wilkins.

Dierks, K. (1927), "Der normale menstruelle Zyklus der Menschlichen Vaginalschleimhaut," *Arch. Gynäk.*, **130**, 46–79.

Dogiel, A. S. (1893), "Die Nervenendigungen in der Haut der aussern Genitalorgane des Menschen," *Arch. mikr. Anat. u. Ent.*, **41**, 585–612.

Dogiel, A. S. (1903), Kapitol Methylenblau zur Nervenfarbung. Berlin, Germany, Urban.

Douglas, J. (1730), *A Description of the Peritonaeum, and of That Part of the Membrana Cellularis Which Lies on Its Outside*, 37–38. London, England: Roberts.

Douglass, M. (1936), "Operative Treatment of Urinary Incontinence," *Am. J. Obstet. Gynec.*, **31**, 268–279.

Duperroy, G. (1953), "L'innervation du Col Utérin Chez la Femme; quelques Particularites Morphologiques," *Gynéc. et obst.*, **52**, 506.

Duperroy, G. (1954), "L'innervation du Col Utérin Chez la Femme: Quelques Particularites Morphologiques," *Bruxelles-méd.*, **34**, 1064.

Egea-Esteban, A. (1953), "Aportaciones a la Innervation Vaginal," *Anal. Anat. (Granada)*, **2**, 355.

Feldmann, N. G. (1935), "Experimentell Morphologische Studien der Innervation der Weiblichen Genitalorganen," *Arch. Russ. d'Anat.*, **14**, 698.

Felix, W. (1912), "The Development of the Urogenital Organs," in *Manual of Human Embryology*. **2**. 752. F. Keibel and F. P. Mall, Eds. Lippincott. Philadelphia. Pa.

Ferrer y Jiménez De Anta, D. (1949), "Observations Complementaries en la Inervacion des Aparate Genital de Oveja," *Arch. Méd. exp.*, **12**, 87.

Finger, E. (1893), *Die Blennorrhöe der Sexualorgane und ihre Complicationen*. 3rd ed. Deuticke. Germany and Vienna, Austria: Leipzig.

Finger, W. (1866), "Über die Endigungun der Wollustnerven," *Z. rat. Med.*, **28**, 222–230.

Frankenhäuser, F. (1865), "Die Nerven der weiblichen Geschlechtsorgane des Kaninchens," *Jena. Z. Med. Naturw.*, **2**, 61.

Gasparini, F. (1952), "Morphologische Befunde an den Pyrenophoren des Ganglion Cervicale Uteri unter Berucksichtigung des Alters und des Funktionszustandes der Geschlechtsorgane," *Acta. anat.*, **15**, 308.

Gawbronski, N. Von (1894), "Ueber Verbreitung und Endigung der Nerven in den weiblischen Genitalien," *Arch. Gynäk.*, **47**, 271.

Geller, F. C. (1922), "Untersuchungen über die Genitalnervenkörporchen in der Klitoris und den kleinen Labien." *Zbl. Gynäk.*, **46**, 623.

Goff, B. H. (1931), "An Histological Study of the Perivaginal Fascia in Nullipara," *Surg. Gynec. Obstet.*, **52**, 32–42.

Goff, B. H. (1948), "The Surgical Anatomy of Cystocele and Urethrocele with Special Reference to the Pubocervical Fascia," *Surg. Gynec. Obstet.*, **87**, 725–734.

Gray, H. (1930), *Anatomy of the Human Body*. 22nd ed. Philadelphia, Pa.: Lea and Febiger.

Gunn, J. A. and Franklin, K. J. (1922–1923), "The Sympathetic Innervation of the Vagina," *Proc. roy. Soc.*, **B94**, 197–203.

Güterbock, P. (1890), *Die Krankheiten der Harnblase*, Part 2. "In Die Chirurgischen Krankheiten der Harn- und Mannerlichen geschlechtsorgane," Leipzig, Germany and Vienna, Austria: F. Deuticke.

Henle, F. G. J., (1866), *Handbuch der systematischen Anatomie des Menschen.*, **2**, 446. Brunswick, Germany: Vieweg.

Hyrtl, J. (1887), *Lehrbuch der Anatomie des Menschen*, 19th ed. Vienna, Austria: Braumüller.

Izquierdo, V. (1879), *Beiträge zur Kenntniss der Endigung der sensiblen Nerven*. Strassburg, Germany: Heitz.

Johnson, F. P. (1922), "Homologue of Prostate in Female," *J. Urol.*, **8**, 13–34.

Jung, P. (1905), "Untersuchungen über die Innervation der weiblichen Genitalorgane," *Mschr. Geburtsh. Gynäk.*, **21**, 1.

Kalischer, O. (1900), *Die Urogenitalmuskulatur des Dammes mit besonderer Berücksichtigung des Harnblasenverschlusses*. pp. 1–184. Berlin, Germany: Karger.

Kantner, M. (1954), "Studien über den sensiblen Apparat in der Glans Clitoridis: I. Die Clitoris der Greisin," *Z. mikr.—anat. Forsch.*, **60**, 388.

Kato, M. (1955), Histology of Clitoris on Dog and its Innervation, Especially Sensory Innervation," *Arch. Hist. Jap.*, **9**, 21.

Kehrer, E. (1907), "Physiologische und Pharmakologische Untersuchungen an den Überlebenden und Lebenden Inneren Genitalien," *Arch. Gynäk.*, **81**, 160.

Kennedy, W. T. (1946), "Muscle of Micturition, its Role in Sphincter Mechanism with Reference to Incontinence in the Female," *Amer. J. Obstet. Gynec.*, **52**, 206–217.

Kimura, S. (1930), "Embryological Investigation of the Nerve Endings Distributed in the External Genitals of the Human Fetus, Especially in the Clitoris and the Labium Minus Pudendi. *Jap. J. Obstet. Gynec.*, **13**, 90.

Klaften, E. (1934), "Vascularization der weiblichen Geschlechtsorgane. *Z. Gynäk.*, **58**, 468.

Kölliker, R. A. von. (1889–1902), *Handbuch der Gewebelehre des Menschen*. 6th ed. 1. Leipzig, Germany: Engelmann.

Kostlin, R. (1894), "Die Nervenendigungen in den weiblichen Geschlechtsorganen," *Fortschr. Med.*, **12**, 411.

Krantz, K. E. (1950), "Anatomy of the Urethra and Anterior Vaginal Wall," *Amer. Assoc. Obstetricians Gynecologists Abdom. Surgeons*, **61**, 31–59.

Krantz, K. E. (1951), "Anatomy of the Urethra and Anterior Vaginal Wall," *Amer. J. Obstet. Gynec.*, **62**, 374–386.

Krantz, K. E. (1958), "Innervation of the Human Vulva and Vagina; a Microscopic Study," *Obstet. and Gynec.*, **12**, 382–396.

Krause, W. (1866), "Über die Nervenendigung in den Geschlechtsorganen," *Z. rat. Med.*, **28**, 86–88.

Krause, W. (1876–1880), *Handbuch der menschlichen Anatomie*. 3rd ed. Hanover, Germany: Hahn.

Krause, W. (1868), "Die Anatomie des Kaninchens," in *Topographischer und operative Ruchsicht*. Leipzig, Germany: Engelmann.

Krause, W. (1876), *Handbuch der menschlichen Anatomie: Allgemeine und mikroskopische Anatomie*, Hanover, Germany: Hahn.

de Lamballe, J. (1841), "Recherches sur la Disposition des Nerfs de l'Uterus; Applications de ces Connaissances à la Physiologie et à la Pathologies de cette Organe," *C. R. Acad. Sci.*, **12**, 882.

Landau, E. (1952), "Contribution à l'Étude de l'Innervation de l'Appareil Génital Féminin," *Gynéc. et. obst.*, **51**, 107.

Landowsky, M. D., and Owsjanikoff, F. V. (1888), *Grundlagen zum Studium der Mikroskopischen Anatomie der Menschen und der Tiere*. St. Petersberg: K. Rikker.

Langley, J. N., and Anderson, H. K. (1896), "The Innervation of the Pelvic and Adjoining Viscera: VI. Histological and Physiological Observations upon the Effects of Section of the Sacral Nerves," *J. Physiol.*, **19**, 372.

Langworthy, O. R. and Hesser, F. H. (1940), "Innervation of Blood Vessels as Observed in the Urinary Bladder," *Bull Johns Hopkins Hosp.*, **67**, 196–209.

Laurentjen, B. J., and Naiditsch, M. S. (1933), "Études Experimentals-Morphologiques Relatives à la Structure du Systeme Nerveux Autonome," *Trav. labor. rech. biol. Univ. Madrid*, **28**, 223.

Lennander, K. G. (1905), "Ueber lokale Anesthesie und Über Sensibilität in Organ und Gewebe; weitere Beobachtungen," *Mitt. Grenzgeb. Med. Chir.*, 15:465.

Long, J. A. and Evans, H. M. (1922), *The Oestrous Cycle in the Rat and Its Associated Phenomena*. Berkeley, Calif.: Univ. Calif. Press.

Loewenstein, M. (1871), "Die Lymphfollikel der Schleimhaut der Vagina," *Zbl. Med. Wiss. Berlin*, **9**, 546.

Lueders, C. F. A. (1892), *Über das Vorkommen von subpleuralen Lymfdrüsen*. Kiel, Germany: Handorff.

Luschka, H. von. (1863–1869), "Die Anatomie des Menschen," in *Rücksicht auf die Bedürfnisse der praktischen Heilkunde*. Tübingen, Germany: Laupp.

Mabuchi, K. (1924), "Morphologische Studien über das Verhalten der Nerven in den weiblichen Geschlechtsorganen des Menschen mit besonderer Berücksichtigung der Veränderungen ihres Verhaltens während der Gravidität und Menstruation und im zunehmenden Alter. Anhang die Nerven in der Nabelschnur und Plazenta," *Mitt. Fakult. Univ. Tokyo.* **31**, 385–495.

McAllister, A. (1889), *A Textbook of Human Anatomy.* p. 458. London, England: Griffin.

Mackenrodt, A. (1894–1895), "Über die Ursachen der normalen und pathologischen Lagen des Uterus," *Arch. Gynäk.*, **48**, 393–421.

Mandt, C. (1849), "Zur Anatomie der Weiblichen Scheide. *z. rat. Med.*, **7**, 1–13.

Marchetto, G. (1955), "Sulle terminazioni nervose de clitoride di neonata. *Monit. zool. ital.*, **63**, 23.

Marcille, M. (1902), Lymphatiques et Ganglions Ilio-pelviens. Paris, France.

Marshall, V. F., Marchetti, A. A. and Krantz, K. E. (1949), "The Correction of Stress Incontinence by Simple Vesicourethral Suspension. *Surg. Gynec. Obstet.*, **88**, 509–518.

Matsuda, T. (1937), "Untersuchungen über die Nervenendapparate der ausseren Geschlechtsorgane mit Hilfe einer neuen verselberings Methode," *Jap. J. med. Sci. and Biol.*, **6**, 146.

Medowar, J. L. (1928), "Die Nerven des Uterus und der Vagina des Hundes," *Z. ges. Anat.*, **86**, 776.

Merkel, F. S. (1880), *Ueber die Endigungen der sensiblen Nerven in der Haut der Wirbelthiere.* Rostack: H. Schmidt.

Miura, Y. (1956), "On the Histology and the Sensory Innervation of the Vagina and the Sinus Urogenitalis of Dog," *Arch. Hist. Jap.*, **10**, 101.

Moench, G. (1894), *De Vaginae Anatomie Physiologia et Pathologia.* Haloe.

Moreau, E. (1896), *Contribution à l'Étude des Abcès Péripharyngiens.* Thesis No. 177. Paris, France.

Morris, H. (1942), *Morris' Human Anatomy: a Complete Systematic Treatise.* 10th ed.: 1555. New York, N.Y.: Blakiston.

Nagel, W. (1896), "Die weiblichen Geschlechtsorgane," in *Handbuch der Anatomie des Menschen.* 7 (Part 2, Sects. 1–2). K. von Bardeleben, Ed. Jena, Germany: Fischer.

Nothnagel, H. (1905), "Zur Pathogenese der Kolik," *Arch. f. Verdau Kr.*, **11**, 117.

Oberdieck, G. (1884), *Uber Epithel und Drüsen der Harnblase und weiblichen und Männlichen Uretra.* Göttingen, Germany: Kaestner.

Oikawa, M. (1954), "Sensory Innervation of Urogenital Organs of Fourth Month Female Embryo," *Thoku J. exp. med.*, **61**, 55–66.

Ozaki, M. (1937), "Histologische Studien über die peripheren Nerven in den weiblichen Geschlichtsorganen des Menschen," *Jap. J. med. Sci. and Biol.*, **6**, 225.

Poirier, P. (1889), "Lymphatiques des Organes Génitaux de la Femme," *Progr. méd.*, **10**, 491, 509, 527, 568, 590.

Poirier, P. (1890), "Lymphatiques des Organes Génitaux de la Femme," *Progr. méd. Paris*, **11**, 41–65.

Poirier, P. and Cuneo, B. (1902), "Les lymphatiques. Traité d'anatomie humaine de Poirier et Charpy," **11**, 4. Paris, France: Delamere. *The Lymphatics, General Anatomy of. The Lymphatics, Special Study of. The Lymphatics in Different Parts of the Body.* Authorized English ed., trans. and edited by Cecil H. Leaf. Chicago, Ill: Keener.

Polle, G. (1865), *Die Nerven-Verbreitung in den weiblichen Genitalien bei Menschen und Saugethieren.* Göttingen, Germany: Huth.

Rakoff, A. E., Feo, L. G. and Goldstein, L. (1944), "Biologic Characteristics of Normal Vagina." *Amer. J. Obstet. Gynec.*, **47**, 467–494.

Retzius, G. (1890), "Ueber die Endigungsweise der Nerven in den Genitalnervenkorperchen des Kaninchens, *Int. Mschr. Anat. Physiol.*, **7**, 323.

Reynolds, S. R. M. (1949), *Physiology of the Uterus* (ed. 2). New York: Hoeber.

Ricci, J. V., Lisa, J. R., Thom, C. H. and Kron, W. L. (1947), "Relationship of Vagina to Adjacent Organs in Reconstructive Surgery; Histologic Study." *Am. J. Surg.*, **74**, 387–410.

Ricci, J. V., Lisa, J. R., Thom, C. H., Jr. and Kron, W. (1949), Vagina in Reconstructive Surgery; Histologic Study of Its Structural Components. *Amer. J. Surg.*, **77**, 547–554.

Riehm, H. (1951), "Das Bindegewebe der Vagina während und nach der Geburt," *Arch. Gynäk.*, **179**, 145–158.

Röhrig, A. (1879), "Experimentelle untersuchungen über die Physiologie der Uterus-bewegungen," *Arch. path. Anat.*, **76**, 1.

Roith, O. (1907), "Zur Anatomie und klinischen Bedeutung der nervengeflechte im weiblichen Becken," *Arch. Gynäk.*, **81**, 495.

Rouvière, H. (1938), *Anatomy of the Human Lymphatic System*, trans. by M. F. Tobias. pp. 159, 161, 162, 194, 234, 236. Ann Arbor, Mich.: Edward Bros.

Sappey, M. P. C. (1888), *Traité d'Anatomie Descriptive.* 3rd ed. Paris, France: V. A. Delahaye.

Sappey, M. P. C. (1874), *Anatomie, Physiologie, Pathologie des Vaisseaux Lymphatiques Considérés Chez l'Homme et les Vertébrés.* Paris, France: A. Delahaye and E. Lecrosnier.

Sappey, M. P. C. (1854), *Recherches sur la Conformation Extérieure et la Structure de l'Urètre de l'Homme.* Paris, France: Baillière.

Schabadasch, A. (1930), Untersuchungen zur Methodek der methylenblau Farbung des vegetativen Nervensystems. *Z. Zellforsch.*, **10**, 221.

Schreiber, H. (1942), "Konstruktionsmorphologische Betrachtungen über den Wandungsbau der menschlichen vagina," *Arch. Gynäk.*, **174**, 222–235.

Seitz, L. and Americh, A. I. (1953), "Biologie und Pathologie des Weibes," 2nd ed. **1**, 170–174.

Seto, H. (1939), "Uber die intraepithelialen Nerven bein Menschen: I. Die afferenthen Nervenendapparate in dem urethralepithel Sowie in der Glans penis resp. Clitoridis und dem Praeputium. Gemeinsamen Epithelplatte." *Arb. anat. Inst. Sendai.*, **22**, 1–25.

Shaw, W. and O'Sullivan, J. (1950), "Fold in Posterior Vaginal Wall; Preliminary Communication," *Lancet.*, **1**, 306.

Shaw, W. (1947), "Study of Surgical Anatomy of Vagina, with Special Reference to Vaginal Operations," *Brit. med. J.*, **1**, 477–482.

Smith, B. G. and Brunner, E. K. (1934), "The Stature of the Human Vaginal Mucosa in Relation to Menstrual Cycle and to Pregnancy," *Amer. J. Anat.*, **54**, 27–85.

Stockard, C. R. and Papanicolaou, C. N. (1917), "The Existence of Atypical Oestrous Cycle in the Guinea-pig, with Study of Its Histological and Psychological Changes," *Amer. J. Anat.*, **22**, 225–283.

Szymonowicz, L. (1921), *Lehrbuch der Histologie und Mikroskopischen Anatomie.* Leipzig, Germany: Kabitzsch.

Tandler, J. (1930), "Anatomie der weiblichen topographische Anatomie der weiblichen Genitalien," in *J. Veit, Handbuch der Gynakologie.* W. Stoeckel, Ed. 3rd ed. ed. 1. Munich, Germany: Bergmann.

Tandler, J. (1913), "Entwicklungsgeschichte und Anatomie der weiblichen Genitalien," in *Handbuch der Frauenheikunde.* 1. Wiesbaden, Germany: Bergmann.

Tello, G. F. (1935), "Contribution à la Connaissance des Terminaisons Sensitives dans les Organes Genitaux Externes et de Leur Development," *Arch. int. Neurol.*, **54**, 521.

Traut, H. F. Bloch, and Kuder, A. (1936), "Cyclical Changes in the Human Vaginal Mucosa," *Surg. Gynec. Obstet.*, **63**, 7–15.

Tubin, I. C. and Novak, J. (1956), *Integrated Gynecology.* **1**, 61–72. New York, N.Y.: McGraw-Hill.

Uhlenhuth, E. and Nolley, G. W. (1957), "Vaginal Fascia, a Myth?" *Obstet. and Gynec.*, **10**, 349–358.

Ullery, C. (1953), *Stress Incontinence in the Female.* p. 10. New York, N.Y.: Grune and Stratton.

Waldeyer-Hartz, H. W. G. von. (1899), *Das Becken.* Bonn, Germany: Cohen.

Walthard, M. (1937), *Die Beziehungen des Nervensystems zu den normalen Betriebsablaufen und zu den funktionellen Storungen im weiblichen Genitale.* München, Germany: Bergmann.

Webster, J. C. (1891), "The Nerve-endings in the Labia Minora and Clitoris with special reference to the Pathology of Pruritus Vulvae," *Edinb. med. J.*, **37**, 35.

Worthmann, F. (1906), "Beiträge zur Kenntniss der Nervenausbreitung in Clitoris und Vagina," *Arch. mikr. Anat.*, **68**, 122.

Yamada, K. (1951), "Studies in the Innervation of Clitoris in Tenth Month Human Embryo," *Tohoku J. exp. med.*, **54**, 151.

Yamada, K. (1951), "On Sensory Nerve Terminations in Clitoris in Human Adult," *Tohoku J. exp. med.*, **54**, 163.

Zimmermann, R. (1909), "Experimentelle untersuchungen über die Empfindungen in der Schlundrohre und im Magen, in der Harnröhre und in der Blase und im Enddarm," *Mitt. Grenzgeb. Med. Chir.*, **20**, 445.

2. THE UTERUS AND CERVIX

D. M. SERR

The morphological changes, physiological processes and biochemical reactions occurring in the uterus and cervix daily and periodically, constitute a preparation for survival and growth. These processes, some of which will be expounded in this chapter, involve hormonal, enzymatic, structural and vascular changes, which occur with regularity yet which differ in the pregnant and the non-pregnant state. This ability for change demonstrates the complexity of the metabolic processes involved in a hollow muscular organ having as its specialty, a part in the reproductive life cycle.

Although basically the uterine body and cervix have similar anatomical layers, yet the outer and inner linings, and the fibromuscular layer differ in form and function in the two portions of the uterus.

The smooth muscle fibres of the myometrium are arranged in cylindrical flat bundles separated by interstitial connective tissue containing isolated smooth muscle cells.

The length of the smooth muscle fibre of the myometrium is about 50 microns, increasing during pregnancy to more than 500 microns. Furthermore, in pregnancy, the number of muscle fibres increases by division (Mark, 1956), and through transformation of the embryonic connective tissue cells and lymphocytes into new muscular elements (Stieve, 1929). The increase in muscular tissue during pregnancy is marked particularly in the body of the uterus and the isthmic portion, whereas there is only a slight increase in the cervix. Using viscometry and fractionated precipitation methods, it has been shown that there is an increase in contractile protein (adenomyosin), adenosine triphosphate and phosphocreatinine in uterine muscle cells during pregnancy, besides changes in intra and extra cellular electrolytes. Studies on the ultrastructure of myometrial cells have also shown changes during pregnancy. Dessouky (1968) showed an increase in both number and size of the myofibrils, and an increase in the number of ribosomes. Electron microscope studies of the muscle cell of the pregnant uterus show features similar to those found in actively secreting cells. There is evidence of increased mitochondrial activity (Peterson and Leblond, 1964). Studies in experimental animals on the arterio-venous differences in glucose concentrations show that in the pregnant uterus not all glucose in the uterine artery is destined for the placenta and fetus, but that some accumulates in the myometrium, mostly as glycogen and glucoprotein. Thus the smooth muscle of the pregnant uterus contains relatively large amounts of glycogen, this probably being the source of energy for muscular contraction during parturition (Battaglia, Hellegers, Heller and Behrman, 1964).

The smooth muscle cells of the cervix are scanty and apparently distributed at random. The cervix has more connective tissue than muscle, but has to be able to remain closed during pregnancy and to relax during labour. There may be more than just passive collaboration with the body of the uterus in these functions. Intra-molecular changes in the collagen may also have some bearing on the ability of the cervix to dilate in labour. The recognition of incompetence of the internal os as a pathological phenomenon in repeated late abortions points to the necessity for more studies on the ultrastructure of the cervix.

Disassociation of the collagen bundles into their fibrillar components is a fundamental change responsible for the increasing effacement and dilatability of the cervix. There are changes in the reticulin fibres and collagen concentrations in the cervix during pregnancy, but there is no apparent change in the natural state of the cervical collagen. It is probable that during gestation there are changes in connective tissue structures not only in the cervix but over all the body (Buckingham, Selden and Danforth, 1962).

These considerations are of importance in discussing the etiology of the incompetent cervical os, as a cause of habitual abortions. Although purely mechanical factors are regarded as the cause of the post-traumatic incompetent cervix, a state of congenital incompetence is not rare. It is possible that an inborn error of collagen metabolism effecting the connective tissues may be involved in this condition.

Endometrial Ultrastructure

The structural changes of the endometrial glands are closely related to the cyclic changes of the ovary. Thus, histological study of the endometrium has been employed for years as an indirect means of estimating ovarian function. A vast amount of information has been accumulated on the cyclic changes of the endometrium as studied by light microscopy (Noyes, 1966). Such morphological studies give an insight, although somewhat limited, into the intrinsic mechanism of the complex function of the endometrial cell. Integration of recent electron microscopy studies of the ultrastructure of the endometrium together with sensitive and specific histochemical and biochemical methods will probably provide a more adequate explanation of the structural changes of endometrial cells during the menstrual cycle. These cells have a single evolutionary cycle in the interval between two menstruations. During this short period the glandular cell undergoes intense proliferation followed by a marked modification of structure and function during the secretory phase. The proliferative and secretory function of the endometrium is governed mainly by ovarian steroids, although other hormones such as thyroxine, hydrocortisone and insulin may influence these processes (Cavazos, Green, Hall, and Lucas, 1967).

The electron microscope picture of the endometrium has revealed two different types of cells, the secretory cell and the ciliated cell (Gompel, 1962). Both types probably play a role in the secretory function of the endometrium. Recently a third type of cell was demonstrated (Colville, 1968) of lesser electron density and sparse cell organelles. No specific function has as yet been attributed to this cell. Cavazos *et al.* (1967) in an extensive study of the ultra-structure of the endometrial glandular cells have described in detail the cyclical changes in the endometrial cells.

The various stages of proliferative activity and secretory function of the endometrial epithelium observed in electron microscope studies can be correlated with and verified by chemical and histochemical studies of the endometrial tissue and intrauterine fluid.

Endometrial Histochemistry

The prominent proliferation of the endometrial cell observed prior to ovulation and the secretory activity noted during the latter part of the menstrual cycle demand an increasing synthesis of DNA and RNA necessary for the producion of proteins and enzymes. Histochemical studies (Hughes, Jacobs, Rubulis and Husney, 1963) show that the endometrial content of DNA and RNA increases gradually throughout the cycle reaching a peak on the 17th–19th day of the cycle. DNA is found in the nuclei of all cells while RNA is more prominent in the cytoplasm of the glandular epithelium. The protein synthesis as evidenced by the nitrogen content of the endometrium increases likewise throughout the cycle reaching a peak during the secretory phase.

Enzyme studies have provided interesting and important information on the metabolic function of the endometrium (Boutselis, De Neef, Ullery and George, 1963). Alkaline phosphatase is present in the endometrium during almost the entire cycle. During the early proliferative phase this enzyme occurs diffusely throughout the entire glandular epithelium and also in the stromal cells and is thought to play a role in the process of regeneration of the endometrium. The largest concentration of alkaline phosphatase is observed around the time of ovulation. During that period the enzyme is present mainly in the cell of the glandular epithelium. Alkaline phosphatase probably plays a role in the metabolism of carbohydrates. However, its main function is changing the permeability of the cell membrane, thus facilitating the transport of glucose or glycogen.

Acid phosphatase, which may also have a function in the detoxicating mechanism of the cell, is present in the glandular epithelium of the endometrium. Its concentration seems to increase with the cycle.

Reduced diphosphopyridine nucleotide (DPNH) and reduced triphosphopyridine nucleotide (TPNH) are the essential coenzymes in the metabolic function of the endometrium. The TPNH activity shows a distinct peak prior to ovulation and DPNH activity increases particularly during the luteal phase of the cycle.

The building up of the endometrial cell during the proliferative phase and the secretory activity during the luteal phase demand vast amounts of energy. This energy is provided mainly by the break-down of carbohydrates. The endometrium is known to be capable of the synthesis

and metabolism of glucose and glycogen. Break-down of these materials by various aerobic and anaerobic pathways has been shown to take place in the endometrium. Glucose-6-phosphatase, the enzyme essential for conversion of the glucose-6-phosphate complex back to free glucose, has been shown to be present in the endometrium. Its concentration increases rapidly between day 8 and 14 of the cycle and reaches a peak during the 14th–16th day. The pattern of glucose-6-phosphatase concentration parallels that of the free glucose content of intra-uterine fluid. The glycogen content of the endometrium rises steadily throughout the first part of the cycle, reaches a peak during the 17–19th day and remains on a relatively constant plateau value thereafter. The lactic acid content and lactic dehydrogenase activity as well as the isocitric and malic dehydrogenases activity are most prominent during the 17th–19th day of the cycle. This indicates that during this period the metabolic activity of the endometrium is at its peak and that aerobic as well as anaerobic pathways of carbohydrate break-down are used to provide the energy required for synthesis and secretion of various materials such as nucleic acids, proteins and lipids. These materials are essential for the subsequent nidation and nutrition of the fertilized ovum.

The clinical significance of these biochemical and metabolic parameters of endometrial structure and function should have application in the future. In sterility and in repeated abortions the nutritional physiology of the endometrium was classified as abnormal in about 80 per cent of the cases examined, and in this particular series was the only pathological finding in otherwise normal couples. (Hughes *et al.*, 1963). Although not yet in general use as a clinical indicator it may be that the larger sterility centers would do well to investigate their sterile but apparently "normal couples" for possible uterine metabolic and enzymatic abnormalities.

Changes in the Endocervix

The uterine cervix participates actively in the menstrual cycle, its morphology and function depending on the level and ratio of sex steroids. Cyclical variations may be observed in the length and diameter of the cervical canal and isthmus, and the appearance of the external cervical os changes strikingly according to the phase of the menstrual cycle (Rabau, David, Insler and Lunenfeld, 1965). It is probable, although not yet proven in the human, that cyclical changes occur in the histologic appearance of the endocervical glands. There is, however, no doubt that the secretion of these glands is stimulated by estrogen and inhibited by progesterone (Zondek, 1957). Recent studies by electron microscopy revealed that each cell of the endocervical canal lining is a glandular unit in itself, releasing mucus of varying quantity and quality depending upon the phase of the cycle (Marcus and Marcus, 1965).

Physical properties and chemical constituents of the cervical mucus change according to the level and ratio of oestrogen and progesterone. Estrogen increases the amount, spinnbarkeit and ferning capacity of the mucus. Under the influence of oestrogen there occurs an increase in the amount of water, sodium chloride and scialic acid, and a decrease in the protein and glucose content.

Observations have been made on 6-phosphogluconate dehydrogenase (6GPD) activity of cervical mucus as compared to the concentration in vaginal fluid in benign and malignant tumours of the body and cervix of the uterus (Brooks and Muir, 1968). This and other enzyme studies in uterine cancer may produce reliable screening tests for invasive cervical carcinoma. In general, however, it seems that as yet there are too many false positives dependent perhaps upon such conditions as trichomonas vaginitis or cervical erosions to justify acceptance of these methods.

A vast amount of clinical and laboratory data on the physical and chemical properties of cervical mucus and their changes during the normal and abnormal menstrual cycle has accumulated. The exact mechanism by which ovulatory cervical mucus aids and enhances the migration of spermatozoa, and the thick, scarce, viscous mucus typical of the luteal phase, creates an impenetrable barrier for sperm, is still unknown. Recent studies (Elstein and Pollard, 1968) indicate that the quantity *and* the quality of proteins of the cervical mucus change under the influence of various steroids. It might well be that the stereoscopic nature of macromolecular chains ultimately determine the ability to penetrate cervical mucus. Recently convenient laboratory methods have been devised for testing the sperm penetration in vitro (Kremer, 1965). The use of these methods together with sophisticated immunoelectrophoretic and chemical studies of the protein content of cervical mucus will perhaps answer the question how cervical mucus enhances sperm penetration during the ovulatory phase of normal menstrual cycle, and consequently provide an explanation why subtle biochemical or immunological changes of cervical secretion may lead to infertility in the so-called "normal" couples.

THE UTERUS AND CERVIX AS A FUNCTIONAL UNIT

Observations on uterine function must of necessity correlate the interaction of numerous parameters affecting one or several aspects of uterine activity, and the periodicity of the reproductive cycle. Estimation of hormonal influence whether local or systemic, endogenous or exogenous, must take into account the pregnant or non-pregnant state, and also the stage of pregnancy, and with this the volume of the uterus. Measurements of uterine activity may differ depending upon the recording method used. There are for instance discrepancies between electrical measurements of uterine activity and mechanical estimations, differences which may be artificial or may have some physiological explanation. There are also variations in recordings made of mechanical uterine activity depending upon the system and site of the recording apparatus.

From studies carried out by many investigators, particularly the teams of Caldeyro-Barcia and Alvarez (1952); Csapo and Lloyd-Jacob (1963b), and Reynolds (1965), basic knowledge of how the uterus as an organ acts, and even how individual fibres work, has evolved. Hendricks

(1966) suggested that the uterine activity of an individual is singular and peculiar to that person as are her fingerprints.

Measuring Uterine Activity

The original observations of Knaus (1929) on kimographic recordings using a simple intra-uterine balloon have been the source of continuous debate. The inconsistent results due to the varying surface:volume ratio of different intra-uterine balloons gave rise to more sophisticated methods for measuring myometrial activity. Simple instrumentation for either direct or indirect methods of measuring uterine activity is now commercially available. Such instruments are known as tocometers or tocodynamometers. The term tocometry should refer solely to the measurement of the expulsive forces of the uterus in labour; however, it is now used in general as a term expressing measurement of any type of uterine contractility.

Direct methods of measuring uterine activity include the simple intrauterine balloon, saline filled open ended polyvinyl catheters (Hendricks, 1964), and the more compound intra-mural micro-balloon system of Caldeyro-Barcia (1958). This latter system by measuring the intra-myometrial pressures at various sites on the uterine wall enables the measurement of an intra-myometrial pressure gradient starting at the fundus and propagating down to the cervix. These measurements were carried out simultaneously with those obtained during pregnancy by the introduction of a thin-open-ended polyethylene catheter introduced into the amniotic sac, through the anterior abdominal wall (Caldeyro-Barcia and Alvarez, 1952), and connected to a pressure transducer coupled to a recording system.

Indirect methods using external tocometers have obvious advantages over internal pressure measurements by means of catheters, balloons and intrauterine pressure transducers, because of their easy clinical application. With a simpler external application of a multi-channel pressure recording from the external abdominal wall, Reynolds, Heard, Bruns and Hellman (1948) have been able to show variations in the type of the pressure gradient obtained during normal and pathological labours. The accuracy of the external tocometer such as that described by Smyth (1957) is in our experience close to that of intraamniotic pressure measurements. This view has recently been expressed also by Turnbull and Anderson (1968), when recording pressures up to 30 mm.Hg. However, Wagner (1965) using Malmstrom's Parturiometer showed discrepancies between the intraamniotic and external measurement which became greater as the pressure rose. Most observers do today accept values obtained by external tocometry as being close enough to internal measurements for all practical purposes.

Various standards have been suggested for the quantitative assessment of uterine contractility. The intensity of each contraction has been defined as the rise in amniotic fluid pressure produced by the contractions; tonus is the lowest pressure between contractions. Expressing the frequency as the number of contractions in 10 minutes, Caldeyro-Barcia (1958) introduced the Montevideo unit which defined uterine activity as the product of the intensity and the frequency of the contractions expressed in mm.Hg/10 min.

Turnbull and Anderson (1968) have suggested the alternative use of an activity index. *Intensity* has been defined for this purpose as the average height above the testing pressure (tonus) of all contractions of 5 mm.Hg or more recorded in one hour. *Frequency* is the total number of such contractions in that hour. The product of intensity and frequency is expressed in "activity units". It is claimed that this excludes possible masking of a real increase in uterine contractility by small contractions (less than 5 mm.Hg) of great frequency.

The Electrohysterogram (EHG)

The method of studying uterine physiology by measuring action potentials began when Du-Bois Reymound described in 1849 that a piece of a non-pregnant rabbit uterus produced a weak electrical current. Bode (1931) examined patients in labour using a string galvanometer and was the first to introduce the term "electrohysterogram" to express the electrical activity of the uterus. Data on observations concerning the electrical activity of the uterus are rather divergent. This is due to the different methods and equipment used by various investigators, and the lack of agreed upon standards and nomenclature. The method of recording whether direct from the uterus or indirect, the mode and place of application and the type of electrodes used, are important in assessing the data given.

Several investigators (Bozler, 1941; Levy-Solal and Morin, 1952; Steer, 1954; Jung, 1958 and Larks, 1960) have described a pattern which can be regarded as a basis for defining the physiological standards of the electrical activity of the uterus. Most observers report distinct low frequency waves of 0·5–2 c.p.s. arising from the uterus, although Sureau, Chavinie and Cannon (1965) have suggested that this type of activity may be an artefact. High frequency waves are sometimes recorded from the uterus of the order up to 70 c.p.s. Often both frequencies are recorded simultaneously. It appears that there are discrepancies regarding the wide frequency range reported by the various investigators of uterine action potentials. This is only to be expected when the wide range of equipment and electrode placing is reviewed. What emerges, however, from the numerous recordings made is a constant description of two types of electrical wave groups. Reference to these types is made by the use of the terms slow or fast waves, or low frequency and high frequency waves.

The duration of the electrical discharge ranges between 20–60 seconds, and characteristically ends abruptly. Following bursts of activity, relatively long-silent intervals are observed (Figs. 1 and 2). The duration of the electrical discharge differs according to the phase of the reproductive cycle, being longer towards the end of pregnancy than during the menstrual cycle. The amplitude of the electrical waves is of some physiological importance but is also dependent upon the electrodes and the method of recording. Simultaneous mechanical registration (pressure recordings) and electrical recordings show that the electrical activity is associated with and precedes the mechanical action of the uterus (Csapo, Takeda and Wood, 1963a; Csapo, Jaffin, Kerenyi, Lipman and Wood, 1963c). There is a correlation between a contraction and clinical hardness of the uterus and the frequency of the action potentials in the EHG (Jung, 1956). The change in frequency in the EHG during a contraction is due to the fact that the whole uterus as a smooth muscle organ produces a synchronous discharge. The change in amplitude in the EHG during a contraction is due to the increase in the number of the fibres contracting simultaneously.

Oxytocin injections into the uterine muscle produce a visible contraction with slow (low frequency) waves in the EHG. Mechanical stimulation of the uterus and emotion or sexual excitement are recorded as an increase in activity in the EHG (Masters and Johnson, 1966, Serr, Porath, Rabau, Zakut and Mannor, 1968). Huiskes (1966) considers the slow electrical activity in the electrohysterogram as the electrical representative of the "tonus" or resting pressure of the uterine musculature. The faster (high frequency) electrical activity, resulting from an increase in the excitability and the conduction of impulses constitutes the electrical equivalent of a tetanic type contraction. The fact that this activity has a higher amplitude in the pregnant than in the non-pregnant uterus, seems to be due to increased stretching of the uterine musculature. It is as yet uncertain what physiological processes in the uterine muscle are represented by the slow and fast waves of the electrohysterogram. It may be that differences in excitability and conductivity resulting from synchronization and coordination at the cellular level may result in these two distinct types of electrical waves. The two frequency types could then be seen as basic elements in the various patterns of bursts of activity and periods of inactivity noted in electrohysterograms during the menstrual cycle, sexual activity, pregnancy and labour.

Menstrual Cycle

During the proliferative phase, electrical waves are found lasting up to one second, with an amplitude ranging from 20–100 μV, depending upon the method of recording. Following a period of electrical activity, long silent intervals are often observed (Liesse, 1947). During the secretory phase of the menstrual cycle, spontaneous low frequency electrical activity disappears (Jung, 1956, Csapo, 1959). At menstruation high frequency biphasic waves of high amplitude up to 500 μV have been described (Liesse, 1947).

Using two types of uterine electrodes Mannor, Zakut and Serr, (1968), have compared the electrical activity of the uterus in various physiological states. A cervical electrode consisting of a vacuum type cap attached to the cervix, has confirmed the basic data on electric potentials during the menstrual cycle, and provide a simple means of measuring it. Electrical activity of the uterus was also shown to be augmented during sexual stimulation and also during pregnancy (Figs. 3 and 4).

An intra-uterine electrode was also developed by the implanting of a platinum iridium wire into a polythene intra-uterine contraceptive device. Behrman and Burchfield

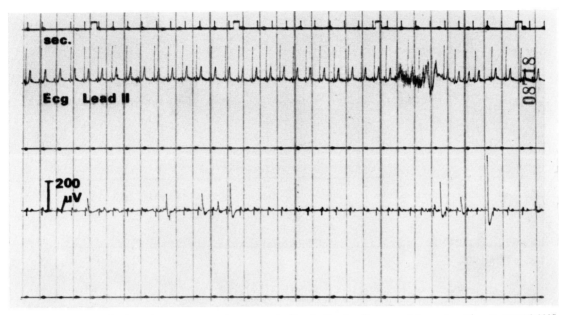

Fig. 1. Electrical activity from the non-pregnant human cervix. Day 6 of cycle. Paper speed 5 mm./sec. Time constant 0·003″. Frequency 70 c.p.s. (Serr *et al.*, 1968).

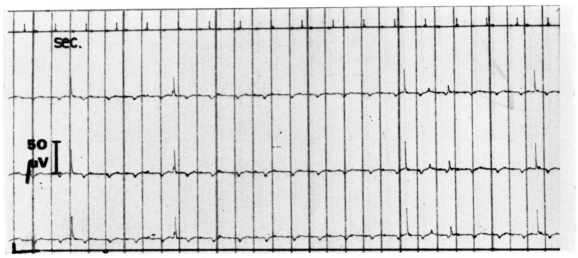

Fig. 2. Typical action potentials recorded from the non-pregnant human cervix. Day 20 of cycle. Paper speed mm./sec. Time constant 0·03″. Frequency 70 c.p.s. The small downward deflections represent patient's ECG. (Serr *et al.*, 1968).

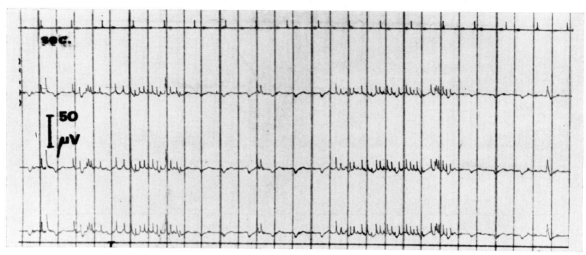

FIG. 3. Increased electrical activity recorded from human cervix following clitoral stimulation. Day 20 of cycle. Paper speed 10 mm./sec. Time constant 0·03″. Frequency 70 c.p.s. (Serr *et al.*, 1968).

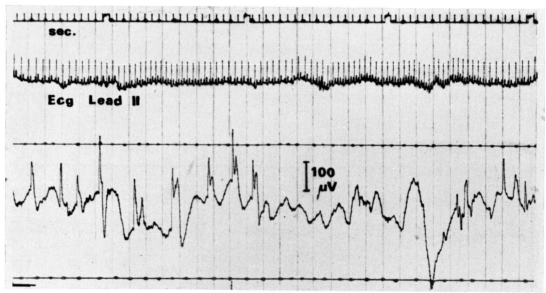

FIG. 4. Irregular type action potentials recorded from the human cervix during pregnancy (20 weeks). Paper speed 2·5 mm./sec. Time constant 0·03″. Frequency 70 c.p.s. (Serr *et al.*, 1968).

(1968) using a pressure transducer attached to an intra-uterine device, have measured mechanical activity of the uterus as compared to our own observations on the electrical activity. Data have been collected on the cyclical changes in the electrical pattern following the introduction of the device. Potentials were recorded between the intra-uterine electrode and a pubic electrode using an 8-channel polygraph.* Recordings were made on alternate days throughout the menstrual cycle. Marked activity was noted immediately following insertion of the device. Three different types of electrical potentials were observed. The first type consists of groups of high frequency activity (Fig. 5). The second type is a simple high frequency peak which recurs rhythmically (Fig. 6). The third type noted consisted of low frequency single waves (Fig. 7).

* Minograph 81, Elema–Schonander, Sweden. Frequency range (D.C.) 0–700 c.p.s. Maximum amplification 20 μV/cm.

During menstruation both types one and two were noted. Activity was low at the end of menstruation and in the early proliferative stage. Around mid-cycle, at the time of ovulation, marked activity was again noted but less than that which was observed during menstruation. In the early secretory phase intermittent low frequency activity was found. Later in the secretory phase the three types of activity gradually increased reaching a maximum during menstruation.

The differences of potential found during the various stages of the menstrual cycle tended to confirm a correlation between bio-electric potentials and the various phases of the cycle. Significantly much more electrical activity is recorded from the IUD electrode as compared to the electrical activity which is recorded from the human cervix, especially during the secretory phase, and menstruation. Since the IUD in itself may give rise to other

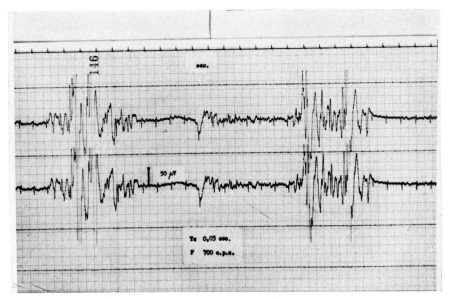

FIG. 5. High frequency potentials (type one) recorded with the intra-uterine device electrode (day 17 of cycle). (Mannor *et al.*, 1968).

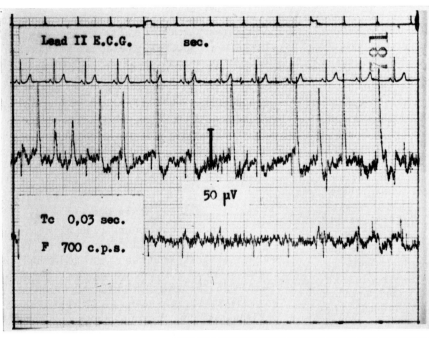

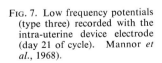

FIG. 6. Rhythmic high frequency potentials (type two) recorded with the intra-uterine device electrode (day 15 of cycle). (Mannor *et al.*, 1968).

FIG. 7. Low frequency potentials (type three) recorded with the intra-uterine device electrode (day 21 of cycle). Mannor *et al.*, 1968).

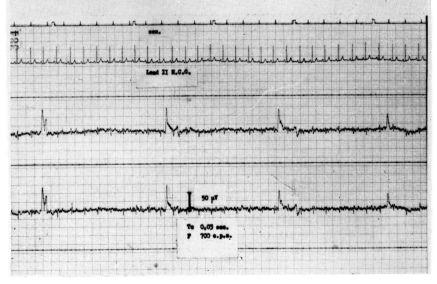

than spontaneous activity, it is felt that the more numerous high frequency waves recorded from the IUD electrode as compared to cervical recording alone may represent the uterine musculatures reaction to the foreign body.

The peak of uterine muscle activity around ovulation time and the gradually increasing potentials later in the secretory phase may represent possible uterine hyper-activity. This could interfere with the passage and nidation of a fertilized ovum and therefore may be a factor in the contraceptive mechanism of the IUD.

Pregnancy and Labour

Low frequency electrical activity can be demonstrated in pregnancy from the 10th week onward, and during labour and the puerperium. Groups of waves may be found alternating with periods of a flat type EHG. During the second half of pregnancy these groups of electrical discharge coincide with palpable uterine contractions.

The fact that during pregnancy some recordings show little or no electrical activity may be due to the physio-logical dominance of progesterone on the myometrium, and it has even been suggested that this effect be used as a test for placental function. A decrease in the progesterone level in pregnancy, possibly combined with other factors, will result in an increase in the low frequency electrical activity and occasionally also in the high frequency activity, especially over the fundal regions (Kloosterman, 1965).

There has not yet been found any correlation between the electrical activity and the duration of pregnancy. An increase in the low frequency electrical activity is accompanied by hypertonicity of the pregnant human uterus. This increase in the low frequency electrical activity is reported to be reduced after administration of progesterone (Huiskes, 1966).

Oxytocin infusions in the pregnant female produce low frequency activity and occasionally some high frequency electrical activity. The same type of activity is observed during labour. However, during pregnancy small amounts of oxytocin will produce the above mentioned type of electrohysterogram without accompanying cervical dilatation.

Towards the end of pregnancy increased spontaneous electrical activity is found. There is an overall increase in the low frequency activity while high frequency activity begins to appear over the fundus. These changes indicate an increase in excitability and conductivity of the uterus towards term. However, this increased activity cannot be suppressed by progesterone.

Huiskes (1966) suggested the term "transitional activity" to describe this super-imposed fast (high frequency) action potential on the slow (low frequency) electrical waves of pregnancy. This effect may be seen about 3 weeks before delivery and is correlated to antenatal preparation of the cervix (Kloosterman, 1959). In cases in which low fre-quency activity predominates over the high frequency activity, pre-labour effacement and dilatation appear to proceed slowly. False labour electrohysterograms are characterized by low frequency activity only, unaccom-panied by high frequency activity. On the other hand in prolonged pregnancy, the EHG shows no low frequency activity.

No constant uniform pattern of the EHG has been found during parturition. Several investigators (Sureau, 1955, Jung, 1956, Kao, 1959, Huiskes, 1966), have described changing EHG patterns during labour. It was found that during the first stage of labour and up to 5 cm. cervical dilatation, low frequency electrical activity was recorded from the lower uterine segment. After 5 cm. dilatation there is a change in the EHG recordings from the lower uterine segment. Superimposed on low frequency waves, faster action potentials are now recorded indicating that the whole uterus is now involved in a tetanic type contrac-tion, the organ now acting as one functional unit. These findings can be correlated with observations that cervical dilatation up to 5 cm is much slower than dilatation from 5 cm. onward and is in keeping with Friedman's division of labour into a latent phase and an active phase (Friedman, 1955).

During labour, absence of low frequency electrical activity from the lower uterine segment has been associ-ated with a hypotonic type of uterine inertia and slow dilatation of the cervix. On the other hand a "hypertonic type inertia" shows increased low frequency activity from the lower uterine segment. This may be interfering with the propagation of the contraction from fundus to cervix. Administration of relaxant drugs such as pethidine, results in a decrease in the hypertonicity of the lower uterine segment. This will be seen in the EHG recordings as a decrease in the low frequency activity and a clinically increased rate of dilatation.

Puerperium

There is no clear-cut boundary in the electrical record-ings from the uterus in the three stages of labour. After delivery the EHG recordings show active high frequency electrical waves for several minutes. Throughout the puerperium rhythmic discharges are recorded, the rate of the faster action potentials decreasing with the length of the puerperium. Beginning about a week after delivery low frequency electrical activity is recorded indicating a shift from the puerperium to the non-pregnant state. Breast feeding and suction of the nipples increase the elec-trical activity during the puerperium.

The EHG and the Pacemaker

Reynolds, Harris and Kaiser (1954) described fundal dominance and Alvarez and Caldeyro-Barcia (1950) described the triple descendant gradient of uterine con-tractions. Jung (1956) on the other hand, using micro-electrodes found that the vaginal end of the uterus is the most active while Kao (1959) found as much electrical activity at the tubo-uterine junction as at the vaginal end of the uterus. Larks (1960) concluded that during labour the uterus is under the hegemony of a single dominant pacemaker, the wave of excitation from the pacemaker being propagated equally in all directions.

In spite of all the data accumulated from investigations on the type and place of uterine pacemakers, no clear-cut evidence is as yet available that there is one pacemaker that can be excited either by mechanical, pharmacologic or electronic means.

Applications of the Electrohysterogram

Contractility of the Uterus

Though there is not an accepted definition for hyper-contractility of the uterus in pregnancy from the stand point of the EHG recordings Serr *et al.*, (1968) showed that well differentiated electrical activity can be continu-ously recorded from leads over the uterus for at least 15 minutes. Other authors consider longer periods up to 30 minutes (Huiskes, 1966) to be normal.

The hypercontractility pattern has been found in preg-nant patients during infections, and even during anxiety states (Rawlings and Krieger, 1959, Huiskes, 1966). Hypercontractile states of the uterus may explain some cases of abortion and premature labour. A drop in the pregnandiol level in the urine has been found to be connected with increased uterine activity. (Kloosterman, 1965). Injection of progesterone into the human uterus is followed after 30 to 40 minutes by a decrease in electrical activity. The potentials gradually obtain a distinctly local character and ultimately disappear completely, causing a "soft" low uterus. Repeated daily EHG recording may possibly serve as a test for the presence of an efficient progesterone block and thereby give some impression of placental function.

Induction of Labour

It may be considered advisable to adapt a conservative attitude to the induction of labour and to avoid oxytocics until it becomes certain that the progesterone block is withdrawn and the patient can go into true labour. This may delay action for a period of 24–48 hours, but the danger would be avoided that the myometrium, only partly recovered from the block, is ineffectively stimulated and exhausted before the uterus as a whole can be put into effective action. When the progesterone block is with-drawn from the myometrium, normal excitability, pro-pagation and pharmacological reactivity return and a normal physiological labour can ensue. However, neither spontaneous activity of the uterus nor its sensitivity to oxytocin give any real warning of the onset of labour during the last days of pregnancy. The pressure tension relationship is affected by both uterine size and hormonal factors. Methods for the assessment of the possibility of successful induction of labour have been described by Muller (1958), Smyth (1958), Caldeyro-Barcia (1959), and Boden (1966).

The electrical activity after administration of oxytocin during the last weeks of pregnancy, depends upon the duration of the pregnancy. It can be assumed that if no spontaneous electrical activity is detectable, a sufficient progesterone block is still maintaining decreased excita-bility and conductivity of the myometrium which is there-fore incapable of functioning. Therefore, a flat EHG together with other sensitivity tests may help in the difficult assessment of when to induce labour.

Further refinements in this method may make the ENG an easily applied and practical source of information in the delivery rooms and become of help to the obstetrician in his evaluation of the progress of labour.

ENDOCRINE EFFECTS UPON UTERINE FUNCTION

The ovarian hormones are known to be the prime endocrine agents controlling uterine activity. Estrogens are involved in the biochemical reactions of the uterine smooth muscle, a system including actomyozin, high energy phosphates, and other enzymes, particularly adenosine triphosphatase. It has been shown that increased activity of the pregnant human uterus follows intravenous administration of estradiol 17β. (Pinto, Votta, Montnovi and Baleiron, 1964). There is however, as yet little other direct evidence that the estrogens are essential for the control of myometrial function.

In pregnancy and labour the ratio between estrogen and progesterone is differentially balanced according to the stage of pregnancy. The ratio of pregnandiol to estriol in pregnancy urine is 100:1 in the early weeks and falls to 3:1 by the 20th week, the period when develop-ment of spontaneous myometrial activity is noticed (Klopper and Billewicz, 1963).

It is known that progesterone has an inhibiting effect upon myometrial activity, in the rabbit. Csapo's studies have contributed much to our knowledge of progesterone effects on uterine activity. The place of progesterone in this system involves more than a direct cause and effect relationship. The site of progesterone production, its concentration in the blood, its metabolism, the systemic and local effects, all are connected in what is a complicated mechanism not yet completely understood. There is how-ever, evidence to-day that the effect of progesterone upon the human myometrium may be as much a local as a systemic action. At the cellular level, the depression of propagation and synchronization of contractions in myometrial cells has been proved in some animals, and may in the human be due to the effect of progesterone on ionic distribution and membrane potential. (Kumar, Wagatsuma, Sullivan and Barnes, 1964). Progesterone blocks sodium transport through the cell membrane (Jung, 1965). The ions of potassium and calcium are also closely linked to membrane potential, and observations by some investigators indicate that the effect of progesterone on the myometrial cell is to increase the membrane potential and stabilize the membrane (Coutinho and Csapo, 1959, Daniel, 1960, Marshall, 1959). Kao and Nishiyama, (1964) have not been able to confirm these results.

The contractility of the myometrium has been shown to be blocked by progesterone when the propagation is measured mechanically or by recording of electrical activity. Csapo's work in this field has been extensive and although the evidence produced holds true mainly for laboratory animals, there is reason to believe that there is a close correlation between findings in animals and humans (Csapo *et al.*, 1963c). Micro-electrodes placed in the myometrium at placental and non-placental sites record differences between the membrane potential (Kuriyama and Csapo, 1961). These differences can be eliminated by administration of progesterone in the animal. Schofield (1963) using wax dummies to replace fetuses in animal pregnancies with intact placentae, demonstrated that there were differences in the myometrium overlying the placenta. There is a general conclusion that progesterone produced by the placenta may have a direct influence on the myometrium, and that towards the end of pregnancy as progesterone declines, a differential develops between the different areas of the uterus. This differential has been spoken of as "the staircase effect".

The Prostaglandins

These are a relatively new class of biologically active substances having an effect upon smooth muscle and may also be modulators of intracellular metabolism. Fourteen types have been isolated and in some instances their chemical identification completed. Found in their highest concentration in human seminal plasma, they have an action particularly on uterine muscle. The main groups of prostaglandins have been extensively studied and the response of the myometrium, whether inhibitory or stimulatory, depends upon which type of prostaglandin is used and the dosage. It appears that discrepancies in the various prostaglandins can be explained by comparing dose response, mode of application and the method used for measuring the response. Deposition of seminal plasma in the vagina has been reported to affect uterine motility only at the time of ovulation and it has been reported that in a small series, males of infertile couples lacked prostaglandins. (Bergstrom and Samuelsson, 1967.) In pregnancy, uterine activity similar to normal labour has been induced by the intravenous injection of small amounts of prostaglandins (Bygdeman, Kwon, Mukherjee and Wiqvist, 1968). It seems reasonable to surmise thst this may be a factor in some cases of spontaneous abortions. The implications of these findings are sufficiently far reaching to warrant further research.

CLINICAL AND THERAPEUTIC EFFECTS OF DRUGS ON UTERINE ACTIVITY

The pharmacological action of various drugs on the uterus can be used for experimental and therapeutic purposes. Often the experimental proof of a compound's effect upon the uterus is not sufficient to justify its clinical use as a pharmacological agent. Freedom from side effects is necessary and proof is often lacking that clinical systemic administration produces the same effect as experimental application to uterine muscle strips.

Progesterone has been used clinically for prevention of abortion and the efficacy of this treatment much discussed. Although there is proof that progesterone reduces both spontaneous and pharamacologically induced uterine activity, on the other hand double blind studies on clinical data have failed to prove the efficacy of such treatment in the human female. (Brenner and Hendricks, 1962, Shearman and Garrett, 1963, Fuchs, 1965.) Although

it appears that systemic progesterone in conventional doses has little effect upon the human uterus as far as prevention of threatened abortion is concerned, its continued use has never been clinically condemned since "it may help and doesn't appear to harm".

The use of high doses of progesterone and of long acting progestational agents has however, been of concern since they appear to have effects of consequence on uterine activity in some cases of threatened abortion. When haemorrhage is threatening miscarriage it may be that even high and sustained levels of progesterone may not be able to prevent the human uterus from expelling its contents if in fact the local placental effect of progesterone is really necessary for the myometrial block. In such cases separation of the young placenta may have already released the uterus from the progesterone block and abortion will inevitably follow. On the other hand, if a high enough dose of progesterone is administered to prevent or inhibit uterine contractility, then the result may be to encourage the development of a missed abortion instead of an inevitable abortion. Furthermore, it has been observed that post-abortal amenorrheas may also result from the continuing action of the long-acting progesterones after the uterus has been cleared of the products of conception. These observations together with earlier reports of the masculinizing effects of some progestagens upon fetal development, when considered against the scanty evidence of the clinical value of systemic progesterone in threatened abortion, may justify reconsideration of the pharmacologic benefits of this group of drugs. Support, however, may be given to the practical application of experiments based upon the local effects of progesterone given by vaginal or transabdominal intramyometrial injection (Coutinho, Fischer and Mascarenhas, 1962; Bengtsson, 1962).

Alcohol in Premature Labour

Although many attempts to prevent premature labour by pharmacologic means have been made and abandoned, recent observations on the effect of ethyl alcohol in humans for this purpose has aroused interest. It has been shown that in rabbits the onset of labour is inhibited, typical contractions are absent, and delivery prolonged by using an infusion of ethyl alcohol (Fuchs and Wagner, 1963). The uterine sensitivity to exogenous oxytocin however, is reported to be unimpaired. This interference with parturition is therefore assumed by Fuchs, Fuchs, Poblete and Risk (1967), to be attributed to a central inhibition of the release of oxytocin. However, it was noted that whenever the membranes were ruptured and/or cervical dilatation was greater than 5 cm. alcohol had no inhibitory effect upon uterine contractions. From tocometric recordings we have been able to confirm the inhibitory action of ethyl alcohol in premature labour, although we have not as yet been able to ascertain whether this effect can be overcome by exogenous oxytocin. The effects of alcohol upon the patient is to cause some restlessness and inebriation and occasionally a sclerosed blood vessel with an intravenous infusion concentration of 10 per cent alcohol in 5 per cent dextrose. Of 19 patients so treated, labour was delayed for periods of 12 hours up to 14 days in 12. However, in

7 patients, labour ensued in less than 12 hours following cessation of the alcohol infusion (Fig. 8).

Although more studies both basic and clinical are required for assessment of this method of treatment, it should be noted that in one case of twins, in which alcohol was administered for 12 hours, labour continued and at 26 weeks pregnancy resulted in the birth of a 620 gram male infant. At birth, although the cord blood was not examined, the mother was semiconscious under the influence of 8 hours of alcohol infusion. This immature infant has survived and is alive and well today at ten months of age (Serr, Zakut and Mannor, 1969). However,

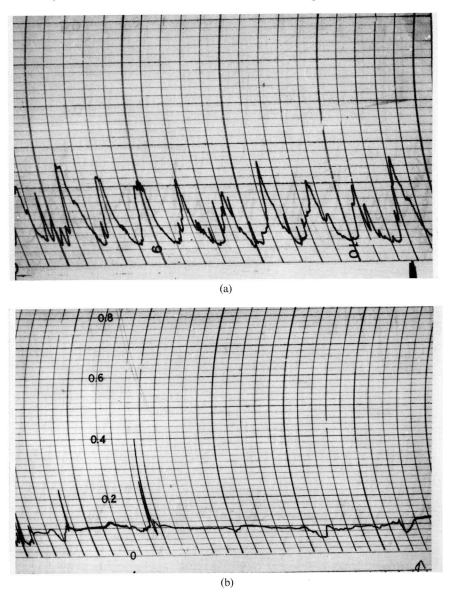

(a)

(b)

FIG. 8. Effect of intravenous ethyl-alcohol infusion on uterine contractility (Twin channel guard-ring tocograph, Stanley Cox Ltd. London). (a) Before alcohol infusion, contraction rate approximately 4/10 min. (b) Quiescence following alcohol infusion. (Serr *et al.*, 1969).

the time of delivery the mother's blood showed an alcohol concentration of 100 mgm per cent. The twins weighing 900 grams and 1130 grams and an Apgar score of 7 and 3 respectively lived for 95 and 12 hours, and the alcohol concentrations measured in the umbilical cord blood at birth were 137 mgm per cent and 168 mgm per cent, both noticeably higher than in the mother. Autopsy showed no liver damage of other findings directly attributed to alcohol. It would be correct to report at this point on another case in this series, where a failed alcohol infusion

we do feel that more observations on the fetal effects of maternally administered alcohol are necessary.

Promethazine and Uterine Activity

The clinical usage of a combination of pethidine and promethazine (Phenergan) has become accepted practice in the labour ward. It has been assumed that besides an antiemetic effect, promethazine may potentiate the effect of pethidine in the parturient. However, at certain dose levels it could be shown that promethazine administered alone had an inhibitory effect upon uterine contractions, even in the presence of an oxytocin infusion.

In an intra-amniotic hypertonic saline induced abortion, regular contractions were suppressed by intravenous administration of 50 mgm. promethazine. In this case was observed in the amplitude of the contractions (Zakut, Mannor, Serr, 1969). Figures 11 and 12 show the time-lag between administration of the drug and its effect upon contractions, and the duration of this effect.

This inhibitory effect of promethazine in large doses

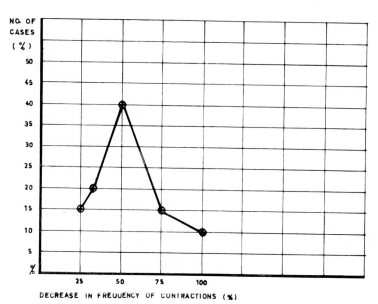

FIG. 9. Range of inhibitory effect of Phenergan (50 mgm. i. v.) on the frequency of contractions in 40 patients. (Zakut *et al.*, 1969).

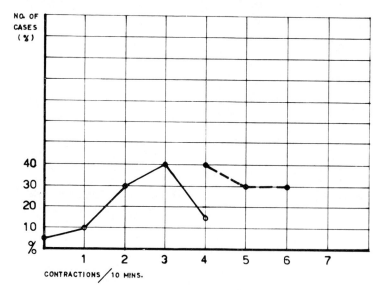

FIG. 10. Effect of Phenergan on frequency of uterine contractions.
. – – – . – – – . – – – . Frequency range before Phenergan;
——— . ——— . ———. Frequency range after Phenergan (50 mgm. i. v.)
(Zakut *et al.*, 1969).

uterine activity did not recur spontaneously and a second intraamniotic injection of saline was performed two days later. In a series of 40 patients studied, 40 per cent of the cases showed a 50 per cent decrease in the frequency of uterine contractions following intra-venous administration of 50 mgm. Phenergan (Figs. 9 and 10). A similar effect should be taken into account in prolonged labour. A cumulative effect may possibly result in further delay due to suppressed uterine activity. In premature labours given in large enough doses some damping effect upon uterine activity has been noted, but not to the extent that is seen when using alcohol or isoxsuprine.

Isoxsuprine

In 1948, Alquist reported a series of experiments on the effects of epinephrine and related compounds upon isolated and intact organs. The conclusion led to the concept that there were two types of adrenergic receptors. The alpha receptor concerned with excitatory functions was connected with myometrial stimulation, whilst the beta reactors would be inhibitory. The best effect upon an organ would be the correlation between the activity of the agent and the population density of alpha and beta receptors in the tissue.

hypotension, which characterize beta-adrenergic agents have prevented the use of this and similar drugs in effective doses. However, recent reports suggest that beta-receptor blocking agents such as propranolol may prevent the systemic disturbances whilst allowing the effect upon the myometrium to continue. These studies which are being carried out *in vitro* may however prove difficult to prove

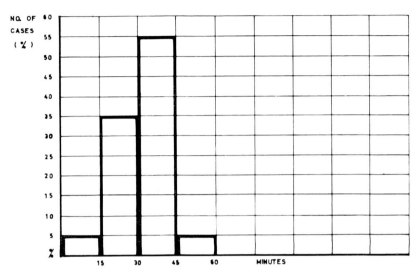

FIG. 11. Time (in minutes) from injection of 50 mgm. Phenergan i. v. until observation of inhibitory effect. (Zakut *et al.*, 1969).

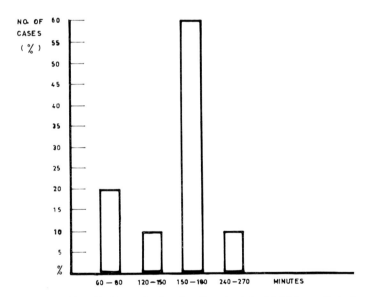

FIG. 12. Range in duration (in minutes) of inhibitory effect of Phenergan upon uterine contractions. (Zakut *et al.*, 1969).

This led to the use of a beta adrenergic stimulating agent such as isoxsuprine (Vasodilan)* for the inhibition of the uterine contractions of premature labour. The maternal cardiovascular effects, chiefly tachycardia and

* Mead Johnson Co., Ewansville, Ind.

in vivo, since there appear to be discrepancies between the actions of these compound on muscle strips *in vitro* and their general effect *in vivo*. Other similar substances with higher inhibitory activity on the myometrium and less cardiovascular effect are being tested (Landesmann, Wilson and Zlatnik, 1966; Landesmann and Wilson, 1968).

The use of these agents has led to theoretic considerations of the relationship of the sympathetic neuro-hormones and receptors, and the myometrial "progesterone block". Shabanah, Toth, Carassavas and Maughan (1968a) and Shabanah, Toth, Omay and Maughan (1968b) have proposed a hypothesis based upon animal experiments showing (1) a link between estrogen and acetyl-choline; (2) a possible link between progesterone and certain catecholamines and (3) the dependence of uterine function on these neuro-hormones and their interaction with the sex-steroids. Experiments show an inter-relationship between progesterone, epinephrine and norepinephrine and demonstrates that the effect upon myometrial activity of the progesterone block is mediated through these amines, by which the effect upon myometrial adrenergic receptors is modified by progesterone. From these and other observations on estrogen primed and hypophysectomized rats, it is possible to arrive at a representation of the factors controlling uterine activity and therefore premature labour, and maybe abortion and delivery. The hypothesis of Shabanah and associates states that estrogen synthesizes acetylcholine and sensitizes the myometrial cholinergic receptors to its effect. Acetyl choline-like compounds stimulate the release of oxytocin which in turn potentiates the effect of acetyl-choline. At the same time estrogen is shown to control the myometrial uptake of catecholamines. This effect upon the myometrium is modulated by progesterone which in small amounts lowers the threshold of alpha receptors and in large amounts lowers the beta receptors. These studies point to a purpose of a sharply rising estrogen level in the last trimester of pregnancy, in order to inhibit the effect of trophic like hormones which diminish the myometrial response to progesterone irrespective of its level. (Bengtsson and Schofield, 1963.)

What Starts Labour?

The suddenness of the onset of labour has given rise to much discussion and a detailed review of the observations on the subject would be beyond the scope of this work. However, in brief it may be stated that although myometrial activity increases towards the end of pregnancy, sudden volume changes, or a sudden outpouring of oxytocin have not as yet been proven as causes for the abrupt change from spontaneous pregnancy contractions of the Braxton-Hicks type, to the labour cervix dilating type.

Volume Changes and Oxytocin Sensitivity

Clinical experience suggests that the pregnant human uterus appears to be an organ which is activated at one time by volume increase such as in hydramnion and twins, and at another time by volume reduction such as in amniotomy, spontaneous or induced.

Csapo et al. (1963a, b) in their model experiments in animals established a relationship between uterine volume and activity. Using rabbits in late pregnancy in which ovarian and placental endocrine function was eliminated (by surgical means) and in which pregnancy was maintained by exogenous hormones they were able to demonstrate that both onset and progress of labour is a function of uterine volume. Rabbits with different uterine volumes deliver at different times, and the same animals deliver at different times from the two uterine horns if their volumes

are different. By simultaneous recording of electrical and mechanical activity of the uterus it was shown that myometrial activity is maximal at an optimum volume. They concluded that the maintenance or termination of pregnancy is determined by the ratio of uterine volume/myometrial progesterone content.

In Csapo et al.'s work (1963c) on the human it was found that the results of model experiments (rabbits) and clinical trials are in close agreement. An increase of uterine volume in normal term pregnancies by intra-amniotic injection of 5 per cent glucose or physiological saline (Portes, Mayer, Granjon and Bommelaer, 1964; Csapo, Jaffin, Kerenyi, de Mattos and de Sousa Filho, 1963d) increases uterine activity and may induce labour. Schofield (1963) has claimed that the volume of a dummy fetus is also another factor influencing the time of delivery. However, Turnbull and Anderson (1968) have recently shown that such an artificial increase in volume at 18 weeks gestation whilst producing increased frequency of low intensity contractions, does not alter the spontaneous activity or oxytocin sensitivity of the uterus at this period. There is, however, a physiological sudden increase in spontaneous activity around the 20th–22nd week of pregnancy followed a little later by an increase in oxytocin sensitivity.

Other parameters have been studied such as the effects of enzymatic changes on the carbohydrate metabolism of the myometrium influencing the start of labour. The role of oxytocin in the onset of labour has been the subject of much controversy. Recently Contractor, Jones and Routledge (1968) have studied the response of human myometrial strips to 5 Hydroxytryptomin (5HT) and the threshold for oxytocin sensitivity. A correlation has been found between the duration of pregnancy and both oxytocin sensitivity and MAO activity. When the duration of gestation is excluded, there is a highly significant correlation between the thresholds for oxytocin and for 5 HT. This shows that irrespective of the duration of pregnancy, the uterine muscle strips that were most sensitive to oxytocin were also the most sensitive to 5 HT.

The endocrine role of the fetus itself in the onset of labour has recently been given more serious consideration. Some evidence that the fetal pituitary adrenal pathway may be involved in the initiation of labour has been presented (Liggins, Holm and Kennedy, 1966). It is known that anencephalic fetuses are often associated with prolonged gestation. Drost and Holm (1968) in a nice series of experiments, have adrenalectomized fetal lambs, and shown prolongation of labour as a result. This strongly suggests that the fetal adrenal may also have something to do with the onset of labour. Ellis, Beck and Currie (1966) have demonstrated the production of growth hormone by the fetal adeno-hypophysis at 19 weeks gestation, and this coincides with an increase at this time of spontaneous myometrial activity. It appears therefore that the fetal endocrine system may be one more parameter involved in the uterine activity of pregnancy and labour along with uterine volume, oxytocin concentrations and myometrial sensitivity, maternal estrogen and progesterone levels, both local and systemic.

In view of these observations and the theories on the relationship between estrogen sensitization of the myometrium and the connection between the neurohormones and the beta and alpha adrenergic receptors, it would appear that the mechanism initiating labour has been given a new complexity. Clinical and basic studies of these considerations are important for a new approach to the dynamics of the uterus. The modern attitude to the safety of mother and fetus and the reduction of perinatal mortality demand deeper understanding of the physiology of the uterus and the processes of labour. Some of the problems connected with this aim have been discussed in the light of biochemical, hormonal and biophysical considerations. It remains to combine these parameters for improved diagnostic aids and therapeutic possibilities.

ACKNOWLEDGEMENT

Appreciation is due to Drs. S. Mannor and H. Zakut who have contributed both in material and thought to this review.

REFERENCES

Ahlquist, R. (1948), "A Study of the Adrenotropic Receptors," *Amer. J. Physiol*, **153**, 586.

Alvarez, H. and Caldeyro-Barcia, R. (1950), "Contractility of the Human Uterus Recorded by New Method," *Surg. Gynec. Obstet.*, **91**, 1.

Battaglia, F. C., Hellegers, A. E., Heller, C. J. and Behrman, R. (1964), "Glucose Concentration Gradients across the Maternal Surface, the Placenta, and the Amnion of the Rhesus Monkey (Macaca mulatta)," *Amer. J. Obstet. Gynec.*, **88**, 32.

Behrman, S. J. and Burchfield, W. (1968), "The Intrauterine Contraceptive Device and Myometrial Activity," *Amer. J. Obstet. Gynec.*, **100**, 194.

Bengtsson, L. P. (1962), "Experiments on the Suppressive Effect of a Synthetic Gestagen on the Activity of the Pregnant Human Uterus," *Acta. obstet. gynec. scand.*, **41**, 124.

Bengtsson, L. P. and Schofield, B. M. (1963), "Progesterone and the Accomplishment of Parturition in the Sheep," *J. Reprod. Fertil.*, **5**, 423.

Bergstrom, S. and Samuelsson, B. (Eds.), (1967), "The Prostaglandins." *Proc. II Nobel Symposium*, Almquist and Wiksell, Uppsala and John Wiley and Sons, Inc., New York.

Bode, O. (1931), "Die Wirkung des Hypophysenhinterlappen hormons auf den schwangeren Uterus im Elektrohysterogram," *Arch. Gynaek.*, **144**, 499.

Boden, W. (1966), "Die praktische Bedeutung der aussern Wehenmessung, insbesondere des Oxytocin Empfindlichkeitstestes fur die klinische Geburtshilfe," *Geburt. u. Frauenheilk.*, **26**, 3.

Boutselis, J. G., De Neef, J. C., Ullery, J. C. and George, O. T. (1963), "Histochemical and Cytological Observations in the Normal Human Endometrium. I. Histochemical Observations in the Normal Human Endometrium," *Obstet. Gynec.*, **21**, 423.

Bozler, E. (1941), "Influence of Estrone on the Electric Characteristics and the Motility of Uterine Muscle," *Endocrinology*, **29**, 225.

Brenner, W. E. and Hendricks, C. H. (1962), "Effect of Medroxyprogesterone Acetate, upon the Duration and Characteristics of Human Gestation and Labour," *Amer. J. Obstet. Gynec.*, **83**, 1094.

Brooks, P. C. and Muir, G. G. (1968), "6-Phosphogluconate Dehydregenase (6PED) Activity in the Cervical Mucus and Vaginal Fluid in Benign and Malignant Gynecological Lesions," *J. Obstet. Gynaec. Brit. Com.*, **74**, 111.

Buckingham, J. C., Selden, R. and Danforth, D. N. (1962), "Connective Tissue Changes in the Cervix during Pregnancy and Labour," *Ann. N.Y. Acad. Sci.*, **97**, 733.

Bygdeman, M., Kwon, S. U., MuKherice, T. and Wiqvist, N. (1968), "Effect of Intravenous Infusion of Prostaglandins E₁ and E₂ on Motility of the Pregnant Human Uterus," *Amer. J. Obstet. Gynec.*, **102**, 317.

Caldeyro-Barcia, R. (1958), "Uterine Contractility in Obstetrics," in *Modern Trends in Obstetrics and Gynecology*. International Congress on Gynecology and Obstetrics, Second World Congress, Montreal, 1958. Montreal, Librairie Beauchemin Limiteé 1959, **1**, 65.

Caldeyro-Barcia, R. (1960), "Oxytocin in Pregnancy and Labour," First International Congress of Endocrinology, Copenhagen, *Acta Endocrinologica (Kobenhavn)*, **34**, (Supplement 50), 41.

Caldeyro-Barcia, R. and Alvarez, H. (1952), "Abnormal Uterine Action in Labour," *J. Obstet. Gynaec. Brit. Emp.*, **59**, 646.

Cavazos, F., Green, J. A., Hall, D. G. and Lucas, F. V. (1967), "Ultrastructure of the Human Endometrium Glandular Cell during the Menstrual Cycle," *Amer. J. Obstet. Gynec.*, **99**, 833.

Colville, A. E. (1968), "The Ultrastructure of the Human Endometrium," *J. Obstet. Gynaec. Brit. Com.*, **75**, 342.

Contractor, S. F., Jones, J. J. and Routledge, A. (1968), "The Response of Human Myometrial Strips to 5-Hydroxytryptamine and Oxytocin and its Monoamine Oxidase Activity at Various Stages of Gestation," *J. Obstet. Gynaec. Brit. Com.*, **75**, 1113.

Coutinho, E. M. and Csapo, A. (1959), "Effect of Oxytocics on Ca-deficient Uterus," *J. gen. Physiol.*, **43**, 13.

Coutinho, E. M., Fischer, G. and Mascarenhas, G. B. (1960), "Local Effect of Progesterone. (1) Intra-myometrial Administration of Small Doses," Brazilian Congress of Obstetrics and Gynecology, October, 1960.

Csapo, A. (1959), "Zur molekular Physiologie und Regulation des Uterus," *Bibl. Gynaec.*, **20**, 27.

Csapo, A. I., Takeda, H. and Wood, C. (1963a), "Volume and Activity of the Parturient Rabbit Uterus," *Amer. J. Obstet. Gynec.* **85**, 813.

Csapo, A. I., Lloyd-Jacob, M. A. (1963b), "Effect of Uterine Volume on Parturition," *Amer. J. Obstet. Gynec.*, **85**, 806.

Csapo, A. I., Jaffin, H., Kerenyi, T., Lipman, J. I. and Wood, C. (1963c), "Volume and Activity of the Pregnant Human Uterus," *Amer. J. Obstet. Gynec.*, **85**, 819.

Csapo, A. I., Jaffin, H., Kerenyi, T., de Mattos, C. E. R. and de Sousa Filho, M. B. (1963d), "Fetal Death in Utero," *Amer. J. Obstet. Gynec.*, **87**, 892.

Daniel, E. E. (1960), "Effect of the Placenta on the Electrical Activity of the Cat Uterus *in vivo* and *in vitro*," *Amer. J. Obstet. Gynec.*, **80**, 229.

Dessouky, A. D. (1968), "Electron Microscopic Studies of the Myometrium of the Guinea Pig," *Amer. J. Obstet. Gynec.*, **100**, 30.

Drost, M. and Holm, L. W. (1968), "Prolonged Gestation in Ewes after Foetal Adrenalectomy," *J. Endocr.*, **40**, 293.

DuBois Reymond, E. (1849), "Untersuchungen uber thierische Elektrizität," cited by Huiskes, J. A. J. in *Slow Potentials of the Human Uterus*, p. 13. Central Drukkerij N. V., Nijmegen, 1966.

Ellis, S. T., Beck, J. S. and Currie, A. R. (1966), "The Cellular Localisation of Growth Hormone in the Human Foetal Adenohypophysis," *J. Path. Bact.*, **92**, 179.

Elstein, M. and Pollard, A. C. (1968), "Proteins of Cervical Mucus," *Nature*, **219**, 612.

Friedman, E. A. (1955), "Primigravid Labour: Graphicostatistical Analysis," *Obstet. Gynec.*, **6**, 567.

Fuchs, A. R. and Wagner, G. (1963), "Effect of Alcohol on Release of Oxytocin," *Nature (London)*, **198**, 92.

Fuchs, F. (1965), "Clinical Considerations on the Use of Progestational Hormones in Pregnancy," in Martini, L. and Pecile, A. (Eds.) *Hormonal Steroids*, Vol. 2, p. 273. Academic Press, New York.

Fuchs, F., Fuchs, A. R., Poblete, V. F. and Risk, A. (1967), "Effect of Alcohol on Threatened Premature Labour," *Amer. J. Obstet. Gynec.*, **99**, 627.

Gompel, C. (1962), "The Ultrastructure of the Human Endometrial Cell Studied by Electron Microscopy," *Amer. J. Obstet. Gynec.*, **84**, 100.

Hendricks, C. H. (1964), "A New Technique for the Study of Motility in a Non-pregnant Human Uterus," *J. Obstet. Gynaec. Brit. Com.*, **71**, 712.

Hendricks, C. H. (1966), "Inherent Motility Patterns and Response

Characteristics of the Non-pregnant Human Uterus," *Amer. J. Obstet. Gynec.*, **96**, 824.

Hughes, E. C., Jacobs, R. D., Rubulis, A. and Husney, R. M. (1963), "Carbohydrate Pathways of the Endometrium," *Amer. J. Obstet. Gynec.*, **85**, 594.

Huiskes, J. A. J. (1966), "Slow Potentials of the Human Uterus. An Electrohysterography Study," *Proefschrift*. Centrale Drukkerij. N. V. Nijmegen, p. 115, 153, 134, 135.

Jung, H. (1956), "Über die Beziehung der Aktionspotentiale des Uterus zur Mechanishen Leistung," *Pflügers Arch. ges. Physiol.*, **263**, 419.

Jung, H. (1958), "Über die Electrophysiologie der Uterusmuskulatur," *Fortschr. Geburts. u. Gynäk.*, **7**, 4.

Jung, H. (1965), "Zur Physiologie und Klinik der hormonalen Uterusregulation," *Bibl. Gynaec.*, **33**. S. Karger (edit.) Basel.

Kao, C. Y. (1959), "Long-term Observation of Spontaneous Electrical Activity of the Uterine Smooth Muscle," *Amer. J. Physiol.*, **196**, 343.

Kao, C. Y. and Nishiyama, A. (1964), "Ovarian Hormones and Resting Potential of Rabbit Uterine Smooth Muscle," *Amer. J. Physiol.*, **207**, 793.

Klopper, A. and Billewicz, W. (1963), "Urinary Excretion of Oestriol and Pregnanediol during Normal Pregnancy," *J. Obstet. Gynaec. Brit. Com.*, **70**, 1024.

Kloosterman, G. J. (1959), "Een langdurige baring," *Ned. T. Geneesk.*, **103**, 2409.

Kloosterman, G. J. (1965), "Hoe lang groeit de menseligke placenta?" *Ned. T. Verlosk.*, **60**, 202.

Kraus, H. H. (1929), "Eine neue Methode zur Bestimmung des Ovulationstermines," *Zbl. Gynäk.*, **53**, 2193.

Kremer, J. (1965), "A Simple Sperm Penetration Test," *Int. J. Fertil.*, **10**, 209.

Kumar, D., Wagatsuma, T., Sullivan, W. J. and Barnes, A. C. (1964), "Studies on the Mechanism of Action of Progesterone on the Human Myometrium. II. *In vitro* Hyperpolarizing Effect of Progesterone on Human Myometrium," *Amer. J. Obstet. Gynec.*, **90**, 1355.

Kuriyama, H. and Csapo, A. (1961), "A Study of the Parturient Uterus with the Microelectrode Technique," *Endocrinology*, **68**, 1010.

Landesman, R., Wilson, K. and Zlatnik, F. J. (1966), "The Myometrial Relaxant Properties of Isoxsuprine and 2 Methanesulfonamido Derivatives," *Obstet. Gynec.*, **28**, 775.

Landesman, R. and Wilson, K. H. (1968), "The Relaxant Effect of Diazoxide on Isolated Gravid and Non-gravid Human Myometrium," *Amer. J. Obstet. Gynec.*, **101**, 120.

Larks, S. D. (1960), *Electrohysterography*. Charles Thomas (edit.) Springfield U.S.A., 1960.

Levy-Solal, E., Morin, P., Zacouto, F. (1952), "Analyse obstetricale des potentiels d'action de l'uterus eu travail (electrouterographie)," *Presse Medicale*, **63**, 60.

Liesse, A. (1947), "A propos de la technique d'enregistrement de l'activite electrique spontanee de l'uterus chez la femme," *Gynéc. et Obstét.*, **46**, 239.

Liggins, G. C., Holm, L. W., Kennedy, P. C. (1966), "Prolonged Pregnancy following Surgical Lesion of the Foetal Lamb Pituitary," *J. Reprod. Fertil.*, **12**, 419.

Mannor, S. M., Zakut, H., Serr, D. M. (1968), "Recording of Electrical Activity of the Human Uterus in the Presence of Intra-uterine Contraceptive Device." The VI International World Congress of Fertility and Sterility, June 1968 (Abstract).

Marcus, C. C. and Marcus, S. L. (1965), "The Cervical Factor in Infertility," *Clin. Obstet. Gynec.*, **8**, 15.

Mark, J. S. T. (1956), "An Electron Microscope Study of Uterine Smooth Muscle," *Anat. Rec.*, **125**, 473.

Marshall, J. M. (1959), "Effects of Estrogen and Progesterone on Single Muscle Fibres in the Rat," *Amer. J. Physiol.*, **197**, 935.

Masters, W. H. and Johnson, V. E. (1966), *Human Sexual Response*. Little, Brown and Company, Boston.

Müller, H. A. (1958). "Erfahrungen mit der elektrischen Wehendruckmessung bei Geburtseinleitungen," *Bibl. Gynaec.*, **17**, 59.

Noyes, R. W. (1966), "Endometrial Dating for the Detection of Ovulation," in *Ovulation*. Ed. by Greenblatt, R. B. J. B. Lippincott Co., Philadelphia, p. 319.

Peterson, M. and Leblond, C. P. (1964), "Synthesis of Complex Carbohydrate in the Golgi Region as shown by Radioautography after Injection of Labelled Glucose," *J. Cell Biology*, **21**, 143.

Pinto, R. M., Votta, R. A., Montuori, E. and Baleiron, H. (1964), "Action of Estradiol 17-beta on the Activity of the Pregnant Human Uterus," *Amer. J. Obstet. Gynec.*, **88**, 759.

Portes, L. Mayer, M., Granjon, A. and Bommelaer, M. (1964), "A propos de la technique de l'avortement therapeutique," *Gynéc. et Obstét.*, **47**, 185.

Rabau, E. David, A., Insler, V., and Lunenfeld, B. (1965), "New Aspects in the Treatment of Chiari-Frommel and Sheehan Syndromes," *Clinica Europea, Suppl.*, 5, **4**, 101.

Rawlings, W. J., Krieger, V. I. (1959), "The Value of the Pregnanediol Excretion Test in the Prognosis of Abortion," *J. Obstet. Gynaec. Brit. Emp.*, **66**, 905.

Reynolds, S. R. M. (1965), *Physiology of the Uterus*. Hafner Publishing Company, New York, 1965.

Reynolds, S. R. M., Harris, J. S. and Kaiser, I. H. (1954), *Clinical Measurement of Uterine Forces in Pregnancy and Labour*. Charles Thomas (edit.) Springfield, U.S.A.

Reynolds, S. R. M., Heard, O. O., Bruns, P. and Hellman, L. M. (1948), "A Multichannel Strain Gauge Tokodynamometer; an Instrument for Studying the Patterns of Uterine Contraction in Pregnant Women," *Bull. Johns Hopk. Hosp.*, **82**, 446.

Schofield, B. M. (1963), "The Local Effect of the Placenta on Myometrial Activity in the Rabbit," *J. of Physiol. (Lond.)*, **166**, 191.

Serr, D. M., Porath, A., Rabau, E., Zakut, H., Mannor, S. M. (1968), "Recording of Electrical Activity from the Human Cervix," *J. Obstet. Gynaec. Brit. Com.*, **75**, 360.

Serr, D. M., Zakut, H. and Mannor, S. M. (1969), "Effects upon Mother and Fetus of Intravenous Alcohol in Premature Labour," In press.

Shabanah, E. H., Toth, A., Carassavas, D. and Maughan, G. B. (1968a), "The Role of the Autonomic Nervous System in Uterine Contractility and Blood Flow. IV. Interrelationship of Progesterone and Certain Catecholamines in the Control of Myometrial Function," *Amer. J. Obstet. Gynec.*, **100**, 974.

Shabanah, E. H., Toth, A., Omay, Y. and Maughan, G. B. (1968b), "The Role of Autonomic Nervous System in Uterine Contractility and Blood Flow. V. Interrelationship of Estrogen, Progesterone and the Pituitary Trophic Hormones in the Control of Myometrial Function," *Amer. J. Obstet. Gynec.*, **100**, 981.

Shearman, R. P. and Garrett, W. J. (1963), "Double Blind Study of Effect of 17-hydroxyprogesterone Caproate on Abortion Rate," *Brit. med. J.*, **2**, 292.

Smyth, C. N. (1957), "The Guard-ring Tocodynamometer," *J. Obstet. Gynaec. Brit. Emp.*, **64**, 59.

Smyth, C. N. (1958), "The Concept of Uterine Irritability and its Clinical Application Exemplified by the Oxytocin Sensitivity Test," *Bibl. Gynaec.*, **7**, 71.

Steer, C. M. (1954), "The Electrical Activity of the Human Uterus in Normal and Abnormal Labour," *Amer. J. Obstet. Gynec.*, **68**, 867.

Stieve, H. (1929), "Das Mesenchym in der Wand der menschlichen Gebermutter," *Zbl. Gynäk.*, **53**, 2706.

Soureau, C. (1955), "Étude de l'activité électrique de l'utérus au cours de la gestation et du travail," *Thése*. Foulon edit. Paris. 19.

Sureau, C., Chavinie, J. and Cannon, M. (1965), "L'electrophysiologie uterine," *Bull. Féd. Gynec. et d'Obstet.*, **17**, 79.

Turnbull, A. and Anderson, B. M. (1968), "Uterine Contractility and Oxytocin Sensitivity during Human Pregnancy in Relation to the Onset of Labour," *J. Obstet. Gynaec. Brit. Com.*, **75**, 278.

Wagner, G. (1965), "Correlation between External and Internal Methods of Recording Uterine Contractions in the Second Trimester of Pregnancy," *J. Obstet. Gynaec. Brit. Com.*, **72**, 976.

Zakut, H., Mannor, S. M. and Serr, D. M. (1969), "Effect of Promethazine on Uterine Contractions," In press.

Zondek, B. (1957). *Cervical Mucus Arborization as an aid in Diagnosis in Progress in Gynecology*. Eds. Meigs and Sturgis, Grune and Stratton, New York, London, p. 86.

3. THE TUBE

L. MASTROIANNI

The fallopian tube (oviduct) is a vital structure interposed between the ovary and the uterus. Its functions may be divided into two broad categories: transport of ova and spermatozoa and provision of a favorable environment for the gametes, for the fertilization process and for the fertilized ovum during early development. Each normally implanted pregnancy is preceded by successful transfer of the ovum from the ovulating follicle into the oviduct and delivery of the fertilized ovum to the uterus after a measured three day interval. Contiguity of the reproductive tract, allowing unobstructed passage of gametes, is a requisite to fertility, but does not in itself insure normal reproductive function at the tubal level. The ability of the tube to create an intraluminal milieu favorable to the proper function and survival of spermatozoa and ova is equally important. Conditions appropriate for the fertilization process and for the development of the ovum through many cell divisions must be maintained.

At this point, we depend heavily upon animal experimentation for much of our understanding of oviductal function. The rabbit, and more recently the subhuman primate, have been favored experimental models for the study of tubal physiology. Both species are endowed with relatively large tubes, and ova, spermatozoa and tubal secretions can be recovered with relative ease. In each the tube has anatomical features reminiscent of those seen in the human. It is equally clear that there are species differences, and data obtained from species other than human must be interpreted with caution. The remarks that follow are, in the main, general observations, interspersed, when possible, with factual information on the human species. References have not been cited for all the various experimental observations alluded to in the text. Those who wish to explore the experimental facets in depth are referred to some of the recent detailed works on the mammalian oviduct (Hafez and Blandau, 1968).

Gross Anatomical Considerations

In general, the mammalian oviduct may be divided into anatomically discrete segments. Its ovarian end, in several species including man, terminates in delicately arranged fronds, the fimbria. These cilia-lined muscular elements are thought to play a major role in the mechanisms of ovum pick-up. They surround the tubal ostium, and this portion of the oviduct constitutes the infundibulum. At a point beyond the ostium, the ampulla, the widest portion of the oviduct, is seen. This occupies the largest linear segment of the tube, and in the human, ends in a gradual narrowing, the tubal isthmus. In the human species the line of demarcation between ampulla and isthmus is not as distinct as it is in the rabbit. In the latter the isthmo-ampullary junction is clearly delineated and plays an important role in the transport of ova In the

human the very narrow isthmus enters the uterus, and the intrauterine portion of the oviduct measures at least 0·5 cm. At this point the lumen is often tortuous.

The tubal mucosa is composed of both ciliated and secretory cells and is surrounded by three discrete layers of musculature. There is a subperitoneal layer which runs a longitudinal course along the tube, a middle or vascular layer whose fibers parallel the vessels encircling the tube, and an inner layer whose fibers are arranged in spirals which originate from different directions and intersect at regular intervals.

The muscular arrangement at the fimbriated extremity has been carefully evaluated (Stange, 1952). Fibers of the subperitoneal layer continue out along the fimbria. They extend further at the upper and lower tubal edge than on either side, creating a fork-like enclosure. At the neck of the infundibulum these fibers are met by and anchored to fibers of the subperitoneal blood vessels. The inner muscular layer ends at the infundibulum where its fibers intertwine with the circular fibres of the vascular layer. The base of the infundibulum is well vascularized. Here the powerful vascular musculature, by a complicated regrouping of its fibers, forms what has been interpreted as a functional sphincter. At one point the fimbria extends longitudinally on to the surface of the ovary to which it is anchored (Fig. 1). This portion of fimbria, the fimbria ovarica, may have important functional significance. A separate muscle bundle runs on a longitudinal course along the fimbria ovarica from the tubal ostium to one ovarian pole. This has been referred to as the tubal attracting muscle or m. tubae attrahens. It originates from the interlacing muscle bundles of the vascular layer and the parallel fibers of the subperitoneal musculature and terminates at the cranial pole of the ovary. Muscular elements, separate from the tube, may also have functional significance. It has been suggested that at the time of ovulation muscles in the paraovarium contract, lifting the ovary toward the tubal ostium. At the same time the m. tubæ attrahens contracts, bringing the fimbriated end of the tube down on the ovary.

These anatomical observations have provided a basis for the earlier observations of Axel Westman whose name is almost as intimately associated with the oviduct as that of Fallopius himself. Westman (1928) viewed the muscular movements of the oviduct during ovulation via an abdominal window in the rabbit and by means of a laparoscope in the monkey. In both species the fimbria actually embraces the ovary during ovulation. In the rabbit the movement of the fimbriated end of the oviduct is dramatic. Recently, this has been documented with cinematography. The fimbria actually moves to and fro over the surface of the ovary and in that way ovum pick-up is practically assured.

The relationship between fimbria and ovary at ovulation

4

time in man has not as yet been satisfactorily assessed. Some observations have been carried out by Decker through the culdoscope, an instrument which permits visualization of the adnexal structures as the patient is in the knee-chest position. A repositioning of the fimbria as well as shortening of the utero-ovarian ligament was observed. Both ovary and fimbria were drawn closer to the uterus into a fossa on the posterior aspect of the broad ligament. Westman suggested that ovum pick-up is assisted by a tubal suction mechanism, a sort of vacuum cleaner action created by a current of fluid within the tube. There is good evidence for such a current in the human.

they are best compared with a carpet sweeper. As they move to and fro over the rupturing follicle the fimbria with their cilia insure transfer of ova into the oviduct.

In the human, although the exact mechanism of ovum pick-up is not thoroughly documented, there is reasonable indirect evidence that the fimbria plays an important role. When it is diseased, when the tubal ostium is partially occluded, or when fimbrial-ovarian relationships are modified by adhesions, there is impaired fertility. On the other hand, pregnancies have been observed in patients with but one oviduct on one side and one ovary on the other. In these circumstances the fimbria is obviously not

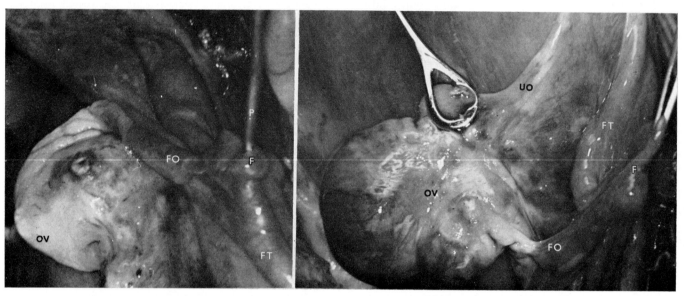

Fig. 1. Normal human adnexa, showing ovary (OV), fallopian tube (FT), fimbria (F), and fimbria ovarica (FO). *Left:* Probe (P) in the ostium. *Right:* Clamp on utero-ovarian ligament (UO) and forceps on fimbria expose fimbria ovarica (FO).

Dye and foreign particles may be recovered at the cervix some hours after they have been placed in the cul-de-sac. A current of fluid coursing along the tubal lumen is not essential to ovum pick-up in the rabbit. In that species transfer of ova is not impaired when the oviduct is occluded by a ligature at the base of the fimbria (Clewe and Mastroianni, 1958). The fimbria itself is capable of ovum pick-up and the cilia lining the fimbria play an important role. When the fimbria is separated surgically from the site of ovulation, ova remain adherent to the surface of the ovary after release from their follicles, unless they are swept away by the mechanical action of the tube. Blandau has demonstrated with cinematography that spheres of inert material the same size as rabbit ova are not efficiently transported by the fimbriated end of the tube (Blandau, 1968). Ova, on the other hand, with their entourage of sticky cumulus cells are, in fact, transported efficiently. The cumulus cells are apparently responsible for the remarkable ability of the cilia to direct the ova toward the tubal ostium. Various observations in the rabbit have prompted Clewe to suggest that the fimbriae do not work as a vacuum cleaner which would suck an egg into the tubal lumen; nor do they resemble a hand which would grasp an egg as it is released from the follicle:

brought into juxtaposition to the rupturing follicle, and a secondary mechanism, possibly involving tubal suction, may be responsible for the ultimate delivery of the ovum. A means by which physiological observations of the action of the fimbria may be carried out in the human is not yet available. The mechanism behind the change in relationship between fimbria and ovary at ovulation is still unclear. We do not know what it is which triggers the vigorous muscular action of the fimbria, resulting ultimately in the delivery of ova into the tubal ostium. The biological events associated with ovum pick-up do not seem to have a parallel in other systems, and the remarkable efficiency with which the oviduct carries out its function as the ovum is released has only recently fired the imagination of those interested in regulatory mechanisms.

Ovum Transport within the Tube

Once ova are within the oviductal lumen they are transported rapidly to a point well within the ampullary portion. This occurs in a matter of minutes in the rabbit. Ova are transported by muscular as well as ciliary action. There is an increase in the rate of ciliary action at the time of ovulation, with the direction of movement toward the uterus. Intraluminal transport of ova has not as yet been studied in humans. The rate of transport of eggs and the influence of various hormonal agents on the rate has been explored extensively in the rabbit. Recently, the use of rabbit ova stained with a vital dye has facilitated evaluation of ovum transport (Harper, 1966). The rate of movement is indeed influenced by estrogen-progesterone balance.

Retention of Ova within the Oviduct

In most mammalian species fertilization occurs in the oviduct and the fertilized ovum is retained there for approximately three days before it is delivered to the uterus. This three day residence in the tube appears to be essential to normal implantation in some species. Chang (1950), in a classical set of experiments, has evaluated the influence of the residence within the fallopian tube in the rabbit. If the ova are transferred from the tube into the uterus one day after fertilization they do not implant. If they are transferred two days after fertilization they may or may not implant. If transfer is carried out after three days, at approximately the time when they would ordinarily be delivered to the uterus anyway, the majority implant. In the rabbit, then, the timing of tubal transfer is important in the economy of reproduction and modifications in timing result in reproductive failure. There is presumptive evidence that the ovum is retained in the human fallopian tube for approximately three days but conclusive experiments to bear this out have not as yet been performed. Although ovum recovery in the human is possible, the presently available means of ovulation timing do not allow even retrospective assessment of the duration of residence in the tube when ova have been recovered.

In the rabbit the basis for retention of ova following fertilization has been established. There is a physiologic closure of the whole isthmus, and ova are retained within the ampullary portion of the tube near the ampulloisthmic junction. This closure is brought about, at least in part, by edema and can be reproduced by administration of high doses of estrogen. The mechanism behind the timing of the closure and the opening of the isthmus has not as yet been elucidated. The duration of the closure in that species has been worked out and occupies an interval of approximately 96 hours.

In the human a different mechanism is probably responsible for the delay in transfer of the fertilized ovum. There is no clear cut evidence for a physiologic closure at the isthmus or the utero-tubal junction. In fact, carbon dioxide and radio-opaque material may be passed from the uterus to the tube at any time in the cycle. Definitive experiments to evaluate the ability of the isthmic portion of the tube to accommodate ova or foreign particles as they are passed in the direction of the uterus have not been carried out. The muscular arrangement as the tube enters the uterus is of some interest (Vasen, 1959). The subperitoneal musculature of the uterus is arranged in a loop around the intramural portion of the tube, as it enters the uterus. There are, in addition, one or two vascular rings within the intramural portion of the tube itself. These are accompanied by muscle bundles. The inner layer of musculature is arranged in spirals which encircle the intramural portion of the tube. All of these layers, separately or in combination, would be capable of constricting the tubal lumen at the uterotubal junction. As yet there is no evidence in favor of a sustained contraction of this musculature during the three day interval following ovulation. The muscular arrangement is, however, of clinical importance in that spasm occasionally results in an incorrect diagnosis of anatomical closure in infertility patients. When closure at the utero-tubal junction is suspected one cannot do enough to confirm this fact before proceeding to operative measures to re-establish patency. It is clear that we do not as yet understand the mechanism responsible for ovum retention in the primate. This area of investigation is of tremendous importance. There is a possibility that one might modify the events surrounding tubal transport of ova when the physiology of the region is better understood.

Cyclic Modifications in Tubal Epithelia

The three day residence of the fertilized ovum within the fallopian tube is a subject of continuing speculation. Is the delay in transit at the tubal level designed merely to allow the ovum to mature before it is ready for implantation, or does it serve yet another more subtle purpose? It is obvious, in any case, that the tube is responsible for the provision of the environment in which early development occurs.

Early attention was given to the cyclic variations in the structure of the human tubal epithelium. The changes in tubal epithelium were emphasized as early as 1928 by Novak and Everett. They described an increasing height of the epithelium in the proliferative phase of the menstrual cycle. Premenstrually, the ciliated cells become lower and the secretory cells project beyond them. They observed the presence of cilia though the cycle and did not subscribe to the theory proposed by earlier workers that ciliated cells are replaced by secretory cells. More recently, the changes in tubal epithelium have been studied by more sophisticated approaches. Fredricsson (1959), using histochemical techniques, has confirmed the variations in cellular height described by earlier workers and has noted an increase in interluminal secretions at ovulation. Secretory development was most pronounced in the mid-luteal phase of the cycle. PAS reactive material was demonstrated throughout the cycle. This was diastase digestible and was thought to represent glycogen. Early in the cycle this material was noted in the supranuclear and infranuclear areas of the ciliated cells. The supranuclear material disappeared in the early luteal phase. Its disappearance coincided with the increased ciliary activity observed following ovulation. In the midluteal phase of the cycle large amounts of PAS-reactive, diastase-resistant material were seen in the tubal lumen.

Recent ultrastructural studies of human tubal epithelium also emphasize the changes which occur during the menstrual cycle. The histochemical and ultrastructural studies of the tubes of various species confirm the fact that modifications in morphology are brought out under endocrine influence. The actual contents of the tubal secretions in the human remain to be explored.

Tubal Secretions

As early as 1891 Woskressensky postulated the presence of an active secretion in the rabbit oviduct. He noted an accumulation of a clear fluid in oviducts ligated at both ends. Conclusive proof of an active secretory process within the rabbit oviduct was provided by D. W. Bishop (1956). He observed that the tubal fluid could be produced against a pressure gradient. Administration of pilocarpine increases the secretion pressure. When the rabbit oviduct is ligated at both ends the rate of fluid accumulation within it is greatest in the estrous animal, less in the pregnant animal and least in the ovariectomized animal.

Using a method for continuous collection of oviduct secretion in the rabbit, the influence of changing hormonal conditions has been studied (Mastroianni et al., 1961). The secretory rate decreases following castration but can be increased to precastration levels by the administration of exogenous estrogens. In intact animals and estrogen-primed castrates the rate decreases following progesterone administration.

The changes in the secretions are physiologically significant only during the first three days of pregnancy. During that interval the secretory rate diminishes to about one-half of the estrous rate (Mastroianni and Wallach, 1961). Lactate and pyruvate levels, which are high in tubal fluid, increase significantly. These substrates may act as nutriments during the early growth phases of the fertilized ovum. The mouse ovum for example, will not develop satisfactorily in vitro in the absence of lactate and pyruvate. It is possible that the high concentrations of these substrates occur as a result of the rather unique metabolic properties of the oviduct itself. Both human and rabbit oviducts in in vitro studies show a preference for the anærobic route of metabolism, and when incubated ærobically with glucose, produce large quantities of lactate. It is likely that the lactate is transferred into the tubal fluid. In his in vitro studies of the mouse ovum Brinster (1967) has found that the ratio between lactate and pyruvate is critical in early development. It is possible that lactate and pyruvate may be among the essential ingredients of tubal fluid which support early development.

Influence of the Tubal Environment on Gametes

Upon ovulation, the ovum is surrounded by a mass of cells, the cumulous oophorus (Fig. 2). When freshly ovulated rabbit ova are exposed to spermatozoa in vitro there is a rapid disintegration of the cumulus mass and a densely packed inner layer of cells, the corona radiata, remains. Some of the early observations of the relationship between the cumulus cells and the ovum were carried out by Swyer (1948). He observed rapid denudation of rabbit ova to the level of the corona radiata when they were placed in a solution of washed rabbit spermatozoa or in the supernatant from diluted, centrifuged semen, with or without spermatozoa. Continued in vitro exposure for as long as 30 hours failed to produce dispersion of the corona radiata itself. The enzyme, hyaluronidase, caused denudation of the cumulus cells in about 10 minutes, but the corona radiata remained intact. Swyer placed ova, denuded to the level of corona radiata, into the oviducts

of estrous rabbits. Untreated ova were placed in the opposite oviducts. The latter were still unchanged at the end of three hours. The previously treated ova were completely denuded. It would appear that in the rabbit complete dispersion of the corona radiata is brought about by some

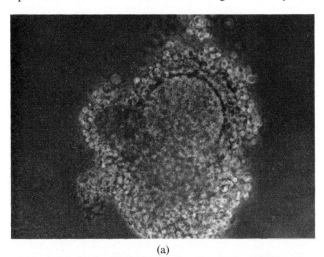

(a)

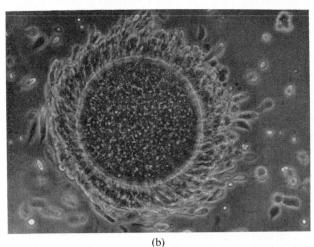

(b)

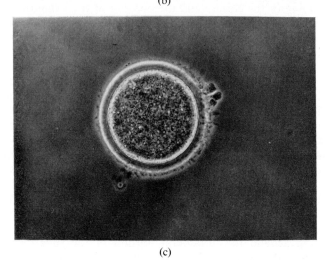

(c)

FIG. 2. (a) Recently ovulated rabbit ovum surrounded by cumulus cells. (b) Hyaluronidase-treated ovum with corona radiata intact. (c) Ovum after exposure to tubal fluid for 2 hours in vitro. Note that the corona cells have been dispersed.

influence within the tube itself. The influence of tubal fluid on the corona radiata cells has recently been assessed further. It is clear that there is a specific property of tubal fluid which brings about a separation of the corona cells from the zona pellucida. The relationship between the corona radiata cells and the zona pellucida changes under the influence of tubal fluid. The pseudopods of the corona cells which normally extend into the zona are withdrawn. Possibly this change precedes fertilization, although macroscopically the corona cells are still seen surrounding

of exposure to the female reproductive tract is a requisite to fertilization. The process through which spermatozoa acquire the ability to fertilize is referred to as capacitation. This phenomenon has been demonstrated in the rabbit, rat, and hamster, and probably occurs also in cattle and sheep. No evidence for or against the occurrence of capacitation has been gathered in man. Although experiments have been carried out which suggest that it is possible to produce capacitation *in vitro*, a definite reproducible system for this has not been developed.

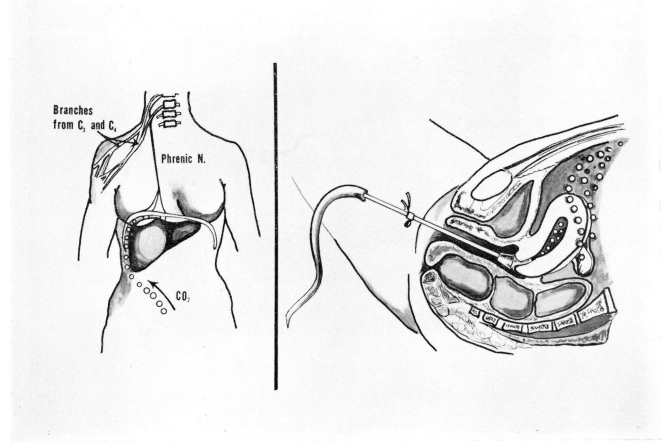

FIG. 3. Schematic illustration of technique for utero-tubal insufflation. If CO_2 is delivered to the peritoneal cavity it causes referred shoulder pain via phrenic nerve when patient assumes the upright position.

the egg shortly after fertilization. Corona cell dispersion is brought about by a non-specific property of tubal fluid which recently has been established as the bicarbonate ion (Stambaugh *et al.*, 1968). Rabbit tubal fluid is rich in bicarbonate, the result of a substantial carbonic anhydrase activity in the epithelium. Corona-zona relationships have not as yet been evaluated in any primate species including man. The availability of techniques for collecting tubal fluid under refrigeration in the monkey has now made it possible to explore its importance in reproductive economy.

In several species tubal secretions have a definite effect on spermatozoa. Following coitus, spermatozoa normally await the arrival of ova in the fallopian tube and an interval

Evaluation of Tubal Function

Clinical techniques for assessing tubal function are directed solely at evaluating the anatomical integrity of the fallopian tube. Methods are not as yet available to evaluate the two dynamic functions of the tube: transport of gametes and secretion. Our efforts are confined to a consideration of tubal patency and of the structural integrity of the periadnexal area, including the fimbria.

In the management of the infertility patient, anatomical abnormalities of the tubes receive concentrated diagnostic attention. Reproductive function is obviously impaired when bilateral tubal occlusion exists. Peritubal adhesions which distort the relationship between the ovary and the fimbria may also cause infertility by interfering with the mechanisms of ovum pick-up. Tubal obstruction or peritubal adhesions usually result from infections or irritative processes in or adjacent to the fallopian tubes. Occlusion can be caused by both salpingitis and peritubal disease. Infections commonly involving the tube include gonorrhea, puerperal sepsis and pelvic tuberculosis. Adhesions may be the result of extra-tubal disease. A ruptured appendix, especially if it has occurred in childhood when the appendix and adnexa are close to one another, diverticulitis, prior pelvic surgery and endometriosis may cause a distortion of pelvic relationships.

actual escape through the tube. Shoulder pain may occur if gas has passed through one tube but not the other. Thus, the presence of shoulder pain indicates only that one tube, but not necessarily both, is patent. Utero-tubal insufflation is useful as a screening procedure, but if infertility persists the tubes should be evaluated further by a means which allows a more detailed evaluation of tubal anatomy. An approach which is frequently used is hysterosalpingography (Fig. 4). Radiopaque material is introduced into the uterus, and its spillage from the fallopian tubes is evaluated radiographically. The test should always be

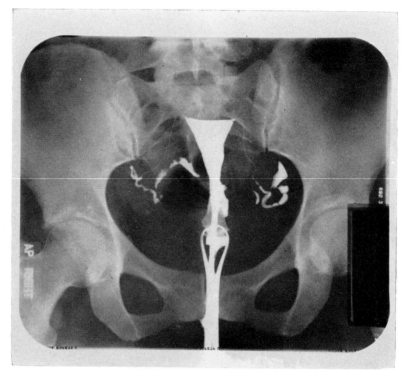

Fig. 4. Normal hysterosalpingogram with bilateral tubal patency.

A simple and therefore popular method of checking for tubal patency is utero-tubal insufflation, or the test of Rubin. It is performed in the office, without anesthesia or elaborate equipment. A cannula is placed at the cervix (Fig. 3), and carbon dioxide is delivered along the uterus and tubes into the peritoneal cavity. Any one of a number of commercially available insufflating apparatuses may be used for the delivery of the carbon dioxide. Carbon dioxide is the gas of choice, and air should never be used because of the danger of air embolism. If there is tubal patency, the carbon dioxide usually passes at a pressure under 100 millimeters of mercury. Immediately following insufflation, the instruments are removed and the patient is instructed to sit up. When carbon dioxide has traversed the tubes and is in the peritoneal cavity, it rises to the under surface of the diaphragm and causes shoulder pain, mediated by the phrenic nerve. Shoulder pain is absolutely necessary for the diagnosis of tubal patency, regardless of the pressure at which the gas has apparently passed. Gas may fill a dilated closed tube at a constant rate of pressure, causing distension without

performed in the preovulatory phase of the menstrual cycle, at a time when there is no risk of exposing an early pregnancy to radiation. The use of fluoroscopy, with an image intensifier, is helpful but not essential in the performance of this test.

The most effective means of exploring the relationship between the fimbriated end of the tube and the ovary is through direct visualization (Decker, 1967). For this, culdoscopy is employed. With the patient in the knee-chest position, a telescope similar to a cystoscope is introduced through the posterior vaginal fornix (Fig. 5). Ordinarily, complete visualization of the adnexal structures is possible. The presence or absence of adhesions or anatomical defects in that area can be evaluated directly. At the same time, dye may be introduced into the uterus, and its spillage from the tubes into the peritoneal cavity observed. There is an increasing trend to proceed directly to culdoscopy to evaluate the infertile patient, and more and more this procedure is being used as a substitute for either utero-tubal insufflation or hysterosalpingography. Culdoscopy should certainly be carried out on any patient with inexplicable infertility. Perviously unsuspected anatomical deficiencies are often recognized.

The management of anatomical abnormalities of the adnexa is surgical. Patients with peritubal adhesions whose tubes are patent can be offered a reasonably good prognosis. When there is tubal occlusion, the prognosis is considerably less favourable. The success rate is greater when the surgeon who approaches the tube has a clear idea of the functional importance of the structure under consideration. It goes without saying that the fimbria deserves special attention. Recently, a plastic prosthesis

Chang, M. C. (1950), "Development and Fate of Transferred Rabbit Ova or Blastocysts in Relation to the Ovulation Time of Recipients," *J. exp. Zool.*, **114**, 197.

Clewe, T. H., unpublished observations.

Clewe, T. H. and Mastroianni, L., Jr. (1958), "Mechanisms of Ovum Pick-up: I. Functional Capacity of Rabbit Oviducts Ligated near the Fimbria," *Fert. and Ster.*, **9**, 13.

Decker, A. (1967), *Culdoscopy*. Philadelphia: F. A. Davis.

Fredricsson, B. (1959), "Histochemical Observations on the Epithelium of the Human Fallopian Tubes," *Acta obstet. gynec. scand.*, **38**, 109.

Hafez, E. S. E. and Blandau, R. (1968), *The Mammalian Oviduct*, University of Chicago Press (in press).

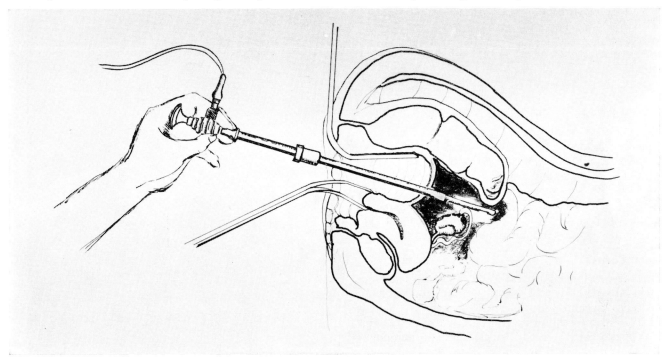

FIG. 5. Schematic representation of culdoscopy technique. Culdoscope is introduced through the posterior fornix with patient in the knee-chest position.

has been used when the tube is occluded at the distal extremity, to protect any fimbria which has been salvaged. This is left in place until the healing process is complete and then removed at the time of the second laparotomy.

On the basis of present evidence, we are justified in viewing the oviduct as more than a transporting passage for ova and sperm. The regulatory mechanisms concerned in the three-day retention of the ovum within the oviduct and the environment provided by the oviduct for the zygote during this interval are worthy subjects for continued investigation. At the clinical level our efforts are still directed at the detection of anatomical abnormalities and at their correction.

REFERENCES

Bishop, D. W. (1956), "Active Secretion in the Rabbit Oviduct," *Amer. J. Physiol.*, **187**, 347.

Blandau, R. (1968), "Gamete Transport—Comparative Aspects" in *The Mammalian Oviduct*, ed. Hafez, E. S. E. and Blandau, R. Univ. of Chicago Press (in press).

Brinster, R. L. (1968), "Mammalian Embryo Culture" in *The Mammalian Oviduct*, ed. Hafez, E. S. E. and Blandau, R. Univ. of Chicago Press (in press).

Harper, M. J. K. (1966), "Hormonal Control of Transport of Eggs in Cumulus through the Ampulla of the Rabbit Oviduct," *Endocrinology*, **78**, 568.

Mastroianni, L. Jr., Beer, F., Shah, U. and Clewe, T. H. (1961), "Endocrine Regulation of Oviduct Secretions in the Rabbit," *Endocrinology*, **68**, 92.

Mastroianni, L. Jr. and Wallach, R. C. (1961), "Effect of Ovulation and Early Gestation on Oviduct Secretions of the Rabbit," *Amer. J. Physiol.*, **200**, 815.

Novak, E. and Everett, H. S. (1928), "Cyclical and Other Variations in the Tubal Epithelium," *Amer. J. Obstet. Gynec.*, **16**, 499.

Stambaugh, R., Noriega, C. and Mastroianni, L. Jr. (1968), "Bicarbonate Ion; the Corona Cell Dispersing Factor in Tubal Fluid," *J. Reprod. Fertil.* (in press).

Swyer, G. I. M. (1947), "A Tubal Factor Concerned in Denudation of Rabbit Ova," *Nature*, **159**, 873.

Strange, H. H. (1952), "Zur Funktionellen Morphologie des fimbrienendes der menschlichen Tube und des Epoophoron," *Arch. Gynäk.*, **182**, 77.

Vasen, L. C. L. M. (1959), "The Intramural Part of the Fallopian Tube," *Int. J. Fert.*, **4**, 309.

Westman, A. (1926), "A Contribution to the Question of the Transit of the Ovum from Ovary to Uterus in Rabbits," *Acta obstet. gynec. scand.*, **5**, 7.

Woskressensky, M. A. (1891), "Experimentelle untersuchungen über die Pyo- und hydrosalpinxbildung bei den Thieren," *Zbl. Gynäk.*, **15**, 849.

4. PELVIC VISCERAL INNERVATION

C. P. WENDELL-SMITH

INNERVATION OF INTERNAL GENITALIA

The older work on the innervation of the uterus in particular was reviewed and supplemented by Davis (1933) and more recently by Krantz (1959). Attempts to produce a synthesis of the anatomical, physiological and pharmacological aspects of uterine innervation have been made by Reynolds (1949) and again more recently by Shabanah, Toth and Maughan (1964a). The following account aims to place these studies in more general perspective.

Central Control

The descending influences of the autonomic nervous system are derived primarily from the hypothalamus which has a controlling influence on centres of tonic activity. Other forebrain structures, including the cerebral cortex, basal ganglia and thalamus, affect the autonomic outflow by means of their connections with the hypothalamus (Shabanah, Toth and Maughan, 1965). Its output is conveyed by a diffuse multisynaptic descending pathway through the reticular formation to brainstem and spinal centres. In the reticular formation the descending pathway interacts with input from the viscera, with other ascending influences and with modulating feedbacks. In this way the sum of multitudinous influences is brought to bear on the brainstem and spinal centres.

Down to this stage the pathway is controlling and concerned with balancing the effects of the two peripheral autonomic divisions, the sympathetic and the parasympathetic nervous systems. The two systems should not be thought of as necessarily antagonistic. In many instances they are synergistic and work harmoniously under the control of the descending pathway to achieve a given effect. The brainstem and spinal centres project fibres beyond the central nervous system into the two divisions separately; they are thus executive and concerned with the activity of one or other peripheral division rather than both.

Sympathetic System

The sympathetic centres for the female reproductive system lie in the lower thoracic and upper lumbar segments of the spinal cord. They project preganglionic fibres via the ventral roots of the corresponding spinal nerves and their rami communicantes, through the ganglia of the sympathetic trunk (usually without synaptic interruption) and through the thoracic, lumbar and sacral splanchnic nerves to reach the autonomic plexuses where they finally synapse.

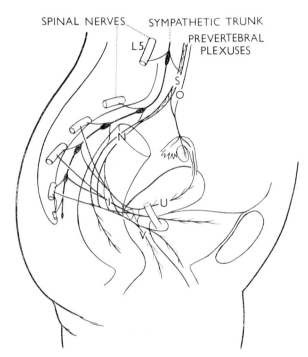

FIG. 1. A schema of pelvic visceral innervation, as though viewed from the right side after removal of the right hip bone. The spinal nerves, sympathetic trunk and prevertebral plexuses form parallel longitudinal arrays following the curve of the vertebral column; their connections and branches of distribution are highly stylized and are, in fact, much more diffuse. Note the continuity of the superior hypogastric plexus (S), the hypogastric nerve (N), the inferior hypogastric plexus (I) and the uterovaginal plexus (U, V). Note also the two routes for innervation of the uterine tube, from the ovarian plexus (0) and the upper part of the uterovaginal plexus (U) respectively.

These plexuses are the ovarian, the superior hypogastric, the inferior hypogastric and the uterovaginal. The ovarian plexus is an extension of the aorticorenal plexus along the ovarian artery; it also receives fibres from the hypogastric plexuses. The superior hypogastric plexus or presacral nerve is the continuation of the aorticorenal plexus down over the bifurcation of the aorta. It divides in front of the sacrum into two trunks, the right and left hypogastric nerves. In front of the lower sacrum each hypogastric nerve is joined by the pelvic splanchnic nerves (parasympathetic; nervi erigentes) of the corresponding side to form the right and left inferior hypogastric or pelvic (Frankenhauser's) plexuses.

The superior hypogastric plexus, the right and left hypogastric nerves and inferior hypogastric plexuses are embedded in a sheet of fascia, the presacral or Waldeyer's fascia, which lies between the fascia propria recti and the superior fascia of the pelvic diaphragm (Roberts, Habenicht and Krishingner, 1964). The inferior hypogastric plexuses and their extensions contain an admixture of sympathetic and parasympathetic elements. The uterovaginal plexus of each side is an extension of the inferior hypogastric plexus along the uterine artery; it also receives some postganglionic sympathetic fibres directly from the lower lumbar and sacral ganglia of the sympathetic trunks.

Postganglionic sympathetic fibres project from neurons in the ganglia of the plexuses or trunks, via the plexuses, to their endings in relation to the smooth muscle of the viscera and the smooth muscle of their vessels. The pharmacological events which follow the arrival of an impulse at postganglionic sympathetic nerve endings are complex and not completely understood. The uterus was one of the first organs for which it was demonstrated that sympathetic stimulation releases acetylcholine as well as adrenergic substances (Sherif, 1935). There is increasing evidence for the view of Burn (1967) that the release of acetylcholine is the first event in the sequence, making the membrane of the sympathetic fibre permeable to calcium ions. The calcium ions enter the fibre and release adrenergic transmitter substances from the bound form in which they are held. Furthermore adrenergic transmitters are not pure substances but are mixtures of adrenaline, noradrenaline (the major component), probably dopamine and possibly other compounds (Vane, 1962). The proportions and amounts of these depend upon the intensity of nervous activity and their synthesis, in the myometrium at least, is promoted by oestrogens (Vander-Pol, 1956). Catecholamines (mainly adrenaline) may, of course, also be released from the adrenal medulla and from chromaffin cells, examples of which are found in relation to the ganglionic neurons of the autonomic plexuses and in the ovary.

Catecholamines, whether released from sympathetic nerve endings or arriving via the blood, act on at least two types of receptor (Ahlquist, 1948). Alpha (α) receptors are most sensitive to adrenaline, least sensitive to the sympathomimetic isopr(opylnoradr)enaline and are blocked by ergot alkaloids and phenoxybenzamine. In most cases the effect of catecholamines on α-receptors is excitation (contraction). Beta (β) receptors are most sensitive to isoprenaline, least sensitive to noradrenaline and are blocked by propranolol. In most cases the effect of catecholamines on β-receptors is inhibition (relaxation).

Progesterone and, indirectly, gonadotrophins may influence the dominance of the excitatory or inhibitory effect on the myometrium. Gonadotrophic hormone of pituitary and possibly of chorionic origin is necessary to render the myometrium responsive to progesterone (Reynolds, 1949). A low level of progesterone activity, as in the nonpregnant state, tends to lower the threshold of the α-receptor and increase the excitory effect (Willems,

Bernard, Delaunois and de Schaepdryver, 1965), whereas a higher level, as in pregnancy, tends to lower the threshold of the β-receptors and increase the inhibitory effect (Shabanah, Toth, Carassavas and Maughan, 1968).

The high ratio of postganglionic to preganglionic fibres, the supplementation of the postganglionic transmitter substances by locally produced and blood-borne catecholamines and the slow deactivation of these compounds in the body, all contribute to the diffuseness and sustained action of the sympathetic nervous system.

Parasympathetic System

The parasympathetic centres for the female reproductive system probably lie only in the sacral segments of the spinal cord, but the possibility of the ovary being innervated via the vagal system cannot be excluded. The parasympathetic centres project preganglionic fibres via the ventral roots and ventral rami of the corresponding spinal nerves, the pelvic splanchnic nerves and the inferior hypogastric plexuses to synapse in ganglia in the uterovaginal and ovarian plexuses, near but probably not in the wall of the innervated organ. Postganglionic parasympathetic fibres are projected from the ganglia to their endings in relation to the smooth muscle of the viscera and the smooth muscle of their blood vessels.

The transmitter substance in the autonomic ganglia (sympathetic and parasympathetic) and at the postganglionic parasympathetic nerve endings is acetylcholine, a substance which affects cell membrane permeability and produces excitation. Acetylcholine is rapidly deactivated by locally occurring cholinesterases so that each discharge is localized and of short duration. However, not all acetylcholine is of nervous origin. Local non-nervous production has been demonstrated in the intestinal wall (Koelle, 1963), and the placenta, which is devoid of nerves, contains more acetylcholine than any other tissue (Chang and Gaddum, 1933). Acetylcholine from this source reaches the general circulation and at term may stimulate the neurosecretion of oxytocin by the hypothalamic nuclei and its release into the capillaries of the neurohypophysis. Acetylcholine is also necessary for the action of oxytocin on the myometrium (Shabanah, Toth and Maughan, 1964). Oestrogens have several important effects on the cholinergic system. They promote the synthesis and activation of acetylcholine, they render the myometrium responsive to it and, by depressing cholinesterase activity and thus acetylcholine breakdown, they permit its accumulation (Reynolds, 1938, 1949; Sauer, Jett-Jackson and Reynolds, 1935).

Sensory System

Sympathetic and parasympathetic efferent fibres are accompanied by sensory (general visceral afferent) fibres with cell bodies in the spinal and cranial ganglia corresponding to the level of origin of the efferent fibres. The input from the sensory fibres is integrated into segmental reflex arcs (the efferent neuron of the arc may be somatic or visceral) which it may activate. It is also relayed, via the ascending multisynaptic reticular system and the lateral spinothalamic tract to higher centres. These include the thalamus, whence the input may reach the level of consciousness, and autonomic centres, into the activity of which it is integrated. The overall level of activity is thus modulated, perhaps leading to the discharge of descending impulses and the completion of a more complicated reflex arc.

In sum, it should be appreciated that since every synapse is a region where input may be modified and since hormones affect the level of nervous activity and the nature of the muscular response, we are dealing with a system which is extremely complex. It is exposed to "extraneous" influences at so many sites that some aspects of it are imponderable and our present knowledge is stochastic. This is not to be defeatist for there is much useful information available and stochastic systems are amendable to modification.

OVARY

Preganglionic sympathetic fibres serving the ovary and outer part of the uterine tube arise from the lower thoracic levels (T_{10} to T_{11}). They pass in splanchnic nerves to the autonomic plexuses where they synapse. Postganglionic fibres arise from cells in the aorticorenal or upper ovarian plexuses and project via the ovarian plexus. They are accompanied by sensory fibres which enter the lower thoracic levels (T_{10}) and probably transmit impulses interpreted as ovulation pain (Mittelschmertz). Preganglionic parasympathetic fibres may arise from the dorsal nucleus of the vagus (X) and project via the vagus nerve and the coeliac, aorticorenal and ovarian plexuses to ganglionic neurons at the hilus of the ovary but this is not established. The ovarian plexus also receives fibres from the hypogastric plexuses and it is possible that the parasympathetic centres for the ovary lie at the sacral level of the spinal cord. Although nerve endings in relation to follicles and corpora lutea have been described, the autonomic innervation of the ovary is probably concerned only with control of its blood supply.

UTERUS

Preganglionic sympathetic fibres serving the remainder of the uterine tube, uterus and vagina arise from the lowermost thoracic and upper lumbar levels (T_{12} to L_2). Most pass in splanchnic nerves and down to or through the superior hypogastric, inferior hypogastric or uterovaginal plexuses to synapse with ganglionic neurons in these plexuses. Some, however, descend in the sympathetic trunks and synapse in their lumbar or sacral ganglia. These ganglia project postganglionic fibres directly into the uterovaginal plexuses where they join postganglionic fibres from the ganglia of the autonomic plexuses. Sensory fibres from the corpus uteri accompany the sympathetic fibres and enter the lower thoracic and upper lumbar levels. They probably transmit those impulses which come into consciousness as referred pain from the iliac crest and groin, regions supplied by the iliohypogastric and ilioinguinal nerves (T_{12} to L_1). Preganglionic parasympathetic fibres arise from the sacral level of the spinal cord (S_2 to S_4) and project via the pelvic splanchnic nerves and the nferior hypogastric plexuses to juxtamural ganglionic neurons in the uterovaginal plexuses. Sensory fibres from the region of the cervix uteri accompany these fibres to the sacral level. Pain produced by stretching the cervix is thus referred to the sacral region.

Denervation

The fact that the uterus may receive its innervation by these alternative routes makes difficult its control and investigation by surgical means. Transection of the cord at any level (Shabanah, Toth and Maughan, 1964a) removes the influences of higher centres and is followed by a period in which uterine contractions are absent. Following this period, however, contractions are resumed under the control of the spinal centres. Transections above or below the sympathetic spinal centres have similar effects although the latter spares some of the sensory input to higher centres, particularly from the corpus uteri. Transection of the cauda equina divides spinal nerve roots thus dividing preganglionic parasympathetic fibres and cutting off some of the sensory input, but with this and with spinal or caudal anaesthesia the same clinical picture presents. It may be noted here that epidural anaesthesia at the lowermost thoracic level will interrupt the sensory input from the corpus uteri without significantly affecting the autonomic output (Bromage, 1961).

Lumbar sympathectomy and presacral neurectomy divide most (but not all) of the sympathetic post-ganglionic fibres and also some sensory fibres. The relief of spasmodic dysmenorrhoea may be due to interruption of these sensory fibres but since the operation also results in a more profuse and more prolonged menstrual flow, the relief may be due to interruption of vasoconstrictor fibres leading to vasodilatation and the abolition of ischaemic pain. Labour, too, may be easy and rapid suggesting the removal of an inhibitory effect. The inhibition of contractions by fear, and the relaxation of constriction rings by adrenaline also suggest that the β-receptors and inhibitory effect predominate in the pregnant(progesterone-primed) uterus. Finally specific β-adrenergic blocking agents will not only increase uterine activity in pregnancy but will also block the uterine inhibitory action *in vivo* of isoxsuprine (Barden and Stander, 1968) and *in vitro* of diazoxide (Landesman and Wilson, 1968) all suggesting that the sympathetic is inhibitory to myometrial activity in pregnancy.

These effects on myometrial activity are not necessarily paralleled by those on the uterine vascular bed. During pregnancy the resting uterine vascular tone is also low, but whereas intrauterine pressure remains essentially the same during direct sympathetic nerve stimulation, uterine blood flow and vascular conductance fall, indicating vasoconstriction (Greiss and Gobble, 1967).

Bilateral pelvic neurectomy or parasympathectomy divides all the preganglionic parasympathetic fibres and some of the sensory fibres. It spares the postganglionic parasympathetic neurons and both preganglionic and postganglionic sympathetic neurons. It may produce abnormal prolonged contractions in the nonpregnant and postpartum uterus, effects which may be abolished by phentolamine methanesulphonate (Shabanah, Toth and

Maughan, 1964b); this compound not only blocks α-adrenergic receptors but has some effect on cholinergic endings and some directly on tissues (Barlow, 1964) so that the interpretation of this abolition is uncertain. Bilateral pelvic neurectomy early in pregnancy may cause much reduced placental transfer and foetal death (Shabanah, Toth and Maughan, 1964b) but apparently produces no significant changes in vascular conductance or myometrial activity (Greiss, Gobble, Anderson and McGuirt, 1967a). Performed near term it may lead to delay in the onset of labour, which may be prolonged (Shabanah, Toth and Maughan, 1964b). Electrical stimulation of the pelvic nerves generally has little effect on uterine contractions or vascular conductance in the nonpregnant or pregnant uterus (Shabanah, Toth and Maughan, 1964b; Greiss, Gobble, Anderson and McGuirt, 1967a).

Combined bilateral sympathectomy and parasympathectomy is said to produce an autonomous uterus with regular contractions. It is not, however, a denervated uterus, for the postganglionic neurons in the uterovaginal plexus remain intact. Bilateral paracervical block picks off the fibres and ganglia of this plexus and if complete produces total functional denervation. Paracervical block is usually an effective method of anæsthesia in the first stage of labour (Alvarado-Duran, Bazan and Peredo, 1967; Jencio, 1968) but may sometimes inhibit uterine activity (Zourlas and Kumar, 1965).

Intrinsic Innervation

Regarding the intrinsic innervation of the uterus, little is known. Nerve fibres enter the substance of the uterus along the blood vessels, the richest innervation being at the isthmus uteri and the sparsest at the fundus uteri. Myelinated, presumably sensory, fibres reach the mucosa and form a subepithelial plexus. Beyond this, the results of electron microscopy, fluorescence microscopy and histochemistry (Silva and Klajn, 1968) are difficult to reconcile and not easy to interpret. This may be a result of the biochemical and pharmacological pecularities of the uterus (Wurtman and Axelrod, 1966). The synthesis of adrenaline requires phenylethanolamine-N-methyltransferase, but the uterus lacks demonstrable activity of this enzyme suggesting that most or all uterine adrenaline is taken up from the circulation and bound rather than being synthesized locally. The binding efficiency and adrenaline content of the uterus increases in pregnancy and falls with the onset of labour. Furthermore, unlike the adrenaline bound in other tissues, uterine adrenaline is not concentrated in the granular vesicles (of sympathetic endings), its uptake is not blocked by cocaine and only a small fraction of it is released by tyramine.

These unusual features, with uncertainties about the specificity and precise actions of pharmacological agents, make the interpretation of experiments involving their use hazardous. Apparent differences in response in various species occur. Some of these are due to methodological differences, other to dose-effect relationships and to differences in sensitivity and mode of action. However, the basic mechanisms controlling myometrial activity are similar in all mammals (Reynolds, 1949; Bengtsson, 1962).

Pharmacological Modification

The immature uterus is inactive and unresponsive to acetylcholine, carbachol and oxytocin; oestrogen-priming induces spontaneous activity after which the uterus becomes responsive to drugs. (Shabanah, Toth and Maughan, 1964b). The drug hemicholinium impedes choline transport and thus acetylcholine synthesis. Following its exhibition to the oestrogen-primed uterus, contractility ceases (Shabanah, Toth and Maughan, 1964b). Acetylcholine also causes vasodilatation of the uterine vascular bed which, beyond priming, may be related inversely to the level of oestrogen secretion (Greiss, Gobble, Anderson and McGuirt, 1967b).

In pregnancy the administration of propranolol, a β-adrenergic blocking agent, augments uterine contractility (Barden and Stander, 1968). A similar effect may be achieved with reserpine, which produces catecholamine depletion (Shabanah, Toth, Carassavas and Maughan, 1968). Patients with hypertension in pregnancy have responded well to a combination of reserpine and phenoxybenzamine (Maughan, Shabanah and Toth, 1967). Presumably the latter α-adrenergic blocking agent "neutralizes" the effect of the reserpine on uterine contractility as well as having an antihypertensive effect. Uterine contractility may also be suppressed by isoxsuprine, a sympathomimetic with β-enhancing effects which is used to arrest premature labour (Maughan, Shabanah and Toth, 1967).

Pregnancy and Labour

The foregoing considerations have led to a possible explanation of the events leading to the onset of labour. During the first and second trimesters of pregnancy, uterine activity is normally inhibited due to the stimulation of β-adrenergic receptors, the threshold of which has been lowered by high progesterone activity in the presence of gonadotrophins. As oestrogen activity rises during the third trimester it promotes the synthesis of catecholamines, activates the cholinergic system and gradually inhibits, the effect of the gonadotrophins (Shabanah, Toth, Omay and Maughan, 1968). The myometrial response to progesterone is thus lowered, regardless of the blood progesterone level (Bengtsson and Schofield, 1963). As a result the threshold of the β-adrenergic receptors rises and that of the α-receptors falls, increasing the excitatory effect of adrenergic stimulation. With the release of oxytocin the stage is set for the production of those strong regular coordinated contractions which characterize the onset of labour.

REFERENCES

Ahlquist, R. P. (1948), *Amer. J. Physiol.*, **153**, 586.
Alvarado-Duran, A., Bazan, T., and Peredo, C. (1967), *Amer. J. Obstet. Gynec.*, **97**, 367.
Barden, T. P., and Stander, R. W. (1968), *Amer. J. Obstet. Gynec.*, **101**, 91.
Barlow, R. B. (1964), *Introduction to Chemical Pharmacology* London: Methuen.
Bengtsson, L. P. (1962), *Acta Obstet. Gynec. Scand.*, **41**, supp. 1, 87.
Bengtsson, L. P., and Schofield, B. M. (1963), *J. Reprod. Fert.* **5**, 423.
Bromage, P. R. (1961), *Canad. med. Ass. J.*, **85**, 1136.
Burn, J. H. (1967), *Brit. med. J.*, **2**, 197

Chang, H. C., and Gaddum, J. H. (1933), *J. Physiol. Lond.*, **79**, 255.

Davis, A. A. (1933), *J. Obstet. Gynec. Br. Commonw.*, **40**, 481.

Greiss, F. C., and Gobble, F. L. (1967), *Amer. J. Obstet. Gynec.*, **97**, 962.

Greiss, F. C., Gobble, F. L., Anderson, S. G., and McGuirt, W. F. (1967a), *Amer. J. Obstet. Gynec.*, **99**, 1067.

Greiss, F. C., Gobble, F. L., Anderson, S. G., and McGuirt, W. F. (1967b), *Amer. J. Obstet. Gynec.*, **99**, 1073.

Jencio, H. J. (1968), *Gynæcologia*, **165**, 369.

Koelle, G. B. (1963), *Handbuch der Experimentellen Pharmakologie*, 15. Berlin: Springer-Verlag.

Krantz, K. E. (1959), *Ann. N.Y. Acad. Sci.*, **75**, 770.

Landesman, R., and Wilson, K. H. (1968), *Amer. J. Obstet. Gynec.*, **101**, 120.

Maughan, G. B., Shabanah, E. H., and Toth, A. (1967), *Amer. J. Obstet. Gynec.*, **97**, 764.

Reynolds, S. R. M. (1938), *Science*, **87**, 537.

Reynolds, S. R. M. (1949), *Physiology of the Uterus*. New York: Paul B. Hoeber, Inc.

Roberts, W. H., Habenicht., J., and Krishingner, G. (1964), *Anat. Rec.*, **149**, 707.

Sauer, J. J., Jett-Jackson, C. G., and Reynolds, S. R. M. (1935), *Amer. J. Physiol.*, **3**, 250.

Shabanah, E. H., Toth, A., Carassavas, D., and Maughan, G. B. (1968), *Amer. J. Obstet. Gynec.*, **100**, 974.

Shabanah, E. H., Toth, A., and Maughan, G. B. (1964a), *Amer. J. Obstet. Gynec.*, **89**, 841.

Shabanah, E. H., Toth, A., and Maughan, G. B. (1964b), *Amer. J. Obstet. Gynec.*, **89**, 860.

Shabanah, E. H., Toth, A., and Maughan, G. B. ((1965), *Amer. J. Obstet. Gynec.*, **92**, 796.

Shabanah, E. H., Toth, A., Omay, Y., and Maughan, G. B. *Amer. J. Obstet. Gynec.*, **100**, 981.

Sherif, M. A. F. (1935), *J. Physiol. Lond.*, **85**, 298.

Silva, D. G., and Klajn, N. (1968), *J. Anat. Lond.*, **103**, 210.

Vander-Pol, M. C. (1956), *Acta physiol. pharmacol. neerl.*, **4**, 445.

Vane, J. R. (1962), Chap. 3, in *Recent Advances in Pharmacology*, Edit. J. M. Robson and R. S. Stacey. London: Churchill.

Willems, J. L., Bernard, A. J., Delaunois, A. L., and Schaepdryver, A. F. (1965), *Arch. int. Pharmacodyn.*, **157**, 243.

Wurtman, R. J. and Axelrod, J. (1966), Chap. 6 in *Endocrines and the Central Nervous System*, Edit. R. Levine. Baltimore: Williams and Wilkins.

Zourlas, P. A., and Kumar, D. (1965), *Amer. J. Obstet. Gynec.*, **91**, 217.

5. THE LYMPHATICS OF THE PELVIS

STANLEY WAY

The lymphatic system as a whole is of enormous importance in modern medicine and, although the topographical anatomy has been well known since the time of Leonardo da Vinci, it is only in the last ten to fifteen years that, largely as a result of organ transplant surgery, the exciting possibilities of the physiology of the lymphatic system have been studied and its ultimate potentiality realized. Even now, the physiology is difficult, confused, and ill-understood.

In gynaecology, it is largely in the field of malignant disease that the lymphatics are of importance. This chapter will, therefore, be divided into three sections. Firstly, a brief description of the minute anatomy and functions of the lymphatic system. Secondly, the topographical anatomy of the groups of lymph nodes and lymph channels of importance to the gynaecologist, and, thirdly, what may be described as "Applied Lymphology" which consists of a consideration of the lymphatic pathways and groups of lymph nodes likely to be of importance in the individual malignancies seen in the genital tract of the female.

The Minute Structure and Function of Lymphatics

As in the blood stream, so in the lymphatic circulation, the smallest entity is the lymphatic capillaries. These are extremely numerous, especially in mucous membranes, and consist of closed networks without valves and with extremely free intercommunications. Their walls consist of endothelial plates whose sole function is to retain lymph. The capillaries join together to form lymphatic trunks which are provided with valves. The walls of these trunks are contractile containing smooth muscle which is abundantly supplied by nerves. These trunks are extremely numerous, diverse, and complex in their course, but all eventually lead to a lymph node in the course of their path.

Lymph nodes consist essentially of a mass of free cells, almost all of them lymphocytes, with a supporting framework of reticulum cells and fibrous and elastic elements. Despite the complexity and profusion of the lymphatic capillaries and the lymph trunks, the same does not apply to the lymph nodes. These are not terribly abundant in number and nature seems to have taken the very economic view of never providing two lymph nodes if one will do. Thus, the lymph nodes draining the sole of the foot also do duty for the lymphatics draining the vulva, and in the lower animals this economy of lymph nodes is even more marked as for instance in the case of the dog where only one lymph node exists in the groin in the place of the several lymph nodes found in the groin of a human being, that of the dog being much larger than the smaller ones found in the human groin.

The efferent vessels entering a lymph node go first to the cortical or marginal sinus, then through the medullary sinuses to the efferents of the hilum, and from there through more lymphatic channels to the next group of nodes. The structure of the nodes is extremely fine and intricate and they form very efficient filters capable of holding up structures larger than $2\,\mu$ in diameter. On account of this very fine structure it was for a long time thought that lymph nodes acted purely as mechanical filters separating unwanted elements which were not required to pass into the blood stream. The recent more enlightened studies of the lymphatic system cast doubt on the truth of this old belief. Lymph may bypass one or two nodes of a specific group, but it is virtually impossible for it to bypass a complete group of lymph nodes.

It is almost certain that once a group of lymph nodes has been excised they hardly ever regenerate but, on the other hand, lymphatic channels can regenerate very quickly and, after excision of a group of lymph nodes, alternate pathways, albeit not so effective as the original one are soon established.

The recent interest in organ transplant surgery and the rejection phenomenon has given a new stimulus to the study of the lymphocyte and, secondly, the lymphatic system as a whole, and it is now clear that there are two distinct types of lymphocyte. Those which are immunologically competent, i.e. they are capable of taking part in an immune reaction and these are found in the lymph nodes, the spleen and the thymus gland; and a second group which are hæmatopoietically competent and these are found in the bone marrow. Immunologically competent lymphocytes are not hæmatopoietically competent and vice versa.

The role of the immunologically competent lymphocyte appears to be that of recognition of the presence of what might be described as a foreign substance, be this in an infective agent (and who has not seen enlarged axillary lymph nodes after a successful vaccination in the upper arm) or a transplanted "foreign" organ. This process apparently consists of the recognition by the lymphocyte of an antigen produced by the foreign substance and the response of the lymphocyte is the production of an antibody to that antigen. It is by this means that a foreign skin graft is recognized by the lymphatic system and promptly rejected, unless that graft be protected by drugs, X-rays, or antilymphocytic serum, all of which are destined to destroy the immunological competence of the lymphocyte. Most of us are well acquainted with the presence of enlarged inguinal lymph nodes in association with a septic lesion on the leg or vulva, and it is a well known fact that patients who have been the subject of organ transplant and are rendered immunologically incompetent by direct attacks upon the lymphocytes are thus rendered immunologically incompetent to infective diseases and may even find the common cold lethal.

It is probable, therefore, that the lymphatic system is not only protective against infections, but against foreign substances in general and may even be protective in the case of cancer itself.

Concomitant with these interesting studies and the role of the lymphatic system in relation to transplant surgery, there has been in the field of gynaecology remarkable success by the means of vaginal cytology in the recognition of early cancer of the cervix. Debate and confusion has existed in relation to this subject as it has in the case of the lymphocyte and many arguments have been raised from time to time as to whether these really early cancerous lesions of the cervix known as dysplasia and preinvasive carcinoma can disappear spontaneously.

I have never seen this occur and I would not accept proof of this unless the following conditions were fulfilled:

1. The vaginal smear must be positive.

2. Biopsy must confirm the presence of a preinvasive lesion.

3. The smear must remain positive for a considerable length of time after biopsy.

4. It must then return to negative and remain so on more than one occasion for at least six months.

5. Hysterectomy must subsequently be performed and serial sectioning of the cervix must show the complete absence of any carcinomatous lesion, preinvasive or invasive.

These conditions are hard to fulfil and would probably lead their instigator to a charge of professional negligence. Nevertheless, in a long experience of preinvasive carcinoma, I have from time to time come across foci in sections from a removed cervix of evidence of attempts by the body to destroy the tumour and I have more than one section of anaplastic cancer cells, differentiating and degenerating cells and foreign body giant cells present together in one focus. All the foci that I have observed in this way have been surrounded by lymphocytes, plasma cells and mast cells. This histological picture is identical with that of progressive destruction of carcinoma by radiation and also of skin graft rejection. Unfortunately, in all the cases that I have observed there has been active lesion and in some invasive lesion present in other parts of the cervix.

I have suggested (Way, 1967) that it may be the case that "everyone has cancer, but few suffer from it, and those who do not are protected by an immune process the success of which we are not at this moment aware and that in the study of even preinvasive cancer we may be too late in the development of malignancy to appreciate the successful immunological approach of the body."

It has been suggested many times in the literature that the prognosis for radiation treatment of a cervical carcinoma is better in those tumours which show a massive surrounding by lymphocytes in their initial biopsies than those which do not. We have never been able to confirm this and Robinson (1967) pointed out that his studies tend to support the theory of an inhibition of the immune response in cancer patients. It could well be that cancer cells being derived from a patient's tissues and although being obviously abnormal by some means render the lymphocyte incapable of immunological recognition. This is supported to some extent by Woodruff (1964) who explained that "Tumours which evoke immunological reaction are destroyed in their early stage, possibly before their presence is even suspected, or they succeed in escaping from control. Possible escape mechanism may be (1) loss of specific antigen, (2) inhibition of immunological response, and (3) non-immunological escape.

Two facts become apparent to me. The first is that the common invasion of lymph nodes by carcinoma is a deliberate attempt on the part of the body to provide protection to the host and it is more than likely that many emboli of tumour reaching the lymphatics are destoyed before metastasis can take place and, secondly, that the progression of the common lesion of carcinoma of the cervix from basal cell hyperplasia to preinvasive carcinoma, microinvasion and, finally, clinical carcinoma of the cervix—stages 1 to 4—represents a progressive decline in immunological response."

Lymphatic Anatomy

The lymphatics which are of interest to the gynæcologist start in the thigh, to which the vulva drains, and extend along the course of the external iliac vessels and the common iliac to the aorta at least as far as the kidney.

The Lymphatics of the Groin

These are usually known collectively as the *superficial inguinal nodes*, but they fall into two groups—those which are situated along the inner two-thirds of the inguinal ligament and those which are clustered around the entrance of the saphenous vein into the femoral vein. These latter are also known as *superficial femoral* or *subinguinal* nodes. The subinguinal nodes can be divided into two groups, the medial which is the larger and situated near the entry of the superficial circumflex iliac, the superficial epigastric and the superficial external pudendal veins into the saphenous, and the lateral group or the smaller which lie on the external side of the saphenous vein. The number of nodes in these combined groups is very variable and may be as small as three or as large as twenty and they communicate very freely with each other. The efferent lymphatic trunks of these nodes pass through the fascia covering the femoral artery and vein to communicate with the external iliac group of nodes.

They are frequently said to pass through the deep femoral lymph nodes. These latter are entirely non-existent and are the figment of some anatomical imagination.

The Lymph Node of Cloquet. This node is said to be the upper of the deep femoral nodes and it has received great prominence in the description of operations for carcinoma of the vulva and I myself subscribed to this in my earlier writings. The lymph node obtained its name from Jules Germaine Cloquet, who was a great anatomist and Professor of Clinical Surgery at the University of Paris in the early part of the 19th Century. He described the node in an account of his researches on hernia, which is one of his earliest works. I pointed out (Way, 1948) the position of this node at the upper end of the femoral canal and Rentschler (1929) pointed out that the upper pole projected into the pelvic cavity. My experience of groin dissection since 1948 has considerably increased and it is now my considered opinion that no separate node exists at the upper end of the femoral canal, but indeed this is the lowest of the external iliac nodes the lower pole which projects into the femoral canal, in relatively few cases.

The myth of the Node of Cloquet should now be dismissed. A small pad of fat frequently lies over the opening of the femoral canal into the femoral triangle and is often thought by the surgeon to be the Lymph Node of Cloquet. So much importance has been attached in the past to this named lymph node that many surgeons operating for cancer of the vulva remove this pad of fat under the mistaken impression that they have removed the all-important Lymph Node of Cloquet and need not progress further.

The External Iliac Lymph Nodes

These lie in three groups.

1. The lateral group. This consists of a lowest node, which is usually very large and lies on the lateral side of the external iliac artery underneath the inguinal ligament. It is the most constant of all the nodes and has a very marked constant blood supply which enters its lateral side and invariably bleeds and needs ligature when removed. The remainder, some two to five in number, are smaller and spread along the lateral side of the external iliac artery.

2. The anterior group. These are the least constant and the smallest. They lie in the sulcus between the external iliac artery and vein and never are more than three in number.

3. The medial group. These are the most important to the gynaecologist and may be up to six in number and never less than three. They are comparatively large and lie inferior and slightly medially to the external iliac vein. The lowest of this group sometimes projects into the femoral canal and has been mis-named in the past The Lymph Node of Cloquet.

The obturator node. This node probably belongs to the external iliac group, although it lies lower and more lateral, and is so named by its close proximity to the obturator nerve which lies immediately beneath it. It is a large and very constant node bounded superiorly by the external iliac vessels, laterally by the pelvic wall and inferiorly by the obturator nerve. The afferent lymph trunks of all these groups of nodes come from the inguinal group and the efferents pass directly to the common iliac group.

Before considering the onward path of the efferents of this group of nodes, it is necessary to consider two other node groups in the pelvis which are important to the gynæcologist and are not concerned in the drainage of lymph from the lower limbs. These are:

1. The *para-cervical* nodes. These nodes, one on each side of the cervix, are inconstant and seldom clinically reconizable, but microscopic examination of the parametrium of the uterus removed at a radical hysterectomy frequently shows complete and well formed lymph nodes of microscopic size. With such an infrequent and minute lymph node it is not possible to be certain of the route which its efferents take, but they are probably mostly into the external iliac nodes, although an alternative route into the hypogastric group cannot be denied.

2. The *hypogastric* nodes. These are variable in existence and also in number and lie on the medial side of the hypogastric artery and lateral to the rectum. They are in direct continuity with the utero-sacral ligament in that some of them are placed at the insertion of that ligament.

The Common Iliac Nodes. The common iliac nodes lie on the lateral side of the common iliac artery. They are very constant in this position and vary in number from one to three. On the medial side of the common iliac vessels are a few inconstant lymph nodes being in direct continuity with the hypogastric group previously described. On the left side, the hypogastric nodes lie directly above the body of the fifth lumbar vertebra and the sacro-iliac joint but, on the right side, they lie immediately in front of the lowermost portion of the inferior vena cava since the junction of the left and right common iliac veins to from the vena cava occurs at a slightly lower level than the bifurcation of the aorta into right and left common iliac arteries.

Peri-aortic Nodes. These are very constant and numerous. The aorta is completely surrounded by a dense lymphatic network. The largest nodes are on either side of the vessel, those on the right overlying the inferior vena cava. The nodes follow the course of the artery rather than that of the vein, but occasionally there are some nodes which follow the lateral border of the inferior vena cava, but these are rare. In addition to the larger nodes on the lateral sides of the aorta, there are anterior aortic groups and retro-aortic nodes. Of these two groups, the anterior nodes are probably the most constant, although both groups are seldom fully absent. The retro-aortic nodes are inaccessible from a surgical standpoint. There is free communication between the various groups of peri-aortic nodes.

These continue up as far as the origin of the renal vessels where they receive lymphatics from the kidneys and further up along the course of the aorta they join with the celiac nodes from the small intestine, from the liver, pancreas and spleen, and then proceed into the chest where they receive efferents from the lungs and heart, eventually combining to form the lymphatic duct which enters the venous system on the left side of the root of the neck.

These then are the anatomical dispositions of the lymph trunks and the lymph nodes which are of interest to the gynaecologist. As will be seen later, all the nodes from the groin to the level of the renal arteries are of potential practical importance to the gynaecological surgeon.

Applied Lymphology

In this section the various groups of lymph nodes likely to be involved by the cancers seen in the genital tract will be discussed. From the surgical standpoint a radical operation for cancer should consist of the wide removal of the affected organ and the dissection of at least the primary lymph node relay of that organ and the secondary relay if possible.

Vulva

Primary node relay: Superficial inguinal nodes.
Secondary node relay: External iliac nodes.

The superficial inguinal nodes are the only nodes likely to be involved in a gynaecological cancer that can be detected by clinical palpation and are therefore of importance in the *pre-operative* assessment of the patient. All the others lie too deep for even an approximate evaluation of their state prior to laparotomy. Even in the case of the easily accessible superficial inguinal nodes errors in diagnosis are only too easy (Way, 1960).

The important finding in Table 1 is the fact that 43 per cent of impalpable nodes in carcinoma of the vulva are involved when the patient is first seen. The decision to allow nodes to remain simply because they are impalpable is therefore wrong and of great hazard to the patient. 53 per cent of cases of cancer of the vulva have involved

nodes when the patients are first seen, and it must further be remembered that although the vulva is frequently regarded as a bilateral organ there is a very free communication of lymph channels from one side to the other. The result of this is that about 5 per cent of patients show contralateral node involvement when the tumour is situated on only one side of the vulva. That is the involved nodes are on the *opposite* side to the tumour; and in 17 per cent of unilateral tumours bilateral node involvement is present.

TABLE 1

CARCINOMA OF THE VULVA
CLINICAL AND HISTOLOGICAL EVALUATION
OF THE INGUINAL LYMPH NODES

	Histologically positive	Histologically negative
Nodes palpable	58 (88%)	9
Nodes not palpable	22 (43%)	29

When the tumour is bilateral or involves the midline (clitoris or perineum) then 35 per cent of such tumours have involved nodes. Operations such as hemivulvectomy or unilateral node dissection are thus illogical and harmful. Although lymphatic trunks may bypass one node in a particular group it is very unusual for a complete group to be entirely bypassed (Yoffey and Drinker, 1938). This did occur in 4 per cent of large series of cases in that the secondary relay namely the external iliac nodes were involved whereas the primary relay was free of tumour.

It has often been said that carcinoma of the clitoris is notorious in this respect in that it frequently drains to the external iliac nodes. This has not been my experience or that of others (Campbell, 1959). Anaplastic tumours in any site carry a higher node involvement and a greater tendency to bilateral node involvement than do differentiated tumours.

In my series anaplastic tumours showed an overall node involvement of 62 per cent compared with 35 per cent for differentiating ones. There was bilateral node involvement in 35 per cent of anaplastic tumours as compared with 12 per cent in the case of differentiating ones, and both the superficial and deep nodes were involved in 22 per cent of anaplastic tumours and only 8 per cent of the differentiating group. The importance of lymph node involvement in this disease cannot be over-estimated. Even after the extended radical vulvectomy the results are much poorer when the nodes are involved than when they are not and after less extensive surgery they are disastrous.

TABLE 2

RESULTS OF EXTENDED RADICAL VULVECTOMY
ACCORDING TO NODE INVOLVEMENT

	Five year survivors	Ten year survivors	Fifteen year survivors
Lymph nodes positive	47%	42%	32%
Lymph nodes negative	70%	38%	27%

Finally the extent of node involvement at the time of treatment seriously affects prognosis. If there are not involved nodes the five year survival rate is 70 per cent. If the superficial nodes only are involved it is reduced to 55 per cent but if the deep nodes (external iliac) are involved as well then the five year cure rate is reduced to 21 per cent. Bilateral superficial inguinal node involvement provided the deep nodes are not involved carries no worse prognosis than unilateral node involvement (Way, S. and Henningan, M., 1966).

Vagina

Lower third. First node relay. Superficial inguinal nodes. Second node relay. External iliac nodes.

Upper third. First node relay. External iliac nodes. Second node relay. Common iliac nodes.

Middle third. The node relays for the middle third of the vagina are either as for the upper or lower third or a combination of both.

Carcinoma of the vagina is a fairly rare disease and many of the patients are elderly and not suitable subjects for surgery, but there is a tendency to forget the existence of a lymphatic drainage of this organ.

The suitability of many cases of vaginal cancer for some form of pelvic exenteration has brought the lymphatics of the vagina into prominence in recent years. It is also of major importance not to forget the lymphatic system when treating a vaginal cancer with radiotherapy.

Cancer of the upper third of the vagina presents the same lymphatic problems as cancer of the cervix.

Cancer of the lower third is managed as for carcinoma of the vulva.

Cancer of the middle third drains similarly to both cancer of the cervix and vulva.

Cervix Uteri

Primary lymph node relay:

1. Paracervical (Inconstant).
2. External iliac nodes.

Alternative primary relay. Hypogastric nodes.
Secondary lymph node relay. Common iliac nodes.

The lymphatic drainage of the cervix is widespread and of importance both in the surgical and radiotherapeutic treatment of cancer of that organ. The node groups involved are almost always impalpable clinically. When the are palpable, the case is almost always very advanced and untreatable. Even with the abdomen open palpation through the intact pelvic peritoneum is an unreliable guide to involvement (Table 3) (Cherry, Glucksmann and Way, 1953).

Even with the pelvic peritoneum open palpation is still liable to a 20 per cent diagnostic error (Henriksen, 1949).

The distribution of metastases is clearly shown in Table 4 which is a study of 169 involved nodes removed from 91 cases of carcinoma of the cervix treated by radical hysterectomy and node dissection.

A few anomalies in the spread of cancer are sometimes encountered. In a few cases the metastases occur in the common iliac nodes and not in the external iliac group

and in two cases we have seen metastases in the aortic nodes only but in both these cases a secondary deposit of cervical carcinoma was found in the ovary.

TABLE 3

MACROSCOPIC ASSESSMENT OF NODE INVOLVEMENT AT LAPAROTOMY

	No.	Percentage of all nodes
Total number of nodes studied	573	—
Palpable and involved with cancer	158	27
Palpable and not involved with cancer	113	20
Impalpable and involved with cancer	73	13
Impalpable and not involved with cancer	229	40

TABLE 4

INCIDENCE OF NODE GROUP INVOLVEMENT

	Right	Left	Total	Percentage	
Paracervical	3	3	6	2	
Obturator	34	31	65	20	
External iliac medial	50	53	103	31	69·0
External iliac anterior	15	17	32	10	47
External iliac lateral	10	9	19	6	
Hypogastric	15	9	24	7	
Common iliac	28	18	46	14	
Peri-aortic	14	17	31	10	
Total number of nodes	169	157	326		

There is little point in discussing the incidence of node involvement in relation to tumour stage. Staging of carcinoma of the cervix exists purely for a comparison of the results of treatment between centres. It is not a basis for treatment and since it is based on clinical examination and the nodes in this disease can almost never be felt it is pointless to pursue this exercise further.

The histological type of the tumour in relation to lymph node involvement is of as great significance in cancer of the cervix as it has been shown to be in relation to carcinoma of the vulva. We found in 213 cases of carcinoma of the cervix an involved node incidence of 31 per cent in differentiating tumours and 49 per cent when the tumour was anaplastic. A further difference between the two groups is that anaplastic cancers when they metastasise do so more frequently to both sides of the pelvis and to more node relays than do differentiating tumours. This difference is statistically significant. Of great interest to those who employ a technique of modified irradiation followed by radical surgery as a method of treating cervical cancer is the difference in node involvement in those cases where residual cancer is found in the cervix of the surgical specimen and those in which it is not. When there is no residual cervical cancer 30 per cent show involved nodes and when cancer persists in the cervix 51 per cent have node involvement and this difference in our series showed a high degree of statistical significance. The evil influence of node involvement on the results of treatment of this disease was shown long ago by Bonney (1941) who had a five year cure rate of 53 per cent when the nodes were not involved and one of only 21 per cent when they were. In my series of early cases the figures were 86 per cent and 19 per cent for the two groups respectively (Way, 1964).

Corpus Uteri

Primary lymph node relay. External iliac nodes.
Secondary lymph node relay. Common iliac nodes.

There is a common belief that cancer of the corpus uteri spreads by a different route to that of the cervix and there are many who would place the primary relay in the common iliac group and the secondary in the aortic group. This has not been our experience. It is only in recent years that attention has been paid to lymphadenectomy in this disease and information is still incomplete. Most surgeons do not remove the pelvic lymphatics in treating endometrial carcinoma. The incidence of lymph node involvement in this disease appears from the available studies to be between 8 and 12 per cent. It is probable that these represent only the more anaplastic types of endometrial cancer and from this it may be argued that surgical dissection would contribute little to the improvement of results. Nevertheless, I have a patient who presented with an advanced corporeal cancer infiltrating the bladder. At operation massive node involvement was encountered in both external iliac groups but she remains well twelve years after anterior exenteration and node dissection.

Fallopian Tube

Cancer of the Fallopian tube is so rare and information so incomplete that it would be presumptuous to state dogmatically what the node relays are. In two of my six cases which had node involvement both the common and the external iliac nodes were involved and it could well be that the common iliac nodes are the primary relay.

Ovary

Primary lymph node relay. Aortic nodes.
Alternative primary relay. External and common iliac nodes and inguinal nodes.

The ovary is developed from the mesonephric ridge along with the kidney and descends during embryonic life to its permanent position in the pelvis bringing its blood supply and lymphatics with it.

Ovarian cancer is often seen so late that by this time the lymphology is of little practical importance. There is one situation, however, where it is of importance and this is in the case of dysgerminoma, a tumour which often spreads by the lymphatics without giving widespread intra-abdominal metastases. Here lymph node dissection is invaluable. These tumours are often radiocurable and aortic lymph node dissection followed by X-ray therapy can give very happy results. One of my patients who was fourteen when treated is now happily married and aged thirty-six.

The round ligament of the uterus is really the gubernaculum of the ovary and drags the ovary into the pelvis in the embryo. Its lymphatics are associated with the ovary and occasionally cancer of the ovary can metastasise primarily to the groin. This is a rare but old diagnostic pitfall leading the patient to a surgical department with a diagnosis of strangulated inguinal hernia with intestinal obstruction. The "hernia" is a mass of metastatic cancer in the inguinal lymph nodes and the abdominal distension is ascites!!

Lymphography

In view of the difficulty of diagnosing the state of the lymph nodes before treatment in all forms of cancer. techniques have been introduced to try and overcome this. All have so far failed. Lymphography has received most prominence. It is performed by first outlining a lymphatic in the foot by an intradermal injection of sky-blue. A lymphatic is then canalized with a very fine needle and iodized poppy seed oil is injected under pressure. This substance is radio-opaque and the lymph channels and nodes become very prominent on X-ray examination. Filling defects it is claimed will reveal the presence of lymph node metastases. We have studied this extensively in my department and have come as a result of combined radiological, clinical and histological examination to the following conclusions:

1. Nodes full of cancer cannot be penetrated by any substance.
2. Filling defects in lymph nodes can be due to fat and not cancer.
3. Even when due to cancer so much depends on the angle of the X-ray picture that it is not always seen.
4. Small metastases such as marginal sinus emboli are not demonstrated.
5. The distribution of oil in the nodes is never uniform.
6. Some normal nodes do not take up the oil at all.

Our conclusions are that this technique which is laborious and consuming of skilled time is valueless in gynaecological cancer. There is one situation in which it can help and this is to assess the efficacy of node dissection at the time of operation. An X-ray picture taken at the conclusion of dissection may reveal a node that has been left behind which can then be removed. It must be remembered, however, that an awkwardly situated node full of cancer will not contain radio-opaque material and may be so inaccessible that it cannot be felt. Further in carcinoma of the cervix it must be remembered that the hypogastric nodes cannot be demonstrated by canalizing a lymphatic on the dorsum of the foot.

It has been seen in this chapter that whereas the lymph nodes in the pelvis are comparatively few the lymph channels are many and widespread. The practice of adding Chlorophyll to lymphography in order to outline the lymph channels has no value. It simply covers the pelvis with "a green mess" which obscures the important extraperitoneal structures. Its use cannot be condemned too strongly and like passing ureteric catheters to assist in finding the ureter is a sign of a lack of proper training in the performance of radical pelvic surgery.

REFERENCES

Bonney, V. (1941), *J. Obstet. Gynaec., Brit. Emp.*, **48**, 41.

Campbell, A. D. (1959). Personal communication.

Cherry, C. P., Glucksmann, A. and Way, S. (1953), *J. Obstet. Gynæc. Brit. Emp.*, **60**, 368.

Henriksen, E. (1949), *Amer. J. Obstet. Gynec.*, **58**, 924.

Rentschler, C. B. (1929), *Ann. Surg. Chicago*, **89**, 709.

Robinson, E. (1967), *The Lymphocyte in Immunology and Haemopoieses*, ed. J. M. Yoffey, p. 309, London: Butterworth.

Way, S. (1948), *Ann. R.C.S. Eng.*, **3**, 187.

Way, S. (1960), *Amer. J. Obstet. Gynec.*, **79**, 692.

Way, S. (1964), *Acta Cytol.*, **8**, 14.

Way, S. and Hennigan, M. (1966), *J. Obstet. Gynaec. Brit. Cmwth.*, **73**, 594.

Way, S. (1967), Victor Bonney Lecture R.C.S. (Eng). In press.

Woodruff, M. F. A. (1964), *Lancet*, **ii**, 265.

Yoffey, J. M. and Drinker, C. K. (1938), *J. Exp. Med.*, **68**, 629.

6. MENSTRUATION

S. LEON ISRAEL

Menstruation entails periodic anabolic and catabolic processes that occur simultaneously in the uterus and ovaries—two organs that differ embryologically, histologically, and functionally. The cyclic changes in the endometrium are governed entirely by the two steroid hormones of the ovary. The rhythmic ovarian changes are regulated solely by the gonadotropic hormones of the anterior pituitary, the release of which is controlled by specific centers in the hypothalamus. It has been suggested that the endometrium itself exerts a feedback hormonal influence upon the ovaries by production of a luteolysin (Denamur, Martinet and Short, 1966); there is, however, not yet proof of its existence in man.

We will deal here with the characteristics of menstruation, including its manner of onset, singular periodicity, and some of the features of its three well-recognized phases.

The Menarche

The first menstrual flow, the menarche, is only one of the many manifestations of puberty in the female. Its appearance usually fits the established pattern of growth for the individual girl. It signalizes the onset of the gonadotropic-stimulating function of the hypothalamus and marks the beginning of stabilization of the pituitary-ovarian-uterine mechanism. The timely inception of menstruation provides an important landmark in the girl's development and represents a constitutional trait of considerable significance. It may appear during the span of years that connotes the transition from childhood to maturity—occasionally as early as 9 years, often as late as 16—depending largely upon complex genetic and environmental factors.

Factors Controlling the Menarche

The inception and maintenance of the ovarian cycle are established and nurtured by hypothalamic-pituitary functions. Man and the great apes are the only mammals to have a lengthy childhood that delays puberty and reproductive function. The earlier belief that the ovaries must grow to a certain stage in order to be responsive to gonadotropic stimulation is not entirely true. Such prerequisite ovarian maturity may take place rapidly, as is clear from some striking examples of constitutional precocious puberty. Once started, the pubertal mechanism, including ovarian maturity, is capable of proceeding to ovulation and reproduction as early as the age of 6 (Escomel, 1939). Many experiments have proved that it is not the pituitary but the hypothalamus which requires the years of childhood to mature (Harris, 1964). However, the entire delaying mechanism is not yet clarified. The challenge remains to explain some of the features of the brain's maturing processes.

There has been during recent times a world-wide tendency for the menarche to appear at an earlier age (Tanner, 1962). This trend has been attributed variously to socio-economic progress, factors of race, and variations in climate. Increased standards of hygiene and diet induce better growth and development, being linked to larger body size which may lead to greater capacity to rise in the social scale (Clements and Pickett, 1954). Few doubt the influence of nutrition in initiating the menarche at an early age. However, the same may not be said of race and climate, the alleged effects of which may not be disengaged from nutritional circumstances (New, 1964).

World-wide opinion holds that the appearance of the menarche before the age of 9 represents precocious puberty and its non-appearance by the age of 17 is abnormal. There is frequently a relation between a delayed menarche and a later occurrence of menstrual disorders. The latter must not, however, be confused with the physiologically irregular pattern of the adolescent's menstrual cycle.

Menstrual Cycles during Early Adolescence

After the menarche, the initial menstrual cycles are frequently irregular in both rhythm and quantity. The length of the menstrual cycle in healthy mature women varies from 21 to 35 days. During early adolescence, before the cyclic mechanism is well established, the length of the menstrual cycle is extremely variable; it is not unusual for the interval between the menarche and second period to be as long as 6 months. As time passes, the cycle becomes steadier but summer oligomenorrhea persists in about 20 per cent of adolescent girls. The quantity of the flow is likewise variable, tending for several years following the menarche to be of longer duration and scantier in quantity.

Anovular menstruation is the rule rather than the exception during early adolescence (Fig. 1). The anovulation tends to disappear gradually during the first 2 or 3 years after the menarche, some cycles being ovulatory, others not. Occasionally, the physiological transference from anovulatory cycles to ovulatory ones is not smooth.

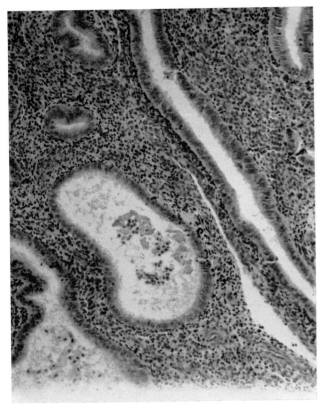

FIG. 1. Anovulatory menstruation. Endometrium showing no progesterone effects obtained 24 hours prior to onset of flow from girl of 15.

Ovulation may be established but the succeeding luteinization is imperfect, little or not progesterone being produced. Such an ovarian derangement constitutes one of the causes of abnormal uterine bleeding in the adolescent girl.

The Established Menstrual Cycle

The interval between the onset of successive menstruations varies considerably even in the same individual. Statistics obtained from women's colleges are not too reliable, inasmuch as the change of environment and its attendant anxieties may disturb the menstrual rhythm. The type of cycle met in gynecologic office patients is likewise not representative of the average; too many of these women have conditions that may alter menstrual rhythm. On the other hand, the gynecologic patient is more likely to keep an accurate record of her menstrual cycles. Similarly, the careful basal temperature charts kept by many regularly menstruating infertile women constitute accurate records. Using information derived from 1,000 such infertility histories, the author found that 80 per cent

of women in good health menstruate at periods ranging from 26 and 34 days, with an average of 28·6 days. Fewer than 3 per cent had cycles of less than 26 days; nearly 17 per cent had irregular cycles. Variations of slight degree from cycle to cycle were present in almost all of the records. The latter observation, in accord with the classical data obtained by others (Gunn, Jenkins, and Gunn, 1937; Arey, 1939; and Vollman, 1956), illustrates the fact that the faultlessly regular cycle is uncommon.

Considering all factors involved, it may be justifiably concluded that menstrual cycles of from 21 to 40 days and bleeding periods of from 3 to 7 days are within physiological limits.

Control of the Menstrual Cycle

The cyclic ovarian actions directly governing the changes of the endometrium culminating in menstruation are under the control of the anterior lobe of the pituitary, which itself is subject to neurohormonal influences. These make the gonad-stimulating function of the anterior hypophysis also cyclic, the rhythm being synchronous with the ovarian and endometrial phenomena.

Studies of the cadence of hypothalamic-pituitary function show that the highest concentration of released FSH prevails between 6 and 9 days after the onset of the menstrual flow, a phase of the cycle when the estrogen level of the blood is relatively low and progesterone not yet present. As the blood level of estrogen rises to a point known to reduce the release of FSH and to augment release of LH as well as LTH (Eik-Nes, 1964; Rothchild, 1965), ovulation occurs. Progesterone, the concentration of which rises in the blood as the corpus luteum blooms, inhibits further secretion of the luteinizing hormone(s) that leads to deterioration of the corpus luteum. As that occurs, the level of both estrogen and progesterone fall, effecting the chain of events that terminates in menstruation and removing the inhibition of the release of FSH. The periodicity of pituitary gonadotropic function is, therefore, at least partly governed by the quantity of estrogen in the circulating blood. The hypothalamic-pituitary unit stimulates the production of estrogen by the ovarian follicle and of estrogen and progesterone by its successor, the corpus luteum. When progesterone causes its reciprocal inhibition of the hypothalamic-pituitary unit, followed by the disintegration of the corpus luteum, menstruation occurs. The cycle rests upon the functional relationship between the ovaries and the central nervous system.

This glib working hypothesis of the inversely related, self-perpetuating, seesaw mechanism of the CNS-pituitary-ovarian axis that controls the menstrual cycle is based upon the evidence at hand now.

THE THREE PORTIONS OF THE MENSTRUAL CYCLE

The menstrual cycle is classically divided into three portions—the menstruating or dismantling part; the proliferative, estrogen, or the preovulatory phase; and the secretory, progesterone, or postovulatory portion.

Menstruation Itself

The menstruating portion of the cycle in the normal fertile woman is characterized by disintegration and exfoliation of the two functional layers of the endometrium, the compacta and spongiosa, embracing approximately three-fourths of the uterine lining. Only the functionless basal layer, wherefrom regeneration and resurfacing of the endometrium occur, remains intact.

As observed by Markee (1950) in endometrial transplants in the eye of a monkey, the dismantling process is initiated about two days prior to the actual appearance of menstrual bleeding—at the time of withdrawal of the growth stimulus from the corpus luteum—by decrease of bloodflow, loss of glandular secretion, pyknosis of the epithelial cells, and disappearance of stromal edema. The increased coiling (buckling) of the spiral arterioles that results from shrinkage of the endometrium creates circulatory stasis, leading to further tissue ischemia. This is followed by an observable vasoconstriction of the spiral arterioles, causing focal necrosis of their walls and bleeding. Not all portions of the shedding endometrium bleed simultaneously. Repair and resurfacing of the endometrium from the cells lining the remnants of the glands in the basal zone—a layer not affected by loss of blood from the spiral arterioles because of the straight artery nourishing it—are microscopically evident in some of the denuded places while other areas of the endometrium are still bleeding (McClennan and Rydell, 1965).

This circulatory concept of the changes in the endometrium leading to menstruation is based solely upon hormonal deprivation, the alterations of the spiral arteriolar system being an essential part of the mechanism. While no one questions the initiatory role of hormone withdrawal, issue has been taken with the essentiality of the spiral arteriole itself (Okkels, 1950).

Components of Menstrual Discharge

The quantity of blood lost in each menstruation is not fixed, varying from woman to woman and even in the same woman from month to month. The average total loss is estimated to be about 60 ml., ranging from 30 to 180 ml. (from 1–6 ounces), an insignificant quantity compared to the total blood volume. A slight increase in menstrual blood loss may cause unwarranted apprehension. Reassurance is attained by learning that the daily number of vulval pads or vaginal tampons and the degree of their saturation are within normal limits. An erythrocyte count and hemoglobin estimation to determine the presence of anemia are of further help in evaluating the degree of blood loss.

Menstrual blood does not clot readily unless it remains in the vagina for a long time. Inasmuch as blood obtained from a stab wound of the cervix during menstruation does clot, it is believed that blood shed in menstrual discharge—like blood serum—lacks prothrombin and fibrinogen, the essential ingredients for coagulation. An alternative explanation proposes that menstrual blood has been clotted and the clots dissolved in the endometrial cavity by an unidentified lytic agent. This viewpoint is supported by the thrombocytopenia observed in menstrual discharge (Pepper and Lindsay, 1960).

From the half to three-fourths of the menstrual discharge is blood; the remainder contains nonblood elements such as mucus, fragments of endometrial tissue with macrophages, histiocytes, mast cells, and desquamated vaginal epithelium. The menstrual discharge contains also cholesterol, estrogen, a variety of lipids, and a euglobulin believed to be formed in necrotic endometrial tissue.

Precise Cause of Menstrual Bleeding

The production of estrogen and progesterone by the corpus luteum depends, as previously stated, upon support from pituitary gonadotropin. The gradually increasing quantity of estrogen or progesterone, or of both, inhibits the further release of the sustaining pituitary hormones, resulting in regression of the corpus luteum, cessation of its steroid secretions, and menstruation.

The precise chain of events in the endometrium itself, initiated by withdrawal of the trophic influences of estrogen and progesterone following deterioration of the corpus luteum, has been investigated in two ways. One line of study, the static, uncovered the histologic minutiæ of both human and simian endometrial specimens collected during all phases of the menstrual cycle. They showed the changing patterns of the development and structure of the endometrial vascular tree (Dalgaard, 1946; Bartelmez, 1957). The other type of investigation, the dynamic, yielded information concerning the growth, bleeding, desquamation and restoration of *living* endometrium transplanted into the anterior corneal chamber in rabbits and monkeys (Markee, 1950). All investigators agree that growth and development of the vascular system of the endometrium, trophic functions of estrogen and progesterone, control integrity of the endometrium locally. However, the immediate regulators of the basic changes in the tissue are probably multiple, several of which are presently moot. They include hormonal deprivation, an unidentified locally produced substance, and the histologic structure of the endometrium itself.

It is not doubted that *withdrawal of estrogen* accounts for disintegration of the endometrium and bleeding. However, this is not true in all mammals, for actual bleeding accompanies the estrogen-withdrawal shrinking process in only a few species. Moreover, both monkeys and women are known to bleed, often rhythmically, while being given low doses of estrogen continuously. For these reasons, it is probably not estrogen alone that controls the menstrual process in the normal cycle.

The fact that both estrogen and progesterone are withdrawn in the normal cycle when the corpus luteum regresses does not invalidate the role of estrogen. Progesterone causes differentiation of an estrogen-reconstructed endometrium. A *fall in the level of progesterone* causes endometrial desquamation and bleeding only if there has been prior or simultaneous action by estrogen. The latter, however, cannot protect the endometrium from the breakdown-effect of progesterone withdrawal. Inasmuch as endometrial bleeding does occur in the absence of progesterone, as shown by the effect of estrogen alone in experimental animals as well as by anovulatory menstruation of women, progesterone likewise cannot possibly be the sole cause of menstruation.

In spite of the dependence of the endometrium upon estrogen and progesterone, a *local tissue agent* is believed to trigger the regressive endometrial changes that follow hormonic withdrawal. According to the Markee theory, the hypothetical tissue factor that is evoked by withdrawal of steroid influence on the endometrium is a potent vasoconstrictor. When this substance affects the coiled spiral arterioles that supply the superficial two-thirds of the endometrium, vascular necrosis and bleeding ensue. The identified tissue substance may be the euglobulin found in disintegrating endometrium by the Smiths (Smith and Smith, 1950). In addition to this "menstrual toxin" of endometrial origin, lethal upon injection in rats, the Smiths found a pseudoglobulin in the circulating blood of women during menstruation, labor, and toxemia of pregnancy. These authors proposed that the pseudoglobulin prolonged the survival of rats given menstrual toxin. Zondek (1953), on the other hand, questioned the validity of the toxic nature of the endometrial substance for he found that rats could be protected from its lethal quality by aseptic precautions in its preparation as well as injection and by the simultaneous administration of penicillin. Whether or not menstrually shed endometrium is toxic to rats is not as important as proving the existence of an endometrial substance, produced as a consequence of hormone withdrawal, that effects the local changes leading to endometrial disintegration.

Markee's idea that increased coiling of the highly specialized spiral arterioles of the superficial two-thirds of the endometrium initiates the tissue changes leading to production of a substance locally that effects menstruation is questioned by some investigators who propose that a *system of arteriovenous anastomoses* exists in the endometrium, the control of which is vested in nerves terminating in contractile elements surrounding the anastomotic areas (Schlegel, 1946; Okkels, 1950). According to this theory, shunting of blood through the A-V anastomoses upon hormonic stimulus, creates large veins. These venous lakes are held to be responsible for the ischemia in the endometrium that takes place before bleeding, rather than the buckling and later vasoconstriction of the spiral arterioles. The existence of such arteriovenous shunts is not accepted by all authorities (Ober, 1949; Markee, 1950). There is agreement about the presence of venous lakes in the upper third of the premenstrual endometrium; the differences between the two viewpoints include the mechanism of the formation of the venous lakes and the importance attached to them.

Bartelmez (1957), in addition to denying the presence of endometrial A-V shunts, does not believe that much tissue is lost during menstruation, a viewpoint partially supported by the studies of menstruating endometrium by McClennan and Rydell (1965). If little of the endometrium is shed and it merely becomes temporarily more compact, the process of menstruation must involve *absorption of stromal elements*, for which the lymphatic system of the endometrium seems to be inadequate

(Wislocki and Dempsey, 1939; Reynolds, 1947). The absorptive theory gains some support from the work of Zuckerman (1949) who believes that rapid resorption of water removes the "fluid scaffolding" upon which the endometrium had been constructed under steroid stimulus; the resorption of water, in his belief, initiates endometrial regression (Fig. 2).

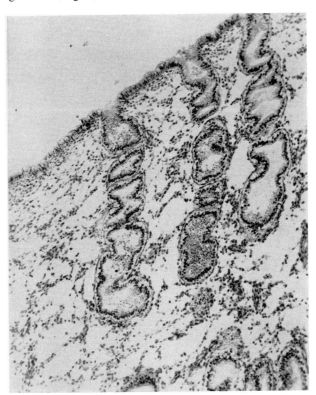

FIG. 2. Well-developed secretory endometrium showing the "fluid scaffolding" of stromal edema. (from S. L. Israel's "Menstrual Disorders and Sterility," 5th ed. Courtesy of Hoeber Medical Division, Harper and Row, New York.)

In summary, the probable immediate cause of menstrual bleeding is withdrawal of the hormonal stimulus for its growth that rapidly affects specialized vascular structures in the endometrium—arteriovenous anastomoses or the coiled arterioles, or both. This leads to regression of the endometrium, a change that initiates local alterations—probably mediated by a substance, or substances, formed in the deteriorating endometrium—eventuating in tissue loss.

Proliferative, Estrogen or Preovulatory Portion of the Cycle

As the function of the corpus luteum regresses, the level of both ovarian steroids diminishes, the inhibition of the hypothalamic-pituitary unit is reduced, and an increasing quantity of FSH becomes available to stimulate the growth of a new crop of follicles in the ovary. The theca interna of these follicles begins to secrete estrogen under the influence of the trace of LH that always accompanies release of FSH. The estrogen evokes regrowth of patches of the endometrium, even while other portions of that tissue are still shedding. Shortly, the preovulatory peak of blood estrogen once again inhibits the release of FSH and, at the same time, causes the release of LH in larger quantity.

The proliferative, estrogen, or preovulatory phase of the menstrual cycle occurs during the period of follicular growth described in the preceding paragraph—from the end of menstruation of the time of ovulation. This is the stage of endometrial reconstruction and growth, a response

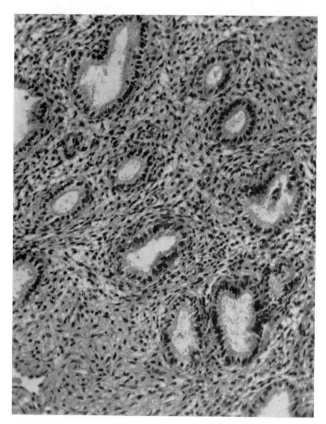

Fig. 3. Early proliferative phase in endometrium. Note tubular glands far apart in dense stroma.

to the estrogen secreted by the theca interna of the developing follicles; the endometrium attains during this time a thickness of more than 3 mm. In the beginning of this phase, the endometrial glands, lined by moderately low columnar cells with irregularly located nuclei, are narrowly tubular and far apart (Fig. 3). Mitotic figures become numerous, and blood vessels begin to run upward from the basal layer toward the subsurface area of the endometrium where a capillary network develops. As ovulation approaches and the terminal portion of this phase of the endometrial cycle is reached, the glands become more numerous and are lined by columnar-type cells with centrally placed nuclei; there is an increase of alkaline phosphatase and ribonucleoprotein in the endometrium, especially in the surface and glandular cells. The latter histochemical and biochemical evidences of protein synthesis are in keeping with the growth of the endometrium (McKay, Hertig, Bardawil and Velardo, 1956). Studies

of the ultrastructure of the endometrium by electron microscopy likewise support this viewpoint (Gompel, 1962).

The mucus-producing glands of the cervix and the vaginal epithelium, likewise responsive to estrogen, participate in the growth process. The increased supply of cervical mucus becomes physically changed, acquiring its preovulatory characteristics. As the layers of vaginal epithelium increase in number, the superficial cells become distant from their blood supply and are shed in cornified fashion. At the height of the proliferative phase of the cycle, the cytoplasm of the desquamated vaginal cells is devoid of granules and the nucleolus is either absent or small and fragmented.

During the proliferative stage of the cycle, two separate processes occur in the ovary: The corpus luteum of the preceding cycle continues to disintegrate and new follicles grow. One of the latter reaches the graafian stage preparatory to ovulation (Fig. 4); the others function actively by secreting estrogen and are later lost by atresia.

Secretory, Progesterone or Postovulatory Portion of the Cycle

Following ovulation, the granulosa cells lining the empty graafian follicle multiply and differentiate into granulosa lutein cells which, together with luteinized theca cells and fresh capillary tufts from the vessels of the surrounding theca interna, form the corpus luteum. This signalizes the onset of the final phase of the menstrual cycle, the secretory portion.

The secretory, progesterone, or postovulatory portion of the endometrial cycle—the differentiative phase—reflects the combined, finely balanced action of estrogen and progesterone. The change in the endometrium is gradual during the course of a week. The glands become increasingly tortuous and filled with secretion; their enlarged size brings them closer together. Viewed in cross-section, the glandular epithelium appears "saw-toothed" because of infoldings resulting from growth (Fig. 5). Each glandular cell increases in size, develops vacuoles, realigns its nucleus in a basal position, and bulges with secretion. In contrast to the proliferative phase, the endometrium now contains little alkaline phosphatase and ribonucleoprotein. There is, however, abundant glycogen, acid phosphatase, and lipids. The intercellular matrix of the now edematous stroma (predecidua) is depolymerized, probably to provide for the anticipated trophoblastic invasion (McKay, 1950). Marked changes of the ultrastructural elements of the glandular cells, as observed by electron microscopy, keep pace with such an expected activity (Schmidt-Matthiesen, 1963).

A progressive increase in vascularization occurs in the endometrium during the secretory phase. The histologic pattern of such secretory endometrium closely resembles that of early decidua (Fig. 6). If it were otherwise, it would not be ready for implantation. This intense preparation has been well summarized in these words: "The cytotrophic phase of embryonic life begins as the ovum implants on the surface epithelium and invades the endometrial stroma. These tissues then become its

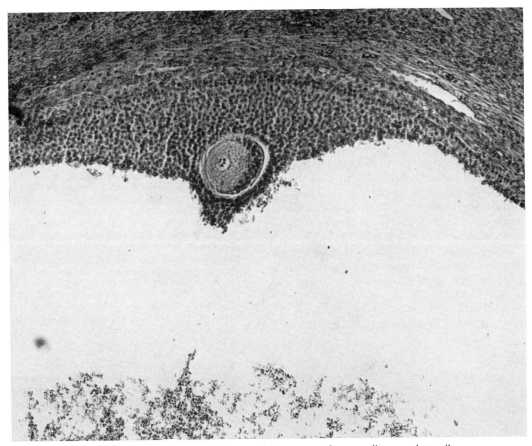

FIG. 4. Portion of graafian follicle containing ovum and surrounding granulosa cells.

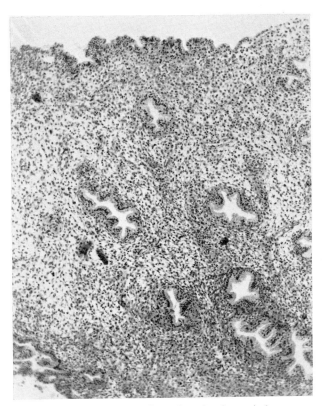

FIG. 5. Premenstrual endometrium showing typical saw-toothed glands.

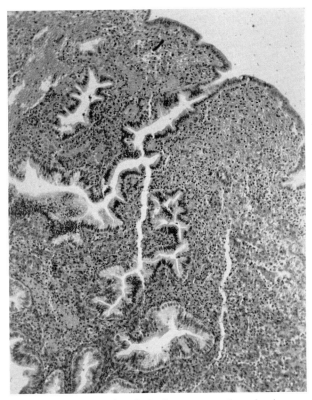

FIG. 6. Endometrium during late secretory phase showing empty glands and predecidual stroma.

immediate environment and source of nutrition . . . On a chemical basis it is of interest to note that implantation begins on endometrium that is at its metabolic peak" (McKay *et al.*, 1956).

The marked influence of estrogen upon the mucus-producing cervical glands and upon the squamous epithelium of the vagina is altered during the secretory phase by progesterone. The quantity of cervical mucus is lessened, and "ferning" as well as other physical changes characteristic of the preovulatory estrogen peak disappear. The vaginal epithelium shows alteration of the process of cornification. The cells desquamated now contain relatively large, vesicular nuclei and granular cytoplasm. In addition, cytologic study shows also an increased number of leukocytes, bacteria, and fragmented cornified cells.

In summary, the postovulatory changes in the endometrium reflect the anticipated reception and maintenance of a blastocyst. If no blastocyst is present, chorionic gonadotropin is not available to support the corpus luteum, no longer stimulated by pituitary hormones. The corpus luteum fails and changes occur in the endometrium that initiate menstruation itself.

REFERENCES

Arey, L. B. (1939), "Degree of Normal Menstrual Irregularity; Analysis of 20,000 Calendar Records from 1,500 Individuals," *Amer. J. Obstet. Gynec.*, **37**, 12.

Bartelmez, G. W. (1957), "The Phases of the Menstrual Cycle and their Interpretation in Terms of the Pregnancy Cycle," *Amer. J. Obstet. Gynec.*, **74**, 931.

Clements, E. M. B. and Pickett, K. G. (1954), "Body Weight of Men related to Stature, Age and Social Status," *Brit. J. Prev. Soc. Med.*, **8**, 99.

Dalgaard, J. B. (1946), "The Blood Vessels of the Human Endometrium; a Histological Study by Means of Injection and Blood Corpuscle Colouration," *Acta obstet. gynec., scand.*, **26**, 342.

Denamur, R., Martinet, J. and Short, R. V. (1966), "Sécrétion de la progestérone par les Corps Jaunes de la Brébis après Hypophysectomie, Section de la Tige Pituitaire, et Hystérectomie," *Acta endocr.*, **52**, 72.

Eik-Nes, K. B. (1964), "Effects of Gonadotrophin on Secretion of Steroids by Testis and Ovary," *Physiol. Rev.*, **44**, 609.

Escomel, E. (1939), "La plus Jeune Mère du Monde," *Presse méd.*, **47**, 875.

Gompel, C. (1962), "The Ultrastructure of the Human Endometrial Cell Studied by Electron Microscopy," *Amer. J. Obstet. Gynec.*, **84**, 1000.

Gunn, D. L., Jenkins, P. M. and Gunn, A. L. (1937), "Menstrual Periodicity; Statistical Observations on a Large Sample of Normal Cases," *J. Obstet. Gynaec. Brit. Emp.*, **44**, 839.

Harris, G. W. (1964), "Sex Hormones, Brain Development and Brain Function," *Endocrinology*, **75**, 627.

Markee, J. E. (1950), "The Endocrine Basis of Menstruation," in *Progress in Gynecology*, Vol. 2, Ed. J. V. Meigs and S. H. Sturgis. New York: Grune & Stratton.

McKay, D. G. (1950): "Metachromasia in the Endometrium," *Amer. J. Obstet. Gynec.*, **59**, 875.

McKay, D. G., Hertig, A. T., Bardawil, W. and Velardo, J. T. (1956), "Histochemical Observations on the Endometrium: I. Normal Endometrium," *Obstet. Gynec.* **8**, 23.

McLennan, C. E. and Rydell, A. H. (1965), "Extent of Endometrial Shedding during Normal Menstruation," *Obstet. Gynec.* **26**, 605.

New, M. L. (1964), "Endocrine Factors in Growth," *Med. Sci.*, **15**, 50.

Ober, K. G. (1949), "Die Zyklischen Veranderungen der Endometrium-gefaesse," *Geburts. u. Frauenheilk.*, **9**, 736.

Okkels, H. (1950), "The Histophysiology of the Human Endometrium," in *Menstruation and Its Disorders*, Ed. E. T. Engle, Charles C Thomas, Springfield, Ill.

Pepper, H. and Lindsay, S. (1960), "Levels of Platelets, Leukocytes, and 17-Hydroxycorticosteroids during the Normal Menstrual Cycle," *Proc. Soc. exp. Biol.*, **104**, 145.

Reynolds, S. R. M. (1947), "Physiologic Basis of Menstruation; Summary of Current Concepts," *J. Amer. Ass.*, **135**, 552.

Rothchild, I. (1965), "Interrelations between Progesterone and Ovary, Pituitary, and Central Nervous System in Control of Ovulation and Regulation of Progesterone Secretion," *Vitamins and Hormones*, **28**, 210.

Schlegel, J. U. (1946), "Arteriovenous Anastomoses in Endometrium in Man," *Acta anat.*, **1**, 284.

Schmidt-Matthiesen, H. (1963), *Das normale menschliche Endometrium*. Stuttgart: Georg Thieme.

Smith, O. W. and Smith, G. V. S. (1950), "Menstrual Toxin," in *Menstruation and Its Disorders*, Ed. E. T. Engle, Charles C Thomas, Springfield, Ill.

Tanner, J. M. (1962), *Growth at Adolescence*, 2nd ed., Charles C Thomas, Springfield, Ill.

Vollman, R. F. (1956), "The Degree and Variability of the Length of the Menstrual Cycle in Correlation with the Age of Woman," *Gynaecologia*, **142**, 310.

Wislocki, G. B. and Dempsey, E. W. (1939), "Remarks on the Lymphatics of the Reproductive Tract of the Female Rhesus Monkey (Macaca mulatta)," *Anat. Rec.*, **75**, 341.

Zondek, B. (1953), "Does Menstrual Blood Contain a Specific Toxin?" *Amer. J. Obstet. Gynec.*, **65**, 1065.

Zuckerman, S. (1949), "Menstrual Cycle," *Lancet*, **1**, 1031.

1. THE OVARY

L. L. FRANCHI

INTRODUCTION

The object of this chapter is to provide an account of the dynamic aspects of ovarian development and structure and the functional significance of the constituents of the ovary in the normal human female. The hormones of the ovary will be mentioned only briefly, however, since they are considered in detail in other parts of this book (Sec. X, Ch. 2).

Much of our current knowledge of ovarian development and functions has been derived from a study of animals under both normal and experimental conditions. Direct information about the human ovary is scanty since there are relatively few opportunities to examine the organ in completely normal women either before or during their reproductive phase of life. There is, however, substantial evidence that the human ovary does not differ from that in other mammals in any fundamental respect and that in many of its developmental and functional aspects the ovary is remarkably uniform in vertebrates in general. For these reasons the present account draws heavily on the results of studies on animals, in so far as they can be confidently applied to the human ovary.

For full reviews of the development and structure of the ovaries in vertebrates reference should be made to Cole & Cupps (1969), Zuckerman, Mandl & Eckstein (1962), and Brambell (1956).

The primary function of the ovary is to produce female gametes which, when fertilized, become diploid cells (zygotes) with the full potential for the production of new individuals. If this were all that was required to ensure the perpetuation of the species, the ovary could be simply a sac whose walls enclose the germ cells[1] during the preliminary stages of their differentiation. This is virtually the situation in many invertebrates and lower vertebrates, although even among these groups there are variable degrees of complexity of the ovary which ensure the survival and union of gametes, both at the correct time and in a closed environment favourable to the development of the zygote.

In the mammal, therefore, the ovary has evolved into a complex organ in which germ cells may be maintained for long periods in a semi-differentiated state, and which also periodically prepares the reproductive tract for the reception and nurture of the zygote. The latter function is performed by hormones produced cyclically by somatic cells in the ovary, under the influence of pituitary gonadotrophic stimulation. As appears to have been the case in evolutionary development of the gonads, the germ cells arise before typical hormone-producing elements. Yet, as will be described, germ cells appear to be predisposed to the influence of hormonal substances, even in the very early stages of differentiation; this is an example of the interaction of cells with their local environment which is typical of the development of the reproductive system as a whole. Many structural and functional abnormalities which are detectable later on in the life of an individual may well stem from disturbances in this relationship which occur during embryonic and early fœtal development.

DEVELOPMENT OF THE OVARY

During development the ovary passes through a series of stages which are usually recognized by their histological features. The first of these is termed the *genital ridge stage*, an important part of which is concerned with the early history of the germ cells. The second, or *indifferent gonad stage*, refers to the general development of the somatic elements. Following this, *sex differentiation* takes place; this is a more protracted stage during which the histological features of the ovary are first defined, specific somatic cell types become established, and oogenesis begins. The morphological changes throughout this period have been fully investigated in a series of human embryos by Witschi (1948) and van Wagenen & Simpson (1965). As indicated earlier, however, an understanding of the dynamics of ovarian development has relied mainly on a study of animal material.

A. Germ Cells and their Origin

In all vertebrate embryos which have been studied, the primitive or *primordial germ cells* are segregated very early in embryonic development from the main mass of cells which form the remainder of the body. It has been claimed, for some species, that part of the cytoplasm of the uncleaved zygote contains groups of organelles ('germ cell determinants') which, as a result of cleavage, are segregated into only a few of the blastomeres.[2] From the latter are formed the primordial germ cells, which can be traced through subsequent embryogenesis by their large size and sometimes by the presence of fatty globules in the cytoplasm. In many instances, however, the germ cells are not

---

[1] The term *germ cells* refers to those cells which, from early cleavage stages in the embryo, are distinct from *somatic cells* and provide the sole source of all future gametes. The term *germ layer*, referring to sheets of cells forming the embryonic endoderm, mesoderm and ectoderm is irrelevant in this context, except in as much as germ cells reside in one or more of these layers prior to organogenesis.

[2] Experiments in which this region of the zygote is damaged by cauterization or ultraviolet radiation result in the production of individuals the gonads of which remain rudimentary and may completely lack germ cells. This and other evidence (see text) gives abundant support to the early concept of "continuity of the germ-plasm" (Weismann, 1885).

distinguishable until the germ layers (see footnote 1) are formed. They are first identified in the primitive endoderm or mesoderm in regions of the embryo quite distinct from that in which the gonads will develop, i.e. germ cells have an *extra-gonadal origin* (see Franchi, Mandl & Zuckerman, 1962). In human embryos, for example, these cells are first seen at about 4 weeks *post conception* (*p.c.*), embedded in the epithelium of the yolk sac stalk, overlying the allantois region (Witschi, 1948). In succeeding days the cells change their location until, at about 5 to 6 weeks *p.c.*, they are found at the root of the dorsal mesentery of the

phosphatase-rich germ cells. Furthermore, the majority of them failed to migrate to the future gonad region, and they were unable to proliferate. These and similar studies have shown that primordial germ cells are not only important in stimulating the development of the gonads, but also that they must give rise to the definitive germ cells, as no others develop if their migratory movement is suppressed (see p. 114). A similar technique has been used to trace the migratory path of primordial germ cells in human embryos (Figs. 1, 2; McKay, Hertig, Adams & Danziger, 1953, 1955).

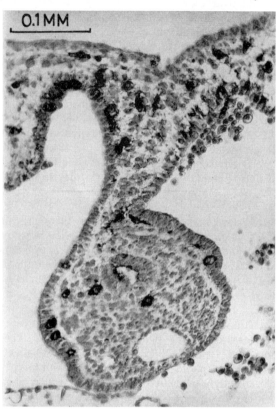

Fig. 1. Transverse section through the dorsal mesentery of a 5 mm. (*ca.* 4½ weeks *p.c.*) human embryo (FHW S-52-1019). The primordial germ cells, deeply stained by the alpha-naphthyl alkaline phosphatase technique, are present in the coelomic epithelium and connective tissue of the mesentery and the presumptive genital ridges.

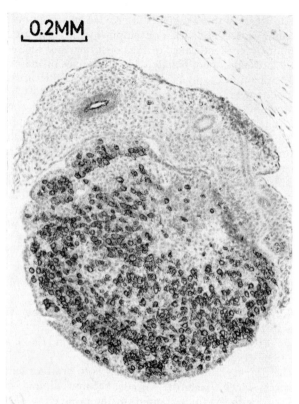

Fig. 2. Transverse section of the developing ovary of a 35 mm. (*ca.* 7 weeks *p.c.*) human embryo (BLI S-52-640). Technique as in Fig. 1. The primordial germ cells reside mainly in the ovarian cortex. The large numbers are due to mitotic division. (Figs. 1 and 2 reproduced by permission from McKay, Hertig, Adams and Danziger (1963); *Anat Rec.* **117**, pp. 208 and 213.)

developing gut, in the region of the embryo where the transitory mesonephric kidney will develop (Fig. 1). They attain this position by active migration, possibly amoeboid in nature and aided by lytic action, as shown by Witschi and more recently confirmed by Pinkerton, McKay, Adams & Hertig (1961).

Studies on the migration of primordial germ cells in the mouse have been aided by the observation that they are rich in alkaline phosphatase, which produces a deeply coloured end-product after the application of the Gomori histochemical technique (Chiquoine, 1954). Following the discovery by Mintz and Russell (1957) that certain mutations in mice result in the production of females with rudimentary, sterile gonads, Mintz (1959) found that the embryos of these mutants possessed very few alkaline

B. The Indifferent Gonad

The early development of the reproductive system is similar in both sexes. The first evidence of gonad formation is a slight hypertrophy of the coelomic or future peritoneal epithelium overlying the developing mesonephroi. These bilateral, elongated thickenings are called *genital ridges*, and they are detectable before the primordial germ cells have completed their migration. According to some authors the further growth of the ridges may be conditioned by the arrival of germ cells. These tend to collect both within the epithelium and in the mesenchyme beneath it, and once there they proliferate by mitosis. The peripheral development of the genital ridge marks the beginnings of the *primary cortex* of the gonad. There is general agreement that the deeper tissue, the *primary medulla*, is derived by a downgrowth of cells from the middle region of the mesonephric blastema (see Witschi, 1951; Franchi *et al.*, 1962). Segmentally arranged cords of cells link this blastema with the gonadal medulla and constitute the presumptive rete apparatus which, in the male, is destined to provide the channels through which spermatozoa enter the reproductive tract proper. It is also considered that the adrenal cortex is derived from the same region as the primary ovarian medulla; subsequent functional activity (i.e. synthesis of steroid hormones) by both adrenocortical and ovarian medullary elements is further evidence of a common origin of these otherwise separate structures (Witschi, Bruner & Segal, 1953).

The result of continuing proliferation of primordial germ cells and of somatic cells in the genital ridges is that the cortex thickens and cord-like ingrowths ('sex-cords') are formed which penetrate the narrow layer of mesenchyme (primary tunica albuginea) into the ovarian medulla. The early gonad thus contains germ cells in both cortex and medulla. Under normal circumstances the pattern of further somatic development is determined primarily by the genetic sex of the embryo. In the genetic male, the medulla will form the basis of a testis and the cortex will later revert to a simple epithelium. In the genetic female, the cortex will proliferate further and the primary medulla will decrease in size and importance. Before this differentiation sets in, both male and female gonads are identical in appearance. This stage is thus termed the *indifferent gonad stage*. The organ contains all the necessary ingredients for the development of either an ovary or a testis. It is now considered by many that the cortex and medulla are the source of two antagonistic inductor substances, 'cortexin' and 'medullarin'. In the indifferent gonad these are at balance. The cortical inductor will, if it becomes predominant, promote the differentiation of oocytes from the primordial germ cells, stimulate development of the paramesonephric (Müllerian) duct and suppress both medullary proliferation and the differentiation of the male reproductive ducts. Conversely, the inductor in the medulla may suppress further cortical proliferation and stimulate the growth of rete tubules and mesonephric (Wolffian) ducts. There is much evidence, particularly from experiments on Amphibia, that the balance is very delicate, and can easily be upset in either direction by surgical means or by adding sex hormones to the local environment (for example, parabiosis of a female embryo in the indifferent gonad stage, with a male where testicular differentiation has begun, will always result in the development of part or whole of a male system in the younger parabiont. The reverse situation has also been shown to occur (see Witschi, 1951; Burns, 1955; Wolff, 1962). Since, however, the results of experimental intervention are by no means identical in all classes of vertebrates, there is as yet no universally accepted hypothesis for the precise mechanisms determining the direction of gonad development. Nevertheless, it is clear that the most important factor which determines whether the germ cells will differentiate into oocytes or spermatozoa is not their genetic sex but the local humoral environment in which they are bathed. The germ cells are thus bipotential.[3]

C. Sex Differentiation

(1) General Histology

During the course of internal organization the developing gonad undergoes changes in shape and size. These are at first similar in both sexes, resulting from continued proliferation of the primordial germ cells and somatic cells, and leading to a marked increase in volume. In mammals there is a concomitant involution of the mesonephros, so that the gonad becomes suspended from the overlying structures by a narrow sheet of tissue. In the female this forms the *mesovarium*, and its point of entry to the ovary, the future *hilus*. Connections of the medulla with the receding mesonephros (Figure 3) are retained in rudimentary form only, since unlike the situation in the male, its duct system plays no part in the eventual transport of gametes. After birth these persist as vestiges known as the *epoöphoron* and *paraoöphoron* associated with the mesovarium, and the *rete ovarii* in the ovarian hilus. It is believed that, at least for a time during development, these structures retain their potentiality for full differentiation, but are normally inhibited by the cortical inductor substance in the ovary. The examples of sex reversal in birds (footnote 3) suggest that when a gonad remains in a rudimentary condition, but later becomes active, the corresponding duct rudiments are no longer sensitive to hormones and remain in a vestigeal condition.

As ovarian differentiation progresses the thickening cortex becomes split up into irregular cords of cells by the ingress of connective tissue and blood vessels from the medulla (Figure 3 and Figure 5). In section, therefore, the tissue appears to consist of islands of germ cells in mitosis with associated somatic cells, separated by a limited amount of connective tissue which will eventually expand to form the stroma in the adult (Figure 4 and Figure 6). The increasing overgrowth of cortical tissue pushes the regressing primary medulla towards the hilar region. The latter becomes reduced in length because of the dwindling connection with the mesonephros. The overall result is a gradual rounding-off of the contours of the organ, although the human ovary remains dorsoventrally flattened for a considerable time. In the testis, on the other hand, cords of germinal and somatic cells in the medulla (the future seminiferous tubules) become separated by centripetal downgrowth of blood vessels from the primary tunica albuginea. By the age of 8 weeks *p.c.* these changes are sufficiently advanced to allow a distinction between developing ovary and testis to be made with confidence.

[3] That bipotentiality amongst germ cells persists into the adult is demonstrated by the situation in those vertebrates where the ovary reaches full development on one side only. For example, most adult female birds possess an atrophic right gonad: the cortex is sterile and feebly represented but a few indifferent germ cells remain in the medulla. If the functional left ovary is destroyed, either surgically or by disease, the right gonad hypertrophies to produce a fully functional testis: sperms develop and the secondary sexual characteristics become those of a male bird. It is also well established that the gonads of cyclostomes and certain fishes are hermaphroditic, producing male or female gametes in successive breeding seasons. For a review of various aspects of the bipotentiality of germ cells see Franchi, (1962): Franchi *et al.*, (1962).

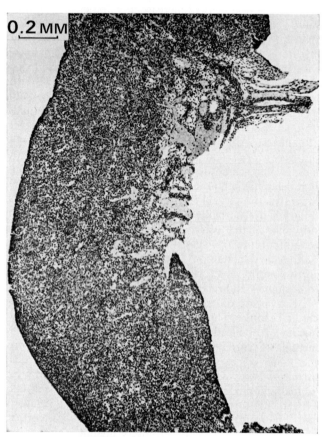

FIG. 3. Section through human ovary (*ca.* 3 months *p.c.*). The cortex appears rather uniform. Part of the primary medulla and regressing urogenital connection is shown at the top right.

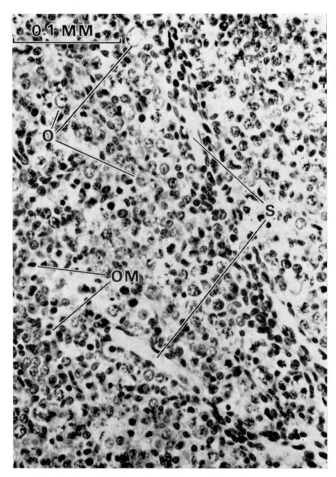

FIG. 4. Cortex of 3 months *p.c.* ovary. Oogonia at rest (O) and undergoing mitosis (OM) are widely scattered amongst the somatic elements. Connective tissue strands (S) have begun to penetrate from the medullary region.

(2) Differentiation of the Oocytes (Oogenesis)

The continued mitotic divisions amongst germ cells during early somatic ovarian differentiation result in the production of many thousands of stem cells which may be termed *oogonia* (Figure 4). The subsequent history of these cells has been the subject of much debate (see below) for almost 100 years, although it is only relatively recently that sufficiently reliable techniques for counting germ cells have been devised. A comprehensive quantitative

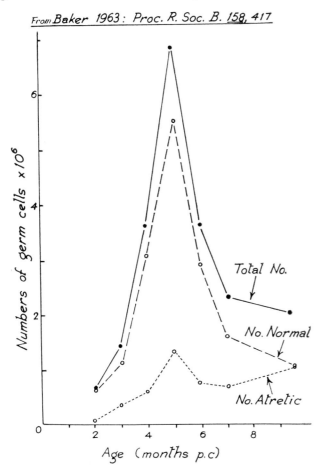

From Baker 1963: Proc. R. Soc. B. 158, 417

Fig. A. Graph showing the total numbers of germ cells (oogonia and oocytes in meiotic prophase) in the human foetus. From Baker, (1963).

and cytological analysis of the ovaries in the human foetus has been carried out by Baker (1963), based on methods used for the rat by Beaumont & Mandl (1962). The cytological study was extended to an electron microscopical characterization of human foetal germ cells by Baker & Franchi (1967a, b). From the age of about 2 months *p.c.* an increasing proportion of the oogonia cease dividing mitotically; they enter the prophase of meiosis,[4] the various stages of which can be identified by specific chromosomal configurations (Figure 6; and Figure 8). These cells are now referred to as *primary*

[4] The prophase of meiosis is that part of the reduction division (see p. 123) during which chromosomes become associated in pairs and interchange of genetic material takes place between them. For a full treatment of the significance of various subphases which are mentioned here the reader should consult a standard text on genetics.

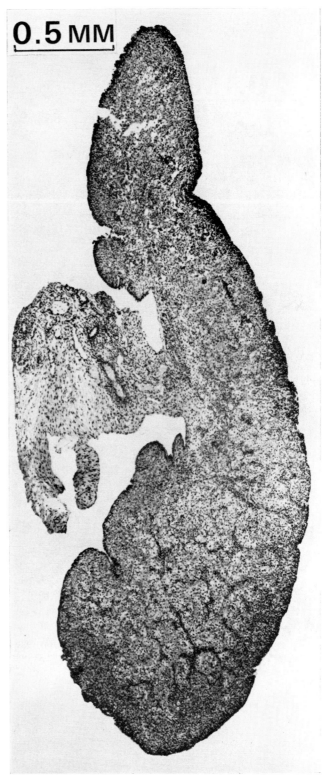

Fig. 5. Section through human ovary ($3\frac{1}{2}$ months *p.c.*). Part of the mesovarium is also shown. The inner part of the cortex has become subdivided into lobules by strands of vascular connective tissue, while the outer zone remains relatively uniform.

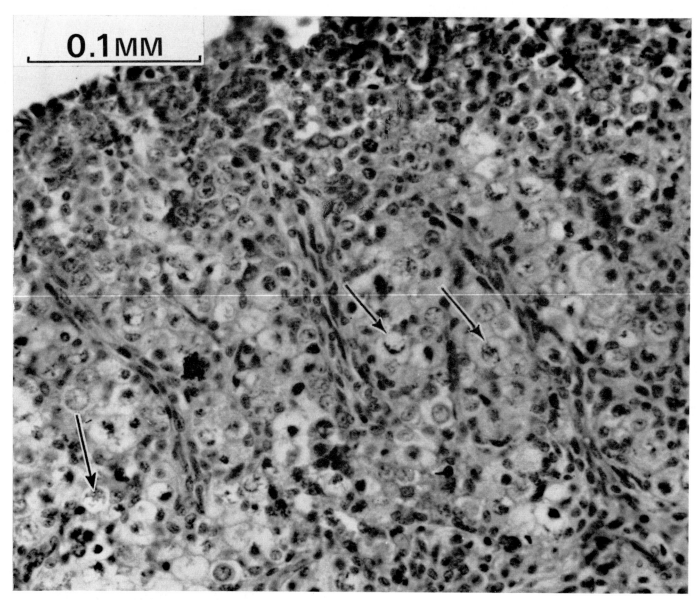

Fig.   6. Cotex of 3½ months *p.c.* ovary. Many of the germ cells lying in the inner cortex have entered the prophase of meiosis and are primary oocytes (arrows). Those towards the outer zone remain as oogonia. The medullary strands are clearly shown.

TABLE 1

THE LIFE HISTORY OF THE FEMALE GERM CELL (HUMAN). CORRELATIONS IN TIME WITH OVARIAN DEVELOPMENT AND FOLLICULAR ORGANIZATION.

The vertical lines in the fourth column represent the persistence in the ovary, with time, of the stages indicated; the line for oocytes at diplotene is shown continuous from *ca.* 5 months *p.c.* into old age, representing the 'stock' of oocytes. Oocytes which are not called upon for ovulation and which do not undergo atresia during this time remain at diplotene indefinitely. The stages following diplotene—diakinesis to zygote—are shown linked to the diplotene stock by an arrow starting at puberty. It should be clear that one or more oocytes pass through all these stages up to and including ovulation at monthly intervals over a period of forty years or more. Only the first of these cyclical events is shown, together with the associated follicular development.

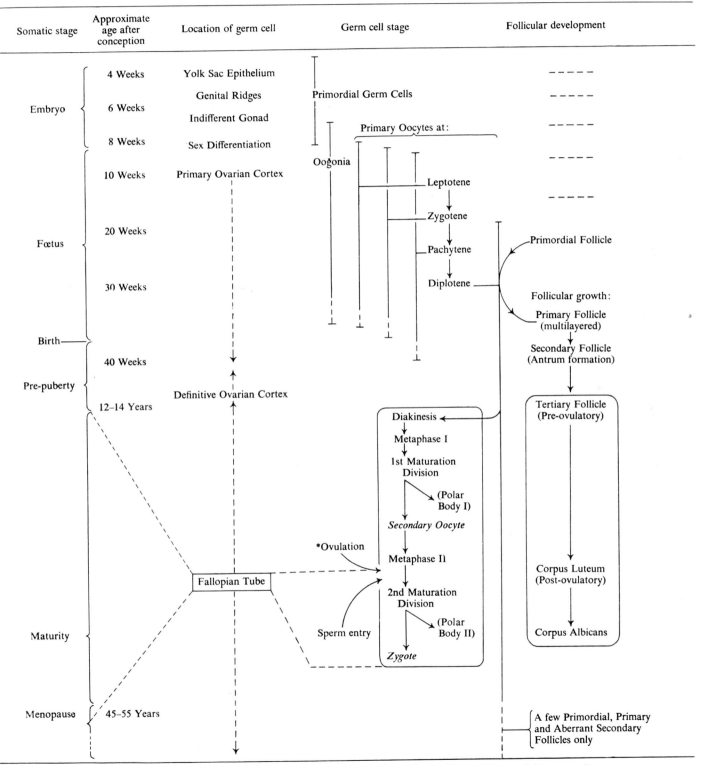

*This monthly event affects a total of approximately 400 oocytes during the entire reproductive lifespan. The remaining germ cells are lost through atresia which starts in the embryo and continues into old age (see text).

5

oocytes (see Franchi *et al*., 1962). The remaining oogonia continue dividing so that their total number reaches a peak at 4½ to 5 months *p.c.* Baker's calculations show that at this time a pair of ovaries contains approximately 2 million oogonia, together with 4·8 million oocytes in various stages of meiotic prophase. It is clear, however, that not all cells are normal: characteristic signs of degeneration are shown by both oogonia and oocytes. During the remaining months of gestation the total number of cells declines markedly as more and more oocytes degenerate, but the decrease is also due to the cessation of mitosis among oogonia and their entry into meiosis (Fig. A). An analysis of the various stages of differentiation shows that between 5 months *p.c.* and term the numbers of oogonia and of oocytes at the leptotene and zygotene stages falls practically to zero. Of oocytes at pachytene, while the total number falls, a higher proportion show atretic changes; those at the diplotene stage increase in number by transformation from pachytene. At birth the oocytes at diplotene constitute about 65 per cent of the germ cell population, the remainder being composed of earlier stages. Within the first few weeks following birth, germ cell stages other than diplotene rapidly disappear (Table 1).

(3) The 'Stock' of Definitive Germ Cells

The ovaries of a new-born child contain only about 2 million oocytes (Baker 1963). At 7 years of age about

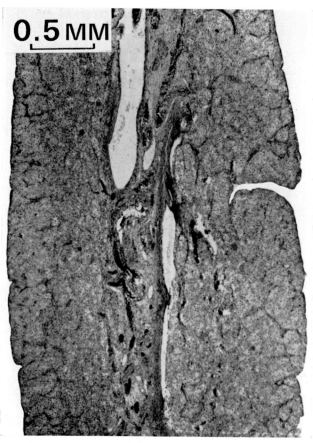

0.5 MM

FIG. 7. Section through human ovary (5 months *p.c.*). Lobulation of the cortex has extended outwards and the vascularity of the medulla has increased.

300,000; and at 45–55 years, perhaps only a few hundreds at the most. It should be apparent, from the above, that the decline from a potential stock of nearly 7 million cells in the foetus is due largely to a degenerative process or 'atresia', the causes of which have not yet been adequately defined. Baker's study makes it clear that oogonia largely succumb during mitotic division, and oocytes during the zygotene, and pachytene stages, so that it is tempting to believe that faults may develop in the actual mechanisms of mitosis or chromosome pairing. Atresia continues to deplete the stock of oocytes when they have reached the long diplotene stage, however, and in all post-natal ovaries there are some 10–30 per cent of primary oocytes undergoing degeneration, either in primordial follicles or during follicular growth (see pp. 115 and 119).

Numerous studies on other species among mammals, birds and some lower vertebrates show that the pattern of germ cell differentiation is both quantitatively and qualitatively similar to that in the human. They lend support to the now widely accepted view (Zuckerman, 1951, 1956)[5] that all definitive germ cells are derived from the primordial germ cells with which the gonads were first populated; that with very few known exceptions among mammals, all oocytes complete their differentiation from oogonia up to the diplotene stage during foetal or early post-natal life; and that *oocytes are derived only from pre-existing oogonia*. These facts are also based on results of experiments which show that once all oogonia are eliminated by transformation into oocytes, no other ovarian elements transform into oogonia to add to the established stock (for review see Franchi *et al*., 1962; Zuckerman, 1965a).

The oocytes which survive early waves of atresia and differentiate as far as the diplotene phase, at the latest soon after birth, thus form the entire definitive stock of cells from which all future female gametes are derived. They remain at diplotene for an indefinite period. The cells are somewhat larger than at earlier stages (35μ cf. 19μ mean diameter at pachytene in human) and the chromosomes form distinct, deeply staining threads. When Graafian follicles begin to form (p. 119) the chromosomes in the enclosed oocytes become somewhat more diffuse,[6] but still

---

[5] Concerning earlier views on oogenesis, it was widely held that *all* oocytes derived from primordial germ cells are destined to disappear and that the ovary is repopulated with oocytes which simply develop from the epithelium covering the organ ("germinal" epithelium). Those who upheld this view (e.g. Allen, 1923; Evans & Swezy, 1931) considered that what are now known to be normal stages in meiotic prophase were cells undergoing degeneration and that all the early oocytes must therefore die off. The concept of a true "germinal epithelium," producing the definitive oocytes from ordinary somatic cells, was undoubtedly due to misinterpretations of the events taking place during the proliferation of the cortical sex-cords in the foetal ovary, and partly also to an unfortunate adherence to views first expressed in 1870 by Waldeyer. There is little point in giving further credit to these older arguments, since the protagonists have consistently failed to provide convincing evidence for the formation of germ cells in the absence of oogonia. It is nevertheless disappointing to discover that several recently published text-books of histology still propose the coelomic epithelial cells covering the ovary as the source of oocytes.

[6] Recent work in the author's laboratory, using electron microscopy and associated techniques, has demonstrated that diplotene chromosomes in human oocytes are similar in form to the "lampbrush" chromosomes characteristic of ovarian oocytes in non-mammalian vertebrates (Baker & Franchi, 1967a, b). Similar studies in progress suggest that this form of chromosome may be widespread in the oocytes of mammals.

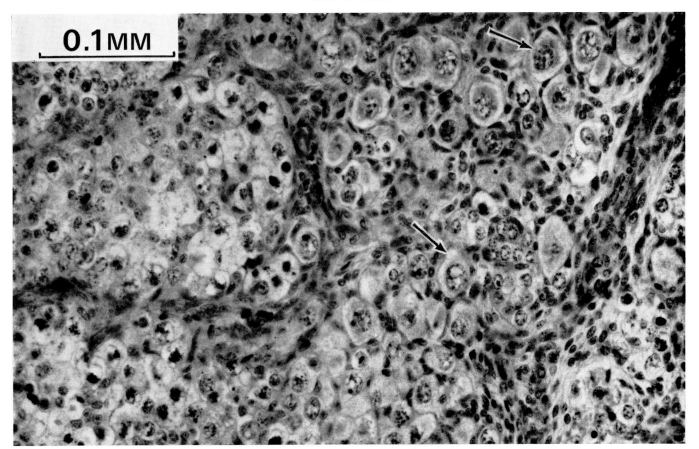

0.1 MM

Fig. 8. Part of the cortex of 5 months *p.c.* ovary. The outer zone (left) contains nests of oogonia and oocytes in the early stages of meiotic prophase. Many of the larger oocytes in the right hand half of this picture (inner cortex) have reached the prolonged diplotene stage and have become enclosed in simple primordial follicles (arrows).

maintain the diplotene configuration. The diakinesis and prometaphase stages which, perhaps many years later, herald the maturation division proper do not ensue until a few hours before ovulation (p. 123 & Table 1; Fig. 8).

4. Origins of Other Cell Types

(a) **Follicular Cells.** All primary oocytes at some time during differentiation become invested by a single layer of flattened epithelial cells. This may occur as soon as the migrating primordial germ cells settle in the genital ridges (Witschi, 1948), although the more recent electron microscopical studies indicate that a complete covering of cells, forming the primary or *primordial follicle*, does not invest oocytes individually until the late pachytene or diplotene stage. Prior to this, groups of oocytes generally share a common covering. Individual primordial follicles first appear in association with the oocytes lying deep in the cortex (Fig. 8).

There is no general agreement about the origin of the follicular cells. They are probably derived from the "germinal" epithelium during the downgrowth of proliferating cells to form the cortical "sex-cords". One piece of evidence that supports this view is that radioactive or particulate substances actively taken up by the superficial cells in young mouse ovaries subsequently appear in

primary follicular cells but, significantly, not in oocytes (Chiquoine, 1960). Another view is that these cells originate from the medullary blastema cells which penetrate the cortex with the blood vessels during sex differentiation. In view of the androgenetic inductor substance associated with the primary medulla, and the fact that follicle cells are intimately associated with the oocyte, this view is less convincing.

(b) **Secretory Cells.** Whilst the major secretory activities of the ovary develop well after birth, human ovaries in the later fœtal and early post-natal periods almost invariably contain a few follicles which have begun to grow and have developed both an antrum and a surrounding layer of thecal cells, which are known to synthesize œstrogenic precursors. In addition, *interstitial cells* are sometimes found scattered in the interfollicular tissue. Although they do not develop generally until after birth, some mammalian ovaries in the fœtal period contain large numbers of glandular interstitial cells which regress after birth. Yet again, there is no general agreement about the source or initial function of these cells. The common derivation of the adrenal cortex and the primary ovarian medulla (p. 109) and the steroidogenic capacity of interstitial cells suggests that they arise from the mesonephric blastema. It has been claimed too, that additional secretory cells do not arise *de novo* but only from pre-existing ones; in this view the first thecal cells may well have arisen from the medulla, but when the associated follicles undergo atresia they form a "pool" from which both interstitial cells and further thecal cells are derived. It is difficult, however, to understand the rather complex mechanisms of dedifferentiation and cellular migration which would be involved in such a scheme (Fig. 10).

In addition to the above cell types, others whose function is possibly secretory are found scattered in the hilar region of the ovary and associated with blood vessels and nerves. They are variously known as chromaffin cells, sympathicotropic or Berger cells, or simply as hilus cells. They can be demonstrated in the human foetus and after puberty, but are difficult to detect in prepubertal ovaries. Their cytological characteristics suggest that they are also derived from the medullary blastema and are homologous to testicular Leydig cells, and similarly secrete androgenic hormones. The exact hormonal status of interstitial cells *per se* is less certain. They appear to exhibit androgenic activity under certain conditions, although there is much evidence for the view that they synthesize oestrogenic hormones. For further information on the origin and significance of ovarian secretory cells the reader should consult the reviews by Eckstein (1962), Harrison (1962) and Young (1961).

(c) Stromal Cells. The characteristic "swirly" stroma of the cortex does not develop in the human ovary until several years after birth. There is as much debate about the origin of the cells as about the other somatic elements in the ovary. It seems logical to believe that the definitive medulla, which also develops after birth, contains cells which eventually contribute to the stroma, although much of it may be derived indirectly from the follicles which undergo atresia.

As can be seen, there is a considerable lack of agreement not only about the derivation but also on the role of the somatic cell types which appear during the development of the mammalian ovary. The uncertainties that exist are only likely to be resolved by careful investigations of the kind used in the study of germ cells.

MORPHOLOGY AND HISTOLOGY; POST-NATAL

The ovaries are situated bilaterally in the pelvic region of the abdomen, where they are attached by the mesovarium to the dorsal aspect of the broad ligament. The medial end of each ovary is further attached to the lateral wall of the uterus by the ligamentum ovarii proprium, and to the pelvic wall at the opposite end by the suspensory ligament, in which run the ovarian blood vessels. Except for cyclical changes, the ovaries are equal in size and superficially similar in shape to a large almond. The surface is generally smooth, although the outline may sometimes be disturbed by the presence of a large Graafian follicle or corpus luteum; pitting and scarring of the surface also becomes more evident in older subjects, due to successive rupturing of follicles during ovulation.

Many of the principal cellular components of the ovary have already received some consideration in the previous section. What follows is a brief description of their interrelationships in the ovary between birth and the menopause. It should be recognized that an examination of the fixed ovary provides only a glimpse at what is structurally the most changeable organ in the body. Important changes, as we have seen, occur during foetal life, and these continue after birth and into old age, although the mechanisms involved may differ. For the mature ovary, as Greep (1963) puts it: ". . . the adult ovary and its retinue of accessory adnexa operate in a cyclical manner that is unique among all systems of the body. Consequently, when we look at the structure of the ovary as seen in histologic sections we are seeing nothing more than a still frame out of a cinema of cyclic anatomic and physiologic events." The author was referring in particular to the developmental history of oocytes and their associated follicles, and the behaviour of the latter following the discharge of the oocyte. Other features of the ovary do not change perhaps so readily, so that we may think of the "germinal" epithelium, stroma and medulla as being relatively static. Nevertheless even these alter, both in composition and prominence, over the course of time, and it is essential to recognize the most important of the changes which take place between immaturity and old age.

A. The Ovary in Childhood

Within the course of the first few weeks following birth all oocytes which have succeeded in differentiating as far as the diplotene phase of meiosis become enclosed in primordial follicles (see p. 115). These are generally widely scattered through the substance of the gonad (Figs. 9, 10) but in time become limited to a relatively narrow peripheral zone. This is due to a number of factors.

1. Formation of the Definitive Tunica Albuginea

A zone of connective tissue, somewhat hyaline in appearance, gradually develops immediately underneath the epithelial covering of the ovary. It is composed largely of elongated cells and interwoven bundles of collagen fibres and, although developing in parallel with the vascular supply in the stroma, remains relatively avascular; (p. 111, testis and Figs. 11, 12). Oocytes disappear slowly from this region either during the course of spontaneous follicular atresia or simply by being pushed deeper into the underlying cortex. The tunica albuginea may be considered well formed by the age of about 10 to 12 years, although it increases in thickness throughout life and merges with the stroma in old ovaries. It forms a tough, resilient layer which is often difficult to cut during dissection; it is all the more remarkable that follicles rupture through it with comparative ease. It should be noted that this tunica differs from the primary tunica albuginea not only in the character of its tissue but also in that the latter, appearing early in development, separates the primary cortex and primary medulla (Fig. 26).

2. Formation of the Definitive Ovarian Medulla

The medulla of the adult ovary is mainly occupied by the large tortuous blood vessels which enter and leave by the

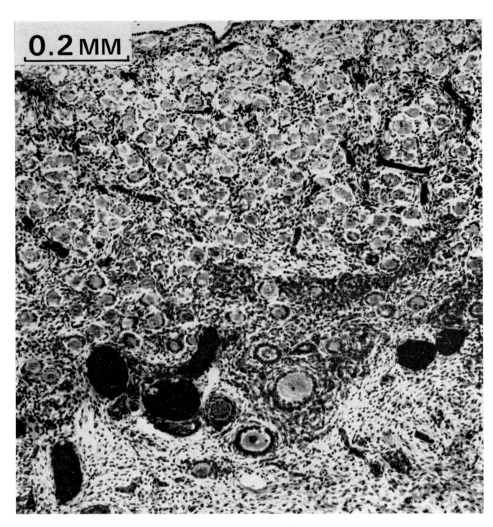

FIG. 9. Section through human ovary (neonatal). The cortex is dominated by oocytes at diplotene, in primordial follicles, and has been extensively invaded by blood vessels and other stromal elements. Large blood vessels in the developing secondary medulla are shown deeply stained. Follicles in the early stages of growth are present in this region.

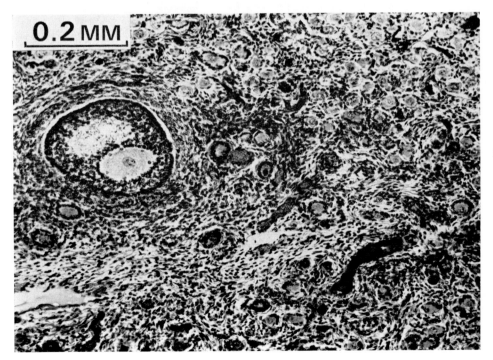

FIG. 10. Section similar to that in Fig. 9, showing a secondary follicle, and the penetration of the cortex by fusiform stromal cells typical of older ovaries. (Material for Figures 3 to 10 loaned by Dr. T. G. Baker.)

hilus, supported by networks of connective tissue. Since the vascular supply of the infant ovary is poor in comparison, this region is inconspicuous and does not reach the proportions seen in the adult until about 7 years of age. At this time the medulla and cortex are distinct regions of the ovary, although connective tissue interconnections make it difficult to draw a sharp line of demarcation between the two.

3. Growth and Atresia of Follicles

As already mentioned, precocious follicular development is not uncommon in late fœtal ovaries and is quite widespread after birth. Usually, it is the more deeply situated primordial follicles which first pass through the normal stages of differentiation and may reach the Graafian follicle stage (p. 119). Since ovulation does not normally begin until about 12 to 14 years of age, all follicles which enter the growth phase will become atretic in the space of a few days. Many growing follicles begin to degenerate

before the antrum begins to form; a drastic reduction in total numbers is due, of course, to atresia in primordial follicles (p. 114). However, the large size and rapid growth of a small proportion tends to push the main mass of primordial follicles out towards the tunica albuginea. The cortex therefore appears to have an outer zone containing many oocytes (Fig. 11) and a relatively sterile inner stroma.

The pattern of atresia of growing follicles is very variable. Either the oocyte or some part of the follicle may show the earliest signs of degeneration. Not uncommonly the nuclear chromatin of the oocyte in growing follicles passes through an abortive reduction division ("pseudomaturation" changes), often well in advance of the normally associated stages of follicular development (see p. 123 and Ingram, 1962). It appears that the somatic cells which survive from atretic follicles are incorporated into the cortical stroma, which gradually increases in amount during prepubertal and early adult life.

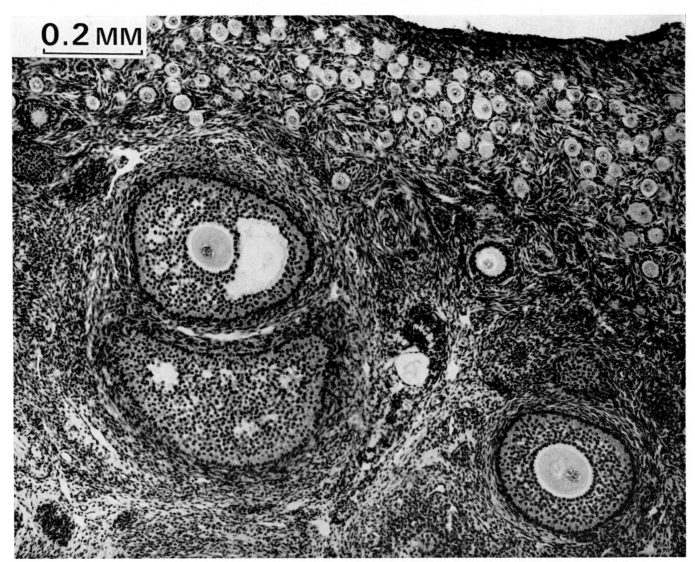

Fig. 11. Section through ovarian cortex (sexually mature rhesus monkey) showing the outer narrowed zone containing many primordial follicles, flanked externally by the sterile tunica albuginea and internally by the deeper cortex which contains follicles in various stages of growth.

B. The Ovary at Puberty

The main distinction between pre- and post-pubertal ovaries lies in the fact that menstrual activity is established, and some follicles which begin their growth phase survive and eventually undergo ovulation. The remnants of each follicle subsequently develop into the yellowish structure called a corpus luteum. An examination of ovaries at various times after puberty will thus reveal additional features which are indicative of active reproductive capacity, and it is possible to follow the complete life history of the oocyte and follicle.

1. Growth of the Follicle (Figs. 11, 13)

During the course of each menstrual cycle a small number of follicles enter a stage of rapid growth, culminating in the process of ovulation. Whilst multiple ovulation occurs in many species of animals, only one oocyte is

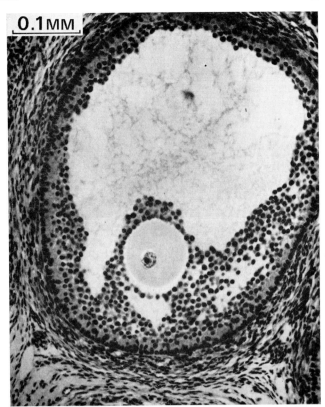

FIG. 13. A Graafian follicle from the monkey ovary. The oocyte is large compared with those in Fig. 12. The unstained zone around the apparently featureless cytoplasm of the oocyte is the zona pellucida (see also Fig. 15). The cumulus oöphorus remains part of the granulosa cell layer in this follicle. Note the epithelial character of the outermost layer of granulosa cells, and the developing theca beyond it. The fluid in the antrum has formed an irregular precipitate upon fixation.

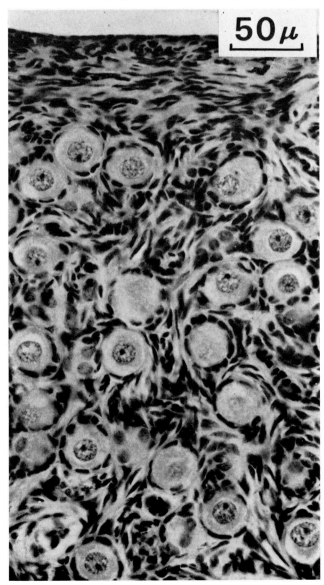

FIG. 12. Outer cortex of monkey ovary at higher magnification. Note the character of the primordial follicles and of the stroma and tunica. The "germinal" epithelium at the top consists of flattened mesothelial cells.

discharged per cycle from the pair of human ovaries as a rule.[7]

Characteristic changes take place both in the oocyte and the surrounding follicle. The flattened cells of the primordial follicle become roughly cuboidal in shape and proceed to divide by mitosis until a compact, multilayered structure, the *membrana granulosa* (or simply, the granulosa), surrounds the oocyte. The outermost layer of cells retains its epithelial character and is supported by a prominent basement membrane. During this time the oocyte itself remains more or less central in the follicle; later, irregular spaces appear between the cells of the granulosa and these merge to form a fluid-filled *antrum*, which pushes the oocyte to one side as it enlarges. Follicles containing an antrum, commonly called Graafian follicles, are also known as

[7] Several follicles in each ovary may grow during the course of a menstrual cycle even although only one normally ovulates. It is generally considered that the process is controlled quantitatively by pituitary hormones and that the amount of oestrogenic hormones produced by the additional follicles satisfies the requirements of the reproductive tract. Follicles which fail to ovulate undergo early atresia (p. 118) or may become luteinized to form accessory corpora lutea, passing through the same cycle of events as in normal corpora lutea (see p. 124) except that they contain a degenerating oocyte. Such accessory structures are not uncommon in primates (see Harrison, 1962).

The factors which condition the particular follicles that ovulate rather than degenerate are not understood.

vesicular or *secondary* follicles, but it should be remembered that the enclosed germ cell is diploid and thus still a primary oocyte. Continued rapid elaboration of follicular fluid further enlarges the follicle, the granulosa of which forms a proportionately thinner wall except in the immediate neighbourhood of the oocyte, which is surrounded by a mound of granulosa cells termed the *cumulus oöphorus* (Figs. 13, 14).

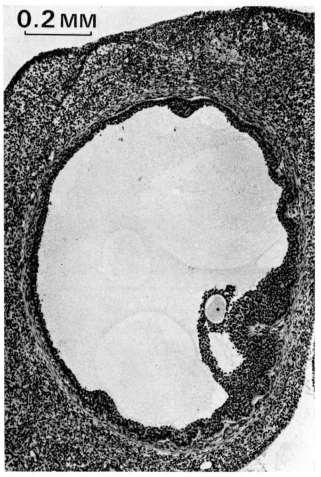

0.2 MM

FIG. 14. Early tertiary follicle (mature rat ovary). Note the proportionately greater size of the antrum, thinning and folding of the granulosa layer and the differentiation of the thecal layers. The chromatin of the oocyte in this follicle has begun to condense prior to the first maturation division (see text).

During the growth of the granulosa layer the follicle acquires two additional features. The first is a jelly-like coat, the *zona pellucida*, immediately surrounding the oocyte. This starts to develop while the granulosa layer is still one cell thick and is probably secreted entirely by the follicle cells. It soon forms a complete layer, reaching a maximum thickness of about 4μ when the follicle is fully developed. The zona is composed of amorphous material rich in mucopolysaccharides. Fine cytoplasmic extensions from the proximal granulosa cells penetrate through it and lie in contact with the oocyte cell membrane, which also sends many short microvilli into the zona, (Fig. 15). There is, however, no evidence from electron microscopical studies that the cytoplasm of the two cells freely communicates,

and the functional significance of the close relationship remains rather obscure (Franchi, 1960; Wartenberg & Stegner, 1960). The second addition is in the form of a sheath or theca, external and concentric to the granulosa. This begins developing before antrum formation, but later differentiates into a vascular *theca interna*, with large glandular cells which produce œstrogenic hormones, and a *theca externa* of fusiform cells which differ little from those of the surrounding stroma. The possible modes of origin of the theca cells were discussed earlier (p. 115) (see Figs. 11, 13, 14).

The relationship between the growth of the follicle and oocyte is an interesting one in that the system exhibits a biphasic pattern (Fig. B; Green & Zuckerman, 1951).[8] It will be noted that the oocyte undergoes a 2- or 3-fold increase in diameter during the pre-antrum phase of follicular growth, but thereafter virtually ceases growing. Curves such as that shown may be constructed for the follicles of many mammals, based on the regression equation: $y = a + bx$, where x and y are the diameters of the follicle and oocyte respectively, and a and b are regression coefficients. The major part of the increase in follicle size during the second phase is due to the accumulation of follicular fluid. This becomes even more pronounced just prior to ovulation, when there is a dramatic increase in the size of the antrum due to the accumulation of a less viscous form of follicular fluid. There is reason to believe that the latter represents, not a sudden spurt in the secretory activity of the granulosa cells, but a sequestration of lymph from the highly vascular theca interna. One of the results of this rapid follicular enlargement is that the follicle forms a conspicuous bulge up to 2 cm. across on the surface of the ovary, and there is a significant thinning out of the overlying tissue.

2. Ovulation (Fig. 14)

(a) Changes in the Follicle. The pre-ovulatory swelling of the antrum marks the beginning of what is often called the *tertiary* follicle stage. It is accompanied by a number of rapidly successive changes in the oocyte and in each of the cellular layers of the follicle wall. Early on, the cumulus oöphorus rounds off and separates from the rest of the granulosa, so that it floats free in the antrum. Its cells become slightly rearranged, those in the inner layer becoming radially disposed. This layer is termed the *corona radiata*. Shortly before ovulation the follicle wall becomes thinner on the side nearest the ovarian surface. At one point, the stigma, rupture will occur to release the oocyte in its envelope of cumulus cells. The stigma develops as a conical protrusion which rapidly penetrates the outer surface of the ovary and persists for a while as a thin membrane until it is ruptured by the egress of follicular fluid. Although it has been shown that the fluid in pre-ovulatory follicles is under a considerable pressure, observations of the actual process show that this is not a major

---

[8] Whereas the second phase of follicular growth is dependent on circulating follicle-stimulating hormone levels, the first phase is largely independent of pituitary stimulation. This has been demonstrated in hypophysectomized animals. The presence of follicles in the second growth phase in the ovaries of the fœtus is probably due to stimulation by maternal gonadotrophins.

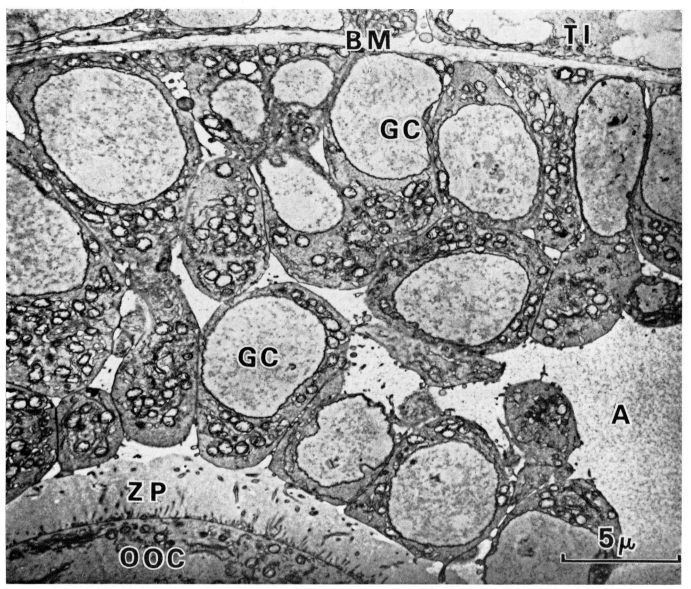

FIG. 15. An electron micrograph of a part of a small secondary follicle (rat ovary). Only a small part of the oocyte is shown (OOC). The zona pellucida (ZP) and the cytoplasmic processes which penetrate it are clearly shown. Also note the granulosa cells (GC), antrum (A), membrana propria (BM) and part of the theca interna (TI).

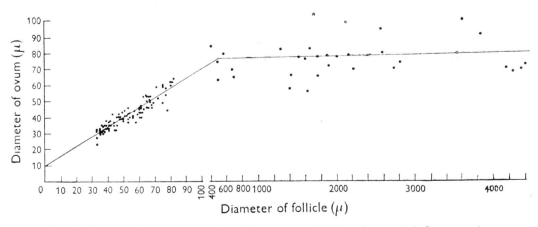

FIG. B. Regression lines relating the size of the oocyte and follicle during growth in human ovaries.
From Green & Zuckerman, (1951).

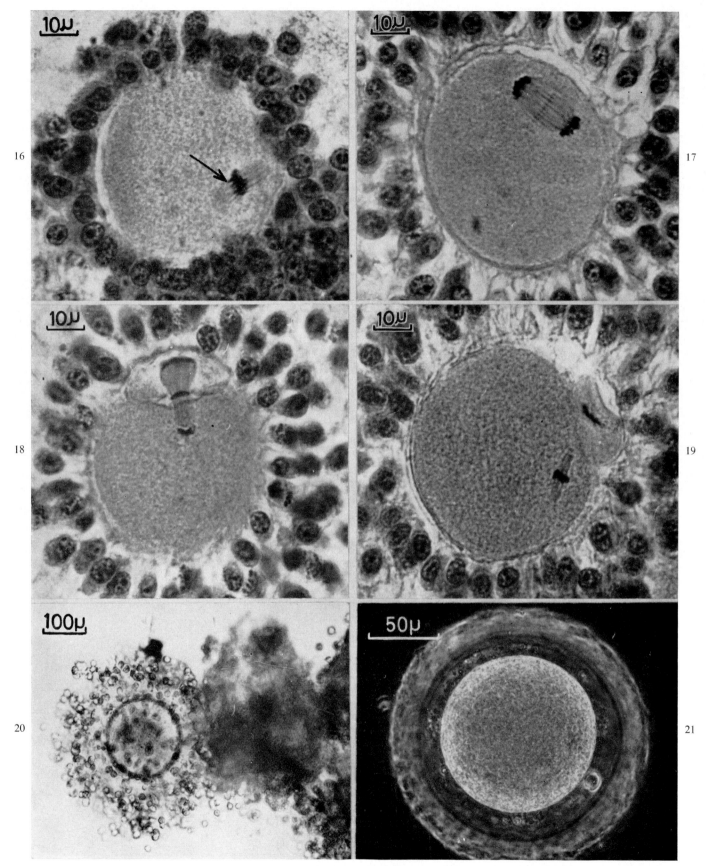

FIGS. 16–21. (See foot of opposite page for legends.)

factor in inducing ovulation. There is little or no sign of an explosive rupture, followed by the immediate collapse of the follicle. The cumulus emerges from the stigma in a slow oozing fashion, followed by a variable amount of fluid. In the human, $1\frac{1}{2}$ to 2 minutes may elapse between the formation of the stigma and the emergence of the cumulus. These recent observations of the phenomenon *in vivo* have largely helped to clarify earlier ideas about the mechanisms involved. Theories which have been advanced to explain ovulation include such factors as osmotic pressure, enzyme action, chemical changes and hormone action, and these have been adequately reviewed by Asdell (1962) and Blandau (1966) (Fig. 20).

Loss of blood from the attenuated theca in the vicinity of the rupture point usually appears to be minimal, since the stigma itself is avascular. Bleeding is probably also reduced by the local constriction of blood vessels. Recent ovulation points on the ovarian surface are marked by a local hyperæmia which gradually dissipates during the formation of the corpus luteum (see below).

(b) Changes in the Oocyte. The most significant changes which occur in the oocyte during follicular growth are not observed until a few hours before ovulation, generally on the 13th or 14th day following menstruation. Prior to this the oocyte nucleus remains in the diplotene configuration which was established near the time of birth, although some changes in chromosomal form may occur during the first phase of follicle growth (see p. 114). The large increase in cytoplasmic volume also occurring then is accompanied by changes in the number and distribution of mitochondria, in the Golgi apparatus and in other cytoplasmic organelles.

During pre-ovulatory follicular changes the chromatin of the oocyte resumes the long-interrupted prophase of meiosis. While the process has been closely studied in mammals other than man, such data as are available for the human oocyte suggests a precisely similar pattern of events. The prominent nucleolus first loses much of its basophilia and the chromosomal strands become condensed around it. In consequence, the nucleus appears rather empty (the so-called "germinal vesicle"). Subsequently the nucleolus and chromosomes contract down to form a highly chromophilic knot of reduced size, the "chromatin mass". This and the following stage, diakinesis, take place very rapidly, for example, in about 2 hours in the rat and mouse (see Mandl, 1963). Diakinesis is marked by the formation out of the chromatin mass of a small rosette of punctate chromosomes. This stage is soon followed by the breakdown of the nuclear membrane and the formation of a spindle at the periphery of the cell (prometaphase). The congression of the chromosomes on to the equator of the spindle marks the first metaphase stage. The anaphase and telophase of this first division are highly significant in the life history of the oocyte, since they result in the production of two haploid cells. One set of chromosomes remains in the oocyte and the other set separates off, together with a small amount of cytoplasm, to form the first polar body. In this manner the oocyte is transformed into the *secondary oocyte* (Table 1). The polar body remains attached to it for a while by a prominent spindle remnant called the mid-body. When it eventually becomes detached it persists inside the zona pellucida and may undergo fission during the subsequent maturation stages of the oocyte (see below), although eventually it degenerates (see Figs. 16–21).

The nuclear changes which have been described take place in the oocyte while it is enclosed in the pre-ovulatory follicle. Those which follow may begin only a few minutes before the actual process of ovulation. The chromosomes in the cytoplasm of the oocyte remain in a highly condensed state (unlike the post-telophase chromosomes of somatic cells, which become extended again) and become arranged on a second metaphase spindle, which is smaller and more barrel-shaped than the first (opposite, Fig. 19). The second maturation division, for which this is a preparation, is a straightforward mitosis, although it is not normally completed unless fertilization takes place. After the entry of a sperm (Table 1) the division continues and one set of the chromosomes is again ejected to form a second polar body. The set which remains in the oocyte is soon enclosed by a membrane and becomes the female *pronucleus*. The presence of the sperm head (male pronucleus) has restored the diploid constitution of the cell, which is therefore the zygote. Actual fusion of the male and female pronuclei does not appear to take place; mingling of maternal and paternal chromosomes is first observed when they are liberated into the cytoplasm at the prometaphase of the first cleavage division.

(c) The Term "Ovum". It seems appropriate to digress at this point in order to clarify an item of terminology which can be the cause of much confusion. Many workers use the term *ovum* to refer to oocytes which have ovulated; it is equally used to refer to oocytes at any stage of their intra-ovarian life. Primary oocytes, as defined above, are

---

Figs. 16–21. Stages in the maturation divisions of mammalian oocytes.

Fig. 16 (top, left). Oocyte in pre-ovulatory follicle of the mouse ovary. First metaphase spindle (arrow).

Fig. 17 (top, right). Same. First anaphase. Each pole of the spindle carries a haploid chromosome complement.

Fig. 18 (middle, left). Late telophase of first maturation division. The membrane of the first polar body has formed, but the spindle is still present, bearing a prominent equatorial mid-body (see text, above). The chromatin of the secondary oocyte and first polar body remain condensed at the spindle poles.

Fig. 19 (middle, right). The stage immediately preceding ovulation. The first polar body has separated from the oocyte. The first spindle has disappeared, and the chromosomes of the oocyte have become arranged at the equator of the second spindle. Completion of this division occurs after ovulation and is dependent upon fertilization.

Fig. 20 (bottom, left). Freshly ovulated secondary oocyte (rhesus monkey). The cell is embedded in a mass of cumulus cells and a small clot of follicular fluid.

Fig. 21 (bottom, right). Similar oocyte, cumulus dispersed. The first polar body and some debris which may be of cytoplasmic origin are present inside the zona pellucida. (Photographic negatives for Figs. 16–21 were kindly loaned by Dr. J. H. Marston.)

diploid cells which are wholly intra-ovarian. Secondary oocytes, similarly, are cells in which the chromosome complement has been halved during the first maturation division. These terms alone suffice to distinguish the major phases in gamete production in the female. The ovum is, theoretically, the cell which results from the completion of the second maturation division (and, therefore, exactly equivalent to the spermatozoon). It will be noted, however, that the existence of the ovum, as here defined, is impossible: either the secondary oocyte is fertilized and becomes a zygote, or it degenerates in the Fallopian tube without completing its maturation.

The author would like to add his wishes to those of Oakberg (1965) that the use of the term ovum should be discontinued when describing female gametogenesis in vertebrates. If it is retained, through convenience, authors should define what they mean, and in any case restrict its use to post-ovulatory oocytes.

3. The Corpus Luteum (see Figs. 22–24)

Following the discharge of the secondary oocyte, the remains of the ruptured follicle undergo changes which convert it into the corpus luteum. This takes place under the influence of pituitary luteinizing hormone. The function of the corpus luteum is to produce progesterone and other hormones, but it is only developed to its full extent in the event of pregnancy. That of a non-pregnant woman may only persist for about two weeks before degenerative changes set in.

The histological changes taking place during corpus luteum formation in the human ovary were described in great detail as early as 1911 by Meyer, whose account is regarded as the classical work on this subject. The development follows along similar lines whether or not pregnancy supervenes; the early onset of cellular degeneration in the latter instance provides a means of distinguishing between the two histologically (see Dubreuil, 1944).

The gradual collapse of the ruptured follicle causes the extended granulosa layer to undergo considerable folding. The rupture point is sealed off both by this means and by the formation of a coagulum of follicular fluid and blood into which stromal and epithelial cells grow. The cells of the granulosa become hypertrophied and the cytoplasm fills with lipid droplets. Such modified cells are known as *granulosa lutein cells*. Cells of the theca interna also undergo hypertrophy but remain in distinct groups at the bases of the folds of the granulosa wall. Histochemical tests have shown that both types of lutein cell contain the precursor substances for steroid hormone synthesis (unlike the situation in the Graafian follicle, where granulosa cells are histochemically rather inert).

An additional cell type, called the "K" cell, has been described. It is thought to originate from the theca interna prior to ovulation. Unlike other theca lutein cells, "K" cells penetrate into the granulosa layer. They are irregular in shape and give an intense histochemical reaction for alkaline phosphatase, lipids and phospholipids (White, Hertig, Rock & Adams, 1951). The nature of these cells is not fully understood. It has been suggested that they are a particular phase in the cycle of normal theca lutein

cells. Their properties indicate that they may be a rich source of progesterone.

During the luteinization process the vascular supply of the corpus luteum becomes more elaborate. Capillaries invade the granulosa layer together with connective tissue elements which pass through into the central cavity. The latter gradually fills with fibroblasts and other cells, the products of which include a high proportion of amorphous

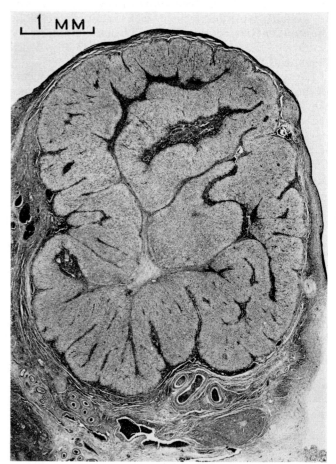

FIG. 22. Corpus luteum of pregnancy (rhesus monkey). The walls of the body show considerably greater thickening and folding than in the menstrual corpus luteum, and the central cavity is almost occluded.

material. This invasive process marks the stage of maturity of the corpus luteum, some 8 to 10 days after ovulation. In the absence of fertilization gradual involution then follows, in which a variety of degenerative processes takes part. Blood is extravasated into the central region, the lutein cells undergo lipolysis and atrophy, and the structure is further invaded by connective tissue cells. Eventually, it is converted into a hyaline body of reduced size called the corpus albicans. The corpora albicantia of recent menstrual cycles are usually apparent in a mature ovary, although they gradually shrink and become dispersed into the ovarian stroma (see Fig. 25).

The corpus luteum of pregnancy does not differ qualitatively from the above either in development or senescence, but it grows to a greater size during the first 6 weeks (2·5 cm. to 5 cm.; cf. 2 cm.). Cellular proliferation,

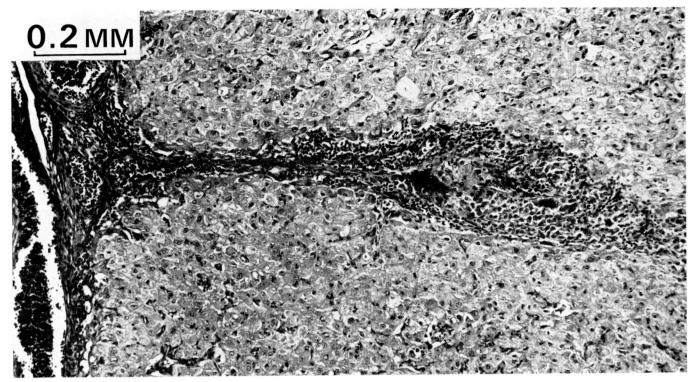

0.2 MM

FIG. 23. Detail from Fig. 22, showing granulosa lutein cells and a deep external fold containing crowded theca lutein cells amongst the vascular connective tissue.

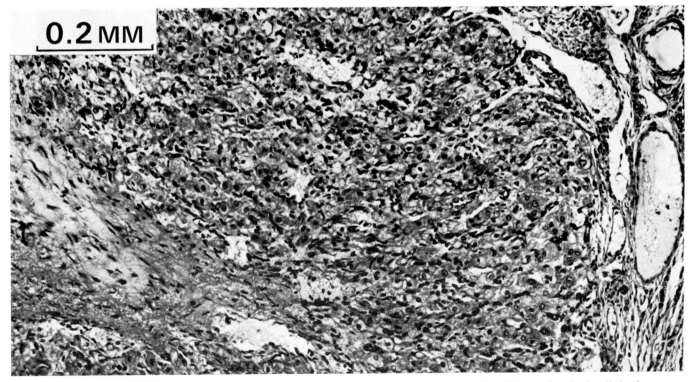

0.2 MM

FIG. 24. Similar region from a corpus luteum of menstruation *ca.* 4 days after ovulation. Hypertrophy of the granulosa lutein cells has been followed almost immediately by luteolysis in some. Thecal elements are poorly represented.

vascular supply and connective tissue framework are all accentuated. The luteal cells also maintain their secretory activity for a relatively long period and may develop large cytoplasmic colloid inclusions; small calcium deposits are also said to be characteristic (Nelson & Greene, 1958). There is ample evidence that the corpus luteum is not essential for the maintenance of pregnancy beyond the

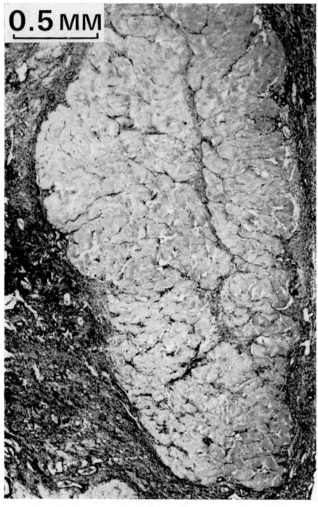

FIG. 25. Corpus albicans (human). Ingressing strands of connective tissue have begun to subdivide the structure.

first three months (Amoroso & Finn, 1962). Its functional importance probably declines well within this period owing to its replacement by placental secretions, but structural deterioration may proceed relatively slowly.

C. The Ovary at the Menopause

A wide variety of abnormalities of genital structure and function, resulting in the absence, impairment or loss of reproductive capacity, have come to light in the course of clinical investigations on women of reproductive age whose menstrual patterns depart from the normal. Infertility may stem from a number of pre- or post-natal developmental errors which affect the structure and function of the reproductive system, or from subsequent changes in the hormonal status of the ovary or another endocrine gland. A

consideration of these derangements is essentially a broad subject in itself, and outside the scope of the present chapter. The interested reader is referred to detailed reviews by Bishop (1962), Orr (1962) and Grady & Smith (1963) and see also Sec. III, Ch. 2 and Sec. X, Ch. 2.

In the normal woman, however, it is characteristic that ovarian function eventually wanes. This may be due simply to an exhaustion of the stock of oocytes (p. 114), although this is commonly preceded by the permanent cessation of menstrual cycles. This condition, which may follow an indefinite period of missed or irregularly timed cycles, is the menopause. It is an outward sign of the cessation of cyclical activity within the ovary itself, since the latter dictates the changes which take place in the wall of the uterus. In the majority of cases there is a concomitant loss of reproductive capacity; in a number of instances, however, women have been known to ovulate and even give birth a year or more after menstrual cycles have ceased (see Sharman, 1962).

The menopause usually occurs in women between the ages of 45 and 55 years. An examination of the ovaries at this time reveals that there are still a remarkable number of primordial follicles, containing apparently normal oocytes. Growing follicles are difficult to find, although commonly there are a few large, anovular cystic follicles, with a thin and atypical granulosa and a fibrous theca. The ovarian stroma is very dense and the tunica albuginea very broad. Occasionally, old corpora albicantia, in various stages of dispersion, persist. The histology of these ovaries suggests that the majority, if not all, of the normal œstrogen-producing structures are absent. Under these circumstances the level of hormone production would fail to influence the uterine endometrium, and thus constitute one of the factors leading to the cessation of menstrual cycles (Swyer, 1954). Further evidence of the decline in ovarian hormonal activity is the marked reduction in the level in circulating oestrogens. Nevertheless, the persistence of a number of oocytes in menopausal ovaries represents a potential for ovulation, fertilization and subsequent development should favourable hormonal conditions recur even on a temporary basis. Except in rare cases, however, ovulation has not been detected in women over the age of 52 years (Sharman, 1962). This indicates that the follicles are no longer sensitive to stimulation by pituitary hormones, even though gonadotrophin levels rise during the menopause. Reproductive capacity generally ceases, therefore, at 52 years of age (see Fig. 26).

The menopause is peculiar to the human race. Other menstruating species among primates, even such closely studied species as the rhesus monkey, do not appear to possess a similar post-reproductive phase of life (Krohn, 1955). Similarly, in lower mammals, cyclical ovarian activity continues into old age, although the ability or desire to mate, or the production of offspring, generally declines in advance. On the other hand, reproductive capacity seems to be influenced to some extent by the number of successful inseminations, particularly in those species where multiple ovulations take place at each cycle and litters of offspring are born. For example, in rats and mice, successive litters tend to be smaller and the more

0.2 MM

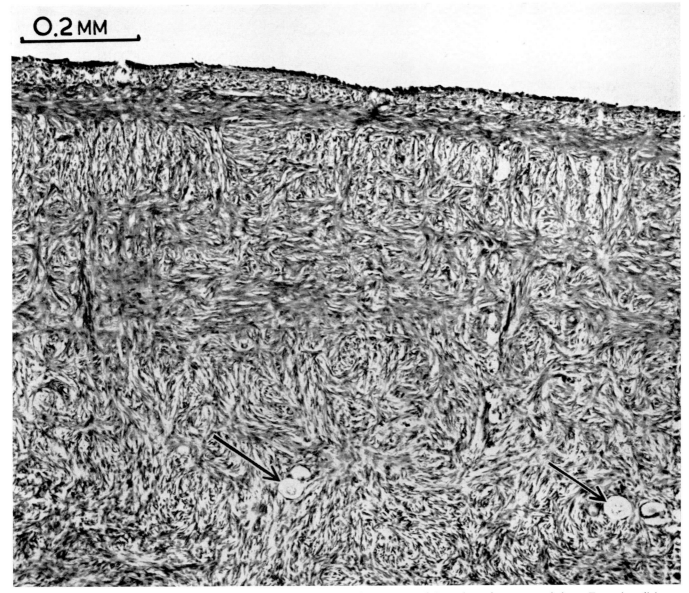

Fig. 26. The cortex of an ovary from a menopausal woman. The dense fibrous nature of the tunica and stroma are obvious. Two primordial follicles (arrows) persist relatively deep down.

frequently litters are produced, the shorter is the reproductive lifespan. Moreover, older females produce smaller first litters and reach an age where they cannot breed (Ingram, Mandl & Zuckerman, 1958; Jones & Krohn, 1960). It is also known that different inbred strains of mice lose oocytes through atresia at different rates. Some strains become devoid of oocytes (i.e. truly sterile) before the end of their lifespan, whereas others retain considerable numbers until the time of death (Jones & Krohn, 1961). Since, however, reproductive ability has declined to zero before this, it is apparent that the total number of oocytes remaining does not have the most profound influence on fertility. There is evidence that infertility in aged animals is a result of failure of the uterus to support the conceptuses. This may be due either to the lack of influence of ovarian hormones on the endometrium, or to gross developmental defects in the embryos, which are aborted.

The first of these two possibilities appears to be important in mice. For example, Talbert & Krohn (1966) have shown that eggs obtained from the Fallopian tubes of aged mice will implant successfully in the endometrium of young recipients of the same strain, although many fail to do so in the uterus of older animals.

D. The Blood Vascular Supply of the Ovary

One of the features which enables the embryologist to distinguish between the ovary and testis during early sex differentiation in the developing fœtus is the internal distribution of the blood vessels. Briefly, in the case of the testis, vessels grow into the developing gonad along with the mesenchyme that fills the cleft between the primary cortex and medulla (primary tunica albuginea). Capillary branches then penetrate from this layer into the medulla, passing in the connective tissue septa which form between the presumptive seminiferous tubules. In the ovary, however, blood vessels which enter via the hilus send out capillary branches centrifugally. The relatively massive growth of the ovarian cortex thus results in the flow of arterial blood towards the surface of the organ. After the oocytes have acquired a simple follicular covering capillary beds develop in the intervening connective tissue. During the growth of individual follicles, an extensive capillary network develops in relation to the theca interna. The granulosa layer remains avascular. During pre-ovulatory growth, the part of the follicle wall which protrudes from the surface of the ovary develops an area, the macula pellucida, which is also avascular.

The medulla of the mature ovary contains characteristically tortuous blood vessels, among which are the so-called spiral arteries. Spiralling of the main ovarian artery before it enters the hilus is not uncommon, although it is not as pronounced as that of the smaller intra-ovarian branches. The condition is known to vary with age, and is often very marked in the late foetus. This is thought by some authors to be due to relatively long-term variations in the level of circulating oestrogens. This special arterial arrangement provides the cortex with a uniform blood supply under somewhat reduced pressure. At the same time, the additional requirements of developing Graafian follicles or corpora lutea are provided for by the relaxation of the spirals in the arterial branches supplying local regions of the cortex.

The distribution of lymphatic channels in the ovary suggests that the system serves not so much for simple drainage of tissue fluid, as for the provision of additional fluid under certain conditions. The possible role of lymph in pre-ovulatory follicular swelling has already been mentioned. It may also contribute to the general hyperaemia and swelling which is observed in the ovary of some mammals prior to ovulation. Fuller accounts of the significance of the ovarian vascular distribution are given by Burr & Davies (1951) for the rabbit, Sauramo (1954) for the human, and a short general review is given by Harrison (1962).

E. Nerve Supply

Although the innervation of the female reproductive tract has been extensively studied, information on that of the ovary itself is relatively sparse. Histologically, the nerves of the ovary are difficult to identify. Recently, however, specific techniques of preparation, combined with fluorescence microscopy, have enabled some workers to detect the presence of monoamines in adrenergic fibres. When applied to the ovary these methods show that nerves arising from the lumbosacral sympathetic chain penetrate the hilus along with the major blood vessels. In the ovarian stroma the nerve bundles split up to form fine networks associated with the periphery of follicles in various stages of growth, but they do not appear to maintain a functional relationship with the arterial branches in the stroma. The vessels of the corpus luteum and those supplying groups of interstitial cells, on the other hand, receive a normal vasomotor innervation. While much of this information derives from studies on laboratory mammals (see Rosen-

gren & Sjöberg, 1967), the innervation of the human ovary is similar (Owman, Rosengren & Sjöberg, 1967).

RADIOSENSITIVITY OF THE OOCYTE

It has long been known that the germ cells of many animals are sensitive to ionizing radiations. The effects produced range from an induction of small genetic changes which may be transmitted to offspring, to a complete destruction of the germ cells, resulting in sterilization of the gonads. The degree to which damage is expressed varies considerably between species and is dependent on the dose of radiation administered. An additional factor which has come to light more recently is that the sensitivity of a germ cell varies at different stages in its life history. Comprehensive reviews on the effects of radiations on structure and function in the ovary are given by Lacassagne, Duplan, Marcovitch & Raynaud (1962), Mandl (1964), Parkes (1966) and Zuckerman (1965b).

Concern about the potential hazards of X-irradiation to the oocytes of the mother and foetus, received during routine radiological examinations, has been expressed from time to time. Whilst it is known that X-rays given in sufficient doses can cause profound disruption in a number of cell systems in man, there is far less certainty about the relative risk to germ cells. The dose received during a roentgenographic examination of the pelvis is usually of the order of 2 to 5 roentgen units (r), spread over an appreciable area of the abdomen. Prolonged examinations may exceed this figure, and repeated exposures have a cumulative effect under some circumstances. The total dose may come close to that which is known to cause genetic disturbances in the oocytes of some laboratory animals (see below), as well as more generalized effects on the developing embryos.

The validity of data obtained from animal experiments in assessing the risks to human oocytes was discussed recently[9], and the remainder of this section will be devoted to a brief consideration of some of the points which emerged.

Radiation biologists are concerned with two different levels of radiosensitivity. The first deals with doses which are sufficient to induce significant changes in genes or in chromosomal behaviour, but which do not necessarily kill the cell. Mutations may therefore be transmitted to daughter cells at meiosis, and may result in some developmental abnormality after fertilization. The second concerns the doses which will destroy the oocytes in a relatively short time. Clearly, the latter relates to sterility in the mother or foetus, while the former may result in infertility (delayed death of oocytes), abortion, still-birth, the birth of visibly abnormal offspring, or of offspring whose own germ cells are the carriers of defects which may be expressed in the following generation.

Faced with this catalogue of potential hazards the radiologist is morally bound to seek ways of reducing the

---

[9] "Symposium on the effects of low radiation doses on the maturation of the developing (human) ovum and foetus; hazards from radiological procedures." Held in May 1967 at the Royal College of Obstetricians & Gynaecologists, London, and sponsored jointly by the R.C.O.G. and the British Institute of Radiology (Br. J. Radiol., **41**, 1968).

doses of radiation received and of limiting the exposure to periods in the menstrual cycle or during pregnancy when they have a minimal effect. It is necessary, therefore, to know the comparative sensitivity of the oocyte or embryo at different stages. At present the only figures available are from studies on common laboratory animals. As will be explained, while these data may be used as a guide, the doses given cannot be reliably applied to studies on human oocytes.

In radiosensitivity experiments it is customary to use species which will breed rapidly and produce many offspring, so that results may be obtained more rapidly and analysed statistically. The mouse is one of the most widely used of mammals. It is known that as little as 15r X-rays delivered to the ovaries of a young mouse will destroy a high proportion of the primordial oocytes in a few days. Oocytes in growing follicles survive this dose, but there is a significant rise in the frequency of chromosomal disorders. The latter are expressed either as "dominant lethals", resulting in the death of the early zygotes, or as known somatic abnormalities in the offspring.

Findings such as this are at first sight discouraging to the gynæcologist, who may have to deliver $3 \times 5r$ to a patient during the course of a diagnostic examination. Recent work on rhesus monkeys, however, shows that the number of oocytes is not appreciably reduced until the ovaries have received doses of the order of 5,000r. It may require 9,000 to 12,000r to effect complete sterilization within a week (Baker, 1966). Further analysis of the results for the mouse, the rat and the monkey shows that primordial and growing follicles differ markedly in their response (Table 2). It will be noted that, whereas oocytes

TABLE 2

COMPARISON OF DOSES OF X-RAYS (r) WHICH DESTROY OOCYTES IN PRIMORDIAL AND GROWING FOLLICLES IN DIFFERENT MAMMALS (POST-IRRADIATION PERIOD: 30 DAYS).

Species	Primordial follicles	Growing follicles
Mouse	15–25	2,000
Rat	315	4,400
Monkey	7,000–12,000	<5,000

in growing follicles in all three species are killed by high doses only, those in primordial follicles in rat and mouse are much more sensitive, and those in the monkey considerably less. The key to this marked difference appears to lie in the precise chromosomal configuration of each stage. The nuclei in primordial oocytes of the rat and mouse enter the diplotene stage at about the time of birth and rapidly proceed to a diffuse chromatin sub-stage known as *dictyate*. Those in the monkey, as in the human, remain at the typical diplotene stage. In growing follicles

of all three species, the chromosomes are of the fuzzy "lampbrush" variety (see footnote 6, p. 114). These observations suggest that certain of the forms assumed by the chromosomes are less susceptible to damage by X-rays, although the possibility that other factors contribute to the death of the cell cannot be ruled out. While there are no comparable radiosensitivity figures for human oocytes, the similarity in chromosomal form to that in the monkey (Baker & Franchi, 1967b) provides grounds for the belief that they are also refractory except to very high doses. Baker & Beaumont (1967) observed that oogonia and pre-diplotene oocytes in the monkey are similarly less sensitive than those in the rat. In both species oogonia in mitosis are the most sensitive cells and irradiation of the fœtus at a crucial time may thus permanently deplete the population of germ cells.

The dose of X-rays received during radiological examinations seem unlikely to result in the loss of oocytes in the way described above. Studies on mice clearly show, however, that cells which are not easily destroyed are genetically more radiosensitive. It follows that mutation rates may be high in irradiated human oocytes. Attempts have been made, using information derived from numerous clinical records, to determine the dose of X-rays which will double the spontaneous mutation rate. Some values which have been suggested are as low as 30r (see Lacassagne et al., 1962). These estimates are open to the criticism that compared with colonies of inbred animals, human populations are genetically heterogeneous. Moreover, the time of appearance of the stages which, in the mouse, are most seriously affected—the secondary oocyte, the zygote and the embryo—cannot be determined with accuracy. Without this knowledge it is difficult to determine the extent to which either the primary oocytes or the later stages have contributed to the production of the overall figures for mutation rates. On the assumption that "the only genetically safe dose of high-energy radiation is *no* radiation" (Israel, 1966), some effort has to be made to restrict exposure without destroying the beneficial aspects of the technique. Measures aimed at reducing exposure include the development of more sensitive radiographic techniques and limitation of the area which is irradiated. In order to further minimize the risk to offspring it is recommended that examinations should be limited to the first 9 or 10 days after the onset of menstrual bleeding. In a typical cycle this should avoid the irradiation of what may be genetically the most vulnerable period for the oocyte and zygote. In view of the potential hazard to the early fœtus, the use of X-rays in the diagnosis of pregnancy should perhaps also be avoided. Techniques employing ultrasound appear to offer themselves as useful alternatives for this purpose (Bourne, see footnote 9, p. 128).

BIBLIOGRAPHY

Allen, E. (1923), "Ovogenesis during Sexual Maturity," *Amer. J. Anat.*, **31**, 439.

Amoroso, E. C. and Finn, C. A. (1962), "Ovarian Activity during Gestation, Ovum Transport and Implantation," p. 451 in *The Ovary* Vol. I (ed. S. Zuckerman, A. M. Mandl and P. Eckstein). New York and London: Academic Press.

Asdell, S. A. (1962), "The Mechanism of Ovulation," p. 435 *ibid.* Vol. I.

Baker, T. G. (1963), "A Quantitative and Cytological Study of Germ Cells in Human Ovaries," *Proc. roy. Soc. B,* **158,** 417.

Baker, T. G. (1966), "The Sensitivity of Oocytes in Post-natal Rhesus Monkeys to X-irradiation," *J. Reprod. Fertil.,* **12,** 183.

Baker, T. G. and Franchi, L. L. (1967a), "The Fine Structure of Oogonia and Oocytes in Human Ovaries," *J. cell Sci.,* **2,** 213.

Baker, T. G. and Franchi, L. L. (1967b), "The Structure of the Chromosomes in Human Primordial Oocytes," *Chromosoma (Berl.),* **22,** 358.

Baker, T. G. and Beaumont, H. M. (1967), "Radiosensitivity of Oogonia and Oocytes in the Foetal and Neonatal Monkey," *Nature, Lond.,* **214,** 981.

Beaumont, H. M. and Mandl, A. M. (1962), "A Quantitative and Cytological Study of Oogonia and Oocytes in the Foetal and Neonatal Rat," *Proc. roy. Soc. B,* **155,** 557.

Bishop, P. M. F. (1962), "Derangements of Ovarian Function," p. 553 in *The Ovary,* Vol. I (ed. S. Zuckerman, A. M. Mandl and P. Eckstein). New York and London: Academic Press.

Blandau, R. J. (1966), "The Mechanisms of Ovulation," p. 5 in *Ovulation: Stimulation, Suppression, Detection.* (ed. R. B. Greenblatt). Philadelphia: Lippincott Co.

Brambell, F. W. R. (1956), "Ovarian Changes," p. 397 in Marshall's *Physiology of Reproduction,* Vol. I, Part 1 (ed. A. S. Parkes). London: Longmans, Green & Co.

Burns, R. K. (1955), "Urinogenital System," p. 462 in *Analysis of Development* (ed. B. H. Willier, P. A. Weiss and V. Hamburger). Philadelphia: Saunders Co.

Burr, J. H. and Davies, J. I. (1951), "The Vascular System of the Rabbit Ovary and its Relationship to Ovulation," *Anat. Rec.,* **111,** 273.

Chiquoine, A. D. (1954), "The Identification, Origin and Migration of the Primordial Germ Cells in the Mouse Embryo," *Anat. Rec.,* **118,** 135.

Chiquoine, A. D. (1960), "Electron Microscopic Observations on the Vitally Stained Ovary of the Mouse," *Anat. Rec.,* **136,** 176.

Cole, H. H. and Cupps, P. T. (eds.) (1969), *Reproduction in Domestic Animals,* 2nd Edition. New York and London: Academic Press.

Dubreuil, G. (1944), "De quelques caractères propres des corps gestatifs de la femme," *C. R. Soc. Biol. (Paris),* **138,** 699.

Eckstein, P. (1962), "Ovarian Physiology in the Non-pregnant Female," p. 311 in *The Ovary,* Vol. I (ed. S. Zuckerman, A. M. Mandl and P. Eckstein). New York and London: Academic Press.

Evans, H. M. and Swezy, O. (1931), "Ovogenesis and the Normal Follicular Cycle in Adult Mammalia," *Mem. Univ. Calif.,* **9,** 119.

Franchi, L. L. (1960), "Electron Microscopy of Oocyte-follicle Cell Relationships in the Rat Ovary," *J. biophys. biochem. Cytology,* **7,** 397.

Franchi, L. L. (1962), "The Structure of the Ovary, B: Vertebrates," p. 121 in *The Ovary,* Vol. I (ed. S. Zuckerman, A. M. Mandl and P. Eckstein). New York and London: Academic Press.

Franchi, L. L., Mandl, A. M. and Zuckerman, S. (1962), "The Development of the Ovary and the Process of Oogenesis," p. 1 *ibid.,* Vol. I.

Grady, H. G. and Smith, D. E. (eds.) (1963), "The Ovary," *International Academy of Pathology Monograph No. 3.* Baltimore: Williams & Wilkins Co.

Green, S. H. and Zuckerman, S. (1951), "Quantitative Aspects of the Growth of the Human Ovum and Follicle," *J. Anat.,* **85,** 373.

Greep, R. O. (1963), "Histology, Histochemistry and Ultrastructure of Adult Ovary," p. 48 in Grady and Smith (1963), *q.v.*

Harrison, R. J. (1962), "The Structure of the Ovary, C: Mammals," p. 143 in *The Ovary,* Vol. I (ed. S. Zuckerman, A. M. Mandl and P. Eckstein). New York and London: Academic Press.

Ingram, D. L. (1962), "Atresia," p. 247 *ibid.,* Vol. I.

Ingram, D. L., Mandl, A. M. and Zuckerman, S. (1958), "The Influence of Age on Litter-size," *J. Endocr.,* **17,** 280.

Israel, S. L. (1966), "Radiation Therapy and Ovulation," p. 91 in *Ovulation: Stimulation, Suppression, Detection* (ed. R. B. Greenblatt). Philadelphia: Lippincott Co.

Jones, E. C. and Krohn, P. L. (1960), "The Effect of Unilateral Ovariectomy on the Reproductive Lifespan of Mice," *J. Endocr.,* **20,** 129.

Jones, E. C. and Krohn, P. L. (1961), "The Relationship Between Age, Numbers of Oocytes and Fertility in Virgin and Multiparous Mice," *J. Endocr.,* **21,** 469.

Krohn, P. L. (1955), "Tissue Transplantation Techniques Applied to the Problem of the Ageing of the Organs of Reproduction," *Ciba Foundation Colloquia on Ageing,* **1,** 141.

Lacassagne, A., Duplan, J. F., Marcovich, H. and Raynaud, A. (1962), "The Action of Ionizing Radiations on the Mammalian Ovary," p. 463 in *The Ovary,* Vol. II (ed. S. Zuckerman, A. M. Mandl and P. Eckstein). New York and London: Academic Press.

Mandl, A. M. (1963), "Pre-ovulatory Changes in the Oocyte of the Adult Rat," *Proc. roy. Soc. B,* **158,** 105.

Mandl, A. M. (1964), "The Radiosensitivity of Germ Cells," *Biol. Rev.,* **39,** 288.

McKay, D. G., Hertig, A. T., Adams, E. C. and Danziger, S. (1953), "Histochemical Observations on the Germ Cells of Human Embryos," *Anat. Rec.,* **117,** 201.

McKay, D. G., Hertig, A. T., Adams, E. C. and Danziger, S. (1955), "Histochemical Horizons in Human Embryos I: Five Millimeter Embryo—Streeter Horizon XIII," *Anat. Rec.,* **122,** 125.

Mintz, B. (1959), "Continuity of the Female Germ Cell Line from Embryo to Adult," *Arch. Anat. micr.,* **48,** 155.

Mintz, B. and Russell, E. S. (1957), "Gene-induced Embryological Modifications of Primordial Germ Cells in the Mouse," *J. Zool.,* **134,** 207.

Nelson, W. W. and Greene, R. R. (1958), "Some Observations on the Histology of the Human Ovary during Pregnancy," *Amer. J. Obstet. Gynec.,* **76,** 66.

Oakberg, E. F. (1965), "The Mammalian Oocyte," World Health Organization Conference on Chemistry and Physiology of the Gametes, Geneva, November 1965.

Orr, J. W. (1962), "Tumours of the Ovary and the Role of the Ovary and its Hormones in Neoplasia," p. 533 in *The Ovary,* Vol. II (ed. S. Zuckerman, A. M. Mandl and P. Eckstein). New York and London: Academic Press.

Owman, Ch., Rosengren, E. and Sjöberg, N. O. (1967), "Adrenergic Innervation of the Human Female Reproductive Organs: a Histochemical and Chemical Investigation," *Obstet. Gynec.,* **30,** 763.

Parkes, A. S. (1966), "Activation of the Gonads," p. 1 in Marshall's *Physiology of Reproduction,* Vol. III, 3rd Edition (ed. A. S. Parkes). London: Longmans, Green & Co.

Pinkerton, J. H. M., McKay, D. G., Adams, E. C. and Hertig, A. T. (1961), "Development of the Human Ovary—a Study using Histochemical Technics," *Obstet. Gynec.,* **18,** 152.

Rosengren, E. and Sjöberg, N. O. (1967), "The Adrenergic Nerve Supply to the Female Reproductive Tract of the Cat," *Amer. J. Anat.,* **121,** 271.

Sauramo, H. (1954), "The Anatomy, Histology and Histopathology and Function of the Ovarian Vascular System," *Acta obstet. gynec. scand.,* **33,** Suppl. 2, 113.

Sharman, A. (1962), "The Menopause," p. 539 in *The Ovary,* Vol. I (ed. S. Zuckerman, A. M. Mandl and P. Eckstein). New York and London: Academic Press.

Swyer, G. I. M. (1954), *Reproduction and Sex,* p. 58. London: Routledge & Kegan Paul.

Talbert, G. B. and Krohn, P. L. (1966), "Effect of Maternal Age on Viability of Ova and Uterine Support of Pregnancy in Mice," *J. Reprod. Fertil.,* **11,** 399.

Wagenen, G. van and Simpson, M. E. (1965), *Embryology of the Ovary and Testis*—Homo sapiens *and* Macaca mulatta, p. 1. New Haven and London: Yale University Press.

Wartenberg, H. and Stegner, H. E. (1960), "Uber die elektronen-mikroskopische Feinstruktur des menschlichen Ovarialeies," *Z. Zellforsch.,* **52,** 450.

Weismann, A. (1885), *Die Continuität des Keimplasmas als Grundlage einer Theorie der Vererbung.* Jena.

White, R. F., Hertig, A. T., Rock, J. and Adams, E. C. (1951), "Histological and Histochemical Observations on the Corpus Luteum of Pregnancy with Special Reference to Corpora Lutea

Associated with early Normal and Abnormal Ova." *Contr. to Embryol Carneg. Instn*, **34**, 55.

Witschi, E. (1948), "Migration of the Germ Cells of Human Embryos from the Yolk Sac to the Primitive Gonadal Folds." *Contr. to Embryol. Carneg. Instn*, **32**, 67.

Witschi, E. (1951), "Embryogenesis of the Adrenal and the Reproductive Glands," *Recent Prog. Hormone Res.*, **6**, 1.

Witschi, E., Bruner, J. A. and Segal, S. J. (1953), "The Pluripotentiality of the Mesonephric Blastema," *Anat. Rec.*, **115**, 381.

Wolff, E. (1962), "Experimental Modification of Ovarian Development," p. 81 in *The Ovary*, Vol. II (ed. S. Zuckerman, A. M. Mandl and P. Eckstein). New York and London: Academic Press.

Young, W. C. (1961), "The Mammalian Ovary," p. 449 in *Sex and Internal Secretions*, Vol. I, 3rd Edition (ed. W. C. Young). Baltimore: Williams & Wilkins Co.

Zuckerman, S. (1951), "The Number of Oocytes in the Mature Ovary," *Recent. Prog. Hormone Res.*, **6**, 63.

Zuckerman, S. (1956), "The Regenerative Capacity of Ovarian Tissue," *Ciba Foundation Colloquia on Ageing*, **2**, 31.

Zuckerman, S. (1965a), "The Natural History of an Enquiry," *Ann. roy. Coll. Surg. Engl.*, **37**, 133.

Zuckerman, S. (1965b), "The Sensitivity of the Gonads to Radiation," *Clin. Radiol.*, **16**, 1.

Zuckerman, S., Mandl, A. M. and Eckstein, P. (eds.) (1962), *The Ovary*, Vol. I. New York and London: Academic Press.

2. OVULATION

CARL GEMZELL

Ovulation is a process whereby an egg is released from the ovary and becomes available for conception to occur. The normal human ovary contains about 400,000 eggs at birth. Only a few of these are released by the process of ovulation during the 3 decades or so of a woman's reproductive life, and the others degenerate. Once the ovarian cycle has been established at the time of menarche it goes on uninterrupted to the time of the menopause when no more eggs are present in the ovary. Ovulation is interrupted by pregnancy and subsequent lactation. Following termination of pregnancy, the cyclic release of eggs is resumed after a variable interval. In women who for various reasons do not ovulate the degeneration of eggs occurs at a similar rate.

Ovulation is under the control of two gonadotrophic hormones from the anterior pituitary, follicle stimulating hormone (FSH) and luteinizing hormone (LH), otherwise known as interstitial cell stimulating hormone (ICSH). At the onset of a cycle and under the influence of FSH, a follicle which has reached the antrum stage of development, ripens and starts secreting estrogens. The rupture of this follicle or ovulation itself is a phenomenon which requires the addition of LH. After ovulation the follicle is converted into a corpus luteum which in the absence of pregnancy starts degenerating after 10 to 14 days. In humans there is nothing to suggest that a third hormone from the anterior pituitary, prolactin or luteotropic hormone (LTH), is intricately involved in controlling the life span or function of the corpus luteum. Induction of ovulation can be induced in a hypophysectomized patient with FSH and LH alone and the subsequent corpus luteum has the normal life span of 2 weeks (Gemzell and Kjessler, 1964).

During the past 20 years a large amount of evidence has been presented which indicates that the release of pituitary gonadotropins is under hypothalamic control. Protein or polypeptide extracts from the hypothalamus are capable of stimulating the release of specific hormones from the anterior pituitary. The pituitary is dependent on these factors to establish the amount and duration of secretion of its gonadotropic hormones. Destruction or dysfunction of the hypothalamus or the removal of the pituitary from hypothalamic control results in disturbances of ovarian function. As yet no hypothalamic extract has been available for clinical use.

The number of follicles developing to maturity and the rate at which follicles mature seem to be constant for each species. By the addition of exogenous FSH the number of follicles can be increased but the rate at which the follicles mature is unaltered. Thus, in order to deliver a certain number of eggs, significant for each species, the amount of FSH released from the anterior pituitary must be constant.

In the human female, during the early part of each menstrual cycle, a group of follicles start to grow. When they have reached a certain size only one goes further to full maturation and rupture while the others became atretic. The mechanism behind this selection of a single follicle is not understood. It may be that the amount of FSH released from the pituitary is only enough to evoke estrogen production in the most receptive follicle. This endocrine response of the follicle might then depress the release of FSH below the reactive threshold of other follicles. An alternative hypothesis is that appreciable amounts of estrogen produced by the dominant follicle may desensitize the other follicles to FSH.

Initially a follicle stimulating effect was obtained by using FSH obtained from animal pituitaries or by hormones extracted from pregnant mare's serum (PMS). In 1958 Gemzell *et al.* reported that FSH from human pituitaries when administered to amenorrheic women produced follicular growth and estrogen excretion and together with human chorionic gonadotropin (HCG) brought about ovulation. In 1960 Lunefeld and collaborators showed that FSH extracted from menopausal urine was also clinically active. This is named human menopausal gonadotropin (HMG) and the purification of this factor has been carried out by Donini, Puzzuoli and Montezemolo (1964).

Roos (1967) has recently purified FSH from human

pituitaries and from urine of menopausal women and compared their physico-chemical and biological properties. The yield of FSH was about 2 μg. per pituitary with a biological activity of 14,000 IU per mg. and about 1 μg. per litre of urine with a potency of 780 IU per mg. The molecular weight of pituitary FSH was 41,000 and approximately 28,000 for urinary FSH. Although the pituitary and urinary FSH are chemically different, their clinical effect seems to be identical. However, final opinion about this point must await the results of extensive clinical trials using pituitary and urinary preparations on the same patients.

There has never been any need to use LH for the induction of ovulation thanks to the luteinizing effect of chorionic gonadotropin which is readily extracted from pregnancy urine. When sufficient supplies of LH are to hand it will be desirable to test it clinically.

Valuable information about human ovulation can be achieved through 3 different means:

1. Assays of FSH, LH, estrogens and pregnanediol in blood and urine during normal spontaneous ovulation;

2. studies of the effect of exogenous FSH and LH on the process of ovulation; and

3. morphological studies of the follicles during different phases of the menstrual cycle.

It seems reasonable to assume that the pattern of FSH, LH, estrogens and progesterone in blood and urine reflects the corresponding changes in their release from the pituitary and the ovaries respectively. A present day concept of the urinary excretion of FSH, LH, the three classic estrogens and pregnanediol during a normal menstrual cycle is shown in (Fig. 1). There are two FSH peaks, one in the early part of the cycle and another in the mid-cycle. LH excretion is low throughout the cycle except for a midcycle rise of 4 days. The three estrogens rise continuously during the first 10 days of the cycle. Thereafter, following a decrease at the time of ovulation, a second rise is noticed with a peak around the 20th day of the cycle. Following the LH peak a rise in pregnanediol excretion is found, which lasts to the time of menstruation.

In assessing follicular status it is of interest to form some impression about the number of follicles stimulated as well as the maturity they have achieved. Brown (1955) measured the 24 hour urinary excretion of estrogen during 10 menstrual cycles of 8 women between 17 and 40 years of age. He found that the total estrogen excretion begins to rise at about 7 days and reaches an ovulatory peak at about 13 days with an average of 56 microg. (range 28–99 microg.) per 24 hours at that time.

Anovulation is often the basic deficit in various disorders of the hypothalamus, anterior pituitary, ovary, adrenal cortex and thyroid. In order to induce ovulation it is therefore necessary to investigate the function of these organs separately and subsequently choose the adequate therapy. Unfortunately, the most important of these organs for the control of ovulation namely the hypothalamus, pituitary and the ovary are closely integrated and a dysfunction of one of them will cause dysfunction of the others.

The most obvious example of hypothalamic dysfunction is when specific emotional disturbances such as fear of pregnancy or infertility are followed by cessation of ovulation.

The first hormone that is interfered with in the pituitary —ovarian dysfunction of hypothalamic origin is LH. Anovulation may, therefore, be the initial effect. Lack of FSH comes second and leads to ovarian arrest while a relative insufficiency of FSH may lead to anovulation.

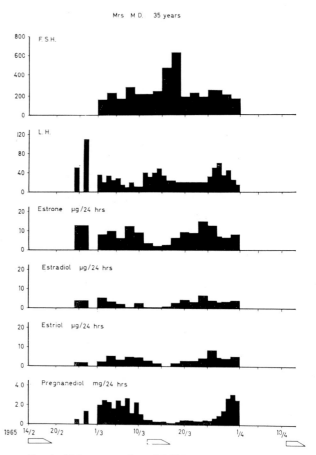

FIG. 1. Urinary excretion of follicle stimulating hormone (FSH), luteinizing hormone (LH), estrone, estradiol, estriol and pregnanediol in a normally menstruating woman. All urine is collected from the middle of one cycle to the middle of the next one.

Clomiphene has proved to be an especially useful drug in patients who do not ovulate due to hypothalamic dysfunction. It is essential that the estrogen excretion is adequate and that the FSH excretion is within normal limits. The dose of clomiphene will vary from patient to patient and depends probably upon ovarian sensitivity. The useful therapeutic procedure involves the administration of 50 to 100 mg. for 5 days starting on the fifth day of a spontaneous or progesterone induced menses.

The precise mode of action of clomiphene is not known. When administered to a woman with adequate estrogen excretion there is evidence of increase LH and eventually FSH excretion. The most important side effects of clomiphene are the formation of ovarian cysts, various vasomotor symptoms, abdominal bloating, transient blurring of vision and slight loss of hair.

The reported results of clomiphene treatment for induction of ovulation vary considerably, probably due to the fact that different criteria have been used for the selection of patients. Usually about 70 per cent are expected to ovulate once or several times and about 25 per cent became pregnant. The rate of abortion runs about 25 per cent.

In cases of anovulation with sufficient release of FSH from the pituitary human chorionic gonadotropin (HCG) can be used to induce ovulation but in general the results are not convincing. The dose of HCG has to be rather large—at least 3,000 IU for 6 days. A group of 42 women with amenorrhea were treated with HCG. Only 3 ovulated, all belonging to a group of 12 with adequate estrogen and FSH excretion. None of the 30 women who had inadequate FSH and estrogen excretion responded.

If in a case of anovulation of hypothalamic origin FSH excretion is lacking or inadequate, neither clomiphene nor HCG alone have any effect. Those cases have to be treated with human pituitary or urinary FSH followed by HCG.

It is often impossible to decide if anovulation is due to a hypothalamic dysfunction or to a pituitary failure. However, as far as treatment is concerned it makes little difference. The choice of treatment depends on the presence of adequate FSH excretion in urine. If there is no FSH in the urine the patient must be treated with human pituitary FSH followed by HCG. If there are subnormal or normal levels of FSH in the urine the patient can be treated with clomiphene or eventually HCG alone. If there is no response to this treatment human FSH and HCG should be the second choice. If the urinary FSH is abnormally high, treatment is usually worthless as the anovulation is due to a primary ovarian failure or to an early menopause.

In the polycystic ovary syndrome anovulation is the basic deficit. Most important is the alteration in steroid synthesis which occurs. The aetiology of this syndrome is unknown. It may either be due to disturbances in the hypothalamo-pituitary mechanism which leads to subnormal non-cyclic release of FSH or LH, to an adrenal cortex hyperfunction with abnormal androgen excretion in urine or to some inherent factor in the ovaries which leads to an abnormal steroid synthesis.

The woman with the polycystic ovary syndrome usually presents herself in the clinic with amenorrhoea or oligomenorrhoea. The cycles are anovulatory. The level of urinary FSH is usually low to normal, estrogen production is adequate as indicated by proliferative endometrial activity and normal to slightly elevated levels of estrogen in urine.

Three different techniques are available for the induction of ovulation in these patients, namely: wedge resection, clomiphene and human FSH followed by HCG.

By wedge resection a part of the ovaries is removed with reduction of estrogen output. As a consequence there is an interruption of the positive feed-back effect of the estrogen and the depletion of pituitary FSH is halted.

A proof of this theory is the finding that the addition of small amounts of exogenous FSH will bring about spontaneous ovulation.

The fact that fertility is corrected less often than anovulation can be due to many non-hormonal factors.

Results of wedge resection yield widely different effects. Regular cycles varies from 10 to 85 per cent and pregnancies from 15 to 90 per cent. The reason for this discrepancy in results may very well be the selection of patients.

Promising results have been reported with the use of clomiphene in patients with polycystic ovaries. Too few reports have appeared, however, for proper evaluation but it is likely that clomiphene under certain conditions in carefully selected cases will be an ideal agent.

Human pituitary FSH and HCG have been administered to a great number of patients with the polycystic ovary syndrome with mixed success. In eight patients a single treatment gave a rather strong response and was followed by spontaneous ovulation and pregnancies within 6 months. A second treatment gave usually a much more normal response than the first one and more patients became pregnant following the second than the first treatment. Two women with oligomenorrhoea, anovulation, hirsutism and obesity were treated with wedge resection without any effect on ovulation. About a year later both responded normally to human FSH and HCG. They became pregnant but aborted in the third and fifth month respectively.

It may be suggested that a single treatment with human FSH and HCG acts as a wedge resection. It brings about rupture of a great number of follicles and in that respect decreases the ovarian estrogen production and interrupts the positive feedback effect on FSH.

Even if the results following treatment with human FSH and HCG seem to be quite good, it is still an open question if this technique should be used in cases of polycystic ovaries. The great risk of treatment is superovulation leading to multiple births and the formation of large ovarian cysts. Under no circumstances should conception be allowed to take place following the first treatment. The second treatment is usually more normal as far as ovarian response is concerned. It may be that treatment with FSH alone, which is less risky, will cause follicles to rupture, and later eventually produce spontaneous ovulation.

The relationship between adrenal cortex hyperfunction and ovarian dysfunction leading to anovulation is well established. Correction of the adrenal disorder will usually improve ovarian function with restoration of ovulation. The effect of cortico-steroids on ovulation is usually rather dramatic. If the treatment is going to work it should work rather quickly. Once the woman resumes regular ovulatory cycles and the 17-ketosteroids in urine are within normal limits, it is advisable to wean her slowly from steroid treatment to determine if she will maintain ovulatory cycles on her own. A useful therapeutic procedure involves the daily administration of 25 to 40 mg. of cortisol.

Disorders of thyroid function are frequently associated with menstrual disorders. Anovulation is common in thyrotoxicosis and treatment of the disease usually results in return of ovulation. In myxoedema if a change in the menstrual cycle occurs, the clinical picture is usually that of metropathia hæmorrhagica and administration of thyroid hormone almost invariably results in the return of ovulation. The manner in which thyroid dysfunction relates to anovulation is not known but relevant observations have been made regarding the relationship between thyroid and ovarian function. In thyroidectomized animals estrogen is ineffective in suppressing pituitary gonadotropins. It is therefore possible that anovulation of patients with myxoedema is the result of persistent FSH stimulation without the interplay of LH. This suggests that HCG could be used cyclically for induction of ovulation in these patients.

An attempt has been made to discuss our present knowledge about human ovulation and our experience of induction of ovulation in patients with various menstrual disorders. Inevitably, facts have had to mingle with conjecture and theory. No excuse is made for the latter, for they must in part form a basis for future experiments, research and progress.

REFERENCES

Brown, J. B. (1955), "Urinary Excretion of Œstrogen during the Menstrual Cycle," *Lancet*, **I**, 320.
Donini, P, Puzzuoli, D. and Montezemolo, R. (1964), "Purification of Gonadotrophin from Human Menopausal Urine," *Acta Endoc.*, **45**, 321.
Gemzell, C. A., Diczfalusy, E. and Tillinger, K. G. (1958), "Clinical Effect of Human Pituitary Follicle-stimulating Hormone (FSH)," *J. clin. Endocr.*, **18**, 1333.
Gemzell, C. A. and Kjessler, B. (1964), "Treatment of Infertility after Partial Hypophysectomy with Human Pituitary Gonadotropins," *Lancet*, **I**, 644.
Lunenfeld, B., Menzi, A. and Volet, B. (1960), "Clinical Effects of Human Postmenopausal Gonadotrophin," *Acta Endocr.*, Suppl., **51**, 587.
Roos, P. (1967), "Human Follicle-stimulating Hormone," *Diss. Uppsala Univ.*

3. FERTILIZATION AND EARLY DEVELOPMENT FROM THE INNER CELL MASS

LANDRUM B. SHETTLES

The formation, maturation, and meeting of the male and female germ cells are all preliminary to their actual union into a combined cell, the zygote, which definitely marks the beginning of a new life. This penetration of ovum by sperm and the coming together and pooling of their respective nuclei constitutes the process of fertilization. It begins with the sperm-egg collision and ends with fusion of the haploid nuclei.

Although it constitutes but a tiny portion of the life span of the individual, no other time is more crowded with important events. Not the least of these is the one which provides that even though several sperm enter the ovum, normally it will be fertilized by only one, Allen (1959), Austin (1953), Blandau and Odor (1952), Shettles (1953).

CHARACTERISTICS OF SPERM AND OVUM

In fertilization the sperm stimulates the ovum to continue development, and it contributes a set of 23 chromosomes embodying the paternal contribution to the genetic make up of the zygote and a central body which is a requisite for cell division, Shettles (1964b).

Both the male and female sex cells have to be in a proper state of maturity if union is to occur. Experimentally it was demonstrated that the changes in the ovary which result in ovulation are normally controlled by the hormones of the adenohypophysis, Smith and Engle (1927). Subsequently, it has been shown that the events of the menstrual cycle are dependent upon the integration of neural and neurohumoral as well as humoral stimuli, Kawakami and Sawyer (1959).

For the human ovum to be fertilizable, it is necessary for the first polar body to be extruded; not until then does penetration by the sperm begin.

Ripening of the follicle (Figs. 1 (a), (b), (c)) normally leads to its rupture (Fig. 2) and release of the mature ovum with the first polar body formed (Fig. 1, (c), (d), (e)). These processes are governed by the gonadotropic secretion of the anterior pituitary gland under the control of the hypothalamus, (Shettles (1962a)).

The follicle-stimulating hormone (FSH) arises from the adenohypophysis and appears in the blood. Follicular maturation in the ovary is dependent on this hormone and is accompanied by the appearance of estrogen secretion in the follicular fluid. After the FSH secretion appears and maturation of the ovum occurs, the initiation of ovulation is associated with a sudden increase in secretion of the luteinizing hormone (LH). Stimulated by the follicle-ripening hormone (FSH) from the hypophysis, the dormant follicle becomes active and in about 2 weeks reaches maturity. During growth increase in blood supply and congestion occur adjacent to the follicle. For the ovum to undergo maturation before ovulation (to be ready for fertilization) the two gonadotropic secretions of the adenohypophysis must be in exact quantitative proportions to each other, but the proportions may show individual fluctuations, Lewin (1950), Shettles (1956a).

It has been observed that the relationship between the growth of the ovum (diameter in microns) and the increase in size of the follicle (diameter in microns) is the same in man as in other placental mammals in which the quantitative aspects of the process have been studied. This growth

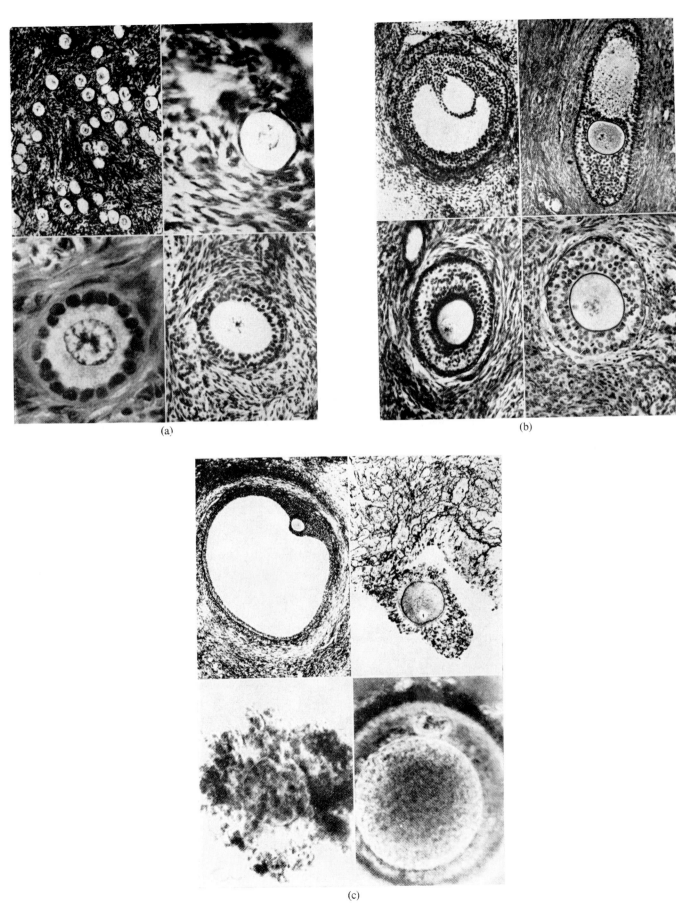

(a)

(b)

(c)

FIG. 1. *ABCDE.* Maturation stages of oocyte and ovarian follicle.

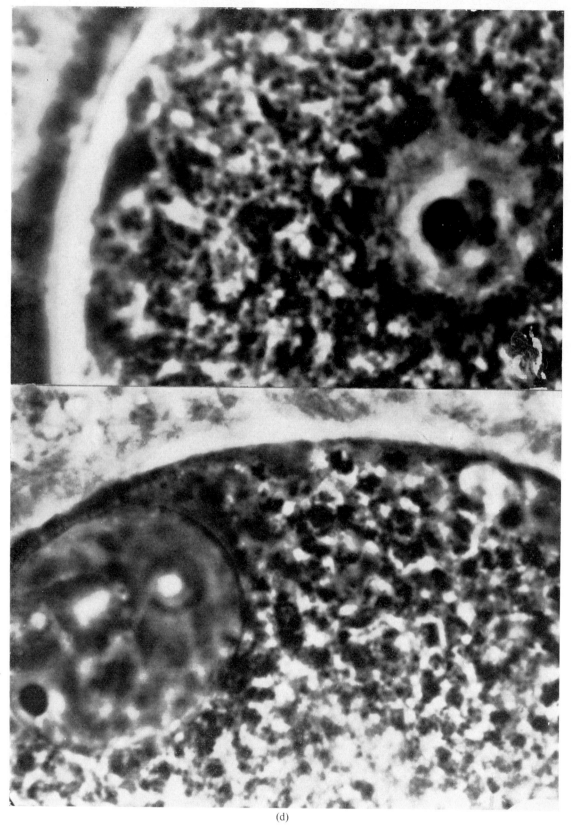

(d)

Fig. 1. (*contd.*)

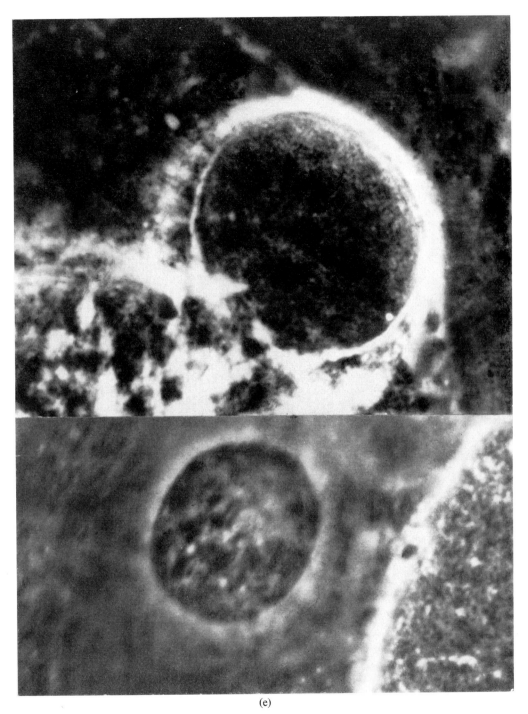

(e)

FIG. 1. (*contd.*)

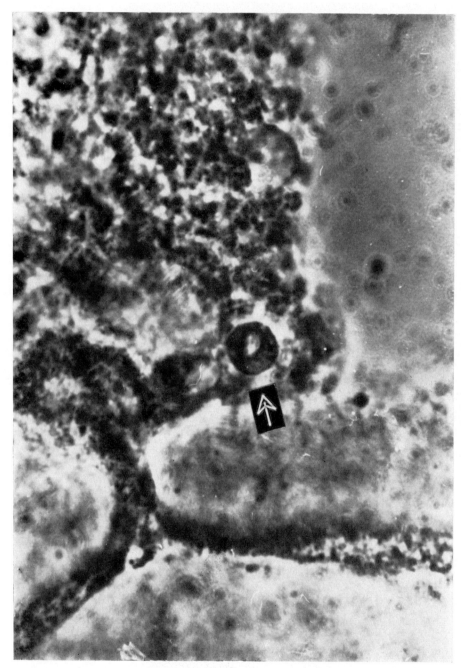

Fig. 2. Recently ruptured follicle with released ovum.

may be divided into two phases; in the first, the regression line relating ovular to follicular size is steep, and in the second the line is practically horizontal (Green and Zuckerman (1951)).

By the time the Graafian follicle reaches 10 to 15 mm. in diameter it extends partly above the ovarian surface. As it grows, the amount of follicular fluid and the intra-follicular pressure increase. If the follicle is punctured through the ovarian tissue with a needle attached to a small syringe, the plunger is displaced appreciably (Fig. 3).

of a stream. Consequently, the contents of all the granulosa cells may eventually pass through the zona pellucida by way of the cannules and empty into the perivitelline space about the developing ovum. By means of vital staining, the granular content of the corona radiata cells may be observed which can be recognized in the superficial part of the ovum within a few hours. The zona pellucida is technically not a part of the egg. It might be termed a receptacle for the nutritive bath of the developing ovum. This highly elastic pellucid membrane normally remains

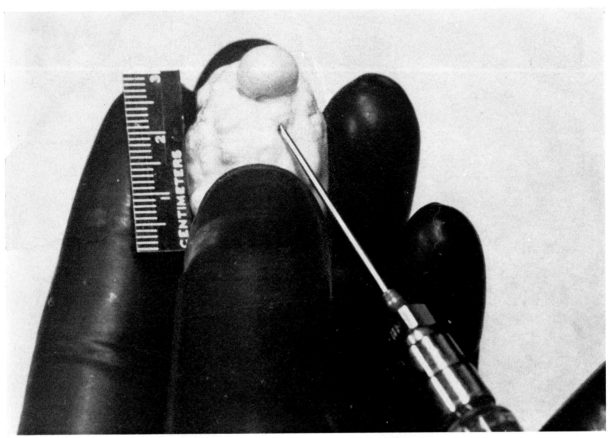

FIG. 3. Aspiration of mature follicle.

The outermost tip of the follicular wall becomes thin and transparent. The mature ovum within the zona pellucida is covered with a cloud of some 3,000 to 4,000 corona radiata cells and is set free in the follicular fluid by an undercleaving of the base of the cumulus oophorus (Fig. 1 (c)).

When observed by means of phase contrast microscopy immediately after ovulation, the living human ovum, washed from the distal part of the fallopian tube, is surrounded by the 3,000–4,000 cumulus and corona radiata cells. Tubular processes or cannules lead from the granulosa cells nearest the zona pellucida; they traverse the entire thickness (8–10 microns) of this pellucid membrane and empty their contents on its inner surface (Fig. 4). Interconnecting tubules or cannules may be noted among the granulosa cells more distant from the zona pellucida, which lead into one another like tributaries

intact around the ovum during its sojourn in and transit through the fallopian tube and through development of the morula and blastocyst stages until nidation in the event of fertilization. Premature rupture of this membrane might increase the likelihood of tubal nidation.

As a result of necrobiotic changes in the follicular wall and of increased follicular pressure, ovulation occurs with a gradual opening of the exposed tip of the follicular wall and release of a viscous mass containing the mature egg into the fimbriated end of the fallopian tube. The fluffy, succulent, gelatinous mass of cumulus and granulosa cells around the ovum facilitates its uptake by the fimbriated end of the tube when ovulation occurs.

At laparotomy, just prior to or at ovulation, the fimbriated end of the fallopian tube may be observed hovering over the follicle and adjacent ovarian surface to facilitate and ensure its reception of the ovum (Fig. 5). The ovary

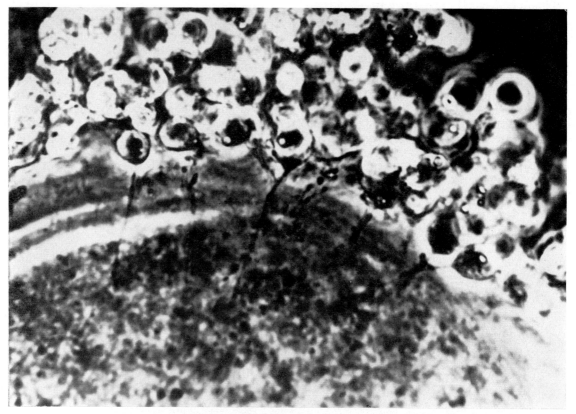

FIG. 4. Tubular processes of corona radiata cells.

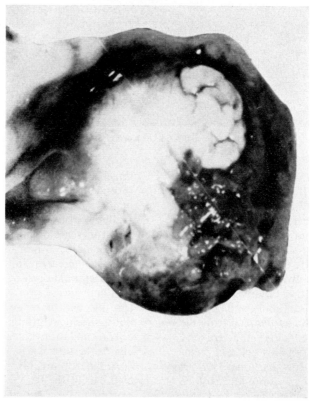

FIG. 5. Fallopian tube hovering over mature ovarian follicle.

is steadied by tautening of the utero-ovarian ligament. This same trophic behaviour may be induced in the fallopian tube by aspirating and gently expressing follicular fluid onto its fimbriated end.

In the mature egg, the second polar spindle is also present but in a state of arrest (Fig. 1 (c)). Only during the preliminary events of fertilization does the second meiotic division go through to completion. To ensure success in its role, a sperm must still possess high motility and, like the egg, must be in the functionally potent phase intermediate between under- and over-ripeness. Studies in human fertility lead to the conclusion that millions of sperm are needed to bring about successful insemination, Shettles (1962b).

Nature equips the sex cells with the basic structure common to most cells: a nucleus containing genetic material, mitochondria to provide energy, a host of enzymes to synthesize the materials needed for growth, and so forth, but each of the two cells is highly specialized for its unique role. The head, midpiece, and tail of the small and active sperm are designed to accomplish four main tasks, all usually within the space of a very short time. First, the sperm must swim to the egg by means of the energy of the mitochondria in the midpiece driving the whiplike tail. Second, the sperm must become oriented to the surface of the egg. Third, it must activate the ovum to begin the processes leading to embryonic development. Fourth, after it has become incorporated in the egg, it must provide the nucleus containing the paternal set of genes.

The egg, in contrast to the sperm, is a huge, immobile cell. Its first function is to be receptive to the fertilizing sperm. For its role in embryonic development, its cytoplasm is loaded with stored foods to provide energy and building materials, and its nucleus contains the maternal genes. Despite its food reserve, the human ovum dies within a matter of some 12–24 hours if it is not fertilized, Shettles (1956b). Studies of early cleavage stages in the human indicate that the ovum is fertilized soon after ovulation, within 12 hours, Rock and Hertig (1944), Rock and Hertig (1948). Thus, for the egg, fertilization is a particularly urgent business.

Human sperm normally live a day or more and reach the tube in less than 1 hour after coitus, Brown (1955). However, freezing in the appropriate medium at extremely low temperatures prolongs the viability of sperm. Four pregnancies have been reported after insemination with frozen semen; two specimens had been frozen for 6 weeks, one for 5 weeks, and one for 48 hours, Bunge, Keettel and Sherman (1954). Another 6 women were impregnated with frozen, preserved semen kept for 2 days to 20 weeks. Four of the these women delivered normal healthy babies, Sawada (1959).

Site of Fertilization

The meeting and union of the human sex cells take place normally in the upper third of the fallopian tube. Shettles (1962b). The average time required for sperm to traverse the cervical canal, uterine cavity, and tube is approximately an hour, Brown (1955). That fertilization may occur in the ovary is indicated by ovarian pregnancies. It is altogether certain that fertilization cannot normally be delayed until the ovum reaches the uterus, since staleness and degeneration occur rather soon. Presumably fertilization does not take place in the lowest levels of the tube, since degenerating human ova have been recovered from the tube, and unfertilized eggs begin to show visible signs of deterioration by the time they approach the uterus. The final fate of unfertilized eggs is dissolution in utero or passage in the cervical mucus.

Process of Fertilization

In vivo, approximately 24 hours after ovulation, the cumulus and corona radiata cells have dropped away from the zona pellucida. *In vitro*, through enzymatic action of the tubal mucosa and semen in the follicular fluid at 37°C for 3 hours, the zona pellucida is completely denuded of cells, revealing the first polar body of the secondary oocyte or mature ovum (Fig. 1 (c)). Hyaluronidase of the sperm also assists in the dissolution of the intercellular cement of the follicle cells. Shettles (1955a, b; 1958a, b; 1960).

Random movements bring the sperm cells in contact with an egg. There is no evidence of a trophic influence of the ovum on the sperm. Although swimming in the closest proximity to the egg, sperm may pass right by it without any apparent attraction. Having arrived at the surface of the unfertilized egg, the sperm tails continue to move vigorously. In time they cover the surface of the denuded zona pellucida completely (Fig. 6). After once accidentally touching the ovum, the vast majority remain in contact with it. The sperm rotate on their longitudinal axes with their heads against the zona pellucida, move their tails synchronously, and often rotate the ovum as rapidly as 360° in 15 seconds for as long as 20–30 hours. The ovum is often moved about within the medium and simultaneously rotated, while other cellular particles are motionless, Shettles (1958b). Such rotary movement could facilitate tubal transport.

The zona pellucida is entered at any point by sperm (Fig. 7). As the sperm enters the zona pellucida, a clear area appears in front of the head (Fig. 8). They may first enter the zona pellucida along the collapsed tubular extensions of the denuded corona radiata cells. After passing into the perivitelline area, the sperm may penetrate at any point on the egg surface (Fig. 8). There is no evidence of fertilization membrane formation and no discernable decrease in egg volume at the moment of fertilization.

In man, as in all other species of mammals investigated, the whole fertilizing sperm enters the ovum, i.e., head, neck and tail. Consequently, there is cytoplasmic as well as nuclear contribution on the part of the male at fertilization to his offspring (Fig. 9). Since the ovum and sperm nuclei are each haploid, fertilization results in the restoration of the normal diploid number of chromosomes. In other words, the male and female haploid pronuclei fuse to form the diploid zygote. Since one of two kinds of sperm successfully penetrates the ovum, fertilization determines the sex of the embryo. Fertilization stimulates

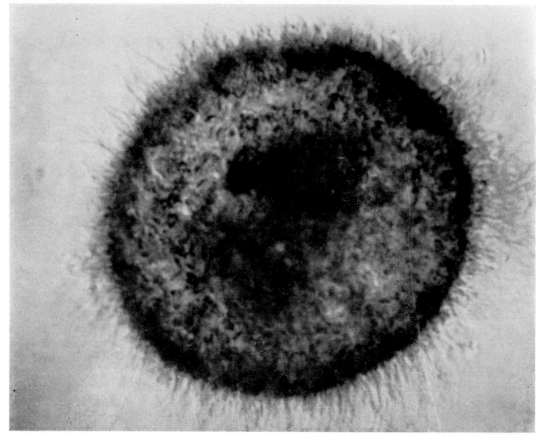

FIG. 6. Zona pellucida completely covered with sperm.

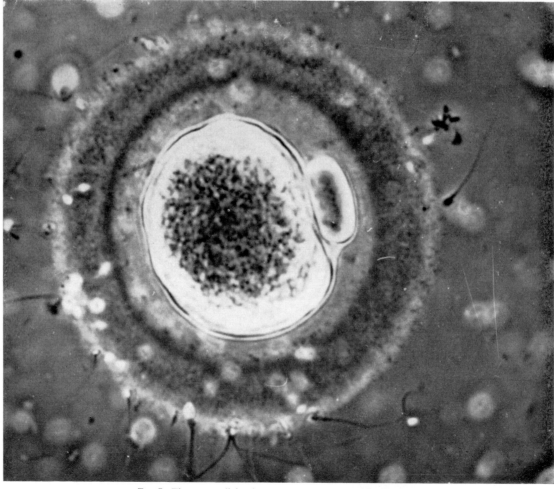

FIG. 7. The mature living human egg at moment of fertilization.

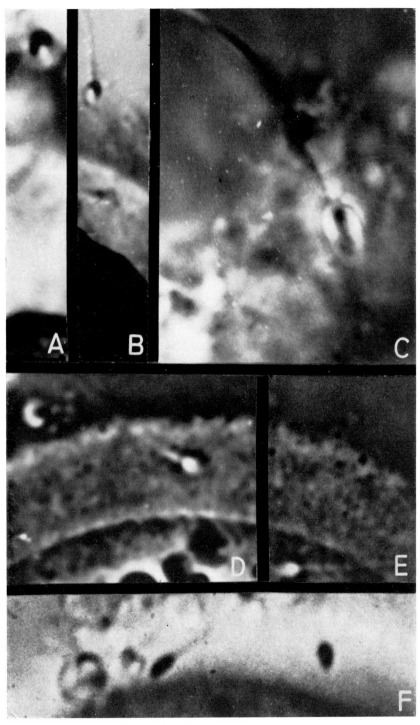

Fig. 8. *A–F.* Steps in sperm penetration.

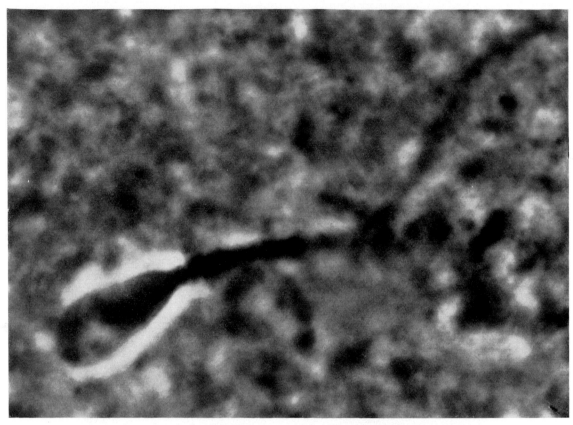

Fig. 9. Whole fertilizing sperm enters egg ooplasm.

the egg so that its cytoplasm becomes rather violently active and completes its maturation and the pronuclei approach each other.

Recent observations indicate that the number of sperm which penetrate the ovum and the degree to which entry occurs are manifestations of the size, shape, number, activity and viability of the respective male germ cells, and the time of insemination in regard to ovulation, Shettles (1961), Shettles (1964a). With sperm penetration of the ooplasm, the second polar body is formed (Fig. 10). Instead of undergoing immediate degeneration, the first polar body may also divide. Each of the resulting polar bodies and the ovum proper contain the haploid number of 23 chromosomes (Fig. 11). Fertilization of the ovum and one or more of the polar bodies would give rise to a multiple pregnancy, with possibly marked difference in the weights of offspring.

Although a number of sperm may penetrate the ovum, only one effects fertilization by the following mechanism: Within the ovum, the frequency and amplitude of beating of the fertilizing sperm tail is now reduced. Due to the viscosity of the ooplasm, the sperm moves forward 10–20 microns by interrupted thrusts, until the head comes into close proximity with the egg pronucleus. During this journey the head swells, becomes open-structured, and converts into the fairly rounded male pronucleus. During the progress of these events, the final maturation division of the egg has been completed and the pronucleus recon-

stituted, ready for union. In the unfertilized ovum, the female pronucleus may be situated almost any place in the cytoplasm, in the center or at the periphery. In the formation of the male and female pronuclei, discrete chromatin bodies can be seen which swell and coalesce in the respective nucleoli. As the sperm head swells in the ooplasm and becomes more open-structured, its lobulated chromatin spiral, or helix, gives rise to the hitherto depicted numerous nuclei in the formation of the male pronucleus, Austin (1951), Blandau (1952), Gresson (1942), Kremer (1924), Lams (1913), Lams and Doorme (1908), Mainland (1930), Noyes et al. (1965), Sobotta (1895), Sobotta and Burckhard (1911). As observed in phase-contrast, the lobulated chromatin helix breaks up, and the chromatin bodies which form are smooth, uniformly dark spheres differing from each other only in size.

The climax of fertilization is reached when the pronuclei approach, meet and unite; they appear to attract each other as the second maturation metaphase is reached (Fig. 12). The fusion of the haploid nuclei gives rise to a new individual with the diploid number of 46 chromosomes. When fertilization is complete, the egg, freed from its previous restraints, divides in the ordinary mitotic way. After union of the pronuclei, the chromosomes appear, split lengthwise and arrange themselves on the mitotic spindle in anticipation of the first cell division. The great disparity in size and consistency of the sperm and egg are not reflected in the genetically important chromosomes of

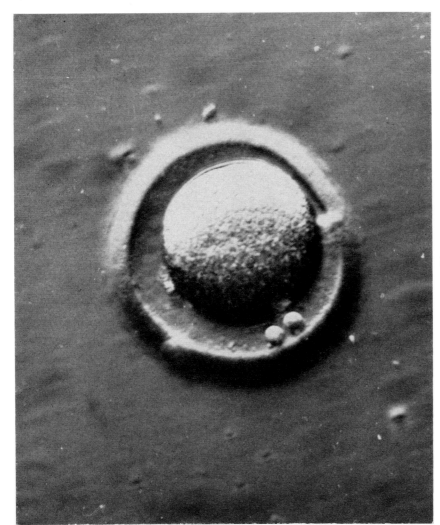

Fig. 10. Fertilized egg with
2 polar bodies.

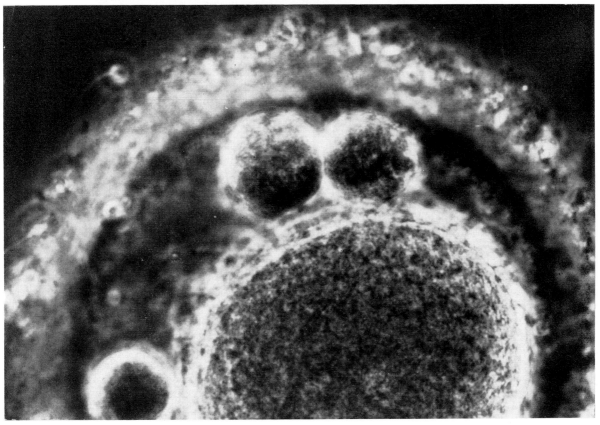

Fig. 11. Mature egg with 3 polar bodies, the 1st having divided.

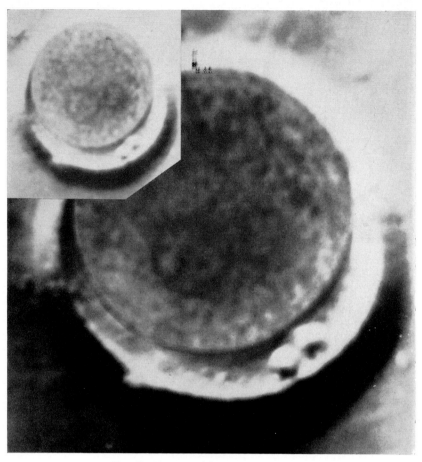

FIG. 12. The pronuclei approach each other.

the nucleus. Each cell has its full complement of chromosomes and each chromosome must find its pair in the other nucleus.

The sperm contributes little or nothing to the nutrition of the early fertilized egg and probably has little to do with the type of cleavage that ensues. It stimulates the dormant ovum to activity, contributes its hereditary influences and then is absorbed as the zygote nucleus readies the stored yolk and cytoplasm of the ovum for the early cleavages.

Cleavage

The early cleavages are total and nearly equal, conditions that are expected in normal isolecithal eggs. After its fertilization in the upper fallopian tube, the ovum spends about 3 days en route to the uterine lumen. During this time it undergoes the first several cleavages. With fertilization *in vivo* or *in vitro*, the first cleavage is accomplished after approximately 30 hours, giving rise to the two cell stage (Fig. 13). There is no explanation for the late timing of the first cleavage except that the maturation of the egg must be accomplished, the sperm head must be transformed into a pronucleus, some degree of zygogenesis (fusion of pronuclei) must take place, the cytoplasm of the ovum must undergo some changes and the apparatus for the cleavage must be set up. Once cleavage begins, it accelerates as the resulting cells become smaller and smaller.

After some 40 hours following fertilization, the four-cell stage may be found (Fig. 14). The morula or mulberry stage and the blastocyst appear about 50–60 hours and 3–4 days, respectively, following fertilization (Figs. 15 (a), (b), 16 (a), (b)). The zona pellucida is still present and will remain until just before implantation. During the first 3 days of its life the human zygote has as its environment the tubal secretions. It may be retained there through the muscular arrangement of the isthmic portion of the tube which functions as a sphincter and through decrease in the isthmic tubal lumen secondary to increased mucosal succulence associated with a rising estrogen level.

Free within the uterus on the 4th day, the developing blastocyst becomes eccentric within the zona pellucida so that some of the blastocyst cells lie in direct contact with its inner surface (Fig. 16 (a)). Nutriment and oxygenated fluid from the maternal uterus may pass through the zona pellucida to these cells. In phase contrast microscopy the zona pellucida appears to contain a number of granules. Upon careful examination these are found to represent the collapsed tubular processes of the previously attached granulosa cells. Approximately 5 to 6 days after fertilization, protoplasmic processes grow out from the cells of the blastocyst in closest proximity to the zona pellucida, traverse this membrane and pass beyond its outer surface. They undergo undulatory, ameboid-like

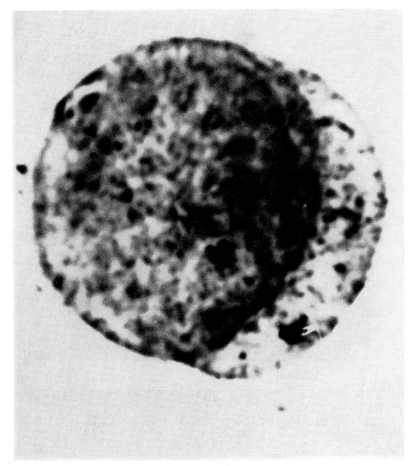

FIG. 13. Two-cell stage of fertilized egg.

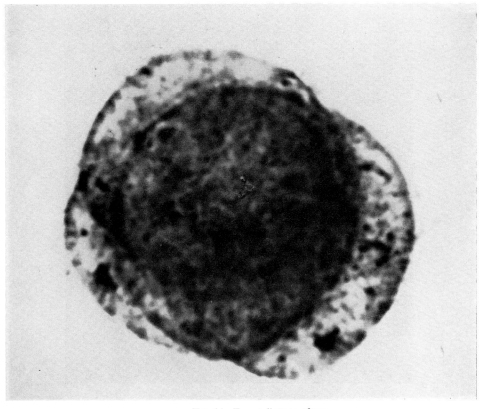

FIG. 14. Four-cell stage of egg.

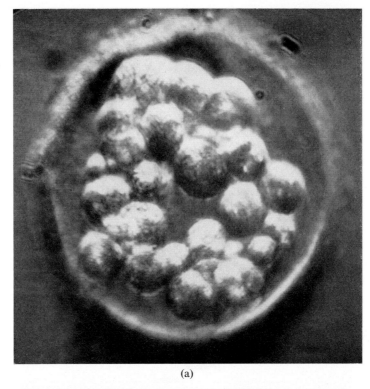

(a)

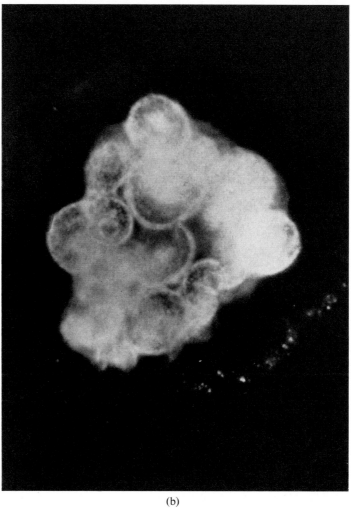

(b)

FIG. 15 (a), (b). Early and late morula stages.

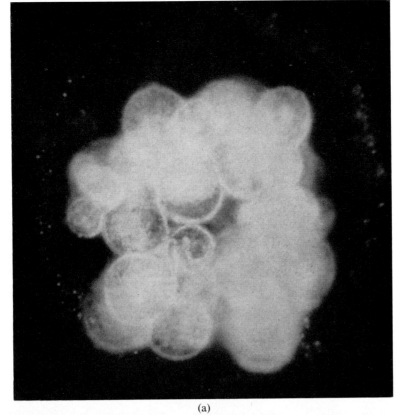

(a)

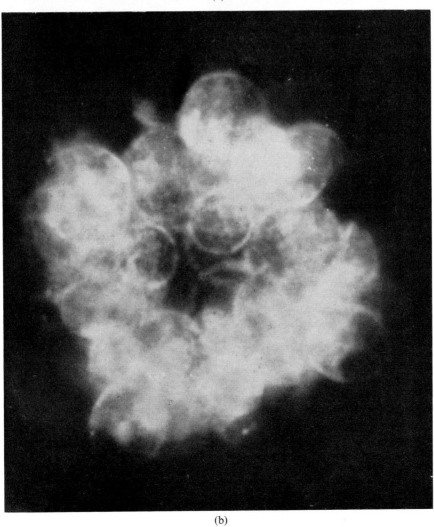

(b)

FIG. 16 (a), (b)   Early and late blastocysts.

movements as though they were in search of an attachment. (Fig. 17). By 6 to 6½ days following fertilization the fully developed blastocyst becomes attached to the uterine mucosa and implantation commences (Fig. 18). By the time attachment of the blastocyst to the endometrium is definitely established the zona pellucida disappears in its entirety, giving freedom for the developing and expanding conceptus, Shettles (1964b). By the ninth or tenth day following fertilization of the egg the blastocyst is entrapped in a mucosal crypt in the dorsal wall of the uterus. Although implantation is possible at almost any point from the ovary to the cervix, an ovarian, abdominal, ampullary, tubal, or cervical implantation is abnormal and such an ovum generally dies or becomes anomalous.

Implantation of the developing human ovum involves loss of the zona pellucida, contact of the embryonic trophoblasts with the uterine epithelium, digestion with the aid of enzymes of the uterine mucosa in preparation

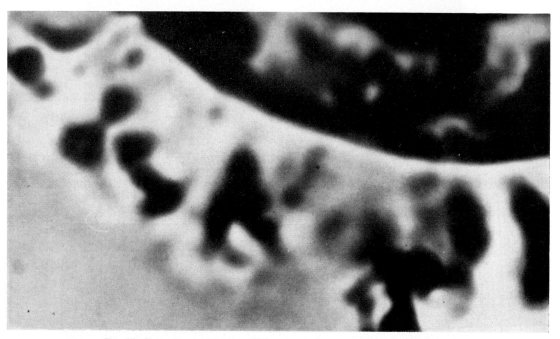

FIG. 17. Protoplasmic processes of blastocyst cells traverse the zona pellucida.

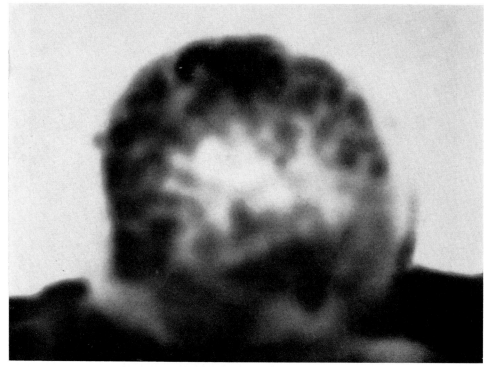

FIG. 18. Implanting blastocyst in uterine mucosa.

for the blastocyst, edema and capillary destruction in the environs of the blastocyst, engulfing of the blastocyst by the mucosa, distinction of the inner cellular and outer syncytial trophoblast, expansion of the latter and differentiation of the uterine mucosal layers. Normally there is no direct connection between the embryonic and maternal circulation.

Early Development from the Inner Cell Mass

The embryonic period is the time of most rapid growth in the life of the human organism. The human embryo increases its size over three million times as it evolves from the fertilized ovum to the newborn; it grows from

to form a single cavity, the blastocyst cavity. As a result of these changes the inner cell mass comes to be related eccentrically to the inner aspect of the outer layer, the trophoblast. As the blastocyst enlarges, the trophoblastic cells become flattened and press against the zona pellucida. As the latter disappears the trophoblast comes to lie in direct contact with the uterine epithelium (Fig. 18). The maternal tissues are invaded in the process of implantation by rapidly dividing trophoblast cells, and this penetration is probably accompanied by erosion involving enzymic action. Certainly the uterine epithelium has become sensitized to the blastocyst, and the trophoblast (Fig. 19) appears to penetrate the maternal tissue aggressively.

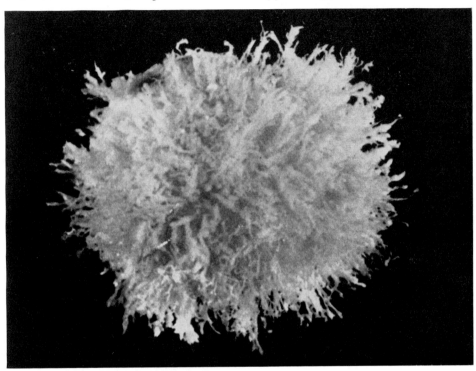

FIG. 19. Trophoblastic processes removed from maternal tissues.
(*Figures* 1, 4, 6, 7, 9, 10–19 *by courtesy of Shettles, L. B.*, Ovum Humanum. Urban and Schwarzenberg, Munich, 1960. The other illustrations are originals.)

the size of a needle point, to some 20 inches in length. During this time the weight increases 6 thousand million times and cellular growth from one to some 200 million cells.

Human development may be conveniently divided into three stages. The first period starts at fertilization of the ovum and ends when the ovum is successfully implanted. The second period extends from the third to the eighth week during which time all major organ primordia appear and the embryo assumes features which make the embryo readily recognizable as a human being. The third is the foetal period from the third month until term.

Just after its entry into the uterus, the morula undergoes modifications which are chiefly of a physical nature. Fluid accumulates in the intercellular spaces between the centrally placed cells, which become the inner cell mass (Figs. 15 (a), (b), 16 (a), (b)). With the increase in the amount of fluid, the spaces on one side become confluent

While the blastocyst is implanting, important morphological changes are occurring in the embryonic tissues derived from the inner cell mass. The first sign of differentiation of the inner cell mass is the appearance of somewhat flattened cells which separate from its inner surface to form the primitive endoderm. The remaining cells of the inner cell mass form the primitive ectoderm in which the cells become arranged into a layer of columnar cells. The primitive ectoderm also forms the floor of the amniotic cavity, while the primitive endoderm forms the roof of the primitive yolk sac.

At the same time as the above changes are occurring in the inner cell mass, stellate mesenchymal cells delaminate from the inner surface of the trophoblastic cells lining the blastocyst cavity. Proliferation of these mesenchymal cells gives rise to the extra-embryonic mesoblast which encroaches on, and reduces the relative size of the blastocyst cavity, which is thus converted into a primitive yolk

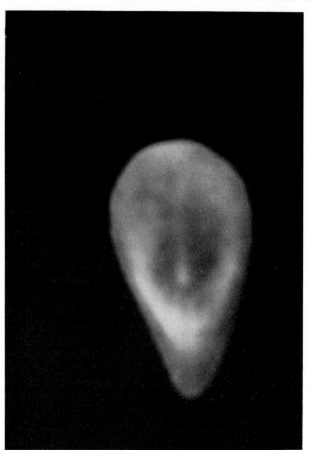

FIG. 20. Embryonic disc showing 14 days of ovum development.

sac. The inner aspect of the mesenchymal cells forms a membrane which has been designated as Heuser's or exocoelomic membrane. This is continuous with the embryonic endoderm. Cells from the embryonic endoderm soon grow round the inner aspect of Heuser's membrane converting the primitive yolk sac into a definitive yolk sac. It must be stressed that the yolk sac does not contain yolk, though for a time the yolk sac endoderm constitutes part of a primitive (yolk sac) placenta which provides nutrition for the embryo by diffusion from the maternal tissues.

At the 8th day a cavity has appeared between the ectoderm and the thin covering trophoblast. This is the beginning of the amniotic cavity. Thus, during the first week following fertilization, cleavage progresses to blastocyst formation with subsequent implantation which is the end of the first period. The embryo is a two-layered disc with the amniotic cavity. It measures on the average 0·3 mm. in length.

The endoderm spreads rapidly to line the trophoblast and form a yolk sac which contains no yolk. The endoderm cells of the yolk sac are cuboid near the ectoderm cells of the inner cell mass and flat and mesothelium-like elsewhere. Some of the cuboid cells become columnar to indicate the impending formation of the prechordal plate and the determination of the anterior-posterior axis of the embryo. As the yolk cavity is thus reduced, the amniotic cavity enlarges. For a time however, the yolk

sac endoderm obtains nutrition for the embryo by diffusion from the maternal tissues. Primitive extraembryonic mesoderm rapidly masses between the yolk sac endoderm and the trophoblast and at least some of it comes from the trophoblast cells. The mesoderm shortly acquires small spaces, lacunæ, which coalesce to form the exocœl or extraembryonic cœlom except a part between the amniotic cavity and the trophoblast. The exocoel splits the mesoderm into two layers, an outer somatic one lining the trophoblast and an inner splanchnic one covering the yolk sac. The somatic mesoderm and the trophoblast constitute the somatopleure, and the splanchnic mesoderm and the endoderm constitute the splanchnopleure. The embryo is suspended from the inner aspect of the chorionic vesicle by the mesoderm not invaded by the exocœl.

The embryonic disc, between the amniotic and yolk sac cavities, is composed of endoderm toward the yolk sac and ectoderm toward the amniotic cavity. Cells within the ectoderm of the disc rapidly proliferate toward its posterior edge, causing a bulge into the amniotic cavity, the beginning of the primitive streak (Fig. 20). Cells from the streak move outward between the ectoderm and endoderm to constitute the extraembryonic mesoderm.

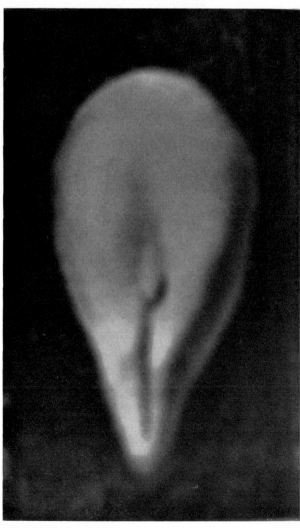

FIG. 21. Embryonic disc showing 16 days of ovum development.

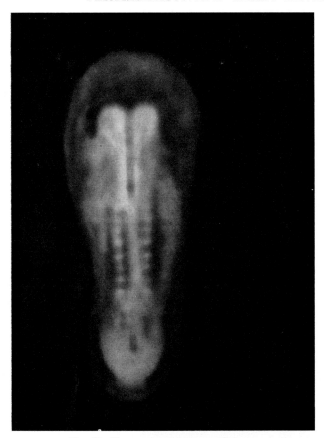

FIG. 22. Human development at 19 days.

The embryonic disc is now triploblastic, having all three primary germ layers. It expands into a pear-shaped mass with mesoderm emanating from its primitive streak in almost all directions. Although the streak remains in the posterior portion of the disc, this outflow of mesoderm may be in part responsible for the elongation and expansion of the disc (Fig. 21).

A primitive groove extends the length of the primitive streak, ending anteriorly in a primitive pit. Just anterior to the primitive pit is the primitive knot. The primitive knot adds mesoderm to that derived from the primitive streak. Anteriorly from the primitive pit to the prechordal plate, cells bud off between the ectoderm and endoderm to form the head process, the precursor of the notochord. The primitive streak shrinks after the head process appears and as it shrinks, the primitive knot moves posteriorly so that the early embryonic axis lengthens. The primitive pit invagination continues into the notochordal mass to form the elongated notochordal canal. This canal sends tributaries through the underlying endoderm into the yolk sac so that, by way of the primitive pit, the amniotic and yolk cavities are for a time connected. The notochordal cells then coalesce into a notochordal plate in the roof of the yolk sac. The notochord is shortly pinched off dorsally from the endoderm and at 18 days after fertilization it is the major axial element of the embryo, with a thickened neural or medullary plate and neural groove forming in the ectoderm above it. The crown-rump length of the embryo is 1·5 mm. (Fig. 22). It is already evident that

weight is gained more rapidly than length. The rate of increase in weight of the fertilized ovum during the first, second, third and last months of development is 1,000,000, 74, 11 and 0·3 times, respectively.

Although some embryonic mesoderm is anterior to the primitive streak, most of it arises from the streak and ultimately merges with the extraembryonic mesoderm between the amniotic ectoderm and yolk sac endoderm. As the streak recedes posteriorly it leaves mesoderm on either side of the extending notochord. The only regions remaining free of this embryonic mesoderm are the streak itself and the node from which it derives. The mesoderm immediately lateral to the notochord and continuous lengthwise is thicker than the adjoining nephrotome or intermediate cell mass and the lateral plate mesoderm. At 18 days development it anticipates the somites, the first of which to appear are the most anterior. A total of about 44 pairs of somites eventually forms.

The lateral plate splits into somatic and splanchnic layers. The nephrotome or intermediate cell mass between these layers and the somites gives rise to much of the excretory system. Some mesenchyme anterior to the prechordal plate and ventral to the notochord becomes cardiac mesoderm. An extension of the exocoel within the embryonic lateral plate forms the intracoel, or true coelom of the embryo. This is continuous with the pericardial cavity in the cardiac mesoderm.

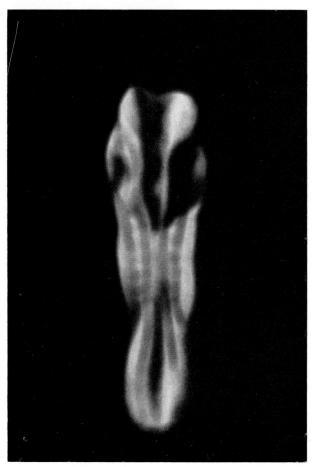

FIG. 23. Human development at 21 days.

After 3 weeks of development the crown-rump measurement is on the average 2·3 mm. (Fig. 23). The neural groove is complete and beginning to close at the center and the neural crests are continuous bands on either side of the forming neural tube. The optic vesicles, auditory placodes, and ganglia are present. The stomadeum is an ectodermal pit and the oral membrane may rupture to form the mouth. An undercutting at the extremities

the cloaca. Part of the coelom closes off as the pericardial cavity and the mesenteries and the septum transversum are evident.

The 4 weeks old embryo measures 5 mm. in length and the body has a C shape owing to the various flexures (Fig. 24). The neural tube has entirely closed, the three primary brain vesicles have formed, and the spinal and cranial nerves are developing. The optic cup induces

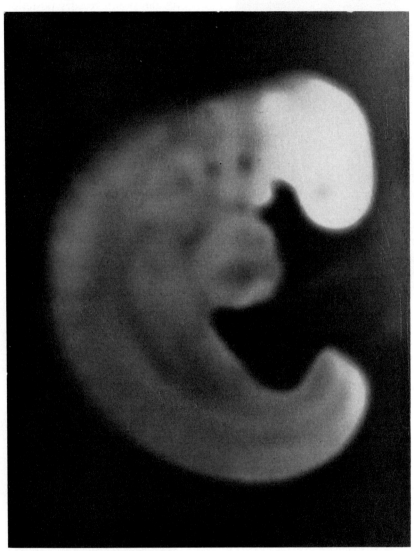

FIG. 24. Human development at 28 days.

starts the separation of the body from the yolk sac producing the foregut and hindgut and yolk stalk, the pharynx is dorsoventrally compressed and gives rise to visceral pouches between externally evident visceral arches, a thyroid pocket forms in the pharyngeal floor and the laryngotracheal groove and liver diverticulum appear. Fourteen pairs of somites the anterior ones with sclerotomes and myotomes, are apparent. The notochord is cellular. Blood vessels containing corpuscles arise in both the embryo and the extraembryonic membranes and connect with an S-shaped heart in which pulsations begin. The pronephros forms and its ducts grow posteriorly to

formation of the lens, the auditory pits close and olfactory placodes and nerves appear. In the endoderm the tongue primordia develop and Rathke's pocket forms, all the visceral pouches are present, a single thyroid diverticulum is in the floor of the pharynx and just behind it and anterior to the short esophagus are the thymus primordia and the future site of the thyroid, paired lung buds grow posteriorly from the trachea, the stomach, liver, pancreas and intestines are defined, and the yolk stalk is a narrow tube. Paired limb buds, most of the somites, all the visceral arches and maxillary processes are apparent. Primitive vertebral organization is evident around the notochord.

Abundant blood is forming in the yolk sac splanchnopleure and circulating through the body vessels and the heart is tubular but shows a sinus venosus, ventricle, atrium, and bulbus arteriosus. The pronephros is degenerating as the mesonephros is developing and the metanephros arises as a diverticulum from the cloaca.

With 5 weeks of embryonic development the length is 5–8 mm., the olfactory pits are prominent, the embryo (Fig. 26). Rathke's pocket moves toward the infundibulum, derivatives of the visceral pouches form, the thyroid loses its connection with the pharynx and becomes bilobed, the bronchial buds develop, the gall bladder and the ductus choledochus arise and a cystic duct forms between them while a hepatic duct forms between the liver and the ductus, the yolk stalk separates from the gut and the intestines elongate. The trunk and appendage muscles develop and

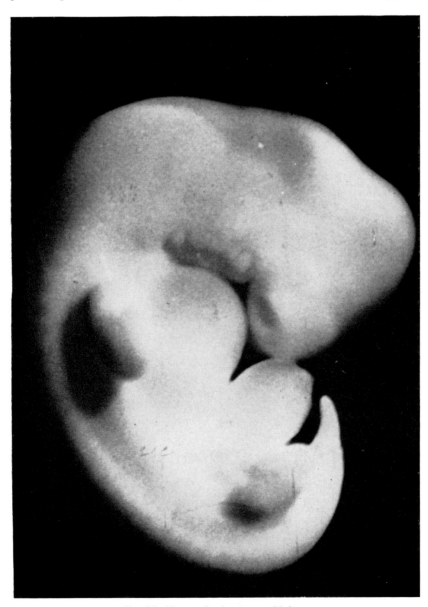

FIG. 25. Human development at 35 days.

has a temporary tail, the umbilical cord is the main channel from the placenta to the embryo and the viscera (mesonephroi, liver, and heart) cause a bulging of the body (Fig. 25). The face is assuming a human appearance with jaws indicated. The ectoderm is a double-layered epidermis, five brain vesicles are present, with obvious cephalization, the eye has a lens and choroid fissure and vitreous humor is forming and endolymphatic ducts are evident bone-forming centers arise. The circulatory system is extensive within the body, the heart begins its final divisions and the spleen primordium appears. The mesonephros is complete, genital ridges form and ureters develop. Membranes begin to divide the cœlom into pericardial, peritoneal and pleural cavities.

The fifth through the eight week is the period of embryo completion. These embryos, ranging between 5 and 30 mm.

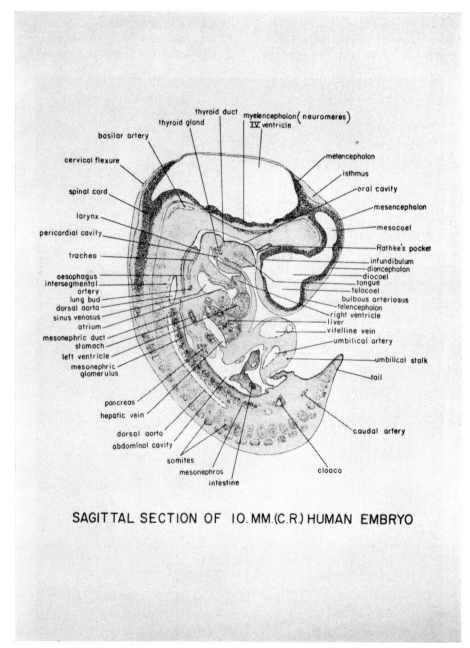

SAGITTAL SECTION OF 10.MM.(C.R.) HUMAN EMBRYO

FIG. 26. Sagittal section of embryo in Fig. 25.

in length, show marked changes. Their external form although quite unfinished, comes to resemble the human (Figs. 27, 28). After the second month the developing young is commonly called the fetus. The external metamorphosis is due principally to the following:

1. Changes in the flexures of the body, the dorsal convexity is lost, the head becomes erect and the body straight.

2. The face develops.

3. The external structures of the eye, ear and nose appear.

4. The limbs organize as such with digits demarcated.

5. The prominent tail of the fifth week becomes inconspicuous both through actual regression and concealment by the growing buttocks.

6. The umbilical cord becomes a definite entity, its embryonic end occupying a relatively diminishing area on the belly wall.

attains sufficient perfection so that spontaneous movements are possible.

Almost all of the internal organs are well laid down at two months. Henceforth, until the end of gestation, the chief changes undergone are those of growth and further differentiation. The rapidly developing cells have not yet

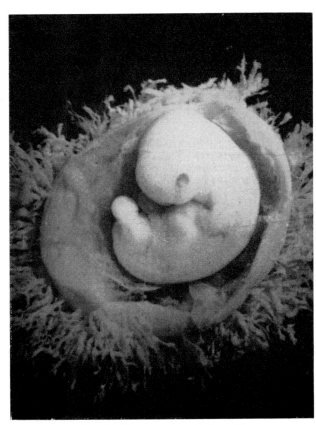

FIG. 27. Human embryo 42 days old.

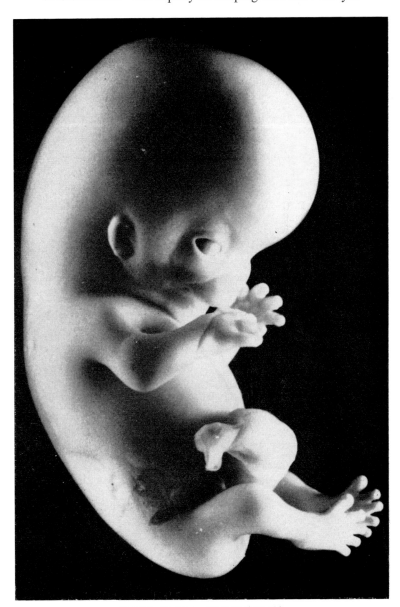

FIG. 28. Human embryo 56 days old.

7. The heart, which was the chief ventral prominence in earlier embryos, now shares this distinction with the rapidly growing liver. These two organs determine the shape of the ventral body until the eighth week when the gut dominates the belly cavity and the contour of the abdomen is more evenly rotund.

8. The neck becomes recognizable due chiefly to the settling of the heart caudad and the effacement of the branchial arches. The external genitalia appear incompletely differentiated. The neuro-muscular mechanism

assumed their final form under the influence of the genes contained in their nuclei. Outside influences can also affect the cells, and during the first three months especially fetal development may be readily influenced by the mother's condition. Certain diseases of the mother, e.g. German measles or even certain drugs, e.g. thalidomide she takes may cause abnormal fetal development. When the comparative development and budding forth of all organs at these early stages are considered, the teaching of Sir William Osler of therapeutic nihilism for adult man becomes all the more fitting for the expectant mother in view of the known toxic effects of certain medications upon early fetal development. The same preventative medicine is equally apropos concerning the injurious effects of certain infectious agents and radiation in the expectant mother upon the very young conceptus. The multifarious embryological intricacies, complexities and sensitivities in the beginning of life are manifest until its end in various and sundry ways. With these in mind and our present knowledge, unless a medication or treatment is known to be safe regarding human development, it should not be given the expectant mother unless it is imperative to do so.

REFERENCES

Allen, R D. (1959), "The Moment of Fertilization," *Sci. Amer.*, **201**, 124.

Austin, C. R. (1951), "The Formation, Growth, and Conjugation of the Pronuclei in the Rat Egg," *J. roy. micr. Soc.*, **71**, 295.

Austin, C. R. (1953), "The Growth of Knowledge on Mammalian Fertilization," *Aust. vet. J.*, **29**, 191.

Blandau, R. J. (1952), "The Female Factor in Fertility and Sterility: I: Effects of Delayed Fertilization on the Development of the Pronuclei in Rat Ova," *Fertil. and Steril.*, **3**, 349.

Blandau, R. J. and Odor, D. L. (1952), "Observations on Sperm Penetration into the Ooplasm and Changes in the Cytoplasmic Components of the Fertilizing Spermotozoon in the Rat," *Fertil. and Steril.*, **3**, 13.

Brown, R. L. (1955), "Rate of Transport of Sperma in the Human Uterus and the Tubes," *Amer. J. Obstet. Gynec.*, **47**, 153.

Bunge, R. G., Keettel, W. C. and Sherman, J. K. (1954), "Clinical Use of Frozen Semen: Report of 4 Cases," *Fertil. and Steril*, **5**, 520.

Green, S. H. and Zuckerman, S. (1951), "Quantitative Aspects of the Growth of the Human Ovum and Follicle," *J. Anat.*, **85**, 373.

Gresson, R. A. R. (1942), "A Study of the Cytoplasmic Inclusions during Maturation, Fertilization and the First Cleavage Division of the Egg of the Mouse," *Quart. J. micr. Sci.*, **83**, 35.

Kawakami, M. and Sawyer, C. H. (1959), "Induction of Behavioral and Electroencephalographic Changes in the Rabbit by Hormonal Administration or Brain Stimulation," *Endocrinology*, **65**, 631.

Kremer, J. (1924), "Das Verhalten der Vorkerne im befruchteten Ei der Ratte und der Maus mit besonderes Berücksichtigung ihrer Nucleoln," *Z. mikr.-anat. Forsch.*, **1**, 353.

Lams, H. (1913), "Étude de l'œuf de Cobaye aux Premiers Stades de l'Embryogenèse," *Arch. Biol. (Paris)*, **28**, 229.

Lams, H. and Doorme, J. (1908), "Nouvelles Recherches sur la Maturation et la Fécondation de l'œuf des Mammifères," *Arch. Biol. (Paris)*, **23**, 259.

Lewin, H. (1950), "Die Ovulation als Physiologischer Vorgang," *Gynaecologia*, **129**, 273.

Mainland, D. (1930), "The Early Development of the Ferret: The Pronuclei," *J. Anat.*, **64**, 262.

Noyes, R. W., Dickmann, Z., Clewe, T. H. and Bonney, W. A. (1965), "Pronuclear Ovum from Patient using an Intrauterine Contraceptive Device," *Science*, **147**, 744.

Rock, J. and Hertig, A. T. (1944), "On Development of Early Human Ovum with Special Reference to Trophoblast of Previllous Stage: Description of Seven Normal and Five Pathologic Human Ova," *Amer. J. Obstet. Gynec.*, **47**, 149.

Rock, J. and Hertig, A. T. (1948), "The Human Conceptus during the First Two Weeks of Gestation," *Amer. J. Obstet. Gynec.*, **55**, 6.

Sawada, Y. (1959), "Studies on Freezing-preservation of Human Spermatoza," *Jap. J. Fertil. Steril.*, **4**, 1.

Shettles, L. B. (1953), "Observations on Human Follicular and Tubal Ova," *Amer. J. Obstet. Gynec.*, **66**, 235.

Shettles, L. B. (1955a), "Further Observations on Living Human Oocytes and Ova," *Amer. J. Obstet. Gynec.*, **69**, 365.

Shettles, L. B. (1955b), "Studies on Living Human Ova," *Trans. N.Y. Acad. Sci.*, **17**, 99.

Shettles, L. B. (1956a), "The Ovum in Fertility, Abortion and Developmental Anomaly," *Fertil. and Steril.*, **7**, 561.

Shettles, L. B. (1956b), in *Handbook of Biological Data*, p. 123. Washington: National Research Council.

Shettles, L. B. (1958a), "Die lebende menschliche Eizelle," *Arch. Gynäk.*, **193**, 278.

Shettles, L. B. (1958b), "The Living Human Ovum," *Amer. J. Obstet. Gynec.*, **76**, 398.

Shettles, L. B. (1960), *Ovum Humanum*. Munich: Urban & Schwarzenberg.

Shettles, L. B. (1961), "Conception and Birth Sex Ratios," *Obstet. and Gynec.*, **18**, 122.

Shettles, L. B. (1962a), *Ovulation: Normal and Abnormal, in the Ovary*, p. 128. Baltimore: Williams and Wilkins Co.

Shettles, L. B. (1962b), "Human Fertilization," *Obstet. and Gynec.*, **20**, 750.

Shettles, L. B. (1964a), "The Great Preponderance of Human Males Conceived," *Amer. J. Obstet. Gynec.*, **89**, 130.

Shettles, L. B. (1964b), "In the Beginning," *Bulletin of the Sloane Hospital for Women*, **10**, 246.

Smith, P. E. and Engle, E. T. (1927), "Experimental Evidence regarding Role of Anterior Pituitary in Development and Regulation of Genital System," *Amer. J. Anat.*, **40**, 159.

Sobotta, J. (1895), "Die Befruchtung und Furchung des Eies der Maus," *Arch. mikr. Anat.*, **45**, 15.

Sobotta, J. and Burckhard, G. (1910), "Reifung und Befruchtung des Eies der Weissen Ratte," *Anat. Hefte*, **42**, 433.

4. TROPHOBLAST

W. D. BILLINGTON

INTRODUCTION

It is often said that an understanding of abnormal function requires recognition of normal function, and this is particularly apposite in the study of trophoblast. It is only comparatively recently that the normal tissue has been investigated from the functional point of view, yet this knowledge is already leading to clinical application in pregnancy and effective treatment of many patients with pathological disorders of the trophoblast.

The trophoblast was first named by A. A. W. Hubrecht in 1889 in a memoir on the placentation of the hedgehog. He described a tissue which he considered to be drawing food from maternal sources to nourish the developing embryo, and therefore named it trophoblast (Gr τροφή, nourishment, βλαστ-ός, bud). It is now apparent that nutrition is not the sole function of trophoblast; in most situations it also mediates the attachment of the embryo to the uterine wall, provides a means for the intimate apposition of maternal and foetal tissues and later develops secretory and regulatory functions essential for the maintenance of pregnancy.

DEVELOPMENT OF THE TROPHOBLAST

Trophectoderm

The cells which give rise to the trophoblast are usually first identified as the wall of the unimplanted blastocyst and are known as the trophectoderm or blastocystic trophoblast. Some investigators distinguish between polar trophoblast covering the inner cell mass (the future embryo), and mural trophoblast composed of the remaining blastocyst wall.

Cytotrophoblast and Syncytiotrophoblast

After implantation the trophectoderm gives rise to a cellular trophoblast, the primitive cytotrophoblast. Subsequent development is species dependent and it may either proliferate by mitotic division to form only cellular tissue or, as in man, later give rise to a syncytium, the syncytiotrophoblast. There has been considerable controversy over the origin of this syncytium, but recent investigations lend unequivocal support for the derivation of syncytial trophoblast from the cellular form, probably by cell division and fusion. It has been suggested that the formed syncytium may be self-reproducing by the mechanism of amitosis and it is significant that throughout the history of trophoblast study the nuclei of syncytial trophoblast have never been seen in mitosis. It seems more likely that it is continuously derived from proliferating basal cytotrophoblast, and electron microscope studies now indicate that cytotrophoblast can persist throughout gestation.

Giant Cells

There is a further basic trophoblast type consisting of the so-called giant cells. These may be uninucleate, but more frequently multinucleate, and may appear at particular stages of placental development or throughout pregnancy.

FURTHER TROPHOBLAST SPECIALIZATIONS

The architecture of the mature placenta has engaged the attentions of many workers and the vast literature accumulated on this topic is testimony to their efforts. It must be remembered that in considering the human placenta we are dealing with but a single type, a chorioallantoic placenta, and only one variation of this, the haemochorial placenta. This is characterized by the outermost foetal layer, the chorion, being bathed directly by maternal blood. The placentation in man may be more fully described as villous haemomonochorial since there is a single layer of syncytial chorionic trophoblast in the form of numerous villi extending into the intervillous space containing pools of maternal blood.

The trophoblast is the very fabric of the placenta and its specializations are many and varied. As pregnancy progresses the syncytium increases greatly in amount and lacunae are formed within it. At this time there is an extension of the cytotrophoblast into the syncytial region forming the villous primordia, and with the development of the lacunae the intervillous space is formed.

Cytotrophoblastic Shell

At the tips of the villi the cytotrophoblast undergoes rapid proliferation and forms columns of cells which progressively extend into the peripheral syncytium. The cytotrophoblast from these columns extends laterally in all directions and eventually joins to form a cytotrophoblastic shell around the whole implantation site. Gaps in this shell allow maternal blood to communicate with the intervillous space. The mature villus consists of a thin syncytium covering a continuous layer of cytotrophoblast (Langhan's layer) with a mesodermal core.

The Placental Barrier

The definitive placental syncytium is that covering the chorionic villi and thus lining the intervillous space. This is the so-called "placental barrier" separating the maternal and foetal blood streams. The syncytium displays remarkable regional variations in its structure and Hamilton and Boyd (1966) consider that there are at least four types: projections from the syncytial surface into the intervillous space (syncytial sprouts); projections into the stroma of the villus (syncytial buds); areas devoid of nuclei (epithelial plates); and areas with nuclear aggregations (syncytial knots or clumps) (Fig. 1).

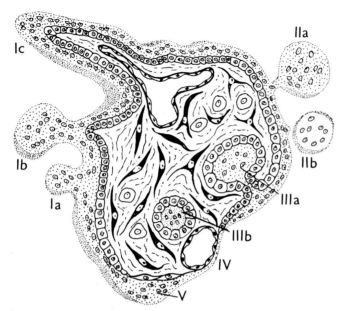

FIG. 1. Schematic diagram to show possible syncytial derivatives of a chorionic villus. Ia, Early syncytial sprout. Ib, Later stage in the development of a syncytial sprout, commencing invagination by cytotrophoblast. Ic, Fully established small chorionic villus branch with stromal core and capillary. IIa, Pedunculated syncytial sprout. IIb, Liberated syncytial sprout in intervillus space. IIIa, An early stage in the development of a stromal trophoblastic bud. IIIb, A stromal trophoblastic bud separated from the suface and situated in the interior of villus. IV, Epithelial plate with underlying capillary. V, Syncytial knot or clump. (Reprinted from the British Medical Journal 1966, Vol I, Page 1501–6 by permission of the Authors, Editor and Publishers.)

PROPERTIES OF TROPHOBLAST

Trophoblast must be considered as the most important single tissue in the placenta since it is involved in most of those functions ascribed to the placenta as a whole. The three main functions are those of invasion, nutrition and regulation.

Nutrition

Nutrition is considered to be the most primitive function and involves not only the uptake of food material to the embryo before the placenta is established but also molecular transport during the remainder of pregnancy. The placenta can no longer be regarded as a simple semipermeable membrane since transfer of material may be carried out by mechanisms involving ultra-filtration, active transport (both by enzyme systems and "carrier" molecules), phagocytosis and pinocytosis. The recent information about the ultrastructure of the placental "barrier," the trophoblastic syncytium, shows that it is well suited for its sophisticated transfer function. It has also been claimed that two morphologically distinct zones can be recognized in the trophoblast of the free chorionic villus in the term placenta—thin alpha zones consisting mainly of syncytium and showing the ultrastructural characteristics of an absorptive and active transport membrane, and thicker

beta zones with both syncytium and cytotrophoblast and having organelles related to cellular synthesis.

Many studies on the transfer of macromolecules, especially γ-globulins, have shown that the syncytium is capable of high powers of selectivity, irrespective of molecular size. This is particularly important with respect to the transplacental transmission of passive immunity from mother to foetus. It is significant that many of the drugs used in obstetrics traverse the placenta and this should perhaps be more thoroughly investigated.

Hormone Production

The regulatory function mainly concerns the production of hormones essential for the maintenance of pregnancy. Proteins and steroids are the two main categories, and these include, at least, chorionic gonadotrophin, human placental lactogen, oestrogens and progesterone. Evidence for the placental production of other hormones is unsatisfactory (See Sec. III, Ch. 10 and Sec. X, Ch. 9.) and many of the clinical findings might be explained by synthesis in the foetus. There is very likely an interplay in hormone production by the foetus and placenta. Many of the earlier studies indicated that the cytotrophoblast was involved in chorionic gonadotrophin secretion, but evidence is now accumulating that both protein and steroid hormones are synthesized by the syncytiotrophoblast.

The precise role of human chorionic gonadotrophin (HCG) is not clear, but it is certainly a most valuable indicator of early pregnancy. It is detectable soon after implantation of the egg and reaches peak levels between the second and third months of pregnancy. There is good evidence for a luteotrophic effect of HCG since it is capable of maintaining the corpus luteum in a functional state during pregnancy. Human placental lactogen (HPL) is a protein hormone immunologically related to human pituitary growth hormone (HGH). It is secreted by the syncytiotrophoblast in steadily increasing amounts during pregnancy. Although the physiological role of this hormone remains to be established it has somatotrophic, lactogenic and luteotrophic effects in test animals, and potentiates the biological effect of HCG and HGH in various experimental situations.

Oestrogens and progesterone are produced by the syncytiotrophoblast supplementary to their initial source in the maternal endocrine tissues. Syncytiotrophoblast becomes the main site of steroid synthesis during pregnancy and these hormones are demonstrable after removal of the ovaries, pituitary and adrenals. The function of oestrogens and progesterone in the maintenance of pregnancy is outside the scope of this chapter and the reader is referred to the review of Ryan (1962).

There are reports of an association between elevated HCG levels and complications of pregnancy, particularly pre-eclampsia, but there appears to be little prognostic value in the findings. HCG is also produced by abnormal trophoblast tissue and moles and choriocarcinoma have been successfully followed using serial determinations of this hormone. It now seems that there are qualitative differences in the gonadotrophins produced by normal and abnormal trophoblast and this may usefully supplement the well-established consecutive quantitative assays. There is as yet no clear diagnostic value in the determination of other hormones excreted in the urine, although there may be some changes in hormone metabolism during molar pregnancy, at least, and choriocarcinoma can produce significant quantities of oestrogen.

Until recently biological assays were widely used for HCG determinations but these are being replaced by immunological techniques which are quicker, at least as accurate, and require smaller samples of serum or urine. Immunological tests are also proving accurate in diagnosing, and assessing the effects of chemotherapy on, hydatidiform moles and choriocarcinoma. Nevertheless advances in the field of hormone chemistry will undoubtedly lead to an even wider application in clinical practice.

Invasive Properties

Perhaps the most spectacular property of trophoblast is its invasiveness. Although all basic types of normal human trophoblast exhibit this property at some stage, it is usually the syncytiotrophoblast which is considered to be the most invasive. The highly invasive mouse trophoblast is now known to be cellular and since this is also true of many invasive tumours any theory of trophoblast invasion must take this into account.

Experiments on laboratory animals have thrown some light on the mechanism of invasion, particularly the relevance of considering the environmental background that apposes the trophoblast. Using the basic techniques of tissue culture and ectopic transplantation it can be shown that trophoblast invasion involves both chemical and physical mechanisms. Studies in our laboratory have demonstrated that ectopically developing rodent trophoblast can invade by phagocytosis or cytolysis, depending upon the nature of the host substrate, and both these mechanisms may be operative in the destruction of the uterine tissues during pregnancy. It is also clear that the endometrium is considerably involved and will normally only be receptive to invasion when the hormonal "climate" is favourable.

Under the experimental conditions of transplantation trophoblast often undergoes an exuberant proliferation and this suggests that some constraint is imposed upon it in the pregnant uterus. This constraint may well be due to the buffering action of the maternal decidual cells which develop at implantation. Transplantation of proliferating mouse trophoblast into a non-decidualized uterus allows the invasion to go unchecked and it may even extend through the uterine wall. This is perhaps comparable to the pathological *placenta accreta* where the trophoblast oversteps its physiological limit and does not readily evacuate at parturition. The condition is usually associated with sparse decidual tissue, a phenomenon seen in ectopic pregnancy where trophoblast penetration is also excessive. How such an anti-invasive action of the decidua might operate is not yet clear.

Other factors controlling trophoblast invasion are unknown, both for the normal and pathological state. A delicate balance must exist since low activity may lead to pregnancy failure and hyperactivity may result in trophoblastic tumours, endangering the life of both mother and embryo. It is becoming increasingly evident that immunological factors must play an important role in the control of trophoblast activity, and these are discussed later.

TROPHOBLAST DISPERSAL DURING NORMAL PREGNANCY

Giant Cells

During placental ontogeny there occurs considerable trophoblastic extension into the maternal organism. The presence of "giant cells" in the decidua basalis and myometrium during pregnancy has been known for many years, and although their origin is still a matter for dispute it seems likely that they are usually trophoblastic. Examination of *in situ* placentæ from selected stages of pregnancy shows an outgrowth of syncytial elements into the maternal tissues and this may be a stage in the development of giant cells. Their structure and staining properties show marked similarities with the placental trophoblast. Giant cells of pregnancy have been observed in many mammalian species and considered by most authors to be of foetal origin.

The presence in large numbers of these giant cells deep within the uterine tissues is of considerable interest. Suggestions for their function have been purely speculative and include enzyme production and hormone synthesis. Although the cells are migratory they do not appear to be invasive in the sense of having a destructive effect on the maternal tissue. Their persistence, even into the post-partum period, invites questions on their immunological status and their apparent preclusion from homograft rejection reactions (see section on antigenicity of the trophoblast).

Intra-arterial Migration

Another type of trophoblast excursion is the migration of cytotrophoblast cells into the terminal portions of the endometrial spiral arteries. These cells are reputed to arise from the cytotrophoblastic shell mainly during midpregnancy. Although their function is unknown it has been suggested that they plug the ends of the arteries and control the arterial pressure before the blood enters the intervillous space. This thesis requires the cells to migrate against the arterial blood flow.

Such intra-arterial cell invasion has been reported in a number of species but most of the authors suggest a maternal origin for the cells. In the hamster, however, there is an undoubted migration of trophoblastic giant cells into the maternal arterial system during normal pregnancy. This phenomenon has recently been demonstrated experimentally by the transplantation of hamster trophoblast to ectopic sites in recipient animals. After transfer beneath the tunica albuginea of the testis or the capsule of the kidney, cells of such trophoblast transplants undergo an active migration and preferentially invade the organ's vascular system. They penetrate the testicular or renal arteries and come to line the endothelial wall

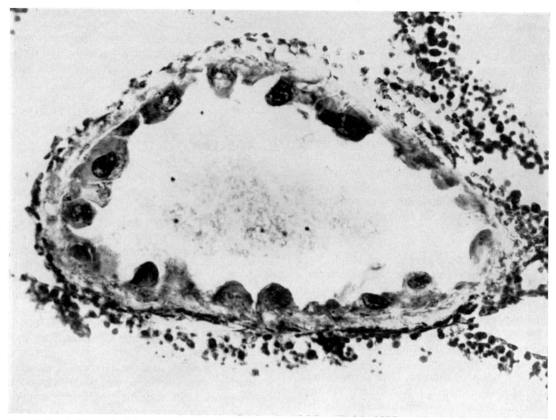

FIG. 2. Trophoblast cells lining the endothelial wall of an artery in the hamster testis, six days following transplantation beneath the tunica albuginea.

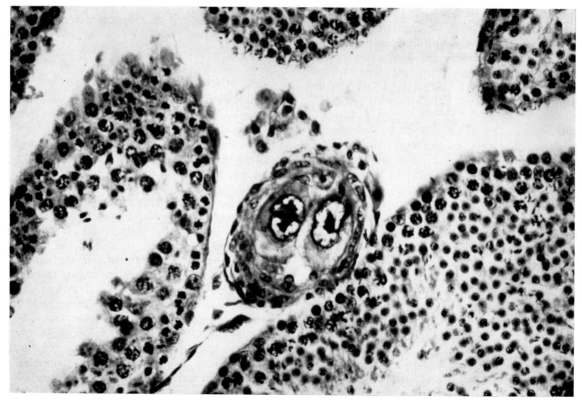

FIG. 3. Trophoblast cells almost completely blocking the lumen of a small artery in the hamster testis.

(Fig. 2), sometimes almost blocking the lumen of the vessel (Fig. 3). This might be regarded as comparable to the situation in human pregnancy and provide a useful experimental model for investigation of the function of trophoblast cells in the intra-arterial site.

Deportation

The most remarkable example of trophoblast excursion into the maternal system is the phenomenon of deportation. It is well established that during normal human pregnancy portions of the syncytium break away from the chorionic villi (usually as syncytial sprouts but, rarely, as villous fragments) and come to lie in the intervillous space. From here they are swept into the maternal veins draining the uterus and can there be demonstrated in large numbers

trophoblast might produce hormones aiding in the maintenance of pregnancy, or enzymes such as thrombokinase, affecting blood coagulation during pregnancy; the trophoblast could be inducing some maternal immunological response to the genetically foreign foetal tissues, perhaps a state of tolerance. There is no convincing evidence for any of these suggestions, but it nevertheless seems unreasonable to regard their regular presence in the maternal system as entirely without purpose.

Whatever function is ultimately assigned to deported trophoblast a causal relationship with known complications of pregnancy, such as toxaemia, is still conceivable. There is certainly an increase of trophoblastic material in the lungs of toxaemic patients, and this is further increased following eclamptic convulsions. The presence

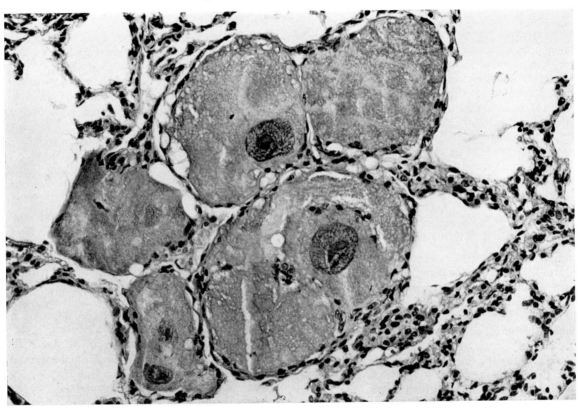

FIG. 4. Deported trophoblast in the lung of a pregnant chinchilla.

throughout most of pregnancy. Although many are subsequently destroyed, possibly by some lytic action of the blood, considerable numbers reach the maternal lungs. It was the finding of trophoblastic material in the lungs of eclamptic patients who had died during or shortly after pregnancy that led the early investigators to believe the phenomenon germane to the eclamptic condition. However, as long ago as 1896, only a few years after Schmorl's famous monograph on eclampsia, Kassjanow asserted that trophoblast embolism of the lungs was a normal physiological occurrence during pregnancy (see Ober, 1959).

The functional significance of deportation is unknown but a number of suggestions have been forwarded. It may be merely a physiological desquamation; the deported

of hydatidiform mole may also influence trophoblast deportation to the lung. Attempts to correlate the number and distribution of trophoblast elements in the blood with obstetrical complications have generally proved unrewarding. There have been a number of attempts experimentally to induce deportation of trophoblast, particularly in the mouse and monkey, but such studies have been of limited value.

It is reported that deportation of trophoblast also occurs in the direction of the foetus. Claim has been made that umbilical cord blood at the time of delivery, and tissues of the newborn, contain syncytial trophoblast. In view of the difficulty in the identification of these syncytial masses and at least two reports of negative findings in cord blood the claim should be noted with caution.

Such deportation might have to involve the passage of syncytial buds from the placental villi through the endothelium into the foetal blood circulation. However, if this can occur it might explain the rare occurrence of choriocarcinoma in both mother and foetus, and those foetal abnormalities thought to result from blockage of foetal blood vessels.

Trophoblast deportation as an event of biological importance has been considered unlikely due to its apparent restriction to human pregnancy. This reasoning may be made less tenable with the finding of a comparable phenomenon during normal pregnancy in the chinchilla, at least with respect to the residence in the maternal lungs of large amounts of trophoblastic material (Fig. 4). This pulmonary trophoblast may persist for some months into the post-partum period, whereas in human pregnancy it usually disappears within a few days following parturition. The essential pathway of deportation has yet to be determined but it seems reasonable to suggest the venous route demonstrated in man. Chinchilla breeders report that animals sometimes die during delivery for no apparent reason, and it has been tentatively suggested that this could reflect an eclamptic condition.

The finding of an animal amenable to investigation and the use of histochemical and electron-microscopical techniques should throw light on the function of trophoblast in this situation. We may well also find that other animal species bearing a comparable placental type to man exhibit deportation of the trophoblast.

TUMOURS OF TROPHOBLAST

Since the classic studies of Marchand and his contemporaries towards the end of the last century a truly awesome literature has accumulated on trophoblastic tumours. Despite this, the present status of knowledge led Bardawil and Toy (1959) to exclaim upon ". . . a tangled confusion of vague clinical histories, equivocal diagnoses, semantic altercations, and fragmentary researches." It is perhaps only fair to add that the last few years have seen considerable increase in our understanding and that effective therapy of many tumours is now commonplace.

Classification

There are usually considered to be three principal categories of trophoblastic tumours; choriocarcinoma, hydatidiform mole, and chorioadenoma destruens, although bizarre differentiation may prevent many cases from falling readily into any one category. The status of these tumours can be flexible in that malignant change in a benign tumour has been reported. The basis for such change is unknown, but the notable number of patients developing choriocarcinoma and chorioadenoma destruens after hydatidiform mole makes investigation desirable. One might ask whether there is any evidence in moles of a propensity for malignant change. It is also now clear that both malignant and benign tumours are capable of metastasis. Clinical diagnosis of trophoblastic tumours appears to depend mainly upon chorionic gonadotrophin determinations and X-ray examination, and therapy effected by radiation, surgery and chemotherapy.

Chemotherapy

Most modern chemotherapy involves the use of folic acid antagonists since both normal and neoplastic trophoblast have a metabolic dependence upon high levels of folic acid. In this context it is interesting that choriocarcinoma of the testis does not readily respond to these antagonists. Chemotherapy by combinations of drugs may be more successful, and is made necessary if resistance to any one type develops. One of the hazards of chemotherapy is toxicity due to the systemic approach, and infusion techniques may be recommended wherever possible, as in localized pelvic trophoblast lesions.

Immunotherapy

The genetic difference between trophoblast tumours and their host, due to the paternal moiety, has provided the rationale for an immunological therapy, but no results leading to wide application have yet emerged. In most cases reported attempts were made to immunize the patient with her husband's antigens (e.g. skin, and white blood cells), but remissions have been rare. Two patients with chorionepithelioma in fact rejected random skin homografts whilst retaining the husband's skin grafts for prolonged periods. This suggested some genetic identity between the tumour and the husband's tissues, and subsequent investigation demonstrated a compatibility of leucocyte antigens of husband and wife in both cases. This genetic identity might be considered to be the cause of the primary "take" of the tumour.

For the future it seems likely that effective therapy of trophoblastic tumours will depend upon the recognition of some tissue characteristic and the means for its specific suppression.

Tumours and Transplantation

Trophoblast tumours are usually considered to have no real counterpart outside man although there are isolated reports of choriocarcinoma in laboratory animals. Attempts to produce them experimentally have proved extremely difficult and this avenue of approach appears unrewarding. Nevertheless, since the natural history of such tumours is inseparable from that of the normal trophoblast a study of this tissue in experimental animals can still yield useful information.

Transplantation of normal trophoblast and tumour tissue demonstrates the similarities of their invasive pattern. Human choriocarcinoma has been transplanted to ectopic sites in the hamster and the invasion shown to compare closely with similarly transplanted murine gestational trophoblast. It has been further shown that mouse trophoblast transplanted into certain tumours in the mouse brings about local destruction of the tumour and may inhibit its growth. In such situations the trophoblast has the strategic advantage of rapid proliferation, but, having an inherent life-span, it later undergoes involution and does not replace the tumour with another invasive growth.

The technique of transplantation into experimental animals has provided information on the basic biology of trophoblast tumours. For example, the electron microscope studies on human choriocarcinoma growing in hamsters have elucidated some of the endocrine functions of this tumour. Lajos and his collaborators have transplanted human trophoblast from therapeutic abortions to the rectus muscle of the abdominal wall of patients (see Park, 1965). Although they reported survival of trophoblast only in those patients with elevated oestrogen levels (either endogenous or exogenous) the infirmity of the patients and the previous therapeutic treatment renders any assessment of the findings difficult.

TISSUE CULTURE

Until recently most studies on the *in vitro* growth of trophoblast were limited to explants of normal and pathological placentæ. Although these often proved equivocal they gave some information on cell types and demonstrated the production of hormones by the placenta. The main difficulty has always been one of identifying the cells in culture with their *in vivo* counterparts. This has been partly overcome by culturing cells in monolayers on glass slides and using histochemical stains to demonstrate their synthetic activities. The increasing use of organ culture techniques is also helping to solve this problem. Explants of trophoblast from ectopic pregnancies and hydatidiform moles have been grown in prolonged culture for quantitative studies on gonadotrophin production and correlation with cytological differentiation.

One profitable field of study using culture techniques lies in the investigation of chromosome abnormalities of trophoblast and its tumours. Sex chromatin studies have already provided a reliable method of determining the sex of abortuses as well as normal early conceptuses, and further cytogenetic investigations may yield useful information on the genesis of neoplastic tissues. In this context it is of interest that most benign trophoblastic tumours seem to have an XX constitution, whereas only about half the choriocarcinomas are sex chromatin positive.

Current research on trophoblast in culture has been directed towards the immunology of the tissue. It has now been shown that both trophoblast and post-gestational choriocarcinoma undergo gross cytolysis when cultured *in vitro* with allogeneic (genetically foreign) lymphocytes, whereas syngeneic tissues are not susceptible. It is suggested that this "allogeneic inhibition" indicates that trophoblast and choriocarcinoma express their antigenicity which is then recognized by the immunologically competent lymphocytes. Since these tissues apparently escape destruction *in vivo* it seems likely that they are there protected by a coating of sialomucin which is normally present but removed by the trypsinization before culturing *in vitro*. This important finding may well explain the apparent non-antigenicity of both normal and pathological trophoblast, a fundamental problem considered in the next section.

Considerable data are also available on the *in vitro*

cultivation of mammalian eggs and these have provided much information on early differentiation of the trophoblast and its role in the implantation process.

IMMUNOLOGY OF THE TROPHOBLAST

The Foetus as a Homograft

From the viewpoint of transplantation immunity the relationship between the mother and foetus represents a unique situation. With the rare exception of highly inbred pregnancies, the foetus not only inherits paternal transplantation antigens which are foreign to the mother but also fails to inherit all of the maternal histocompatibility factors. This genetically alien foetus develops in most intimate association with the maternal tissues during the whole of gestation without eliciting any apparent homograft rejection reactions. Naturally occurring instances of foetal death from maternal homograft incompatibility have never been recorded, although it is possible that early foetal deaths, at present etiologically uncertifiable, could be due to some such reaction.

Most of the investigations concerning this immunological problem of pregnancy have been within the philosophical framework proposed by Medawar in 1953. He suggested that the apparently unqualified success of the foetus *qua* homograft could be due to either an antigenic immaturity of the foetal tissues, an immunological inertness of the mother during pregnancy, or to an anatomical barrier between maternal and foetal tissues. There is the further possibility that the uterus may to some extent be an immunologically privileged site, although there is some experimental evidence and the relative success of ectopic pregnancies to argue against this. It is also now generally accepted that transplantation antigens develop very early in foetal life and that the mother is perfectly capable of reacting against such antigens (see review by Billingham, 1964). This has led to consideration of a barrier hypothesis, and this refers the problem to the placenta.

Antigenicity of Trophoblast

It must be emphasized that the foetus is not in actual physical contact with the mother; it is only the placenta, or more precisely, *foetal trophoblast* which is in intimate and prolonged contact with the maternal uterine tissues, and it is at this interface that the tissue reactions of transplantation immunity might be expected to occur. Nevertheless, such immunological reactions have not been detected within the placenta, and this brings into focus the question of trophoblast and its antigenicity.

In every mammalian species that has been critically examined foetal trophoblast has been detected in apposition to the maternal tissues. The placental barrier must surely involve this trophoblast, and to fulfil the barrier role the trophoblast must be non-antigenic. Since the trophoblast is unquestionably foetal in origin it should possess similar transplantation antigens to the foetus, yet most experiments designed to demonstrate the antigenic capacity of trophoblast have proved negative. Trophoblast appeared neither to induce, nor be susceptible to, a state of specific immunity in the mother.

In experimental animals allogeneic transplantation of gestational trophoblast can be carried out with impunity, even between different host species, whilst the embryonic tissue from the same conceptus is relentlessly destroyed. Earlier reports of induction of homograft sensitivity by placental extracts do not demonstrate antigenicity of the trophoblast since such extracts contain many non-trophoblastic cell types which are antigenic. Growths of pure trophoblast can be attained by the transplantation of ectoplacental cones (the proliferative portion of the early murine trophoblast) or tubal eggs to ectopic sites in the mouse. This trophoblast not only exists unharmed in genetically alien environments but may even show greater exuberance than in genetically similar environments.

The evidence so far indicated that trophoblast was either lacking in transplantation antigens or that there was a deficiency in their expression. In this context it is of interest that most investigators have failed to demonstrate the presence of A and B blood group substance (antigens) on human trophoblast, although there is one recent report claiming the presence of A substance localized by rabbit antiserum.

Recent experiments show that ectopically transplanted mouse eggs fail to develop in highly immunized hosts and this is interpreted as demonstrating that immunological reactions are directed against histocompatibility antigens present in the trophectoderm of the eggs. When ecto-placental cone trophoblast is transplanted under similar conditions no such reactions occur and the trophoblast develops unharmed. This may be explained by the presence of a characteristic "fibrinoid" material shown to be present around trophoblast cells, both in the placenta and in extra-uterine sites, and particularly conspicuous at the junction between these cells and the host tissues. It now seems likely that trophoblast contains transplantation antigens but that they are normally masked by a non-cellular envelope described as fibrinoid or sialomucin.

The idea of a barrier (acting either physically or electro-chemically) was developed from observations on fibrinoid around the trophoblast in the mouse placenta, but reference to this type of material can be found in reports on the placentae of many other species, including man. If this is a universal phenomenon it could explain the apparent non-antigenicity of trophoblast, the lack of immune reactions in the placenta, and the survival of the foetus and placenta as a homograft.

Antitrophoblast Antibody

Hulka and his colleagues have studied the appearance of antibodies to human trophoblast in the post-partum period, both in normal and toxaemic pregnancies. They interpret evidence of specific binding of fluorescein-tagged serum globulin by the cytoplasm of the syncytiotrophoblast as indicating the presence of antitrophoblast antibody (and hence antigens in the trophoblast), although the reaction was not specific to the patient's own placenta. They suggest that the appearance of antibody during pregnancy is suppressed by some mechanism such as elevated levels of adrenocorticosteroids, and this must be given some consideration in any explanation of the reports of unsuccessful attempts to detect antibodies to placenta during pregnancy. It is possible that trophoblast antigens are only exposed by the placental commotion at parturition and hence antitrophoblast antibodies would appear solely in the post-partum period. A similar explanation would account for the recent finding of antitrophoblast antibodies in the serum of women with incomplete abortion and also of those in the post-abortive puerperium.

Immunological Competence

There is some indication that mouse trophoblast is immunologically competent, although variability in control experiments and the possibility of mesenchyme cell contamination makes the results difficult to accept without reservation. There is also the intriguing report by Good and Zak of a woman with agammaglobulinaemia who raised antibody titres to the injection of typhoid bacilli in the latter part of pregnancy, and again became non-responsive after delivery of a baby with no demonstrable antibody. This strongly suggests immunological competence of the placenta, and most likely the trophoblast component.

CONTROL OF TROPHOBLAST ACTIVITY

It has been considered that there is a balance between the activity of the gestational trophoblast and the defensive mechanisms of the maternal organism, such that the development of trophoblastic tumours represents a failure of this balance allowing the trophoblast to overstep its normal physiological limit. In the light of recent information on the immune status of trophoblast and mother this balance could have an immunological basis. The placenta itself shows many progressive degenerative changes which might be consistent with an immune response. Trophoblast deportation might be a phenomenon with immunological importance. It has long been claimed that otherwise unexplained regressions of trophoblast tumours could involve immunological mechanisms, and that some spontaneous abortions are homograft rejections. The birth of malformed foetuses following thalidomide administration might reflect the immunosuppressive property of this drug which prevents the immune rejection of an abnormal conceptus. Likewise, immunosuppressive therapy might actually prevent the organism from calling into play immunological processes to reject tumours of the trophoblast.

Some evidence for the implication of maternal antibody systems in the control of trophoblast comes from the findings that choriocarcinoma is much more likely to occur when maternal and foetal blood groups are compatible on the ABO system, and that there is a higher incidence of this tumour amongst women from inbreeding communities. Abnormal trophoblast activity may here be stimulated by a lack of normal maternal responses.

In the mouse genetic dissimilarity between mother and offspring appears to evoke a reaction which influences the size of the placenta. Hybrid foetuses have larger placentae than inbred foetuses in mothers of the same strain of mouse, larger placentae develop when pure-bred eggs are transferred to the uterus of a genetically *dissimilar* foster mother, and placental size may be further influenced by rendering the mother immune or tolerant to the paternal antigens. The most likely explanation is that trophoblast invasiveness is affected by the immunological disparity and that this controls the ultimate size of the placenta.

From the clinical point of view the most urgent question is whether trophoblast tumours have histocompatibility antigens which are expressed, and whether an immunological attack can be directed against such antigens effectively to destroy the tumour. The few previously mentioned cases where immunotherapy appeared to be causally related to trophoblast tumour remission would argue in favour of this, although most opinions agree on the effective non-antigenicity of such tumours. It must be considered possible that the antigenic expression of trophoblast may undergo changes such that it is sometimes vulnerable to immunological attack.

Under normal circumstances it would appear that the trophoblast and its tumours contain histocompatibility antigens, but a coating material may effectively allow the tissue to escape recognition by the maternal immunological mechanisms. Currie and Bagshawe (1967) have recently suggested that a pericellular sialomucin material provides an effective electrochemical barrier to immunologically competent cells, whereas Kirby, Billington, Bradbury and Goldstein (1964) considered a similar "fibrinoid" envelope as a barrier primarily preventing the release of antigen into the maternal circulation. On the basis of these findings a direct immunotherapeutic approach to the tumours of trophoblast seems unlikely to prove rewarding, unless accompanied by a means for disrupting such a barrier.

The whole question of the immunological inter-relationship of mother and foetus is being widely explored at the present time, and it is becoming increasingly evident that immunological mechanisms play an important role in the reproductive process (see Billington, James and Kirby, 1968).

ACKNOWLEDGEMENTS

I am indebted to Dr. D. R. S. Kirby for many helpful discussions, and to those other colleagues who kindly read the manuscript.

SELECTED BIBLIOGRAPHY

Billingham, R. E. (1964), "Transplantation Immunity and the Maternal-foetal Relation," *New Eng. J. Med.*, **270**, 667 and 720.

Billington, W. D., James, D. A. and Kirby, D. R. S. (1968), "Some Effects of Genetic Dissimilarity between Mother and Foetus," *J. Reprod. Fertil. Suppl.*, 3.

Billington, W. D. and Weir, B. J. (1967), "Deportation of Trophoblast in the Chinchilla," *J. Reprod. Fertil.*, **13**, 593.

Bradbury, S., Billington, W. D. and Kirby, D. R. S. (1965), "A Histochemical and Electron Microscopical Study of the Fibrinoid of the Mouse Placenta," *J. Roy. micros. Soc.*, **84**, 199.

Currie, G. A. and Bagshawe, K. D. (1967), "The Masking of Antigens on Trophoblast and Cancer Cells," *Lancet*, **1**, 708.

Enders, A. C. (1965), "A Comparative Study of the Fine Structure of the Trophoblast in several Haemochorial Placentas," *Amer. J. Anat.*, **116**, 29.

Good, R. A. and Zak, S. J. (1956), "Disturbances in Gamma Globulin Synthesis as 'Experiments of Nature'," *Pediatrics*, **18**, 109.

Hamilton, W. J. and Boyd, J. D. (1966), "Specializations of the Syncytium of the Human Chorion," *Brit. Med. J.*, **1**, 1501.

Hulka, J. F. and Brinton, V. (1963), "Antibody to Trophoblast during Early Postpartum Period in Toxaemic Pregnancies," *Amer. J. Obstet. Gynec.*, **86**, 130.

Hulka, J. F., Brinton, V., Schaaf, J. and Baney, C. (1963), "Appearance of Antibodies to Trophoblast during the Postpartum Period in Normal Human Pregnancies," *Nature*, **198**, 501.

Kirby, D. R. S., Billington, W. D., Bradbury, S. and Goldstein, D. J. (1964), "Antigen Barrier of the Mouse Placenta," *Nature*, **204**, 548.

Ober, W. B. (1959), ed. "Trophoblast and its Tumours," *Ann. N.Y. Acad. Sci.*, **80**.

Park, W. W. (1965), ed. *The Early Conceptus, Normal and Abnormal.* Edinburgh and London: E. & S. Livingstone, Ltd.

Ryan, K. J. (1962), "Hormones of the Placenta," *Amer. J. Obstet. Gynec.*, **84**, 1695.

Thiede, H. A. (1961 and 1963), ed. *Transcripts of the 1st and 2nd Rochester Trophoblast Conferences.* Rochester, N.Y.

Wislocki, G. B. and Padykula, H. A. (1961), "Histochemistry and Electron Microscopy of the Placenta," in *Sex and Internal Secretions*, vol. II, ed. W. C. Young. Baltimore: The Williams & Wilkins Co.

Wynn, R. M. (1967), "Fetomaternal Cellular Relations in the Human Basal Plate: An Ultrastructural Study of the Placenta," *Amer. J. Obstet. Gynec.*, **97**, 832.

5. RHESUS IMMUNIZATION

T. E. CLEGHORN and ELLIOT E. PHILIPP

Nearly a quarter of a century elapsed between discovery of the rhesus blood group system with its relationship to haemolytic disease of the newborn (Levine and Stetson, 1939; Landsteiner and Wiener, 1940) and development of a credible means of prophylaxis (Clarke *et al.*, 1966). Landmarks in this progress have been: early induction of labour calculated to remove the foetus from the maternal antibody environment, combined with correction of any anaemia by simple blood transfusion (1941): replacement, or exchange, transfusion with the dual purposes of lowering bilirubin and maternal antibody levels in the infant's circulation, and of replacing its antibody-coated red cells by neutral rhesus negative blood (1943): in 1963, the dramatic and desperate measure of intra-uterine transfusion of red cells into the foetal peritoneal cavity, calculated to maintain the haemoglobin content above cardiac failure level until delivery of a viable infant was possible.

Levine and Stetson (*loc. cit.*) had investigated a case of severe transfusion reaction in the mother of a stillborn infant. The ABO groups were not involved and they concluded that the mother lacked a new antigen and had become immunized against this by her foetus which had inherited it from its father. They were able to show that this new antigen was not part of the ABO, MN or P groups, the only blood group systems known at that time. The maternal antibody agglutinated 80 out of 104 random ABO-compatible samples. An attempt to immunize rabbits against the antigen was unsuccessful.

A few months later, Landsteiner and Wiener (*loc. cit.*) reported work on immunization of rabbits against the red cells of rhesus monkeys. The antibody so produced reacted strongly with 85 per cent of New York random cell samples; weak reactions with the remaining 15 per cent were discounted and so delayed discovery of LW, one of the "background" antigens of the rhesus system, for many years (Levine *et al.*, 1963). They designated the 85 per cent positive reactors Rh positive and the remainder Rh negative. Wiener and Peters (1940) then demonstrated antibodies with identical reactivity in the sera of patients who had suffered severe transfusion reaction not due to ABO incompatibility. The Levine and Stetson antibody was soon shown to be identical with Landsteiner and Wiener's anti-Rh, and Levine and his associates (1941) established conclusively that erythroblastosis foetalis was due to rhesus blood group incompatibility between mother and foetus.

Elementary Genetic Terms

Before proceeding with a description of the further development of our knowledge of the rhesus blood groups, it is necessary to define a number of genetic terms which will be used.

First, the position occupied by a gene on its chromosome is called the *locus* and alternative forms at a particular locus are *alleles*. Re-arrangement of alleles can take place between a matching pair of chromosomes during the first meiotic division in gametogenesis and is known as *crossing-over*. If two loci are on different chromosome pairs, then the apparent cross-over rate will be 0·5 (50%). Values significantly below this figure indicate *linkage*; that is, both loci are on the same chromosome pair. The lower the cross-over rate, the closer the linkage and the shorter the distance between the two loci on the chromosome. An individual who has received an identical allele from each parent is *homozygous* at that locus; *heterozygous* if the alleles differ.

Development of Knowledge of the Rhesus Groups

Other antibodies clearly related to anti-Rh were soon identified and Fisher and Race (1944) published a synthesis built round the reactions of anti-Rh and three such related antibodies. Of these, two were noticed to be giving antithetical reactions and it was postulated that they were defining two alleles *C* and *c*. It was further suggested that the observed facts of inheritance of the groups could all be accommodated within a theory of a closely-linked triplet of alleles. Thus, to *C* and *c* were added *D*, the original Rh antigen, and *E* defined by one of the new antibodies, with postulation of their respective alleles, *d* and *e*. Eight different triplets are theoretically possible and seven of these were identified by Race and Fisher in family studies by use of the four antisera. They considered that linkage between the elements of the triple alleles must be very close, since no example of crossing-over was seen and, further, the genotype frequencies observed were not those which could be expected if crossing-over were other than a very rare event.

The seven triple alleles identified were *CDe*, *cDE*, *cde*, *cDe*, *Cde*, *cdE* and *CDE*. The other theoretical possibility, *CdE*, was described some years later (van den Bosch, 1948) and numerous examples have been recorded since then. Further confirmation of the theory came when Mourant (1945) identified anti-*e* defining the allele of *E*. Early reports of discovery of anti-*d* have been discounted and serious doubts as to its existence are now entertained (Race and Sanger, 1968).

Frequency of the Rh Gene Complexes

Fisher (1953) noted that there were three orders of gene frequency, namely:

First order:	*CDe*, *cDE* and *cde*	12% and over
Second order:	*Cde*, *cdE*, *cDe* and *CDE*	Less than 3%
Third order:	*CdE*	Very rare indeed, and not discovered until later.

He suggested that on statistical grounds these were compatible with the sequence *DCE* along the chromosome and that the second order of frequency could have arisen by occasional crossing-over from the common hetero-zygotes in the first. The great rarity of *CdE* could also be explained by its origin as a result of further crossing-over from a genotype involving a second order complex.

The gene frequencies* in Caucasians are as follows with Wiener's symbols in parenthesis. (After Race and Sanger *loc. cit.*, 1968.)

Rh (*D*) Positive			Rh (*D*) Negative		
CDe	(*R¹*)	0·41	*cde*	(*r*)	0·39
cDE	(*R²*)	0·14	*Cde*	(*r'*)	0·01
cDe	(*R⁰*)	0·03	*cdE*	(*r''*)	0·01
CDE	(*Rᶻ*)	Less than 0·01	*CdE*	(*rʸ*)	Less than 0·001
Combined		0·59	Combined		0·41

Nomenclature of the Rhesus Groups

A voluminous literature has accumulated stressing real and imaginary differences between the Fisher–Race interpretation and that of Wiener and his associates who favoured a theory of multiple alleles at a single locus. Race withdrew from this controversy some years ago with the statement that "the work of the bacterial geneticists on the fine structure of genes shows that we are unlikely to be dealing with one mutational site or with three, but more probably with hundreds" (Race and Sanger, 1962). On the basis of practical understanding, the CDE nomen-clature has much to commend it and little against. On the other hand, some of the shorthand evolved from Wiener's views has the merit of simplicity and convenience in everyday use. The facts are admittedly identical and it is unfortunate that such an exciting chapter in human genetics should have been clouded by what is virtually now a "non-controversy". A noble attempt to introduce neutrality came from Rosenfield and his colleagues (1962) following a lead from Murray (1944) but their proposals are more for discussion between computers than clinicians.

The ABO Groups

A brief statement of the basic facts concerning the ABO blood groups is not inappropriate at this stage. There are three main alleles, *A*, *B*, and *O* and the antisera are anti-A, anti-B, and anti-A + B. No true example of anti-O has been found, so that group O is defined by default of reaction with any of the antisera. Consequently, hetero-zygotes *AO* and *BO* may only be recognized as a result of family studies and homozygotes *AA* and *BB* almost always only on the basis of statistical probability.

A feature of these groups is the invariable presence of naturally-occurring antibodies, the iso-agglutinins, in the plasma of healthy individuals and these are directed against any antigens not present on the cells; thus:

Cells (Antigens)	*Serum* (Antibodies)
A	Anti-B
B	Anti-A
AB	No antibody
O	Anti − A + B.

* The frequency of a homozygote may be obtained by squaring the appropriate gene frequency; that of a heterozygote by doubling the product of the two gene frequencies.

The Rhesus Antibodies

The early discoveries within the system were made with saline agglutinins but it was soon found that a number of cases of undoubted haemolytic disease of the newborn disclosed no antibodies on investigation. Independent work in 1944 by Diamond, Race and Wiener led to recognition of a second category of Rh antibody which could be shown to react with Rh positive cells in such a way as to prevent their agglutination by the saline agglu-tinins, the so-called "blocking" reaction. These blocked cells were found to agglutinate in the presence of a variety of substances of high molecular weight including bovine albumin, polyvinyl pyrrolidine and even fish glue. Coombs, Mourant and Race (1945) re-discovered the Moreschi test (1908) and demonstrated that the blocked cells were coated with antibody globulin and would agglutinate after addition of a rabbit anti-human globulin reagent. This Coombs' test has been widely applied to laboratory diagnosis of haemolytic disease of the newborn by cord blood tests, as well as to antibody estimation and cross-matching of blood for transfusion, and has been instru-mental in identification of a number of the newer, un-related blood group systems.

It is now recognized that the saline-agglutinating anti-body, also called complete, belongs to the IgM, 19S fraction of gamma globulin, while the "blocking", albumin-reactive or incomplete ones are IgG, 7S in type. Work initiated by Pickles (1946) has demonstrated that incomplete antibodies may readily be detected when the appropriate test cells have been treated with certain en-zymes, which include papain, trypsin, bromelin, pronase and neuraminidase. These all have in common the ability to remove sialic acid from the red cell membrane with consequent alteration in the net electrical charge (*see* Whittam, 1964).

In general, IgM antibodies are formed as the early response to Rh immunization and seem unable to cross the placental barrier. Later response is of the IgG type which readily passes into the foetal circulation to sensitize the cells of the Rh positive infant and bring about their destruction. Many Rh antisera retain some proportion of saline agglutinating antibody and recent work (Murray, 1967; Hopkins, 1969) suggests that this persistence, or recall, may be of ill-omen for the foetus although the mechanism is not understood.

The Mechanism of Rhesus Immunization

It has long been known that a single transfusion of rhesus positive blood to a rhesus negative recipient will result in formation of Rh antibodies in about 50 per cent of cases (Diamond, 1947). Considerable evidence exists on the experimental side, however, for equal effectiveness of much smaller doses; for example Freda and his col-leagues (1966) demonstrated Rh antibodies in the sera of 6 of 13 volunteers who were given a single dose of 1·0 ml. Even doses as small as 0·1 ml. of red cells have been shown to be effective (Zipursky), and an antibody may appear within one month of injection (Lehane). Repeated in-jections will increase the number who respond and there is some evidence to suggest that a long interval between injections is more effective than a short one (*see* Chown, 1968). About one third of all individuals seem to be highly resistant to repeated attempts at immunization (Wiener, 1949; Clarke, 1963).

Levine (1943) noted that there was a significant excess of ABO compatible husbands of women who had borne infants with haemolytic disease and numerous studies subsequently have confirmed this observation (for references, *see* Mollison, 1967). Stern and his associates (1956) in their studies of experimental immunization found that ABO-compatible cells were more effective in stimulating antibody formation than were cells which were ABO incompatible with the recipient's serum. The precise mechanism of this group effect has not been elucidated.

There seems to be little doubt that maternal Rh immunization is the result of transfer of rhesus positive foetal red cells into the rhesus negative mother's circulation. Such foetal haemorrhages have been reported at all stages of pregnancy, but it seems certain that they occur most frequently during the third trimester. Obstetric interference and manipulation causes a sharp increase in the percentage of maternal samples showing foetal blood, as does delivery itself (*see* Woodrow and Finn, 1966). There is a strong positive correlation between the estimated volume of foetal blood present in a woman's circulation immediately after delivery and the probability that she will form antibodies. On this basis, the Liverpool school divided parturient women into high-risk (22%) and low-risk (78%), categories (Clarke *et al.*, *loc. cit.*, 1966).

It is generally agreed that antibody formation is rarely seen during the first pregnancy, perhaps only in 1–2 per cent of cases. However, during the six months postpartum, antibodies have been demonstrated in 20 per cent or more of cases, but there are wide variations between different population groups perhaps due to differences in obstetric practice or even in sexual habits (*see* Chown *loc. cit.*, 1968). There is no doubt however that second pregnancies differ greatly from first ones and represent the period of maximum antibody manifestation. From then onwards the number of newly immunized cases diminishes sharply and approximates to zero in fifth and subsequent pregnancies (Nevanlinna and Vainio, 1960). Mollison (*loc. cit.*, 1967) compares results from these workers with those of Wiener (1949) in respect of the much greater effectiveness of immunization by injection and suggests that maternal tolerance may play a part. In comparison of results from different laboratories, it must be borne in mind that there are great differences in sensitivity of the laboratory techniques in routine use.

Rhesus Genotypes of Husbands of Immunized Women

The two common rhesus positive genes in Caucasians are *cDE* (R^2) and *CDe* (R^1) and there is considerable evidence to suggest that foetuses which carry the former are more likely to stimulate formation of Rh antibodies and to be at greater risk from these (Murray, Knox and Walker, 1965). This accords with the observation by Rochna and Hughes-Jones (1965) that the number of D

antigen sites on the red cells was 14,500–19,300 for *CDe/CDe* and 15,800–33,300 for *cDE/cDE*.

It is also important to know the husband's genotype, and hence zygosity, in order to advise on the probable outcome of future pregnancies. The blood typing reagents available for this purpose are anti-C, -D, -E, -c and -e, and it should be borne in mind that in the absence of anti-d, true genotyping is not possible. Results of these tests are, or should be, given as the most probable interpretation of the laboratory findings. As will be seen below, the three common genotypes apparently homozygous for D have a 5–10 per cent chance of being heterozygous; similarly, there is a 5 per cent chance that the two common apparent heterozygotes will actually be homozygous for D. These facts should be studied carefully before any sterilization procedure is advised for immunized women and investigation of the groups of the husband's family should be carried out wherever possible in these cases and may be most informative.

Genotype	Apparent	Zygosity	Probability
CDe/CDe	R^1R^1	DD	0·95
CDe/cDE	R^1R^2	DD	0·89
cDE/cDE	R^2R^2	DD	0·86
CDe/cde	R^1r	Dd	0·94
cDE/cde	R^2r	Dd	0·94
cDe	R^0 (phenotype)	Dd	0·97

The proportion of *D* heterozygotes in a Caucasian population is 0·48 (2 × 0·59 × 0·41); that of *D* homozygotes 0·35 (0·59 × 0·59); the remaining 0·17 (0·41 × 0·41) being rhesus negative. It follows that rhesus positive husbands will be homozygous with a probability of 0·42 compared with 0·58 for heterozygosity. Offspring of the former will all be rhesus positive, probability 1·0; on average, 50 per cent of children of the latter will be rhesus positive, probability 0·5. From this it will be seen that the mating of a rhesus positive man with a rhesus negative women will result in a rhesus positive foetus with a probability of 0·59 (0·35 × 0·48 × 0·5); the probability of two successive rhesus positive foetuses from this mating is 0·47 (0·35 × 0·48 × 0·5 × 0·5). It is important to note that the incidence of formation of anti-Rh and haemolytic disease of the foetus is only about one-tenth of this figure of 0·47 (Mollison, *loc. cit.*, 1968).

Detection of Foetal Bleeds

Foetal cells may be detected in the maternal blood by a variety of different techniques but the most useful by far is the acid-elution method. Alcohol-fixed blood films are treated with an acid buffer (pH 3·3) in which adult, but not foetal, haemoglobin is soluble (Betke and Kleihauer, 1958). The foetal cells stand out prominently from a background of adult ghosts in a counter-stained preparation, and an estimate of the extent of foetal bleeding can be made from their number. Considerable experience with the test is necessary.

Measurement of Antibody Concentration

Until recently, Rh antibody quantitation involved titration of the serum against rhesus positive indicator cells, using one of the several recognized techniques for demonstrating antibodies. Most frequently, doubling dilutions of the serum were made, the titre being the reciprocal of the greatest dilution at which antibody was still detectable.

Methods which have been found to give the most consistent results involved either agglutination of enzyme treated cells, or the indirect Coombs' technique using un-modified cells. This latter consists of incubation together of standard volumes of indicator cells and of the different dilutions of serum, followed by washing away the excess serum and demonstration of antibody uptake by means of the anti-human globulin reagent.

Hughes-Jones (1967) developed a more sophisticated version of this test for his quantitative studies and was able to express the antibody content of sera in terms of microgrammes per millilitre. The newer automated techniques using enzyme-treated cells for antibody detection (Spurgeon, Cedergren and McQuiston, 1963) have recently been calibrated against standards evaluated by the Hughes-Jones' technique, and allow of reports of antibody quantitation in absolute terms. This is now standard practice in a number of specialist laboratories. An indirect Coombs' titre of 1 was shown by Hughes-Jones to be equivalent to 0.02 ± 25 per cent microgrammes of antibody per millilitre of serum (*loc. cit.*). Although this range may appear at first sight large, it should be viewed in comparison with the accepted one-tube variation either way in a doubling dilution titration, where the true range is between one half and double the value given.

Antibody Quantitation and Antenatal Assessment of Severity

The conditions of antibody quantitation *in vitro* differ greatly from those *in vivo* and it is hardly surprising that the correlation is poor between maternal antibody titre and the state of the foetus. A titre of 64 or less by the indirect Coombs' technique usually means that treatment will not be needed, while 256–512 is of ill omen and indicates a severely affected infant. These latter values correspond to 5–10 microgrammes of antibody per millilitre of serum in quantitation by Hughes-Jones' method.

The Role of Amniocentesis

Intraperitoneal transfusions are nothing new. The first experimental ones in animals were done over a hundred years ago and human beings seem to have received them as long ago as 1875 (Ponfick, 1875), but transuterine intraperitoneal transfusions are new, and were first described in 1963 by Liley (1963), whose technique is still the standard one throughout the world.

In 1956 Bevis first described the inspection of liquor by amniocentesis (Bevis, 1956). The first step is to place a needle through the abdominal wall into the pregnant uterus and withdraw some amniotic fluid. If the tap is not blood-stained and the liquor looks very yellow it can be assumed that the child is likely to be affected; for in the process of the destruction of red blood cells bilirubin is liberated and some of this is excreted in the child's urine into the liquor. As simple inspection of the liquor is not accurate enough spectrophotometry is used.

A word about liquor is not out of place here. It seems likely, according to the work of Gordon Bourne (1962) and others including Plentl and Hutchinson (1953) carried out in England and the United States, that the whole volume of liquor can be changed in three hours. This means that if the volume of liquor is nearly two pints, every hour about two thirds of a pint will be absorbed from the bag of membranes into the foetal or maternal circulation. The infant *in utero* swallows some of the fluid, which by an indirect mechanism, returns to the mother via the placenta.

There are other ways in which the liquor is adsorbed through the wall of the uterus, through the placenta directly and possibly even through the umbilical cord. The liquor is replaced by the child passing urine, possibly by its sweat and by transudation through the amnion yet once more. In this way toxins that the child passes in its urine are eventually excreted by the mother in her urine possibly after being detoxicated in her liver. If a child is unable to swallow because of a defect in the oesophagus, such as atresia, hydramnios will occur. This is a well-known clinical feature of foetal defects of the upper digestive tract. On the other hand, if the child's kidneys are maldeveloped or not developed at all then there may be a deficiency of liquor and this is also well recognized.

If some of the liquor surrounding a rhesus-affected baby is placed in a spectrophotometer it is possible for the distortion of the spectrum of light passing through the liquor to be measured and from this the quantity of bilirubin in the liquor can be estimated (Liley, 1963). It is on the results of the spectrophotometric analysis of the amniotic fluid that the decision is taken whether to attempt intraperitoneal foetal blood transfusion. The optical density as measured at 450 A on the spectrophotometric machine gives most information because that is the wavelength of bilirubin. Several samples are withdrawn at different intervals in the pregnancy, very often starting soon after 20 weeks; by the measurement of optical density rise at 450 A compared with the normal graph for that particular stage of gestation, the degree of severity of the disease can be ascertained. Skilled observers using for comparison graphs of normal and abnormal liquor optical properties can predict whether a child is likely to die *in utero* within the next week or two, and decide whether to give it an intraperitoneal transfusion. Naturally in a case where the baby is rhesus negative there should be little or no rise in bilirubin as the pregnancy continues and therefore no indication for intrauterine transfusion, and we can reassure the mother of the outcome.

If the curve shows that the baby is likely to die in spite of all measures one might even consider terminating the pregnancy to avoid further suffering for the mother. If on the other hand there seems a reasonable possibility that the intraperitoneal transfusion will prolong the survival of the child in the uterus until such time as it is unlikely to die of prematurity, then such transfusion will be made. The survival rate for babies receiving intrauterine transfusions is in the region of 40 to 50 per cent.

Prevention of Rh Immunization of Pregnancy

Attention has been drawn above to the comparative inefficiency of the ABO incompatible cells in immunizing mothers or volunteers to the rhesus factor. This fact led the Liverpool workers to suggest that passively-administered Rh antibodies of high titre might in similar manner bring about rapid elimination of ABO compatible Rh positive foetal bleeds and so reduce the incidence of immunization. This work has proved to be brilliantly successful although the ABO protection model is almost certainly not relevant. While passive administration of anti-Rh at, or shortly after, delivery of a mother or injection of a volunteer is almost 100 per cent successful in suppressing antibody response, rapid clearance of rhesus positive red cells from the circulation may be only a minor part of the process (Pollack, 1968).

It is known that in other immune systems simultaneous administration of specific antibody with antigen can inhibit completely primary antibody response (for references, *see* Mollison *loc. cit.*, 1967). The IgG type of antibody is by far the more efficient and the Liverpool workers even suggested that IgM might have an enhancing effect. While this suggestion has yet to be put to more critical experimental test, there is no doubt as to the effectiveness of IgG antibody globulin. Rosenfield (1968) reported on a symposium on Rh immunological suppression held in New York in 1967 with figures showing that only 4 out of 2,602 protected primiparae developed Rh antibodies within 6 months of delivery compared with 160 out of 1,918 unprotected controls. Subsequent work confirms the almost complete success of this treatment.

It is agreed that doses of 200–300 microgrammes of antibody globulin given by the intramuscular route within 36–48 hours of delivery are adequate. Restriction on the category of case which merits such prophylaxis come only from difficulties of supply which will soon be resolved.

REFERENCES

Betke, K. and Kleihauer, E. (1958), "Fetaler und Bleibender Blut-farbstoff in Erythrozyten und Erythroblasten von Menschlichen Feten und Neugeborenen," *Blut*, **4**, 241.

Chown, B. (1968), "On Rh Immunization and its Prevention: Observations and Thoughts," *Vox Sang.*, **15**, 259.

Clarke, C. A. and many others (1966), "Prevention of Rh Haemolytic Disease: Results of the Clinical Trial. A combined Study from Centres in England and Baltimore," *Brit. med. J.*, **ii**, 907.

Clarke, C. A. and many others (1963), "Further Experimental Studies on the Prevention of Rh Haemolytic Disease," *Brit. med. J.*, **i**, 979.

Coombs, R. R. A., Mourant, A. E. and Race, R. R. (1945), "Detection of Weak and 'Incomplete' Rh Agglutinins: A New Test," *Lancet*, **ii**, 15.

Diamond, L. K. (1944), "Progress Report to Committee on Medical Research of the Office on Scientific Research and Development," *OEM.* cmr. 384, Jan. 1st.

Diamond, L. K. (1947), "Erythroblastosis Foetalis or Haemolytic Disease of the Newborn," *Proc. Roy. Soc. Med.*, **40**, 546.

Fairweather, D. V. I. and Walker, E. (1965), "Current Views on the Management of Rhesus Iso-immunization," *Ob. Gyn. Digest*, **7**, 49.

Fisher, R. A. *see* Race, R. R. (1944).

Fisher, Sir Ronald (1953), "Population Genetics," *Proc. Roy. Soc. B.*, **141**, 510.

Freda, V. J. (1963), "The Rh Problem in Obstetrics and a New Concept of its Management using Amniocentesis and Spectrophotometric Scanning of Amniotic Fluid," *Amer. J. Obstet. Gynec.*, **92**, 341.

Freda, V. J., Gorman, J. G. and Pollack, W. (1966), "Rh Factor: Prevention of Immunization and Clinical Trial on Mothers," *Sci.*, **151**, 828.

Hopkins, D. F. (1969), "Saline Anti-Rh (D) and Haemolytic Disease of the Newborn," *Vox. Sang.*, **16**, 32.

Hughes-Jones, N. C. (1967), "The Estimation of the Concentration and Equilibrium Constant of Anti-D," *Immunology*, **12**, 565.

Landsteiner, K. and Wiener, A. S. (1940), "An Agglutinable Factor in Human Blood Recognized by Immune Sera for Rhesus Blood," *Proc. Soc. exp. Biol. (N.Y.)*, **43**, 223.

Lehane, D. Personal Communication to Chown, B. (1968).

Levine, P. and Stetson, R. E. (1939), "An Unusual Case of Intra group Agglutination," *J. Amer. Med. Ass.*, **113**, 126.

Levine, P., Burnham, L., Katzin, E. M. and Vogel, P. (1941), "The Role of Isoimmunization in the Pathogenesis of Erythroblastosis Fetalis," *Am. J. Obst. Gynec.*, **42**, 925.

Levine, P. (1943), "Serological Factors as Possible Causes in Spontaneous Abortions," *J. Hered.*, **34**, 71.

Levine, P., Celano, M. J., Wallace, J. and Sanger, Ruth (1963), "A Human 'D-like' Antibody," *Nature (Lond.)*, **198**, 596.

Liley, A. W. (1961), "Liquor Amnii Analysis in Management of Pregnancy Complicated by Rhesus Sensitization," *Amer. J. Obstet. Gynec.*, **82**, 1359.

Mollison, P. L. (1967), *Blood Transfusion in Clinical Medicine*, 4th edition, p. 321, Oxford, Blackwell.

Moreschi, C. (1908), "Neue Tatsachen uber die Blutkorperchen-agglutination," *Zbl. Bakt.*, **46**, 49.

Mourant, A. E. (1945), "A New Rhesus Antibody," *Nature (Lond.)*, **155**, 542.

Murray, J. (1944), "A Nomenclature of Subgroups of the Rh Factor," *Nature (Lond.)*, **154**, 701.

Murray, Sheilagh, Knox, G. and Walker, W. (1965), "Haemolytic Disease and the Rhesus Genotypes," *Vox. Sang.*, **10**, 257.

Murray, Sheilagh (1967), "Rh Antibody Type in Haemolytic Disease of the Newborn," *Vox. Sang.*, **12**, 81.

Nevanlinna, H. R. and Vainio, T. (1960), "An Attempt to Calculate the Probability of Rh Immunization during Pregnancy," *Commun. 8th Cong. Int. Soc. Blood Transf. (Tokyo)*.

Pickles, Margaret M. (1946), "Effects of Cholera Filtrate on Red Cells as Demonstrated by Incomplete Rh Antibodies," *Nature (Lond.)*, **158**, 880.

Pollack, W., Gorman, J. G., Hager, H. J., Freda, V. J. and Tripodi, D. (1968), "Antibody-mediated Immune Suppression to the Rh Factor: Animal Models suggesting Mechanism of Action," *Transfusion*, **8**, 134.

Race, R. R. (1944), "An 'Incomplete' Antibody in Human Serum," *Nature (Lond.)*, **153**, 771.

Race, R. R. and Sanger, Ruth (1962), *Blood Goups in Man*, 4th edition, p. 138, Oxford, Blackwell.

Race, R. R. and Sanger, Ruth (1968), *Blood Groups in Man*, 5th edition, p. 173. Oxford: Blackwell.

Rochna, Erna and Hughes-Jones, N. C. (1965), "The Use of Purified 125 I-labelled Anti-γ Globulin in the Determination of the Number of D Antigen Sites on Red Cells of different Phenotypes," *Vox Sang.*, **10**, 675.

Rosenfield, R. E. (1968), "Immunological Suppression of Primary Rh Antibody Formation," *Transfusion*, **8**, 125.

Rosenfield, R. E., Allen, F. H., Swisher, S. N. and Kochwa, S. (1962), "A Review of Rh Serology and Presentation of a New Terminology," *Transfusion (Philad.)*, **2**, 287.

Stern, K., Davidsohn, I. and Masaitis, Lillian (1956), "Experimental Studies on Rh Immunization," *Amer. J. Clin. Path.*, **26**, 833.

Sturgeon, P., Cedergren, B. and McQuiston, Dorothy (1963), "Automation of Routine Blood Typing Procedures," *Vox Sang.*, **8**, 438.

Van den Bosch, Clara (1948), "The very Rare Rh Genotype Ryr (CdD/cde) in a Case of Erythroblastosis Foetalis," *Nature (Lond.)*, **162**, 781.

Walker, W., Fairweather, D. V. I. and Jones, P., "Examination of Liquor Amnii as a Method of Predicting Severity of Haemolytic Disease of the Newborn," *Brit. med. J.*, **ii**, 140.

Whittam, R. (1964), *Transport and Diffusion in Red Blood Cells.* Monographs of the Physiological Society. London: Arnold.

Wiener, A. S. (1944), "A New Test (Blocking Test) for Rh Sensitization," *Proc. Soc. exp. Biol. (N.Y.)*, **56**, 173.

Wiener, A. S. (1949), "Further Observations on Isosensitization to the Rh Factor," *Proc. Soc. exp. Biol. (N.Y.)*, **70**, 576.

Wiener, A. S. and Peters, H. R. (1940), "Haemolytic Reactions following Transfusions of Blood in the Homologous Group, with Three Cases in which the same Agglutinogen was Responsible," *Ann. int. Med.*, **13**, 2306.

Woodrow, J. C. and Finn, R. (1966), "Transplacental Haemorrhage," *Brit. J. Haemat.*, **12**, 297.

Zipursky, A. Personal Communication to Chown, B. (1968).

6. FOETAL SEX AND DEVELOPMENT OF GENITALIA

C. J. DEWHURST

Any consideration of foetal sex is hampered by a lack of a single criterion by which an individual's sex may be judged. Broadly speaking there are four separate criteria of sex which appear in this order.

1. Chromosomal sex: females have an XX arragement of sex chromosomes, males an XY arrangement.

2. Gonadal sex: females possess ovaries, males testes.

3. Genital sex: females, in addition to ovaries, have a vulva, vagina, uterus and two fallopian tubes; males, in addition to testes, have a penis, prostate, seminal vesicles, vasa differentia and epididymes.

4. Pyschological sex: females have a characteristic feminine psyche and a sex drive directed towards males; males have a characteristic masculine psyche and a sex drive directed towards females.

Normally all four criteria agree but not always, for each of these stages is not inexorably followed by the next. Disregarding psychological sex as inappropriate to our present considerations, a foetus may for instance have XY sex chromosomes and testes yet may develop female external genitalia (the testicular feminizing syndrome): or XY sex chromosomes, rudimentary "streak" gonads and female genitalia (pure gonadal dysgenesis); or XX sex chromosomes and ovaries but female internal and male external genitalia. Clearly the relationship between these factors is important and must be studied further.

If a zygote forms as a result of union between an ovum and a spermatozoom bearing a Y sex chromosome the XY zygote will develop testes and then male genitalia. If the sex chromosomes are XX testes will not appear which suggests that a Y chromosome is necessary for testicular development. A Y chromosome alone however is not sufficient for no YO zygote has ever been found and this combination must be considered non-viable. Provided there is an X present more than one Y chromosome still permits testicular formation for XYY individuals appear to have normal testes and to be fertile (Ricci and Mallacarne, 1964; Sandberg, Koepf, Ishihara and Hauschka, 1961; Jacobs, Brunton, Melville, Brittain and Mc-Clemont, 1965). One or more Y chromosomes in association with two X chromosomes (XXY, XXXY) again allows testicular formation although the subsequent development of the testes in later life is unlikely to be normal (Jacobs and Strong, 1959; Overzier, 1963; Lennox, 1963).

If the zygote is XX ovaries will normally develop. As we have seen a Y chromosome present as well will determine testicular development. If one X chromosome only is present the embryo will not be non-viable as in the case of the YO arrangement for an XO individual may be born alive and may live a normal life span although the percentage of XO foetuses which are aborted is high (Carr, 1965). Such an XO foetus will not develop normal ovaries but mere streaks of tissue at the usual ovarian sites (Turner, 1938; Miller, 1964). The presence of one or more extra X chromosomes (XXX, XXXX, etc.) is compatible with normal ovarian development both in utero and at puberty (Close, 1963; Miller, 1964).

The relationship of the sex chromosomes to foetal sex may therefore be summed up as follows—*the presence of a Y chromosome in combination with one or more X chromosomes will determine testicular development in the early embryo. The presence of two or more X chromosomes without a Y will determine the development of ovaries.*

We must next examine the fascinating relationship between the formation of gonads and the development of the other genital organs. The XO individual referred to above will possess only "streak" ovaries but otherwise normal female genital organs. Normal genital development therefore does not appear to depend upon normal ovarian development. The relationship which does exist between the development of the gonad and that of the other genital organs was established by Jost (1947) in a series of remarkable experiments which demonstrated that the testes of the early embryo have a twofold function to perform:

1. that of promoting the development of Wolffian structures;

2. that of inhibiting the development of Mullerian structures, both systems being present in the early embryo and capable of development.

Removal of the testes from the early embryo in the rabbit permitted the growth of female genital organs without any development of male ones. Removal of the testes at a later stage did not prevent male differentiation.

Removal of ovaries in the early female embryo had no effect on the subsequent growth of female genital organs. The relationship between the nature of the gonad and the development of the remaining genital organs may therefore be summed up as follows: if testes are present and fulfilling their normal intra-uterine function male differentiation of the genital tract takes place. If testes are not present or are not fulfilling their normal intra-uterine function female differentiation of the genital tract takes place whatever the nature of the sex chromosomes and whether ovaries are present or not.

We may say therefore that the nature of the sex chromosomes determines the nature of the gonad which in turn determines the differentiation of the other genital organs.

Normally the development of the external genitalia is the criterion by which the sex of an individual is judged and as we have seen it is dependent on the nature of the gonads in the early embryo. But this is not the only factor concerned in external genital development. Mention must be made of two circumstances in which external genital development is inappropriate to gonadal and chromosomal sex. The first of these is when excessive androgen stimulation affects the female foetus during early development. The adreno-genital syndrome in the female foetus may give rise to masculinization of external genitalia although internal genitalia are normal; androgenic drugs given to the mother in early pregnancy may have a similar effect. A male foetus would be unaffected by either event since male differentiation would occur anyway. These instances suggest that the testicular substance or substances giving rise to the twofold action noted above are not known androgens which although they may masculinize external genitalia never inhibit mullerian duct formation. The second condition characterized by inappropriate external genital development is the testicular feminizing syndrome. In this condition XY patients with testes nevertheless develop a normal looking vulva and a short blind vagina; the uterus is rudimentary or absent. Moreover these patients undergo normal secondary sex development at puberty. The explanation of this syndrome is unknown but it may be concerned with an abnormal response of end organs rather than an abnormal production of hormones.

Development of the Genital Tract

Since suitable human embryos at different stages of development are comparatively scarce and the nature of the work involved in their examination is extremely specialized few people have the opportunity of personally studying the development of the foetus. Most embryological accounts agree however on the principles of development of the genital tract as a whole although different views are held on gonadal and vaginal development.

The genital organs develop in close association with those of the urinary tract. Both systems arise in the intermediate mesoderm lying on each side of the root of the mesentery beneath the coelomic epithelium. The pronephros appears first as a few transient excretory tubules in the cervical region. These quickly degenerate but the duct, which begins at the caudal end of the pronephros,

persists and passes down the body to open at the cloaca. Connection will ultimately be established between this duct and some of the tubules of the mesonephros presently to appear; the duct is accordingly known as the mesonephric (Wolffian) duct. The mesonephros, a second primitive kidney, develops as a long prominent swelling bulging into the dorsal wall of the coelom in the thoracic and upper lumbar regions. The mesonephros later degenerates to a different extent in each sex: in the male portions of it persist as the excretory system of the male genital system, in the female a few vestiges only survive (Fig. 3).

Two structures of great importance become evident on the coelomic surface of the mesonephros. The first, the genital ridge from which the gonad in each sex is to develop, is visible as a swelling on the medial aspect of the mesonephros; this ridge at first extends throughout the length of the mesonephros but later becomes condensed to the central portion only. The second structure of importance is the paramesonephric (Mullerian) duct from which much of the female genital tract will develop; this forms as an ingrowth of coelomic epithelium on the lateral aspect of the mesonephric bulge. The ingrowth becomes a groove and then sinks below the surface to form a tube; its subsequent development will be followed presently.

The Development of the Gonads

The first signs of the primitive gonad are evident in embryos of 5·5 to 7·5 mm. crown rump (5 weeks). Gillman (1948) gives a detailed account of the development of the gonads in man. He believes the gonad to be of triple origin from:

1. the coelomic epithelium of the genital ridge;
2. underlying mesoderm;
3. the primtive germ cells which come from some extra gonadal source (see later).

The gonad begins as a bulge on the medial aspect of the mesonephric ridge. The earliest changes are a proliferation of the cells of the coelomic epithelium beneath which is a concentration of mesenchymal cells. Beneath this again is a zone containing scanty mesenchymal cells separating the developing gonad from the mesonephros proper. By 7 to 9 mm. (5–6 weeks) stage cords of coelomic epithelium are seen projecting into the substance of the developing gonad breaking up the mesenchyme into loose strands interdigitating with these cords. Rapid development of the cords follows and in the deeper layers of the developing gonad they become branched and complex. During these early stages large numbers of big, primitive germ cells can be seen lying between the cords. Gradually the primitive germ cells become evident within the sex cords and the cells themselves become reduced in size. This is the indifferent stage of gonadal development which is alike in the male and the female. It may be seen that the coelomic epithelium gives rise to the sex cords and the primitive mesenchymal tissue gives rise to the supporting tissue between. The germ cells (as will be seen shortly) arise extragonadally.

Gonadal differentiation is first evident in the testes. In embryos of some 14 to 16 mm. crown rump length

(7 weeks) early differentiation is visible by great prominence of the sex cords, a decrease in number and size of the cells of the outer cellular layer and of wide separation of cords by mesenchymal tissue. Primitive germ cells first disappear from the peripheral region. The epithelial cells of the outer layer then become smaller and separated from each

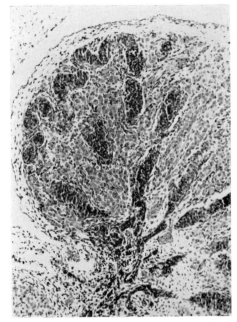

FIG. 1. The testis of a 14 week foetus. The tunica is visible; the sex cords, separated by mesenchyme, are continuous into the hilar region. × 144 (from Willis, 1962).

other by oedematous matrix; they later become differentiated into spindle-shaped fibroblasts and ultimately form the tunica albuginea. The rete testis, the straight and seminiferous tubules arise from the sex cords; the interstitial cells develop from the mesenchymal portion of the genital primordium (Fig. 1).

The ovary is not positively identifiable until some time later than the testes, the first indication that the gonad will develop into an ovary being failure of the testicular changes already outlined to make their appearance. The gonad that is to become an ovary passes from the indifferent stage into one of differentiation and growth and later into the stage of follicle formation and stromal development. By the 17 mm. stage sex cords beneath the outer cellular layer increase greatly in size and are sometimes called the secondary sex cords; those which have formed during the indifferent stage, and are so important in the male, are thus displaced centrally into the hilum of the developing gonad. The mesenchymal cells between these secondary sex cords become inconspicuous so that, instead of an outer zone without primitive germ cells and with loose cells later to become spindle shaped as in the testis, there is a very thick active cellular zone in which many germ cells persist (Fig. 2). The epithelial cells of these secondary cords are called by Gillman (1948) the pregranulosa cells. These early differentiation changes are followed by a very active growth phase. This is characterized by a proliferation of pregranulosa cells and

germ cells the latter being considerably reduced in size. This growth phase continues until the embryo has a crown rump length of about 100 mm. or so (14 weeks) and as a result of it there is a great increase in bulk of the developing gonad.

The stage of follicle formation and stroma development follows. Recognizable foetal stroma cells develop from the mesenchyme in the region of the ovarian hilum at first. They are seen in embryos of 150 to 180 mm. crown rump length (20–24 weeks) and they gradually spread peripherally until they permeate the whole ovary by 280 to 300 mm. (32–34 weeks). In advance of the developing stroma the oocytes become encapsulated by a ring of pregranulosa cells. An interesting feature of the formation of follicles and the development of stroma is the disintegration of many oocytes. Those which do not succeed in encircling themselves with a capsule of pregranulosa cells degenerate as the advancing stroma reaches them, suggesting that the stroma does not provide the satisfactory support for them or is lethal to them. Once the stroma has spread throughout the primitive ovary the primary follicles develop a capsule of stroma cells and the pregranulosa cells become granulosa cells. The granulosa cells secrete a fluid which is first retained within the cell membrane but ultimately accumulates in the follicular cavity. The stroma cells of the follicular capsule differentiate into theca cells. Many follicles at this stage are seen to be atretic.

As mentioned at the outset the interpretation of changes in early embryos is specialized and difficult and other workers although observing similar changes to those reported by Gillman (1948) have put somewhat different interpretations on them. Willis (1962) summarizes these differing views.

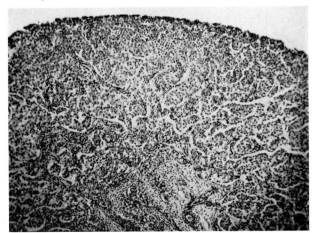

FIG. 2. Ovary of a 13 week foetus. There is no tunica but continuation of the outer cellular zone into underlying tissue. Compare Fig. 1. × 60 (from Willis, 1962).

The Origin of the Ova

Over many years there have been conflicting views expressed concerning the origin of the germ cells. Their origin is now generally accepted to be in the endoderm before the formation of the mesoderm of the lateral plate and before somite formation (Pinkerton et al., 1961) although Willis (1962) believes this to be not yet proved. Witschi (1948) studying a 3·5 mm. (4 weeks) embryo found primitive germ cells in the epithelium of yolk sac. According to Pinkerton and his colleagues germ cells migrate along the endoderm of the yolk sac into the gut, through the mesenchyme of the root of the mesentery and into the medial aspect of the mesonephros at the site of the primitive gonad. Using histochemical techniques these workers demonstrated germ cells at the 3·7 mm. stage in the area where the genital ridge would shortly develop. Indeed, it seems probable that the presence of the germ cells is necessary for the subsequent development of the gonad. There is rapid proliferation of germ cells thereafter until about the 15th week when maturation, as judged by chemical methods, becomes evident; the germ cells then become surrounded by granulosa cells as described above and become oocytes. At this stage mitotic division by which the germ cells have been increasing in number, ceases and they enter the first stage of meiosis.

The number of oocytes is maximal sometime before birth and steadily declines thereafter. Pinkerton *et al.* say the number is greatest during the last trimester; by the 28th week they believe the ovary has acquired a majority of its oocytes, some of which will degenerate before they acquire the granulosa layers as described above, others by follicle atresia later. Baker (1963) observed similar changes. He found that the total population of germ cells increased from some 600,000 at 2 months to a peak of 6,800,000 about 5 months. By the time of birth the number had fallen to 2,000,000 of which 50 per cent were atretic. During the later weeks of intra uterine life a moderate degree of follicular development is evident in the ovary. Follicles in various stages of development and of various sizes are seen; indeed the size of many is greater at this time and during the first few weeks of life than it will be again until just before puberty.

The Development of the Uterus and Fallopian Tubes

The formation of the paramesonephric (Mullerian) duct from the lateral side of the mesonephros begins in embryos of some 10 mm. crown rump length (5–6 weeks). The duct extends caudally until it reaches the urogenital portion of the now sub-divided cloaca about 9 weeks. The blind end of the ducts projects into the posterior wall of the urogenital sinus as the Mullerian tubercle. By the beginning of the third month the Mullerian and the Wolffian ducts with associated mesonephric tubules are both present and capable of development (Fig. 3 (a)). The genital tract has not yet become differentiated into male or female although differentiation of the gonad has occurred some time previously. From this point onwards in the male the Wolffian system proliferates and the Mullerian system degenerates (Fig. 3 (c)). In the female with whom we are here concerned the opposite occurs and degeneration of the Wolffian system is associated with a period of marked growth of the Mullerian system (Fig. 3 (b)). The lower portions of the Mullerian ducts approach each other in the mid-line and fuse to form the uterus and cervix, the cephalic portion of the ducts remaining separate to form the fallopian tubes. A little later during the fourth month

marked proliferation of mesenchyme around the fused portion of the ducts leads ultimately to the development of the thick muscular walls of the uterus and cervix.

The Development of the Vagina

There is more or less agreement about the events described so far but less about vaginal development now to be considered.

It has been seen that the mesonephric ducts reach the urogenital sinus and their solid tips protrude into the dorsal wall of the sinus as the Mullerian tubercle about the 30 mm. stage (9 weeks). The Mullerian system which beyond doubt gives rise to the formation of the cervix, uterus and tubes is then closely adjacent to the sinus epithelium. From this stage onwards in this region there is a marked growth of tissue from which the vagina will ultimately form.

According to Koff (1933) the important event is the formation of the paired sino-vaginal bulbs, which are posterior evaginations of the urogenital sinus, in association with stratification of the cells lining that part of the sinus so that the Mullerian tubercle becomes obliterated. At the same time degenerative changes are evident in the Wolffian ducts. The sino-vaginal bulbs become solidified by further proliferation of epithelium and they fuse with the lower solid end of the Mullerian ducts; the fusion of the, now, solid sino-vaginal bulbs and the Mullerian duct tips forms the vaginal plate. The vaginal plate grows rapidly in all dimensions greatly increasing the distance between the cervix and the urogenital sinus and carrying the degenerating remnants of the Wolffian duct cranially. By the 130 mm. stage the central cells of this plate begin to break down to form the vaginal lumen. Koff concludes that the upper part of the vagina (approximately $\frac{4}{5}$th) is formed from the Mullerian ducts, the lower part of the vagina (approximately $\frac{1}{5}$th) being formed upon the urogenital sinus by the growth of the sino-vaginal bulbs; the hymen is formed passively as a result of invagination of the posterior wall of the urogenital sinus by expansion of the lower end of the vagina and therefore is totally derived from the sinus epithelium.

Others, notably Vilas (1932) and Bulmer (1957), have formed a somewhat different opinion. They are not in doubt about the upgrowth from the urogenital sinus, although in Bulmer's recent account the sino-vaginal bulbs are known as the dorsal lateral projections; the uncertainty is whether the sinus upgrowth fuses with the Mullerian component as Koff suggests, or extends up to the cervix displacing the Mullerian component completely. Vilas (1932) and Bulmer (1957) believe the latter to be true the vaginal epithelium thus arising totally from the endoderm of the urogenital sinus.

It seems certain that part at least of the vagina is formed from the urogenital sinus; it is, at the moment, uncertain whether the Mullerian component is involved and to what extent.

The Development of the External Genitalia

The primitive cloaca becomes divided by a transverse septum into an anterior uro-genital portion and a posterior

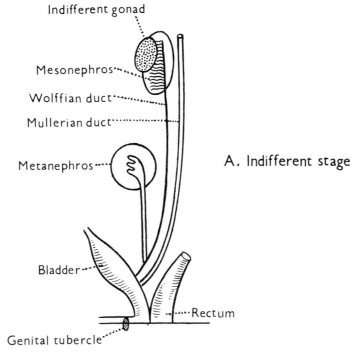

A. Indifferent stage

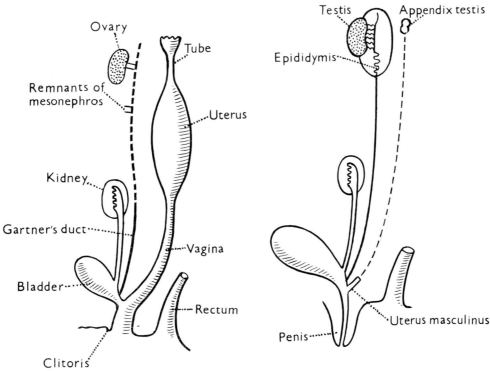

B. Female development   C. Male development

FIG. 3. Diagrammatic representation of the development of the male and female reproductive system.

rectal portion. This subdivision begins about 5 mm. and is complete in embryos of 15 mm. crown rump length, when this uro-rectal septum extends caudally as far as the cloacal membrane and fuses with it. Stephens (1953) maintains that this form of division extends only as far caudally as the Mullerian tubercle: below this an inward growth of mesoderm from the sides of the embryo fuses with the uro-rectal septum and completes the closure. The urogenital portion of the cloacal membrane breaks down shortly after division is complete.

The urogenital sinus soon shows three portions (Fig. 4 (a)). Externally there is an expanded *phallic* portion, then a deeper narrow *pelvic* portion between it and that part of the sinus where the Mullerian ducts meet it; above this point is the vesico-urethral part connected, at its superior aspect, with the allantois.

On the external surface of the embryo in this region may be seen the genital tubercle which is a conical projection encircling the anterior end of the cloacal membrane; the genital tubercle is evident before cloacal division is complete. Two pairs of eminences, a medial pair called the genital folds and a lateral pair called genital swellings, are then formed by proliferation of mesoderm around the lower end of the urogenital sinus. Up to this time, when the embryo is approximately 50 mm. crown rump length (10 weeks), the development just described will be alike for male and female and it will not be possible to be certain by external examination what sex the child will be.

Differentiation then occurs. The bladder and urethra are formed entirely from that portion of the vesico-urethral division of the urogenital sinus above the Mullerian tubercle. The pelvic and phallic division of the sinus then become increasingly shallow to lead ultimately to the formation of the vestibule (Fig. 4 (b)). The genital tubercle undergoes little enlargement and becomes the clitoris. The genital folds remain separate as the labia minora and the genital swellings enlarge to become the labia majora. In male embryos enlargement of the genital tubercle forms the penis; further growth of the genital folds takes place and they finally fuse over a deep groove formed between them to give rise to the phallic portion of the male urethra; the genital swellings also enlarge and fuse to form the scrotum.

Further mention must be made briefly about the growth of the mesoderm in this area. This proliferating mesoderm extends ventrally round the body wall raising up the genital folds and genital swellings and uniting with its fellow from the opposite side to complete the development of the clitoris or penis and to give rise to the anterior surface of the bladder and the anterior abdominal wall below the umbilicus.

MALFORMATIONS

So numerous are the congenital malformations of the genital tract which may occur in clinical practice that only brief mention is possible.

Gonadal Anomalies

Streak gonads may be found in patients with gonadal dysgenesis whether XO, XX or XY or XX/XO or XY/XO mosaics. Gonadal development in mosaic patients is dependent upon the percentage and distribution of normal and abnormal cells in the early embryo so ovarian development of any degree between a normal ovary and a rudimentary streak may be found in one or both gonads in XX/XO patients; similarly variable testicular development may be found in XY/XO patients. Partial failure of testicular formation may itself be associated with imperfect male differentiation of the genital tract and with a degree of development of the vagina, uterus and tubes the individual being known as a male intersex (Dewhurst, 1967).

Testes, abdominal, inguinal or labial in position may be found in apparent females with other features of the testicular feminizing syndrome (Morris, 1953; Dewhurst, 1967).

Testicular and ovarian tissue may both be present in certain individuals termed hermaphrodites. Their other genital development will be a mixture of male and female genital organs. The full explanation of hermaphroditism is as yet unknown but might be associated with the passage of male-determining genes from the Y to the X chromosome during the first meiotic stage of spermatogenesis (Ferguson Smith, 1966).

Agonadism in which no vestige of gonadal tissue is to be found has been described. Patients recently reported have been shown to be XY, the female differentiation of the genital tract being presumably associated with total testicular failure (Dewhurst, 1967).

Mullerian Duct Anomalies

Absence of the uterus is, with few exceptions, the rule when the vagina is also absent; uterine absence with partial or complete development of the vagina is, for practical purposes, confined to the testicular feminizing syndrome.

Fusion anomalies are comparatively common. These may be minor, such as the arcuate or sub-septate uterus, or major, two separate uteri and two cervices being present; any degree of failure of fusion between these two may be found. In clinical practice these anomalies are generally of relatively limited significance. Imperfect development of one half of the Mullerian system may lead to rudimentary horn formation. Uterine rupture may follow the implantation of a pregnancy in such a rudimentary horn.

Vaginal Anomalies

Absence of the vagina is usually associated with absence of the uterus although in a minority of cases the uterus is present and capable of child-bearing if an artificial vagina can be constructed.

Septate vagina, a septum in the sagittal plane may exist throughout the whole length of the vagina or over a limited distance only.

An imperforate membrane occluding the vagina may be evident at various levels but is commonest just deep to the hymen which may often be distinguished as a separate structure. Retention of menstrual flow above such an imperforate membrane (haematocolpos) may produce important clinical features at or after puberty; less

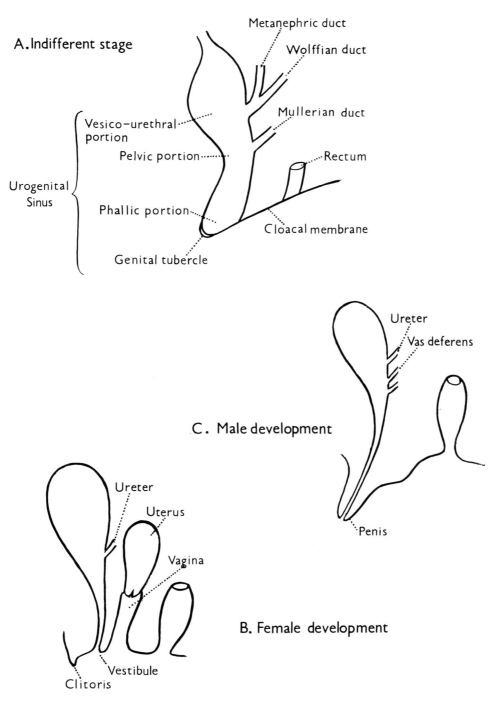

IG. 4. Diagrammatic representation of the development of the lower genital tract.

commonly collections of watery fluid may produce similar features shortly after birth (hydrocolpos) (Dewhurst, 1963; Stephens, 1963).

Vulval Deformities

Partial masculinization of the external genitalia may occur as a result of hermaphroditism or partial testicular failure as already mentioned but also as a result of increased androgenic stimulation of a female foetus by adrenal hyperplasia or by androgenic drugs having been given to the mother during early pregnancy. The clitoris is enlarged,

A variety of abnormalities exists in which the genital tract communicates with the bowel. Figure 5 indicates some of these. Normal development may be arrested at a very early stage, the cloaca persisting as a common orifice for bowel, uterus and bladder. At a slightly later stage incomplete division of the cloaca may lead to a high or low rectovaginal fistula. Later still incomplete formation of the perineum may produce an ectopic anus opening alongside the vagina; excessive fusion of genital folds may cover the anus projecting the orifice forwaids to produce a similar abnormality (Stephens, 1963).

ANOMALIES OF THE UTERO-VAGINAL CANAL

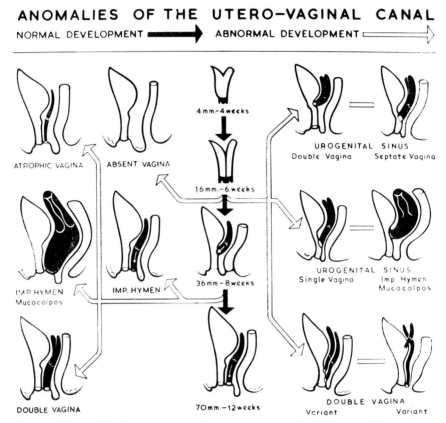

FIG. 5. Scheme of development of anomalies of the uterovaginal canal. Normal development is indicated by black arrows, abnormal development by white arrows. (After Stephens, 1963.)

the labial folds are fused to cover the vaginal introitus and the skin of the labia majora becomes pigmented and rugose.

Wolffian Duct Remnants

Remnants of the Wolffian duct system may be evident as vaginal cysts (Gaertner's cyst) or as thin walled cysts within the layers of the broad ligament (parovarian cysts).

Anomalies Associated with other Systems

Genital tract anomalies are not uncommonly associated with congenital malformations of the urinary tract such as a pelvic kidney, a double renal element, ectopic ureters and others. Similarly gross bladder defects, such as bladder exstrophy, may have genital tract associations which are of course minor compared with the severity of the vesical lesion.

REFERENCES

Baker, T. G. (1963), "A Quantitative and Cytological Study of Germ Cells in Human Ovaries," *Proceedings of Royal Society (London)*, **158**, 417.

Bulmer, D. (1957), "The Development of the Human Vagina," *Journal of Anatomy*, **91**, 490.

Carr, D. H. (1965), "Chromosome Studies in Spontaneous Abortion," *Obstetrics and Gynaecology*, **26**, 30B.

Close, H. G. (1963), "Two Apparently Normal Triple X Females," *Lancet*, **II**, 1358.

Dewhurst, C. J. (1963), *The Gynaecological Disorders of Infants and Children*, p. 39. London: Cassell & Co. Ltd.

Dewhurst, C. J. (1967), "The XY Female," *Journal of Obstetrics and Gynaecology of the British Commonwealth*, **74**, 353.

Ferguson Smith, M. (1966), "X–Y Interchange in the Aetiology of True Hermaphrodites and of XX Klinefelters Syndrome," *Lancet*, **II**, 475.

Gillman, J. (1948), "The Development o the Gonads in Man: Contributions to Embryology," No. 210, *Carnegie Institute of Washington Publication 575*, Vol. 32, p. 83.

Jacobs, P. A. and Strong, J. A. (1959), "A Case of Human Intersexuality having a Possible Sex Determining Mechanism," *Nature (London)*, **183**, 302.

Jacobs, P. A., Brunton, M., Melville, M. E., Brittain, R. P. and McClemont, W. F. (1965), "Aggressive Behaviour, Mental Subnormality and the XYY Male," *Nature (London)*, **208**, 1351.

Jost, A. (1947), "Recherches sur la Differenciation Sexuelle de l'Embryon de Lapin, III," *Arch. Anat. Microscop. Morphol. Exptl.*, **36**, 271.

Koff, A. K. (1933), "Development of the Vagina in the Human Foetus: Contributions to Embryology No. 140," *Carnegie Institute of Washington Publication* 443, Vol. 24, p. 61.

Lennox, B. (1963), "Possible Fertility in Klinefelters Syndrome," *Lancet*, **I**, 611.

Miller, O. J. (1964), "The Sex Chromosome Anomalies," *Obstetrics and Gynaecology*, **90**, 1078.

Morris, J. M. (1953), "Syndrome of Testicular Feminization in Male Pseudohermaphrodites," *Amer. J. Obstet. Gynec.*, **65**, 1192.

Overzier, C. (1963), *Intersexuality*, p. 277. London and New York: Academic Press.

Pinkerton, J. H. M., McKay, D. G., Adams, E. C. and Hertig, A. H. (1961), "Development of the Human Ovary—A Study using Histochemical Techniques," *Obstetrics and Gynæcology*, **18**, 152.

Ricci, N. and Mallacarne, P. (1964), "An XYY Human Male," *Lancet*, **I**, 721.

Sandberg, A. A., Koepf, G. F., Ishihara, T. and Hauschka, T. S. (1961), "An XYY Human Male," *Lancet*, **II**, 488.

Stephens, F. Douglas (1963), *Congenital Malformations of the Rectum, Anus and Genito-urinary Tracts*, p. 4. Edinburgh and London: E. & S. Livingstone Ltd.

Turner, H. H. (1938), "A Syndrome of Infantilism Congenital Webbed Neck and Cubitus Valgus," *Endocrinology*, **23**, 566.

Vilas, E. (1932), "Uber die Entwicklung der menschlichen Scheide," *Z. Anat. Entwicklungsgeschichte*, **98**, 263.

Willis, R. A. (1962), *The Borderland of Embryology and Pathology*, 2nd Ed., p. 47. London: Butterworth.

Witschi, E. (1948), "Migration of Germ Cells of Human Embryos from the Yolk Sac to the Primitive Gonadal Folds: Contributions to Embryology," *Carnegie Institute of Washington Publication* No. 32, p. 67.

7. THE MEMBRANES

GORDON BOURNE

The Amnion

The human amnion, which was for many years thought to be a simple epithelial lining for the uterine contents, is now accepted as a complicated tissue constructed histologically of five different layers (Bautzmann and Schroder, 1955; Schmidt, 1956; Petry and Damminger,

1. The Epithelium

The epithelium is composed of a single layer of simple, non-ciliated cuboidal cells. It is not yet known (Leonardi and Rigano, 1966) if the amniotic epithelial cells are engaged in absorption or formation of amniotic fluid, but the exchange of amniotic fluid between the foetal and

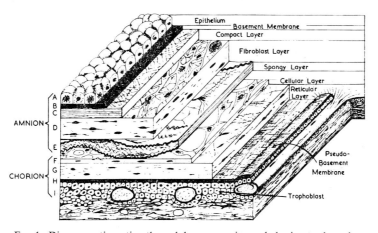

FIG. 1. Diagrammatic section through human amnion and chorion to show the various layers. (Reproduced with permission, from "The Human Amnion and Chorion" by G. L. Bourne, published by Lloyd-Luke, London.)

1956; Bourne, 1960; Bourne, 1962; Leonardi and Rigano, 1966) which are illustrated in Figure 1. This illustration shows in diagrammatic form the layers as they are seen in both cut vertical section and in membrane preparation.

The five layers of the amnion consist, from within outwards, of:

maternal compartments has been established beyond doubt (Hutchinson *et al.*, 1959; Jeffcoate and Scott, 1959; Vosburgh *et al.*, 1948).

2. The Basement Membrane

This is a narrow band of reticulous tissue lying along the base of the epithelial cells to which it is securely adherent by means of fine fibrils and half desmosomes (Thomas, 1965). The basement membrane consists of very fine fibrils adjacent to the epithelial cell, then a layer of coarse fibrils without periodicity and also coarse collagen fibrils.

3. The Compact Layer

This layer is a relatively dense, aceilular layer immediately subjacent to the basement membrane (Fig. 2). This layer

Nerve supply of the amnion. A nerve supply has been described in the amnion by Russian workers but these findings have not been confirmed.

Lymphatic vessels. There are several reports of lymphatic vessels being present in the amnion (Hanon et al., 1955). Very large spaces may be present between the bundles of reticular fibres, especially in the spongy layer of the amnion, but examination at high magnification has failed to confirm the presence of actual lymphatic vessels.

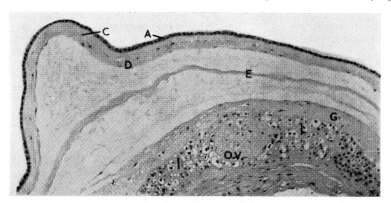

FIG. 2. Human amnion and chorion. A vertical histological section through amnion (above) and chorion (below). Compare with Fig. 1. A = epithelium. C = compact layer. D = fibroblast layer. E = spongy layer. G = reticular layer. I = trophoblast. OV = obliterated villus. Note the fine reticular tissue connecting the spongy layer with its adjacent structures. Haematoxylin-eosin (×90). (Reproduced with permission, from "The Human Amnion and Chorion" by G. L. Bourne, published by Lloyd-Luke, London.)

shows a marked resistance to leucocytic infiltration so that its boundaries can be easily observed in membranes suffering from a severe inflammatory response.

4. The Fibroblast Layer

This is by far the most complex of all the amniotic layers, consisting of fibroblasts and Hofbauer cells buried in a reticulin mesh. The thickness of this layer varies considerably in different parts of the amnion and this layer would appear to play quite a considerable part in the transmission of fluid between the foetal and maternal compartments, although exactly how this transfer takes place is inadequately understood.

5. The Spongy Layer

The spongy layer is composed of the reticulum of the extra-embryonic coelom. It is capable of considerable distension and it contains large quantities of mucus. The greatest importance of this layer is that it allows movement of the amnion upon the underlying chorion, so that as the lower segment of the uterus forms toward the end of pregnancy the amnion is not automatically ruptured but is allowed a considerable degree of movement and is thus able to remain intact. If the amnion were firmly attached to the chorion premature rupture of the membranes would doubtless occur much more frequently and at a much earlier stage in pregnancy.

Blood supply of the amnion. Blood vessels have not been demonstrated within the layers of the amnion at any stage of pregnancy, although there is an unsupported Russian report of amniotic blood vessels in early pregnancy.

The Chorion

The chorion is made up of four layers of cells, shown diagrammatically in Figure 1. This chapter is concerned only with the extra, or non-placental, chorion but the placenta obeys the same basic anatomical criteria that are set out below.

6. The Cellular Layer

This is the innermost layer of the chorion, consisting of a thin layer of interlacing fibroblasts, and is more easily demonstrated in the earlier embryo.

7. The Reticular Layer

The recticular layer forms the major part of the reticular tissue of the chorion. It consists of a reticulin network containing fibroblasts and Hofbauer cells. The blood vessels in the early embryo lie within this layer, which dips down to make the core of either the obliterated villi in the non-placental chorion or in the villi themselves in the placenta. It is also a direct extension with the connective tissue that surrounds the vessels in the umbilical cord.

8. The Pseudo-Basement Membrane

This is for the overlying trophoblast.

9. The Trophoblast

In a non-placental chorion this consists of a layer of trophoblast cells varying in thickness from two to ten cells. It lies immediately adjacent to the maternal decidua, with which it is in intimate contact. Syncytio-trophoblast is not normally present in the non-placental chorion, although various degenerative changes may be seen in the non-placental trophoblast. Atrophic, or ghost chorionic villi are easily recognized in sections taken from the non-placental membranes, and when cut in cross section they are recognized as oval bundles of reticulin tissue embedded between trophoblast cells. These bundles contain blood vessels in the early embryo but these vessels are absorbed when the placenta develops and cannot be recognized in later pregnancy.

Blood supply of the chorion. The recticular layer of the chorion at term contains the vessels as they pass from the umbilical cord to the chorionic villi of the placenta. The remainder of the reticular layer of the chorion also contains blood vessels in very early pregnancy, but after the end of the first trimester a capillary blood supply cannot be demonstrated in the chorion (Bourne, 1962).

Nerve supply of the chorion. Recent Russian literature has suggested that the chorion has a nerve supply, but these findings have not been confirmed.

Lymphatic vessels. No actual lymphatic vessels have been observed within the layers of the chorion.

THE ELECTRONMICROSCOPIC APPEARANCE OF MATURE AMNION

The main interest during recent years has been centred upon the structure of the amniotic epithelial cell (Danforth & Hull, 1958; Bourne, 1960; Bourne & Lacey, 1960;

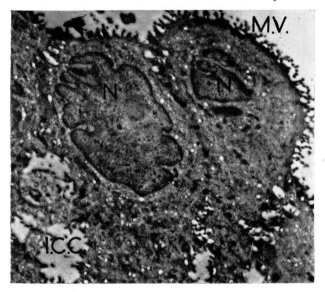

FIG. 3. Amnion epithelium. The upper, or free, margin of a portion of two columnar shaped epithelial cells from the placental amnion at term. Microvilli (M.V.) cover the surface of the cells. The nuclei (N) are irregular in outline. Intracellular canals (I.C.C.) extending from the free surface are dilated in places to form vacuolar-like spaces. Many smaller vacuoles are present in the cell cytoplasm. (×6,500). (Reproduced with permission, from "The Human Amnion and Chorion" by G. L. Bourne, published by Lloyd-Luke, London.)

Bourne, 1962; Hadeck, 1963; Leonardi et al., 1966; Thomas, 1965).

The epithelial cells are cuboidal or columnar in shape (Fig. 3). Microvilli are produced on the surface of the cell in fairly early pregnancy and as maturity advances the microvilli become more complex and numerous. Intercellular canals pass between the lateral aspects of the two membranes of adjacent cells. In the basal region the cell membrane forms irregularly shaped processes of varying size (basal processes) which efficiently increase the surface area of the base of the cell, just as the intercellular canals increase the surface area of the lateral aspect of the cell and the microvilli the surface area of the foetal aspects of the cell.

Surface Microvilli

Surface microvilli can be recognized during the first trimester of pregnancy, although at this stage they are relatively simple (Fig. 4). The microvilli are bordered by

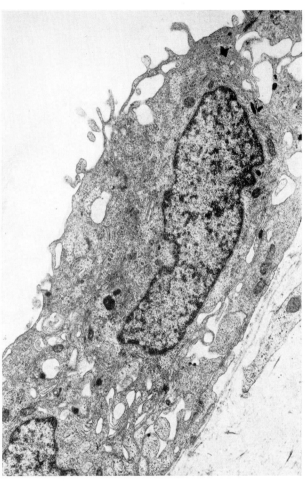

FIG. 4. Human amniotic epithelium at the 13th week of pregnancy. Note the complex intercellular canal together with the large intracellular vacuoles. The surface microvilli are comparatively simple and not yet numerous. Mitochondria are present as well as endoplasmic reticulum. (×93,500).

two closely applied membranes and occasionally they appear to contain a 9 + 2 arrangement, found in cilia and flagella (Bradfield, 1955; Bourne and Lacy, 1960; Thomas, 1965). The exact function of the surface microvilli is yet uncertain, but as better methods of fixation and examination become available their complexity increases.

Basal Processes

The epithelial cell is attached to its basement membrane by a series of half-desmosomes, and the finer tissue of the basement membrane protrudes in between the basal processes and even extends for a considerable distance up the intercellular canal.

Lateral Vacuoles

The lateral vacuoles which invaginate into the side walls of the cell are part of the intercellular canal system. They form a very complex and complicated system of spaces

Nucleus

This is a large, dense, relatively simple object in early pregnancy, but as pregnancy advances it becomes indented and sometimes fenestrated.

VARIATIONS IN CELL TYPES

It has long been postulated that some epithelial cells secrete whilst others absorb. Differences in the characteristics of epithelial cells can be seen in various conditions such as amnion nodosum, hydramnios (Leonardi *et al.*, 1966), intrauterine death, etc.

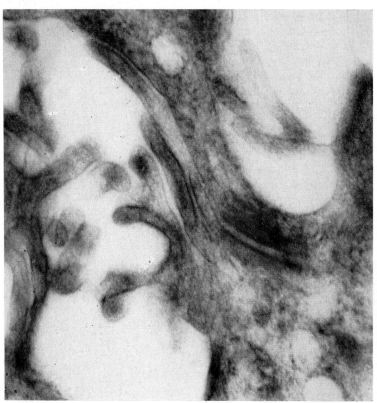

Fig. 5. Term amnion. High magnification of a portion of the intercellular canal. Many microvilli protrude into the canal, the dilatations (or vacuoles) of which are joined by fine channels, usually about 170 Å (but varying from 100 Å to 200 Å) internal diameter and lined by a double membrane. (× 75,000). (Reproduced with permission, from "The Human Amnion and Chorion" by G. L. Bourne, published by Lloyd-Luke, London.)

bounded by the lateral cell membranes, into some of which microvilli protrude and this protrusion of microvilli becomes more noticeable as pregnancy advances (Fig. 5). The intercellular canals are present in very early pregnancy but they rapidly assume a complex pattern (see Fig. 4).

Cytoplasm

The components of the cytoplasm vary as pregnancy advances. Mitochondria are present throughout pregnancy but tend to diminish in number towards term. Numerous vacuoles are present, some of which appear to be "empty" and others contain fat. The number of vacuoles varies from cell to cell. Very active endoplasmic reticulum is present in some cells and a Golgi apparatus can be demonstrated in nearly all epithelial cells (Thomas, 1965).

Thomas, in a very interesting article, states "Human amnion epithelial cells may be divided into two types on the basis of ultra-structural characteristics. One type exhibits a cytoplasm which shows membrane-bounded vacuoles, a highly developed Golgi complex, and distended cisternæ of rough endoplasmic reticulum; it has been named the 'Golgi type' cell. The second type has a cytoplasm filled with coarse fibrils, a small Golgi complex, and a few cell organelles; it has been named the 'fibrillar type' cell. These may represent two distinct cell types or only one cell type in different physiological phases. The placental and reflected portions of the amnion show some variation in cell forms, although the same two cell types are demonstrated. In general, the placental portion of the membrane is characterized by high, closely spaced, columnar cells, whereas the reflected portion shows lower, more cuboidal cells with areas of degenerate cells. The possible secretory activity of one of these cell types is discussed. The observations were made on membranes delivered by caesarean section, and also after a normal labour."

The exact function, however, of the amnion remains uncertain. It can, however, be assumed that such an active epithelial cell is engaged in an extensive physiological activity and it is only a question of time before someone satisfactorily defines the action of these complicated cellular structures.

The remainder of the layers of both the amnion and chorion conform to connective tissue layers in most structures, consisting of reticular tissue together with fibroblasts and macrophage cells.

REFERENCES

Bautzmann, H. and Schroder, R. (1955), Z. Anat. Entwickl. Gesh., 117, 166.

Bourne, G. L. (1960), Amer. J. Obstet. Gynec., 79, 1070.
Bourne, G. L. (1962), Human Amnion and Chorion. London: Lloyd-Luke.
Bourne, G. L. and Lacy, D. (1960), Nature (Lond.), 186, 952.
Bradfield, J. R. G. (1955), Symp. Soc. Exp. Biol., 9, 306.
Danforth, D. N. and Hull, R. W. (1958), Amer. J. Obstet. Gynec., 75, 536.
Hadeck, R. (1963), J. Ultrastruct. Res., 9, 445.
Hanon, F., Coquin-Carnot, M. and Pignard, P. (1955), Le Liquide Amniotique. Paris: Masson et Cie.
Hutchinson, D. L., Gray, M. J., Plentl, A. A., Alvares, H., Caldeyro-Barcia, T., Kaplan, E. and Lind, J. (1959), J. Clin. Invest., 38, 971.
Jeffcoate, T. N. A. and Scott, J. S. (1959), Canad. Med. Ass. J., 80, 77.
Leonardi, R. and Rigano, A. (1966), Arch. Ost. Gin. Vo. 71, No. 5, p. 549.
Leonardi, R and Rigano, A., Riv. Ost. Gin., 21/1, p. 33, 1966.
Petry, G. and Damminger, K. (1956), Z. Zellforsch., 44, 235.
Schmidt, W. (1956), Anat. Entwickl. Gesch., 119, 203.
Thomas, C. E. (1965), J. Ultrastruct. Res., 13, 65.
Vosburgh, G. J., Flexner, L. B., Cowie, D. B., Hellman, L. M., Proctor, N. K. and Wilde, W. S. (1948), Amer. J. Obstet. Gynec., 56, 1156.

8. DEVELOPMENT OF THE HUMAN PLACENTA

W. J. HAMILTON AND J. D. BOYD

I. INTRODUCTION

This chapter is based, in the main, on the publications by us in the Journal of Anatomy, 1960, and in the Journal of Obstetrics and Gynaecology, 1967. It is therefore presented in two parts; an attempt has been made to obviate certain repetitions. It has been necessary to clarify and modify some of the earlier statements in the light of further information. Some of the illustrations in both papers have been omitted. The process of implantation has been summarized. It must be appreciated that if this chapter had been presented *de novo*, the arrangement would have been considerably modified. Owing to the death of one author (J.D.B.) and to the present commitments of the other (W.J.H.) it was not possible to produce this chapter other than in the present form.

In spite of an extensive literature, going back to the eighteenth century, our knowledge of the details of the structure of the human placenta is still most fragmentary. This is due partly to the fact that much of the work published on its histology has been concerned with late stages of its development and predominantly with placentae separated from the uterus. So far as the earlier stages are concerned, individual investigators have had access only to a very limited number of specimens. We have in our possession an extensive collection of pregnant uteri at all stages of gestation from about the 11th day after fertilization to full term. In addition, we have available a large number of *in situ* specimens in which, alone, the precise relationships obtaining between maternal and foetal tissues can adequately be determined. Serial sections of a

part or the whole of the implantation sites and placental areas of these specimens have been examined. Consequently the authors have been able to make a full survey of the structure of the human placenta throughout the period of gestation. This chapter deals with the establishment of the placenta and with its development up to full term.

In a classical review, published in 1927, Grosser summarized the then existing knowledge of implantation and development of the placenta in Man. The early stages of human development available for study at that time were unsatisfactory. Many of the specimens were incomplete, fragmentary or even pathological (e.g. T.B.I., Bryce and Teacher, 1908; and Davies, 1944). Since Grosser's review there have been outstanding contributions on the early stages of human implantation and placental development. Especially noteworthy are the investigations of Hertig and Rock since 1941 (summarized by Hertig, Rock and Adams, 1956). To a lesser extent, a number of other investigators have also added descriptions of specimens at these stages (see Hamilton and Boyd, 1950; Hamilton, Boyd and Mossman, 1952; and Mazanec, 1959, for summaries). Additions in the last thirty years to knowledge of stages of human placental development later than the 18th post-ovulational day and especially of the fully established *in situ* placenta have been much less extensive. Indeed, as indicated in earlier communications (Boyd and Hamilton, 1950; Hamilton and Boyd, 1951), there is still disagreement and doubt on a number of fundamental points relating to the structure and function of the human placenta at all stages of its development.

The numerous contributions from the Carnegie Laboratory of Embryology on implantation of the blastocyst and on placental development in the macaque monkey (Wislocki and Streeter, 1938; Heuser and Streeter, 1941; Ramsey, 1949, 1954b) have provided a remarkably clear picture of foetal-uterine relationships in this primate. It must be stressed, however, that, as Ramsey (1954a) has stated with regard to placental circulation in the two species, the findings in the macaque are not replicas of those found in Man.

A special problem in the description of the development of the foetal components of the placenta is posed by the various appearances presented by the trophoblast at different stages of development and in different regions of the blastocyst wall. Part of the difficulty resides in the variety of terminologies used by investigators in their descriptions. Recently, the authors (Boyd and Hamilton, 1960) have discussed this terminological problem, and it is not considered necessary to review the matter in detail in the present chapter. As the suggestions on terminology put forward by us, however, will be used in our subsequent descriptions, a brief summary of them is required. It must at once be stressed that this terminology is essentially a topographical and descriptive one. Briefly, those cells constituting the wall of the unimplanted blastocyst, and which are individual cellular units, together constitute the *blastocystic trophoblast*. All of the trophoblast of later stages is derived from it. During the early stages of implantation the blastocystic trophoblast differentiates into *primitive syncytiotrophoblast* and *primitive cytotrophoblast*. The former, receiving increments over a considerable period from the latter, is, by the development of the cytotrophoblastic, or trophoblastic, shell, separated into two varieties. First, there is the *definitive syncytium* which forms a covering for the villi and lines the lacunar and, later, the intervillous spaces. Secondly, there is syncytium on the maternal side of the shell which we call *peripheral syncytium*. Both varieties of syncytium are augmented until late stages of placental development by further contributions from the related cytotrophoblast (Boyd and Hamilton, 1966b). This last named tissue gives origin to: (1) the *villous cytotrophoblast* (Langhans layer); (2) proliferations at the tips of the villi which constitute the *cytotrophoblastic columns*; and (3) the *trophoblastic shell* itself.

Until the contribution of Spanner (1935) it was generally accepted that, for the most part, the decidual arteries open into the intervillous space, at or near the margins of the septa which separate the cotyledons, and that the uterine veins communicate with the intervillous space through orifices in the interseptal zones of the basal plate. Indeed, Bumm (1893) considered that the openings of the decidual arteries are usually situated quite far down the septa and well away from the basal plate itself. Spanner, however, as a result of observations on placentae injected *in situ*, concluded that the arteries open into the intervillous space solely through the basal plate and that the blood is only drained away from this space through a specialized peripheral region of it called the marginal sinus. Stieve (1942) and we, ourselves (Hamilton and Boyd, 1950; Boyd,

1956), have criticized Spanner's concept of the intervillous circulation and have denied the existence of a constant marginal sinus in Spanner's sense of the term. In particular, it can be shown that there are frequent venous openings through the whole of the basal plate. Ramsey (1954b, 1956a, b) has also shown that uterine venous connections with the intervillous space can be found in all regions of the uterine surface of the macaque placenta. She points out, indeed, that, in this monkey, such connections are even less prominent at the margin of the placenta than in Man; she attributes this difference to the superficial implantation in the macaque which "precludes contact between the placental margin and the endometrium when vascular connections are being established". Data on the number of villi at these stages and on the chorionic villous trunks and their branches are discussed in the light of our views on placental lobes and septa (Boyd and Hamilton, 1966a).

In view of the physiological and clinical importance of the circulation in the intervillous space, and of the conflict of opinion on it, special attention has been given to the morphology of the circulatory arrangements in the placenta at all stages of our study.

II. MATERIAL AND METHODS

The material available includes *in situ* specimens from the 11th day of development until full term: these comprise six specimens at the early stages from the 11th day until the 26th day, and a complete series of *in situ* placentae from the 10 mm. stage until term. We have 188 *in situ* placentae and over 400 immature separated specimens. Further details of the history of these specimens are given subsequently. In these earlier stages, the embryonic age has been estimated from the coital and menstrual history and from the general state of development of the trophoblast and embryo. In the older specimens, the crown-rump measurement has been used in the assessment of the age.

In addition to the *in situ* material we have an extensive collection of sections through placentae at all stages of gestation. For certain histological and cytological purposes this disparate material has proved very useful as a supplement to our *in situ* specimens.

The histories of the patients from whom the placentae, associated with embryos of between 10 mm. and full term, were obtained, do not require special comment.

In some of the *in situ* material the maternal uterine arteries were injected with coloured gelatine or India ink. In yet other specimens the foetal vessels were injected following opening of the amniotic cavity and cannulation of an umbilical vessel. When conditions permitted the sizes and weights of the foetuses and of the corresponding placentae and the volumes of the associated amniotic fluid were recorded. Some attention has also been given in the *in situ* material to the site of attachment of the placenta to the uterine wall. To clarify relationships between placental and neo-natal size and weight, data from a series of 1,000 pregnancies at term were collected. In this material one of the umbilical arteries in each cord was injected with coloured gelatine to establish the pattern of its placental distribution and its connection with its fellow artery. The frequency of occurrence of a single umbilical artery was noted. For the investigation of the blood supply to the foetal villi the umbilical vessels of over 100 other placentae were injected with radio-opaque coloured solutions (Chromopaque) and X-rayed. Comparison of the radiographs with photographs of these specimens enabled an assessment to be made of the average number of villous trunks in the placental lobes. In yet other material the umbilical vessels were injected with latex or with a setting plastic and then rendered apparent by acid corrosion or enzymatic digestion.

Data from a parallel electron-microscopic study of placental structure have been included when clarification could be added to the findings with light microscopy. The electron-microscopic observations are based on the examination of a wide range of placentae from the sixth week (6 mm. C.R. length embryo) to the late sixth month (210 mm. C.R. length foetus) of pregnancy and from full-term (Caesarian section) specimens. Unfortunately there is a gap in the series in the seventh and eighth months when we have been unable to acquire chorionic villi in a state fresh enough to permit electron-microscopic study.

III. DESCRIPTION OF SPECIMENS

At the time of implantation of the blastocyst the human endometrium shows a distinct division into a superficial *stratum compactum* and a deep, oedematous, *stratum spongiosum*. It measures about 4–5 mm. (see Krafka, 1941, for details) in thickness and is, of course, under the influence of the luteal hormone secreted by the ovary. After implantation, the endometrial oedema becomes even more marked, particularly in the region underlying, and round, the blastocyst. The oedema, which is presumably to be attributed to alterations in the walls of the blood vessels or in the flow through them, results in an eosinophilic exudate which separates the endometrial cells from each other. The blood vessels near the implantation site are hyperaemic and sinusoidal vascular spaces become apparent; such spaces may be dilated venules or capillaries.

PRESOMITE STAGE
11- to 12-day Stage

The Barnes embryo. The earliest developmental stage at our disposal is the Barnes embryo, of which a brief description has already been published (Hamilton, Barnes and Dodds, 1943). This specimen was found in a uterus obtained by hysterectomy on the 25th day of a menstrual cycle. Previous cycles were regularly 28 days in duration and the menstrual periods lasted 2–3 days. A history which appears to be reliable establishes that coitus had taken place on the 10th and on the 12th days previous to the operation. Consequently, the maximum conceptional age is not more than 12 days. On examination an elevation (Fig. 1) was seen on the posterior uterine wall as a slightly raised translucent area, clearly demarcated from the surrounding endometrium. After sectioning, the dimensions of the chorionic sac were approximately 0·931 × 0·770 × 0·737 mm.

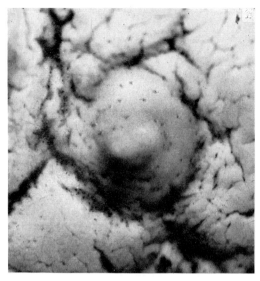

Fig. 1. Photograph (×12) of the surface view of the implantation site of the Barnes embryo. The implantation site itself appears as a slightly elevated area of the endometrium on which openings of the uterine glands can be seen. The surface of the endometrium shows characteristic shallow and irregular furrows.

The embryo is almost completely implanted, the site of entry being covered with a thin layer of endometrium though the flattened uterine epithelium has not extended entirely over it (Fig. 2). The regional differentiation of the trophoblast is not uniform. Both primitive syncytium and cytotrophoblast are present but no definite indications of transitional cell types between the two have been seen. In the abembryonic region, towards the uterine cavity, the blastocyst wall is thin and composed almost exclusively of cytotrophoblast with only a small amount of syncytium, and here there is no lacunar formation. Elsewhere, however, the main mass of trophoblast is clearly differentiated into a cytotrophoblastic component and a spun-out primitive syncytium in which the intercommunicating lacunae, containing a small number of maternal blood corpuscles, are well established (Fig. 3). A wax-plate reconstruction of the implantation site indicates that the majority of the lacunae are in free communication with each other. When compared with the maternal blood cells elsewhere in the sections those in the lacunar spaces stain very poorly; presumably some influence operating on them in the spaces has markedly diminished their tinctorial affinities. The primitive syncytium possesses a granular cytoplasm; where it is in contact with the maternal endometrial tissue the latter frequently shows marked oedema (Fig. 4). Where the syncytium forms the boundary of the lacunae it is usually irregular with surface projections of vacuolated protoplasmic fronds and streamers. In some regions, however, there is the appearance of a not very well defined brush border. In no part of the primitive syncytium are any mitotic figures observed. No evidence for amitotic division is found but frequently syncytial nuclei are closely apposed or clumped together (Fig. 5), although long stretches of protoplasm may be devoid of them (Fig. 4). The syncytial nuclei vary

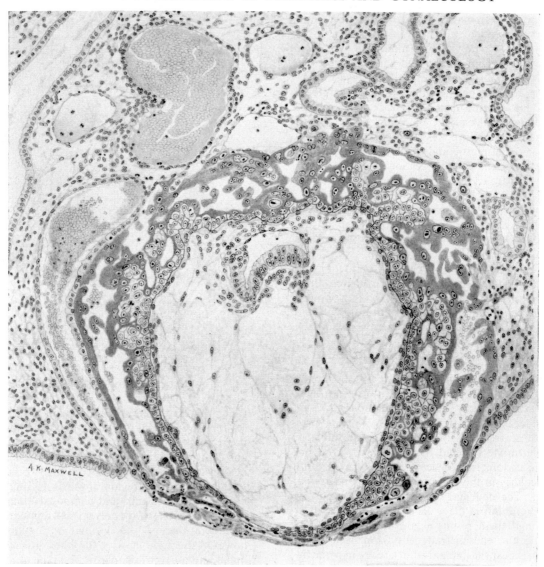

FIG. 2. A drawing (×150) of a section through the middle of an implantation site at the 11th–12th day of development
(Barnes embryo). The surface view of the implantation site is shown in Figure 1. The blastocystic trophoblast has
differentiated into primitive syncytium and cytotrophoblast: the latter surrounds the primitive mesoblast which almost
completely fills the original blastocyst cavity. At intervals the cytotrophoblast has proliferated to form projections
which are the forerunners of the 'primary villi'. The primitive syncytium, which has not yet extended completely round
the superficial aspect of the implantation site, shows an extensive development of intercommunicating lacunae containing some maternal blood cells. The endometrium surrounding the implanted ovum is oedematous and there is
haemorrhage into a uterine gland in contact with the syncytium. Photomicrographs of selected portions of the
trophoblast of this specimen are illustrated in Figs. 3–5.

considerably in size. The cytotrophoblast completely
covers the embryonic mesoderm, which is, in fact, separated
from this covering by a space which is a fixation artefact.
There are in addition, however, aggregates of cytotrophoblastic cells, particularly round the equator of the chorion,
which project into the syncytium. These aggregates may
represent regional proliferative activity of the cytotrophoblast though no sign of special mitotic activity is shown by
them. The cytotrophoblastic proliferations are always
covered by syncytium and are similar in appearance to
those described in other embryos at this stage of development (Stieve, 1936; Dible and West, 1941; Hertig and
Rock, 1941, 1944; Wilson, 1954). Such proliferations have
often been regarded as forming the early primordia of

the chorionic villi and they will be discussed later. The
presence of the lacunae within the syncytium gives the
latter a sponge-like structure. Consequently, the system
of lacunar spaces is primarily labyrinthine and, as there
are no free villi, the term "intervillous space" is not quite
appropriate.

The endometrial stroma, immediately round the implantation site, shows the predecidual reaction, and is
markedly oedematous (Fig. 2). In view of the findings by
Hertig et al. (1956) on a number of early specimens, this
oedema must be regarded as a normal feature of the
endometrium. The endometrial cells themselves do not
yet show the histological changes distinctive of later stages.
The intercellular spaces are distended with a slightly

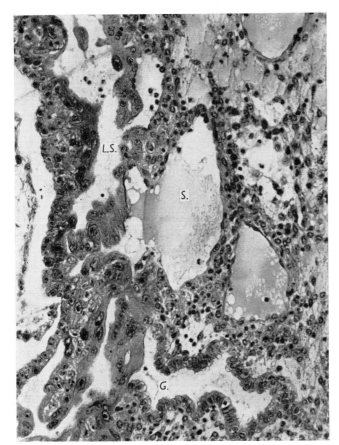

FIG. 3. Photograph (×230) of a section through the deep central portion of the implantation site of the Barnes embryo; maternal tissue is on the right of the illustration. The intercommunicating lacunar spaces (*L.S.*) are shown surrounded by syncytial trophoblast. Uterine venous sinusoids (*S.*) communicate with these. A plug of syncytium can be seen in direct contact with the lumen of the uterine gland (*G.*).

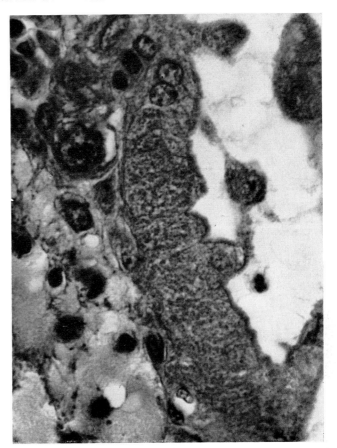

FIG. 4. Photomicrograph (×950) of a section through the primitive syncytium and adjacent oedematous endometrium in the Barnes embryo; maternal tissue is on the left of the illustration. Note the texture of the syncytial cytoplasm, a long stretch of which is devoid of nuclei. In the upper part of the figure there is an irregular projection of syncytium, containing a very large nucleus, into the endometrium; elsewhere the foetal-maternal junction is smooth.

eosinophilic exudate containing occasional blood cells. The uterine glands are tortuous and dilated with large amounts of secretion. Those adjacent to the implantation site are deflected aside by the proliferating trophoblast. Glands near and in contact with the trophoblast show degenerative changes. In some instances the glandular epithelium has disappeared at the point of contact with the trophoblast which thus comes to plug the glandular lumen. Maternal blood corpuscles are present in the lumina of many of the glands but the precise source of such blood cells is not apparent (Fig. 2).

Round the implantation site, and especially on its deep surface, a number of thin-walled, intercommunicating sinusoids, lined with endothelium, are in free communication with the lacunar spaces. At the points of communication the primitive syncytium is directly continuous with the endothelium lining the sinusoids. There is no evidence at these points of junction of endothelial reaction to the syncytium. The sinusoids can be traced to veins in the deeper part of the endometrium. Typical coiled arteries are found in the endometrium; they are surrounded by regions of specialized, non-oedematous, decidua. Several

of the arteries approach and become intimately related to the implantation site. Many of the arteries appear to end blindly in the endometrium. No evidence of alterations in the walls of the coiled arteries was observed in this specimen. Hertig and Rock (1941), in their description of a human implantation of the 11th day, have described the related sinusoids as being arterio-venous in nature, considering that there is an arterio-venous anastomotic connection between an adjacent spiral artery and the sinusoids. We have been unable to identify any such anastomoses, and the work of Bartelmez (1957) makes their presence unlikely. It seems to us, therefore, that the first maternal vessels to be "tapped" by the lacunae are slightly dilated venules or capillaries in the stratum compactum of the decidua. With further extension of the invading syncytium, and more dilatation of the blood vessels, the supply of blood to the lacunae comes from venous sinusoids.

14- to 18-day Stages

The Missen embryo. The maximum diameters of the chorionic sac (measuring from the edge of the trophoblastic

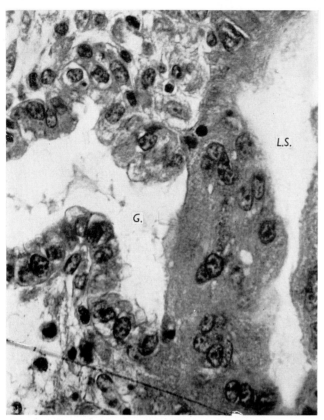

L.S.

G.

Fig. 5. Photomicrograph (×720) of the foetal-maternal junction of the Barnes embryo. A mass of primitive syncytium is in direct contact with the lumen of a uterine gland (*G.*) in which secretion can be seen. The syncytium separates this lumen from a lacunar space (*L.S.*).

shell) are 1·66 × 1·43 mm. The embryonic disc, which is cut obliquely, measures 0·280 × 0·214 mm. The primitive streak is differentiating and the first indication of Hensen's node and the primordium of the head process have appeared. The specimen, therefore, corresponds in state of development to such early embryos as Carnegie 1801 (Heuser, Rock and Hertig, 1945) and the Edwards–Jones–Brewer (Brewer, 1937, 1938); these embryos fall into the period of 13½–15 days of development.

The general arrangement of the trophoblast and related endometrium in this embryo is shown in Figure 6. It will be seen that the cytotrophoblast has increased very considerably in amount when compared with the 12-day specimen. The trabeculae of peripheral syncytial trophoblast of the previous stage have been invaded by the cytotrophoblast or have been transformed partially into it; certainly the latter tissue now forms a more or less continuous trophoblastic shell round the conceptus. In this peripheral shell there are to be found many spaces of varying size and shape. Some of these spaces contain maternal blood, others possess variously shaped masses of syncytium which is often vacuolated and shows phagocytosis of maternal blood cells. The nuclei of the syncytial masses frequently possess extremely large eosinophilic nucleoli. The spaces in the trophoblastic shell communicate only infrequently with the main portion of the lacunar system. On the maternal side of the trophoblastic shell

many strands of peripheral syncytium are present; they extend as streamers into the surrounding endometrium making contact with the sinusoids, the coiled arteries and the glands. The presence of these syncytial streamers makes the external aspect of the trophoblast irregular. On the embryonic side of the trophoblastic shell, many of the trabeculæ ("villi"), separated by the dilated lacunæ, can be traced to the chorionic plate. These trabeculæ are mainly arranged radially and are covered by a thin layer of syncytium. They now possess a mesodermal core. At the periphery of those of the radial strands which reach the trophoblastic shell there is a concentration of small, darkly staining, cytotrophoblastic cells which may well be the original source of the existing shell and which are doubtless the source of subsequent additions to it. The appearance of cytotrophoblast and of mesoderm within the trabecular syncytium does not alter the fundamentally labyrinthine nature of the lacunar spaces of earlier stages. Not all of these trabeculæ, however, reach the trophoblastic shell for a number of them arise from the chorionic plate, or even from the main trabeculæ, to terminate as *free* villi. It is such finger-like proliferations of trophoblast, with the contained mesoderm, that lay the basis for the subsequent villous structure of the placenta. At this stage, however, the human placenta clearly presents a combination of labyrinthine and villous characters. It must be stressed that the main trabeculæ, which we will call primary villous stems, were never free villi. From this stage forwards, however, it would be pedantic to avoid calling the lacunar system the intervillous space.

The endometrium adjacent to the trophoblast in this embryo shows a well marked decidual reaction. Portions of the uterine glands in the immediate vicinity of the trophoblast are eroded or destroyed. Other glands, situated more remotely, show degenerative changes and maternal blood in their distended cavities. The endothelially lined maternal sinusoids in the implantation region are dilated and filled with plasma and some maternal blood cells. At a number of points, especially in the basal region, the intervillous space communicates with the sinusoids by way of channels through the trophoblastic shell (Fig. 7). Some of these channels are in part lined by syncytium but many of them possess walls formed by cytotrophoblast alone. The sinusoids can be traced away from the implantation site to become continuous directly with endometrial veins. As it is only the superficial part of the endometrium that is available in this specimen few details can be provided for the coiled arteries. Several of them, however, could be traced through the endometrium adjacent to the trophoblastic shell and into the latter where they terminate blindly. None was found to enter directly into the intervillous space; indeed, none could be traced into the spaces in the cytotrophoblast. In the walls of several arteries in the decidua compacta, which were separated by several hundreds of microns from the trophoblastic shell, there were signs of degeneration. A number of cells of syncytial origin were found in close relation to these endometrial arteries.

The Gar embryo. This embryo with its implantation site has been described in considerable detail by West (1952).

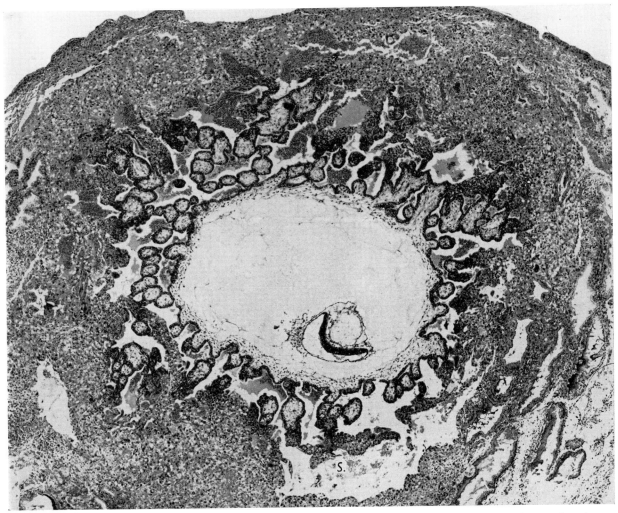

FIG. 6. Photomicrograph (×52) of a section of the implantation site of a 14-day embryo (Missen). Chorionic villi with mesodermal cores are now well established round the whole of the chorionic sac. There is an extensive intervillous space which, in this section, communicates at two points with a large venous sinusoid (S.). Details of the differentiation of the trophoblast in this specimen are shown in Fig. 7.

Here we restrict observations on it to points directly relevant to placental development.

From the menstrual and coital history, West concluded that the embryo was 18 days old. The developmental state of this specimen corresponds closely to that of other embryos known to be of this age. The chorionic sac was embedded in the anterior uterine wall close to the ostium of the left uterine tube. It appeared as a hemispherical hæmorrhagic swelling 5 mm. in diameter and raised 4 mm. above the surface of the adjacent endometrium. In the sections the chorionic sac is somewhat triangular in shape, tapering to a blunt point towards the myometrium. The widest internal measurement of the sac is 2 mm. The external measurement at this level is 4·1 mm. The embryonic disc measures 0·56 mm. antero-posteriorly and 0·6 mm. from side to side.

The chorionic villi in this specimen are of two types. There are, first, those which have free endings in the intervillous space and which take their origin from the chorionic plate or from other villi near to their chorionic attachment. Many of these villi are well developed and branch as often as three or four times. The second villous type includes those which extend from the chorionic plate to the trophoblastic shell with which they are continuous. Such primary villous stems are, at least in part, persistent portions of the original trabeculae of the earlier stages. Apart from the small syncytial sprouts, which are attached to each type, the villi possess a well-developed core of mesoderm. They are covered by syncytial trophoblast deep to which a layer of cytotrophoblastic cells (Langhans cells) can be identified. Early embryonic blood vessels are now present in the mesenchymal cores. At the periphery of the primary villous stems, the cytotrophoblast has broken through the syncytial layer and, by lateral expansion and fusion, constitutes a thick trophoblastic shell (Fig. 8). In the shell there are many labyrinthine irregular spaces, the walls of which are formed for the most part by cytotrophoblast alone. In these spaces there are many maternal blood corpuscles and such elements can also be found lying between the loosely arranged cytotrophoblastic cells themselves. The peripheral cells of the trophoblastic shell are intimately intermingled with the decidua and it is

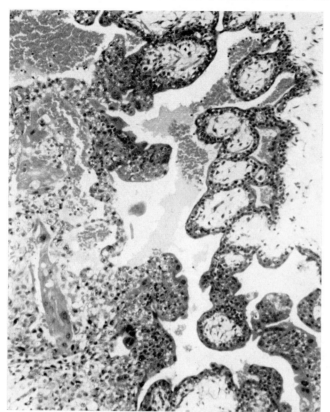

FIG. 7. Photomicrograph (×113) of part of a section (H. and E.) through the foetal-maternal junction of a 14-day embryo (Missen). The chorionic villi (to the right of the illustration) possess mesodermal cores but as yet no definitive blood vessels are present. The villi possess a covering of definitive syncytium overlying Langhans layer. At the tips of some of the villi cytotrophoblastic columns, by proliferation, are contributing to the trophoblastic shell. On the maternal side of this shell a number of persisting masses of primitive syncytium can be identified. In the intervillous space there are maternal blood vessels and at about the centre of the figure an isolated syncytial sprout in the intervillous space; maternal blood cells are also present in the intervillous space.

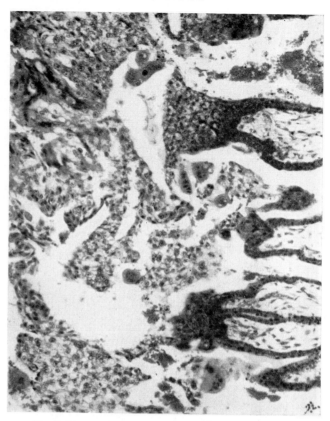

FIG. 8. Photomicrograph (×110) of a section (H. and E.) of an 18-day embryo (Gar). Marked proliferation at the tips of the villi (to the right) has resulted in the production of a trophoblastic shell which now extends completely around the foetal tissue. The villi are covered except at their tips by a Langhans layer of cytotrophoblast and a superficial layer of definitive syncytium. At one point a syncytial sprout can be seen arising from the definitive syncytium. Remnants of the primitive syncytium lie within and on the maternal aspect of the trophoblastic shell. Early vasculogenesis is present in the mesodermal cores of the villi.

impossible to define a distinct foetal-maternal junction. Syncytial streamers from the trophoblast are occasionally found amongst the decidual cells. The syncytium frequently shows active phagocytosis (Fig. 9). The decidua basalis in this specimen is oedematous and, adjacent to the implantation site, blood corpuscles in large numbers are found amongst the endometrial cells. Coiled arteries can be seen in the deeper parts of the endometrium. As they approach the implantation site the walls of these arteries show necrotic changes; none was, in fact, found to open directly into the cytotrophoblastic lacunar spaces, nor into the intervillous space. The arteries adjacent to the implantation site have apparently been pushed laterally by the expanding chorion; some of them can, however, be traced to the decidua capsularis.

Large venous sinusoids lie adjacent to the implantation site; they anastomose freely with each other and receive a number of communications from the lacunar labyrinth by way of clefts in the trophoblastic shell. The most

conspicuous communications between the intervillous space and the maternal veins in the Gar specimen are situated round the equatorial region of the trophoblastic shell. The uterine glands in the region of the implantation site are frequently invaded by the trophoblast with resultant destruction of the glandular epithelium.

Owing to the nature of placental expansion, however, the glands at the margin of the placenta are much less affected than those in the central region; consequently, well-preserved glands can be found in the marginal zone of the decidua basalis throughout the period with which we are at present concerned. Glandular secretion is apparent in many of the persisting basal glands until comparatively late stages (Hamilton and Boyd, 1951).

Possibly as a result of the glandular penetration by the destructive action of the trophoblast, maternal blood cells are early apparent in many of the glands. Such extravasated blood is already present in several glands in the 12-day specimen (Fig. 2) and is a striking feature in the central

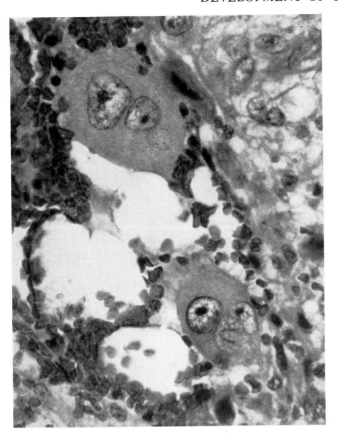

FIG. 9. Photomicrograph (×450) of a section (H. and E.) through a uterine gland near the implantation site of an 18-day embryo (Gar). The lumen of the gland possesses maternal red blood corpuscles and two masses of multinucleated syncytium.

part of the decidua basalis of the 28-somite specimen (Fig. 10). From the accounts in the literature on early implantations it would seem that such haemorrhage into the glands does not occur earlier than the 12th day. Even in later stages it may be absent (for discussion, see Krafka, 1941). Blood in the glands, however, has been described in so many older specimens that its presence must be considered a normal feature of human implantation from 12 days onwards. Haemorrhage into the uterine glands has also been described in the neighbourhood of the implantation site in the macaque by Wislocki and Streeter (1938); they found that the blood was not present in the glands until the 17th post-ovulational day and that it persisted until the end of the first month of conception. Haemorrhage into glands which are not yet occluded by the pressure of the expanding trophoblast is probably the explanation for the slight external haemorrhage, in both women and the macaque monkey, now well known to occur at, or about, the time of the first "missed" menstruation. This blood loss constitutes the so-called "placental sign" to which attention was first directed by Hartman (1928, 1932).

The Shaw embryo. This specimen has already been described in some detail (Hamilton and Gladstone, 1942). They originally estimated it from the coital history to be 20–23 days old. From its general development, however,

we consider that its age is distinctly younger than this estimation and that it is about 18 days old. A small elevation about 1 cm. in diameter was observed on the posterior uterine wall. The measurements of the chorionic sac are as follows: maximum external diameter, 11 mm.; maximum internal diameter, 8 mm. The embryonic disc measured 1·05 × 1·34 mm.

Part of the decidua capsularis had been damaged previous to fixation and there is some distortion in the region of the decidua basalis. Notwithstanding these deficiencies, the specimen shows certain features relevant to understanding the development of the villi and the trophoblast. On the deep aspect of the chorionic sac, the wall of the implantation cavity is formed by an incomplete trophoblastic shell in which spaces containing small masses of syncytium are present (see Pl. 3, Fig. 6, in Hamilton and Gladstone, 1942). On its embryonic side, the shell is continuous with the cytotrophoblastic cell columns proliferated from the tips of anchoring villi, some of which are presumably villous stems. Freely ending villi, similar to those found in the Gar embryo, are also present. Syncytiotrophoblast of varying thickness covers the cell columns and the intervillous aspect of the trophoblastic shell. The mesenchymal cores of the villi are in the form of a loose reticulum in which there are some, for the most part empty, endothelially lined vascular spaces. These spaces, which are the precursors of the foetal villous vessels, are best developed in the region of attachment of the connecting stalk to the chorionic plate.

A wide space, the basal sinus (which may, in this specimen, be partly artefact), separates the decidua basalis from the trophoblastic shell and communicates very freely with the intervillous space. Owing to the small amount of maternal tissue removed with the conceptus, it has not been possible to trace the endometrial arteries or to determine with accuracy their mode of termination.

The examination of presomite embryos, such as the Edwards–Jones–Brewer (Brewer, 1937), the HR 1 (Johnston, 1940), the Shaw (Hamilton and Gladstone, 1942), the Torpin (Krafka, 1941) and the Gar (West, 1952) has shown that there are no direct arterial openings into the intervillous space; this would seem to indicate that the flow of blood into the spaces is a "controlled seepage", as Krafka has suggested. It can further be pointed out that, in the macaque monkey (Wislocki and Streeter, 1938), it is not until the 17th day that maternal vessels discharge their contents into the lacunae. A continuous flow of blood through the intervillous space was not considered likely until the 3rd week. These investigators, however, go further for they state: "We have no absolute information as to when the maternal blood actually begins to flow through the intervillous space, but it may safely be assumed as occurring gradually and as probably being completed in the main before the time that the fetal circulation is established."

Whether the blood in the syncytial lacunae is simply "pooled" or is subject to a slow ebb and flow circulation cannot be decided on the evidence. We have already recorded, however, that the maternal blood cells in the lacunae of the 12-day specimen show staining characteristics

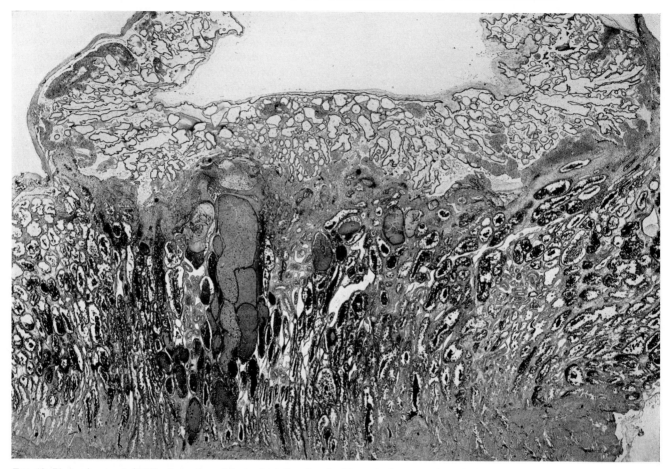

FIG. 10. Photomicrograph (×12) of a section of the implantation site of a 28-somite human embryo (Camb. H. 710). Villi which cover the whole of the chorionic sac are well established, and possess numerous foetal vessels. There is no indication of a marginal sinus in the intervillous space; there is, however, venous drainage from the left margin of this space. The decidua basalis is thick and contains many dilated glands; several of the central ones show haemorrhage into their lumina. The effect of expansion of the chorionic sac on the uterine glands is particularly well shown on the right of the illustration where their necks are constricted and stretched, thus damming back the products of secretion. Veins and spiral arteries can be identified at intervals in the decidua basalis.

suggesting that the circulation is, in fact, very sluggish. Mossman (1956) has suggested that, as the perforation into a single sinusoid (he actually instances a capillary) elongates, two openings, an inlet and an outlet, can be achieved. With increase in the trophoblastic invasion, Mossman considers that the maternal vessels would disappear progressively back to the level of true arterioles and venules, thus permitting a "through" circulation.

TROPHOBLASTIC DIFFERENTIATION

Reference has been made in the introduction to certain difficulties in the terminology used to describe the different varieties of trophoblast. In particular, we have avoided terms such as "implantation trophoblast" and "resorptive syncytium" that attribute specific functions to parts of the trophoblast at successive periods of development. There can, of course, be no doubt that there is a functional specialization on the part of the different regions of the trophoblast; until more is known about the details of trophoblastic function, however, terms implying a particular activity by a given region should be avoided.

Moreover, as Wislocki and Streeter (1938) have stated, such an adjective as "resorptive" can apply "equally well to the entire development of the trophoblast and should not be restricted to any particular stage".

In the 7½-day human ovum described by Hertig and Rock (1945) the blastocystic trophoblast has already differentiated at the implantation pole into a thick plaque of proliferating, and intermingled, syncytium and cytotrophoblast. The remaining part of the blastocyst wall is constituted by a thin "mesothelial" membrane which consists of a single layer of flattened blastocystic cells. In the junctional region between the latter and the plaque itself cells intermediate in character between the two are found. In specimens several days older (Hertig and Rock, 1945, 1949), when implantation is nearly achieved, differentiation into primitive cytotrophoblast and primitive syncytiotrophoblast is much clearer. Both of these are alike derived from the blastocystic trophoblast but the syncytium arises indirectly in the sense that it stems from cells which are uninucleate and which, consequently, cannot initially be distinguished from other cytotrophoblastic cells. How the syncytium actually takes its origin is an important question to which, so far, there is no compelling answer. Either certain cytotrophoblastic cells undergo nuclear division—mitotic or otherwise—without cellular division, or adjacent cytotrophoblastic cells unite and, by their fusion, constitute a multinucleate mass of cytoplasm (for details see Boyd and Hamilton, 1966b). We have given much attention, throughout the study of all of our material, to the method of syncytial formation in the trophoblast and have been unable to decide between the two possibilities. The syncytium presents a histological structure quite strikingly different from the cytotrophoblast. Hence, if elements of the latter are included by fusion in the former the cytotrophoblastic cytoplasm must rapidly change in character during the assimilation. On the other hand, if there is nuclear multiplication in the syncytium, the absence of signs of mitosis in the multinucleate cytoplasm suggests the not very satisfactory explanation of amitotic division. Whatever factors do, in fact, cause the appearance of the syncytium, contact with the endometrial tissues does not seem to be an absolutely determining one, for primitive cytotrophoblast is found in direct apposition to the maternal cells. Once it has appeared, however, the primitive syncytium seems to be mainly responsible for the local destruction of the maternal tissues.

Soon after its first appearance the syncytium of the trophoblast shows marked vacuolation. The vacuoles become confluent and by the 12th day a well-established system of lacunar spaces is present throughout the syncytium. Moreover, some of the dilated maternal sinusoids are now in open communication with the lacunæ and maternal blood is present in them. The method whereby the sinusoids are tapped is not apparent. It does not appear to be a disordered destruction of maternal tissue that is responsible; the endothelium of the maternal vessels, at the points of communication, is in neat apposition to the peripheral syncytium (Fig. 3) and there is no sign of maternal hæmorrhage into the decidua surrounding this part of the trophoblast. The maternal blood cells in the lacunar spaces in the 12-day specimen are very palely stained. The difference in the degree of eosinophilia between them and the maternal erythrocytes in blood vessels away from the implantation site is quite striking. It is, therefore, possible that the cells in the lacunar spaces in this stage, due to the stagnant nature of the circulation or to the effect of syncytial secretion on them, are in a special physiological state.

In the 12-day specimen the primitive syncytium covers the cytotrophoblast and the latter is present only in some of the trabecular columns which incompletely separate the lacunæ from each other (Fig. 2). There is no sign, at this stage, of villus formation by the extension of separate syncytial "streamers" into a maternal blood space. The traditional picture of "primary villi" is one that must be dismissed. It was based on conclusions arrived at from the study of badly fixed material and on an absence of understanding of the method of formation of the lacunar spaces and of the relationship of the trophoblast to them. Already at the 12th day the human placental arrangement is haemo-chorial, to use Grosser's terminology, but at this stage it quite obviously possesses not a villous structure but a labyrinthine one.

In the period from the 14th to the 20th day there is intense proliferative activity in the trophoblast; this activity results in the appearance of the definitive structure of the placenta and in the full establishment of the circulation in the rearranged lacunar spaces which now, collectively, constitute the intervillous space. The first result of the growth processes is that the trophoblastic trabeculae, instead of being arranged quite irregularly become more and more radially arranged. The cytotrophoblastic cells then proliferate and extend into the syncytial trabeculae which thus gradually assume the histological characteristics of the so-called "primary villi". The primary villous stems do not arise as individual and separate sprouts from the chorion. In due course chorionic mesoderm invades, or differentiates *in situ* within, such primary villi converting them into "secondary villi". By the appearance within these mesodermal cores of embryonic blood vessels, these villi are, in turn, gradually transformed into "tertiary villi". Thus, when applied to the villi, the adjective *primary*, *secondary* and *tertiary* do no more than define stages in the elaboration of their histological structure. The newly formed mesodermal cells of the cores of the villi do not come into direct contact with the syncytium on their surfaces. Proximally (i.e. at their chorionic ends) the villous stems preserve a single layer of cytotrophoblastic cells which, as Langhans layer, separates the mesodermal core from the overlying syncytium. Distally the cytotrophoblastic cells, as the cytotrophoblastic columns, form the full thickness of each villous stem. On their free surfaces the columns are covered by definitive syncytium which separates them from the enlarging intervillous space. At their decidual ends, however, active proliferation of the cytotrophoblastic columns results in an expansion of the cytotrophoblast beyond the distal ends of the villous stems where their cells extend into the primitive syncytium. In this position they mushroom outwards from the maternal end of each villous stem with the result that, eventually, they meet equivalent cells from adjacent primary villous stems to form an irregularly complete cytotrophoblastic layer, known as the trophoblastic shell, round the whole conceptus. This shell was first described and named by Siegenbeek van Heukelom (1898) and his description was amplified by Peters (1899). The term is a useful one for it ascribes to the expanded and fused tips of the primary villous stems precisely that feature which is most characteristic of the resulting cytotrophoblastic layer—that it forms a shell for the developing conceptus and placenta.

Any decidual cells included within the trophoblastic shell are soon destroyed, for our own observations confirm those of Jones and Brewer (1935) and Brewer (1937) that no maternal cells persist within it. Immediately on the decidual side of the trophoblastic shell there is the special transformation of the endometrial stroma to which Merrtens (1894) first directed attention, and which has variously been known as the "boundary zone", the *Durchdringungszone, Umlagerungszone* and the "trophosphere". It is the compact decidua, immediately surrounding the trophoblastic shell, which presents a different histological picture from the more remotely situated endometrium. In it are the terminations of the maternal

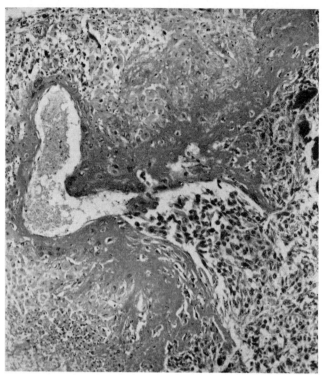

FIG. 11. Photomicrograph (×95) of a section through the termination of an endometrial artery in the *in situ* placenta of a 50 mm. embryo (C.X. 111). The arterial wall shows marked degeneration and cytotrophoblastic cells are extending into the vessel. At each side of the arterial opening Nitabuch's membrane can be seen.

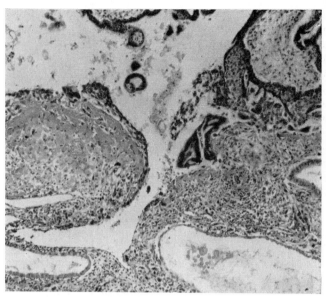

FIG. 12. Photomicrograph (×85) of a section of the central region of an *in situ* placenta of a 50 mm. embryo (C.X. 111) showing communication between the intervillous space and a maternal vein. Note the continuity between cytotrophoblastic cells and unaltered venous endothelium. There is no cytotrophoblast within the lumen of the vein but a sectioned syncytial sprout can be seen.

blood vessels and through it the blood must pass to reach the intervillous space. In the region of junction between the boundary zone and the shell there appears the fibrinoid deposit which is called Nitabuch's membrane and which is shown in our 28-somite stage and in all of the older specimens (Figs. 11 and 12). The boundary zone is traversed by the maternal blood vessels on their way to and from the intervillous space and, in the younger stages, uterine glands pass through it to open into spaces in the trophoblastic shell or even into the intervillous space itself (Frassi, 1908; Boyd, 1959).

By the method of its formation the trophoblastic shell splits, in an irregular fashion, the initial primitive syncytium into a part on the intervillous space aspect of the shell and a part on its decidual aspect. The former of these two portions of the primitive syncytium becomes the lining of that part of the intervillous space in contact with the basal plate of the placenta. The residual syncytium on the decidual side of the shell persists only in part and in an irregularly distributed fashion until late developmental stages; this persisting peripheral syncytium probably gives origin to some of the giant cells of foetal origin which become so widely distributed in the decidua basalis and the adjacent part of the myometrium (Boyd and Hamilton, 1960). The cells of the trophoblastic shell itself, however, also appear to be able to differentiate into syncytial giant cells. Indeed, after it has apparently reached a stage of full differentiation the cytotrophoblast retains the potency to produce syncytium throughout pregnancy.

The trophoblastic shell, though in general consisting of closely packed cells (Pl. 1, fig. 1) possesses many variously shaped, and occasionally quite large, intercellular spaces and gaps to which attention was first drawn by Jung (1908). Many of these spaces come to communicate with the peripheral part of the intervillous space, and some of them do so with the lumina of the uterine glands. In the spaces (Fig. 13) detritus, glandular secretion and, eventually, maternal blood cells are found, often accompanied by portions of syncytium. In our opinion these spaces are of considerable importance in the earlier histiotrophic phase of embryonic nutrition and they are also important in that many of the endometrial spiral arteries will communicate with the intervillous space by way of them. It must be stressed that the cells of the cytotrophoblastic shell never develop mesenchymatous derivatives equivalent to the mesodermal cores of the villous stems and the villi. Hence, when the foetal blood vessels develop in the mesenchymal cores to produce the "tertiary villi", they do not penetrate the shell and do not come into contact with the maternal decidua or blood.

By the establishment of the trophoblastic shell a mechanism is apparently provided, through its interstitial growth, for a rapid circumferential extension of the whole implantation site. The surrounding decidua, including the glands, is encroached upon and, at the same time, the side of the implantation site in contact with the decidua capsularis bulges out into the uterine lumen. Generally the trophoblastic shell becomes markedly thinned from the 10 mm. stage onwards, and, at the same time, the related fibrinoid material increases in amount. In the regions overlying the attachment of the villi, however, its attenuation is much less marked.

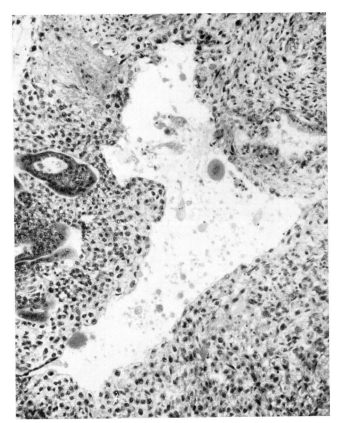

FIG. 13. Photomicrograph (×70) of a section (H. and E.) through the tips of the chorionic villi and trophoblastic shell of a 28-somite human implantation site (Camb. H. 710). The portion of the trophoblastic shell illustrated contains a typical irregularly shaped space in which glandular secretion and cellular detritus can be identified. There are several masses of primitive syncytium related to the cytotrophoblast. One of these shows extensive vacuolation and an inclusion within one of the vacuoles.

As a result of the expansion of the trophoblastic shell the area available for the intervillous space is considerably augmented. Into this enlarged area extend sprouts from the surface of the primary villous stems and also, we think, from the surface of the chorion itself. These sprouts are initially formed of definitive syncytium alone. Soon, however, they increase in size and pass through the stages of villi possessing cytotrophoblastic, mesodermal and, eventually, vascularized mesenchymal cores. Such sprouts are undoubtedly true villi and their presence justifies the ascription of a villous character to the human placenta. Nevertheless, these true villi are a secondary addition to the structure of the placenta. Some of them later become joined together at their free ends by syncytial fusion, but we doubt if this fusion involves more than the syncytium for we have never observed unequivocally the junction, described by Stieve (1941), of separate villi by the fusion of their mesodermal cores or of their constituent blood vessels. We have not, by direct observation, been able to decide if some of the villi arising from the chorionic plate manage to reach the basal plate and to fuse with it. As the placenta grows extremely rapidly in the period between the 5 mm. stage and the 60 mm. stage it seems likely that new major villous stems are continuously added. There

may, however, be some longitudinal splitting of the initial primary villous stems. Certainly there is rapid growth in their length and marked branching at their basal extremities. The accounts of the placentation in primates by Hill (1932), Wislocki and Streeter (1938) and Starck (1956) add strength to the interpretation which denies the presence of initially independent villi in the human placenta.

SOMITE STAGE

Embryo H. 712 (7 somites, c. 23 days)

The embryo measured 1·8 mm. in total length and possessed seven somites. We place it about the 23rd day of gestation. Only a portion of the implantation site of this embryo is available. The trophoblastic shell is thinner than in the earlier specimens but in parts it can be seen to possess spaces. Villi are well developed over the whole of the chorionic sac. In those villi which reach and fuse with the cytotrophoblast the average length is about 1·5 mm. The villi are more branched than heretofore and consequently the intervillous space possesses a more complicated structure. The glands in the decidua show signs of secretory activity. The available portions of the specimen, unfortunately, do not permit of comment on either the spiral arteries or the uterine veins.

Embryo H. 710 (28 somites, c. 26 days)

The ovulational age of this specimen is estimated to be about 26 days; comparison with the histories of the few other described somite embryos at comparable stages of development suggests that, in fact, H. 710 may be a little older than this. A pronounced swelling projected from the posterior wall of the uterus near the fundus.

The implantation site in this specimen is shown in Figures 10 and 14. The embryo was removed by way of a cruciate incision through the decidua capsularis. On the deep aspect of the chorion the main villi have an average length of about 1·75 mm. They are also present, although less well developed, in the region of the decidua capsularis. All of the villi are covered by a continuous band of syncytium deep to which a fully established Langhans layer of cytotrophoblast is present (Fig. 13). Well established blood vessels are found in many of the villous mesodermal cores. The intervillous space contains some maternal blood. Peripherally many of the villi are attached to the attenuated trophoblastic shell by columns of cytotrophoblast. There are also islands of cytotrophoblast scattered, in an apparently random fashion, throughout the villous tree. The trophoblastic shell shows many spaces (Fig. 13). Some of these communicate with each other and others can be seen to open into the adjacent intervillous space. The spaces often contain cellular debris, glandular secretion and, occasionally, maternal blood cells. Many of these spaces also contain masses of syncytium which are often markedly vacuolated. The cytotrophoblastic cells of the shell are loosely arranged; debris and maternal corpuscles can frequently be seen between these cells.

The peripheral margin of the trophoblastic shell is intimately related to the decidua compacta and it is difficult to establish the precise line of junction between

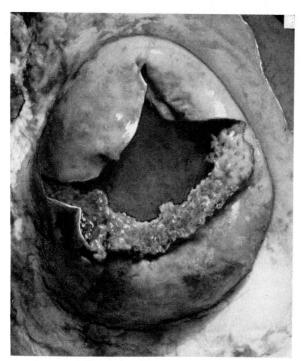

FIG. 14. Photograph (×3·5) of the surface view of the partially opened implantation site from which a 28-somite embryo (Camb. H. 710) had been removed. Chorionic villi are seen on the everted cut surface of the decidua capsularis. Photomicrographs of sections through this implantation site are illustrated in Figs. 10 and 13 and Pl. 1, Figs. 1 and 2.

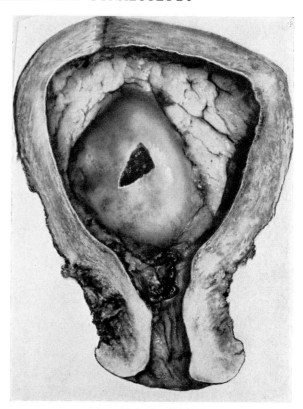

FIG. 15. Photograph (×1·1) of a general view of the interior of the uterus containing the implantation site of a 10 mm. embryo (C.X. 100). A small opening has been made through the central part of the decidua capsularis. Note the smoothness of this portion of the decidua in comparison with the furrowed decidua vera (parietalis).

the two tissues. The decidual cells are surrounded by collagenous and reticular fibrils; the cytotrophoblastic cells, however, have no fibrillar material between them (Pl. 1, fig. 1). Apart from some stray strands of decidual collagen which are apparently being digested by the cytotrophoblastic cells there are no intercellular fibrils in the trophoblastic shell. In the decidua basalis there are many dilated glands, often with large amounts of maternal blood in their lumina. Those in the marginal zone of the implantation site are distorted as they pass to their openings situated on the decidua capsularis (Fig. 10). The glands situated directly below the implantation, in the decidua basalis, have had their connections with the uterine lumen interrupted. They terminate blindly in the junctional zone and many of them have their cavities invaded by cytotrophoblast. The secretion of such glands can in some instances be traced into the interstices between the cytotrophoblastic cells. Frequently, however, the appearance is presented of the damming back of secretion owing to the pressure exerted by the expanding conceptus. In those glands which flank the lateral margins of the implantation site there are frequently marked signs of degeneration. That part of a gland wall closer to the trophoblast shows cellular destruction while the opposite wall may possess a lining of intact glandular epithelial cells. (Illustrations of the relationship of the glands to the trophoblast can be found in Boyd, 1959.)

Many coiled arteries are found in the decidua adjacent to the implantation site. These vessels can be traced through the junctional region to the peripheral cytotrophoblast where most of them terminate, apparently blindly. Some of the arteries, however, have open endings which give the appearance of having permitted the escape of maternal blood into the interstices between the cells of the trophoblastic shell. None of the arteries, in spite of most careful search, could be found to discharge directly into the intervillous space itself. The walls of the terminal arteries show signs of degeneration with disappearance of their muscle cells and marked swelling of their endothelium (Pl. 1, Fig. 2). Such striking changes in the endothelium can be found in loops of the coiled arteries quite remote from the junctional zone. Openings from the intervillous space to endometrial veins are present over the basal surface of the implantation site; several large communications drain its equatorial region.

Specimens of *in situ* Placentae with Embryos of the 10 mm. Stage (37–38 days)

Implantation sites of four embryos at this stage of development are available (Figs. 15 and 16). The general features of the utero-placental junction and of the chorionic villi are very similar in all four specimens. A photomicrograph (Fig. 17) of a section through one of them shows that, in comparison with earlier stages, the decidua basalis is now distinctly reduced. The decidua parietalis, however, is if anything even thicker than in younger specimens.

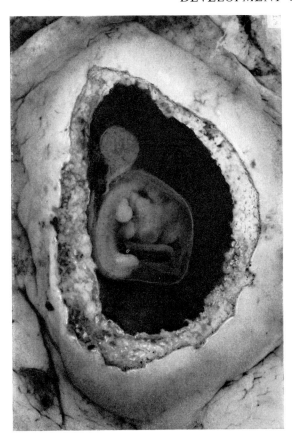

FIG. 16. Photograph (×3·5) of the implantation site of a 10 mm. embryo (C.X. 100) with the decidua capsularis removed to an extent sufficient to show the embryo, within the collapsed amnion, and the yolk sac. Note the extent of development of the chorionic villi related to the decidua capsularis. This photograph has been rotated in relation to Fig. 15. to show the embryo in a suitable orientation. A section through the placenta of this specimen is illustrated in Fig. 17.

The trophoblastic shell varies in thickness. Over extensive areas of the basal plate it has become attenuated; deep to such areas there is a fibrinoid deposit in the most superficial part of the decidua. In some regions this fibrinoid material shows a lymphocytic invasion. The shell still remains thick, however, where the well-developed cellular columns at the tips of the main villous stems are attached. No clear distinction can, in fact, be made, in such regions, between the cytotrophoblastic cells of the shell and those of the villous extremities. Between such cytotrophoblastic cells there are many of the spaces to which attention has already been drawn. Some of these spaces are in communication with the intervillous space, but most of them are isolated small cavities. Villi, both attaching and free, are distributed over the entire surface of the chorion. Opposite to the decidua basalis they have a slightly greater average length and are more luxuriant and better vascularized than those in relation to the capsularis. The cytoplasm of the trophoblastic components of the basal villi is generally more basophilic than that of the equivalent cells in the capsular villi.

Aggregations of cytotrophoblastic cells, in the form of the so-called cytotrophoblastic islands, are present in relation to the villi. Such islands are not restricted to, but are much larger on, the basal side. These islands will become increasingly apparent in later stages. Their superficial cells are in direct contact with the contents of the intervillous space.

The glands in the decidua basalis are very much distorted and the long axes of most of them are now orientated at an angle to the myometrium. They still show signs of secretory activity, however, and their lumina are frequently distended. Evidence of glandular breakdown in the neighbourhood of the implantation site is still apparent. There are many coiled arteries in the decidua and those in the basal part can be traced into the junctional zone. The walls of the dilated terminal parts of these vessels show a very marked fibrinoid degeneration with complete disappearance of the histological features of an artery. Some of these terminal arterial segments extend up to the trophoblastic shell and here the continuity of the vessel wall is often interrupted. Blood from these arteries and secretion and debris from the glands can be traced through gaps in the peripheral part of the shell to the cytotrophoblastic lacunae and, thence, to the intervillous space. Communications from the intervillous space to the endometrial veins are evident over the whole of the basal plate but, in one of the specimens, there is a preferential drainage from the zone of transition between the decidua basalis and decidua capsularis (Fig. 17). When the uterus of this 10 mm. specimen was opened, it was seen that the decidua capsularis projected across the uterine lumen and made contact with the decidua parietalis of the opposing wall. Here there was no fusion of the two deciduae but, as subsequent section showed, the epithelium of the decidua parietalis in the area of contact had become markedly thinned and the underlying endometrial capillaries and veins were markedly dilated.

Specimen of an *in situ* Placenta with an Embryo of the 15 mm. Stage (41–43 days)

The implantation site associated with a 15 mm. embryo is shown in Figure 18. A section through the central part of the implantation site of this specimen is shown in Figure 19. The diameter of the actual attachment area measures 26 mm. The thickness of the placenta proper varies between 3 and 6 mm. The combined thickness of the chorion and decidua capsularis is about 2 mm. and there are well-developed capsular villi. By this stage there is a striking reduction in the thickness of the decidua basalis but its glands continue to show secretory activity. Many of them open directly into the intervillous space and it is noteworthy that these are, for the most part, empty. Other glands, however, which do not communicate with the space, are distended with secretion; their cells are flattened and a number of them contain maternal blood. Except at the site of attachment of the cytotrophoblastic columns at the villous tips the thickness of the trophoblastic shell has become much reduced, often to a single layer of cells. On the decidual side of the shell there is frequently a fibrinoid deposit which is scattered in an irregular fashion over the surface of the basal plate.

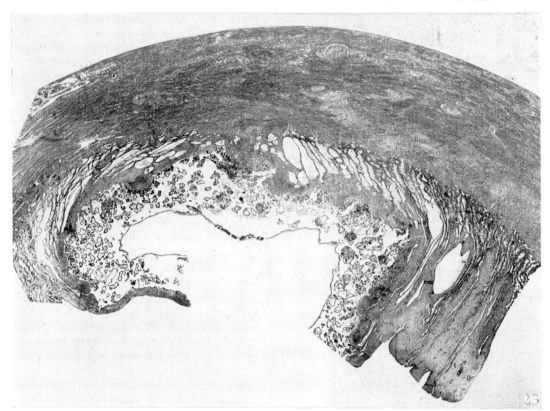

FIG. 17. Photomicrograph (×6) of a section through the uterus and *in situ* placenta of a 10 mm. embryo (C.X. 100). The villi are more or less equivalently developed round the whole of the chorionic sac. The decidua capsularis is still relatively thick. The distortion and dilatation of the glands in the decidua basalis, which has been irregularly penetrated by the trophoblast, are clearly shown. The thick decidua vera is well shown on the right of the illustration.

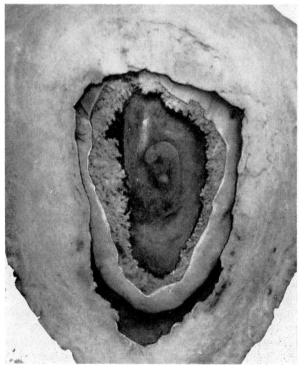

FIG. 18. Photograph (×1) of a coronal section of a uterus containing a 15 mm. embryo (C.X. 102). The decidua capsularis has been opened to show the amnion containing the embryo. A section of the placenta of this specimen is illustrated in Fig. 19.

Numerous arteries ensheathed by decidua can be traced from the myometrium towards the intervillous space. The terminal portions of these vessels show the hyaline degenerative changes described for earlier specimens and all of them are being invaded by cytotrophoblast. There is also a marked thickening of their endothelial linings in the deeper part of the decidua. The actual terminations of the arteries are in communication with spaces in the thickened parts of the trophoblastic shell. No direct arterial communications with the intervillous space itself have been observed. It would appear, therefore, that, at this stage, blood from these arteries could only have reached the intervillous space by percolation through the interstices situated between the cytotrophoblastic cells (Fig. 20). A striking feature of this specimen is the paucity of maternal veins underlying the central area of the implantation site. Consequently the main drainage of the intervillous space is through communications which open into veins in the region of junction of the decidua capsularis with the decidua parietalis. The villi themselves are clothed by both syncytium and cytotrophoblast; their mesodermal cores contain well differentiated foetal blood vessels.

Specimens of *in situ* Placentae with Embryos of between 20 and 30 mm. Stages (48–60 days)

Figure 21 shows the implantation site associated with a 29 mm. embryo. Sections through the whole uterus

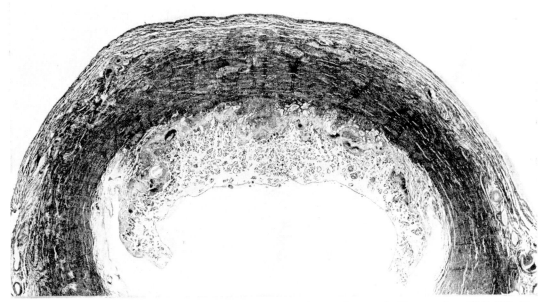

FIG. 19. Photomicrograph (×6) of a section through the uterus and *in situ* placenta of a 15 mm. embryo (C.X. 102). The chorionic villi are now distinctly better developed in relation to the decidua basalis and the decidua capsularis is much attenuated. The uterine glands are less apparent than in the specimen illustrated in Fig. 17. The very irregular decidua basalis and the decidua vera are both much thinned.

showing the developing placenta of the 29 mm. stage and of the 30 mm. stage are shown in Figures 22 and 23 respectively. The placentae of these two specimens have diameters of approximately 40 and 47 mm. respectively. It will be seen from these illustrations that there are villi on the part of the chorion related to the decidua capsularis. The latter is now projecting deeply into the uterine lumen but has not yet fused with the decidua parietalis. Indeed, as will be seen from the account of later stages, such fusion does not occur until later. The trophoblastic shell is now very thin except in the regions of attachment of the terminal cytotrophoblastic cell columns of the anchoring villi. Extensions of syncytium into the decidua basalis are a striking feature of these stages. Such extensions frequently reach the myometrium and isolated syncytial masses can be found in its inner part. Other irregularly shaped plates of syncytium, often highly vacuolated, are present along the basal plate, particularly in the regions near the attachment of the villi.

The villi possess a structure similar to that of earlier stages. They are, however, more branched with resulting increase in the complexity of the intervillous space. The connective tissue in the villi is further differentiated and numerous Hofbauer cells are present.

As in previous stages, the walls of the terminal parts of the spiral arteries show fibrinoid and hyaline degenerative changes. Thickening of the endothelium is still present and in the portions of the vessels nearest to the intervillous space plugs of cytotrophoblast can be identified. Small irregular clefts can be followed from the arterial lumina through the interstices situated between the cytotrophoblastic cells. In some instances, indeed, as, for example, in a 22 mm. specimen, such clefts are represented by narrow, but straight, channels passing directly from the vessels to the intervillous space. Venous drainage from the intervillous space now occurs from point to point over the

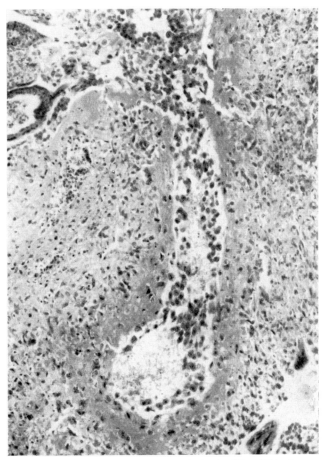

FIG. 20. Photomicrograph (×126) of a section (H. and E.) of the termination of an endometrial spiral artery in the *in situ* placenta of a 15 mm. embryo (C.X. 102). Cytotrophoblast cells are invading and plugging the lumen of the vessel. The wall of the artery shows marked degenerative changes. A portion of syncytium can be seen to the right of the illustration.

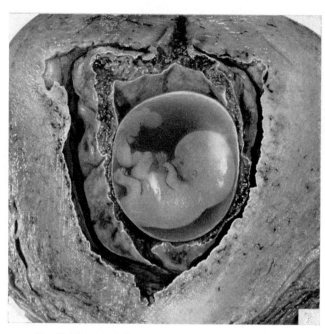

FIG. 21. Photograph (×1·4) of a coronal section of a uterus containing a 29 mm. embryo (C.X. 105). Note that the uterine lumen is still widely patent. A section through the uterus and *in situ* placenta of this specimen is illustrated in Fig. 22.

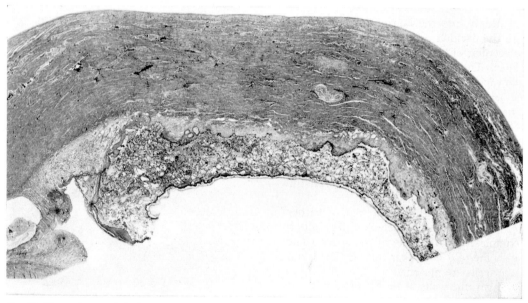

FIG. 22. Photomicrograph (×2·5) of a section through the uterus and *in situ* placenta of a 29 mm. embryo (C.X. 105). The foetal-maternal junction is now very distinct and the decidua basalis is thin. The implantation in this specimen was low on the posterior uterine wall and the cervix can be seen to the left of the illustration. On the right there has been some separation of the chorionic villi from the decidua.

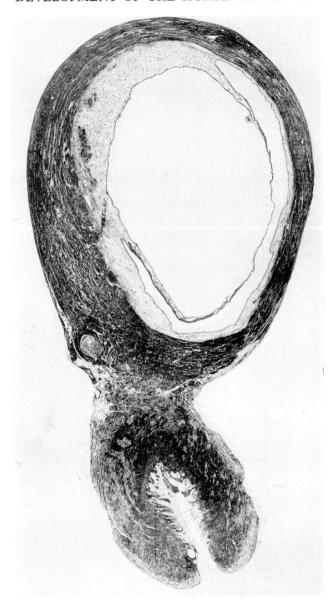

FIG. 23. Photograph (×1·5) of a uterus which contained a 30 mm. foetus (C.X. 106). The decidua capsularis, which is very thin, approaches but does not make contact with the decidua vera. Note the complete absence of any indication of a marginal sinus in the intervillous space.

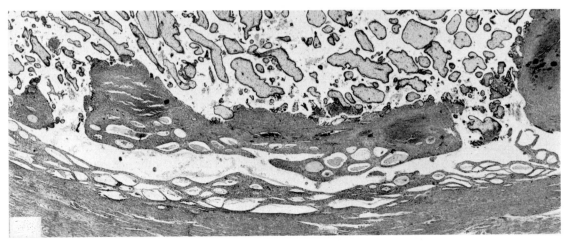

FIG. 24. Photomicrograph (×18) of a section through the central portion of the *in situ* placenta of a 30 mm. foetus (C.X. 106). Two large openings from the intervillous space into uterine veins are shown. A plug of villi can be seen in the right of these communications.

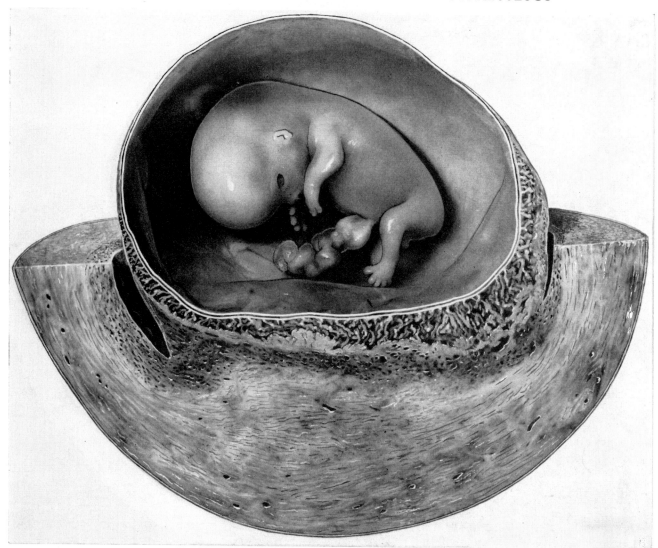

FIG. 25. Photograph (×2·3) of section through a portion of the uterus to show the placenta and chorionic sac containing a 36 mm. foetus (Camb. H. 789.). The basal placental plate separating the chorionic villi and the intervillous space from the decidua basalis appears as a thin band across the greater part of the attachment area. The decidua basalis, though of variable thickness, is still very distinct. The placental (i.e. lower) half of the decidua capsularis has chorionic villi related to it projecting into an associated extension of the intervillous space. The upper part of the decidua capsularis, together with the abembryonic portion of the chorion, is markedly attenuated. Consequently in this region the interior of the chorionic sac is separated from the uterine lumen by only a very thin double layer of foetal and maternal tissue. The decidua vera can be seen on either side of the placenta extending up to the cut margin of the uterine wall. Note the presence of uterine veins throughout the decidua basalis and the absence of any region of the intervillous space which could be identified as a marginal sinus.

whole of the basal plate. By the end of this period of development centrally placed communications between the intervillous space and the decidual veins are numerous and often very large ((Fig. 24).

Specimens of *in situ* Placentae with Foetuses of between 31 and 60 mm. Stages (60–90 days)

We have sixteen specimens of *in situ* placentae which, on maternal history and foetal size, can be considered to belong to the third month of gestation (Figs. 25, 26 and 27). The shape of these placentæ is variable but the average transverse diameters range from 50 to 70 mm. There is also considerable variation in placental thickness from specimen to specimen and even in different regions in a given placenta. Although the chorionic sac becomes much

larger during this period the increasingly thinned and stretched decidua capsularis has not, in any of the specimens, yet fused with the decidua parietalis. The villi related to the decidua capsularis, however, show marked signs of retrogression. This retrogression, in the earlier specimens, is most apparent at the pole opposite to the placenta. As older specimens are examined the disappearance of villi is seen gradually to spread from this pole in an equatorial direction so that by the end of the third month nearly the whole of the decidua capsularis is related to a part of the chorion in which the villi are represented only by little stumps. Accompanying the villous retrogression there is a disappearance of the associated intervillous space. The villi in the placenta itself become much more numerous in this period. The main villous stems become thicker and

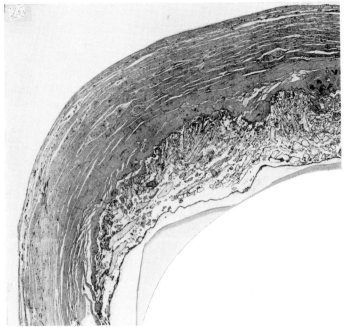

FIG. 26. Photomicrograph (×3·5) of a section through rather less than half of the *in situ* placenta of a 42 mm. foetus (C.X. 110) and the related uterine wall.

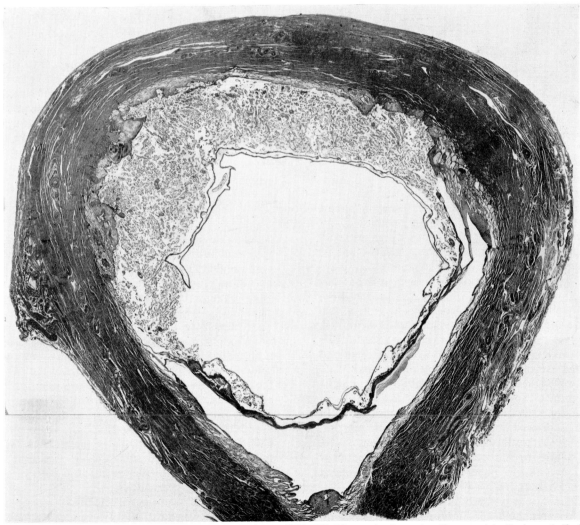

FIG. 27. Photograph (×1·8) of a uterus which contained a 60 mm. foetus (C.X. 112). The uterine lumen is still apparent in the lower half of the uterus. The decidua basalis is very thin. Distorted and dilated uterine glands are present in the decidua vera to the right of the area of placental attachment.

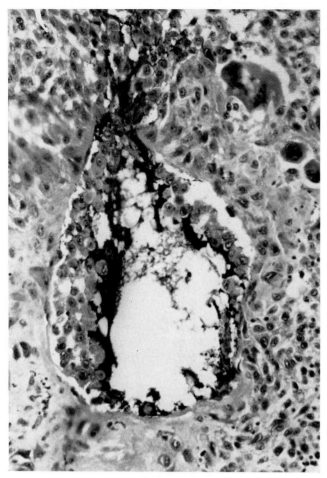

FIG. 28. Photomicrograph (×510) of a section through the termination of a spiral artery. The percolation of ink between the cytotrophoblastic cells is clearly seen. Note the highly modified arterial wall and the cytotrophoblastic cells within the arterial lumen.

the specimens. A striking feature is marked development of the uterine glands in the decidua parietalis at the angle of junction of the decidua basalis with the decidua capsularis. Occasional haemorrhage into the basal glands can be detected in all of the specimens. Erosion of some of these glands by cytotrophoblast is also shown in most of them. The decidua basalis in every specimen contains many masses of multinucleated cytoplasm which, on the basis of orientation, distribution and cytology, we (Boyd and Hamilton, 1960) consider to be of trophoblastic origin. Such syncytial masses are often arranged radially as they penetrate through the decidua to reach the inner part of the myometrium where they come to lie between the muscle cells.

Spiral arteries can be traced through the decidua to the cytotrophoblast. These arteries show the degenerative changes in their walls to which attention has been directed in the descriptions of the earlier stages. In all the specimens these arteries terminate in a mass of cytotrophoblast and cells of foetal origin can be traced up most of the vessels. In no specimen have we found spiral arteries to open freely into the intervillous space. There are always interposed plugs of cytotrophoblast. Such plugs become more loosely arranged as development proceeds and in the oldest specimens in this period (Fig. 11) they give the appearance of being much less capable of acting as an impediment to blood entering the intervillous space. Sections were available of a specimen into which India ink had been injected into a uterine artery in the broad ligament before the uterus was opened. Such sections (Fig. 28) show ink in the lumina of the spiral arteries from whence it can be traced through intercellular cytotrophoblastic spaces into the intervillous space. In all of the specimens of the third month uterine veins are found to communicate freely with the intervillous space over the whole of the basal plate (Figs. 12 and 24).

PLACENTAE FROM THE END OF THE THIRD MONTH OF GESTATION

Accurate and reliable details of the menstrual histories were not forthcoming for all specimens and, as there are considerable differences in the crown-rump (C.R., sitting height) measurements and the weights of foetuses at a given gestation age, it has not been possible to give reliable estimates of the conception age for all the available material. Up to the time (approximately the end of the sixth month of gestation) when the foetus measures 200 mm. in C.R. length, the specimens have been arbitrarily presented in the order of this length, but the weight of the foetus and its placenta and the presumptive menstrual age have also often been recorded; weights, of course, cannot be given for *in situ* placentae. After the sixth month, however, owing to difficulties in establishing the C.R. length, the presentation of the material is largely in terms of the foetal weight. When available, placental diameters have also been given. The data presented are from singleton pregnancies.

The material has been collected from a large number of sources; the weighings and measurements were made as soon as possible after the termination of the pregnancy

there are more numerous side branches. In the initial part of the third month the cytotrophoblast on most of the villous surfaces constitutes a continuous Langhans layer. By the middle of the period, however, areas in which this layer cannot be identified by light microscopy have become apparent and in the oldest specimens it has disappeared in most of the villi.

The trophoblastic shell is very attenuated in all the specimens except in the area of villous attachments. In certain regions the shell may be reduced to a single layer of cells. Throughout the whole period fibrinoid material is distributed irregularly over the whole of the basal plate. Attached to the apical portions of the villi there are many syncytial sprouts. Some of these sprouts are also distributed from point to point throughout the villous tree. In some of the older specimens in this period there are projections from the basal plate into the intervillous space. These projections are the forerunners of the cotyledonary septa which become such important features in the placenta of the second half of pregnancy.

The decidua basalis is slowly but continuously reduced in thickness throughout the third month of gestation. Nevertheless, glandular activity can be detected in all of and in general under the immediate supervision of one or other of the authors. There were, however, many occasions when neither of us was available which may explain some discrepancies in the data. The variability is greater for placental weights, at a given age, than for those of the foetuses; this difference can be attributed to several factors. Firstly, variable amounts of tissue, foetal and maternal, are separated during placental dehiscence; villi may remain attached to the decidua or parts of the latter may be adherent to the basal plate. Secondly, differing amounts of maternal blood will have been present in, or adherent to, the specimen. Thirdly, part or all of the chorion laeve, of the amnion or of the umbilical cord may have been included in the weighing of the placenta. Usually, the older placentae were weighed after trimming off the chorion laeve and cutting the cord near the chorionic plate. Blood clots were removed from the basal plate but no attempt was made to wash out the blood in the IVS.

For descriptive convenience the placental material has been divided into four groups: (1) specimens in the *fourth* lunar month of gestation (foetuses of 61–100 mm. C.R. length); (2) specimens in the *fifth* lunar month of gestation (foetuses of 101–150 mm. C.R. length); (3) specimens in the *sixth* lunar month of gestation (foetuses of 151–200 mm. C.R. length); and (4) specimens from the

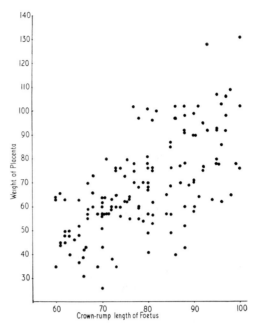

FIG. 29. Graph showing the relationship between the placental weight in grams and crown-rump length of the foetus in millimetres in the fourth lunar month of gestation.

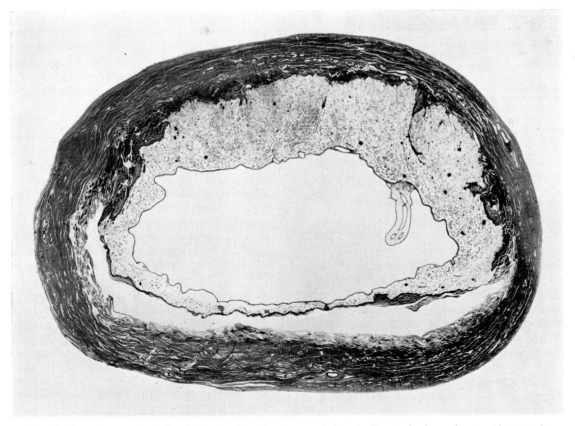

FIG. 30. Photomicrograph of a longitudinal section of a uterus and placenta. The uterine lumen is present between the capsularis and the decidua vera. Well developed villi are established in the placental region and retrogressing ones can be identified in relation to the peripheral part of the decidua capsularis. Some incipient septa can be recognized but the cotyledonary nature of the placenta is not yet clearly apparent. (Foetus, 61 mm. C.R. length; menstrual age, 11 weeks.) × c. 0·75.

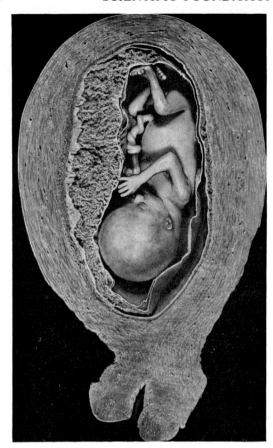

FIG. 31. Photograph of a sagittal section of a uterus containing a 68 mm. C.R. length foetus. The capsular villi have almost completely disappeared and the resulting chorion laeve, with its thin covering of decidua capsularis, is still separated from the decidua vera by the patent uterine lumen. The decidua basalis is of variable thickness and there is only slight indication of septal formation. (Menstrual age, 12 weeks.) × c. 0·75.

beginning of the *seventh* month of gestation (foetuses of 201 mm. C.R. length, and weighing *circa* 750 g.) until term.

1. Placentae in the Fourth Lunar Month of Gestation

In this period, which extends approximately from the 84th day to the 112th day* after the first day of the last menstrual period, there are available 52 *in situ* and 144 separated placentae. The crown-rump lengths of the foetuses measured from a little less than 60 mm. to about 100 mm. The foetal weights ranged from 16·5–130 g., and the extremes of placental weight were 25 and 131 g. The diameters (average of maximum and minimum) and thicknesses of the individual placentae included in the group showed considerable variation, the former extending from 60–110 mm. and the thickness from 10–20 mm. In view of a particular interest in the growth of the placenta (Boyd and Hamilton, 1950), we have analysed its dimensions carefully in the 34 specimens in which within this period accurate measurements were possible. The average diameter for 20 specimens associated with foetuses between 61 and 80 mm. C.R. length was 76 mm.; the corresponding average for the 14 specimens between 81 and 100 mm.

C.R. length was 85 mm. It is obvious therefore that, neglecting the extremely variable thickness of the placenta (measurements of which are not recorded here in detail owing to uncertainty on their accuracy), a significant increase in the superficial area of the placenta occurs in this period.

In Figure 29 the weights of the placentae in this period are plotted against the C.R. lengths of the corresponding foetuses. Though, for reasons indicated earlier, there is a wide scatter of points in the graph, the increase in placental weight with increase in foetal size is clear.

The general topography of the placenta at the beginning of this period is shown in Figures 30–32. The basal decidua is now so reduced in thickness that the villi of the chorion frondosum extend almost to the myometrium. The villi themselves (Fig. 33) possess a very loose texture; they are separated by the intercommunications of the intervillous space (IVS) which shows some indication of subdivision through the development of the placental septa (Fig. 30). The decidua capsularis, not yet fused with the relatively thick decidua vera, appears as a thin darkly staining layer covering the portion of the chorion which bulges into the uterine lumen. In the section illustrated scattered retrogressing chorionic villi are still present on the inner aspect of the capsular decidua. In sections nearer the abplacental pole, however, villi and the IVS have completely disappeared; as a result there is a chorion laeve covered by the decidua capsularis. An incipient chorion laeve is in fact already apparent in some of our earlier specimens (30 mm. and 36 mm.). There is considerable variation in the rapidity with which the abplacental villi retrogress and, consequently, in the time taken for establishment of an extensive chorion laeve; the appearance shown in a section will necessarily depend upon its plane in relation to the poles of the sac.

In a macroscopic preparation of a uterus containing a foetus of 68 mm. C.R. length (Fig. 31) the thin central portion of the decidua capsularis is more extensive owing to marked villous retrogression and a concomitant disappearance of the related IVS. As a consequence the chorion laeve also becomes thin for its "basal" (outer) and "chorionic" (inner) layers become apposed to each other and gradually fuse. By the end of this period the decidua capsularis and the attenuated chorion laeve have also become intimately fused (Fig. 34) and there is difficulty in identifying the decidual cells on the outer side of the chorion. The decidua vera, however, remains relatively thick though its epithelial surface shows retrogressive changes. A narrow chink of persisting uterine lumen is still apparent in the sections through this 90 mm. (*circa* 100 days) specimen; *in vivo*, however, contact of the capsular decidua with the decidua vera had probably already been established.

2. Placentae in the Fifth Lunar Month of Gestation

This group includes 44 *in situ* and 88 separated placentae, the menstrual ages extending from 112–140 days. The foetuses ranged from 101–150 mm. C.R. length and their weights from below 100 to a maximum of 350 g. The extremes of placental weight were 73·5 and 180 g.; in

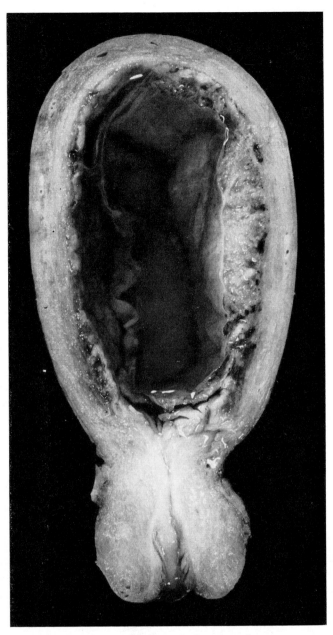

FIG. 32. Photograph of a sagittal section of a uterus, placenta and membranes associated with a 61 mm. C.R. length foetus. Note the combined decidua capsularis and chorion laeve separated from the decidua vera by the persistent uterine lumen. The "dependent" decidua is above the internal os. (Menstrual age, 11 weeks.) × c. 1·0.

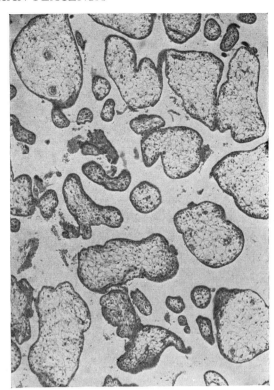

FIG. 33. Photomicrograph of sections of chorionic villi. Note the loose texture of the intervillous stroma. (Foetus, 80 mm. C.R. length.) × c. 55.

Figure 35 the placental weights are plotted against the C.R. lengths of the foetuses. The average diameters of 22 placentae in this group could be accurately determined; associated with foetuses of 101–110 mm. C.R. length averaged 88 mm., those with foetuses of 111–120 mm. C.R. length averaged 98·5 mm., whilst the diameters of the older placentae in the period averaged 117 mm. Clearly there has been a distinct increase in the superficial extent of the placenta during the fifth month.

Owing to growth of, and greater connective tissue differentiation in, the villi, the placenta now shows a more consolidated structure (Figs. 36–38). Moreover, in fixed specimens, the IVS in a given microscopic field occupies less of the area and thus is relatively less apparent than in earlier stages. It would seem (see later discussion) that the diminution in size of the IVS relative to the villous volume is in part the result of a gradual increase in the number of the small villous branches—the terminal or fringe villi—which have arisen from the already established villi (Fig. 38). It is during this period that the so-called "subchorial lake" is established; this is a region of the placenta adjacent to the chorionic plate where the IVS is more extensive than elsewhere (Fig. 36). When fully developed the subchorial lake may occupy from one-sixth to one-third of the thickness of the placenta (Fig. 39). Placentae in the group show striking differences in thickness, differences which may also be found regionally in a single placenta (Fig. 40). The placental septa become more evident in this period (Boyd and Hamilton, 1966a).

The basal decidua is now usually thinner than in younger specimens; in it, however, the remains of many uterine glands can still be identified. There is often some thickening of the endometrium in the region of junction of the decidua basalis with the decidua vera—that is, at the rim of the placenta (*decidua marginalis* of Bühler, 1964; Fig. 37). Beyond this junctional zone the decidua vera can be traced round the interior of the uterus. It is in this period that the uterine cavity is obliterated by the fusion of the retrogressing decidua capsularis with the decidua vera. Consequently the non-placental chorion laeve becomes, in effect, apposed to the decidua vera for,

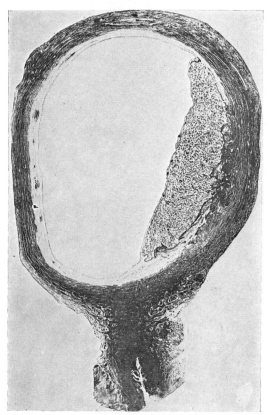

FIG. 34. Photomicrograph of a sagittal section of a uterus with an *in situ* placenta. The uterine lumen is still patent. The decidua basalis is markedly reduced in the central placental region; the dedidua vera, however, is still relatively thick. On the surface of the chorion laeve the decidua capsularis is vestigial. Note absence of a marginal sinus and the gaps in Nitabuch's membrane. (Foetus, 90 mm. C.R. length; menstrual age, 14 weeks.)

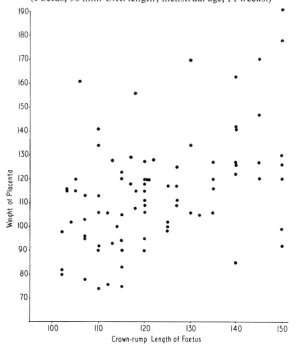

FIG. 35 Graph showing the relationship between the placental weight in grams and the crown-rump length in millimetres of the foetus in the fifth lunar month of gestation.

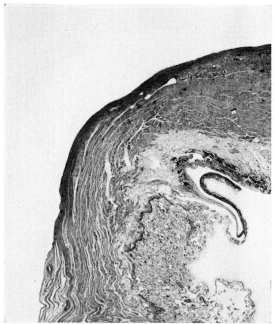

FIG. 36. Photomicrograph of the margin of a placenta in the early fifth month of gestation. Histological fixation was effected after the uterus had been opened. There is still some patency of the uterine lumen at the placental margin In this specimen absence of villi in the marginal region has produced a narrow marginal sinus, their sparseness elsewhere results in a limited subchorial lake. Note gaps in Nitabuch's membrane and attenuation of the basal decidua. (Foetus, 125 mm. C.R. length.) × c. 2·5.

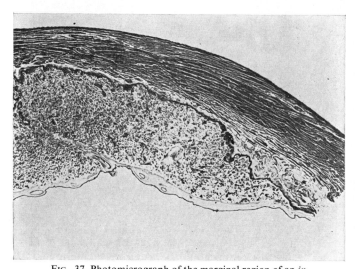

FIG. 37. Photomicrograph of the marginal region of an *in situ* placenta in the fifth month of gestation. Histological fixation effected before opening the uterus. The uterine lumen is obliterated, there is no marginal sinus and several intercotyledonary septa are apparent. At the margin of the placenta the decidua basalis is relatively thick; elsewhere it is generally thin and represented mainly by venous spaces. There is no trace of a centralwards extension of the marginal decidua on the chorionic plate. (Foetus, 118 mm. C.R. length.) × c. 3.

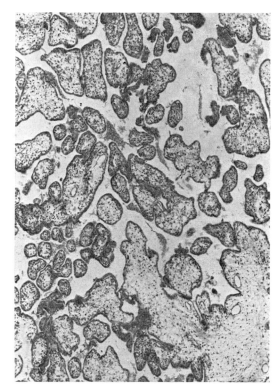

FIG. 38. Photomicrograph of sections of chorionic villi. The villi are more compactly arranged than in Fig. 33. (Foetus, 113 mm. C.R. length; menstrual age, $4\frac{1}{2}$ months.) × c. 55.

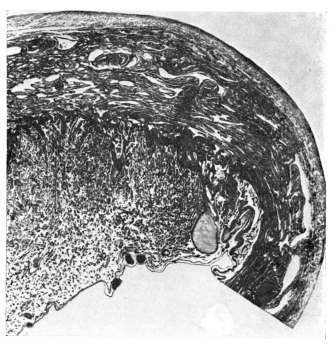

FIG. 39. Photomicrograph of the margin of an *in situ* placenta. Note the subchorial lake. Near the placental margin there is a colloid-containing cyst. (Foetus, 135 mm. C.R. length; menstrual age, 20 weeks.) × c. 1·25.

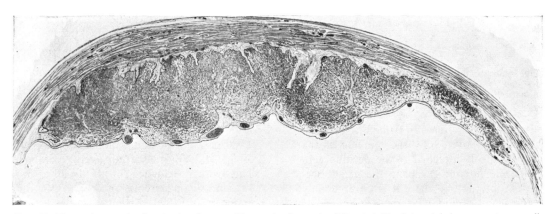

FIG. 40. Photomicrograph of an *in situ* placenta. The uterine lumen is obliterated. The intercotyledonary septa are well established and are continued into persistent parts of the decidua basalis. There is variability in placental thickness and in the degree of development of the subchorial lake. (Foetus, 140 mm. C.R. length, menstrual age, 20 weeks.) × c. 1·5.

over much of the area, it is difficult to identify any persisting capsular decidua. In whole chorionic sacs from cases of hysterotomy or abortion, however, a thin layer of darkly staining material is usually found covering the chorion laeve; this layer is presumably at least in part of capsular decidual origin.

3. Placentae in the Sixth Lunar Month of Gestation

In this period we have 19 *in situ* and 29 separated plaentae. The ages (as judged from L.M.P.) of the specimens extended from approximately 140–168 days; the foetuses ranged from about 151–200 mm. in C.R.

length, and the foetal weights from 304–820 g. The extremes of the placental weights in this group were 134 and 290 g. The association of placental weight and foetal size is given in Figure 41. The average diameter of the placentae in the group is 135 mm., the extremes being 110 mm. × 115 mm. for the placenta of a 165 mm. C.R. length foetus and 170 mm. × 170 mm. for that of a 200 mm. C.R. length specimen.

The basal decidua is now characterized by great dilatation of numerous endometrial veins. It is usually even thinner than in the fifth month, but there is variability and when there has been marked myometrial contraction

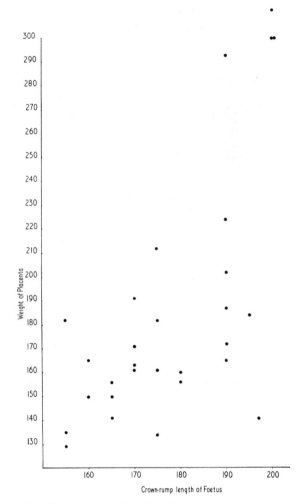

FIG.41. Graph showing the relationship between the placental weight (in g.) and crown-rump length of the foetus (in mm.) in the sixth lunar month of gestation.

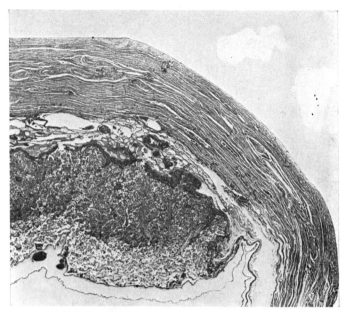

FIG. 42. Photomicrograph of the margin of an *in situ* placenta. There is some artefactual separation of the now attenuated decidua capsularis from the endometrium. Gaps in Nitabuch's membrane permit communication between the IVS and the basal venous plexus. Note the subchorial lake and the absence of a marginal sinus. (Foetus, 170 mm. C.R. length; menstrual age, six months.) × c. 1·5.

during uterine opening it is often surprisingly thick (Fig. 42). The chorion laeve, covered by the remains of the decidua capsularis, is firmly attached to the decidua vera over the whole uterine interior except in the neighbourhood of the cervical internal os where it is covered only by capsular or dependent decidua (Bourne, 1962).

The placental septa are now well established; macroscopically, they divide the placenta into larger lobes and smaller lobules (the so-called maternal cotyledons, see later). The degree of subdivision by the septa, however, varies considerably from placenta to placenta and in different regions of a single specimen, a variation which is the explanation for the differences in placental lobulation (Boyd and Hamilton, 1966a).

A subchorial lake is found in the IVS of all placentae of this period though it may be present only in restricted regions along the chorionic plate (Fig. 42) and, often, it does not extend to the placental margin.

4. Placentae in the Last Four Lunar Months of Gestation

The material in this group falls into two categories. Firstly, there are the 101 specimens which are estimated

or known to be younger than term and in 36 of which the associated placenta was still *in situ*, and, secondly, the much more extensive collection of over 1,000 placentae delivered at term. In the former category the foetuses ranged upwards from 201 mm. C.R. length, their weights extending from 764–2,500 g. As many of the placentae in this category were *in situ* weights for only 65 of them are available (Fig. 43); they ranged from 170 g. up to weights corresponding to those of term specimens. The average diameter of the placenta associated with foetuses up to 1,000 g. in weight was 140 mm., that for foetuses of up to 2,000 g. was 160 mm., and the older placentae (foetuses of up to 2,500 g.) had an average diameter of 172 mm. The average diameter for all placentae in the period was 158 mm. with extremes of 85 and 215 mm. The average diameter of 1,000 placentae delivered at term (i.e., the second category in this group) was 185 mm. with extremes of 105 and 245 mm. The average weight of these term placentae was 508 g. with extremes of 310 g. and 880 g. (Armitage *et al.*, 1967).

Early in this period of gestation the definitive structure of the mature placenta has been fully established. The septa have become more obtrusive, clearly dividing the organ into its characteristic lobes (Figs. 44 and 45) which show much variation in surface extent and, to a lesser degree, in thickness. The smaller lobes, perhaps better called lobules, usually contain only one truncus chorii (main stem villus) whereas the larger lobes often possess several of these trunci. Apart from the variably developed subchorial lake the IVS during this period shows a continuation of the diminution in its volume relative to the space occupied by the villi. The resulting more compact

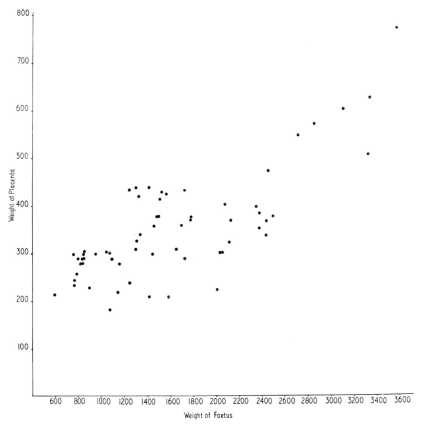

FIG. 43. Graph showing the relationship between the weight of the placenta (in g.) and the crown-rump length (in mm.) of the foetus in the last four lunar months of gestation.

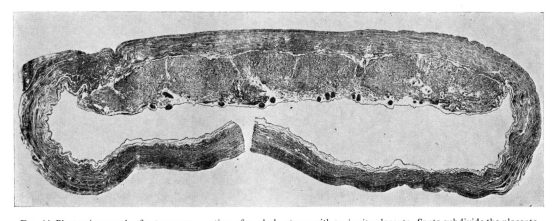

FIG. 44. Photomicrograph of a transverse section of a whole uterus with an *in situ* placenta. Septa subdivide the placenta into a number of cotyledons. The basal decidua is now very thin; at the abplacental pole residual decidua vera is fused with the chorion and the vestigial capsularis. (Foetus, 260 mm. C.R. length; weight 849 g.; menstrual age, 7 to 8 months.) × c. 0·75.

placental structure (Figs. 44, 46–48) is due, it would seem, to the presence of a larger number of smaller villous branches (cf. Figs. 33 and 38). No well established marginal sinus in Spanner's sense of the term was found in any of the *in situ* specimens of placentae in this period (Fig. 49).

Except over the internal os (Fig. 50), the uterine lumen in this period is completely obliterated (Fig. 44); amnion and chorion can both be followed round the whole interior of the uterus, the chorion being fused to the

decidua vera either directly or through the intermediary of some residual capsular decidua. The decidua itself is now everywhere very thin. As gestation advances the myometrium becomes much thinner (Figs. 34, 40 and 44). If, however, the uterus has been opened shortly after its surgical removal, and without the precaution of thorough preliminary fixation, the myometrium often shows marked contraction, and, hence, becomes thickened. Such residual contractile power can often cause marked shortening of the diameter of the basal plate with resulting distortion of

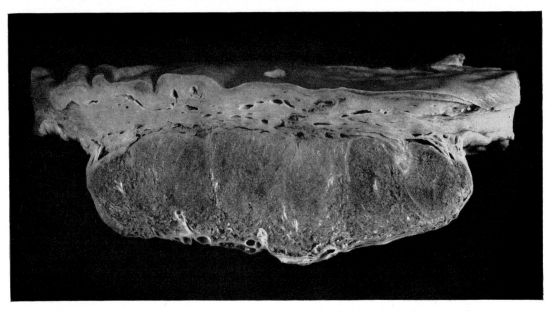

FIG. 45. Photograph of a macroscopic section through an *in situ* placenta. The lobulation is clearly seen. Note the presence of many large endometrial and myometrial veins and the absence of a marginal sinus. This placenta is much thicker than the one of equivalent age shown in Fig. 46. (Foetus, 210 mm. C.R. length; menstrual age, 24 weeks.) × c. 1·5.

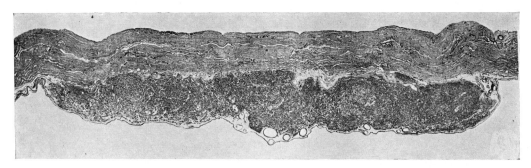

FIG. 46. Photomicrograph of a section of an *in situ* placenta. (Foetus, 205 mm. C.R. length; weight, 859 g.; menstrual age, 22 weeks.) × c. 0·75.

the placenta and, particularly, an apparent increase in its thickness (Figs. 46 and 51).

FEATURES OF PLACENTAL GROWTH AND STRUCTURE IN THE SECOND AND THIRD TRIMESTERS

In the brief description just presented of the available material in the periods concerned emphasis has been placed on general placental features only; it is not possible within reasonable bounds to deal with all the aspects of placental structure and development shown by the specimens. Subsequent sections of this chapter, therefore, restrict detailed consideration to certain selected topics. These are: growth of the placenta; structure, growth and terminology of the placental lobes and chorionic villi; placental histology, including placental barrier, interlobar septa and islets; fibrin and fibrinoid; maternal vessels and intervillous space.

GROWTH OF THE PLACENTA

Few detailed accounts are available for the growth and weight of the placenta throughout gestation. Quantitative

data on the weight and dimensions of the full-term placenta have, of course, been given by a large number of investigators (see Zangemeister, 1911; Kjölseth, 1913; Adair and Thelander, 1925; Grosser, 1927; Shordania, 1929; Calkins, 1937; Dow and Torpin, 1939; Milz, 1946; Sinclair, 1948a and b; Hosemann, 1949; Pitkänen, 1949; Schmid, 1951; Walker, 1954; Snoeck, 1958; Crawford, 1959; Gruenwald and Minh, 1961; Solth, 1961; Gerlach, 1962; Zschiesche and Gerlach, 1963; and Hytten and Leitch, 1964). In their accounts Zangemeister and Hosemann included some reference to placental growth, and further information and discussion on this topic are provided by Streeter (1920b), Stieve (1940), Hamilton and Boyd (1950), McKeown and Record (1953a and b), Walker (1954), and Hendricks (1964). Most of the data, however, relates to placental growth occurring in the later part of pregnancy. A meagre literature exists on certain quantitative aspects of mature placental structure (such as the surface area of the villi, their volume, and that of the IVS) but little information is available on quantitative changes in placental structure and proportions during development, most of the published data relating to specimens at, or

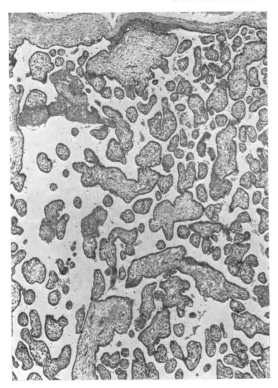

FIG. 47. Photomicrograph of sections of chorionic villi. Many small villi are now present. (Foetus, 230 mm. C.R. length; menstrual age, 7 months.) × c. 55.

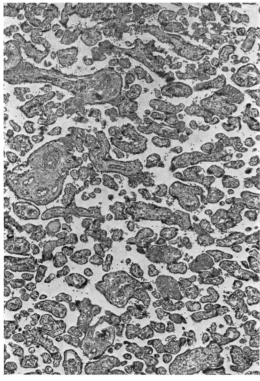

FIG. 48. Photomicrograph of sections of full-term chorionic villi Note the large number of small terminal villi. × c. 55.

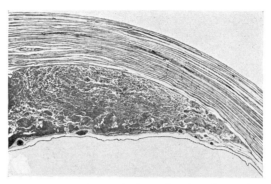

FIG. 49. Photomicrograph of a section through a portion of a uterus with an *in situ* placenta. Note the absence of a marginal sinus and the thinnesss of the basal decidua which is, in effect, replaced by the endometrial venous plexus. (Foetus, 280 mm. C.R. length; at full-term.)

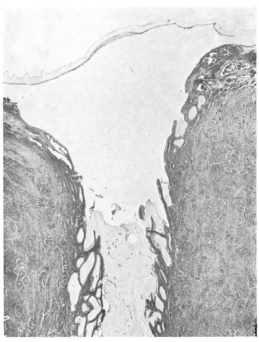

FIG. 50. Photomicrograph of a section through the upper part of the cervix, combined "dependent" decidua and chorion of a near full-term pregnancy. Note the residual uterine lumen lying above the internal os and the mucous plug which obliterates the cervical canal. × c. 14.

near, full-term (see Wilkin, 1958, 1965a and b; Jaroschka, 1959; Knopp, 1960; and Aherne and Dunhill, 1966a and b).

In this chapter we cannot present a detailed statistical analysis of all our data on the size, weight and volume of the placenta in the periods of gestation under consideration. In summary, however, as briefly indicated above in the accounts of the placentae in the individual periods considered, our data show clearly that placental growth continues throughout pregnancy but that the increase becomes progressively slower in the last trimester. Figures 29, 35, 41 and 43 indicate the increase in the weight of the placenta as pregnancy advances. As the rate of placental growth diminishes as maturity is approached there is some

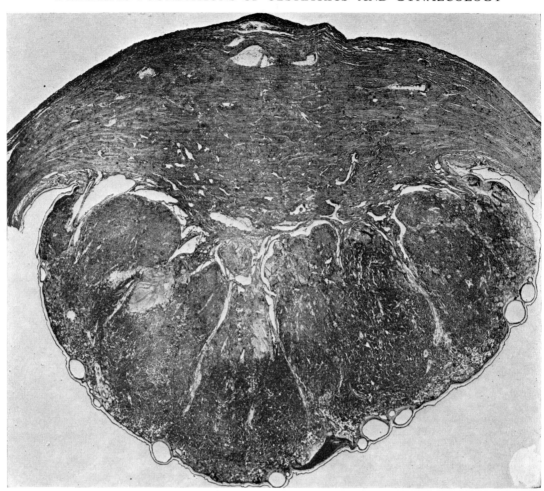

FIG. 51. Photomicrograph of a section of a full-term *in situ* placenta which may represent a stage in the early normal separation. The uterus was opened before fixation with resulting placental distortion due to myometrial contraction. The cotyledons are thickened and the elongated septa are approximated. × c. 1·25.

uncertainty on the weight increase in the last few weeks of pregnancy and especially in postmaturity. Our own data give no grounds for a positive statement on placental growth in these last weeks.

On increase during gestation in placental diameter, surface extent or area, and volume there is surprisingly little information recorded in the literature. Grosser (1927) indicated that by the fourth month of pregnancy the human placenta had reached its maximum extent, occupying about half of the uterine interior. In later development he considered that increase in the placental surface area lagged markedly behind that of the uterine lumen. Fischel (1929) stated that after the fourth month the human placenta grows more slowly than the uterus but, nevertheless, increases two or three times in thickness. Spanner (1935) accepted these interpretations stressing a marked increase in placental thickness during the third, fourth and fifth months; he associated the formation of the septa with this increase. As Stieve (1940) pointed out, however, it is not apparent how Spanner arrived at this conclusion for his youngest recorded specimen stemmed from the fifth month. Stieve's own observations on placentae fixed *in situ* indicated that up to the end of the third month they grew in thickness and circumference.

During the fourth month Stieve found them to be 18 to 21 mm. thick with no later effective increase in this dimension. From the fifth month until the end of pregnancy he recorded an increase in placental circumferential extent and attributed it to marginal growth *pari passu* with that of the attached portion of the uterine wall. At the fourth month Stieve found the placental diameter to be 82 mm. (surface extent, 5,300 mm.^{2}); at full-term the average diameter was 194 mm. (surface, 29,540 mm.^{2}). As the total surface extent of the interior of the uterus at the fourth month is about 20,000 mm.^{2}, Stieve concluded that a placenta with a superficial area corresponding to that of the normal full-term organ could not be accommodated in a uterus of this earlier period. Our measurements (Fig. 52) for placental diameters and surface area respectively are:

beginning of fourth month, 76 mm. and 4,538 mm.^{2} (A);

middle of fourth month, 85 mm. and 5,991 mm.^{2} (B);

late fourth month, 88 mm. and 6,084 mm.^{2} (C);

middle of fifth month, 100 mm. and 7,859 mm.^{2} (D);

late fifth month, 117 mm. and 10,971 mm.^{2} (E);

middle of sixth month, 135 mm. and 14,533 mm.^{2} (F).

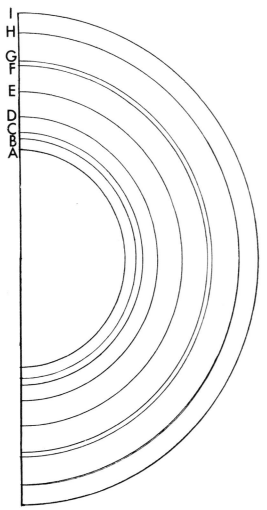

FIG. 52. Diagram to illustrate the average diameters of the placenta at successive gestational stages.

Figure 52 demonstrates a continuation of increase in placental diameter during the last four lunar months of pregnancy:

foetuses of 1,000 g. weight—average diameter, 140 mm., surface area, 15,400 mm.^{2} (G);

from 1,000–2,000 g.—average diameter, 160 mm., surface area, 20,114 mm.^{2} (H);

from 2,000–2,500 g.—average diameter, 172 mm., surface area, 23,245 mm.^{2} (I).

These last figures are smaller than those at full-term, the average diameter of our 1,000 mature placentae being 185 mm. (surface area, 26,920 mm.^{2}).

Owing to distortion during separation and delivery there is much variability in the thickness of placentae of different ages; even after in situ fixation we are reluctant to draw firm conclusions from our measurements. The data indicate a trend towards an increase in thickness up to the sixth month but none is apparent in the last four months. Of 765 freshly delivered full-term placentae the average thickness was 23 mm., the greatest thickness being

41 mm. and the least 11 mm. The average volume of 500 consecutive specimens was 497 ml. (range 200–950 ml.).

Like Stieve we find that, in surface extent the in situ placenta is somewhat smaller than a delivered specimen of corresponding age. The measurements for some of our fixed in situ placentae (before embedding and sectioning) are:

foetus C.R. length

mm.	mm.
68	45 × 75 × 15
90	90 × 90 × 10
90	100 × 100 × 10
106	75 × 75 × 20
140	120 × 120 × 18
150	140 × 108 × 18
180	85 × 85 × 35
230	170 × 170 × 30
240	150 × 150 × 20
280	175 × 175 × 20
285	145 × 110 × 30
Term	220 × 220 × 20

For the earlier specimens the data show that approximately up to the end of the fourth lunar month of gestation (when the foetus has a C.R. length of almost 100 mm. and weighs about 100 g.) the placental weight is greater than that of the associated foetus. Later, however, foetal growth rate exceeds that of the membranes and, consequently, the weight of the foetus rapidly becomes greater. Nevertheless, though our material is relatively restricted in amount for the sixth to the tenth months, it demonstrates a continuous increase in weight and size (both diameter and thickness) of the placenta.

STRUCTURE, GROWTH AND TERMINOLOGY OF PLACENTAL LOBES AND CHORIONIC VILLI

Lobes

The mature human placenta is a lobulated organ. When separated and viewed from the uterine surface it shows a variable number (usually 10–38) of slightly elevated convex areas called lobes, or, when small, lobules. The lobes are separated, often incompletely, by irregular grooves of variable depth (Fig. 53) which, on section, are found to be occupied by the interlobar tissue that constitutes the placental septa (Figs. 44, 45 and 51). The placental lobes are often called cotyledons but confusion has resulted from different usages of the term, some investigators applying it to foetal and others to maternal components of the placenta.

Before considering the number of the lobes and their role in placental growth, it is necessary to summarize how they are established and to consider certain terminological points relating to them. Briefly, the intervillous space is partially subdivided by the interlobar septa into a variable number of incompletely separated compartments; it is into these compartments that the foetal villous systems (trunci chorii, etc.; see later), which constitute the so-called "foetal cotyledons", project. For the placentae of

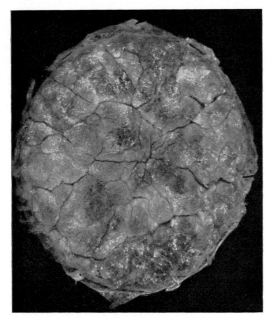

FIG. 53. Photograph of the maternal surface of a mature placenta to show lobes and lobules. × c. 0·33.

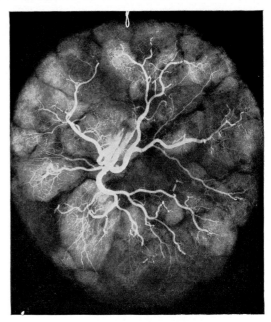

FIG. 54. X-ray photograph of the placenta shown in Fig. 53 after injection of an umbilical artery with Chromopaque.

many species, Bonnet (summarized in 1907) used the term *placentome* to designate the combination of maternal unit (*uterine caruncle* or *maternal cotyledon*) and the collection of foetal chorionic villi (*foetal cotyledon*) associated with it. Caruncles, of course, are not present in the human uterus. Nevertheless, reciprocally related "maternal" and "foetal" cotyledons of the human placenta can together conveniently be regarded as a placentome. The smallest macroscopic subdivision, or unit, of the human placenta is a *lobule* which, in our opinion, can be regarded as corresponding to a single placentome and possesses one foetal cotyledon. On this interpretation the larger placental lobes are compound placentomes and represent fusions, or at least associations, of a variable number of individual lobules. In such lobes, therefore, a number of foetal cotyledons (foetal villous systems—trunci chorii; see later for details) project into a single compartment of the IVS.

In arriving at the opinion just expressed we specifically investigated the placental lobes and lobules in 100 full-term separated and in a number of immature placentae. In these specimens an umbilical artery, the umbilical vein or both an artery and the vein were injected with Chromopaque. After photographing, often in colour, both surfaces of the specimens they were X-rayed stereoscopically. The number of lobes and lobules were recorded for each placenta and correlated with the counts of the trunci chorii (primary villous stems or foetal cotyledons) revealed in the X-ray photographs (cf. Figs. 53 and 54). In these enumerations considerable difficulties were encountered; boundaries between lobes are frequently obscure or incomplete, and even in stereoscopic X-ray photographs it is often difficult to determine if a given foetal blood vessel and its branches represent the complete vasculature of an independent truncus chorii. But while completely accurate counts are difficult or impossible to make, the investigation

has shown quite clearly that the number of primary villous stems (i.e., foetal cotyledons) is distinctly greater than the number of lobes. The average number of lobes for the series is 22 (extremes of 10 and 38) while the corresponding figure for the foetal cotyledons, or trunci chorii (see later), is considerably greater so that it can reasonably be concluded, therefore, that more than one placentome is included in each of the larger lobes.

Chorionic Villi

As already stated the villi have long been recognized as the essential structural feature of the human placenta. There is, however, much terminological confusion in the descriptions of them and of their subdivisions and considerable uncertainty on their number, their method of branching and their mode of attachment to the basal plate. It is not even clear what relationship the individual villi bear to each other; consequently the very nature of the IVS is uncertain (see later).

The villi are at first situated round the whole periphery of the chorion. Rapid growth of the cytotrophoblastic columns causes an increase in the length and complexity of the individual villi especially those adjoining the decidua basalis. Concomitant enlargement and confluence of the lacunae leads to the formation of the extensive and complicated IVS. As the circumference of the chorionic plate is less than that of the cytotrophoblastic shell, the latter provides a greater area for the attachment of each villus to this shell. Consequently, when traced peripherally, there is an increase in villous calibre.

Although villi are initially present round the whole chorion they are always better developed towards the decidua basalis than in relationship to the decidua capsularis. Indeed, in the latter position they retrogress and, by the end of the third month of gestation, have disappeared completely or are mere prejections on the surface of the chorion laeve. In the basal region, however, by becoming increasingly longer and more complex, each of the villi constitutes a *truncus chorii* or main stem villus (*Zottenstamm, tronc villositaire de premier ordre*) of the definitive placenta.

Each truncus chorii continues to lengthen, the increase being due, it would seem, not only to general interstitial growth but also to proliferation of the cells of the apical ends of the cytotrophoblastic columns. While such an increase in length of the trunci is taking place there is a concomitant longitudinal splitting of their distal ends into a variable number of subdivisions. These are the *rami chorii* or villous stems of second or third order (*Zottenaste, troncs villositaires de deuxième ordre*). When traced towards the basal plate the rami chorii in turn subdivide (possibly several times) to constitute the *ramuli chorii* or minor villous stems. As the ramuli terminate peripherally in the substance of the cytotrophoblastic shell and adjacent decidua they are often called *anchoring villi* (*Haftzotten, villosites crampons*). Like the rami, the ramuli chorii probably also owe their origin to a longitudinal division by "splitting" of pre-existing villous-like structures rather than to free outgrowth; the splitting process may be facilitated by the greater volume possessed by the peripheral (basal plate) extremity of each initial truncus chorii.

If this interpretation of the origin of the chorionic villi is correct, their major subdivisions (i.e., the trunci, rami and ramuli chorii) arise essentially from differentiation and growth changes in the early syncytial trabeculae. It is from the surfaces of these subdivisions that an extensive system of syncytial sprouts (*Knospen, Sprossen*) will later proliferate and project freely in all directions into the IVS where they will become the *free*, or *terminal*, villi (*fringing villi, absorption villi, Endzotten, Gitterzotten* or *Resorptionzotten*).

The trunci chorii, with their subdivisions and the associated fringing villi, constitute the essential structural units of the placenta. Their numbers, individual sizes and their relationships to each other, to the placental lobules and lobes, and to the chorionic and basal plates at successive stages of pregnancy must be taken into consideration in the analysis of placental growth and function. In fact, however, few data are available on villous number, and descriptions in the literature on the size of the villi and their relationships are often obscure. Moreover, terminology has tended to vary from one author to another with resulting uncertainty and even confusion (for discussion, see later and Boyd and Hamilton, 1966a). Some investigators (e.g. Crawford, 1956b; Strauss, 1964) use the term *cotyledon* in a way corresponding closely to what we call a truncus chorii; such a cotyledon can be regarded as the foetal component of a placentome. It must be stressed, however, that, as explained above, it is not usual for a single truncus chorii to be the sole occupant of the IVS within a given placental lobe (or maternal cotyledon corresponding to the uterine caruncle of certain mammalian placentae). When there is a one-to-one relationship the situation is, in fact, a placentome in Bonnet's sense of

the term. We would restrict the designation, placental lobule, to such an individual single placentome. Crawford considered that a foetal cotyledon can be formed in a number of different ways and can be of variable size depending on the site of origin of the artery which supplies it. The small cotyledons which in Crawford's opinion continue to be formed for a considerable period we believe to represent part of the progressive branching and growth of the trunci chorii during gestation.

A point of major importance would be to determine whether the number of trunci chorii increases, decreases or remains constant in the course of gestation. Crawford (1959, 1962), from counts on specimens in which the foetal vessels were injected with coloured solution and then studied after controlled selective digestion with trypsin (Crawford and Fraser, 1955), concluded that a normal human placenta is composed of some 200 separate "foetal cotyledons" of different sizes. Basing his opinion on material derived from the twelfth week of gestation until full-term, Crawford considered that the number of these cotyledons remains relatively constant throughout pregnancy though "a placenta at 12 weeks can have more cotyledons than one at 40 weeks". It seems to us that Crawford included branches of foetal vessels within trunci chorii as separate cotyledons and which would have been classified by us as rami or ramuli chorii. Reynolds (1966) states that there are 40–50 "cotyledons" and 150 undeveloped rudimentary ones; it is not apparent how these numbers were established.

We have been able to find only a few reports on the number cf villi in early pregnancy. It will be appreciated that it is difficult to estimate this number precisely without reconstruction and careful definition as to what is to be regarded as a villus. Thus the inclusion of transient syncytial trabeculae during the formation of the IVS can falsely increase an assessment of the number of villi present. Meyer (1924) recorded 411 villi in a conceptus of estimated 18 days age. Stieve (1926) counted 941 villi in a 19-day specimen, and the Boerner-Patzelt-Schwarzacher embryo of allegedly the same age had 430. Ortmann (1938) in an 8-somite specimen found no fewer than 1,131 (± 20 per cent) villi distributed uniformly over the whole chorion. Torpin (1958) states that at the thirteenth day of development the "human fertilized egg" has approximately 80 little trophoblastic buds equally distributed over its entire surface. Of these buds Torpin considers that, in normal development, only 20 grow into decidua vascularized enough to produce placental tissue; the remainder retrogress in the decidua capsularis. This account of Torpin implies that there are 20 major villous stems (trunci) in the normal placenta, but it is not clear, from his account, how he arrived at this figure. Lemtis (1955/56) describes the functions of the placenta as being carried out by 500 villous stems and their branches. Snoeck (1962) states that after retrogression of the capsular villi "all that remains of the chorion frondosum is some 1,000 villi, which result from the subdivision of 14–30 villous pedicles". Strauss (1964) also states that there are 1,000 villi in the mature placenta but does not indicate the manner in which this figure was computed;

by implication it would appear to refer to terminal villi for which, however, this number seems as inadequate an estimate as it would be excessive for trunk villi.

From reconstructions based on serial photographs we have estimated that there are 850 "villi" on the chorion of a 14-day embryo and 428 on that of an 18-day specimen. With older placentae direct counts were made of the trunci chorii (Table I) in delivered placentae by indivi-

TABLE I

Number of Trunci Chorii

	C.R. length mm.	Trunci Chorii
H.1131	14	370
C.X.	45	342
H.1122	45	250
C.X.	70	323
H.1111	73	388
H.1126	77	280
C.X.	90	268
H.1118	95	318
H.1125	107	248
H.1124	110	137
H.1112	117	406
H.1123	132	160
C.X.	140	225
H.1119	145	302
C.X.	172	440
H.1127	180	213
H.1128	Full-term	68
H.1129	Full-term	60

dually enumerating each truncus as it was plucked or snipped with fine scissors and removed from the chorionic plate. Stages in the preparation of the material for the enumeration of the trunci are illustrated in Figs. 55 and 56, showing with striking clarity the general arrangement of the villi.

It will be seen from the Table that, in general, the counts of the number of trunci decrease with advancing gestation. This diminution during early development can in part be explained by retrogression of some villi that are

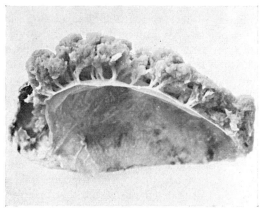

FIG. 55. Dissection of a portion of the chorion with attached villi. Note the separation of the attachments of the individual trunci to the chorionic plate. (Foetus, 60 mm. C.R. length.) × c. 1·1.

assimilated into the chorion laeve. In many older placentae there are appearances suggesting some villous retrogression but the changes are not sufficiently widespread to explain the great reduction in number of trunci. Growth changes in the region of the chorionic plate may result in trunci that initially were closely grouped at their origins becoming assimilated into each other with resulting diminution in their number. Our counts for full-term placentae, giving the number of trunci to be about 60, were supplemented by observations on placentae X-rayed stereoscopically after injecting the foetal blood vessels with radio-opaque material (Fig. 54); examination of these radiographs showed the number of trunci to be of the order of 40 (extremes of 22 and 76; 68 specimens). On the other hand, in material prepared by Crawford's technique, the counts ranged up to 200 villi but about one-half of these were small, or tiny, vascular projections from the chorionic plate. Crawford (1962) has stated that all the divisions of the foetal placental arteries, no matter how small, end in foetal cotyledons.

When the terminal villi first appear they are essentially proliferations or sprouts of the syncytium (Hamilton and Boyd, 1966a) covering the major villous subdivisions (and possibly to a small extent of that on the chorionic plate). Soon, however, most of these sprouts come to contain cores of cytotrophoblast, then mesoderm and finally blood vessels, and thus successively pass through the histological stages of primary, secondary and tertiary villi. Since terminal villi are continually being formed throughout later placental development, some with the histological characteristics of primary and secondary villi can be found in full-term placentae. Indeed, Zhemkova and Topchieva (1964) considered that there is the formation of new villi in post-mature placentae against a background of ageing in other parts of the placentae. As the individual free villi grow they give off side branches which in due course may produce yet further villi. In this manner each truncus chorii and, particularly, its rami and ramuli come to possess an extensive system of branches. As development proceeds the trunci and rami chorii become thicker and tougher; they probably take little part in metabolic exchange, acting chiefly as vessel-transmitting structures (see later). Hörmann (1951), amongst others, has stressed that it is upon the free or terminal villi, which he calls *resorptiv tätigen Bauelements* (the *frei, sog. ernährende Zotten* of Stieve, 1952), that the growing embryo primarily depends for interchange between the foetal capillaries and the maternal blood in the IVS.

There has been considerable debate on whether or not the separate terminal villi can fuse with each other. As this is a matter of some importance in determining the nature of the IVS further consideration must be given to it. Langhans (1870), Strahl and Beneke (1910), Lazitch (1913) and Grosser (1922) all considered that there are varying degrees of junction between the terminal villi, and as early as 1870 Hyrtl described occasional anastomoses between vessels of separate villi. Stieve (1940, 1952) and his pupils (Bien, 1943, and Gluschka, 1945) have amplified such descriptions of villous fusion. Stieve (1940) considered that there are not only syncytial but connective

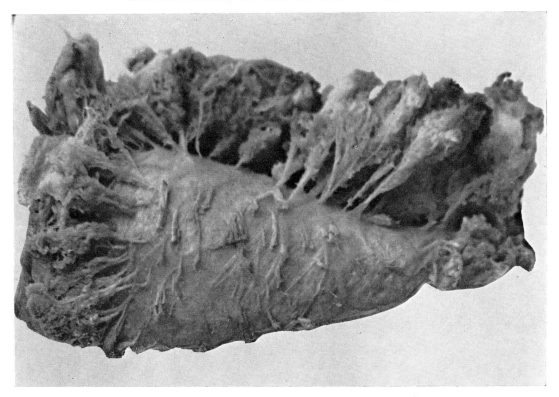

FIG. 56. Dissection of a portion of the chorion with attached villi. Compared with Fig. 55 the trunci have become elongated. (Foetus, 100 mm. C.R. length.) × c. 1·5.

tissue, and even vascular fusions between the villi, converting them into a three-dimensional lattice work (*Raumgitter*), and the placenta into a labyrinth. Peter (1943), from the study of reconstructions of portions of two *in situ* placentae (with embryos of 188 mm. and 235 mm. respectively), found only syncytial fusion between villi. Moreover, as free villi were more frequent in the younger specimen he concluded that syncytial fusion is more common in later pregnancy. Peter considered that no transfer of connective tissue fibres occurs between one villus and another, nor did he observe vascular anastomoses between the villi. Both Stieve and Peter believed that the trauma which the placenta undergoes during separation and expulsion in labour, in contradistinction to specimens examined *in situ*, may lead to the breaking of fusions between the villi.

From the examination of serial sections of placentae in the fourth and fifth months, Ortmann (1941) found syncytial connexion between only a small proportion of the villi, stating that 97 per cent of the villous branches, regardless of size, may be traced from their origins to their free ends. Later (1960) he suggested that fixation artefact may lead to an overestimation of the number of villous adhesions. Spanner (1941) considered that villous syncytial connexions were less frequent than claimed by Stieve and he maintained that the older concept of a "villous tree" (*Zottenbaum*) is valid. A further contribution to this problem is that by Lemtis (1955/56) who studied the foetal placental arteries radiographically after their injection with contrast media. In no instance did he find evidence for anastomoses which would suggest a three-

dimensional vascular network. Hamilton and Boyd (1951) recorded syncytial fusion between the villi as not infrequent in sections of *in situ* placentae; connective tissue and vascular connexions between the villi were occasionally found. The current observations have verified these findings (Figs. 57 and 58; Pl. 1, Figs. 3 and 4). Radiological investigations, however, have provided us with no clear evidence for anastomoses between the vessels of separate trunci chorii. Ishizaki (1960), who confirms the presence of syncytial fusion between villi, considers that they indicate foci of healed placentitis. Extensive villous fusion can result from the presence of fibrin or fibrinoid (Pl. 2, Fig. 5).

Marked variations exist in the size and the shape of individual trunci chorii and in their subdivisions (the rami and ramuli), and the true (terminal) villi. Consequently it is difficult to make and to record, for purposes of comparison, quantitative measurements of their dimensions. Contributions to the technical problems raised in making the measurements and to the analysis of the data themselves, are presented by Hörmann (1951), Vokaer and Vanden Eynden (1957, 1958), Jaroschka (1959), Knopp (1960, 1962) and Aherne and Dunnill (1966a and b).

For mature placentae, Spanner (1935) gave diameters of transversely cut villi as ranging from 25–110 μ, but with most lying between 40 and 60 μ. These were measurements for terminal or fringing villi. Stieve (1940) stated the diameters for such villi as lying between 40 and 70 μ. Hörmann (1951) recorded extensive quantitative data on villi from 116 placentae; he measured villous diameters of fixed, sectioned, and unfixed, teased, villi from different

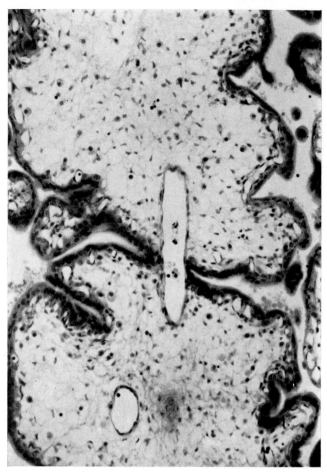

FIG. 57. Photomicrograph of a transverse section of adjacent villi in the placenta of a 96 mm. C.R. length foetus to show capillary anastomosis in the region of fusion. × c. 250.

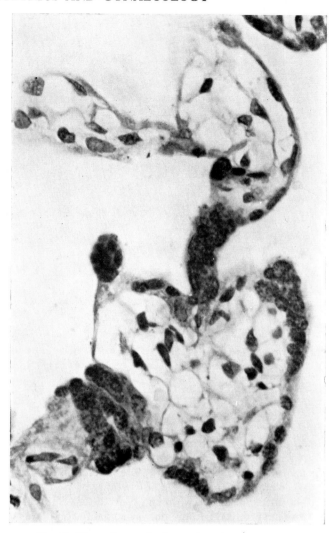

FIG. 58. Photomicrograph of a portion of a full-term placenta to show a syncytial bridge between two adjacent villi. Stained—Luxol fast blue, P.A.S., haematoxylin. × c. 720

regions of placentae for each month of pregnancy. He found that unfixed villi gave more reliable values. Hörmann's graphs show there is a regular decrease in average villous diameter up to the tenth month of pregnancy. The average diameters for the early months of pregnancy were: fixed, 170 μ, unfixed, 140 μ. For the tenth month placentae the corresponding figures were: fixed, 70 μ, unfixed, 50 μ. Knopp (1960), who applied the statistical method elaborated by Linzbach (1947) to the problem of the growth of the "chorionic villi", also demonstrated the marked decrease in the diameter of the terminal villi as they increase in number during gestation. Recently Aherne and Dunnill (1966a and b) have produced frequency distribution histograms at various gestation ages (18, 34 and 40 weeks) showing a modal diameter of the villi to be constant at 40–49 μ. Our own data are all based on fixed material and although we have not yet applied to our measurements the elaborate statistical techniques used by Hörmann and Knopp, none of our measurements fall outside the ranges indicated by these investigators. The decrease in individual diameters and increase in total number of the terminal villi of the human placenta in the course of its maturation are doubtless to be associated with an enhancement of their functional

capacity, as an essential part of the exchange mechanisms between foetus and mother. The resulting increase in surface area is to be associated with such other age changes as trophoblastic thinning and increased villous vascularity. In our opinion none of these changes in the terminal villi can readily be accepted as degenerative in character.

There are fewer data on the diameters of the trunci chorii. Stieve (1940) states that, at the beginning of the haemotrophic placental phase, the stem villi (*Stammenzotten*) have diameters that range between 110 and 140 μ. At the third and fourth months the range is between 300 and 500 μ. In the full-term placenta the equivalent measurements are 500–1,500 μ. For stem villi of the second and third orders (i.e., our rami and ramuli) Stieve records diameters of 300–700 μ. In our own material increase in the average diameter of the trunci, rami and ramuli chorii in the last six months of pregnancy is readily apparent. This increase is, of course, associated with the general growth of the placenta and of the large foetal vessels in the trunci. Indeed, the trunci and rami

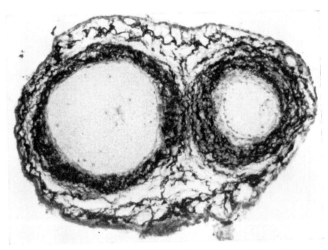

FIG. 59. Photomicrograph of a transverse section of a ramus chorii to show reticular fibres in the stroma and in the vessel walls. (Foetus, 150 mm. C.R. length.) Long's reticular stain. × c. 200.

function principally as "transmitters" or "carriers" of these vessels (Fig. 59). An added factor is, however, the large amount of connective tissue which is laid down in the stroma of the villous trunks to form the tough skeleton of the mature placenta (Tenzer, 1962; and Fig. 60).

PLACENTAL HISTOLOGY, INCLUDING PLACENTAL BARRIER, INTERLOBAR SEPTA AND ISLETS

The best established histological knowledge on the human placenta relates to the "villi" on which there is an extensive literature, a classical account having been given by Wislocki and Bennett (1943). In the past ten years the fine structure of the placenta, as revealed by the electron microscope, has been described by, among others, Boyd and Hughes (1954), Wislocki and Dempsey (1955), Bargmann and Knoop (1959), Hashimoto et al. (1960), Wislocki and Padykula (1961), Rhodin and Terzakis (1962), Sermann and Rigano (1962), Lister (1963a and b, 1964, 1965, 1966), Robecchi et al. (1963), Terzakis (1963), Panigel and Anh (1964), Enders (1965a), Becker and Seifert (1965), Ashley (1965), Anderson and McKay (1966), Okudaira et al. (1966) and Boyd and Hamilton (1966b). In recent years there has also been a considerable contribution from histochemistry to knowledge of villous structure.

In this section the structure and, so far as we have information on them, the age changes in the trophoblast, the stroma and the foetal vessels of the chorionic villi are briefly considered.

In spite of the marked structural similarities between selected portions of the specimens of different ages the growth of the placenta during gestation is accompanied by certain maturational alterations in the microscopical structure of the villous trunks and their branches. These changes involve the trophoblast itself, its basement membrane (basal lamina) and the villous stroma with its contained foetal vessels, and include such phenomena as thinning of the syncytial trophoblast, diminution in the

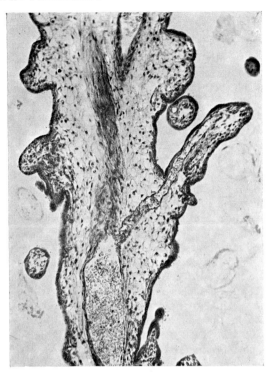

FIG. 60. Photomicrograph of a longitudinal section of a ramus chorii and associated villi. Note blood vessel with capillary branch and the central bundle of collagen fibres. (Foetus, 113 mm. C.R. length.) Masson's trichrome stain. × c. 135.

number of cytotrophoblastic cells with the interruption of Langhans layer, attenuation of the basement membrane, increased stromal fibrosis, fibrin deposition, infarction and so-called endarteritis. Many authorities (for discussion, see Burstein et al., 1956, and Becker, 1962) consider that these placental changes represent a process of precocious ageing. They have also been widely accepted as part, at least, of the explanation for the variation in permeability shown by the placenta during pregnancy (see, for example, Flexner et al., 1948; Hamilton and Boyd, 1950; Snoeck, 1958; and Hagerman and Villee, 1960). Some investigators, however, have tended to regard the structural age changes as degenerative processes; they seem to consider the mature placenta to be an effete, senile or even a pathological structure. In our opinion such an interpretation of a fully functioning organ is hard to accept. Moreover, many statements in the literature on the pathological nature of these age changes do not carry conviction as they have been based on limited numbers of inadequately spaced specimens. Differences in the methods whereby the placentae were obtained (e.g., hysterectomy, Caesarean section or vaginal delivery) and in the techniques of preparation often result in histological sections that are difficult to compare. Whether the cord is ligated or not after delivery, and the precise time when it is tied, can strikingly affect the final histological appearances of the villi.

Our own material indicates in a general way that histological alterations in the chorionic villi do occur and are progressive with maturation but it is difficult to quantitate them. Thus, we found that there are often striking differences in villi of a comparable stage from different regions of a given placenta, an observation stressed also by Fox (1964a). Secondly, successive phases in the histological differentiation of the villi merge so that distinctions between the phases are blurred and cannot be clearly defined. Thirdly, the age changes involve villous and non-villous trophoblast to different degrees. Finally, though pathological changes (e.g., infarcts) and quasi-pathological changes (e.g., increased fibrin or calcium deposits) tend to increase as pregnancy advances, being particularly frequent in post-mature placentae (Becker, 1960, 1962; Zhemkova and Topchieva, 1964), they are so variable that it is difficult to draw conclusions as to placental age from them.

Becker (1959, 1962) has summarized the placental age changes into four "indices of maturity" (*Reifezeichen*). These are: (1) decrease in the villous diameter with increase in the surface of the individual villi; (2) increase in the foetal vascular spaces in the villi; (3) diminution of the peripheral intravillous connective tissue with increase in the number of syncytial bridges (Getzowa and Sadowsky, 1950; Peter, 1950/51; Hamilton and Boyd, 1951); and (4) marked increase in the connective tissue sheaths of the vessels in the trunci chorii.

It is such changes as these, with several others discussed below, that constitute normal placental ageing. We stress their essential normality and agree with Becker (1962) when he writes: "Die Ausreifung der Placenta ist am Schwangerschaftsende auf eine Höhe getrieben, die nicht überboten werden kann." Wilkin (1965a) has also commented cogently on the so-called placental ageing. He writes: "diverses modifications microscopiques qui sont habituellement décrites comme les témoins du vieillissement de l'organe mais qui, à notre avis, traduisent plutôt sa maturation. En effet, la plupart de ces modifications apparaissent très précocement au cours de l'organogenèse et, si elles s'accentuent progressivement en fonction de la durée de la gestation, sont néanmoins le plus souvent contemporaines non d'une diminution mais bien d'un accroissement de l'activité placentaire."

Trophoblast

The trophoblast (Figs. 61–66; Pl. 1, Fig. 4; Pl. 2, Figs. 6–8) covering the terminal villi is an integral part of the "barrier" (placental membrane) interposed between the maternal and foetal circulations and, as such, is primarily involved in the process of placental transmission. The basement membrane (basal lamina; Fig. 65; Pl. 1, Fig. 4; Pl. 2, Fig. 8), of the trophoblast also has a role to play in the materno-foetal exchange mechanism. Moreover, the membrane as, at least in part, a product of trophoblast can conveniently be considered together with it.

The non-villous trophoblast (that of the basal and chorionic plates and of the cell islands) is obviously concerned very little with foetomaternal interchanges. Both villous and non-villous trophoblast, however, are presumably involved in the elaboration of the placental hormones though probably to different degrees (see later).

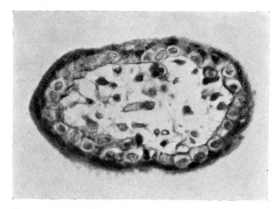

Fig. 61. Photomicrograph of a section of a terminal villus to show a continuous layer of palely staining cytotrophoblast. (Foetus, 61 mm. C.R. length.) Haematoxylin and eosin. × c. 350.

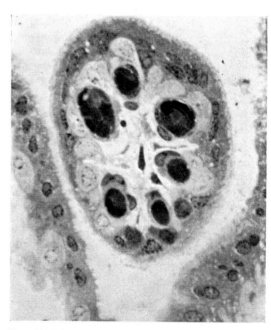

Fig. 62. Photomicrograph of a very thin section of a terminal villus. Note terminal capillary loops in relation to Langhans cells. The syncytium, with a well developed brush border, is of variable thickness. In adjacent larger villus Langhans layer shows interruptions. (Foetus, 76 mm. C.R. length.) Stained—methylene blue. × c. 630.

Cytotrophoblast

The primitive cytotrophoblast is derived from the cells of the wall of the blastocyst and from it stem all varieties of later trophoblastic tissue (Hamilton and Boyd, 1960; Boyd and Hamilton, 1960, 1966b). These varieties include: (1) the villous cytotrophoblast—Langhans layer—which constitutes the *cellular* (as opposed to *syncytial*) investment of the villi. This layer is continuous with the cytotrophoblast of the chorionic plate which, in turn, through a

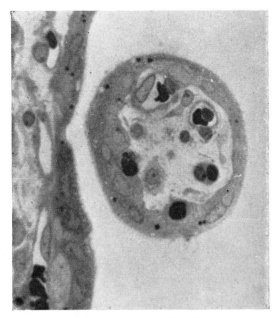

FIG. 63. Photomicrograph of an ultra thin section of a terminal villus and part of an adjacent larger villus. Note capillary loops and interrupted Langhans layer. The syncytium is foamy and possesses osmiophile granules. (Foetus, 150 mm. C.R. length.) Stained—methylene blue. × c. 700.

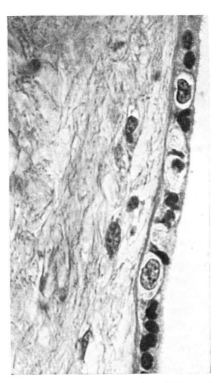

FIG. 64. Photomicrograph of a section of the trophoblast of a truncus chorii to show the presence of palely staining cytotrophoblastic cells. (Foetus, 230 mm. C.R. length; last trimester of pregnancy.) Haematoxylin and eosin. × c. 720.

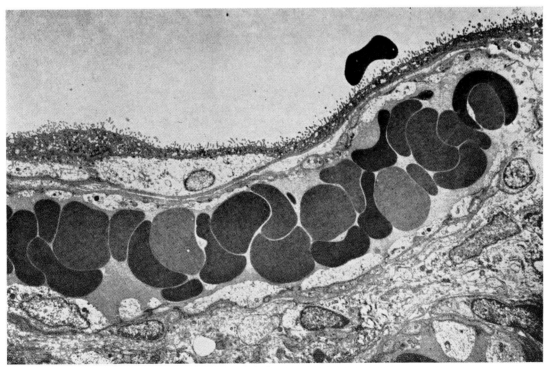

FIG. 65. Montage of two electron micrographs of a portion of a terminal villus. Note the continuous brush border of the syncytium and the thin Langhans cells and the proximity of the foetal capillary to the epithelial plate. Two flattened Langhans cells separate the basal lamina from the syncytium. The syncytium contains two nuclei, one of which is closely related to a plump degenerating Langhans cell. (Full-term foetus.) Glutaraldehyde fixation, post-fixation with Daltons' fluid and double staining. × c. 4,200.

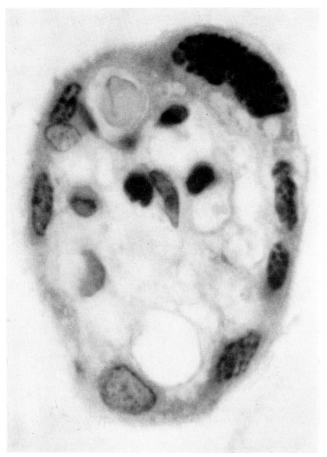

FIG. 66. Photomicrograph of a transverse section of a terminal villus to show a syncytial knot and an adjacent epithelial plate with underlying capillary. Note loose stroma. (Full-term placenta.) Haematoxylin and eosin. × c. 2,100.

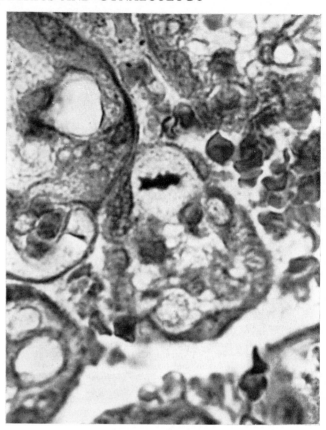

FIG. 67. Photomicrograph of a transverse section of terminal villi, one of which shows mitosis in a cytotrophoblastic cell. (Full-term placenta.) × c. 1,280.

marginal transitional region, passes into that of the chorion laeve; (2) the syncytium; (3) the cytotrophoblastic cell columns at the peripheral extremities of the villi; (4) the cells of the cytotrophoblastic shell which later become part of the so-called boundary zone (*Umlagerungszone* or *Durchwachsungszone*, the *Niemandsland* of Hörmann, 1966) of the basal plate and contribute to the interlobar septa (Boyd and Hamilton, 1966a, and see later); the shell contributes to the peripheral syncytium and to the placental site giant cells (Boyd and Hamilton, 1960); (5) the cells of the so-called cytotrophoblastic islands which become increasingly evident during the second trimester of gestation. The cells found in the lumina of the spiral arteries of the decidua may represent yet a sixth variety of cytotrophoblast (Boyd and Hamilton, 1956; Ortmann, 1960; Hamilton and Boyd, 1966b).

The cytotrophoblastic cells show variations in shape depending on their situation; arranged as a continuous layer they are cuboidal or columnar (Fig. 61), when single they tend to be irregularly ovoid, but in the columns they are polymorphic and often enlarged. The cytotrophoblastic cell columns are often said to disappear by the end of 3½ months (Baker *et al.*, 1944) but traces of them persist until much later in pregnancy.

In our material the cytoplasm of the Langhans cells and of those in the columns is much less basophilic than is the syncytium and the cytotrophoblastic nuclei have less affinity for basic dyes (Pl. 2, Fig. 7). These observations agree with those of Wislocki and Bennett (1943), Ortmann (1960) and Wislocki and Padykula (1961) and are in contrast with the views of Thomsen (1955) and Bargmann (1957) who may possibly have confused the Langhans cells with other varieties of cytotrophoblast. From light microscopy, Wislocki and Bennett (1943) described the cytoplasm of the cytotrophoblastic cells to be enclosed in a slightly denser, more deeply staining, surface membrane. Grosser (1925) had already indicated that there may be such a "capsule" which becomes blue tinged after Mallory's staining technique and which he suggested may be "fibrinoid" in nature. Such "fibrinoid" is, indeed, to be found in relation to Langhans cells in isolated regions of the villi and in the cytotrophoblastic islets, but electron microscopy (Fig. 65) demonstrates quite conclusively that Langhans cells do not possess capsules; they are separated from each other, and from the syncytium, by a narrow space obliterated at intervals by desmosomes but often dilated and containing microvillous projections from the opposed cellular surfaces. A definite basement membrane or basal lamina, however, always separates the cytotrophoblast from the villous stroma; the membrane is well demonstrated in electron micrographs (Figs. 65 and 68) and in sections stained specifically for reticulin (Fig. 59).

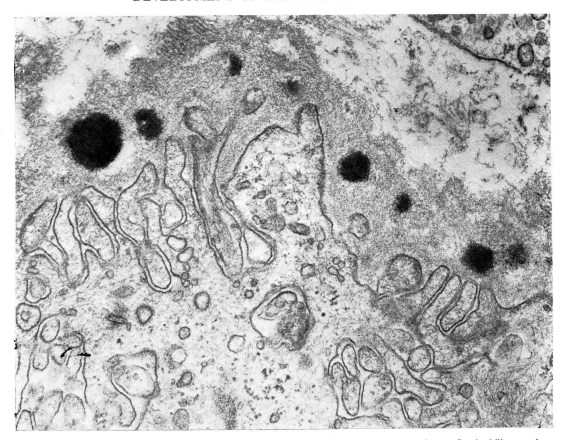

FIG. 68. Electron micrograph of a portion of a villus with the trophoblastic basement membrane. Osmiophilic granules are present in the membrane and many microvilli from the overlying Langhans cells project into it. The appearances are not inconsistent with an interpretation of the membrane as being, at least in part, a secretory product of the Langhans cells. (Foetus, 76 mm. C.R. length) × c. 60,000.

The membrane, which may contain osmiophilic granules, is constituted by an amorphous granular substance, of moderate electron opacity, in which a fine filamentous feltwork can be identified (Figs. 68 and 69). Occasionally the ends of collagenous fibres extend into it from the villous stroma (Fig. 70) and not infrequently (Fig. 68) processes from the trophoblastic cells are in its substance. In the regions of the epithelial plates, with their attenuated syncytium, the inner part of the basement membrane may be fused with the outer fibrils of the membrane covering the foetal capillary endothelium; Getzowa and Sadowsky (1950) and Hörmann (1951) consider that such regions form the effective metabolic barrier which they call the vasculo-syncytial membrane (VSM). In younger placentae, a trophoblastic basement membrane is also present (especially in the trunci and rami chorii) in those regions where the syncytium extends to the villous stroma in a tongue-like fashion between the Langhans cells. In such regions, and increasingly so as gestation proceeds, no more than five structural elements are interposed between maternal and foetal blood, viz.: the syncytium itself (which may possess a brush border or be anucleate), the trophoblastic basement membrane, the stromal connective tissue, the vascular basement membrane and the capillary endothelium (Fig. 71). Metabolites which traverse the placenta through no more than these five layers must, of

course, by-pass the Langhans cells. Where the cytotrophoblast persists as a continuous cellular layer up to full-term, however, a sixth layer is present.

Some investigators consider that the trophoblastic basement membrane increases in thickness in the last few weeks of pregnancy, a finding that has been correlated with a decrease in the permeability of the placental "barrier". In our presumably normal placentae the average thickness of the membrane is from 0·15–0·2 mm.; there is, however, great variability from specimen to specimen and in different regions of the same placenta. In general, however, our material shows an increase in membrane thickness as the placenta matures (Table II). The thickening has been stated to be more marked in the basement membrane of placentae of patients with toxaemia or diabetes (Lister, 1965; Okudaira et al., 1966); it is also thickened in postmaturity. Osmiophilic granules are frequently present in the basement membranes (Figs. 68 and 69) of normal placentae of the fourth to sixth months.

It has been widely believed that the cells of Langhans layer disappear relatively early in pregnancy (Schröder, 1930; Stöhr, 1959; Ortmann, 1949, 1955). In the second half of pregnancy we find the number of Langhans cells in the trunci, the rami and the ramuli chorii to be markedly reduced (Fig. 64). During this period, indeed, they often cannot be identified in these regions. The cytotrophoblast

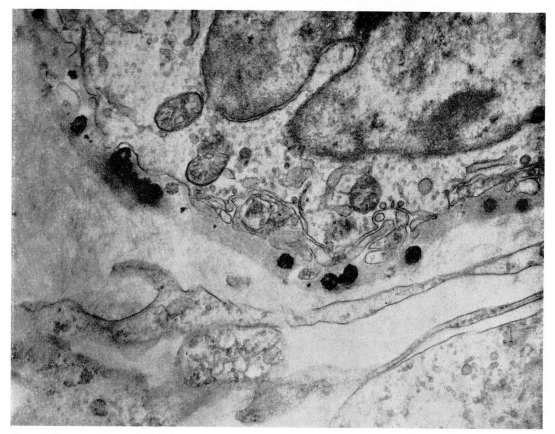

FIG. 69. Electron micrograph of the basement membrane with granules of osmiophilic material at the base of a Langhans cell. Note the complicated foldings of the base of the Langhans cell. (Foetus, 98 mm. C.R. length.) × c. 30,000.

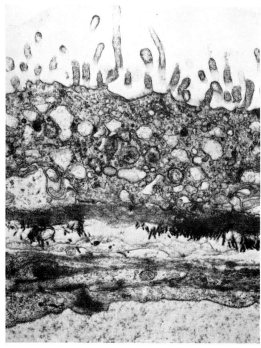

FIG. 70. Electron micrograph of a portion of a chorionic villus of a full-term placenta. The syncytium extends between the Langhans cells to the basement membrane, and shows numerous short microvilli. Note the collagen fibres deep to the basement membrane. × c. 15,000.

in the terminal villi, however, persists throughout gestation and is found in full-term placentae as isolated cells, as small groups of cells, or even as a more or less continuous layer of the Langhans type (Fig. 67; and see also Wislocki and Bennett, 1943; Baker *et al.*, 1944; Uchida, 1957; Thomsen and Blankenburg, 1956; Sauramo, 1961; Wigglesworth, 1962; Hamilton *et al.*, 1962; and Strauss, 1964). Mitotic activity is found in the Langhans cells throughout pregnancy and even at full-term (Fig. 67). Sauramo (1951, 1961) states that in postmature placentae cytotrophoblastic cells are not usually seen. Our own material also shows a diminution in the number of Langhans cells in postmature placentae and the persisting ones often show degenerative changes. On the other hand, there is some evidence for an actual increase in the number of such cells near the end of gestation when they constitute the so-called "X" cells (Wilkin, 1965a). As already stated, the cytotrophoblastic cell columns at the tips of attachment of the anchoring villi can also be identified in relatively late placentae. Wigglesworth (1962) has suggested that Langhans cells were not identified in older placentae by earlier investigators because fixation in formal saline resulted in destruction of the cytoplasmic details upon which their recognition depended; he considers that they can more readily be recognized after fixation in Helly's fluid and staining with Iron Haematoxylin. They can, however, be readily identified in all our material.

Our electron micrographs are in accord with those of

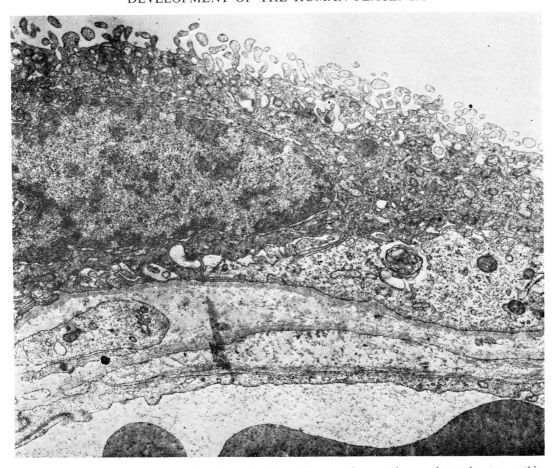

FIG. 71. Electron micrograph of a portion of a terminal villus. The syncytium contains a nucleus and rests on a thin basement membrane. A small portion of a Langhans cell is also present. A portion of a pericyte is applied to the surface of the very thin capillary endothelium. Fixed in 40 per cent glutaraldehyde, phosphate buffered. (Full-term foetus.) × c. 24,000.

Wislocki and Dempsey (1955) in demonstrating flattened Langhans cells in full-term placentae (Figs. 65 and 71). Other investigators (Hashimoto *et al.*, 1960; Rhodin and Terzakis, 1962; Lister, 1963a and b; Becker and Seifert, 1965; and Wynn, 1965) have also confirmed this finding; indeed the Langhans cells are often large and plump, showing no signs of flattening. The cytoplasm of these persisting Langhans cells, however, may show vacuolation or even, in postmature specimens, signs of frank degeneration. Lister, however, has shown us micrographs of placental villi from a fully authenticated case of postmaturity which show well preserved Langhans cells.

Throughout pregnancy most of the cells of Langhans layer possess ultrastructural features which distinctly distinguish them from the overlying syncytium. Thus, compared with the latter, the cytotrophoblastic cytoplasm usually possesses only moderate electron density, the endoplasmic reticulum is poorly developed possessing few attached ribosomes, the mitochondria are large with regular cristae, their Golgi apparatus is extensive but uncomplicated and inclusions are much less common. Moreover, the cytotrophoblastic nuclei are larger with a more homogeneous nucleoplasm which shows less peripheral chromatin condensation. All of these cytotrophoblastic features are those of undifferentiated cells. But

some of the cytotrophoblastic characteristics are not those to be expected of "stem" cells. Thus, at their junctions with adjacent cytotrophoblastic cells and with the overlying syncytium the Langhans cells possess desmosomes and their cytoplasm often shows well developed microfibrillae. Moreover, particularly round their periphery, in relation to the basement membrane, they often show marked surface folding.

In haematoxylin-stained sections Langhans cells are pale when compared with the overlying syncytium (Fig. 67). More refined staining techniques demonstrate that their cytoplasm exhibits very faint basophilia and that it has little affinity for acid dyes and shows no metachromasia. The faint basophilia can be correlated with poor development of the endoplasmic reticulum. Although present in large amounts in Langhans cells of normal villi in younger specimens, glycogen is either completely absent from these cells or present only in small traces in the older placentae with which we are here concerned. Glycogen can, however, be identified in the persistent cytotrophoblastic cells of the chorion laeve up to full-term, and, though variable in distribution and amount, is also found in the equivalent cells of the basal plate and in the placental septa until the seventh or eighth months. In ischaemic villi glycogen may be present in Langhans cells even at full-term although in our material there is considerable variation in its distribution in such villi. We are unable to persuade ourselves that, as alleged by Wislocki and Dempsey (1948), the distribution of trophoblastic glycogen is to be correlated with a local diminution in oxygen supply. There is usually little staining of Langhans cells with the PAS technique after treatment with diastase but occasionally we have seen them stained a magenta (*kardinalrot*) colour as described by Szontágh and Traub (1962). Small amounts of acid and alkaline phosphatase are present in the cytoplasm of the Langhans cells. A moderate amount of succinic dehydrogenase activity is presumably to be correlated with the large mitochondria. Lipids are present in only very small amounts though, occasionally, droplets are to be observed in electron micrographs.

Syncytium

The mode of origin of the trophoblastic syncytium, and indeed of its subsequent growth, has been long disputed. As stated earlier, the cells of the blastocyst wall are uninucleate and it is from them that the syncytium is initially derived. As early as 1885 Kastschenko realized that there was a genetic connexion between the multinucleate and the uninucleate tissues covering the chorionic villi. Mistakenly, however, he derived the cytotrophoblast from the syncytial layer (his "protoplasmic stratum"). Most subsequent investigators have considered that the gradual disappearance of Langhans layer without obvious cellular degeneration supports the view that the cytotrophoblast covering the villi is mainly transformed into syncytium. As stated earlier there is frequent mitotic activity in the cytotrophoblastic cells. The absence of mitotic activity in the syncytial nuclei is a fact generally accepted by all placentologists; we have never observed mitotic activity in these nuclei at any developmental stage in our extensive placental material. Partly on the basis of the occasional dumb-bell shaped appearance of these nuclei, however, Florian (1928) and Bucher (1959), amongst others, have postulated the occurrence of amitosis in the syncytium. More recently, Bargmann and Knoop (1959), from electron microscope studies, expressed the opinion that both origin and nature of the multinucleate placental cytoplasm are still in doubt; they suggest that it is really a plasmodium, arising not from coalescence of originally separate cells but from the multiplication of nuclei within an increasing cytoplasmic mass which itself has not shown division. Such a plasmodium would not, of course, form an uninterrupted and continuous covering over the whole extent of the villi, for there would result a number of plasmodial masses equivalent to the original number of separate blastocyst (later cytotrophoblastic) cells undergoing the multinucleate transformation. Most embryologists who have investigated this problem, however, support the view that the multinucleate state results from cell fusion; studies with optical microscopy have not produced unequivocal evidence for the presence in the resulting syncytium of traces of the cellular boundaries which might be expected if there is cell fusion. Using the electron microscope, however, Enders (1965), Boyd and Hamilton (1966b) and

Okudaira *et al.* (1966) have produced evidence in support of the origin of the multinucleate state through the confluence of individual cytotrophoblastic cells, and have described cells considered to be metamorphosing from Langhans cells into syncytium. This interpretation is supported by experiments using tritiated thymidine in organ cultures of the human placenta (Hertig, 1962; Tao and Hertig, 1965) and by studies on the deoxyribonucleic acid content of syncytial and cytotrophoblastic nuclei (Galton, 1962). Yet further support is given by the immunofluorescence and electron microscope investigations of Pierce and Midgley (1963) on the origin of the syncytium from cytotrophoblast in choriocarcinoma. A cell-type showing characteristics transitional between cytotrophoblast and syncytium can be found in hydatidiform moles (Wynn and Davies, 1964), an observation consistent with the concept of the derivation of the latter type of trophoblast from the former. Ortmann (1960), however, considers that the evidence for the derivation of syncytium from cytotrophoblast is inconclusive; he quotes Howorka's (1956) tissue culture observations as evidence for syncytial independence, and Ashley (1965) notes that transitional cellular types with features suggesting the origin of the syncytium from the cytotrophoblast were not shown by his electron micrographs. Ashley, however, only included one nine-weeks specimen among his otherwise full-term material. Although we find some suggestion of a continuing recruitment of cytotrophoblasts into the syncytium in mature placentae the evidence for the process is much more convincing in younger material.

In placentae with foetuses of about 60 mm. C.R. length, and procured at the commencement of the fourth month of gestation, a superficial layer of syncytium and a deeper Langhans layer of cytotrophoblast are present over the whole extent of the villous trunks and the free terminal villi. Except in relation to the trophoblastic cell islands (see later), the villous syncytium persists as a continuous layer throughout subsequent development. An identifiable membrane never separates the syncytium from the cytotrophoblast but, as pointed out earlier, a distinct reticular basement membrane (basal lamina) persists between the latter and the stroma.

In the first three months of gestation the syncytium is markedly vacuolated (Streeter, 1920a; Stieve, 1926; Florian, 1928; Johnston, 1941; Hamilton and Gladstone, 1942; Wislocki and Bennett, 1943; Baker *et al.*, 1944; Boyd, 1959; and Hamilton and Boyd, 1960), and in older specimens still shows varying degrees of vacuolation, often in different areas of the villous system of a given placenta. The vacuolation is least marked on the trunci, rami and ramuli; it is most frequent on the terminal villi however, especially where a brush border is well developed; it frequently has a foamy appearance (Fig. 63) and the vacuoles are much smaller. Different opinions have been expressed on the nature of the vacuoles. Earlier investigators, e.g., Langhans, believed them to be degenerative in nature. Fujimura (1921) interpreted those in the villi as secretion products of mitochondrial origin, but the opinion of Wislocki and Bennett (1943) that this interpretation is unlikely has been confirmed by electron micro-

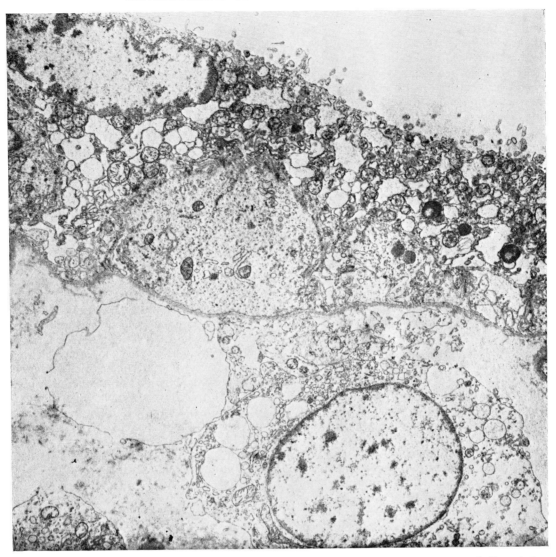

Fig. 72. Electron micrograph of the trophoblast and peripheral stroma of a chorionic villus. A markedly vesicular Hofbauer cell is situated immediately deep to the basement membrane. Portions of several Langhans cells form an interrupted layer on the basement membrane separating it in part from the syncytium; in the latter there is a large nucleus with peripheral concentration of chromatin, markedly dilated endoplasmic reticulum, osmiophile granules and mitochondria. Syncytial microvilli are poorly developed but pits lead into widely dilated canaliculi. (Foetus, 88 mm.) × c. 9,600.

scopy. Wislocki and Streeter (1938) suggested that, in the macaque placenta, there is an association in time between the appearance of the syncytial vacuoles and the establishment of the embryonic circulation and that the vacuolation may be evidence for syncytial pinocytosis.

The nuclei of the syncytium on the trunci, rami and ramuli are markedly basophilic (Fig. 64); in those on the terminal villi and especially in the syncytial clumps the chromatin is in the form of small granules usually aggregated near the nuclear membrane (Pl. 1, Fig. 3; Pl. 2, Figs. 6–8; and Figs. 58 and 66). The syncytial cytoplasm is more basophilic than that of the cells of Langhans layer and wide distribution of the syncytial ribonucleic acid is apparent in our *in situ* material stained with methyl-green-pyronine. This syncytial basophilia usually is more marked in its deeper portion and may often be intense round the nuclei. Occasionally an acidophilic band can

be seen near the surface especially when the syncytium possesses a brush border.

With light microscopy it is often found that part of the syncytial villous surface has a well developed brush border (Fig. 62) when in adjacent regions such a border is absent; this regional specialization probably indicates periodic alteration in syncytial structure and function. Wislocki and Bennett (1943) concluded that, from time to time in life, there is fluctuation in the degree of development of the brush border in a given villous region, emphasizing that the pleomorphic and plastic structure of the syncytial surface reflects the dynamic nature of its activity; such fluctuations may diminish with increase in placental age. Nagy (1960) has stated that the syncytium at full-term possesses no brush border. In our material, however, though it varies in height and regularity in different villi (cf. Figs. 65, 70–72) and in adjacent parts of a given villus, a brush border can be readily demonstrated, with both light and electron microscopy, on extensive areas of the syncytium of the free villi at all stages of gestation. Even on the trunci and rami chorii a brush border can often be recognized in the last half of gestation.

One of the most striking features of electron micrographs of the syncytium is the complex of microvilli which constitute the brush border (Boyd and Hughes, 1954; Wislocki and Dempsey, 1955; Bargmann and Knoop, 1959; Hashimoto et al., 1960; Lister, 1963b; Panigel and Anh, 1963; and Figs. 65, 70 and 71). These microvilli may be up to 2 μ in height, but can, especially in older placentae, be much shorter so that there are regions where they are effectively absent. Between the bases of the microvilli are numerous indentations and pits (Figs. 71 and 72) which appear to communicate with a canalicular system in the syncytial endoplasm; the canaliculi, which may be up to 150 μ in shortest diameter, extend widely throughout the syncytium. The endoplasmic reticulum itself is often concentrated in the deeper portions of the syncytium and the outer portions of its cisternae and canaliculi often possess small microvilli projecting into their lumina (Fig. 72). Moreover, in material exhibiting only slight basophilia, the cisternae of the endoplasmic reticulum are widely dilated, giving a honeycomb effect and, as a consequence, the local concentration of ribosomes is diminished. In syncytium of the third and fourth months, ribosomes, as isolated clusters or attached to the endoplasmic reticulum, are usually numerous. In the full-term placenta, however, the RNA granules are markedly decreased in number. Mitochondria are extremely common in the syncytium and persist into full-term; they are distinctly smaller and appear, per unit volume, to be more numerous than those in the cytotrophoblast but we have no quantitative assessment of their numbers. A Golgi apparatus in the form of a network is frequently to be found in the syncytium of the younger specimens. Lysosomes are variable in distribution and number. Between the cisternae of the endoplasmic reticular system at least several varieties of granules can be observed; the largest of these are markedly osmiophilic and may be of a steroid nature and associated with the production or storage of oestrogen and progesterone hormones (Terzakis, 1963). The smaller granules are usually less osmiophilic and may, in part, be transitional stages in the development of the larger ones. Many investigators have considered them to be lipid particles absorbed from the maternal plasma. The finely granular flocculum in the endoplasmic cisternae may be further indication of absorption from the IVS or a manifestation of the production by the attached ribosome granules of a protein secretion, possibly chorionic gonadotrophin. As already stated, microvilli may project into the canalicular spaces of the endoplasmic systems; this appearance is consistently found near syncytial surfaces with a brush border. Small vesicles which do not, it would seem, form part of the canalicular or endoplasmic reticular systems are present in the syncytium, and may be indications of pinocytotic activity. Not infrequently the appearance of the endoplasmic reticular cisternae suggests that the multinucleate

(i.e., syncytial) condition has resulted from fusion of individual cells. The syncytial nuclei are often very dense, especially in their periphery (Fig. 72), where clumps of dark chromatin are often found in contrast to much paler central areas; well defined nucleoli are usually present. The appearance, indeed, is not unlike that shown by the nuclei of other cells (e.g., late erythroblasts) which will show no further mitotic activity. The cytoplasmic cisternae often show a dilatation in a juxtanuclear position.

Syncytial Structural Specialization

Already in the fourth month of gestation the syncytium shows much regional variation in average thickness from about 2 μ as a minimum on the trunci and the rami to 10 μ, or more, on the free villi (Fig. 62, Pl. 2, Figs. 6 and 7). In the last four months of pregnancy there are extensive regions where, including its brush border the syncytium is much attenuated but even in the mature placenta there are many villi on which it remains thick (Fig. 66). Knopp (1960) gives 6·5 μ as the mean value for syncytial thickness in the tenth month. Our own electron microscopic measurements are given in Table II; the findings are selective but confirm the impression from light microscopy that with advance in foetal age much of the syncytium becomes progressively thinner. The attenuation is often particularly obvious over stromal capillaries, where the thinned syncytial areas, devoid of nuclei, constitute what Bremer (1916) called the "epithelial plates".

In addition to the regional variations in thickness there are at least four other varieties of syncytial modification, variously known as "sprouts", "buds", "knots" and "proliferation nodes" or "les bourgeons syncytiaux" or "syncytiale Knospen". Two of these are syncytial projections which extend for varying distances from the surface of the villi into the IVS and usually possess a concentration of clumped syncytial nuclei; though their eventual fates are quite different, it seems appropriate to use the term "syncytial sprout" for either of them. The stromal trophoblastic buds (Boyd and Hamilton, 1964), consisting of syncytium with clumped nuclei, surrounded by cytotrophoblastic cells, and situated in the substance of the villous stroma, constitute a third variety. Finally, lying between the anucleate epithelial plates, there are syncytial regions with a high concentration of nuclei; these regions, which have been called "syncytial knots" (Fox, 1965a; Hamilton and Boyd, 1966a), bulge slightly into the IVS (Figs. 58 and 66), when they may resemble early syncytial sprouts and, indeed, have been confused with them. Our consideration of these syncytial specializations commences with the sprouts.

Initially, a syncytial sprout possesses no Langhans cells; as growth proceeds, however, cytotrophoblast may penetrate its base, followed in due course, by stromal tissue. Subsequent vascularization of the latter will result in the establishment of a new villus of the "free" or "terminal" type. The development of yet further sprouts from the syncytium covering this terminal villus will, in turn, convert it into a pre-terminal villus on the surface of which another generation of terminal villi is established. In this manner

TABLE II

Average Thickness (in microns) of Syncytium, Cytotrophoblast and Basement Membrane in Electron Micrographs of Placental Villi

C.R. length	Syncytium	Syncytium and Cytotrophoblast	Basement Membrane
13 mm.	10 extremes, 4–25	17·5	0·22 extremes, 0·2–0·3
28 mm.	5·5 extremes, 3·5–7·5	26·0	0·22 extremes, 0·15–0·5
44 mm.	6·33 extremes, 2·4–7·4	15·0	0·24 extremes, 0·2–0·32
88 mm.	5·2 extremes, 3·2–8·1	9·4	0·26 extremes, 0·2–0·28
113 mm.	6·6 extremes, 2·0–8·2	14·0	0·28 extremes, 0·21–0·3
Full-term	2·4 extremes, 1·5–7·0	—	0·8 extremes, 0·4–0·95
Full-term	1·67 extremes, 1·0–4·2	—	0·31 extremes, 0·2–0·7

The data in this Table are based on ten separate measurements of electron micrographs from each placenta. The averages recorded are to be regarded as merely indicative of the thickness of the syncytium and basement membrane at successive stages of development. Obviously the measurements depend on the size of the villus sectioned and on the obliquity of section relative to its long axis. Sections were selected in which it was considered that the plane was perpendicular to the syncytial surface. We have been thwarted in our attempts to get significant data on the thickness of the cytotrophoblast. Langhans layer is extremely variable, the thickness of its cells varies along their length, and at interruptions in the layer syncytium only is present. The data, in our estimation, indicates two distinct trends. Firstly, the average thickness of the syncytium diminishes with advancing placental age and, secondly, the basement membrane increases in thickness in older specimens. Both trends, however, can be reversed by selected measurements at any stage in pregnancy.

the villous systems of the placenta extend and grow; the syncytial projections concerned can, therefore, be called "growth sprouts". There is, however, a second variety of sprout which, though it appears to arise in the same fashion as the growth sprouts just described, never acquires a Langhans layer or stromal core. These purely syncytial sprouts become detached from the villi and pass through the IVS into the maternal circulation where, as "transportation" or "deportation" sprouts, they undergo cytolysis or are eventually trapped in the pulmonary capillary system (Schmorl, 1893; Veit, 1905; Park, 1958, 1965; Douglas *et al.*, 1959; Boyd, 1959; Hamilton and Boyd, 1960, 1966a; Alvarez *et al.*, 1962; Desai and Creger, 1963; Iklé, 1964; and Olivelli and De Palo, 1964).

The projections from the deep aspect of the syncytium into the villous stroma have been called *syncytial trophoblastic buds* (Boyd and Hamilton, 1964) and *syncytial globules* (Alvarez, 1964; Alvarez *et al.*, 1964). Ishizaki

(1960) had referred to such isolated masses of syncytium in the stroma of the chorionic villi as "orphan bodies"; he considered them to be pathological vestiges of placentitis. The significance of the stromal trophoblastic buds is not yet apparent; they may be the explanation for the alleged presence (Salvaggio *et al.*, 1960) of trophoblast in the foetal blood vessels. In agreement with Alvarez (1964) we find that the syncytial buds decrease in number during pregnancy.

The epithelial plates, as already stated, are thinned areas of syncytium overlying the stromal capillaries; the plates are devoid of nuclei but the adjacent syncytium often contains the clumped nuclei of a syncytial knot (Figs. 65 and 66; Pl. 1, Figs. 3 and 4). The nuclear displacement has been attributed to their active migration or to the pressure exerted by the underlying capillaries. Shanklin (1958), however, has suggested that lysis of the nuclei may account for their absence in the plates. On the other hand, Fox (1965a) believes that syncytial knot formation is due to a proliferation of syncytial nuclei by amitosis. This explanation appears unlkely in view of what is known about the behaviour of syncytial nuclei (see earlier). Getzowa and Sadowsky (1950) distinguished between simple anuclear areas (which, confusingly, they called spaces) without relationship to foetal capillaries, and those anuclear areas in which the syncytium is fused with the subjacent vessels to constitute vascular syncytial membranes (VSM). They stated that the latter become distinct in the fifth month and increase in number with advancing pregnancy. Bremer (1916) considered that the plates on the older villi gradually disappeared as they were replaced, and augmented, by others on the developing free villi. Like Fox we find the epithelial plates to be located in great numbers near the basal plate; this distribution was correlated by Fox (1964b) with a presumptively higher oxygen content of the blood in the juxta-decidual part of the IVS.

The syncytial knots have also been referred to as syncytial clumps or sprouts; in our opinion there is little justification for, and some confusion resulting from, this use of the term. While the aggregation of syncytial nuclei related to the plates just described can constitute small protuberances on the villi they are, in fate and function, very different from the syncytial sprouts discussed earlier. Therefore we follow Fox (1965a) in restricting the term syncytial knot to them though "syncytial clump" might be considered more appropriate. Even with the restriction, however, a terminological difficulty remains since many regional aggregations of syncytial nuclei cannot, except arbitrarily, be classified as either syncytial knots or syncytial sprouts. Fox states that in his normal specimens derived from the 37th week and later, there is an increased knot formation with advancing pregnancy.

The presence of a brush border on the surface of the syncytium is generally believed (Wislocki and Bennett, 1943; Boyd and Hughes, 1954; Amstutz, 1960) to be indicative, as elsewhere in the body, of resorptive activities. Ashley (1965) has drawn special attention to the syncytial canalicular system and has stated that when excised placental fragments are incubated in serum containing

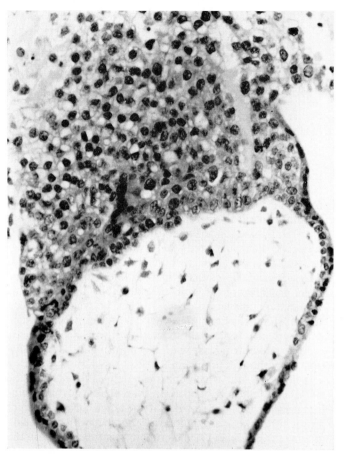

FIG. 73. Photomicrograph of a cell column attaching a villus to the trophoblastic shell. The shell is partially separated from decidual tissue by fibrinoid (Nitabuch's stria) in the junctional zone. (Foetus, 61 mm. C.R. length.) Haemotoxylin and eosin. × c. 1,000.

particles of thorium or ferritin these substances are taken up by the canals. Moreover, the appearances along the length of the canaliculi and vesicles suggest specialized absorptive functions. Thus Sawasaki *et al.* (1957) showed that in the superficial part of the syncytium the vacuoles and vesicles may contain microvilli; our material confirms this fact (see earlier, and Fig. 71). Ashley's investigations were on full-term placentae though he does mention the presence of pits and vesicles in the syncytium from a nine-weeks gestation specimen. Throughout the second and third trimesters we find extensive, though variable, development of this canalicular system (Figs. 65, 70 and 71). Whether the canaliculi should be regarded as a specialized part of the endoplasmic reticulum is uncertain, in most specimens it can be distinguished from the membrane-bounded cisternal system to the outer walls of which ribosomes are attached and in which a flocculent deposit is frequently found.

From the above discussion, the syncytium is obviously more highly specialized in structure and shows more differentiation than the cells of Langhans layer. In addition, however, there is presumptive evidence for the existence of special metabolic activities restricted to, or localized in, specialized syncytial regions. Many investi-

gators regard the epithelial plates as possessing a specific role in placental transmission (Weinbeck, 1936; Wislocki and Bennett, 1943; Getzowa and Sadowsky, 1950; Hörmann, 1951, 1953; and Amstutz, 1960). Transport of gases is more likely to occur in the syncytium of the epithelial plates of the terminal villi than in that covering the villous trunks. Bremer (1916) believed the epithelial plates to be excretory rather than respiratory in function on the basis that all embryos from very early periods require oxygen, yet in many mammalian classes the plates are never developed and in many others they appear relatively late, long after the need for oxygen arises. The epithelial plates are considered by Amstutz (1960) primarily as areas for the exchange of gases by diffusion. He finds that in addition to their characteristic morphological structure, the plates are distinguished by the absence of alkaline phosphatase. In his opinion those syncytial areas that are rich in alkaline phosphatase, and with a brush border, may be concerned with other functions. Thomsen and Lorenzen (1956) assumed the localization of sudanophilic substances in the syncytium to be a further proof of its high metabolic activity. Hörmann (1951, 1953), however, considered that in addition to diffusion processes other activities are also localized in the epithelial plates. Finally, it should be noted that there is almost certainly a waxing and waning of the metabolic and functional activities of different regions of the syncytium during placental growth.

Other Varieties of Trophoblast

Cytotrophoblast (Langhans layer) and associated syncytium are found covering the whole of the chorionic plate and, generally, their history in this position parallels that of the equivalent villous trophoblast; a special problem however, is presented by the trophoblast of the villi on the free (IVS) surface of the basal plate and the chorionic plate margin.

Elsewhere, detailed accounts have been given of certain other varieties of peripheral syncytial trophoblastic tissue. These include the so-called giant cells (Boyd and Hamilton, 1960; Hamilton and Boyd, 1966a) which we have described as foetal in origin. Schramm (1962) has supported this interpretation but Brettner (1964) and Park (1965), however, have been critical of it; no further discussion of this problem will be given here.

There remain for consideration three other groups of cellular elements which, in spite of some opinions to the contrary, we consider to be of cytotrophoblastic origin; these are the cells of (a) the cytotrophoblastic columns, (b) the trophoblastic shell, and (c) the cytotrophoblastic cell islands. The cells found in the terminal portions of the endometrial spiral arteries may constitute yet a further variety of cytotrophoblast (Hamilton and Boyd, 1966b).

Cytotrophoblastic Cell Columns. Some investigators (Ortmann, 1960, and Wilkin, 1965b) restrict the cytotrophoblastic cell columns at the basal plate (distal) ends of the trunci, rami and ramuli chorii to the first four months of gestation. Certainly the columns are relatively much better developed in the early months of pregnancy but, attached to the basal plate (Fig. 73) and also to

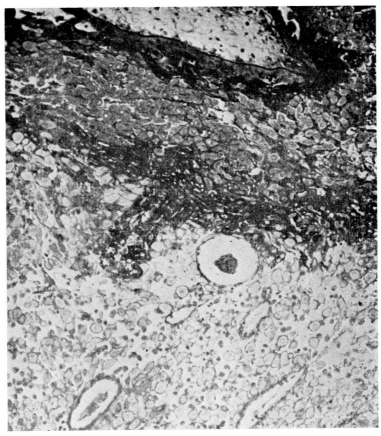

FIG. 74. Photomicrograph of the basal plate to show persisting elements of the cytotrophoblastic shell and their relations. From above downwards in the illustration there can be identified: (a) the tip of a villus with its stroma and basement membrane; (b) residual cells of the cytotrophoblastic column; (c) Rohr's fibrinoid stria (darkly stained); (d) cytotrophoblastic cells of the shell; (e) Nitabuch's fibrinoid stria (darkly stained); and (f) decidual cells in loose stroma with vestiges of uterine glands. (Foetus, 175 mm. C.R. length. × c. 130).

the interlobar septa, they can be identified throughout pregnancy over the stroma at the tips of the attached, or anchoring, "villi" which represent the peripheral (decidual) ends of the trunci and rami chorii. In the earlier stages the polymorphic cells of the columns show numerous mitoses, a fact which, when associated with the abundance of ribosomes and of glycogen in their cytoplasm, suggests special proliferative activity. It has not been determined whether the resulting cells migrate in the foetal direction, thus elongating the villous system, or towards the basal plate where, by increasing the number of cells in the trophoblastic shell, they contribute to the expansion of the chorionic sac. There is, of course, no *a priori* reason why cells from the columns should not migrate in each direction.

In general appearance and structure these cells, though more basophilic, closely resemble those of Langhans layer, the resemblance extending to such histochemical features as the small lipid content. Until the end of gestation, there is usually an uninterrupted layer of cytotrophoblast at the junction of each column with the villous stroma. Here the basement membrane is always very well developed (Fig. 74); vascularization of the adjacent stroma, however, is usually less marked than in other regions of the villi. At many villous attachments

coarse strands of dense collagenous fibres appear to perforate the tips of the columns. Careful examination, however, shows that such strands are usually, if not always, surrounded by foetal cells. Intercellular spaces in the columns of earlier stages may erupt through the ensheathing syncytium and communicate with the IVS. These intercellular spaces can be identified until quite late in pregnancy; they often contain cellular detritus or fibrinoid (Fig. 75; and see later).

Cytotrophoblastic Shell. The method of establishment of the trophoblastic shell has been described in detail elsewhere (Hamilton and Boyd, 1960a). Some investigators consider that the cellular elements of the shell retrogress, or even disappear, early in gestation. Thus Wilkin (1965b) states that the shell becomes thinned and after the fourth month consists only of scattered, though readily recognizable, foetal cells mixed with decidual elements. Our material, however, shows that the cellular elements of the shell persist in the basal plate until term in that region of intermingling of foetal elements with the decidua that has been variously designated as the "junctional", "transitional", "penetration" or "boundary" zone (*Durchdringungszone, Umlagerungszone, Niemandsland*). Considerable mitotic activity is shown by the cells of the shell in the period of rapid placental growth in the first

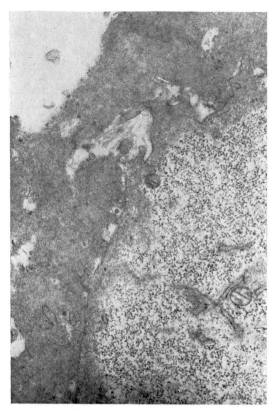

FIG. 75. Electron micrograph of a portion of a cytotrophoblastic cell column at the apex of a villus. The fibrinoid
which is present in an intercellular space is closely
related to the surface of a cytotrophoblastic cell possessing a large amount of glycogen and some rough E.R.
The cytoplasm adjacent to the plasma membrane of
the cell is devoid of organelles. It is, however, more
electron-dense than the remainder of the cytoplasm and
possesses microvilli which extend into the fibrinoid.
The appearances are not inconsistent with an interpretation that this fibrinoid is a product of cytotrophoblastic
secretion. (Foetus, 76 mm. C.R. length.) × c. 55,000.

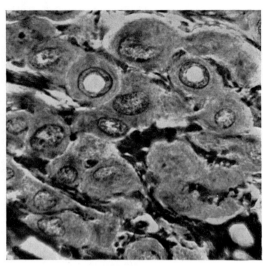

FIG. 76. Photomicrograph of a portion of the basal plate
to show cytotrophoblastic shell cells enmeshed in
fibrinoid. Vacuolation is seen in some of the nuclei; this
is taken as indicative of nuclear secretion. × c. 1,000.

half of pregnancy. In the second half, however, there is
little evidence of multiplication of its cells. On its foetal
aspect, exposed to the IVS, there is initially a transformation of cells of the shell into a thin syncytial layer. Later,
however, many apparently uninucleate, though very
elongated, cells can be found bounding the maternal
periphery of the IVS, and in part replacing the multinucleate syncytium. From an analysis of the Barr bodies
in placentae of male foetuses (Ludwig and Wanner, 1964;
Wanner, 1966) it has been concluded that these uninucleate
cells are of maternal origin. We have tentatively suggested
(1966a) that they may be cells derived from the endothelial
lining of the endometrial veins which, as the result of
dilatation of these vessels during the expansion and
growth of the placenta, become exposed to the IVS
between the septa and the attachments of the anchoring
villi to the basal plate.

Our histological observations on the cytotrophoblastic
cells of the basal plate itself correspond closely with those
of Dallenbach-Hellweg and Nette (1963a and b, 1964).
These cells are markedly basophilic elements which lie
freely in a loose ground-substance (Fig. 76), unencapsulated
by reticular fibres in the manner so characteristic for

endometrial cells; they tend to be spherical, though
radially arranged spindle-shaped ones are not uncommon.
Fibrinoid is early associated with these basal plate cytotrophoblastic cells and as gestation progresses it becomes
markedly increased in amount and arranged to form what
are traditionally described as two layers—that of Rohr
near to the IVS, and that of Nitabuch (Figs. 74 and 78),
further from it. The layers are in fact only incompletely

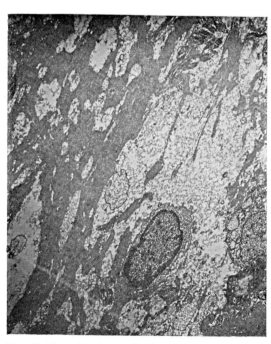

FIG. 77. Electron micrograph of a portion of the basal
plate with Nitabuch's stria. The fibrinoid constituting the
membrane consists of interconnecting trabeculae, in the
interstices of which are remains of both decidua and
trophoblast. (Foetus, 86 mm. C.R. length.) × c. 6,600.

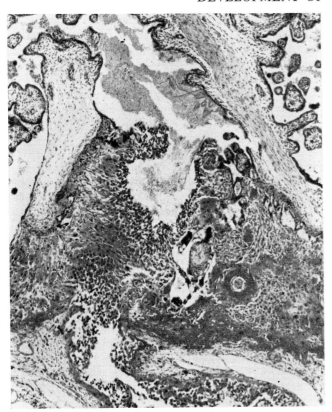

FIG. 78. Photomicrograph to show an opening of a spiral artery into the IVS. Note the massive invasion of the lumen by cytotrophoblastic cells, Nitabuch's membrane and the obliterated vessel with fibrinoid degeneration of its wall. (Foetus, 118 mm. C.R. length.) Haemotoxylin and eosin. × c. 48.

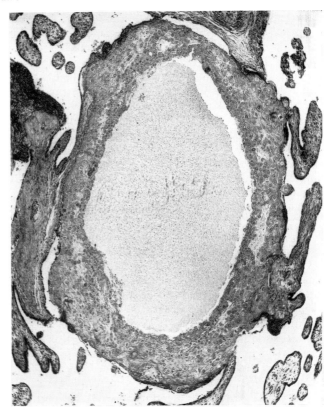

FIG. 79. Photomicrograph of a placental cyst surrounded mainly by cytotrophoblastic cells. The cyst is situated either in a cell island or in the apical region of a septum. (Foetus, 230 mm. C.R. length.) Stained—Masson. × c. 60.

separated from each other; both are frequently perforated by bands of peripheral syncytium and shell cytotrophoblasts (Fig. 74).

Ortmann (1949, 1955, 1960) has described nuclear secretion in the persisting cells of the shell and in the islands. Much of our material (Fig. 76; Pl. 3, Fig. 9), shows appearances (nuclear indentation, nuclear inclusions, nucleolar vacuolation) in these cells which can be similarly interpreted, and which, with their intense basophilia and high lipid content, distinguish them from Langhans cells. Dallenbach-Hellweg and Nette (1964) have also given detailed accounts of the cytological features and histochemical reactions of these basal plate trophoblastic cells, with their cytoplasmic inclusions; they describe a pale variety of cell considered to be derived from the columns, whereas the basophilic cells are more closely associated with the peripheral syncytium. These investigators have suggested that both varieties of basal cytotrophoblast may produce hormones throughout pregnancy and Ortmann (1955) has pointed out that, in the aggregate, the total volume of such cells is at least equivalent to that of the adenohypophysis. Conte (1965) has shown that glycoprotein, identified histochemically, increases in the peripheral cytotrophoblast during the second and third trimesters of pregnancy; he suggests that these cells may gradually replace the villous syncytium as the source of chorionic gonadotropin.

Cytotrophoblastic Cell Islands. These, in our opinion, are derivatives of the cytotrophoblast; they are found attached to villi of different sizes throughout the placenta. Ortmann (1960) described the islands as usually appearing in the fourth month at the time when the intercotyledonary septa are becoming apparent. We have found them, however, at much earlier stages as small collections of cells, resembling those of Langhans layer, which project from the surface of villous trunks often quite close to their attachment to the chorionic plate. By the beginning of the second trimester some of the islets have increased in size and their constituent cells in number (Pl. 3, Figs. 10 and 11) They now often project into the IVS without an apparent covering of the syncytium. Stieve (1952) described them as being situated principally on the periphery of the villous systems; he considered (and has been supported by Wilkin, 1965b, in this opinion) that such cytotrophoblastic groups fuse together to constitute the septa which, thus, are of purely foetal origin. Elsewhere we have supported the view that the septa are partly of maternal origin (Boyd and Hamilton, 1966a). On the other hand, many observers from Kölliker (1879) to Hörmann (1966) have described septa and islands as derivatives of the decidua. From sex chromatin studies, Klinger and Ludwig (1957), and others, also consider these placental structures to be mainly of maternal origin. Whatever their ultimate nature the cells of the cytotrophoblastic islets (and some of those in the septa) show much the same cytological features as those described for the basal plate cytotrophoblasts. Like the septa the islands possess, often quite large, intercellular cystic spaces (Fig. 79). These spaces, the so-called "pseudo-cysts" of Hörmann (1966), may contain a colloid substance giving staining reactions for mucoprotein; lipid is also found in these cysts and they may possess a precipitate resembling fibrinoid. Tips of adjacent villi, their stroma often showing mucoid degeneration, are usually attached to the islands; Hörmann considers that this relationship demonstrates that the insular cells are part of the *Nie-mandsland* of the *Durchwachsungszone*. Such an interpretation, however, does not necessarily indicate a decidual origin for them and, in our opinion, like many elements in the basal plate the insular cells and those related to cysts and retrogressing villi are cytotrophoblasts (Pl. 3, Figs. 9–11). This view is supported by the signs of nucleolar secretion so often shown by cells in all these situations.

Possibly related to the cellular elements, interpreted here as cytotrophoblastic in nature, of the basal plate, of the cell islands and of parts of the septa is a group of cells found in relation to the surface of the periphery of the chorionic plate where they constitute the so-called "sub-chorial closing ring" (*subchorialer Schlussring*) or "mar-ginal structures" (*Randbildungen*) of the placenta. Grosser (1909, 1952), Spanner (1935), Stieve (1936, 1940, 1952) and Ortmann (1960) have all ascribed a trophoblastic origin to the cells of the closing ring. Bühler (1964), however, has recently argued strongly in favour of a decidual origin for its cells basing his conclusion on the study of freshly delivered full-term placentae, and of five specimens between the 7th and 14th weeks of gestation, and support-ing his interpretation with sex chromatin analysis. From our own investigations of *in situ* placentae we are unable to persuade ourselves that Bühler's interpretation is alto-gether correct. There may be some contribution by the marginal decidua to the extreme periphery of the marginal plate, which we find to be extremely variable in develop-ment, but most of the constituent cells possess cytological appearances identical with those of the cell islands and which, as already indicated, we consider to be of foetal origin. Moreover, our sex chromatin analysis of the marginal plate cells does not provide such convincing evidence for their maternal origin as do the data advanced by Bühler.

Mesenchymal Components of Villi, including Foetal Blood Vessels

The villous cores are established when mesenchymal elements invade the primary villi thus converting them into those of the secondary type. The invading stromal mesenchyme is generally assumed to be of extra-embryonic origin, derived from the somatopleuric lining of the chorion, but Hertig (1935) has argued in favour of a cytotrophoblastic origin for some of it, including perhaps, in part, the associated blood vessels. The mesenchyme, however, appears always to be separated from the over-lying trophoblast by the basement membrane (basal lamina). The stromal cells are essentially fibroblasts and form a loose network in the meshes of which are found an intercellular fluid (Figs. 33, 38, 47 and 48) and the special-

ized cells named after Hofbauer (Fig. 80, Pl. 2, Fig. 6). Electron micrographs show that the fibroblasts possess a considerable development of both smooth and rough surface endoplasmic reticulum the cisternae of which are often markedly dilated. The fibroblastic nuclei are of an irregular shape and usually possess a distinct nucleolus. From an early stage the fibroblasts and their processes are supported by reticular fibres which develop within the intercellular matrix. These fibres can often be traced into the basement membrane (Figs. 68 and 69); in silver-impregnated sections they surround the stromal cells as a delicate meshwork (Fig. 59). Vascularization of the stroma converts the secondary villi into those of the tertiary variety; the latter first appear in late presomite embryos but even up to full-term new villi continue to develop. Early villi possess only the reticular network but with growth and differentiation collagenous fibres appear successively in the trunci, rami and ramuli chorii and in the anchoring villi where they thicken into large trabeculae (Fig. 60) and eventually constitute a felt-like collagenous core frequently arranged in bundles parallel to the long axis of these major villi and close to their major blood vessels. The fibres appear to act as supports for the larger vessels which, in the trunci chorii, possess a well defined media. The main function indeed of the larger villous stems is to serve as conduits for the, usually paired, villous arteries and veins.

Depending upon the level in the "villous tree" (trunci, rami or ramuli chorii or free villi) at which sections are examined the villous cores may vary considerably in their structure. There are also differences in the cores of com-parable villi at different times in gestation (cf. (Figs. 33, 38, 47 and 48). When attention is given to ensuring that comparison is made between comparable homologous villi, however, the age differences are not so striking as is sometimes assumed. In the free terminal villi, indeed, the general histological appearances shown by their cores are remarkably similar throughout gestation. Nevertheless, four progressive and quite distinct differences may be observed in them. Firstly, in general, the older the villi the smaller are their average diameters (cf. Figs. 33, 38, 47 and 48), and also Hörmann, 1951; Knopp, 1960; and Alvarez, 1964). Secondly, terminal villi in mature placentae are more richly vascularized than in younger ones, and their blood vessels are more closely related to the overlying trophoblast. Thirdly, as the placenta ages there is an increase in the stromal connective tissue, collagen in-creasingly replacing the reticulin (Costero, 1931; Tenzer, 1962). Fourthly, the fine network of reticular fibres in the terminal villi shows much smaller meshes in the older placentae. As Stieve (1940, 1952) has pointed out, the extent of the intercellular spaces in the terminal villi largely depends upon whether the capillaries are full or empty; when the vessels are distended the intercellular spaces disappear almost completely. The spaces in which the Hofbauer cells are situated often constitute a com-municating system which presumably allows of the free passage of fluid, and possibly of the contained cells, along the villous elements (Figs. 60 and 73). The communications become much less obvious in older placentae.

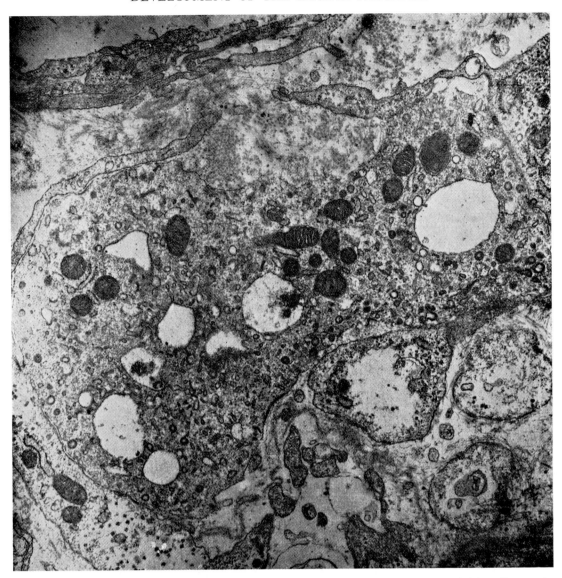

FIG. 80. Electron micrograph of stroma of a full-term placenta showing a Hofbauer cell surrounded by collagen and processes of fibroblasts. The nucleus of the Hofbauer cell is not sectioned but its cytoplasm shows dense mitochondria, a number of large vesicles, some containing a precipitate, many small vesicles and some identifiable rough endoplasmic reticulum. × c. 24,000.

Several investigators have presented histometric data on the relative development of the trophoblast and connective tissue of the villi at different gestational ages. Vokaer and Vanden Eynden (1957) and Ortmann (1960) indicate that about two-thirds of placental tissue consists of connective tissue, the remainder of trophoblast. Neither the Belgian authors nor Ortmann found any fundamental shift in the relative amounts of these tissues between the second and ninth months of pregnancy. Jaroschka (1959) states that, as a percentage of its total mass, the mature placenta contains 19 per cent trophoblastic and 15 per cent connective tissue nuclear substance and indicates that during placental maturation there is a moderate but significant reduction in the proportion produced by the trophoblastic epithelium.

A detailed account of the foetal placental blood vessels or of the related literature (see Grosser, 1927; Stieve, 1940,

1941; Bøe, 1953 and 1954; Crawford, 1956a, b and c, 1959, 1961, 1962; Florange and Hoer, 1958; Mayer et al., 1959; Arts, 1961; Smart, 1962; and Becker, 1963) cannot be given here; we have had to restrict it to a summary of our observations on the villous vessels. The ramifications of the villous vessels parallel those of the rami and ramuli chorii. In the terminal villi, however, arterioles and venules arising from axially orientated larger trunks supply and drain the extensive sub-epithelial capillary network.

Newly formed free villi are at first avascular, the core of each consisting merely of a few mesenchymal cells. Soon, however, a capillary, as an endothelial sprout or as a loop, comes to be included within the core. In the primary villi of presomite or somite embryos these capillaries arise from the blood vessels of the chorion. In the placentae in the age groups in the last half of pregnancy newly established vessels accompany the growth of new villi either as branches of the variably developed capillary plexus of the trunci, rami or ramuli chorii or as loops between villous arterioles and venules (Figs. 62 and 63; Pl. 1, Fig. 4). In the smaller villi, however, there are frequently a number of short vascular loops in which the histological distinctions between artery and vein are absent. These loops are generally referred to as capillaries but they frequently range up to 60 μ in diameter which is considerably in excess of what is usually taken to be that of a capillary. Whether such vessels should be considered a type of arterio-venous anastomosis is a moot point; certainly their shortness and wide calibre will cause less fall in the pressure of blood passing through them than that found in capillary systems generally. In many placentae, indeed, especially in older ones, the looped capillaries are ballooned out to form sinusoidal spaces. The appearance presented is often such as to suggest that the villous capillary has become varicose and, at the apex of the free villus, such regions often show marked vascular congestion. The capillaries, as our injected specimens demonstrate, within the ambit of a major villous system normally do not anastomose with capillaries of terminal villi of adjacent major stems, that is to say between vessels of adjacent foetal cotyledons. In this regard our conclusions correspond to those of Lemtis (1955/56). Stieve (1940) described extensive anastomoses by way of adhesions between villi. Some such vascular communications are found rarely in our material and most of these are probably between adjacent villi irrigated from a common stem. The material injected with Chromopaque and X-rayed, and the latex and Perspex preparations, substantiate that, normally, there are no (or at least very few) communications between the respective territories of distribution of the two umbilical arteries (Fig. 54). As already indicated, mature free villi are more richly vascularized than younger ones. The vessels in the former, especially in the region of the epithelial plates also tend to be more intimately related to the syncytium. Structurally the vessels of the terminal villi, although of larger diameter, closely resemble capillaries elsewhere. They are frequently accompanied by pericytes with which they may be closely associated by a reticular network or by fusion of their basement membranes.

In electron micrographs the villous capillary endothelium is of the type that does not possess pores; at the level of their nuclei the endothelial cells may be as thick as 5 μ but, especially in dilated vessels, their peripheral parts can be extremely thin (Figs. 65, 70 and 71). The endothelial cytoplasm possesses the usual organelles, including Golgi apparatus, and often shows signs suggesting pinocytosis, with foveolae on both the luminal and external surfaces (Fig. 81). A striking feature in many micrographs is the presence in the endothelial cells of innumerable fine fibrillae which may be contractile. Junctions between adjacent endothelial cells are marked by the presence of maculae adhaerentes and other desmosome-like structures. Flap-like projections into the lumen of the capillaries are frequently seen and often seem to be concerned in the formation of microvesicles. A basement membrane usually surrounds the capillary endothelium and, as

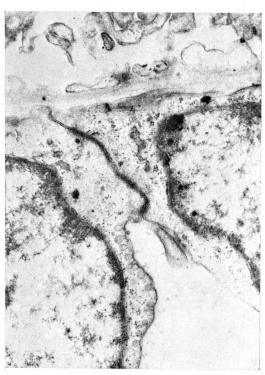

FIG. 81. Electron micrograph of the junction of two endothelial cells in a stromal capillary; elongated desmosomes are present along the line of fusion. On the luminal surface of one of the cells there are numerous foveolae indicative presumably of surface transport. On the external surface of the cells there is a poorly defined basement membrane separating them from the base of the syncytium which consists of cytoplasmic processes lying in a space (artefact?). (Foetus, 98 mm. C.R. length.) × c. 44,000.

already discussed may be fused with the basal lamina of the trophoblast to form a syncytio-vascular membrane. The cytoplasm of the pericytes may contain an abundance of the endoplasmic reticulum and there may be a high concentration of ribosomes. The pericyte nuclei are usually irregularly notched and may be electron dense. At full-term some of the free villi (presumably those most recently formed) are still devoid of capillaries; avascular villi, indeed, are present at all stages commonly in, or near, regions of placental infarction but sporadically in otherwise apparently normal placentae. Such avascular villi often show a mucoid degeneration of their stroma and, particularly in anchoring villi or ramuli, they possess a well developed central core of collagen (Pl. 3, Fig. 12).

Hofbauer Cells

These cells were first fully described in the villi of normal placentae by Hofbauer (1903a and b, 1905); attention had earlier been drawn to them in the stroma of hydatid moles by Chaletzky (1891) and Neumann (1897). Kossmann (1892) referred to them as "wandering cells" and figured them in the stroma of normal placentae. Hofbauer cells are circular or ellipsoidal in shape, possessing a circular nucleus with dense chromatin, a well developed nucleolus and a vacuolated cytoplasm; the vacuoles may be separated or show coalescence. The cells often possess

PLATE 1.

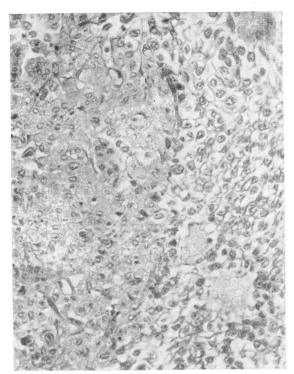

Fig. 1. Photomicrograph of a section (Masson's trichrome stain) of the foetal-maternal junction of a 28-somite implantation site. The foetal tissue (below) shows the trophoblastic shell, the tip of a villus with a cytotrophoblastic column and some residual syncytium. Interspersed among the typical cytotrophoblastic cells of the shell are darkly staining fusiform cells. In the upper portion of the figure the decidua is surrounded by blue-staining collagen in striking contrast to the appearance presented by the cytotrophoblast. × c.150.

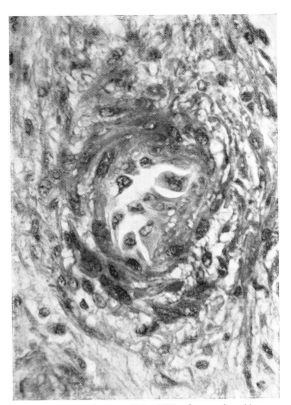

Fig. 2. Photomicrograph (× 350) of a section (Azan stain) through an endometrial spiral artery close to the implantation site of a 28-somite embryo. The cells of the endothelium of the vessel are markedly hypertrophied.

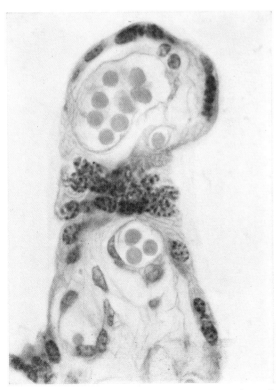

Fig. 3. Photomicrograph of a transverse section of two terminal villi showing syncytial fusion. The endothelium of the dilated capillary is in close contact with the syncytium particularly at the epithelial plates. (Full-term placenta.) Haematoxylin and eosin. × c. 1,000.

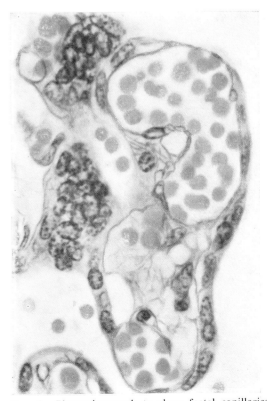

Fig. 4. Photomicrograph to show foetal capillaries and epithelial plates in terminal villi. There is syncytial fusion between three adjacent villi. (Full-term placenta.) Luxol fast blue, P.A.S., haematoxylin. × c. 1,000.

PLATE 2.

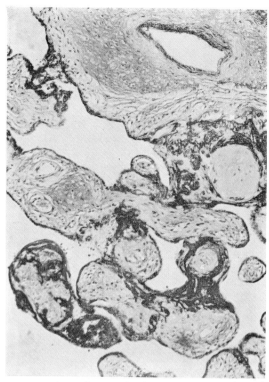

FIG. 5. Photomicrograph of a transverse section of villi with related fibrinoid. (Foetus, 210 mm. C.R. length.) × c. 100.

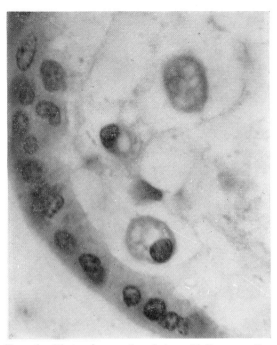

FIG. 6. Photomicrograph of two Hofbauer cells. Note the vacuolated cytoplasm of the cells and the loose texture of the stroma. Haematoxylin and eosin. × c. 1,000.

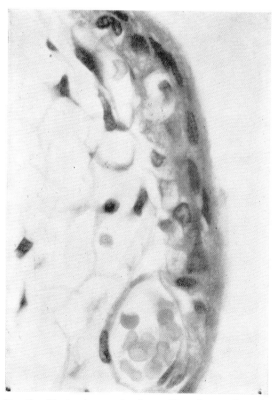

FIG. 7. Photomicrograph of a section of a portion of a villus to show a capillary in contact with flattened Langhans cells; another small capillary is present near a Langhans cell. (Foetus, 61 mm. C.R. length.) Haematoxylin and eosin. × c. 1,000.

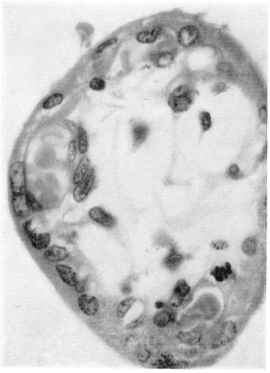

FIG. 8. Photomicrograph of a transverse section of a villus. A capillary wall is in contact with the syncytium which in some regions is still relatively thick and its nuclei are aggregating to form syncytial knots. Cytotrophoblast is present and shows mitotic activity. (Foetus 230 mm. C.R. length.) Haematoxylin and eosin. × c. 1,000.

PLATE 3.

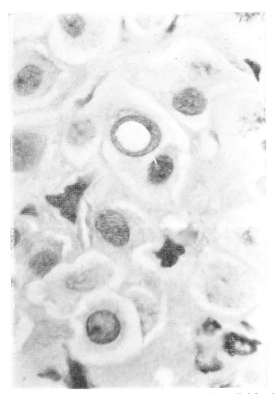

FIG. 9. Photomicrograph of part of the cell island illustrated in Plate 3, Fig. 10. The cytotrophoblastic cells have a finely granular cytoplasm; their nuclei show evidence of nuclear secretion and one of them possesses a large secretory vacuole. Picro-Mallory. × c. 600.

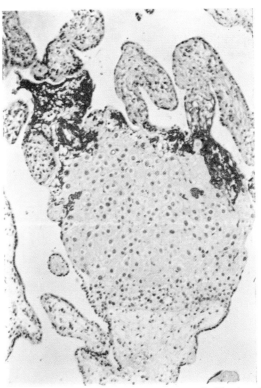

FIG. 10. Photomicrograph of a cytotrophoblastic cell island; villi are attached to it by fibrinoid. (Foetus, 115 mm. C.R. length.) Picro-Mallory. × c. 130.

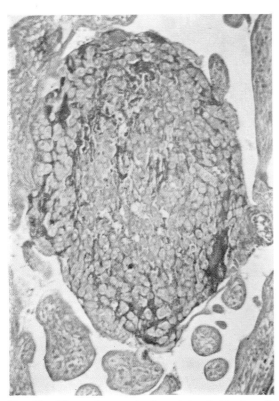

FIG. 11. Photomicrograph of a cytotrophoblastic cell island of which many of the cells are enmeshed by fibrinoid. (Foetus, 135 mm. C.R. length.) Haematoxylin and P.A.S. × c. 100.

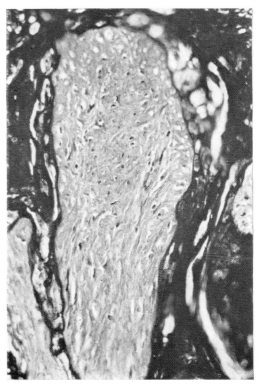

FIG. 12. Photomicrograph of a section of an anchoring villus penetrating the fibrinoid stria of the basal plate. Only a few degenerating cytotrophoblastic cells remain (Foetus, 280 mm. C.R. length.) × c. 250.

PLATE 4.

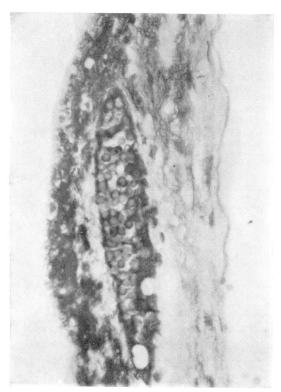

FIG. 13. Photomicrograph of a section of a portion of the chorionic plate to show the deposition of fibrin. (Foetus, 65 mm. C.R. length.) × c. 400.

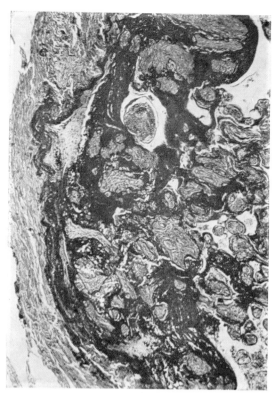

FIG. 14. Photomicrograph of a section of a portion of the basal plate to show villi with degenerating cytotrophoblast enmeshed in fibrinoid. (Foetus, 280 mm. C.R. length.) × c. 60.

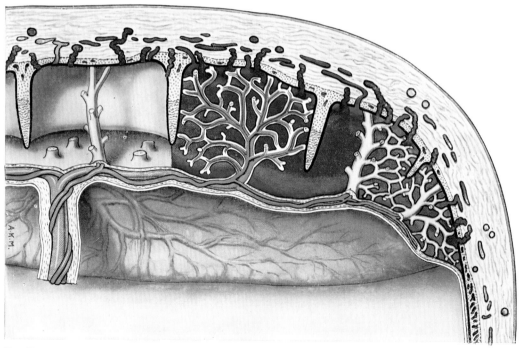

FIG. 15. Scheme to show the essential features in placental structure which are found after the 60 mm. stage. Three cotyledons, including a marginal one, are illustrated; the cotyledons are separated from each other on the maternal side by the septa. They each contain the group of villi which constitute the associated 'foetal' cotyledon. The villi branch freely and there are many adhesions between adjacent ones so giving a partially labyrinthine nature to the intervillous space. Such villi are shown in relief in the marginal cotyledon and in section in the adjacent one. The third cotyledon has been dissected to show the arrangement of the septa. The openings of the endometrial arteries and veins into the intervillous space through the basal plate are indicated and an attempt has been made to show the probable degree of oxygenation of the maternal blood in the intervillous space. A marginal sinus in the intervillous space has not been included in the scheme as our material does not show such a feature.

irregular surfaces and, from presomite stages onwards, are located in the interstices of the reticular meshwork of the villous stroma; not infrequently several Hofbauer cells are found in a single loculus of this meshwork (Pl. 2, Fig. 6). An extensive literature on them (summarized by Bleyl, 1962b, and Horky, 1964), has not yet clarified the functional significance of the Hofbauer cells. They are generally considered to be of mesenchymal origin and, owing to their reactions to vital dyes, allied to histiocytes or macrophages. More recently it has been suggested that they play a part in the transport of substances between the basement membrane of the trophoblast and the foetal capillary endothelium. Some investigators have considered that the Hofbauer cells may, in whole or in part, be derived from Langhans layer (Durst-Zivkovic, 1965). At different stages of development we have occasionally seen indications of a cytotrophoblastic origin for stromal elements. As stressed above, however, a basal lamina separating completely the trophoblast from the stroma is a striking feature of placental histology.

Mitotic figures have been observed in Hofbauer cells in our material; Horky (1964), however, was unable with certainty to demonstrate mitosis in them. Histochemical tests indicate the presence of mucopolysaccharides, mucoproteins and lipids in the Hofbauer cell vacuoles. We have located both acid and alkaline phosphatase in the cells but the reactions for the latter are variable. A number of investigators, including Hofbauer (1925) himself, have considered that these cells are only found in placentae up to the fourth or fifth month of gestation. Bleyl (1962a and b) and Becker and Seifert (1965), however, have described them in older specimens and we find them up to full-term (Fig. 80), although relatively fewer in number than in the middle trimester. Hofbauer cells are also found in the mesenchyme of the chorionic plate but we are unable to verify statements that they are present in the decidua and myometrium; Horky (1964) considers that their numbers increase in cases of maternal diabetes mellitus.

Electron micrographs show that the Hofbauer cells have large numbers of mitochondria and that the characteristic vacuoles often contain an electron-opaque precipitate (Fig. 72). In mature villi they still possess many vesicles, mitochondria and well developed ergastoplasm (Fig. 80) similar to the organelles described for earlier specimens by Bargmann and Knoop (1959), Lister (1963) and Panigel and Anh (1964).

Intercotyledonary Placental Septa

The placental lobes of mature placentae are incompletely separated from each other by projections into the IVS from the basal plate. These projections, called the placental septa, first become apparent in the third month; they gradually increase in height as pregnancy continues, but their free margins never normally reach the chorionic plate. The authors (Boyd and Hamilton, 1966a) have recently given a detailed account of their views on the origin, histology, and possible functional significance of the septa. Notwithstanding statements, based on sex chromatin analysis (Klinger and Ludwig, 1957; Serr

et al., 1958) and on histological observations (Waidl, 1963; Hörmann, 1966), that the septa are of maternal origin, and the many descriptions in the literature alleging a purely foetal origin for them, we concluded that they possess both maternal and foetal elements. Moreover, especially in older placentae, the septa are more attenuated and irregular in arrangement than is generally appreciated. It does not seem likely that they can have the role assigned to them by many investigators of acting as effective partitions between the placental cotyledons. The central parts of some septa may become cystic ("septal cysts" of Fox, 1965b; "Pseudocysten" of Hörmann, 1966), sometimes early in pregnancy, but in general our material supports Fox's conclusion that the cysts increase in number with placental ageing. Similar cysts are also found in cell islands (Fig. 79).

FIBRIN AND FIBRINOID

Through implantation the foetal tissues are brought into intimate contact with the cells of the endometrium and into direct relationship with maternal blood, lymph and interstitial tissue fluids. As these maternal fluids contain fibrinogen in varying amounts it is not surprising that fibrin comes to be laid down in the developing placenta. Indeed, in the IVS, maternal blood is in direct contact with trophoblastic syncytium and it is, perhaps, surprising that more coagulation than is usually found does not occur in this space. The syncytium may possess (like the endothelium of maternal blood vessels) qualities which inhibit clotting or it may augment fibrinolytic activity and so tend to keep the clotting at a minimum. There is, however, a general increase in fibrin deposition in the placenta during gestation. Wilkin (1958), for example, states that in surface extent at full-term there is seven times as much of it as at the end of the first trimester.

In addition to such coagulation in the IVS, there is a deposition in placental structures of a material termed "fibrinoid", with marked resemblance to fibrin. The term was introduced by Neumann (1880) to describe certain substances found in degenerative conditions of connective tissue. There has been much discussion on the nature, source and method of origin of fibrinoid. Its relationship to fibrin has been widely accepted and many histologists regard the two as essentially identical. Fibrinoid, however, also possesses resemblances to certain other substances such as hyalin and amyloid which can be classified as products of colloidal degeneration (Fullmer, 1965).

Langhans* and his pupils, Nitabuch and Rohr, first described the placental fibrinoid deposits, which in fact they called fibrin. Langhans himself (1877) described a layer, or stria, of "canalized connective substance", later named "canalized fibrin", on the chorionic plate in the IVS (Pl. 4, Fig. 13). As this region is junctional he suggested that the layer might be of foetal or maternal origin and he distinguished two components in it—a juxta-chorionic compact zone and a lamellar zone adjacent to the blood in the IVS. In 1887 Nitabuch described an equivalent

---

* An interesting account of Langhans' work and that of his pupils in Placentology is given by Dr. F. Strauss in *Mitt. d. Naturforsch. Gesellschaft in Bern*, band 14.

layer in the substance of the basal plate and considered it to separate the maternal from the foetal cells. In the following year Wolska (1888) drew attention to similar material in the basal plate but lying nearer to the IVS; Rohr (1889) added details to the description of this layer and his name has come to be associated with it. He recognized, however, that it is less constantly present than Nitabuch's stria. In our own material at all stages the two layers in the basal plate do not constitute completely separate entities; strands of the deposit of which they are constituted can frequently be traced from one layer to the other through the interstices between the cells of the cytotrophoblastic shell and round the termination of the anchoring villi.

The term fibrinoid was not used in connexion with the placental deposits until Hitschmann and Lindenthal (1903) introduced it in the description of the so-called "white infarcts". A resulting long dispute on terminology led to Grosser (1909, 1925, 1927, 1952) proposing definitions distinguishing between fibrin and fibrinoid substances. Fibrin is the fibrous protein precipitated from the fibrinogen in blood, lymph or tissue fluids and is entirely of maternal origin. Fibrinoid was defined as a non-cellular non-fibrous homogeneous substance derived from heterogeneous sources, partly as a trophoblastic secretion, and partly as a product of degeneration of trophoblast and, possibly, of maternal tissues; it is blue when stained with Mallory's technique. In spite of its diverse origin, Grosser considered that fibrinoid was a definite entity to be distinguished from fibrin which, as stated above, he believed to be entirely of maternal origin. Wislocki and Bennett (1943) agreed with Grosser that fibrin and fibrinoid could be distinguished histologically and that fibrinoid could have either a foetal or a maternal origin. Later, however, Singer and Wislocki (1948) found that the affinities of fibrin and (placental) fibrinoid to certain colloidal dyes were remarkably similar. They concluded that chemically the two substances are identical or closely related, and indicated that when clotted under different conditions fibrinogen may yield two morphologically distinct types of precipitate—one (fibrin proper) reticular and fibrillar, the other (fibrinoid) homogeneous and compact. Busanny-Caspari (1952), Jobst (1955), Ludwig (1959), Shanklin (1959), Ortmann (1960), Huber et al. (1961) and Benirschke (1962) have all also indicated that there is no fundamental distinction between fibrin and fibrinoid; this opinion has become generally accepted.

There are, however, good reasons for considering that the question is not yet finally resolved. Thus, Geller (1959) has suggested that, in Langhans layer, the compact and more homogeneous stria is fibrinoid derived from foetal cells of the chorionic plate, whereas the "canalized fibrin" stems from the maternal blood. Horn and Horalek (1961), using a number of staining methods on placentae of different ages, identified two components in fibrinoid—one of placental origin, arising from degeneration of decidua and villi, and consisting mostly of glycoproteins, the other, plasma protein from maternal blood. Hughes (1961) and Wilkin (1965a) have also indicated histochemical differences between fibrin and fibrinoid. Fullmer

(1965) has summarized a number of possible origins other than fibrin for fibrinoid; these include: necrosis of collagen, combination of mucopolysaccharides with basic proteins, accumulation of abnormal proteins, degeneration of smooth muscle, gamma globulin, serum albumin and the so-called rheumatoid factors. Fullmer stresses that assessment of origin even by highly specific immunohistochemical methods does not necessarily implicate the identified protein in the production of a deposit or lesion to which it may be secondarily attracted. Brzosko et al. (1965), using such methods, however, have identified serum albumins and globulins in fibrinous placental foci; they consider that the proteins have penetrated into the placental tissues from both maternal and foetal circulations as the result, perhaps, of permeability changes or fibrinolytic disturbances. Hörmann (1966) considers fibrinoid to be a product of chorionic epithelium, its production being associated with hypoxia, hypercapnia and acidosis, and he interprets the substance as a "Konstructionsprinzip" of the placenta. He writes that fibrinoid "hat zum Fibrin des mutterlichen oder kindlichen Blutes wahrscheinlich keine Bezeihung".

If fibrin and fibrinoid have similar compositions they show different morphological characters in the placenta. The differences may, in part, be due to regional blood flow (Kretschmann, 1965) but, as stressed by Grosser (1925) and Wilkin (1965a), their sites of origin are different. Placental fibrin, of undoubted nature, in the form of lamellae between which are erythrocytes undergoing lysis is frequently found in the IVS. According to Wilkin such fibrin is preferentially located round infarcts in placental ischaemic necrosis. In addition, though not considered by Wilkin, the lamellar component of Langhans striae is undoubtedly fibrin as is also much of the deposit round individual villi (Fox, 1963). Fibrinoid, according to Wilkin, is localized in five regions: (1) as Nitabuch's membrane; (2) in the chorionic plate as the juxta-chorionic component of Langhans striae; (3) in the basal plate adjacent to the IVS—Rohr's striae; (4) in the truncus chorii and free villi; and (5) related to the cytotrophoblastic islands and comparable regions in the septa. To these regions we add the extensive deposits of fibrin and fibrinoid in the obliterated IVS related to the decidua capsularis. In many of the sites, e.g. Nitabuch's membrane, the fibrinoid is deposited in an extravascular position. Wilkin has stressed, and our own observations tend to make us agree, that fibrinoid related to the truncus chorii and villi is not initially produced on the external surface of the syncytium. When present in small amounts it usually lies between the cytotrophoblast and the syncytium, always separated by the latter from the maternal blood. When the syncytium degenerates the fibrinoid then comes into direct contact with this blood and it is in this way that Wilkin explains the fibrinoid sheaths investing the villi. On this exposed fibrinoid we consider that fibrin can be deposited. Figures 39, 42, 49 and 79, and Pl. 2, Fig. 5; Pl. 3, Figs. 10 and 11; and Pl. 4, Fig. 14 illustrate some aspects of such fibrinoid deposits as is shown in our material. As with so many aspects of placental histology the extensive variability in the amount and extent of fibrin

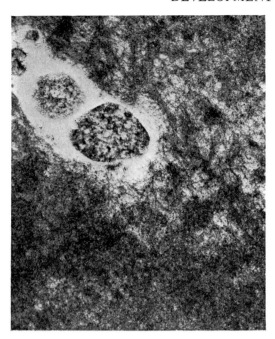

FIG. 82. Electron micrograph of canalized fibrin on the surface of a chorionic villus. Sections of villiform projections of syncytium are surrounded by fibrin (fibrinoid). Note indication of periodicity in fibrils. (Foetus, 170 mm. C.R. length.) × c. 44,000.

and fibrinoid deposits in different normal placentae, and even in different regions of a given placenta, must be stressed. In many areas fibrinoid comes to encapsulate within it cytotrophoblastic cells (the so-called "X" cells of Wilkin) and even isolated portions of syncytium.

Pappas *et al.* (1958) identified fibrin by electron microscopy in the fibrinoid lesions of the Schwartzman phenomenon. To our knowledge, however, there have been no specific electron microscopic observations on human placental fibrinoid. Fibrin (fibrinoid) has frequently been observed in our electron micrographs (Figs. 75, 77, 82 and 83) as close networks of thin filaments which cross each other to form a three-dimensional lattice, in the interstices of which blood platelets have occasionally been identified; presumably these have been associated with the clotting process itself and the subsequent contraction of the clot. Rarely is cross-striation found in the fibrin filaments; when present the periodicity of the striations is less than that found in collagen. In addition to the fibrin we have also observed osmiophilic deposits interpreted as fibrinoid (Figs. 82 and 83). Unlike those interpreted as fibrin, these fibrinoid deposits are only partially, if at all, fibrillar in nature; they often appear as a matrix of osmiophilic material surrounding circular profiles of degenerate cytoplasm, which can be identified as filiform projections from the surface of the cytotrophoblast or

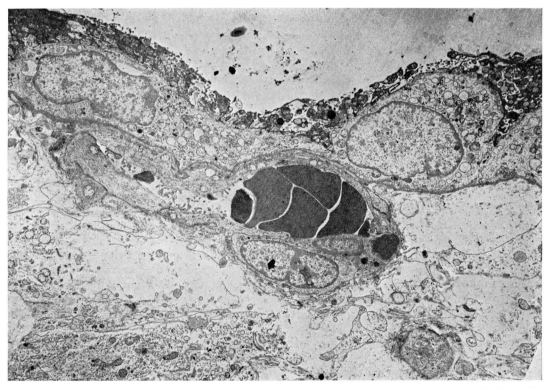

FIG. 83. Electron micrograph of a portion of a chorionic villus. The syncytium is almost completely replaced by fibrinoid. Langhans layer is well preserved and continuous in this portion of the villus. A foetal capillary is present under the basal trophoblastic lamina. The appearances in the syncytium are considered to represent the development of canalized fibrin. (Foetus, 170 mm. C.R. length.) × c. 5,400.

syncyutim (Fig. 82). Not infrequently such fibrinoid material is continued into areas of true fibrin.

Our material indicates that placental fibrin and fibrinoid increase during the last six months of pregnancy. Nevertheless, in many young specimens the deposits of these substances are distinctly greater than in much older and even in mature placentae. It is difficult to quantitate the differences in the extent of the deposits; amongst other things there is much regional variation. We have the general impression that "fibrin" is much commoner in the older specimens and that the amount of placental "fibrinoid" diminishes with age. The latter may be progressively converted into fibrin as development continues; it may, however, represent a stage in the discharge of secretory products from the cytotrophoblast. This latter possibility is particularly relevant in relation to the cells of the trophoblastic islands and of the basal decidua (Dallenbach-Hellweg and Nette, 1964).

O'Meara and Jackson (1958) describe fibrin deposits in relation to neoplasms and considered that the tumour cells may release a thromboplastic substance which coagulates the fibrinogen in the extra-cellular fluid. O'Meara and Thornes (1961) and Boggust et al. (1963) later demonstrated a thermolabile thromboplastic in the normal chorion and Clarke (1965) has indicated that this substance may be located as minute particles in the chorionic cells of full-term placentae.

Our own specimens (Hamilton and Boyd, 1960), and those described by a number of other investigators (Ludwig, 1959), demonstrate that fibrin is deposited very early in relation to human implantation sites; this fibrin is extra-cellular in position. Ludwig, who accepts the identity of fibrin and fibrinoid, has suggested that such deposits protect the decidua from syncytial cytolytic activity; indeed, he indicates that where the chorionic villi meet fibrin the syncytium retrogresses and thus cytotrophoblast comes into direct contact with fibrin. It is in this fashion that Ludwig explains the anchoring of villous branches to the basal plate. Owing to the first adherent villi being outstripped in growth by adjacent ones, he believes that islands of basal decidua become detached from the basal plate and remain attached to villi in the IVS. Ludwig attributes the increase in fibrin deposition in older placentae to the loss in endometrial fibrinolytic activity described by Albrechtsen (1956) and to decrease in syncytial cytolytic activity which, according to the old observations of Gräfenberg (1910), ceases after the fourth month; Ludwig considers that, by then, active growth of the placenta has terminated. The observations described earlier in the present communication demonstrate that Ludwig's conclusion on the relationship of fibrin deposition to placental growth can hardly be accepted. His other conclusions, however, must be kept in mind in any analysis of fibrin deposition.

Fluctuating fibrinolytic activities may be involved in the waxing and waning of the deposit of fibrin and fibrinoid during pregnancy. More knowledge on the histology of early stages of clotting and of the fibrinogen-fibrin transition is necessary for an explanation of early fibrin deposition. In particular it is desirable to have observations on placental fibrin deposition in conditions where there is a reduction in the maternal circulating fibrinogen. Nilsen (1963) has summarized information supporting the conclusion that hypofibrinogenaemia of abruptio placentae is the result of extensive fibrin deposition in the retroplacental region. After an extensive survey of the literature and our own material we are left with the impression that there are sufficient differences between placental fibrin and fibrinoid to justify the retention of the latter term.

MATERNAL VESSELS AND INTERVILLOUS SPACE

Uterine Spiral Arteries

The endometrial vascular system constitutes one of the most reactive in the body (Schmidt-Matthiesen, 1963) and the spiral arteries are continually changing in response to the hormonal and local manifestations of the uterine cycle. In pregnancy and the puerperium the uterine vessels generally undergo even more spectacular alterations. Whatever the explanation of the precise method whereby the spiral arteries themselves come to open into the intervillous space we have not been able to find communications of the arteries with the space until the 10 mm. stage. Even at this stage the communications are only by way of gaps in the trophoblastic shell. Doubtless capillaries have been tapped long before this stage and as their blood pressure is presumably higher than that of the veins a proper circulation through the intervillous space then becomes possible. In our 28-somite specimen, for example, the probability that such a circulation existed in life seems most likely. Indeed, Ortmann (1938) has described spiral arteries opening directly into the intervillous space in a 9-somite embryo originally described by Veit & Esch (1922). In our well-fixed 28-somite specimen, while we have found appearances very similar to some of those illustrated by Ortmann, we have been unable to convince ourselves that the spiral arteries themselves actually open into the intervillous space. But whether they do or do not so communicate already in the 28-somite specimen, the walls of the terminal portions of the spiral arteries show marked alteration and, in particular, a marked hypertrophy of their endothelial linings (Pl. 1, Fig. 2). In subsequent stages the changes in the walls of the arteries become much more marked so that, for long stretches of their length, back from the implantation site, they show a striking degenerative appearance, with disappearance of their muscle cells, hyaline alterations in their walls, and dilatation of the terminal parts of their lumina. Further, from the period when the spiral arteries can actually be found to communicate with the intervillous space, there is the appearance of cells within their lumina (Boyd & Hamilton, 1956). Some of these intrusive cells are certainly of foetal origin for they possess the same histological characteristics as the cytotrophoblast and, indeed, can be traced directly from the shell into the arteries (Figs. 11 and 20). It is possible that some of the intravascular cells in the more proximal part of the spiral arteries are of maternal origin, being derived from the hypertrophied endothelium, the muscle cells, or, even, migrating elements from the adjacent decidua. Our strong impression, however, is that most of the intravascular intrusive cells are of trophoblastic origin.

Up to the 43 mm. stage such cells are found in all of the arteries that pass through the transitional zone and they are also present in many of these vessels until much later stages (see illustrations in Boyd, 1956). The presence of these cells within the spiral arteries during human pregnancy has been recorded by a number of investigators (for summary, see Grosser, 1927). Similar intravascular cells have been reported in the pregnant uteri of other mammals (for summary, see Orsini, 1954). The discussion in the literature has chiefly related to the possible origin of these intra-arterial cells; little consideration has been given to their possible functional import. The constancy with which they are present in the human subject seems to us to justify the conclusion that they play some part in the placental mechanism, probably by cutting down very considerably the pressure in the blood which reaches the intervillous space. In several of our specimens in which we injected India ink into the main uterine arteries, subsequent histological examination of the placentae showed that the ink passed from the spiral arteries through the restricted spaces between the intravascular cells and then by way of very narrow chinks in the cytotrophoblast before reaching the intervillous space itself (Fig. 28). Under such conditions the pressure of the blood reaching the intervillous space must be very much reduced. The extension of the trophoblast into the arteries is obviously not due merely to the growth of this foetal tissue. The invasion of the arteries is selective for it can be affirmed quite dogmatically that, in the human placenta, the veins draining from the intervillous space never show such an invasion.

As has been stated previously, the sinusoids draining the early trophoblastic lacunae can readily be traced to the basal endometrial veins. As development continues the sinusoids increase in number and, indeed, cannot be distinguished from veins. In our earlier specimens the veins are found draining at irregular intervals from the whole of the basal surface of the developing placenta. Ortmann (1938), in his somite specimen, describes and figures the venous drainage as being exclusively from the central part of the basal plate. In our somite specimens, however, the drainage is both central and from the margin. As development proceeds the central veins are retained (Fig. 24) and are progressively added to in number as the placenta increases in size. In none of our placentae up to the 60 mm. stage is there an exclusive venous drainage from the marginal placental zone.

From our observations on the arterial supply to, and the venous drainage from, the intervillous space it seems to us justifiable to conclude that the circulation of maternal blood through the early placenta is under conditions which suggest that the pressure of the blood is low and its rate of flow slow. Moreover, as the maternal arteries and veins are connected with the intervillous space at

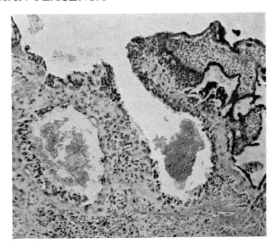

Fig. 84. Photomicrograph of the terminal loop of a spiral artery and of its slightly constricted opening into the IVS between the attachments of two villi. Cytotrophoblastic cells are present attached to the vessel lining and extending into the adjacent wall. (Foetus, 115 mm. C.R. length.) Haematoxylin and eosin. × c. 55.

random over the whole of the basal plate, the circulation in the space cannot be one that follows a fixed path. There may, perhaps, be some preferential channels through the intervillous space but our attempts to establish their presence have been quite unsuccessful. This overall picture of blood entering and leaving the intervillous space at random is not very satisfying, particularly if one is looking for an optimum method for gaseous exchange between the maternal and the foetal organism. Nevertheless, we consider that it corresponds with what is to be found from an unprejudiced survey of the *in situ* placenta.

In the older specimens numerous direct openings of the spiral arteries into the IVS are found, scattered apparently at random, over the basal plate (Figs. 78, 84–86). Photomicrographs of such openings have already been published (Boyd, 1956, 1960; Hamilton and Boyd, 1960). Not infrequently the openings of several such arteries are grouped closely together, and they may be near or actually in the basal part of a developing placental septum. The openings are usually at the terminal end of an artery; not infrequently, however, the trophoblastic erosion may involve several coils or turns of a closely wound, or of what was originally a closely wound, spiral artery. As a consequence multiple openings into the vessel may be present; later these can become separated by the unwinding of the coils and the straightening out of the artery during placental growth. In this fashion as many as five openings into the IVS may be established from a single spiral artery (Fig. 86). Usually, however, only one or two such communications are found. When there are multiple openings the segment of the artery between them often shows complete obliteration of its lumen by thrombosis.

The endothelial cells of the arteries become hypertrophied, often projecting in a striking manner into the lumen of the vessel, and, at the same time, their muscle cells show marked degenerative changes, the interstitial matrix

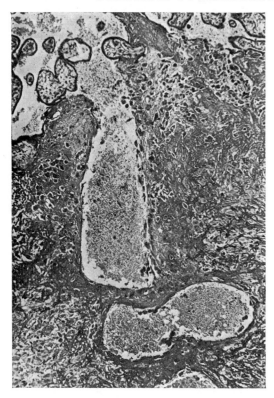

FIG. 85. Photomicrograph to show the opening of a spiral artery into the IVS. The artery wall shows marked degenerative changes. The intraluminal cytotrophoblastic cells are diminished in number. Nitabuch's stria is attached to the vessel wall. (Foetus, 175 mm. C.R. length.) Haematoxylin and eosin. × c. 50.

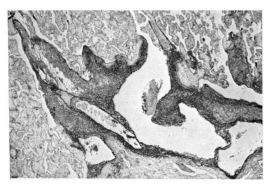

FIG. 86. Photomicrograph to show the terminal coils of a spiral artery at the base of an intercotyledonary septum. There is one free communication with the IVS, another is closed by the attachment of a villus, and yet another small third branch extending into the septum is obliterated by terminal thrombus. (Foetus, 210 mm. C.R. length.) × c. 15.

becoming altered to give the staining reactions of fibrinoid. As a result extensive stretches of spiral arterial wall become completely devoid of cellular elements and, presumably, quite incapable of contractility. Indeed, where such an artery pierces Nitabuch's membrane it may be impossible to define its margin (Fig. 85). Accompanying the degeneration of the media there is

usually a dilatation of the vessel lumen and the appearance in its wall of large round, or polyhedral, cells which, in some instances, seem to have arisen *in situ* from endothelial, muscle or connective tissue elements. Brettner (1964) has summarized the related literature and concludes that the arterial changes are part of the decidual reaction. Many investigators, however, have considered them to be pathological in nature and associated with maternal hypertension (Brosens, 1963; Brosens and Dixon, 1966). A further peculiarity of the spiral arteries is that there is a remarkable extension of cells (Figs. 78, 84 and 85) from the cytotrophoblastic shell along the lumina of many of them (Grosser, 1927; Boyd, 1956; and Hamilton and Boyd, 1960, 1966b). It is from such extensions that some trophoblastic cells may invade the arterial walls.

The alterations in the walls of the spiral arteries are already established throughout the basal plate region at the beginning of the second trimester and become progressively more apparent until about the end of the sixth month of gestation; later the intraluminal trophoblastic cells diminish in numbers, eventually disappearing from most of the vessels. As already stated, the changes in the walls of the terminal segments of the spiral arteries are of such a nature that they must have lost their contractility; consequently, control of the flow of blood to the IVS cannot be attributed to local vasomotor activity. The persistence for a considerable time of the plugs of trophoblastic cells in the lumina of many of the spiral arteries suggests that the blood pressure in them during this time cannot be very high, otherwise the plugs would be dislodged. A number of workers (Zeek and Assali, 1950; Marais, 1962c and d, 1963; Brosens, 1964; Brosens and Dixon, 1966) who have described the changes in these arteries interpret them as arteriosclerotic in nature. Much of our material from normal pregnancies regularly shows these quasi-arteriosclerotic changes; we consider, therefore, that care must be exercised to avoid confusing the changes in these vessels during normal pregnancy with alterations that are, in fact, pathological. Marais (1962b) would appear to share this opinion; he writes, "A certain degree of decidual spiral arteriosclerosis must be regarded as normal."

Counts or estimates of the number of spiral arteries opening into the IVS have been made by few investigators. The earliest assessment we have found is that given by Klein (1890) who stated that two or three endometrial veins drain the centre of each "maternal cotyledon" while 3–5 endometrial arteries are related to their margins. Bumm (1893) interpreted Klein as indicating that in the average placenta there are some 84 freely communicating vessels of which 31 are veins and 53 arteries. Much later, Spanner (1934, 1935) made counts on human placental spiral arteries in an injected specimen at the middle of the eighth month of gestation (?*in situ*) and found 94 spiral endometrial arteries communicating with the IVS. As individual arteries, however, had a number of terminal mouthpieces opening into the IVS the total counts of openings was 488. Spanner did not indicate clearly his criteria for regarding a vessel as an individual spiral artery. Moreover, other aspects of his work (e.g. his denial of generalized venous openings) leave doubt about his conclusions. Franken (1954), on whole fresh placentae, found an average of 263 arterial and 79 venous openings in a whole placenta; for a separate cotyledon the figures were 24 and 7 respectively. Brosens (1965) found 48 spiral arteries in two-fifths of a placenta, and therefore estimated that the total number in the basal plate was of the order of 120, i.e. approximately one artery to every two square centimetres of the plate. Reynolds (1966) states that the number of "endometrial arterioles" entering the IVS is 40–50 without, however, indicating how his assessment was made.

One of us (Boyd, 1956, 1960), from counts in known areas of three placentae in the third and fourth months of pregnancy, estimated that the total number of arterial communications into the IVS varied between 102 and 156; for three term placentae the figures were 180, 310 and 320. Marais (1962a) found 105 to be the largest number of spiral arteries to enter the IVS of a mature placenta but regarded this figure as minimal since the technique he employed did not permit of an accurate quantitative assessment. Boyd had also stressed that his counts could only be regarded as a first approximation; amongst other difficulties it was often impossible to determine if a single endometrial artery possessed multiple orifices. We (Hamilton and Boyd, 1960, 1966b) have shown that in the course of gestation portions of the spiral arteries may be obliterated by cytotrophoblast or thrombosis. The obliteration may involve areas at a distance from the IVS itself, hence fully functional arteries are fewer in number than histologically identifiable vessels.

From studies on the macaque monkey, Ramsey (1959, 1962) estimated that some 40 veins and 20 arteries (the outside limit being 50 veins and 30 arteries) communicate with the IVS. Ramsey et al. (1963), from a cineradioangiographic study in this species found no more than 17 arteries opening into the definitive (primary and secondary) placenta. Ramsey's estimates were based on serial sections of material embedded in toto from animals in the third trimester of pregnancy; hence these counts are presumably more reliable than those available for the human placenta. They are, however, smaller than would be expected from the comparative sizes of the placental areas in the monkey and the human if the number of openings of spiral arteries in the latter, as estimated by Spanner, Boyd, Franken and Marais, is correct.

Boyd's initial computations suggested an increase in the number of spiral arteries opening into the IVS in the course of human pregnancy. According to Ramsey (1954) the number of such openings in the monkey decreases in the later stages of pregnancy. There may be a species difference underlying the lack of agreement between Ramsey's and Boyd's counts; differences in the methods used for computing the number of openings may possibly explain the discrepancy. It should perhaps be pointed out that apart from the size difference, pregnancy is distinctly longer in Man than in the monkey. This greater length could conceivably have an effect on the number of openings of spiral arteries into the IVS.

In the preparation of the present work, Boyd's (1956) material was resurveyed, particular attention being given to multiple openings and thrombosed vessels. It is apparent that while the counts suggest much the same numbers as given in 1956 a considerable proportion of the arterial openings could not have been functional communications. We are not yet able to give a satisfactory assessment of the number of *functional* communications in the normal human placenta; we consider, however, that it is distinctly greater than that indicated by Ramsey and her colleagues in the macaque monkey. Smart (1962) and Wilkin (1965a and b) have suggested that there may be a one-for-one relationship between the number of spiral arteries and the number of placental "subcotyledons" (in our terminology, lobules). Although we have been unable to produce definite evidence in support of this suggestion our tentative estimate of about 100 functional openings (including single and multiple ones) of spiral arteries into the IVS in the mature placenta makes their suggestion a not unreasonable one.

The radioangiographic studies of the maternal circulation in primate and human placentae by Borell et al. (1952, 1964), 1965a and b), Fernström (1955), Ramsey et al. (1960, 1963), Donner et al. (1963) and Eskes et al. (1965) have all shown that maternal blood enters the IVS of the villous haemochorial placenta in the form of discrete "spurts" from, it would seem, the patent orifices of only a few of the spiral arteries. What determines which orifices are in fact used at any given time is not apparent. In at least some of the macaque material, as studied by Ramsey and her colleagues, probably most of the orifices were, in fact, revealed by the technique. In human pregnancy, however, owing to limitations imposed by radiological risk, the total number of orifices has not been established. In one full-term case examined arteriographically Borell et al. (1965b) described 25 IVS openings of spiral arteries; these were derived from three "main branches" (presumably radial uterine arteries). Eskes et al. (1965), in a pregnancy of 26 weeks (hysterectomy for cervical carcinoma), record a total of only six arterial openings; the foetus in this instance weighed 890 grams. In in situ placentae of equivalent age, however, we have found as many as three arterial openings in a single section. In hysterectomies in which the uterine arteries were injected with India ink or Chromopaque we have observed darker areas in the IVS which may correspond to the "spurts" or jets described by Ramsey and her colleagues. The number of such regions is considerably in excess of the six recorded by Eskes et al. (1965). There are, of course, many factors that may cause artefacts in such radiological investigations. Nevertheless, it is remarkable that so few "spurts" from endometrial arteries into the IVS were found in a 26-week pregnant uterus. Borell et al. (1964) have described the influence of uterine contractions on the blood supply to the IVS from the 18th to the 20th week of gestation. The same group (1965a), in three full-term pregnancies with abnormal features, found a marked retardation of blood flow through the endometrial arteries during uterine contractions. This retardation was attributed, in part, to local compression of the arterial wall

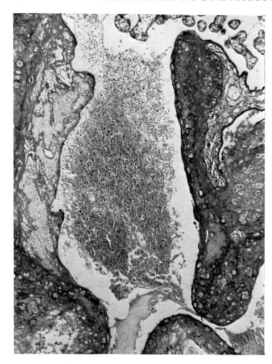

FIG. 87. Photomicrograph of the opening into the IVS of a maternal artery in a full-term pregnancy. Note the marked degeneration of the artery wall and the deposition of fibrin. × c. 200.

by the myometrium; contraction of arterial musculature and compression of the efferent veins, however, were also considered to play a part in the phenomenon.

Our material clearly shows that as full-term is approached the spiral arteries become more dilated but shorter and much less whorled than earlier (Fig. 87). Marais (1962a), in postpartum placentae, has described the arteries as being straight for as long as 2 cm. before entering the IVS. The decrease in the curling is, no doubt, due in part to the stretching of the uterine wall but can also be attributed to a gradual absorption of the arterial walls in a retrograde direction from their IVS extremities. Accompanying this shortening there is a dilatation of the regions of communication with the IVS (Ramsey, 1954a; Boyd, 1956; Wilkin, 1965b). The calibres of the communications are variable. In the fourth, fifth and sixth months they are frequently 500 to 1,000 μ in diameter but in this period are often partially obliterated by cytotrophoblast. It may be that such partial obliteration led Spanner (1935) to describe the arteries as possessing narrow nozzle-like extremities. Such terminal narrowing has also been recorded in plastic-injected vessels by Debiasi et al. (1963). In the last three months of pregnancy, however, both by an actual increase in calibre and by a diminution in the amount of cytotrophoblastic plug, we consider the size of the functional communications between the spiral arteries and the IVS is considerably increased. We have found them up to 2 mm. in diameter. William Hunter described them as possessing the diameter of a goose quill. A scheme of position of the placenta is shown in Plate 4, Fig. 15.

Intervillous Space (IVS)

The blood in the IVS, though maternal, is in contact with the foetal syncytium and ouside the confines of the endothelium of the mother's vascular system. Recognition of the space as an essential characteristic of the villous haemochorial placenta and interpretation of it as an extensive and complicated lacuna in the trophoblast represent great achievements of nineteenth-century placentologists. But although the general nature of the IVS has been understood for nearly one hundred years there is still uncertainty concerning many of its features (Martin, 1965; Freese, 1966). Most studies of it suffer the disadvantage of having been made on delivered placentae at or near term; indeed, even in specimens in situ we have found the nature of the IVS to vary with the fixative used and the method of fixation. Artefacts are probably minimal when fixation has been effected through injection of the uterine arteries and replacement of the amniotic fluid by the fixative before opening the uterine cavity; any injection technique, however, no matter how carefully carried out, must cause some distortion of the IVS. In life, contraction of the uterine musculature, alterations in the maternal and the chorionic villous circulations and variation in the volume of the amniotic fluid all probably contribute to periodic changes in the nature of the IVS. Hörmann (1951, 1953, 1958) and Lemtis (1955/56) consider the space to be an extremely attenuated one, of capillary dimensions, which they call the Zwischenzottenspaltsystem. Nielsen (1961) and Becker (1963) adopt a similar view; their views were based on a technique of injecting milk into the umbilical vein of delivered placentae at a pressure of 33 mm. Hg at which level placental turgor is, they consider, restored to its prevailing physiological value (the assessment of umbilical venous pressure was 35–40 mm. being the one made by Runge and Hartmann, 1930, that of the umbilical arteries being 70 mm. Hg). The placenta was then frozen in liquid nitrogen and sectioned at −27°C. According to Nielsen and Becker in specimens prepared in this manner only a striate cleft is present between the villi and no extensive space is visible; neighbouring villi cling closely to one another, the tips of some fitting into notches of others as in a jigsaw puzzle. Becker (1963) explains the appearance of a wider IVS in the material treated with routine histological techniques as the result of differential shrinkage of the various tissue components. Except for the subchorial lake, Freese (1966) also failed to demonstrate intervillous spaces of larger than capillary dimensions. But although parts of the IVS may, from time to time, be reduced to exiguous dimensions it seems to us unlikely that Hörmann's interpretation can hold regularly for the whole of it. The relatively high pressure of 70–80 mm. Hg (Alvarez and Caldeyro, 1950), of the maternal blood entering the space, the circulation (as indicated by radioangiography) of the blood within it and the effect of intermittent uterine contractions on it all demand a view of the IVS different from that of a network of fixed capillary diameter. Moreover, the presence of a subchorial "cyst" (of Kölliker) or "lake" (of Spanner) is contrary to Hormann's interpretation; Stieve (1952) considered dilation of the IVS adjacent to the chorionic plate to form the lake to be less marked than accepted by most investigators, but throughout pregnancy our specimens always show some indication of it (Figs. 39, 42 and 45). Becker (1963) does accept the existence in the IVS of larger gaps affording passage for the "jets" from the spiral arteries and permitting the blood to reach the chorionic plate whence it trickles back to the basal plate *via* narrower clefts with larger surface areas. But Becker indicates, and here we are in agreement with him, that the villous system is in constant movement as a consequence of which and of changes in the blood pressure (both villous and maternal) the channels in the IVS fluctuate in size and, thus, little rivulets can become main streams.

We agree with Martin (1965) in considering it unlikely that preformed and static channels for maternal blood exist within the IVS. Reynolds (1966) and Freese (1966) have recently supported the Wilkin (1954, 1958, 1965b) description of an intracotyledonary space in the IVS lying within a "*couronne d'implantation*" of the villi of a cotyledon. We have given much attention to Wilkin's interpretation but, as yet, have not been able to substantiate it.

While unable to commit ourselves to a view of the IVS that would make it as exiguous as Hörmann and his supporters believe, our frozen sections show that the IVS is less conspicuous than in paraffin wax embedded material. Moreover, in our *in situ* placentae the IVS is much more extensive if fixation had been effected by injection of the uterine arteries. With the existing imprecision in views on the nature of the IVS, it is obviously difficult, especially in delivered specimens, to be dogmatic on its total volume. We have some estimates for *in situ* placentae at different stages of pregnancy and find that throughout the second and third trimesters the values fall between 20 and 40 per cent.; the younger specimens showing relatively the larger volumes. For the whole placenta the average volume of 500 specimens was 497 ml. (range, 200–950 ml.). In 1922, Dodds gave 63 per cent. as the proportion of the placenta occupied by the IVS, Jonen (1927) recorded that, in 30 full-term specimens, this proportion lay between 30 and 41 per cent., while Vokaer and Vanden Eynden (1958) indicated for it an almost constant value of 35 per cent. Ortmann (1960) considered that the size of the space depends on several uncontrollable factors and probably varies between 17 and 33 per cent. Aherne and Dunnill (1966a and b) found the mean value for the volume of ten normal full-term placentae to be 488 ml. (range, 391–723 ml.) the corresponding mean absolute value for the IVS volume in their specimens being 144 ml. In 44 placentae the volume of the IVS had an average value of 37·5 per cent. of that of the placenta. Strauss (1964) has concluded that the normal full-term IVS volume falls between 175 and 250 ml.; he points out that if the figure of 600 ml. given by Browne and Veall (1953) as the minute volume is accepted there must be a lively circulation in the IVS. Wilkin (1965b) in an *in situ* specimen found the IVS ("*la chambre intervilleuse*") to have approximately double that of its average volume in expelled placentae (60 per cent. compared with 37·7 per cent.). Wilkin also records that, in a hysterectomy specimen at the eighth month, a plastic cast of the IVS

showed it as occupying more than half of the global placental volume. Measurements in our own material in the course of pregnancy also indicate that an *in situ* placenta possesses an IVS of greater volume than that of a comparable separated specimen though not to the extent found by Wilkin. Nevertheless, it seems not unlikely that in its physiological state the IVS of an *in situ* placenta is distinctly larger than can be assumed from measurements on delivered specimens. But, once again, we would stress that, in life, it seems highly likely that a given space is continuously varying in size.

Venous Drainage of the Intervillous Space

Between the basal placental plate and the myometrium in all our *in situ* material there is an extensive plexus of dilated veins which surrounds the residual portions of the uterine glands and obscures the relations of the basal decidua. These veins show extensive atrophy of their media, and indeed often appear to possess only an endothelial wall. From an early stage of development they communicate freely with the IVS (Hamilton and Boyd, 1960). Since the late nineteenth century many investigators have considered that the portions of this endometrial venous plexus related to the margin of the placentae have a special significance in the drainage of the IVS. Spanner (1935, 1941), in particular, included this peripheral venous ring within the IVS and adopted the term marginal sinus for it. He considered that essentially all the drainage from the IVS was by means of endometrial veins communicating exclusively with this marginal sinus.

A number of investigators (e.g., Stieve, 1940, 1941, 1952; Hamilton and Boyd, 1951, 1960; Kladetsky-Haubrich, 1952; Ramsey, 1956a and b; Wilkin, 1958, 1965b) have demonstrated, however, that there are numerous openings into the decidual venous plexus all over the basal plate. The number of the communications between the IVS and the veins is not yet well established; Spanner (1935), who restricted such openings to the periphery of the placenta, recorded 170 in a single specimen; Franken (1954) gave 79 as this average number. Though, individually, larger, often much larger, than those of the arteries, the venous openings do not appear to be as numerous. We have found it extremely difficult to attempt to enumerate them as they frequently open into "bays", or extensions, of the IVS itself and we have suggested (Boyd and Hamilton, 1966a) that, in fact, some of these extensions may be dilated venous openings. Some investigators, e.g., Stieve (1952), have described sphincteric arrangements in the walls of the venous plexus, but we have been unable to confirm their presence.

Bøe (1953), Franken (1954) and Wilkin (1965b) consider that the venous openings are concentrated principally in the periphery of the maternal cotyledons and therefore near the septa. Examination of our own material suggests that such openings have a random distribution though there is, perhaps, some tendency for them to be concentrated near the placental margin where there may be some variable dilatation of the IVS, apparently as a lateral extension of the subchorial lake. But we find that those regions which show some marginal dilatations usually represent no more than the areas between the peripherally situated cotyledon and the placental margin proper. Such regions often extend laterally, and irregularly, into that obliterated portion of the IVS related to the decidua capsularis and the chorion laeve.

Circulation in the Intervillous Space

The IVS is a space, the diameters of which in life are continuously varying but which, notwithstanding Hörmann's opinion to the contrary, are, for the most part, larger than of capillary dimensions. Into this extensive space open an insufficiently determined but large number of maternal arteries (or large arterioles) with diameters up to 1 mm. or even greater, and the venous drainage is through numerous orifices of diameters even greater than those of the arteries. Burwell (1938) suggested that the maternal circulation in the placenta represents an arterio-venous shunt. The blood pressure at the level of the utero-placental arteries is 70–80 mm. Hg. After entering the IVS the pressure rapidly diminishes, from the basal plate along the length of the "arterial jets", to reach a mean value of about 10 mm. Hg in the relaxed uterus and 30–50 mm. Hg during uterine contractions. The maternal blood finally passes into the utero-placental veins where the pressure is not more than 8 mm. Hg. As both arterial and venous orifices are scattered over the basal placental plate, the question arises as to why there is not short-circuiting of the maternal blood. Observations from a number of sources (Ramsey, 1954a, 1959; Ramsey et al., 1963, 1965; Borell et al., 1958, 1963; Nelson et al., 1961; and Martin, 1965) indicate that the arterial pressure, being much higher than that in the IVS, propels the entering blood towards the chorionic plate and that, thus, short-circuiting is prevented. Freese (1966) and Reynolds (1966), indeed, consider that the haemodynamic pressure of the entering blood arranges the villi into the "intracotyledonary crown" pattern described by Wilkin. When the momentum of the entering blood is much diminished, it spreads laterally amongst the villi whence it passes to the venous openings, being moved by the *vis a tergo* of the blood from subsequent "jets". This is the so-called "physiological concept" of the placental circulation which is supported by recorded mesurements of IVS and pelvic venous pressures. In women the IVS pressure approximates to that within the amniotic cavity and during myometrial relaxation lies between 6 and 10 mm. Hg (Caldeyro-Barcia, 1957; Hendricks et al., 1959; Hytten and Leitch, 1964). The pelvic venous pressure is slightly lower.

The blood flow to the uterus during pregnancy is partitioned between placenta (choriodecidual circulation, Dixon et al., 1963) and myometrium, that passing to the latter not participating in materno-foetal exchange. Available techniques do not permit of an easy or reliable quantitative estimate of the respective volumes of these two components of uterine blood flow. There is a great increase in non-placental uterine tissue during pregnancy and a significant part of the total uterine flow must be devoted to the myometrium and cervix. Nevertheless, the products of conception increase in mass even more rapidly and their share of perfusing blood is believed to increase proportionately; most of the uterine blood flow in the second half of pregnancy seems destined for passage through the IVS. Consequently variations of the uterine circulation will be directly reflected in the IVS circulation. Romney et al. (1959) found the average flow in thirteen women with single pregnancies to be 490 ml. per minute; in one woman with a twin pregnancy the flow was 1,150 ml. Assali et al. (1953) gave a flow rate of 750 ml. per minute in full-term pregnancy, and later Assali et al. (1960) indicated that uterine blood flow increased from 50 ml. per minute to 180 ml. per minute at 28 weeks. Martin (1965) has pointed out that the wide range of values given by investigators of uterine blood flow suggests that in addition to long term regulation (i.e., keying into the size and requirements of the metabolism of the uterus) there may be short term adjustments in the flow. With regard to long range regulation there is unfortunately, as has been explained earlier, little dependable information on the numbers, sizes and patency of spiral arteries throughout pregnancy. Martin quotes Crawford (1959) to the effect that after the twelfth week few maternal *vascular stems* are added to the placental complement. The spiral arteries are the site of the greatest fall in pressure in the maternal placental circulation. As the number of arterial orifices are presumed to remain nearly constant and cardiac outflow falls while uterine blood flow more than doubles, a regular and considerable decline in vascular resistance must occur throughout pregnancy; this decline may be explained by the increase in calibre of the arterial orifices and the gradual disappearance of the trophoblast within their lumina, which we have described above.

Ramsey (1962) has indicated that the placental blood flow is markedly diminished or actually abolished by myometrial compression of the utero-placental arteries. The whole situation is still confused and obscure; the trophoblastic cell plugs in the spiral arteries, the alleged venous sphincters, compression of the veins by myometrial contractions of an intermittent nature (first suggested by Braxton Hicks, 1872), and the descriptions of myometrial and endometrial arteriovenous anastomoses (Heckel and Tobin, 1956; Debiasi et al., 1963) all conspire to complicate an analysis of the blood flow through the placenta. Non-homogeneity of the IVS also probably contributes to variation in the flow (Fuchs et al., 1963). As pointed out by Winner (1965), however, the available information suggests that the interpretation of the placenta as a variety of arterio-venous shunt is probably not physiologically valid.

REFERENCES

Adair, F. L. and Thelander, H. (1925), *Amer. J. Obstet. Gynec.*, **10**, 172.
Aherne, W. and Dunnill, M. S. (1966a), *Brit. med. Bull.*, **22**, 5.
Aherne, W. and Dunnill, M. S. (1966b), *J. Path. Bact.*, **91**, 123.
Albrechtsen, O. K. (1956), *Acta endocr. (Kbh)*, **23**, 207.
Alvarez, H. (1964), *Obstet. and Gynec.*, **23**, 813.

Alvarez, H., Alvarez Santin, C., and De Bejar, R. (1962), *Arch. urug. Ginec. Ostet.*, **20**, 58.

Alvarez, H., and Caldeyro, R. (1950), *Surg. Gynec. Obstet.*, **91**, 1.

Alvarez, H., De Bejar, R., Aladjem, S., Alvarez Santin, C., Remedio, M. R. and Sica Blanco, Y. (1964), *Cuarto. Cong. urug. Ginec.*, **1**, 190.

Anderson, W. R. and McKay, D. G. (1966), *Amer. J. Obstet. Gynec.*, **95**, 1134.

Armitage, P., Boyd, J. D., Hamilton, W. J. and Rowe, B. C. (1967), *Hum. Biol.*, **39**, 430.

Ashley, C. A. (1965), *Arch. Path.*, **80**, 377.

Amstutz, E. (1960), *Acta anat. (Basel)*, **42**, 12.

Arts, N. F. T. (1961), *Amer. J. Obstet. Gynec.*, **82**, 147 and 159.

Assali, N. S., Douglass, R. A., Jr., Baird, W. M., Nicholson, D. B. and Sugemoto, R. (1953), *Amer. J. Obstet. Gynec.*, **66**, 248.

Assali, N. S., Rauramo, L. and Peltonen, T. (1960), *Amer. J. Obstet. Gynec.*, **79**, 86.

Baker, B. L., Hook, S. J. and Severinghaus, A. E. (1944), *Amer. J. Anat.*, **74**, 291.

Bargmann, W. (1957), *Geburtsh. u. Frauenheilk.*, **17**, 865.

Bargmann, W. and Knoop, A. (1959), *Z. Zellforsch.*, **50**, 472.

Bartelmez, G. W. (1957), *Contr. Embryol. Carneg. Instn.*, **36**, 153.

Becker, V. (1959), *Med. Ges. Kiel*, 23.7.59, *Ref. Klin. Wschr.*, 1204.

Becker, V. (1960), *Verh. dtsch. path. Ges.*, **44**, 256.

Becker, V. (1962), *Verh. dtsch. path. Ges.*, **46**, 309.

Becker, V. (1963), *Arch. Gynäk.*, **198**, 3.

Becker, V. and Seifert, K. (1965), *Z. Zellforsch.*, **65**, 380.

Benirschke, K. (1962), *Amer. J. Obstet. Gynec.*, **84**, 1595.

Bien, C. S. (1943), *Das Zottenraumgitter in der Placenta von Pithecus fascicularis Raffl.* Thesis, Univ. Berlin.

Bleyl, U. (1962a), *Z. Zellforsch.*, **56**, 404.

Bleyl, U. (1962b), *Arch. Gynäk.*, **197**, 364.

Bøe, F. (1953), *Acta obstet. gynaec. scand.*, **32**, Suppl. 5, 1.

Bøe, F. (1954), *Cold Spring Harb. Symp. Quant. Biol.*, **19**, 29.

Boggust, W. A., O'Brien, D. J., O'Meara, R. A. Q. and Thornes, R. D. (1963), *Irish J. med. Sci.*, **447**, 131.

Bonnet, R. (1907), *Lehrbuch der Entwickslungsgeschichte.* Berlin: P. Parey.

Borell, U., Fernström, I., Lindblom, K. and Westman, A. (1952), *Acta radiol. (Stockh.)*, **38**, 247.

Borell, U., Fernström, I. and Ohlson, L. (1963), *Amer. J. Obstet. Gynec.*, **86**, 535.

Borell, U., Fernström, I., Ohlson, L. and Wiqvist, N. (1964), *Amer. J. Obstet. Gynec.*, **89**, 881.

Borell, U., Fernström, I., Ohlson, L. and Wiqvist, N. (1965a), *Amer. J. Obstet. Gynec.*, **93**, 44.

Borell, U., Fernström, I., Ohlson, L. and Wiqvist, N. (1965b), *Acta obstet. gynec. scand.*, **44**, 22.

Borell, U., Fernström, I. and Westman, A. (1958), *Geburtsh. u. Frauenheilk.*, **18**, 1.

Bourne, G. L. (1962), *The Human Amnion and Chorion.* London: Lloyd-Luke.

Boyd, J. D. (1956), *Trans. Second Conference on Gestation*, p. 132. New York: Macy Foundation.

Boyd, J. D. (1959), *Ulster med. J.*, **28**, 35.

Boyd, J. D. (1960), *Utero-placental arteries* (Russian text). Moscow.

Boyd, J. D. and Hamilton, W. J. (1950), *Trans. Internat. Anat. Congr.*, *Oxford*, p. 30. London: C. U. P.

Boyd, J. D. and Hamilton, W. J. (1956), *J. Anat. (Lond.)*, **90**, 595.

Boyd, J. D. and Hamilton, W. J. (1960), *J. Obstet. Gynaec. Brit. Emp.*, **67**, 208.

Boyd, J. D. and Hamilton, W. J. (1964), *J. Obstet. Gynaec. Brit. Cwlth.*, **71**, 1.

Boyd, J. D. and Hamilton, W. J. (1966a), *Z. Zellforsch.*, **69**, 613.

Boyd, J. D. and Hamilton, W. J. (1966b), *J. Anat. (Lond.)*, **100**, 535.

Boyd, J. D. and Hughes, A. F. W. (1954), *J. Anat. (Lond.)*, **88**, 356.

Braxton-Hicks, J. (1872), *Trans. obstet. Soc. (Lond.)*, **14**, 149.

Bremer, J. L. (1916), *Amer. J. Anat.*, **19**, 179.

Brettner, A. (1964), *Acta anat. (Basel)*, **57**, 367.

Brewer, J. I. (1937), *Amer. J. Anat.*, **61**, 429.

Brewer, J. I. (1938), *Contr. Embryol. Carneg. Instn.*, **27**, 85.

Brosens, I. (1963), *Bull. Soc. roy. belge. Gynéc. Obstét.*, **33**, 61.

Brosens, I. (1964), *J. Obstet. Gynæc. Brit. Cwlth.*, **71**, 222.

Brosens, I. (1965), *The placental bed.* Thesis, Univ. London.

Brosens, I. and Dixon, H. G. (1966), *J. Obstet. Gynaec. Brit. Cwlth.*, **73**, 357.

Browne, J. C. M. (1954), *Cold Spring Harb. Symp. Quant. Biol.*, **19**, 60.

Browne, J. C. M. and Veall, N. (1953), *J. Obstet. Gynaec. Brit. Emp.*, **60**, 141.

Bryce, T. H. and Teacher, J. H. (1908), *Contributions to the Study of the Early Development of the Human Ovum*, pp. 7–66. Glasgow: Maclehose.

Brzosko, W., Nowoslawski, A. and Pisarski, T. (1965), *Ginek. pol.*, **36**, 121.

Bucher, O. (1959), in *Protoplasmatologia. Handbuch der Protoplasmaforschung*, **6**, *Kern- und Zellteilung*, E., *Amitose*, **1**, p. 1, eds. Heilbrunn and Weber. Berlin: Springer.

Bühler, F. R. (1964), *Acta anat. (Basel)*, **59**, 47.

Bumm, E. (1893), *Arch. Gynäk.*, **43**, 181.

Burstein, R., Handler, F. P., Soule, S. D. and Blumenthal, H. T. (1956), *Amer. J. Obstet. Gynec.*, **72**, 332.

Burwell, C. S. (1938), *Amer. J. med. Sci.*, **195**, 1.

Busanny-Caspari, W. (1952), *Virchows Arch path. Anat.*, **322**, 452.

Caldeyro-Barcia, R. (1957), in *Physiology of Prematurity; Trans. First Conf.*, p. 128, ed. Lanham. New York: Macy Foundation.

Calkins, L. A. (1937), *Amer. J. Obstet. Gynec.*, **33**, 280.

Chaletzky, Eva. (1891), *Hydatidenmole.* Thesis, Univ. Bern.

Clarke, N. (1965), *Nature (Lond.)*, **205**, 608.

Conte, D. (1965), *Attual. Ostet. Ginec.*, **11**, 705.

Costero, I. (1931), *Z. Anat. Entwickl. -Gesch.*, **96**, 766.

Crawford, J. M. (1956a), *J. Obstet. Gynaec. Brit. Emp.*, **63**, 87.

Crawford, J. M. (1956b), *J. Obstet. Gynaec. Brit. Emp.*, **63**, 542.

Crawford, J. M. (1956c), *J. Obstet. Gynaec. Brit. Emp.*, **63**, 548.

Crawford, J. M. (1959), *J. Obstet. Gynaec. Brit. Emp.*, **66**, 885.

Crawford, J. M. (1961), *J. Obstet. Gynaec. Brit. Cwlth.*, **68**, 378.

Crawford, J. M. (1962), *Amer. J. Obstet. Gynec.*, **84**, 1543.

Crawford, J. M. and Fraser, A. (1955), *J. Obstet. Gynaec. Brit. Emp.*, **62**, 896.

Dallenbach-Hellweg, G. and Nette, G. (1963a), *Virchows Arch. path. Anat.*, **336**, 528.

Dallenbach-Hellweg, G. and Nette, G. (1963b), *Z. Zellforsch.*, **61**, 145.

Dallenbach-Hellweg, G. and Nette, G. (1964), *Amer. J. Anat.*, **115**, 309.

Davies, F. (1944), *Trans. roy. Soc. Edinb.*, **61**, 315.

Debiasi, E., Damiani, N. and Capodacqua, R. (1963), *Minerva ginec.*, **15**, 539.

Desai, R. G. and Creger, W. P. (1963), *Blood*, **21**, 665.

Dible, J. H. and West, C. M. (1941), *J. Anat. (Lond.)*, **75**, 269–281.

Dixon, H. G., Browne, J. C. M. and Davey, D. A. (1963), *Lancet*, **2**, 369.

Dodds, G. S. (1922), *Anat. Rec.*, **24**, 287.

Donner, M. W., Ramsey, Elizabeth M. and Corner, G. W. Jr. (1963), *Amer. J. Roentgenol.*, **90**, 638.

Douglas, G. W., Thomas, L., Carr, M., Cullen, M. N. and Morris, R. (1959), *Amer. J. Obstet. Gynec.*, **78**, 960.

Dow, P. and Torpin, R. (1939), *Hum. Biol.*, **11**, 248.

Durst-Zivkovic, B. (1965), *Commun. 8th Internat. Anat. Congr., Wiesbaden*, p. 32. Stuttgart: Thieme.

Enders, A. C. (1965a), *Amer. J. Anat.*, **116**, 29.

Enders, A. C. (1965b), *Obstet. and Gynec.*, **25**, 378.

Eskes, T., Stolte, L., Seelen, J. and Lamping, P. (1965), *Arch. Gynäk.*, **200**, 735.

Fernström, I. (1955), *Acta radiol. (Stockh.)*, Suppl. 122, 3.

Fischel, A. (1929), *Entwicklung des Menschen.* Berlin: Springer.

Flexner, L. B., Cowie, D. B., Hellman, L. M., Wilde, W. S. and Vosburgh, G. J. (1948), *Amer. J. Obstet. Gynec.*, **55**, 469.

Florange, W. and Hoer, P. W. (1958), *Ann. Univ. sarav. Med.*, **6**, 1.

Florian, J. (1928), *Anat. Anz.*, **66**, *Erg. Heft.*, 211.

Fox, H. (1963), *J. Obstet. Gynaec. Brit. Cwlth.*, **70**, 980.

Fox, H. (1964a), *J. Obstet. Gynaec. Brit. Cwlth.*, **71**, 749.

Fox, H. (1964b), *J. Obstet. Gynaec. Brit. Cwlth.*, **71**, 885.

Fox, H. (1965a), *J. Obstet. Gynaec. Brit. Cwlth.*, **72**, 347.

Fox, H. (1965b), *J. Obstet. Gynaec. Brit. Cwlth.*, **72**, 745.

Franken, H. (1954), *Zbl. Gynäk.*, **76**, 729.

Frassi, L. (1908), *Arch. mikr. Anat. Entwick.*, **71**, 667.

Freese, U. E. (1966), *Amer. J. Obstet. Gynec.*, **94**, 354.

Fuchs, F., Spackman, T. and Assali, N. S. (1963), *Amer. J. Obstet. Gynec.*, **86**, 226.

Fujimura, G. (1921), *J. Morph.*, **35**, 485.

Fullmer, H. M. (1965), in *Internat. Rev. Connective Tissue Res.*, **3**, 1, ed. by Hall. London: Acad. Press.

Galton, H. (1962), *J. Cell. Biol.*, **13**, 183.

Geller, H. F. (1959), *Arch. Gynäk.*, **192**, 1.

Gerlach, H. (1962), *Statistich Untersuchungen über das Gewicht der Placenta und ihrer Anhange sowie über das Verhaltnis von Placentagewicht und Fruchtmasszahlen*. Thesis, Univ. Halle.

Getzowa, S. and Sadowsky, A. (1950), *J. Obstet. Gynæc. Brit. Emp.*, **57**, 388.

Gluschka, W. (1945), *Bindegewebige Zottenverbindungen einer menschlichen Plazenta aus dem Anfang des 8 Schwangerschaftsmonats*. Thesis, Univ. Berlin.

Gräfenberg, E. (1910), *Z. Geburtsh. Gynäk.*, **65**, 1.

Graham-Jones, O. and Hill, W. C. O. (1962), *Proc. Zool. Soc. (Lond.)*, **139**, 503.

Grosser, O. (1909), in *Lehrbuch Stud. Aertze*. Vienna: Braumüller.

Grosser, O. (1922), *Z. Anat. Entwickl. -Gesch.*, **66**, 179.

Grosser, O. (1925), *Z. Anat. Entwickl. -Gesch.*, **76**, 304.

Grosser, O. (1927), *Frühentwicklung, Eihautbildung und Placentation des Menschen und der Säugetiere*. Munchen: Bergmann.

Grosser, O. (1952), in *Biologie und Pathologie des Weibes*. **7/1**, 1, eds. Seitz and Amreich. Berlin: Urban and Schwarzenberg.

Gruenwald, P. and Minh, H. N. (1961), *Amer. J. Obstet. Gynec.*, **82**, 312.

Hagerman, D. D. and Villee, C. A. (1960), *Physiol. Rev.*, **40**, 313.

Hamilton, W. J., Barnes, Josephine, and Dodds, Gladys H. (1943), *J. Obstet. Gynaec. Brit. Emp.*, **50**, 241.

Hamilton, W. J. and Boyd, J. D. (1950), in *Modern Trends in Obstetrics and Gynæcology*, p. 114, ed. by Bowes. London: Butterworth.

Hamilton, W. J. and Boyd, J. D. (1951), *Proc. roy. Soc. Med.*, **44**, 489.

Hamilton, W. J. and Boyd, J. D. (1960), *J. Anat. (Lond.)*, **94**, 297.

Hamilton, W. J. and Boyd, J. D. (1966a), *Brit. med. J.*, **1**, 1501.

Hamilton, W. J. and Boyd, J. D. (1966b), *Nature (Lond.)*, **212**, 906.

Hamilton, W. J., Boyd, J. D. and Mossman, H. W. (1952), *Human Embryology*, 2nd edition. Cambridge: Heffer.

Hamilton, W. J., Boyd, J. D. and Mossman, H. W. (1962), *Human Embryology*, 3rd edition. Cambridge: Heffer.

Hamilton, W. J. and Gladstone, R. J. (1942), *J. Anat. (Lond.)*, **76**, 187.

Hartman, C. G. (1928), *J. Mammal.*, **9**, 181.

Hartman, C. G. (1932), *Contr. Embryol. Carneg. Instn.*, **23**, 1.

Hashimoto, M., Kosaka, M., Shimoyama, T., Hirasawa, T., Komori, A., Kawasaki, T. and Akashi, K. (1960), *J. jap. Obstet. Gynaec. Soc.*, **7**, 122.

Heckel, G. P. and Tobin, C. E. (1956), *Amer. J. Obstet. Gynec.*, **71**, 199.

Hendricks, C. H. (1964), *Obstet. and Gynec.*, **24**, 357.

Hendricks, C. H., Quilligan, E. J., Tyler, C. W. and Tucker, G. J. (1959), *Amer. J. Obstet. Gynec.*, **77**, 1028.

Hertig, A. T. (1935), *Contr. Embryol. Carneg. Instn.*, **25**, 37.

Hertig, A. T. (1962), *Obstet. and Gynec.*, **20**, 859.

Hertig, A. T. and Rock, J. (1941), *Contr. Embryol. Carneg. Instn.*, **29**, 127.

Hertig, A. T. and Rock, J. (1944), *Amer. J. Obstet. Gynec.*, **47**, 149.

Hertig, A. T. and Rock, J. (1945), *Contr. Embryol. Carneg. Instn.*, **31**, 67.

Hertig, A. T. and Rock, J. (1949), *Contr. Embryol. Carneg. Instn.*, **33**, 169.

Hertig, A. T., Rock, J. and Adams, E. C. (1956), *Amer. J. Anat.*, **98**, 435.

Heuser, C. H., Rock, J. and Hertig, A. T. (1945), *Contr. Embryol. Carneg. Instn.*, **31**, 85.

Heuser, C. H. and Streeter, G. L. (1941), *Contr. Embryol. Carneg. Instn.*, **29**, 15.

Hill, J. P. (1932), *Phil. Trans. B.* **221**, 45.

Hinselmann, H. (1925), *Biol. und Path. des Weibes* (Halban and Seitz), **6**, 241. Berlin: Urban and Schwarzenberg.

Hitschmann, J. and Lindenthal, O. T. (1903), *Arch. Gynäk.*, **69**, 587.

Hofbauer, J. (1903a), *Wien. klin. Wschr.*, **16**, 871.

Hofbauer, J. (1903b), *Die Fettresorption der Chorionzotte*. Wien: Holder.

Hofbauer, J. (1905), *Grundzüge einer Biologie der menschlichen Plazenta mit besonderer Berucksichtigung der Fragen der fötalen Ernährung*. Vienna: Braumüller.

Hofbauer, J. (1925), *Amer. J. Obstet. Gynec.*, **10**, 1.

Horky, Z. (1964), *Zbl. Gynäk.*, **86**, 1621.

Hörmann, G. (1948), *Zbl. Gynäk.*, **70**, 625.

Hörmann, G. (1951), *Arch. Gynäk.*, **181**, 29.

Hörmann, G. (1953), *Arch. Gynäk.*, **184**, 109.

Hörmann, G. (1958), *Arch. Gynäk.*, **191**, 297.

Hörmann, G. (1966), *Z. Geburtsh. Gynäk.*, **165**, 125.

Horn, V. and Horalek, F. (1961), *Zbl. allg. Path. path. Anat.*, **102**, 514.

Hosemann, H. (1949), *Arch. Gynäk.*, **176**, 453.

Howorka, E. (1956), *Poznan. Towarzy. Przyjac. Nauk., Wydz. lek., Prace Kom. Med. doswiad.*, **13**, no. 5, 1.

Huber, C. P., Carter, J. E. and Vellios, F. (1961), *Amer. J. Obstet. Gynec.*, **81**, 560.

Hughes, E. C. (1961), *Amer. J. Obstet. Gynec.*, **81**, 571.

Hyrtl, J. (1870), *Die Blutgefässe der menschlichen Nachgeburt in Normalen und Abnormalen Verhältnissen*. Vienna: Braumüller.

Hytten, F. E. and Leitch, I. (1964), *The Physiology of Human Pregnancy*. Oxford: Blackwell.

Iklé, F. A. (1964), *Bull. schweiz. Akad. med. Wiss.*, **20**, 62.

Ishizaki, Y. (1960), *Obstet. and Gynec.*, **15**, 602.

Jaroschka, R. (1959), *Z. mikr. -anat. Forsch.*, **65**, 434.

Jobst, K. (1955), *Acta morph. Acad. Sci. Hung.*, **4**, 333.

Johnston, T. B. (1940), *J. Anat. (Lond.)*, **75**, 1.

Johnston, T. B. (1941), *J. Anat. (Lond.)*, **75**, 153.

Jonen, P. (1927), *Arch. Gynäk.*, **129**, 610.

Jones, H. O. and Brewer, J. I. (1935), *Surg. Gynec. Obstet.*, **60**, 657.

Jung, P. (1908). Berlin: Karger.

Kastschenko, N. (1885), *Arch. Anat. Physiol. Lpz., Jahrg.* **1885**, 451.

Kermauner, F. (1912), *Arch. Anat. Physiol., Lpz.*, p. 189.

Kjölseth, Marie. (1913), *Mschr. Geburtsh. Gynak.*, **38**, Erg. Heft., 216.

Kladetsky-Haubrich, A. L. (1952), *Acta Anat. (Basel)*, **14**, 168.

Klein, G. (1890), in *Die Menschliche Placenta. Beiträge zur Normalen und Pathologischen Anatomie derselben*, ed. by Hofmeier. Wiesbaden: Bergmann.

Klinger, H. P. and Ludwig, K. S. (1957), *Z. Anat. Entwickl. -Gesch.*, **120**, 95.

Knopp, J. (1960), *Z. Anat. Entwickl. -Gesch.*, **122**, 42.

Knopp, J. (1962), *Verh. dtsch. path. Ges.*, **46**, 306.

Kölliker, A. (1879), *Entwicklungsgeschichte des Menschen und der höheren Thiere*. Leipzig: Englemann.

Kossmann, R. (1892), in *Fetsch. z. 70 Geb. R. Leuckarts*, 236. Leipzig: Englemann.

Krafka, J. (1941), *Contr. Embryol. Carneg. Instn.*, **29**, 167.

Kretschmann, H. J. (1965), *Commun. 8th Internat. Anat. Cong. Wiesbaden*, p. 66. Stuttgart: Thieme.

Langhans, T. (1870), *Arch. Gynäk.*, **1**, 317.

Langhans, T. (1877), *Arch. Anat. Physiol., Anat. Abt.*, 188.

Lazitch, Emilie. (1913), *Les villosites choriales humaines. Leurs formes, leurs modes de ramification*. Thesis, Fac. Med. Geneva. Nancy. Berger-Levrault.

Lemtis, H. (1955/56), *Anat. Anz.*, **102**, 106.

Linzbach, A. J. (1947), *Virchows Arch. path. Anat.*, **314**, 534.

Lister, Ursula M. (1963a), *J. Obstet. Gynaec. Brit. Cwlth.*, **70**, 373.

Lister, Ursula M. (1963b), *J. Obstet. Gynaec. Brit. Cwlth.*, **70**, 766.

Lister, Ursula M. (1964), *J. Obstet. Gynaec. Brit. Cwlth.*, **71**, 21.

Lister, Ursula M. (1965), *J. Obstet. Gynaec. Brit. Cwlth.*, **72**, 203.

Lister, Ursula M. (1966), *J. Obstet. Gynaec. Brit. Cwlth.*, **73**, 439.

Ludwig, K. S. (1959), *Acta Anat. (Basel)*, **38**, 323.

Ludwig, K. S. and Wanner, A. (1964), *Experientia (Basel)*, **20**, 687.

McKeown, T. and Record, R. G. (1953a), *J. Endocr.*, **9**, 418.

McKeown, T. and Record, R. G. (1953b), *J. Endocr.*, **10**, 73.

Marais, W. D. (1962a), *J. Obstet. Gynaec. Brit. Cwlth.*, **69**, 1.

Marais, W. D. (1962b), *J. Obstet. Gynaec. Brit. Cwlth.*, **69**, 213.

Marais, W. D. (1962c), *J. Obstet. Gynaec. Brit. Cwlth.*, **69**, 944.

Marais, W. D. (1962d), *S. Afr. Med. J.*, **36**, 678.

Marais, W. D. (1963), *J. Obstet. Gynaec. Brit. Cwlth.*, **70**, 777.

Martin, C. B. Jr. (1965), *Anesthesiology*, **26**, 447.

Mayer, M., Panigel, M. and Tozum, R. (1959), *Gynéc. et Obstét.*, **58**, 391.

Mazanec, K. (1959), *Blastogenese des Menschen*. Jena: Fischer.

Merrtens, J. (1894), *Z. Geburtsh. Gynäsk.* **30**, 1.

Meyer, R. (1924), *Zbl. Gynäk.*, **48**, 354.

Milz, K. (1946), *Über das Gewicht der Placenta und seine Beziehungen zu Schwangerschaft und Geburt.* Thesis, Univ. Gottingen.

Mossman, H. W. (1956), *Gestation: Trans. 2nd. Conf.* (Villee, ed.), p. 135. New York: Macy Foundation.

Nagy, M. (1960), *Acta Morph. Acad. Sci. Hung.*, **9**, 263.

Nelson, J. H. Jr., Bernstein, R. L., Huston, J. W., Garcia, N. A. and Gartenlaub, C. (1961), *Obstet. Gynec. Surv.*, **16**, 1.

Neumann, E. (1880), *Arch. mikr. Anat.*, **18**, 130.

Neumann, J. (1897), *Mschr. Geburtsh. Gynäk.*, **6**, 17.

Nielsen, Ingrid, (1961), *Über Blutumlauf und Ausdehnung des intervillösen Raumes der menschlichen Placenta.* Thesis, Univ. Kiel.

Nilsen, P. A. (1963), *Acta obstet. scand.*, **42**, Suppl. 2.

Nitabuch, Raissa. (1887), *Beitrage zur Kenntniss der menschlichen Placenta.* Thesis, Univ. Bern.

Okudaira, Y., Hirota, K., Cohen, S. and Strauss, L. (1966), *Lab. Invest.*, **15**, 910.

Olivelli, F. and De Palo, G. M. (1964), *Attual. Ostet. Ginec.*, **10**, 656.

O'Meara, R. A. Q. and Jackson, R. D. (1958), *Irish J. med. Sci.*, **391**, 327.

O'Meara, R. A. Q. and Thornes, R. D. (1961), *Irish J. med. Sci.*, **423**, 106.

Orsini, Margaret W. (1954), *Amer. J. Anat.*, **94**, 273.

Ortmann, R. (1938), *Z. Anat. Entwickl. -Gesch.*, **108**, 427.

Ortmann, R. (1941), *Z. Anat. Entwickl. -Gesch.*, **111**, 173.

Ortmann, R. (1949), *Z. Zellforsch.*, **34**, 562.

Ortmann, R. (1955), *Z. Anat. Entwickl. -Gesch.*, **119**, 28.

Ortmann, R. (1960), *Verh. Anat. Ges.*, (*Jena*) *56th Vers. Anat. Anz.*, Suppl., 27.

Panigel, M. and Anh, J. N. H. (1963), *C.R. Acad. Sci.* (*Paris*), **257**, 3669.

Panigel, M. and Anh, J. N. H. (1964), *Path. et Biol.*, **12**, 927.

Pappas, G. D., Ross, M. H. and Thomas, L. (1958), *J. exp. Med.*, **107**, 333.

Park, W. W. (1958), *J. Path. Bact.*, **75**, 257.

Park, W. W. (1965), *The Early Conceptus, Normal and Abnormal.* Edinburgh: Livingstone.

Peter, K. (1943), *Z. mikr. -anat. Forsch.*, **53**, 142.

Peter, K. (1950/51), *Z. mikr. -anat. Forsch.*, **56**, 129.

Peters, H. (1899), *Ueber die Einbettung der menschlichen Eies und das früheste bisher bekannte menschlichen Placentations-stadium.* Vienna and Leipzig: Deuticke.

Pierce, G. B., Jr. and Midgley, A. R., Jr. (1963), *Amer. J. Path.*, **43**, 153.

Pitkänen, H. (1949), *Ann. Chir. Gynec. Fenn.*, **38**, 356.

Ramsey, Elizabeth M. (1949), *Contr. Embryol. Carneg. Instn.*, **33**, 113.

Ramsey, Elizabeth M. (1954a), *Amer. J. Obstet. Gynec.*, **67**, 1.

Ramsey, Elizabeth M. (1954b), *Contr. Embryol. Carneg. Instn.*, **35**, 151.

Ramsey, Elizabeth M. (1956a), *Trans. Second Conference on Gestation*, p. 229. New York: Macy Foundation.

Ramsey, Elizabeth M. (1956b), *Amer. J. Anat.*, **98**, 159.

Ramsey, Elizabeth M. (1959), *Trans. Fifth Conference on Gestation*, p. 77. New York: Macy Foundation.

Ramsey, Elizabeth M. (1962), *Amer. J. Obstet. Gynec.*, **84**, 1649.

Ramsey, Elizabeth M., Corner, G. W., Jr. and Donner, M. W. (1963), *Science*, **141**, 909.

Ramsey, Elizabeth M., Corner, G. W., Jr., Donner, M. W. and Stran, H. M. (1960), *Proc. nat. Acad. Sci.* (*Wash.*), **46**, 1003.

Ramsey, Elizabeth M., Martin, C. B., Jr. and Donner, M. W. (1965), *Obstet. and Gynec.*, **25**, 417.

Reynolds, S. R. M. (1966), *Amer. J. Obstet. Gynec.*, **94**, 425.

Rhodin, J. A. G. and Terzakis, J. (1962), *J. Ultrastruct. Res.*, **6**, 88.

Robecchi, E., Cremona, G. and Giardinelli, M. (1963), *Minerva ginec.*, **15**, 2336.

Rohr, K. (1889), *Virchows Arch. path. Anat.*, **115**, 505.

Romney, S. L., Metcalfe, J., Reid, D. E. and Burwell, C. S. (1959), *Ann. N.Y. Acad. Sci.*, **75**, 762.

Runge, H. and Hartmann, H. (1930), *Arch. Gynäk.*, **139**, 51.

Salvaggio, A. T., Nigogosyan, G. and Mack, H. C. (1960), *Amer. J. Obstet. Gynec.*, **80**, 1013.

Sauramo, H. (1951), *Ann. Chir. Gynec. Fenn.*, **40**, 164.

Sauramo, H. (1961), *Ann. Med. exp. Fenn.*, **39**, 7.

Sawasaki, C., Mori, T., Inoui, T. and Shinmi, K. (1957), *Endocr. Jap.*, **4**, 1.

Schmid, H. H. (1951), *Zbl. Gynäk.*, **73**, 1714.

Schmidt-Matthiesen, H. (1963), in *Das normale menschliche Endometrium*, p. 225. Stuttgart: Thieme.

Schmorl, G. (1893), *Pathologische-anatomische Untersuchungen über Puerperal-Eklampsie.* Leipzig: Vogel.

Schramm, B. (1962), *Gynéc. et Obstét.*, **61**, 423.

Schröder, R. (1930), in *Handbuch d. mikr. -anat. d. Menschen*, ed. by von Möllendorff, **7**, pt. 1, p. 329. Berlin: Springer.

Sermann, R. and Rigano, A. (1962), *Arch. Ostet. Ginec.*, **67**, 523.

Serr, D. M., Sadowsky, A. and Kohn, G. (1958), *J. Obstet. Gynaec. Brit. Emp.*, **65**, 774.

Shanklin, D. R. (1958), *Obstet. and Gynec.*, **11**, 129.

Shanklin, D. R. (1959), *Obstet. and Gynec.*, **13**, 325.

Shordania, J. (1929), *Arch. Gynäk.*, **135**, 568.

Siegenbeek van Heukelom, D. E. (1898), *Arch. Anat. Phys. Lpz.*, *Anat., Abt.*, p. 1.

Sinclair, J. G. (1948a), *Texas Rep. Biol. Med.*, **6**, 168.

Sinclair, J. G. (1948b), *Anat. Rec.*, **102**, 245.

Singer, M. and Wislocki, G. B. (1948), *Anat. Rec.*, **102**, 175.

Smart, P. J. G. (1962), *J. Obstet. Gynaec. Brit. Cwlth.*, **69**, 929.

Snoeck, J. (1958), *Le Placenta Humain.* Paris: Masson.

Snoeck, J. (1962), *Triangle*, **5**, 178.

Solth, K. (1961), *Zbl. Gynäk.*, **83**, 1558.

Spanner, R. (1934), *Anat. Anz.*, **78**, *Erg. Heft.*, 127.

Spanner, R. (1935), *Z. Anat. Entwickl. -Gesch*, **105**, 163.

Spanner, R. (1941), *Morph. Jb.*, **86**, 407.

Starck, D. (1956), *Ergebn. Anat. Entwickl. -Gesch.*, **35**, 133.

Stieve, H. (1926), *Anat. Anz.*, **61**, *Erg. Heft.*, 138.

Stieve, H. (1936), *Z. mikr. -anat. Forsch.*, **40**, 281.

Stieve, H. (1940), *Z. mikr. -anat. Forsch.*, **48**, 287.

Stieve, H. (1941), *Z. mikr. -anat. Forsch.*, **50**, 1.

Stieve, H. (1942), *Biol. und Path. des Weibes* (*Seitz and Amreich*), **7**, 109. Berlin: Urban and Schwarzenberg.

Stieve, H. (1952), in *Biologie und Pathologie des Weibes*, (Seitz and Amreich), **7**, p. 109. Berlin: Urban and Schwarzenberg.

Stöhr, P. (1959), *Lehrbuch der Histologie und der mikroskopische Anatomie des Menschen.* Jena: Fischer.

Strahl, H. and Beneke, R. (1910), *Ein junger menschlicher Embryo, untersucht von H. Strahl und R. Beneke.* Wiesbaden: Bergmann.

Strauss, F. (1964), *Fortschr. Geburtsh. Gynäk.*, **17**, 3.

Streeter, G. L. (1920a), *Contr. Embryol. Carneg. Instn.*, **9**, 389.

Streeter, G. L. (1920b), *Contr. Embryol. Carneg. Instn.*, **11**, 143.

Szontágh, F. E. and Traub, A. (1962), *Z. Geburtsh. Gynäk.*, **159**, 68.

Tao, T. W. and Hertig, A. T. (1965), *Amer. J. Anat.*, **116**, 315.

Tenzer, W. (1962), *Graphische Rekonstruktion des bindgewebigen Stutzskeletts der menschlichen Placenta.* Thesis, Univ. Kiel.

Terzakis, J. A. (1963), *J. Ultrastruct. Res.*, **9**, 268.

Thomsen, K. (1955), *Arch. Gynäk.*, **187**, 264.

Thomsen, K. and Blankenburg, H. (1956), *Arch. Gynäk.*, **187**, 638.

Thomsen, K. and Lorenzen, C. (1956), *Arch. Gynäk.*, **187**, 462.

Torpin, R. (1958), *Missouri Med.*, **55**, 353.

Uchida, K. (1957), *Acta Anat. Nippon.*, **32**, 287 and 295.

Veit, J. (1905), *Die Verschleppung der Chorionzotten* (*Zottendeportation*). *Ein Beitrag zur geburtshilflichen Physiologie und Pathologie.* Wiesbaden: Bergmann.

Veit, O. and Esch, P. (1922), *Z. ges. Anat. 1. Z. Anat. EntwGesch.*, **63**, 343.

Vokaer, R. and Vanden Eynden, A. (1957), *C.R. Assoc. Anat.*, 44th Reun., 806.

Vokaer, R. and Vanden Eynden, A. (1958), in *Le Placenta Humain*, p. 81, ed. by Snoeck. Paris: Masson.

Wagner, G. A. (1929), *Arch. Gynäk.*, **137**, 699.

Waidl, E. (1963), *Geburtsh. Frauenheilk.*, **23**, 757.

Walker, J. (1954), in *The Mammalian Fetus: Physiological Aspects of Development*, Cold Spring Harb. Symp. Quant. Biol., **19**, 39.

Wanner, A. (1966), *Acta Anat.*, **63**, 545.

Weinbeck, J. (1936), *Z. mikr. -anat. Forsch.*, **39**, 135.

West, C. M. (1952), *J. Obstet. Gynæc. Brit. Emp.*, **59**, 336.

Wigglesworth, J. S. (1962), *J. Obstet. Gynaec. Brit. Cwlth.*, **69**, 355.

Wilkin, P. (1954), *Gynéc. et Obstét.*, **53**, 239.

Wilkin, P. (1958), in *Le Placenta Humain*, ed. by Snoeck, p. 23. Paris: Masson.

Wilkin, P. (1965a), *Pathologie du Placenta*. Paris: Masson.

Wilkin, P. (1965b), in *Organogenesis*, p. 743, ed. by DeHaan and Ursprung. New York: Holt, Rinehart and Winston.

Wilson, K. M. (1954), *Amer. J. Obstet. Gynec.*, **68**, 63.

Winner, W. (1965), *Obstet. Gynec. Surv.*, **20**, 545.

Wislocki, G. B. and Bennett, H. S. (1943), *Amer. J. Anat.*, **73**, 335.

Wislocki, G. B. and Dempsey, E. W. (1948), *Amer. J. Anat.*, **83**, 1.

Wislocki, G. B. and Dempsey, E. W. (1955), *Anat. Rec.*, **123**, 133.

Wislocki, G. B. and Padykula, H. A. (1961), in *Sex and Internal Secretions*, p. 883, ed. by Young. Baltimore: Williams and Wilkins.

Wislocki, G. B. and Streeter, G. L. (1938), *Contr. Embryol. Carneg Instn.*, **27**, 1.

Wolska, W. (1888), *Über die von Ruge beschriebene foetale Vaskularisation der Serotina*. Thesis, Univ. Bern.

Wynn, R. M. (1965), *J. Obstet. Gynaec. Brit. Cwlth.*, **72**, 955.

Wynn, R. M. and Davies, J. (1964), *Amer. J. Obstet. Gynec.*, **90**, 293.

Zangemeister, W. (1911), *Z. Geburtsh. Gynäk.*, **69**, 127.

Zeek, P. M. and Assali, N. S. (1950), *Amer. J. clin. Path.*, **20**, 1099.

Zhemkova, Z. P. and Topchieva, O. I. (1964), *Nature (Lond.)*, **204**, 703.

Zschiesche, W. and Gerlach, H. (1963), *Arch. Gynäk.*, **199**, 199.

9. THE LIQUOR AMNII

R. LISLE GADD

INTRODUCTION

The use of radio-active isotopes demonstrated that the water element of the liquor changes every three hours with the result that amniotic fluid is no longer regarded as a stagnant pool contaminated by foetal excreta. It is now known that a continuous interchange of the liquor constituents takes place between the amniotic sac and the maternal and foetal circulations so that variations in the foetal mechanism affect the composition of the liquor.

This new concept stimulated research into the composition, volume and circulation of the amniotic fluid which can be sampled before birth by amniocentesis.

COMPOSITION

Physical Properties

The amniotic fluid is a solution in which undissolved material is suspended. This material is a mixture of cellular and unorganised insoluble matter which gives the liquor a turbid appearance. Its specific gravity and viscosity are slightly greater than water.

Chemical Properties

As pregnancy progresses the composition of the liquor is changed by foetal excreta but in the early months it resembles the interstitial portion of the extra-cellular fluid consisting of 1–2 per cent solution of approximately equal portions of organic and inorganic substances in 98–99 per cent water. The inorganic substances resemble the constituents of extra-cellular fluid in that the concentration of sodium, chloride and CO_2 are high with only small amounts of potassium, calcium, magnesium and phosphate.

Organic Constituents

Half of the organic constituents is protein, the other half consists of carbohydrate, fats, enzymes, hormones and pigments.

Protein and Protein Derivatives

The reported estimations of the amount of total protein and protein fractions in the amniotic fluid vary considerably so that only general observations on these results can be made. The total concentration of protein is about 1/20th of that in serum. The liquor proteins are electrophoretically and immuno-chemically largely the same as those of serum proteins. Fibrinogen appears to be absent. Amino-acids are present in the same concentration as in maternal plasma. The concentration of urea, creatinine and uric acid is believed to be higher in amniotic fluid as pregnancy progresses than in the maternal serum because they are excreted into the liquor by the foetus.

Carbohydrates

Glucose is present in a lower concentration than in maternal serum.

The lactic acid content is variable and its level depends on whether foetal distress has occurred.

Lipids

The total lipids of amniotic fluid have been reported as 480 mg./litre with half of this fatty acid.

Enzymes

A wide variety of enzymes occur in the amniotic fluid. Alkaline phosphate levels increase with gestational age up to the 7th month and then remains constant unless the amniotic fluid is contaminated by meconium when the levels may increase to 10 to 35 times those observed in maternal serum.

Hormones

Oestrin, oestradiol, oestriol, chorionic gonadotrophin, pregnanediol, progesterone, 17-ketosteroids and other hormones are all present. The study of the hormonal levels in the liquor is a fruitful source for research.

Pigments

The amount of bilirubin in the liquor has probably been studied more than any other constituent of liquor because the amount indicates the degree of severity of Rhesus isoimmunization. In normal pregnancy bilirubin is present and decreases with foetal maturity until it disappears at 36 weeks.

ORIGIN AND DISPOSAL OF LIQUOR

The circulation of liquor has been much discussed and is still imperfectly understood. There are two types of circulation, biophysical and mechanical, which maintain the liquor volume at a normal level for the gestational age. The biophysical circulation operates throughout pregnancy and is selective. It consists of the movement of large volumes of fluid in both directions between the amniotic cavity and maternal circulation via the amniotic epithelium particularly that portion which overlies the highly vascular placenta. The cells of the deepest layer of the amnion have a brush border of microcilli and inter and intra-cellular canals which indicate the potential ability to transfer large quantities of fluid and other substances in solution (Bourne, 1962).

The mechanical circulation is of lesser importance and functions later in pregnancy when foetal swallowing and micturition have developed sufficiently to affect the volume. The swallowing of liquor by the foetus removes all the constituents at the rate of 500 ml. per day whilst the volume is augmented by foetal micturition. Possible minor subsidiary routes of circulation are by the foetal lungs and skin.

Volume

Antenatally the volume can be assessed clinically by abdominal palpation. This gives a rather vague diagnosis of either excessive (hydramnios) or reduced amounts (oligohydramnios).

Estimation of the Volume

1. The volume can be measured directly in intact gestational sacs removed at hysterotomy or passed as complete abortions. This method has provided our knowledge about the liquor volume during the first half of pregnancy (Fig. 1).

2. **Dye Dilution Technique** (Gadd, 1966). This method can be used during the second half of pregnancy without danger of premature termination. If necessary it can be repeated after 48 hours when the first injection of dye has cleared. After the patient empties her bladder, the position of the foetus is noted and the presence or otherwise of the placenta on the anterior uterine wall is determined with the doptone ultrasound. After infiltration of the skin with local anaesthesia a $3\frac{1}{2}$-inch spinal needle with a tap incorporated in the shaft is inserted into the amniotic cavity to avoid the placenta and foetal head. 5 ml. of liquor are withdrawn for control purposes and then 0·5 ml. of Coomassie blue dye are injected with a Mantoux syringe to obtain an exact amount. The Mantoux syringe is discarded and the dye lodged in the spinal needle is flushed into the amniotic cavity by withdrawing and injecting liquor using a fresh syringe. Samples of liquor are withdrawn at 5 minute intervals for 20 minutes. The mean of the samples taken from 15 to 25 minutes is used. The optical density of the liquor extract of dye is read on a spectrophotometer and the volume calculated from a formula using the optical density of the standard compared with the optical density of the test.

The results are accurate to within ±8 per cent, but the test is unreliable with small volumes below 200 ml.

Charles and Jacoby (1966), whilst using the dilution technique, prefer to use sodium aminohippurate as the agent. This substance which is colourless, is converted by a diazo reaction into a coloured solution in the laboratory and the dilution read on a spectrophotometer.

The dilution technique has provided much of our detailed knowledge about the liquor volume in the second half of pregnancy (Fig. 1), and can be used clinically.

Normal Pregnancy

After a slow rise up to 15 weeks the volume rises sharply to 30 weeks when it reaches a plateau extending to 37 weeks. It then falls sharply. (Fig. 1.)

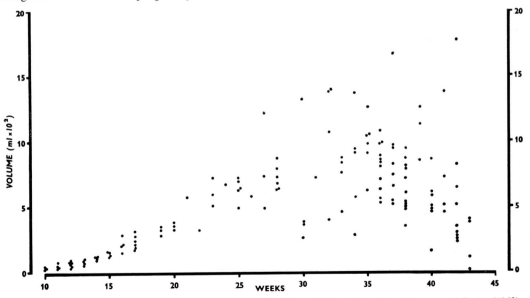

FIG. 1. Volume of liquor in normal pregnancy by gestational age. Values taken from Wagner and Fuchs (1962) and Gadd (1966) for the first half of pregnancy (40 readings) and Gadd (1966) 44 readings and Charles *et al.* (1965) 59 readings for the second and third trimester.

Breech Presentation

No significant difference is found in the volume of liquor with persistent breech presentation where external version has failed. Previously it was believed that a diminished quantity of liquor was the cause of these persistent presentations.

Parity

The volume in parous patients is similar to that found in primigravida. The previous impression and belief that parous patients had greater quantities of liqour probably arose from the general laxity of the abdominal musculature making palpation and movement of the baby relatively easy.

Pre-eclamptic Toxaemia

In mild and moderate cases of toxaemia the liquor volume is normal whilst in severe toxaemia oligohydramnios occurs. Certain conditions found with toxaemia, i.e. diabetes mellitus, twins and hydrops foetalis probably accounted for the mistaken belief that toxaemia and hydramnios were associated. Excluding these three conditions toxaemia alone does not have any particular association with hydramnios.

OLIGOHYDRAMNIOS

Investigation of a large number of normal and abnormal cases by dye dilution technique indicates the conditions found with oligohydramnios. (Fig. 2.)

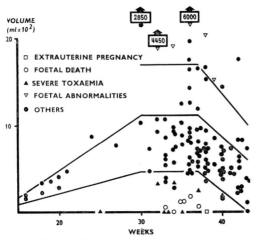

FIG. 2. Volume of liquor by gestational age in normal and abnormal pregnancies. (Reproduced from *Proc. Roy. Soc. Med.*, 1966, 59, 1131 with permission of the Editors.)

Volumes below 400 ml. are found with:
1. Severe pre-eclamptic toxaemia with persistent albuminuria.
2. Foetal death in utero of at least three days duration.
3. Normal cases after 41 weeks duration.
4. Extra-uterine abdominal pregnancy.
5. Retarded intrauterine foetal growth (Elliot, 1967).
6. Renal agenesis (Potter's syndrome).

Causes of Oligohydramnios

In the last condition the absence of foetal urine is believed to cause the low liquor volumes. Placental in-sufficiency with diminished placental blood flow is thought to be the cause in the first five conditions. In extrauterine abdominal pregnancy the poor blood supply to an unusual placental site is believed to cause oligohydramnios.

HYDRAMNIOS

Diagnosis

Unless the volume is measured by dye dilution there is no guide to the degree of hydramnios and in fact the actual diagnosis may be incorrect. In 50 cases of clinical hydramnios with a single foetus the diagnosis was verified by dye dilution (Table 1). In four (8 per cent) of these cases the

TABLE 1

50 CASES WITH A SINGLE FOETUS, OF CLINICAL HYDRAMNIOS (NON-CONSECUTIVE) INVESTIGATED BY DYE DILUTION TECHNIQUE

		Volume in ml. by dye dilution
Normal volume	4	600 to 1100
Anencephaly	6	2300 to 6000
Duodenal atresia	1	4450
Hydrocephalus	2	2950 to 2900
Maternal diabetes	1	1980
Achondroplasia	1	2300
Normal foetus	34	>1700 up to 5000

clinical diagnosis was incorrect, a normal volume with a large foetus being the usual cause for error. The volume which constitutes hydramnios varies as the upper limit of the normal volume varies throughout pregnancy. The lower limit for hydramnios is 1,700 ml. from 30 to 37 weeks and then descends to 1,000 ml. at 43 weeks. (Fig. 2.)

Mechanism of Production

Attention has been focussed on defects in the mechanical circulation as the cause of hydramnios because these are more readily detectable, but minor variations in the biophysical circulation have the same effect. This became clear when the various factors involved in 100 cases of clinical hydramnios were examined (Table 2). In 45 per

TABLE 2

CONDITIONS FOUND WITH 100 CONSECUTIVE CASES OF CLINICAL HYDRAMNIOS

1. *Foetal abnormality*			39
Anencephaly	23	Hydrocephalus	3
Oesophageal atresia	3	Achondroplasia	2
Duodenal atresia	1	Unusual skin condition	1
Hydrops Foetalis	3	Spina bifida	1
Tumour in chest causing kinking of oesophagus			1
Occipito-cervical meningocele			1
2. *Multiple pregnancy*			9
3. *Diabetes mellitus*			7
4. *Normal foetus, normal mother*			45

cent of cases, where there was neither maternal nor foetal abnormality, the hydramnios probably arose from a slight alteration in the biophysical circulation, as yet undetectable by any means. The causes of hydramnios with foetal abnormality, maternal diabetes and twins are now discussed.

I. Foetal Abnormality

(a) **Anencephaly.** The hydramnios which occurs with this gross foetal abnormality is believed by many to arise from absence of the foetal swallowing reflex. The belief is based on the absence in a small number of cases of squames or radio opaque or active material from the foetal gut after its natural or artificial presence in the amniotic sac. The fact that 10 per cent of cases of anencephaly have normal liquor volume is attributed to the presence of sufficient brain tissue to allow foetal swallowing, but all anencephalics appear the same on naked eye inspection.

After 20 ml. of 100 per cent Barium Sulphate were introduced into the amniotic sacs of five anencephalics with proven hydramnios, labour was induced. X-ray of the delivered foetuses 48 hours after the amniogram showed, in four cases, barium in the stomach and concentrated in the gut. In the fifth case barium was not visible in the foetal stomach, probably because the foetus was dead at the time of the amniogram.

These findings indicate that in anencephaly with hydramnios liquor does pass down the foetal gut. Whether the hydramnios arises from delayed gastrointestinal mobility or from transudation of fluid from the exposed meninges is uncertain.

(b) **Alimentary Atresia.** As the foetus is believed to dispose of 500 ml. per day by swallowing, any atresia of the oesophagus or duodenum will produce hydramnios. A similar mechanism operates when a tumour of the thorax or a diaphragmatic hernia compresses the oesophagus. When normal volumes occur with an oesophageal atresia there is invariably a fistula to by-pass the obstruction.

(c) **Hydrocephalus.** The occurrence of hydramnios with hydrocephalus is rare considering that the incidence of anencephaly and hydrocephalus is almost equal. The explanation for this was illustrated by a study of six cases of hydrocephalus, with and without hydramnios, by dye dilution method (Table 3). Hydrocephalus may give an

TABLE 3

ANALYSIS OF THE LIQUOR VOLUME IN CASES OF HYDROCEPHALUS
(6 cases)

Clinical hydramnios	Volume by dye dilution in ml.	Associated abnormalities
+	2950	Oesophageal atresia + hare lip
+	2900	Oesophageal atresia + Spina bifida
+	945	—
—	1513	—
—	876	—
—	1020	—

erroneous impression of hydramnios due to its large bulk. In those cases with a proven hydramnios there was an associated abnormality of oesophageal atresia which accounted for the hydramnios.

II. Multiple Pregnancy

Hydramnios with twins means an excess of liquor in a single sac—not merely in the uterus, for by that standard almost all cases of multiple pregnancy would be graded as hydramnios. Accepting this criterion it is doubtful whether an increased incidence of true hydramnios occurs with binovular twins except for the double chance of a foetal abnormality in one of the sacs causing hydramnios. With uniovular twins there is no doubt that acute hydramnios can develop at a very early stage of pregnancy and often leads to abortion or premature labour. The explanation generally accepted is that in some way a haemodynamic imbalance occurs due to a crossed foetal circulation, one foetus becoming dominant.

III. Maternal Diabetes Mellitus

The evidence regarding hydramnios and maternal diabetes mellitus is contradictory. Peel and Oakley (1948) found no relationship between maternal diabetic condition and the development of hydramnios, based on a clinical impression, nor did the increased sugar content of the liquor found in diabetic pregnancies bear any relationship to the presence of hydramnios. Today, Peel (1967), believes that the amount of hydramnios can be reduced by strict diabetic control, and found that when diabetic control was excellent normal liquor volume measured by dye dilution, was present in 26 cases. We recorded similar findings in the pregnancy diabetic clinic at St. Mary's Hospital, Manchester, but when diabetic control was poor, hydramnios by dye dilution was present in three cases. This implies that the hydramnios with diabetes is related to the maternal blood sugar. Foetal blood sugar would be correspondingly raised with resultant foetal diuresis and hydramnios.

Management of Hydramnios

An X-ray of the foetus is essential to exclude gross foetal abnormality.

Attempts to reduce the maternal discomfort by amniocentesis in cases of acute hydramnios with uniovular twins rarely serves any useful purpose. The reduction in volume usually causes premature labour and in any case the liquor is replaced again very rapidly.

When the foetus is normal, radiologically, an oesophageal tube should be passed immediately after delivery to detect any oesophageal atresia as immediate surgery is indicated if it is present.

Hydramnios with diabetes mellitus is a bad prognostic sign and calls for immediate admission to hospital and maintenance of the blood sugar below 160 mgm./100 ml.

INDUCTION OF ABORTION OR LABOUR BY INTRA-AMNIOTIC INJECTION OF HYPERTONIC SOLUTION

Principle

This method of stimulating the uterus to contract depends on removing the liquor and injecting an equal quantity of a hypertonic solution, which by its osmotic pressure drains water from the maternal, foetal and placental tissues into the amniotic sac. The liquor volume increases by 30 per cent during the first three hours and results in dehydration of the foetus, umbilical cord placenta and decidua. As the cord becomes bloodless and collapsed death of the foetus invariably occurs.

Technique

Two solutions commonly used are 50 per cent glucose and 20 per cent saline. Glucose should be avoided because it has no obvious advantages over saline and may cause an anaerobic infection. The method should never be used before 15 weeks when the liquor volume is low and the cavity relatively inaccessible. Between 15 and 20 weeks the vaginal approach is favoured, after 20 weeks the abdominal approach is more popular. The method is not without danger to the mother if by accident the injection is given intravenously.

[This method can be extremely dangerous and one of the editors has lost a patient from pontine and intra-cerebral haemorrhage following it.—Eds.]

EXAMINATION OF LIQUOR AMNII

(a) Visual without sampling (Amnioscopy)

Saling (1966) recommends inspection of the liquor amnii six to four weeks before birth by means of an amnioscope passed through the cervical canal in certain cases. Normally the liquor is clear or opaque. Absence of liquor or discolouration with meconium or bile indicate impending danger. It is not possible to establish conclusively whether the foetus is in danger by this method but if abnormal signs are present the membranes should be ruptured and the chemical state of the foetus determined by foetal blood sampling.

Technique

Under sterile conditions the cervix is palpated and according to the width of the canal, an amnioscope of 12, 16 or 20 mm. diameter is introduced. After passing the internal os the instrument is advanced a cm. into the uterus. The obturator is removed and the amnioscope brought down into the horizontal position to visualize the amniotic sac, with the light attachment which shines down the side of the metal amnioscope.

Indications for its use are:

1. Suspected postmaturity

Amnioscopy is carried out 10 days after the expected date of delivery and then every other day until (a) spontaneous onset of labour (most common event), (b) meconium staining of the liquor occurs, or (c) oligohydramnios is found.

2. Pre-eclamptic toxaemia

Amnioscopy is advocated from 36th week in mild and moderate toxaemia and from 34th week in severe toxaemia. The procedure is repeated on alternate days until labour ensues or the liquor becomes meconium stained.

There are several disadvantages of amnioscopy which have retarded its acceptance in Britain.

The main criticisms are that the presence of meconium in the liquor is not necessarily an indication for immediate delivery, as it may result from a transient past episode of foetal distress. Also the membranes are accidentally ruptured in about 2 per cent of cases with possible serious consequences for a premature foetus with negative findings.

(b) Sampling of Liquor Amnii for Diagnostic Purposes

1. **Rhesus isoimmunization.** Antibodies develop in the maternal circulation under the stimulation of Rhesus *positive* foetal erythrocytes escaping from the foetal blood in utero. They then pass back into the foetal circulation

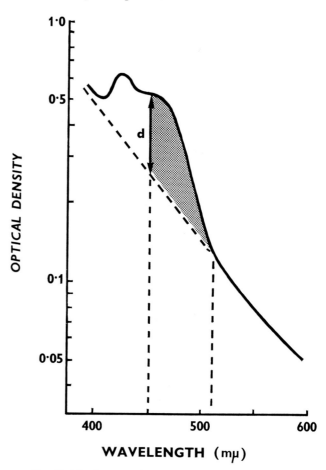

FIG. 3. The interpretation of the absorption curve in a severely affected baby. The stippled area is the "bulge" due to bilirubin. Liley's criterion "d" is the difference in optical density at 450 mu between the curve and a tangent drawn between 550 and 375 mu. Freda measures the difference in optical density at 450 and 525 mu.

to destroy the foetal Rhesus positive erythrocytes with the formation of bilirubin.

Antibody titres have proved unreliable in forecasting the severity of the haemolytic anaemia so that reliance is placed now on the amount of bilirubin present in the liquor (Walker and Jennison, 1962). This calls for the most careful interpretation with emphasis on the gestational age. In the early months of *normal* pregnancy bilirubin is present in the liquor and the amount falls as pregnancy progresses. The presence of significant quantities of bilirubin in the later stages of pregnancy is assumed to be evidence of a haemolytic process in the foetus, particularly if the bilirubin level is rising rather than falling on repeat sampling. The amount present may be measured by biochemical means but the usual method is by the spectral absorption curve which is plotted between 375 and 700 mu. at 10 mu. intervals. The presence of bilirubin makes a peak on this curve with a maximum at 450 mu. (Fig. 3). The size of the peak reflects quantitatively the amount of bilirubin present and can be measured by dropping a vertical line from the apex of the peak to a line drawn as a tangent to the curve at 365 mu. and 550 mu. The interpretation of these readings has been carefully worked out by Liley (1963) and Freda (1965). (Fig. 4.)

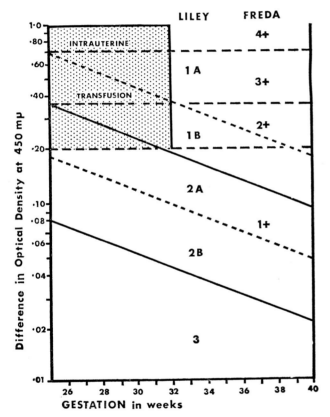

FIG. 4. Assessment of treatment from absorption curve. Liley: 1A, condition critical, immediate delivery or transfusion. 1B, delivery or transfusion urgent; 2A, delivery 35–37 weeks; 2B, delivery 37–39 weeks; 3, delivery at term. Freda: 4+, foetal death imminent, immediate delivery or transfusion; 3+, foetal death within 3 weeks, delivery or transfusion as soon as possible; 2+, foetal survival for 7–10 days, repeat test; 1+, no danger.

2. Genetic information from amniotic fluid constituents.

Now therapeutic abortion is legal if the foetus is believed to be abnormal any technique which clarifies the diagnosis early in pregnancy is valuable. It is now possible to diagnose the foetal sex by examination of liquor removed by amniocentesis early in pregnancy and thereby permits the diagnosis of sex linked hereditary disorders such as haemophilia and muscular dystrophy.

The liquor sample is centrifuged and the sediment transferred to a protein coated slide which is fixed by immersing in equal parts of ether and 95 per cent alcohol. The slide is stained with cresyl echt violet. Examination for the presence or absence of sex chromatin in the cell nuclei is done by alternating low and high magnification. The chromatin negative cells are found in male foetuses and their presence is an indication for termination of pregnancy. The selection of cases for abortion by this technique will increase the number of carriers. Some of these unfortunate mothers are willing to accept this in order to give birth to a healthy child. If the daughter subsequently proves a carrier the same procedure can be carried out when she herself becomes pregnant if by that time it is still not possible to prevent or treat these disorders.

Similarly, as foetal urine blends with the liquor, study of enzyme systems, abnormal amino-acids, hormones and other substances in the liquor should theoretically permit diagnosis of inborn errors of metabolism before birth. This may be of practical value if treatment is indicated immediately after birth.

REFERENCES

Bourne, G. (1962), *The Human Amnion and Chorion*. London: Lloyd-Luke.

Charles, D. and Jacoby, H. E. (1966), "Preliminary Data on the Use of Sodium Aminohippurate to Determine Amniotic Fluid volume," *Amer. J. Obstet. Gynaec.*, **95**, 266.

Elliott, P. (1967), "Foetal Salvage in Retarded Intrauterine Growth of the Foetus," *Aust. N.Z. J. Obstet. Gynaec.*, **7**, 13.

Freda, V. J. (1965), "The Rhesus Problem of Obstetrics," *Amer. J. Obstet. Gynaec.*, **92**, 341.

Gadd, R. L. (1966), "The Volume of the Liquor Amnii in Normal and Abnormal Pregnancies," *J. Obstet. Gynaec. Brit. Cwlth.*, **73**, 11.

Liley, A. W. (1961), "Liquor Amnii Analysis in the Management of Pregnancy Complicated by Rhesus Sensitisation," *Amer. J. Obstet. Gynaec.*, **82**, 1359.

Peel, J. H. and Oakley, W. G. (1949), *Proceedings 12th British Congress Obstetrics and Gynaecology*, p. 161. London: Austral Press.

Peel, J. H. (1966), *Recent Advances in Obstetrics and Gynaecology*, p. 211. London: J. and A. Churchill.

Saling, E. (1966), "Amnioscopy," *Clin. Obstet. Gynaec.*, **9**, 472.

Walker, A. H. C. and Jennison, R. F. (1962), "Antenatal Prediction of Haemolytic Disease of Newborn," *Brit. med. J.*, **2**, 1152.

10. FOETAL ENDOCRINOLOGY

G. C. LIGGINS

The inaccessibility of the human foetus severely limits the extent to which the standard investigational techniques of adult endocrinology can be applied to the study of foetal endocrinology. Nevertheless, within the last few years progress has been rapid and exciting.

The interest which this subject has attracted is not altogether surprising. The physiology of the foetus is not simply a mini-version of adult physiology but has a number of unique biosynthetic pathways and hormonal functions which are peculiarly suited to its intrauterine needs and in particular to its parasitic mode of existence.

Of necessity, much of what is taught about the function of the various human foetal endocrine glands is extrapolated from experiments in animals, always a dangerous practice and particularly so in reproductive physiology where species variation is so great. Nevertheless, such experiments provide working hypotheses to be tested in the human when the opportunity presents itself, often in the form of congenital malformations such as anencephaly or maternal endocrine disorders which affect the foetus. For this reason, animal data will be extensively used in this chapter so that the interested reader may have a basis for the interpretation of the oddities of foetal endocrinology which come his way in the course of his clinical practice.

The foundations of foetal physiology were laid by Alfred Jost who published the results of his first experiments in 1947. Using decapitation of foetal rats and rabbits as his main tool, his work has provided much of our knowledge of endocrine function in relation to foetal growth and development. Jost worked with species in which the corpus luteum of the mother provided the hormonal environment of pregnancy. Thus he had no opportunity to observe the contribution made by the foetoplacental unit of higher species, including man, to the biosynthesis of oestrogen and progesterone. This aspect of foetal endocrinology remained largely unexplained until attention was focussed upon it by the research work of Ryan (1959).

Another aspect of foetal endocrinology which escaped the notice of Jost was the role played by the foetus of some species in determining the time of onset of labour. Although suspected for many years, it was not until 1957 when Kennedy, Kendrick and Stormont described the syndrome of prolonged pregnancy in cows carrying malformed foetuses with adenohypophyseal aplasia that this important aspect of foetal endocrine function became an undeniable entity. These and other major advances in the last few years leave little doubt that equally unexpected and fundamental endocrine functions remain to be discovered.

THE FOETAL HYPOTHALAMUS AND PITUITARY GLAND

The influence of the foetal pituitary gland on other endocrine organs has been extensively investigated in several species (Jost, 1966a), and a wide range of trophic disturbances have been demonstrated in decapitated foetal rats and rabbits. There has been a reluctance to accept most of these as being relevant to the development of the human foetus for the anencephalic human foetus shows relatively few signs of a major endocrine disturbance. Since, however, most, if not all, anencephalics have anterior pituitary tissue present and correspond more closely to a stalk-sectioned preparation than to a hypophysectomised one it becomes necessary to revise opinions on the functions of the human foetal pituitary.

The few apparently pituitary-less infants who have been described do not appear to have endocrine changes different from those of the anencephalic but there is the possibility that ectopic pituitary tissue has escaped notice despite thorough sectioning of the bone surrounding the pituitary fossa.

Growth Hormone

Decapitation experiments in rats and rabbits have generally failed to reveal any evidence that foetal growth is retarded by decapitation. The short gestation period of these animals and the necessarily brief time which can elapse from decapitation to birth limits the opportunity for deficiency of hormones with prolonged biological activities to cause measurable retardation of growth. When a species with a longer gestation period was investigated, clear-cut signs of a pituitary influence on growth was apparent (Liggins and Kennedy, 1968). Foetal lambs which were hypophysectomized by electrocoagulation showed arrest of osseus maturation within 10–14 days of operation and were smaller than their intact twins. Goitrous lambs whose mothers were given thiouracil have similar changes suggesting that thyrotrophic hormone was at fault.

The measurement of human growth hormone in pregnancy was confused until recently by the presence of placental lactogen which has immunological similarities to growth hormone and cross-reacts with it in immunoassays unless special techniques are used. This problem will be considered further in the section dealing with hormones secreted by the trophoblast. Despite the difficulties of assay, it is accepted that growth hormone does not cross the placenta; growth hormone present in foetal plasma arises from the foetal pituitary.

Radioimmunoassay of growth hormone in the cord plasma of human infants reveals levels about twice those of the mother. There is little doubt that a considerable quantity of growth hormone is secreted by the foetal pituitary but its function is unclear. The response of plasma growth hormone levels in neonates to hypoglycaemia may be paradoxical, the plasma concentration falling rather than rising as it does in older children and adults.

The normal birthweight of many human anencephalics is often cited as evidence against the foetal pituitary providing a stimulus to growth. As already pointed out, these abnormal foetuses have pituitary tissue which may be capable of autonomous function. Furthermore, while some anencephalics reach normal or even large proportions at term, those born 2 or 3 months beyond term are not usually disproportionately large. At the present time

of ACTH into the foetus prevents adrenal atrophy in these animals. Cortical hypoplasia is also the rule in human anencephalics, the degree of atrophy correlating with the amount of pituitary tissue present. Hypertrophy of the adrenal cortex is readily induced by injection of ACTH into normal foetal animals (Fig. 2).

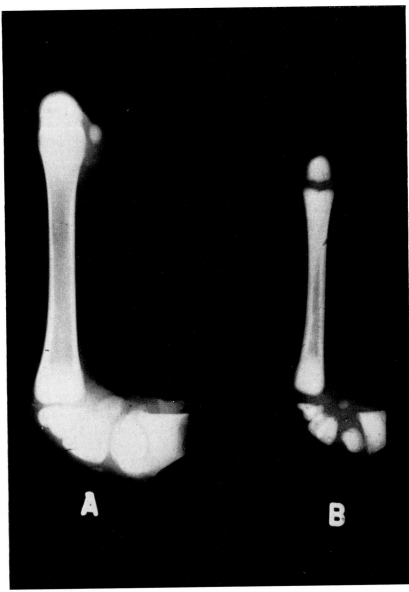

FIG. 1. Radiograph of metatarsal and tarsal bones from twin lambs. The hypothalamus of twin A was destroyed at a gestational age of 93 days; twin B was hypophysectomised at the same time. Ossification of bones of twin A shows no retardation while that of twin B is markedly retarded.

the relation of the human foetal pituitary to growth remains uncertain.

Corticotrophin

There is good evidence in several species that corticotrophin (ACTH) is secreted by the foetal pituitary (Jost, 1966b). Hypoplasia of the adrenal cortex occurs in foetal rats and rabbits following decapitation and in foetal lambs following destructive lesions of the pituitary. The injection

The secretion of ACTH is probably influenced, as it is in the adult, by plasma corticosteroids. The administration of ACTH to the mother has been shown to result in foetal adrenal hypoplasia in rodents, sheep, and monkeys. This paradoxical observation is explained by the transplacental passage of maternal corticosteroids which suppress the foetal pituitary. ACTH crosses the placenta slowly, if at all. In the human, suppression of foetal ACTH secretion by corticosteroids administered to the mother is suggested by reduced urinary oestrogen excretion following doses of dexamethasone. Surprisingly, acute adrenal insufficiency has been described rarely in neonates whose mothers were treated with corticosteroids throughout pregnancy. The outer zones of the human foetal cortex are less dependent on pituitary function than the inner zone for although in anencephalics the inner, foetal zone of the cortex is atrophic the glomerulosa and fasciculata are present.

Despite the ability of corticosteroids to cross the placenta, there is evidence that cortisol in the foetus is regulated by its own pituitary. Thymic development serves as a sensitive indicator of cortisol levels, being inversely related. It is therefore of significance that hypertrophy of the thymus has been described in the human anencephalic and in rabbit foetuses after decapitation, suggesting that corticosteroid levels in the foetus cannot be maintained at normal levels by transfer from the mother under physiological conditions.

Thyroid Stimulating Hormone

Studies of the pituitary-thyroid relationships in various species including the human indicate that normal development and function of the foetal thyroid depends upon stimulation by a foetal pituitary hormone. Thyroid hypoplasia has been observed in decapitated foetal rats and rabbits while human anencephalics have been found to have small thyroids showing histological evidence of reduced activity. Since hypoplasia following decapitation can be prevented by injecting thyrotrophic hormone (TSH) into the foetus, it is likely that TSH is the pituitary hormone normally responsible for regulating the growth and function of the thyroid.

Feed-back mechanisms operate in rat, rabbit, guinea pig, sheep and human foetuses. The administration of antithyroid drugs to the mother causes thyroid hypertrophy which can reach enormous proportions in the lamb and human foetus. Hyperplasia does not occur when foetal rats are decapitated prior to exposure to propylthiouracil, demonstrating that the action of this antithyroid drug depends upon increased secretion of TSH. When antithyroid drugs are used in human pregnancy, tri-iodothyronine, which crosses the placenta more readily than thyroxine, is commonly administered simultaneously to suppress foetal TSH release; foetal goitre from antithyroid treatment has become a rarity.

Gonadotrophic Hormones

According to Jost (1966a) sexual development occurs in 3 major periods.

Period I. Differentiation of the gonads
Period II. Differentiation of the sexual structures
Period III. Growth of the sexual structures.

In the human, Period I begins at 5 weeks and Period II begins at 7 weeks; Period III continues from approximately 10 weeks until term. Before considering the influence of foetal pituitary gonadotrophic hormones on sexual differentiation in the human, it will be helpful to discuss the findings in the rabbit where their role is unequivocal.

Male rabbit foetuses decapitated during Period I have abnormalities of the genital tract which are distributed according to the distance of the particular tissue from the testis. Thus, the epididymis is normal, the prostate is smaller than normal while the external genitalia are feminine in type. These changes can be prevented by giving gonadotrophin to the foetuses at the time of decapitation. The release of gonadotrophin from the pituitary occurs during a brief but critical period. The testis responds with hyperplasia of its interstitial cells and secretion of a hormone or organiser which stimulates differentiation of the genital tract, apparently by spreading locally rather than systemically.

Differentiation of the female genital tract apparently is independent of an influence from either the ovary or the pituitary. In neither the male nor the female rabbit foetus is it known whether pituitary gonadotrophins play any part in differentiation of the gonads.

Unlike rabbit foetuses, rat and mouse foetuses show no abnormality of sexual organogenesis following decapitation. In the human foetus too sexual development appears to be largely independent of pituitary influence. The male anencephalic has either no abnormality of the genital tract or at the most some reduction in size of the penis and testes. The Leydig cells of the testes are however markedly reduced in number and size (Zondek and Zondek, 1965). It is uncertain whether sexual differentiation in male human foetuses is the result of testicular secretion which occurs independently of gonadotrophic stimulation or whether the gonadotrophic stimulus in this instance is provided by chorionic gonadotrophin which reaches maximum levels at the critical period of organogenesis.

Hypothalamic Releasing Factors

The hypophyseal portal system develops in the human foetus about half way through pregnancy. Concurrently with the appearance of the portal system of vessels, neurosecretory material can be identified in the hypothalamus. Thus the potential for hypothalamic regulation of anterior pituitary function is present at a relatively early stage of human pregnancy. There is little evidence available, however, which would indicate that the human foetal pituitary is dependent on its hypothalamic connections. The observation that the anencephalic usually has pituitary tissue present but lacks a hypothalamus might suggest that changes in target organs are the result of absence of hypothalamic stimulation. Unfortunately, the amount of pituitary tissue present in anencephalics is variable and there is no assurance that it is capable of normal function. Moreover, no marked developmental differences are apparent between foetuses which are anencephalic and those which lack a pituitary. On the other hand, large doses of corticosteroids given to the mother undoubtedly reduce foetal adrenocortical activity, an effect which is likely to be mediated by usual feed-back mechanisms operating on the hypothalamus. The question of hypothalamic function in human foetuses thus remains unclear.

In foetal rats and foetal sheep, experiments in which the hypothalamus was removed (rats) or the pituitary stalk was sectioned (lambs) have demonstrated impaired secretion of some anterior pituitary hormones. Jost (1966b) found that encephalectomy of foetal rats, an operation which preserves the pituitary but removes the hypothalamus, caused a degree of adrenal hypoplasia as great as that following decapitation; injections of crude extracts of rat hypothalami prevented hypoplasia.

Observations in foetal lambs (Liggins, unpublished observations) in which the pituitary stalk had been sectioned and the pituitary separated from the hypothalamus by a silicone membrane suggested that the release of some anterior pituitary hormones was dependent on intact hypothalamic connections while the release of others occurred autonomously. As in the foetal rat, the pituitary of the foetal lamb is not dependent on blood supply through the stalk for its survival. Adrenocortical and testicular hypoplasia occurred after stalk section as it did after hypophysectomy, but thyroid hypoplasia was absent, growth was not retarded (Fig. 1) and liver glycogen was not depleted. These findings suggest that ACTH and gonadotrophin release from the foetal pituitary is dependent on hypothalamic connections while TSH and possibly growth hormone release can occur autonomously. Nevertheless, this does not mean that TSH secretion is normally free from hypothalamic influence, only that the basal secretion rates can be maintained in the absence of the hypothalamus. The induction of huge goitres in foetal lambs receiving propyl thiouracil points to the existence of thyroidhypothalamic interrelationships in the intact animal.

Posterior Pituitary

Nothing is known of posterior pituitary function in the human foetus. Vasopressor and oxytocic activity have been detected in extracts of pituitary glands of foetuses from 70–110 days (Benirschke and MacKay, 1953) but it is not known whether these hormones are released and if so, whether they have any function during foetal life. This problem has not yet been investigated in experimental animals but examination of foetuses of various species in which anomalous development led to absence of the posterior pituitary has not demonstrated effects attributable to deficiency of either vasopressin or oxytocin.

THE FOETAL ADRENAL

Adrenal Medulla

Both adrenaline and noradrenaline have been identified in the adrenal medulla of foetuses of a number of species. In general, noradrenaline predominates early in gestation but with increasing age there is a gradual increase in the proportion of adrenaline, possibly which may be related to the stimulation of methylation by corticosteroids. The conversion of noradrenaline to adrenaline is catalysed by the enzyme phenylethanolamine-N-methyl transferase. Marked reduction in activity of this enzyme follows foetal decapitation, the reduced activity being restored to normal by ACTH or cortisol. The observation that the adrenal medulla of anencephalic human foetuses contains only large amounts of noradrenaline is consistent with this hypothesis.

The factors causing release of pressor amines from the adrenal medulla have been studied in foetal lambs and calves (Comline and Silver, 1966). In both these animals, the effective stimulus at early maturities is local hypoxia, the secreted amine being mainly noradrenaline. At birth the direct response to anoxia has almost disappeared, being replaced by a response mediated by the splanchic nerves. The secretion which follows nervous stimulation contains large amounts of both adrenaline and noradrenaline.

It has been proposed that in the human foetus the organs of Zuckerkandl which contain large amounts of noradrenaline but probably lack nervous connections have properties similar to those of the adrenal medulla in the immature calf. This chromaffin tissue may supplement the secretion of pressor amines from the adrenal medulla by means of a direct response to hypoxia. Little is known of the part which adrenaline and noradrenaline play in regulating the haemodynamics of the asphyxiated newborn infant or in preventing hypoglycaemia during the neonatal period.

Adrenal Cortex

The foetal zone of the human adrenal cortex. The enormous size of the human adrenal glands at the time of birth was known to Morgagni (1682–1781) who also recognized the abnormally small adrenals of anencephalic foetuses. Two hundred years were to elapse before their function was discovered and even now many aspects of foetal adrenal physiology remain a mystery.

The main bulk of cortical tissue consists of a layer of great thickness lying between the definitive or adult cortex and the medulla. The presence of this layer, usually called the foetal zone, distinguishes the adrenals of the human foetus from those of other mammals apart from a few such as the ape, armadillo, leopard, lion and tiger. Although the foetal zone can be recognized histologically by the characteristic appearances of the large eosinophilic cells, the clearest distinction is made by incubation of fresh adrenal slices in a medium containing diformazan and a $\Delta 5$, 3β-hydroxysteroid as substrate. In this system, formazan deposition occurs at the site of the enzyme 3β-hydroxysteroid dehydrogenase. The adult layers of cortex show marked formazan staining while the foetal zone is clearly distinguished by absence of formazan granules. As will be seen later, this observation is of great significance in relation to the function of the foetal zone.

There is considerable unresolved speculation about trophic factors responsible for the development of the foetal zone. Lanman (1960) has made a convincing argument for ACTH being responsible, supporting his case by citing the atrophic foetal zone of the anencephalic foetus. He gave ACTH to such a foetus from the 3rd day until death on the 13th day. At autopsy adrenals were as large as those in the normal newborn infant. More recently, ACTH has been shown to stimulate steroidogenesis in foetal adrenal slices *in vitro*. Conversely corticosteroids administered to pregnant women will reduce urinary oestriol excretion presumably by inhibiting foetal adrenal secretion of 16-hydroxy dehydroepiandrosterone (16-hydroxy DHEA) which is the main precursor of oestriol. Thus there is strong evidence in favour of ACTH being a trophic hormone of the foetal adrenal but it is difficult nevertheless for a number of reasons to accept it as being the only trophic hormone. Firstly, the regression of the toetal zone which occurs after birth must be explained; since it proceeds simultaneously with growth of the definitive zones, a trophic factor which is withdrawn at

When HCG is administered to neonates in doses of 3,000–10,000 i.u., there is a substantial increase in excretion of dehydroepiandrosterone; oestrogen is known to cause an increase in adrenal size in rodents. However neither HCG nor oestrogen maintains adrenal size when given to the neonate. Thus, while the circumstantial evidence

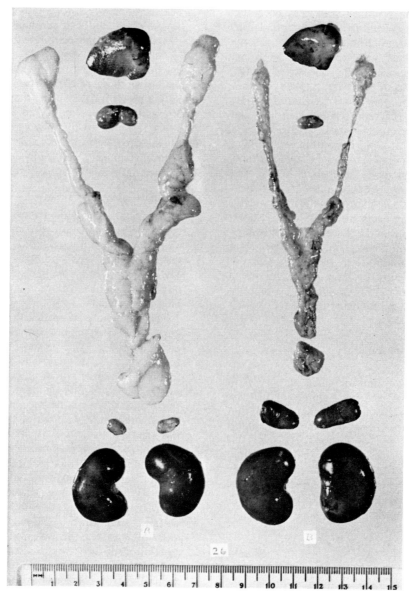

Fig. 2. Organs from twin lambs which were delivered by caesarean section at a gestational age of 111 days. Twin B was infused with ACTH for 10 days prior to birth. From above downwards the organs are spleen, suprascapular lymph gland, thymus, adrenals and kidneys. Hyperplasia of adrenals and hypoplasia of thymus of infused lamb are apparent.

birth is suggested. Secondly, cortical hyperplasia resulting from excessive levels of ACTH, either exogenous or endogenous, does not show the absence of $3\,\beta$-hydroxysteroid dehydrogenase activity characteristic of the foetal zone. Lastly, foetal zone involution follows the usual pattern in infants dying from congenital adrenal hyperplasia. Other hormones which have been proposed as adrenocorticotrophic are chorionic gonadotrophin (HCG) and oestrogen.

supports a second trophic hormone which is synergistic with ACTH and which disappears when the foetoplacental unit is dissociated at birth, its nature is unknown.

The secretory products of the foetal zone are $\Delta 5$, 3β-hydroxysteroids, particularly dehydroepiandrosterone and its sulphate. These steroids, which are the main precursors of oestrogen will be considered in detail in the section describing oestrogen biosynthesis.

The definitive zone of the foetal adrenal cortex. The definitive zone comprises the layers of cortex outside the foetal zone which persist after birth and enlarge to form the adult gland. The zone is made up of the glomerulosa, the fasciculata and the reticulosa, the boundary between the latter and the foetal zone being ill-defined.

The glomerulosa, which is responsible for the secretion of aldosterone in the adult, has an appearance of inactivity when examined histologically. Aldosterone is not known to have any important functions in the foetus, the assumption usually being made that the placenta regulates water and electrolyte balance since babies dying soon after birth from salt-losing congenital adrenal hyperplasia are apparently normal at birth.

The fasciculata and reticulosa are the sites of cortisol and corticosterone synthesis. Although the rate of secretion of cortisol has not been measured in the human foetus, the secretion rate in newborn infants has been shown to be as great as that of the adult when related to surface area. Functions of cortisol in the foetus include regulation of development of the thymus and peripheral lymphoid tissue, and glycogen storage in the liver.

The pattern of corticosteroids in foetal plasma is different from that of the adult. There is a relative increase in corticosterone and a reversal of the ratio of cortisol to cortisone. The latter is probably related to the high activity of the enzyme, 11 β-hydroxy-dehydrogenase in the trophoblast. Since cortisone is biologically inactive, the mechanism may be a method of cortisol disposal which is peculiar to the foetus.

THE FOETAL THYROID

The developing thyroid of the human foetus suddenly achieves the ability to trap iodine and to synthesize thyroxine at a gestational age of about 74 days. Thereafter it makes an essential contribution to the thyroxine requirements of the foetus. Although thyroxine can cross the placenta, it does so at a rate which is incapable of maintaining plasma thyroxine concentration at levels which allow normal development of the skeleton and brain. Athyreotic foetuses have retarded epiphysial development; mental retardation is likely to appear in later life.

Protein bound iodine (PBI) levels in the normal foetus are low relative to the mother. However low PBI values do not reflect low availability of thyroxine since free thyroxine levels reach maternal levels by the 16th week of pregnancy. The low levels result from reduced affinity of foetal thyroid binding globulin for thyroxine. As the maturity of the foetus advances, affinity increases until at term it is nearly that of the mother (Myant, 1963).

The hypothyroid foetus often appears normal at birth, an enlarged tongue and jaundice being only occasionally present. Surprisingly, birthweight is usually above normal, and the body length is increased proportionately. This observation, which cannot be accounted for by postmaturity, remains unexplained. Treatment with thyroxine soon after birth results in normal somatic growth and development but mental retardation persists in about 50 per cent of children.

THE FOETAL GONADS

The foetal ovaries appear to have no endocrine function. The testes, on the other hand, are necessary for normal differentiation and development of the male reproductive tract. The organizer secreted by the testes which is responsible for differentiation is probably not testosterone since injection of this hormone into decapitated male rabbit foetuses does not cause normal differentiation. Nevertheless, as shown by *in vitro* experiments in which labelled acetate or cholesterol was incubated with portions of foetal testes, all the enzymes necessary for testosterone synthesis are present, a finding consistent with secretion of testosterone *in vivo* (MacArthur, Short and O'Donnell, 1967).

The secretory tissue of the human testis, the Leydig cells, start to regress prior to term. Further regression occurs after birth. It is likely that the Leydig-cell hyperplasia is the result of stimulation by HCG; the degree of hyperplasia is increased in conditions such as toxaemia of pregnancy in which HCG secretion is increased. In animals such as the rabbit, rat and lamb which do not secrete chorionic gonadotrophin, Leydig-cell hyperplasia persists throughout foetal life, suggesting that the human foetal testis receives less stimulation from gonadotrophins of pituitary origin, perhaps because of relatively high oestrogen levels. However, since anencephalics have reduced numbers of Leydig-cells, the human pituitary probably makes some contribution to testicular development.

THE FOETAL PANCREAS

Insulin has been demonstrated in the pancreatic islet cells by histochemical and fluorescent antibody techniques in human foetuses at the 15th week of gestation. There is no doubt that the foetal pancreas secretes insulin, but little is known of the factors which regulate it. Following hypophysectomy of foetal lambs pancreatic development continues normally as it does in human anencephalic foetuses. Moreover, the insulin content of the islets and the plasma concentration of insulin are not reduced. Islet cell hyperplasia and increased insulin content is a usual finding in stillborn foetuses from diabetic mothers, suggesting that the foetal pancreas responds to high blood glucose levels. Less explicable is the islet cell hyperplasia which accompanies Rh haemolytic disease. The recent observation that babies salvaged by foetal transfusion have abnormally high birth-weights raises the possibility of a diabetogenic action from increased secretion of growth hormone or placental lactogen.

The glucose tolerance of the normal human infant (and probably the foetus also) is impaired during the first 3 days of life, the blood sugar being equivalent to that of a mildly diabetic adult. Paradoxically, although not unexpectedly in view of the hyperplasia of its pancreatic islet cells, the newborn infant of a diabetic mother has a more "normal" glucose tolerance curve. (Spellacy, Gall and Carlson, 1967.)

THE PINEAL GLAND

The pineal gland in the foetus of various species including the human has an appearance of metabolic activity and the parenchymal cells contain secretory granules.

Little is known, however, of its functions. The gland contains a relatively large concentration of certain mono-amines including 5-hydroxytryptamine and melatonin. The only function which has so far been demonstrated is in the regulation of absorption of macro-molecules by the lower ileum of the foetal rat (Owman, 1964). Human foetuses with gross central nervous system abnormalities which include absence of the pineal gland show no metabolic defects attributable to pineal deficiency.

THE TROPHOBLAST

By far the most active of all the foetal endocrine organs, the trophoblast secretes 4 varieties of hormones, all in enormous quantities. Two of them, the oestrogens and progesterone, are steroid hormones. The other two, HCG and placental lactogen (HPL) are protein hormones. The placental hormones have a common function—to modify metabolism in such a way that the sustenance of the growing conceptus is ensured. Almost without exception, the physiological changes which occur in the mother during pregnancy are induced by these hormones.

Chorionic Gonadotrophin

HCG is a glycoprotein which has been shown by fluorescent-labelled antibodies to arise solely in the syncytiotrophoblast. By immuno assay methods it has been detected in plasma 7 days after conception. Thereafter, there is a rapid increase in the rate of secretion so that when the maximal rate is reached at about the 70th day of pregnancy, the urine contains up to 100,000 i.u./L. Throughout the remainder of pregnancy the excretion of HCG is fairly constant at approximately 20,000 i.u./L. Since urinary HCG probably represents less than 10 per cent of that secreted, the daily production by the trophoblast is at least 100,000 i.u.

The primary function of the HCG is undoubtedly the maintenance of the corpus luteum until the time, usually at about 6–8 weeks of pregnancy, when placental progesterone production is sufficient to maintain pregnancy. In animals such as the pig, sheep and guinea pig, corpus luteum maintenance depends upon inhibition by the conceptus of the endometrial luteolytic factor which is responsible for corpus luteum regression when conception does not occur. The luteolytic factor appears to play little or no part in regulating corpus luteum function in the human; instead the presence of the conceptus is communicated to the corpus luteum by the luteotrophic effects of HCG.

The reason for the abundant secretion of HCG after the need for corpus luteum maintenance is past is not understood. As described in previous secretions, HCG may be important in stimulating the foetal testis at the critical period of sexual differentiation. It may also have a trophic influence on the foetal zone of the foetal adrenal cortex. In addition it has been proposed that HCG is a "placental trophin", influencing the synthesis of steroid hormones in the trophoblast.

Human Placental Lactogen

HPL is a recently discovered protein hormone secreted by the syncytiotrophoblast in even greater quantities than HCG. It has been estimated that the daily production is of the order of 3–12g. HPL has both weak growth hormone-like activity and weak prolactin-like activity. The similarity to growth hormone is not solely biological for it also cross-reacts with HGH anti-serum. The hormone is found in high concentration in maternal serum, in the placenta, and in amniotic fluid but is barely detectable in foetal plasma (Grumbach and Kaplan, 1964).

The function of HPL is thought to be concerned with the mobilization of nutrient materials in the mother for transmission to the foetus. The growth hormone-like action of HPL may be responsible for several of the well-recognized metabolic changes in pregnancy including the rise in circulating free fatty acids, altered utilization of glucose, increased insulin response and increased nitrogen storage.

Progesterone

In the first month of pregnancy the amount of progesterone secreted daily is about 10 mg.; at term the secretion rate is about 250 mg. This tremendous increase is achieved by synthesis of progesterone in the trophoblast. By 6–8 weeks, the maintenance of human pregnancy is no longer dependent on progesterone from the corpus luteum which can be removed without provoking abortion.

The biosynthetic pathways involved in the biosynthesis of progesterone have been investigated by incubating placental tissue with various isotopically-labelled steroid substrates and by perfusing labelled steroids into previable foetuses and in situ placentae (Solomon, 1966). Such studies have shown that the main precursor of progesterone is cholesterol derived from the maternal circulation. Cholesterol is converted in the trophoblast to pregnenoline thence to progesterone (Fig. 3). Apart from the trophoblast, foetal tissues have extremely limited ability to synthesize progesterone since the enzyme, 3 β-hydroxy-steroid dehydrogenase, which is necessary for the conversion of pregnenolone to progesterone is restricted mainly to the trophoblast. Localization of this enzyme to the placenta is of fundamental importance to the maintenance of the correct ratios of progesterone production to oestrogen production since its absence in the foetus allows pregnenolone from the placenta to be kept available for the synthesis of precursor steroids for oestrogen production.

Little is known of factors regulating progesterone secretion in human pregnancy. Although a rough correlation exists between placental mass and urinary pregnanediol there is no evidence of homeostatic control between either the foetus or the mother and the placenta; progesterone secretion continues at unchanged levels for some time after foetal death if the placenta is healthy and undisturbed.

Progesterone is the "pregnancy hormone" as its name suggests. It is responsible, together with oestrogen, for the growth and increased vascularity of the myometrium which allows the uterus to accommodate and nourish the growing conceptus. At the same time, myometrial activity is inhibited by progesterone so that distension of the uterus does not lead to abortion. Progesterone also causes growth of the alveolar tissue of the mammary gland and reduces

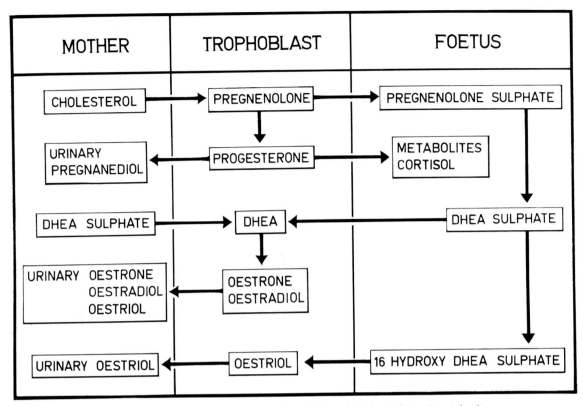

FIG. 3. Simplified outline of pathways of steroid biosynthesis in the foeto-placental unit.

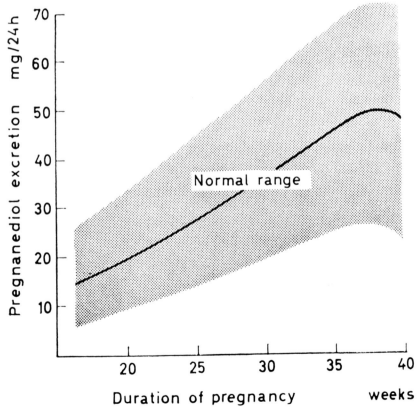

FIG. 4. Urinary pregnanediol excretion in normal pregnancies (Adapted from Russell, C. S., Coyle, M. G. and Dewhurst, C. J. (1957). *Journal of Obstetrics and Gynaecology of the British Commonwealth*, **64,** 649.)

smooth muscle tone throughout the body; ureteric dilatasion, varicose veins and constipation are characteristic consequences of its action. In addition to its action on the maternal tissues, progesterone may be important to the foetus. It has been estimated that near term approximately 75 mg. of progesterone goes to the foetus each day. Much of this is hydroxylated to various metabolites of progesterone in the foetal liver and to cortisol and corticosterone in the foetal adrenal.

maternal compartment since labelled oestradiol is metabolized and excreted after injection into the pregnant woman in the same way as the non-pregnant. The difference lies in the pattern of biosynthesis of oestrogen in the foetal compartment.

Oestrogen biosynthesis by the foetus follows pathways which are more complicated than those of any other hormone secreted by the human body since it involves 3 organs, (the placenta, the foetal adrenal and the foetal liver) with a

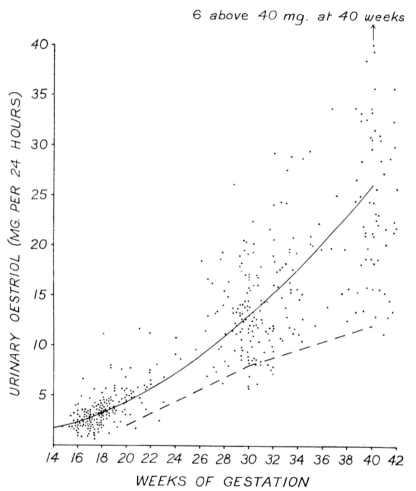

FIG. 5. Urinary oestriol excretion in normal pregnancies. (Beischer, Brown, MacLeod and Smith, 1967).

Normal urinary pregnanediol values throughout pregnancy are shown in Fig. 4. The flattening of the curve during the last month of pregnancy limits the usefulness of pregnanediol excretion as a measure of placental function in late pregnancy complications.

Oestrogen

Not only does oestrogen secretion by the trophoblast increase more than 100-fold during pregnancy but the ratio of oestrone (E1), oestradiol (E2) and oestriol (E3) alters markedly. The ratio in the non-pregnant urine is

$$E1:E2:E3 = 1·1:0·3:1·1$$

while at the end of pregnancy the ratio is $1·0:0·4:22$. The change in ratio is not due to altered metabolism in the

"shuttle service" operating between them. Although some details remain obscure, the general scheme proposed by Frandsen and Stakeman (1961) has been confirmed by recent work reviewed by Siiteri and McDonald (1967).

Pregnenolone, which is synthesized in the trophoblast from cholesterol derived from the maternal circulation, is secreted into the foetal circulation. Within the foetal adrenal, pregnenolone of placental origin together with some synthesized by the foetal adrenal cortex is conjugated with sulphuric acid and hydroxylated at C17, forming 17-hydroxypregnenolone sulphate.

The next step involves side-chain splitting of 17-hydroxypregnenolone sulphate by desmolase to form dehydroepiandrosterone sulphate (DHEAS) which is secreted into the foetal blood stream. Part of the DHEAS returns directly to the placenta but the greater part is transformed to 16-hydroxy-DHEAS by hydroxylation at C16 during passage through the foetal liver before passage to the placenta. Sulphated steroids, although water soluble, pass across the placenta with difficulty. However, the trophoblast contains a highly active sulphatase system capable of hydrolyzing sulphoconjugates to free steroids. Thus free DHEA and 16-hydroxy DHEA are made available for transformation in the placenta to oestrone and oestriol respectively.

The maternal and foetal adrenal contribute approximately equal amounts of DHEA to placental biosynthesis of oestrone and oestradiol; oestriol on the other hand arises largely from 16-hydroxy DHEA derived from the foetal circulation, only a small proportion arising by 16-hydroxylation of oestradiol in the foetal and maternal circulation. It is apparent from this greatly simplified account that the large amount of oestrogen synthesized in human pregnancy stems from the combined activities of the trophoblast and foetal adrenal while the preponderance of oestriol is the result of high activity of 16-hydroxylase in the liver and other foetal tissues.

Oestrogen lowers the threshold of excitability of myometrium, thereby opposing the inhibitory effect of progesterone; this is the most important action of oestrogen since apart from delayed onset of labour, marked impairment of oestrogen biosynthesis due to enzyme defects in the foetus does not lead to abnormal progress of pregnancy (France and Liggins, 1968).

PARTURITION

There is circumstantial and experimental evidence to show that in some species, including the human, the foetus plays a major role in determining the time of onset of parturition and consequently the duration of pregnancy. The human anencephalic foetus may be retained alive in the uterus for 3 months or more beyond term. Recent experimental work with the foetal lamb has shown that when the foetal hypothalamus, pituitary or adrenal are destroyed, parturition is delayed until foetal death occurs weeks beyond term (Liggins, Kennedy and Holm, 1967). Premature parturition, on the other hand, can be provoked by infusing ACTH into the foetus; when the foetal adrenals reach the size of those in a normal term lamb, spontaneous delivery occurs up to 8 weeks before term. Further experiments have demonstrated that the secretory product of foetal adrenal activity which is responsible for the initiation of parturition in the sheep is a corticosteroid but the mechanism by which the corticosteroid acts on the myometrium is unknown.

Mechanical factors such as uterine distension undoubtedly play a greater part in stimulating uterine activity in the human than they do in the sheep. Nevertheless, the human foetus probably makes a significant contribution to the various influences which initiate the onset of labour; whether it does so by mechanisms comparable to those in the lamb is not yet known.

FOETAL ENDOCRINE DISORDERS

A number of disorders of the endocrine system of the human foetus have been recognized prior to birth. The anencephalic foetus which is the best known example has been a rich source of information about pituitary and hypothalamic function and about the contribution of the foetal adrenal to oestrogen biosynthesis. Maternal urinary hormone excretion has characteristic features in anencephaly; pregnanediol excretion is normal while the excretion of oestriol is reduced to about 10 per cent of normal values. The abnormal hormonal pattern is different in placental insufficiency, both oestrogen and progesterone excretion being reduced. In normal pregnancy, urinary excretion of oestriol continues to rise until term (Fig. 5). Serial measurements of urinary oestriol have proved to be of great value in assessing foetal welfare in pregnancy complications such as diabetes and pre-eclamptic toxaemia. Deficiency of a specific placental enzyme, sulphatase, has been diagnosed during pregnancy from an extremely low oestrogen excretion which was elevated by infusion of free dehydroepiandrosterone but not by the infusion of the sulphated steroid (France and Liggins, 1968).

Congenital adrenal hyperplasia has been recognized in the antenatal period by demonstrating an abnormal pattern of adrenocortical hormones in the amniotic fluid. Studies of the amniotic fluid may be fruitful in diagnosing other foetal endocrine disorders since many hormones of foetal origin can be identified there.

Disorders of foetal endocrine function are possibly partly responsible for some of the pathological features of erythroblastosis and maternal diabetes. The foetuses in both conditions are larger than normal and there is hyperplasia of pancreatic islets and adrenal cortices. It remains to be seen to what extent the foetal endocrine system can be implicated in disorders such as foetal growth retardation, pre-eclamptic toxaemia and some cases of premature labour.

REFERENCES

Benirschke, K. and McKay, D. G. (1963), "Histochemical Observations with special reference to Amniotic Fluid Formation," *Obstetrics and Gynecology*, **1**, 638.

Beischer, N. A., Brown, J. B., MacLeod, S. C. and Smith, M. A. (1967), "The Value of Urinary Oestriol Estimation in Patients with Antepartum Vaginal Bleeding," *Journal of Obstetrics and Gynaecology of the British Commonwealth*, **74**, 51.

Comline, R. S. and Silver, M. (1966), "The Development of the Adrenal Medulla of the Foetal and New-born Calf," *Journal of Physiology*, **183**, 305.

France, J. T. and Liggins, G. C. (1968), "Placental Sulphatase Deficiency," *Journal of Clinical Endocrinology and Metabolism*, in press.

Frandsen, V. A. and Stakeman, G. (1961), "The Site of Production of Oestrogenic Hormones in Human Pregnancy. Hormone Excretion in Pregnancy with Anencephalic Foetus," *Acta endocrinologica*, **38**, 383.

Grumbach, M. M. and Kaplan, S. L. (1964), "In vivo and in vitro Evidence of the Synthesis and Secretion of Chorionic 'Growth Hormone—Prolactin' by the Human Placenta: Its purification, immuno assay and distinction from Human Pituitary Growth Hormone," *International Congress Series No. 83*, p. 691. Excerpta Medica Foundation, London.

Jost, A. (1966a), In *The Pituitary Gland*, Vol. 2, p. 9, Butterworths, London.

Jost, A. (1966b), "Problems of Foetal Endocrinology: The Adrenal Gland," *Recent Progress in Hormone Research*, **22**, 541.

Kennedy, P. C., Kendrick, J. W. and Stormont, C. (1957), "Adeno-hypophyseal Aplasia, an inherited defect associated with Abnormal Gestation in Guernsey cattle," *Cornell Veterinarian*, **47**, 160.

Liggins, G. C. and Kennedy, P. C. (1968), "Effects of Electrocoagulation of the Foetal Lamb Hypophysis on Growth and Development, "*Journal of Endocrinology*, **40**, 333–344.

Liggins, G. C., Kennedy, P. C. and Holm, L. W. (1967), "Failure of initiation of Parturition after Electrocoagulation of the Pituitary of the Foetal Lamb," *American Journal of Obstetrics and Gynecology*, **98**, 1080.

Lanman, J. T. (1960), *The Human Adrenal Cortex*, p. 547, E. & S. Livingstone, Edinburgh.

MacArthur, E., Short, R. V. and O'Donnell, V.J. (1967),"Formation of Steroids by the Equine Foetal Testis," *Journal of Endocrinology*, **38**, 331.

Myant, N. B. (1963), "The Supply of Thyroid Hormone to the Foetus," *Journal of Endocrinology*, **27**, i.

Owman, C. (1964), "Further Studies on Prenatal functional relations between Rat Pineal Gland and Epithelium of lower Ileum," *Acta endocrinologica*, **47**, 500.

Russell, C. S., Coyle, M. G. and Dewhurst, C. J. (1957), "Pregnanediol Excretion in Normal and Abnormal Pregnancy," *Journal of Obstetrics and Gynaecology of the British Commonwealth*, **64**, 649.

Ryan, K. J. (1959), "Biological Aromatization of Steroids," *Journal of Biological Chemistry*, **234**, 268.

Solomon, S. (1966), "Formation and Metabolism of Neutral Steroids in the Human Placenta and Fetus," *Journal of Clinical Endocrinology and Metabolism*, **26**, 762.

Siiteri, P. K. and Macdonald, P. C. (1966),' 'Placental Estrogen Biosynthesis during Human Pregnancy," *Journal of Clinical Endocrinology and Metabolism,* **26**, 751.

Spellacy, W. N., Gall, S. A. and Carlson, K. L. (1967), "Carbohydrate Metabolism of the Normal Term Newborn: Plasma Insulin and Blood Glucose Levels during an intravenous Glucose Tolerance Test," *Obstetrics and Gynecology*, **30**, 580.

Zondek, L. H. and Zondek, T. (1965), "Observations on the Testis in Anencephaly with special reference to the Leydig Cells," *Biologia Neonatorum*, **8**, 329.

11. THE FOETAL CIRCULATION

J. W. SCOPES

The isolation of the mammalian foetus in his environment of the uterus protects him from many of the dangers and vicissitudes of life and at the same time poses problems in the direct study of his physiology. The general principle that observation is difficult if not impossible without altering that which one wishes to observe has particular applicability to the foetus. Nonetheless an understanding of the foetal circulation, quite apart from academic interest, is essential for the scientific care of the unborn child and for determining the physiological and pathological changes which occur at birth. Much of our knowledge has been inferred from anatomical study of autopsy material but in the last few decades the foetus of the experimental animal has had his isolation invaded by the questing scientist. With improving techniques some direct observation has been possible in the living human foetus.

Historical

The interest in the foetal cardiovascular system goes back at least to the time of Galen in the second century A.D. From then until the present century all research on the course of the blood consisted of anatomical dissection and piecing together hypotheses. The suggestion supported by Sabatier (1774) that blood did not mix in the right atrium caused great controversy which was not resolved until the cineangiographic studies of Barclay, Barcroft, Barron and Franklin (1939). Perhaps the most masterly early account of the foetal circulation is that of William Harvey (1628) when he proposed an hypothesis, based on his own and previous workers observations, that was remarkably close to the truth as we understand it. Pohlman (1907) and Kellogg (1928) made some observations on alive but dying piglets (retrieved from the abat-

toir) but the period of direct experiment started in 1927 when Huggett delivered a foetal goat and kept it in good physiological condition while it was still attached to the mother by an intact umbilical cord. In 1939 the normal course of the blood flow in the lamb was demonstrated by cineangiographic techniques (Barclay *et al.*, 1939). The book by Barclay, Franklin and Pritchard (1944) published during World War II is a superb account of the use of these techniques and contains a scholarly and detailed review of the history of research into the foetal circulation. Since the studies of Lind and Wegelius (1954) showed that in the human foetus the course of the blood was essentially that described for the lamb, research in the last three decades has been directed toward the factors controlling the circulation rather than the qualitative direction of the passage of the blood.

The Cardiovascular System and the Course of the Blood

The main differences of the foetal circulation from that of the adult derive from the fact that the placenta, rather than the lung, is the organ of gaseous exchange, and from the existence of foetal channels. The atria are linked by the foramen ovale and the two ventricles work in parallel to pump blood from the great veins to the pulmonary trunk and aorta which are linked by the ductus arteriosus.

The human placenta is haemochorial, the maternal blood being in direct contact with the chorion of the foetus (Grosser, 1927). Blood arriving from the foetus along the two umbilical arteries is carried into successively branching vessels until the capillaries carried in the villi project into the intervillous space where they are bathed in maternal blood. Wigglesworth has recently confirmed that this branching results in a tree which is shaped as a hollow bush rather than the traditionally illustrated Christmas tree shape. The mouth of the hollow is directed at the outflow of one of the maternal spiral arteries. This vascular pattern has important implications (Wigglesworth, 1967). Richly oxygenated maternal blood comes into intimate contact with terminal villi for exchange and the dense masses of villi are likely to provide sufficient resistance to allow a substantial arterial pressure to be achieved in the intralobular space before the blood escapes to the uterine veins. The fronds of the bush therefore constitute what may be thought of as a functional intervillous capillary space.

Blood from the placenta is carried back to the foetus by the umbilical vein, or in the case of some species, veins. After traversing the cord, the vein enters the umbilicus usually at the cranial edge of the umbilical ring and empties into the portal sinus. A major portion of the blood passes directly through the ductus venosus to the inferior vena cava, though some of the blood in the human (Lind and Wegelius, 1954) and all of the blood in other species, e.g. mature horse foetus (Barclay *et al.*, 1944) passes through the liver in the portal and hepatic veins.

The course taken by the inferior vena caval blood is the subject of the old Sabatier controversy. That blood from the superior and inferior venae cavae should pass through a single chamber via the right atrium without mixing is difficult to imagine and indeed was stoutly denied by many e.g. Pohlman (1909), Kellogg (1930). However, as the old anatomists had shown, to consider the right atrium as a single chamber in this respect is unreasonable, as the inferior caval flow ends directly at the foramen ovale and is separated by the crista dividens from the flow of the superior vena cava, which is directed at the tricuspid valve. Thus it is anatomically reasonable to assume a streaming of flow and direct experimentation has confirmed this. Huggett (1927) showed that the arterial oxygen content was greater in the carotid than the umbilical artery which must mean streaming has occurred and Barclay *et al.* (1944) resolved the problem in the lamb by cineangiographic studies. Blood from the inferior vena cava passes through the foramen ovale and thus to the left atrium, left ventricle and aorta. Blood from the superior ven cava passes the tricuspid valve to the right ventricle, pulmonary trunk and ductus arteriosus (and lungs). That the findings in lambs are reasonably applicable to the human is shown by cineangiography of the early human foetus after therapeutic abortion (Lind and Wegelius, 1954, Peltonen and Hervonen, 1965). That some mixing occurs is not denied and in the case of the lamb quantitative information is available (see below).

When pumped from the ventricles blood is distributed to the body and placenta. In general the proportion taken by the placenta is large (40–60 per cent) and that by the lungs is small (4–15 per cent). Thus, as Dawes (1961) concludes, the placenta is a relatively low resistance circuit and the lungs a high resistance circuit both in parallel with the foetal tissues.

Blood leaving the aorta above the ductus is distributed to the head and forequarters. Such blood has a higher oxygen saturation as described above. It will return to the heart as venous blood in the superior vena cava directed in such a way that on recirculation it will now pass the ductus arteriosus to the lower aorta. From the lower aorta arise the umbilical arteries carrying blood to the organ of exchange, the placenta.

The umbilical vessels are highly contractile with thick muscular layers but are devoid of a nervous apparatus (Spivak, 1943). The muscular layers of the umbilical arteries, like the ductus arteriosus are arranged in a helical fashion (Von Hayek, 1935). A fifty per cent contraction of a simple circular muscle will merely *reduce* the lumen, a fifty per cent contraction of a helically arranged muscle will cause complete occlusion leaving a star shaped occluded lumen. As Barclay *et al.*, 1944 have said, the umbilical arteries, like the ductus arteriosus are prepared during development for a single post natal performance and are allowed no rehearsal for it. They constrict when exposed to a raised pO_2 or to sympathetic amines and relax when exposed to a raised pCO_2 or to hypoxic solutions (Rech, 1925, Kennedy and Clark, 1942, Kovalčik, 1963).

It should perhaps be pointed out that although the system of parallel circulations and streaming leads to carotid blood having a higher oxygen saturation than femoral blood the advantages to the foetal brain in the normal condition are probably marginal. The difference is not great (Fig. 1). Nonetheless, the system provides a capacity for increasing flow and oxygen content to one part at the expense of another and given a degree of functional control such a system might in certain circumstances confer a considerable advantage.

Distribution of Blood and Rates of Flow in the Foetal Circulation

After the qualitative problems of anatomy and direction of flow had been resolved, the quantitative problems of distribution have engaged research workers. In 1954, Born, Dawes, Mott and Widdicombe published data on oxygen saturation of blood in major foetal vessels sampled simultaneously (Fig. 1). The figures enable one to calculate the contribution of two streams that have mixed. By measuring umbilical blood flow one can calculate approximate blood flows in major foetal vessels and channels, and this led to the general conclusions of the previous section above (*see* Dawes, 1961).

The measurement of umbilical blood flow is an important basic measurement and various methods have been used. Cooper, Greenfield and Huggett (1949) used plethysmographic methods on the exteriorized lamb foetus and found rates of 173 ± 10 SEM ml./kg./min. Dawes and Mott at Oxford have used flow meters inserted into the umbilical vein. In 1959, using a density flow meter they found a rather low rate of 104 ml./kg./min. in near term lambs (Dawes and Mott, 1959). In 1964 using an electromagnetic flow meter they found rates of 217 ± 12 SEM ml./kg./min. in foetus of approximately 90 days gestation and 170 ± 14 SEM ml./kg./min. in near term foetus. In their work the foetus was exteriorized and the ewe anaesthetized. Meschia, Cotter, Makowski and Barron (1967) have used a constant infusion technique and employed the Fick principle to measure umbilical flow rates *in utero* in an unanaesthetized foetus. They found higher rates of 233 ± 19 SEM ml./kg./min., rates confirmed by Rudoph and Heyman (1967). The latter authors state that there was no significant difference in flow per kilogram of foetal weight at different gestational ages. A possible explanation of the earlier low rates, especially in the near term foetus,

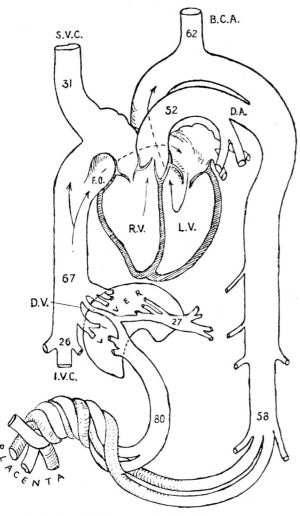

FIG. 1. The Foetal Circulation in the Lamb. (Born, Dawes, Mott and Widdicombe, 1954 by permission of Cold Spring Harbor Symposia on Quantitative Biology.) I.V.C., inferior vena cava; S.V.C., superior vena cava, R.V., right ventricle; L.V., left ventricle; D.V., ductus venosus; F.O., foramen ovale; D.A., ductus arteriosus; B.C.A., brachiocephalic artery. The figures indicate the mean O_2 per cent saturation of blood withdrawn simultaneously and averaged from estimations on six lambs.

may lie in partial separation of the placenta of the exteriorized foetus, despite its good physiological condition. The advantages of an infusion method such as that of Meschia *et al.*, or of Rudolph and Heymann is that the state of the foetus is more physiological whereas the electromagnetic fluorometer has the advantage that rapid changes, for instance in an experimental situation, can be assessed.

The approximate figures for blood flow in various foetal vessels and channels achieved by measuring saturation

have now been amplified by the work of Rudolph and Heymann (1967). They injected "carbonized" microspheres labelled with nuclides into different venous sites in the foetus. These microspheres are held in the precapillary vessels of any capillary bed and are not recirculated. Their distribution pattern therefore was used to determine the relative distribution of blood flow. With simultaneous measurement of umbilical blood flow by the antipyrine method it is possible to calculate cardiac output and organ flow in the foetus. For details of their techniques and findings the reader is referred to their paper. Some of their conclusions are summarized here.

A variable proportion of blood returning in the umbilical vein passes through the ductus venosus (34 per cent to 91 per cent). In general the larger the umbilical flow the greater the proportion that passed through this foetal channel. Blood returning to the heart in the superior vena cava was only minimally shunted through the foramen ovale, if the foetus's pH was normal. Blood from the inferior vena cava was distributed to the whole foetal body. If the foetus was hypoxic or acidaemic, however, superior caval blood was shunted through the foramen ovale and a greater proportion of the inferior caval blood was distributed to the upper body.

Cardiac output was calculated by the sum of superior and inferior vena caval flows, together with coronary and pulmonary venous returns. The numbers of foetuses studied was only twelve and general conclusions were tentative. Total cardiac output and output per kilogram body weight were high in the earlier gestational periods. In the two foetuses near term the output per kilogram body weight was lower—390 and 280 ml./kg./min. respectively. The distribution of this output to various organs was also studied. Umbilical flow was, as Born *et al.* (1954) had found, a large part of the output, varying from 23 per cent to 60 per cent (mean 42 per cent). The proportions received by other organs were, on average: heart 4·6 per cent, lungs 3·9 per cent, gastrointestinal tract, 5·4 per cent, brain 4·9 per cent, upper carcass 4·9 per cent, lower carcass 19·9 per cent, kidneys 2·2 per cent, spleen 1·6 per cent, and liver (from hepatic artery) 1·6 per cent. Whether there is a systematic variation with foetal gestational age is not clear from the small numbers but more numerous data will probably resolve this question. Blood flow in terms of ml. per gm. weight shows high rates for spleen and heart (6 and 3 ml./gm./min. respectively), and, perhaps surprisingly, unremarkable rates for brain (approximately 1·5 ml./gm./min.) and placenta (approximately 1·2 ml./gm./min.).

The details which emerge from this work need amplification and corroboration but even with the small numbers this work is important. The techniques have been applied only to the sheep foetus but the rhesus monkey is being increasingly studied. For a number of reasons, including the anatomy of the uterine veins in the rhesus monkey, the species is more difficult to study. Some differences in absolute figures are to be expected—e.g. Behrman, Parer and Novy (1967), found monkey umbilical blood flows in the order of 90 m./kg./min., considerably lower than in the lamb. However, apart from absolute figures for flow and distribution, interest from the point of view of applied physiology is inherent in the study of the changes in distribution and flow which occur in natural and experimental conditions.

Automatic Nervous Control and Pulmonary Circulation

Despite suggestions as recently as 1939 that autonomic nervous control is deficient in the foetus and newborn (e.g. Clark, 1935, Bauer, 1939) evidence is accumulating that automatic reflexes and controls are sophisticated by the time of birth. Arguing teleologically, it is obviously important to control a circulation with many shunts *in utero* and important to have cardiovascular homeostasis at and after birth. It might be more surprising if there were no evidence of autonomic activity before birth.

The blood pressure of a number of species of animals rises during gestation and after birth (Dawes, 1961) which suggests but does not prove that cardiovascular responses are present. The carotid sinus depressor reflex has been shown to be active near term (Cross and Malcolm, 1952), the mature foetal lamb reacts to anoxaemia with complicated autonomic and cardiovascular responses (Born, Dawes and Mott, 1956), vagal slowing of the heart can be shown in the lamb as early as the 88th day of gestation (Barcroft, 1946) and in the newborn rabbit (Downing, 1960) and monkey (Dawes, Jacobson, Mott and Shelley, 1960), baroreceptor reflexes are active. Foetal chemoreflex activity is shown in various species early in gestation both by the effect of cyanide or CO_2 and by measuring sinus nerve activity (see review by Purves and Biscoe, 1966). At the same time the foetus responds to sympathomimetic and parasympathomimitic drugs in a manner qualitatively similar to their later pharmacological effects (Barclay *et al.*, 1944, Barcroft, 1946, Dawes and Mott and Rennick, 1956). In general the foetal adrenal gland contains a high proportion of noradrenaline compared with adrenaline. Catechols can be released early in gestation in the lamb by asphyxia and by acetyl choline and in the last 20 days of gestation by splanchnic nerve stimulation. There are quantitative differences in the various means of release between the lamb and the calf—the animals most studied (see review by Comline and Silver, 1966).

In the lamb autonomic activity has been more clearly shown after about 80 days gestation than in very early foetal life. More work is needed on species differences of the onset and importance of various reflexes. In the human foetus, evidence of autonomic activity is necessarily more indirect, stemming mainly from (1) extrapolation from work applying in many other species, (2) extrapolation from reflexes found in premature babies after birth and (3) deductions from observations on foetal heart rate e.g. Mendez-Bauer, Poseiro, Arellano-Henandes, Zambrana and Caldeyro-Barcia (1963) deduce that vagal tone is concerned in the slowing of heart rate after contractions in labour.

The pulmonary blood flow in the foetus, as described above, is rather low, taking only a small percentage of the total cardiac output. Because of the profound changes which occur at birth, factors which affect pulmonary

vascular resistance and pulmonary flow have excited much interest. In 1953 Dawes, Mott, Widdicombe and Wyatt, in experiments on the exteriorized foetus with the chest open showed a large fall in pulmonary vascular resistance on positive pressure ventilation with gas (air, oxygen and nitrogen) but not on expansion with saline. Later, from the same unit it was shown that the fall in resistance was greater when the gas used was air rather than nitrogen (Born, Dawes and Mott, 1955). Cook, Drinker, Jacobson,

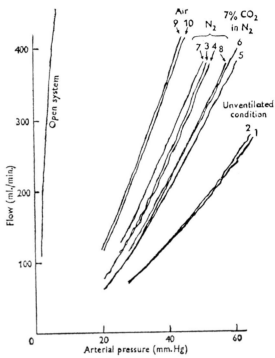

FIG. 2. Left pulmonary pressure-flow curves from the mature foetal lamb. (Cassin, Dawes, Mott, Ross and Strang, 1964 by permission of *Journal of Physiology*.) Curves traced by an X–Y recorder, from the foetal lung in the unventilated state (1 and 2), during ventilation with 7 per cent CO_2 in N_2 (5 and 6), with N_2 only (3, 4, 7 and 8) and with air (9 and 10), and also with the cannula removed from the left pulmonary artery (open system).

Levison and Strang (1963), found that static, as opposed to rhythmic, gaseous inflation of the lung caused only slight vasodilation and emphasized the importance the oxygen and carbon dioxide contents of the expanding gases.

In 1962 Dawes and Mott reported large increases (up to sixfold) of pulmonary blood flow after injections of small doses (2–10 μg.) of acetyl choline or histamine into the pulmonary artery and after a brief period of ischaemia had produced a reactive hyperaemia. Sometimes large increases of flow occurred "spontaneously" in their preparations suggesting other factors, as yet undiscovered, might be operating. They also showed that raising foetal arterial O_2 saturation caused a considerable vasodilatation, and asphyxia caused intense vasoconstriction in unexpanded partal lungs. Thus mechanical ventilation and oxygen and CO_2 tensions in alveolar gases or in pulmonary arterial blood profoundly affected the degree of dilation of pulmonary vessels.

More precise measurements of changes in pulmonary vascular tone have since been measured by generating pressure-flow curves for a pulmonary artery *in vivo* (Fig. 2, Cassin, Dawes, Mott, Ross and Strang, 1964). Displacement of a curve from Right to Left and increasing slope signify a decrease in vascular resistance. The figure confirms the dilatation which occurs with ventilation with N_2, the further dilation which occurs in an oxygen enriched gas (air) and the constricting effect of a CO_2 containing gas mixture. Campbell, Dawes, Fishman and Hyman (1967a) showed that, in immature lambs, the effect of asphyxia in causing pulmonary vasoconstriction was mainly by a local action within the lungs. In ingeneous cross circulation experiments Campbell, Cockburn, Dawes and Milligan (1967) showed that although the main effect was from local action, there was a demonstrable nervous component to the vasoconstriction in foetal lambs of greater than 98 days gestation.

The foetal pulmonary circulation, therefore, has been shown to be extremely reactive. The following factors cause pulmonary vasodilation; a rise in arterial or alveolar pO_2, a fall in arterial or alveolar pCO_2, rhythmical ventilation with a gas, acetyl choline, histamine, thoracic sympathectomy (Colebatch, Dawes, Goodwin and Nadeau, 1965) isoprenaline (Dawes, 1966) bradykinin (Dawes, 1966) and probably other yet undiscovered factors. Adrenaline and noradrenaline and sympathetic stimulation cause vasoconstriction (Dawes, 1966). There is suggestive evidence that there is some sympathetic vasoconstrictor tone in the unexpanded foetal lung but a negligible parasympathetic tone (Dawes, 1966).

Response of the Foetal Circulation to Asphyxia

All foetuses are exposed to some degree of asphyxia at birth; even *in utero*, although the uterine environment protects them against most acute stresses, the stress of asphyxia is one which frequently occurs. The foetus is able to withstand total asphyxia of a duration which would kill or damage an adult (Mott, 1961). This ability depends on a number of special attributes of the foetus the most important of which is the relatively large reserve of carbohydrate contained in the heart (Dawes, Mott and Shelley, 1958, Mott, 1961). The clinical implications of detecting, treating and preventing serious asphyxia in the unborn or newly born child have made the study of the many aspects of foetal asphyxia particularly imperative. This chapter is concerned only with the changes in the foetal circulation.

Heart Rate

Total asphyxia caused by occlusion of the umbilical vessels leads, after a period of up to 30 seconds, to a precipitous fall in the heart rate (e.g. Dawes, Jacobson, Mott, Shelley and Stafford, 1963, Dawes, 1965). This bradycardia is delayed by a few seconds and slightly less profound after vagotomy (Barclay, 1946). Even in the presence of total anoxia some acceleration may then occur but thereafter the rate gradually falls and arrhythmias develop before death. This response to total asphyxia occurs in a number of species e.g. lamb (Born, Dawes and

Mott, 1956), rabbit (Cross, 1961), monkey (Dawes *et al.*, 1963), and in mature and immature foetuses. Should the anoxia be relieved there is a compensatory tachycardia (Britton, Nixon and Wright, 1967).

Less severe degrees of anoxaemia such as those produced by Born *et al.*, 1956 by allowing the ewe to breath hypoxic mixtures lead to a persistent tachycardia in mature foetal lambs. The heart does not slow until the foetal carotid saturation is less than 20 per cent. In the very immature foetus (less than 72 days) this tachycardia is not observed.

In the human foetus, measurement of the heart rate has been a standard clinical tool. Its usefulness has often been underestimated because the usual method of counting tends to mask abrupt or short lived changes. For instance upon auscultation with a foetal stethoscope and counting for half a minute one may find a rate of 140 beats per minute. Such a result could be the result of a basal rate of 160, together with a transient drop to 110 during the period but which was not recognized. A cardiotachometer, which displays beat by beat rates, is theoretically more sound and practically more useful. However, there is general agreement that total asphyxia leads to a profound bradycardia and that severe tachycardia is associated with degrees of asphyxia (Wood *et al.*, 1967).

In clinical practice the foetal heart is not always easy to hear and record. Various stethoscopes and microphones have been developed and have their adherents, but each has its difficulties especially when one wishes to have a permanent record or differentiate beat by beat rates. A comparatively recent and useful device utilizes the Doppler effect. A beam of ultrasound is directed into the patient. Some of this is reflected at every density gradient that the beam traverses, but stationary structures reflect ultrasonic beams at a frequency different from moving structures. This difference in frequency is utilized with the result that movements can be displayed as a visual or audible record. With such a device heart "sounds" can be detected as early as the 10th–12th week of gestation. It is perhaps important to realize that these "sounds" are an artificial noise emitted by the device when the regular heart *movements* are detected.

However, most *recordings* of the foetal heart have employed the foetal electrocardiogram. As long ago as 1906, Cremer recorded the foetal ECG while obtaining an electrocardiogram on a woman at term. External abdominal leads have been used since then but it is difficult to obtain reliable, noise free tracings. In an attempt to improve the quality of the tracing electrodes have been placed in the rectum, vagina, cervix, uterus and on various parts of the foetus (Figueroa-Longo, Poseiro, Alvarez and Caldeyro-Barcia, 1966). The quality of tracing is usually best if at least one electrode can be attached directly to the foetus, the scalp during a vertex presentation being the usual site. Figueroa-Longo *et al.* obtained extremely good tracings with one electrode on the foetal scalp and a needle electrode inserted through the abdominal wall into the foetal buttock. Provided the waves obtained are of reasonable amplitude it is possible to choose a wave, usually the R wave, to measure electronically the time between successive waves, and to display the inverse of this time as a rate in a cardiotachometer tracing. Thus for every beat a rate is displayed and abrupt or short lived changes are easily recognized. The duration and amplitude of the various components of the foetal ECG are the same as for a newborn baby (Figueroa-Longo, *et al.*, 1966).

There is an extensive literature on the use of such apparatus (*see* e.g. Wood *et al.*, 1967; Hon, 1962; Mendez-Bauer *et al.*, 1967). The normal foetal heart rate is about 140 ± 20 beats per minute and there is a normal irregularity of ± 5 per minute occurring three to five times in any minute which tends to disappear in abnormal states. As Hon has suggested the most useful information is found if the heart rate is monitored during uterine contractions. Transient drops in heart rate coincident with contractions are frequently seen in babies whose foetal acid-base status is normal and who are normal at delivery. More sustained and more profound drops in heart rate occurring just after (30–40 seconds) the height of labour contractions and with a slower recovery phase are associated with babies whose acid base status and whose condition at birth suggests moderate to severe asphyxia.

Blood Pressure

The immediate response to total asphyxia by occluding the cord in all species studied is a rise in blood pressure. This raised pressure is maintained for a few minutes and then the pressure gradually falls until arrhythmias and death supervene (*see* Dawes, 1965). Rendering the foetal lamb hypoxic without occluding the cord (by administering hypoxic mixtures to the ewe) causes a rise in blood pressure in mature foetal lambs. Provided the hypoxaemia is not too profound this rise in blood pressure is well maintained over a period of many minutes. In foetal lambs below 88 days gestation blood pressure progressively falls with hypoxaemia even if the heart rate rises temporarily (Born *et al.*, 1956).

Umbilical Blood Flow and Redistribution of Cardiac Output

Umbilical blood flow increases, in foetal lambs who respond to hypoxaemia with a rise in blood pressure; that is, in mature foetal lambs but not in those less than 88 days gestation (Born *et al.*, 1956). Teleologically it would seem desirable to increase the flow to the organ of gas exchange and this is sustained in the particular circumstances of these experiments.

During hypoxaemia the rich saturation of carotid blood compared with femoral blood becomes more important both in relative terms and in terms of absolute difference. A greater proportion of inferior vena caval blood is distributed to the head and upper body (Rudolph and Heymann, 1967). At the same time a profound vasoconstriction occurs in the lungs and in the hindquarters (Campbell, Dawes, Fishman and Heymann, 1967). More detailed experimental work is needed on this subject but the established work shows therefore that the first results of asphyxia lead to the best oxygenated blood being distributed in increased flow to the head (at the expense of the lung and hindquarters) and an increased flow towards the placenta. It is worth noting that during foetal asphyxia the lungs (whose metabolic rate is not inconsiderable, Campbell *et al.*, 1968) fare badly, receiving a lowered flow rate of poorly oxygenated blood.

Conclusion

The advance on the front of foetal and neonatal physiology has been so rapid in the last years that a chapter of this length can only be a summary. It is also unsatisfactory that many infringing aspects of prenatal life cannot be discussed in relation to the foetal circulation because to do so would involve writing at least one whole book. The interested reader would do well to read Dr. Geoffrey Dawes recent book "Foetal and Neonatal Physiology." Most of the work in this field has been done on the lamb, especially on the exteriorized foetus. The advances to be expected in the next few years will almost certainly be from experiments conducted *in utero* and from experiments on the rhesus monkey; a species closer to man is desirable from the point of view of applied physiology. That which is already clear, however, is that study of the foetus is practicable and that the results can have immediate application in human medicine.

REFERENCES

Barclay, A. E., Barcroft, J., Barron, D. H. and Franklin, K. J. (1939), "A Radiographic Demonstration of the Circulation through the Heart in the Adult and in the Foetus and the Identification of the Ductus Arteriosus," *Brit. J. Radiol.*, **12**, 505–17.

Barclay, A. E., Franklin, K. J. and Pritchard, M. M. L. (1944), *The Fetal Circulation*. Oxford: Blackwell Scientific Publication.

Barcroft, J. (1946), *Researches on Prenatal Life*. Oxford: Blackwell.

Bauer, D. J. (1939), "Vagal Reflexes appearing in Rabbits at different Ages. *J. Physiol.*, **95**, 187.

Behrman, R. E., Parer, J. T. and Novy, M. J. (1967), "Acute Maternal Respiratory Alkalosis (Hyperventilation) in the Pregnant Rhesus Monkey," *Pediat. Res.*, **1**, 354.

Born, G. V. R., Dawes, G. S. and Mott, J. C. (1955), "The Viability of Premature Lambs," *J. Physiol.*, **130**, 191.

Born, G. V. R., Dawes, G. S. and Mott, J. C. (1956), "Oxygen Lack and Autonomic Nervous Control of the Foetal Circulation in the Lamb. *J. Physiol.*, **134**, 149–66.

Born, G. V. R., Dawes, G. S., Mott, J. C. and Widdicombe, J. G. (1954), "Changes in the Heart and Lungs at Birth," *Cold. Spr. Harb. Symp. Quant. Biol.*, **19**, 93.

Britton, H. G., Nixon' D. A. and Wright, G. H. (1967), "The Effects of Acute Hypoxia on the Sheep Foetus and some Observations on Recovery from Hypoxia," *Biol. Neonat.*, **11**, 277.

Campbell, A. G. M., Cockburn, F., Dawes, G. S. and Milligan, J. E. (1967), "Pulmonary Vasoconstriction in Asphyxia during Cross-circulation between Twin Foetal Lambs, *J. Physiol.*, **192**, 111–21.

Campbell, A. G. M., Dawes, G. S., Fishman, A. P. and Hyman, A. I. (1967a), "Pulmonary Vasoconstriction and Changes in Heart Rate during Asphyxia in Immature Foetal Lambs," *J. Physiol.*, **192**, 93–110.

Campbell, A. G. M., Dawes, G. S., Fishman, A. P. and Hyman, A. I. (1967b), "Regional Redistribution of Blood Flow in the Mature Fetal Lamb," *Circ. Res.*, **21**, 229.

Cassin, S., Dawes, G. S., Mott, J. C., Ross, B. B. and Strang, L. B. (1964), "The Vascular Resistance of the Foetal and Newly Ventilated Lung of the Lamb," *J. Physiol,*, **171**, 61.

Clark, G. A. (1935), "Development of Blood Pressure Reflexes," *J. Physiol.*, **83**, 229.

Colebatch, H. J. H., Dawes, G. S., Goodwin, J. W. and Nadeau, R. A. (1965), "The Nervous Control of the Circulation in the Foetal and Newly Expanded Lungs of the Lamb," *J. Physiol.*, **178**, 544.

Combine, R. S. and Silver, M. (1966), "Development of Activity in the Adrenal Medulla of the Foetus and Newborn Animal," *Brit. med. Bull.*, **22**, 16.

Cook, C. D., Drinker, P. A., Jacobson, H. N., Levison, H. and Strang, L. B. (1963), "Control of Pulmonary Blood Flow in the Foetal and Newly Born Lamb," *J. Physiol.*, **169**, 10.

Cooper, K. E., Greenfield, A. D. M. and Huggett, A. St. G. (1949), "The Umbilical Blood Flow in the Foetal Sheep," *J. Physiol.*, **108**, 160.

Cross, K. W. and Malcolm, J. L. (1952), "Evidence of Carotid Body and Sinus Activity in Newborn and Foetal Animals," *J. Physiol.*, **118**, 10P.

Dawes, G. S. (1961), "Changes in the Circulation at Birth," *Brit. med. Bull.*, **17**, 148.

Dawes, G. S. (1966), "Pulmonary Circulation in the Foetus and Newborn," *Brit. med. Bull.*, **22**, 61.

Dawes, G. S. (1968), *Foetal and Neonatal Physiology—a Comparative Study of the Changes at Birth.* Chicago: Year Book Medical Publishers Inc.

Dawes, G. S., Jacobson, H. N., Mott, J. C. and Shelley, H. J. (1960), "Some Observations on Foetal and Newborn Rhesus Monkeys," *J. Physiol.*, **152**, 271.

Dawes, G. S., Jacobson, H. N., Mott, J. C., Shelley, H. J. and Stafford, A. (1963), "The Treatment of Asphyxiated Mature Foetal Lambs and Rhesus Monkeys with Intravenous Glucose and Sodium Carbonate," *J. Physiol.*, **169**, 147.

Dawes, G. S. and Mott, J. C. (1959), "The Increase in O_2 Consumption of the Lamb after Birth," *J. Physiol.*, **146**, 295.

Dawes, G. S. and Mott, J. C. (1962), "The Vascular Tone of the Foetal Lung," *J. Physiol.*, **164**, 465.

Dawes, G. S. and Mott, J. C. (1964), "Changes in O_2 Distribution and Consumption in Foetal Lambs with Variations in Umbilical Blood Flow," *J. Physiol.*, **170**, 524.

Dawes, G. S., Mott, J. C. and Rennick, B. R. (1956), "Some Effects of Adrenaline, Noradrenaline and Acetylcholine on the Foetal Circulation in the Lamb," *J. Physiol.*, **134**, 139.

Dawes, G. S., Mott, J. C. and Shelley, H. (1958), "The Ability of the Foetal and Newborn Animal to withstand Total Anoxia," *J. Physiol.*, **144**, 18P.

Dawes, G. S., Mott, J. C., Widdicombe, J. G. and Wyatt, D. G. (1953), "Changes in the Lungs of the Newborn Lamb," *J. Physiol.*, **121**, 141.

Downing, S. E. (1960), "Baroceptor Reflects in Newborn Rabbits," *J. Physiol.*, **150**, 201.

Figueroa-Longo, J. G., Poseiro, J. J., Alvarez, L. O. and Caldeyro-Barcia, R. (1966), "Fetal Electrocardiogram at Term Labour obtained with Subcutaneous Fetal Electrodes," *Am. J. Obstet. Gynec.*, **96**, 556.

Grosser, O. (1927), *Fruhentwicklung, Eihautbildung und Placentation des Menschen und Des Säugetiere.* Munich: Bergman.

Hervey, William (1928), *Exeratatio anatomica de motre cardis et sanguinis in animalibus*, quoted by Barclay, Franklin and Pritchard.

Hayek, H. von (1935), "Der Functionelle Bau Der Naberlarterien und des Ductus Botalli," *Z. Anat. EntwGesch.*, **105**, 15–24.

Hon, E. H. (1962), "Electronic evaluation of the foetal heart rate," *Am. J. Obstet. Gynec.*, **83**, 333.

Huggett, A., St. G. (1927), "Fetal Blood Gas Tensions and Transfusion through the Placenta of the Goat," *J. Physiol.*, **62**, 373–84.

Kellogg, H. B. (1928), "The Course of the Blood Flow through the Fetal Mammalian Heart," *Anat. Rec.*, **42**, 443–65.

Kellogg, H. B. (1930), "Studies on the Fetal Circulation of Mammals," *Amer. J. Physiol.*, **91**, 637.

Kennedy, J. A. and Clark, S. L. (1942), "Observations on the Physiological Reactions of the Ductus Arteriosus," *Amer. J. Physiol.*, **136**, 140–47.

Kovalčik, V. (1963), "The Response of the Isolated Ductus Arteriosus to Oxygen and Anoxia," *J. Physiol.*, **169**, 185.

Lind, J. and Wegelius, C. (1954), "Human Fetal Circulation: Changes in the Cardiovascular System at Birth and Disturbances in the Postnatal Closure of the Foramen Ovale and Ductus Arteriosus," *Cold. Spr. Harb. Symp. quant. Biol.*, **19**, 109.

Mendez Bauer, C., Arnt. I. C., Gulin, L., Escarcena, L. and Caldeyro-Barcia, R. (1967), "Relationship between Blood pH and Heart Rate in the Human Fetus during Labor," *Am. J. Obstet. Gynec.*, **97**, 530.

Mendez-Bauer, C., Poseiro, J. J., Arellano-Hernandez, G., Zambrana, M. A. and Caldeyor-Barcia, R. (1963), "Effects of Atropine on the Heart Rate of the Human Fetus during Labor," *Am. J. Obstet. Gynec.*, **85**, 1033.

Meschia, G., Cotter, J. R., Makowski, E. L. and Barron, D. H. (1967), "Simultaneous Measurements of Uterine and Umbilical Blood Flows and Oxygen Uptakes," *Quant. J. Exptl. Physiol.*, **52**, 1.

Mott, J. C. (1961), "The Ability of Young Mammals to Withstand Total Oxygen Lack," *Birt. med. Bull.*, **17**, 144.

Peltonen, T. and Hirvonen, L. (1965), "Experimental Studies on Fetal and Neonatal Circulation," *Acta Pediat. (Uppsala).* Supp. **161**, 1965.

Pohlman, A. G. (1907), "The Fetal Circulation through the Heart," A review of the more important theories, together with a preliminary report on personal findings. *Johns Hopk. Hosp. Bull.*, **18**, 409–12.

Pohlman, A. G. (1909), "The Course of the Blood through the Heart of the Fetal Mammal, with a Note on the Reptilian and Amphibian Urculabious," *Anat. Rec.*, **3**, 75–109.

Purves, M. J. and Biscoe, T. J. (1966), "Development of Chemoreceptor Activity," *Brit. med. Bull.*, **22**, 56.

Rech, W. (1925), "Untersuchungen uber den physiologischen verschluss der nabelschnurarterien," *Z. Biol.*, **82**, 487.

Rudolf, A. M. and Heyman, M. A. (1967), "The Circulation of the Fetus in Utero: Methods for Studying Distribution of Blood Flow, Cardiac Output and Organ Blood Flow," *Circulation Res.*, **21**, 163–84.

Sabatier (1774), "Memoire sur les Organes de la circulation du sang du Fœtus," Paris edn. published 1778, *Mem. Acad. Royal Sci., Paris*, 198–208.

Spivack, M. (1943), "On the Presence or Absence of Nerves in the Umbilical Blood Vessels of Man and Guinea Pig," *Anat. Rec.*, **85**, 85–109.

Wigglesworth, J. S. (1967), "Vascular Organization of the Human Placenta," *Nature*, **216**, No. 5120, 1120–21.

Wood, C., Ferguson, R., Leelon, J., Newman, W. and Walker, A. (1967), "Fetal Heart Rate and Acid Base Status in the Assessment of Fetal Hypoxia," *Am. J. Obstet. Gynec.*, **98**, 62.

12 ACID BASE METABOLISM IN THE MOTHER AND ITS EFFECT ON THE FOETUS

HEINZ BARTELS

There is hardly any mammalian organ whose function is so difficult to investigate *in vivo* than the foetus in utero. We depend mainly on the belief, generally justified, that almost all foetuses develop normally; if the development is in any way inhibited or disordered we are not aware of this in about 99 per cent of all cases until after birth, or perhaps in a smaller number of cases some days before birth.

The foetal heart is virtually the only signal the foetus gives which can be understood. Questions which a doctor can ask a foetus may sometimes be answered by palpation of the uterus or by an X-ray.

Nevertheless the great variety of changes in the mother during pregnancy will presumably affect the foetus; among these changes those of acid base metabolism are well understood in the mother. We have some information about the influence of such changes on the foetus, mainly during birth, but also some which have been found during Caesarean section in the weeks before term.

We have a great deal of knowledge from experimental studies of other mammals, but extrapolating these data for man should be done with care, because they differ considerably in placental structure and function.

This article discusses (a) acid base metabolism in the mother during pregnancy, (b) the acid base metabolism of the foetus, (c) the effects of the maternal acid base status on that of the foetus and (d) experimental and pathological changes of the acid base metabolism in the mother and its effect on the foetus.

It is assumed that the reader of this chapter is familiar with the scientific basis of acid base metabolism. Those who wish to read further about this subject are recommended to study the articles of Davenport (1963) and Siggaard-Andersen (1965).

(a) Acid Base Metabolism in the Mother during Pregnancy

It is well known that maternal ventilation is increased during pregnancy. This was quantitatively studied by Hasselbalch (1912), and later on in greater detail by Plass and Oberst (1938), Loeschcke and Sommer (1944) and others. The increase is in the range of 40 per cent by the end of pregnancy (Cugell, Frank, Gaensler and Badger, 1953), and mainly consists in an increase of the tidal volume, and to a lesser extent in a rise in the rate of respiration. The increase is mainly of the alveolar ventilation.

The idea that increased ventilation is a result of a rise in basal metabolism can be rejected, because the alveolar carbon dioxide tension is decreased during pregnancy; the mother is definitely hyperventilating. The hyperventilation sets in at the beginning of pregnancy. Hasselbalch and Gammeltoft (1915) observed that after ovulation the alveolar carbon dioxide tension is decreased, and this early observation was confirmed by Döring and Loeschcke (1947). Figure 1 taken from these authors, illustrates the course of the alveolar carbon dioxide pressure during the whole duration of pregnancy in one mother.

Loeschcke and his group showed that hyperventilation was correlated with the increase of progesterone. Hyperventilation could be produced in male subjects by injection of progesterone and oestradiol (Döring, Loeschcke and Ochwadt, 1950). These results were confirmed by Goodland, Reynolds, McCoord and Pommerenke (1953).

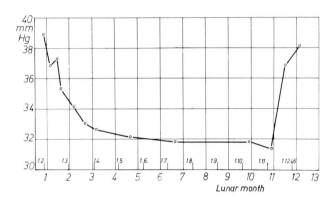

Fig. 1. Alveolar carbon dioxide tension during human pregnancy (one subject), after Doering and Loeschcke (1947).

In terms of acid base balance physiology the mother has a respiratory alkalosis and, as in non-pregnant women and in male subjects the kidney compensates by an increased bicarbonate excretion. The level of standard bicarbonate is consequently diminished, a regulation which tends to restore the blood pH to normal and thus there is a compensatory metabolic acidosis. According to most publications compensation seems not to be complete, that is, the arterial pH is elevated during pregnancy.

Table 1 shows recent data on carbon dioxide tension, pH and standard bicarbonate values in the arterial blood of pregnant women at term. For comparison, the figures of non-pregnant women during the first part of the menstrual cycle before ovulation and values of maternal blood at the intervillous space are given. Hellegers *et al.* (1959) have shown that even at high altitudes where the alveolar carbon dioxide tension in non-pregnant women is 28 mm. Hg., the tension in pregnant women is decreased to 24 mm. Hg.

Hyperventilation not only decreases carbon dioxide tension in the alveolar air, but also increases oxygen tension in the same way. Since while breathing air, the diffusion resistance of the lung for carbon dioxide as well as for oxygen is negligible, arterial blood leaving the lung can be assumed to have the same gas tension as the alveolar gas. Uneven distribution of ventilation and perfusion of the lung and small extra-alveolar right-left shunts produce a diminution in the arterial tension against the alveolar oxygen tension (5 to 10 mm. Hg.). On the other hand the effect on the carbon dioxide pressure is smaller than 1 mm. Hg. and can be neglected.

TABLE 1

CARBON DIOXIDE TENSION (P_{CO_2}), pH AND STANDARD BICARBONATE IN MATERNAL ARTERIAL AND INTERVILLOUS BLOOD AT TERM
(n = number of measurements)

P_{CO_2} (n) mm. Hg.	pH (n)	Stand. Bicarbonate m.Eq./l. (n)	Authors
1. Arterial pregnant			
36·4 (55)	7·435 (58)	20·9 (20)	Wulf (1962)
30·8 (85)	7·463 (85)		Rooth and Sjöstedt (1962) (capillary blood)
32·1 (305)	7·443 (305)	21·4 (305)	Sjöstedt (1962) (capillary blood)
32·3 (10)	7·405 (10)		Schreiner et al (1962)
2. Arterial nonpregnant			
40	7·40	24·3	Bartels (unpublished)
3. Intervillous			
38·0 (16)	7·41 (26)	23·2 (16)	Rooth et al. (1961a)

The foetus receives its oxygen from the maternal arterial blood and gives off carbon dioxide into the maternal venous blood; increased oxygen tension and decreased carbon dioxide can thus be expected to be favourable for gas exchange in the foetus. Later on it will be shown that this is true only for the giving off of carbon dioxide.

Maternal blood at the site for exchange with foetal blood is obtained by puncture of the maternal intervillous space. The most extensive investigations with this method have been undertaken by Rooth, Sjöstedt and Caligara (1961). Their results appear in Table 1. Carbon dioxide tension is higher and pH lower than in the arterial blood. Information obtainable from blood in the intervillous space is however difficult to interpret since in the multi-villous stream bed system of the human placenta (Bartels and Moll, 1964) the maternal blood changes the character of its gas tension from the arterial to the venous state.

Blood samples from the intervillous space are taken at random and *therefore will give gas pressures between arterial and venous values.* The idea of taking blood from the intervillous space in order to measure maternal exchange gas pressures is based on the theoretical existence of a maternal blood pool. This, however, is no longer justified.

(b) The Acid Base Metabolism in the Foetus

The partial pressure of CO_2 in the venous blood of the umbilical artery has been reported as between 45 and 60 mm. Hg. after delivery (Table 2), while in the intervillous space measurements of 35–38 mm. Hg. have been obtained (Table 1). In blood from the uterine vein, CO_2 pressures are approximately 40–45 mm. Hg. Saling (1963) succeeded in drawing blood samples from the hyperaemic scalp of the foetus at the beginning of delivery. He found a value of 44 mm. Hg. This value is confirmed by Beard and Morris (1965). Fischer (1965) found lower values. All values of these authors are calculated from pH and bicarbonate content. Consequently it is appreciated that there is a partial pressure difference between foetal and maternal blood in the placenta, and this represents the removal of carbon dioxide from the maternal blood.

The carbon dioxide formed by the metabolism of foetal cells diffuses into the capillaries. There, it is to a great extent in the red cells, and under the catalytic action of the enzyme carbonic anhydrase. It is now hydrated into H_2CO_3 and then dissociated into (H^+) and bicarbonate (HCO_3^-) ions. The H^+ ions are mainly buffered by the haemoglobin in the red cells, so that only a comparatively small decrease in the blood pH occurs. The buffer effect of haemoglobin acts in two ways:

1. Through its buffer activity as a protein.
2. Through the changing isoelectric point resulting from the deoxygenation of haemoglobin which happens at the same time as carbon dioxide is taken up from the tissues (Christiansen-Douglas-Haldane-effect).

TABLE 2

CARBON DIOXIDE TENSION (P_{CO_2}), pH AND STANDARD BICARBONATE IN FOETAL BLOOD AFTER DELIVERY
(n = number of measurements)

VENA UMBILICALIS			ARTERIA UMBILICALIS			
pH (n)	P_{CO_2} (n) mm. Hg.	Stand. Bicarbonate (n) m.Eq./l.	pH (n)	P_{CO_2} (n) mm. Hg.	Stand. Bicarbonate (n) m.Eq./l.	Authors
7·32 (11)	44·9 (11)	17·0 (11)	7·24 (9)	60·4 (9)	16·5 (11)	Beer et al. (1955)
7·32 (11)	41·6		7·28 (28)	52·9		Goodlin and Kaiser (1957)
7·35 (40)	43·6 (46)	17·5 (21)	7·30 (36)	49·0 (36)	16·5 (11)	Wulf (1958–1960), quoted from Bartels and Wulf (1965)
7·32 (19)	39·7 (19)	17·6 (6)	7·21 (19)	57·0 (17)	14·8 (25)	Rooth et al. (1961b), Rooth (1963)

The second effect is more pronounced than the first; formed bicarbonate leaves the red cells by diffusion in exchange for plasma chloride ions, in this way promoting further dissociation of carbonic acid and further buffering of hydrogen ions within the red cells.

About 30 per cent of transferred carbon dioxide is bound as carbaminohaemoglobin directly by the haemoglobin and about 8 per cent is dissolved as carbon dioxide in equilibrium, whereas the remaining part is bound as bicarbonate.

The carbonic anhydrase in adult blood increases the reaction rate of carbon dioxide with water approximately 13,000-fold, in this way decreasing the time for 90 per cent completion of the reaction to 0·02 sec. This is short enough for a sufficient rapid reaction of H_2CO_3 as opposed to $H_2O + CO_2$. The contact time in the lung is in the range of 0·1–0·5 sec. (Roughton, 1945; Schlosser, Heyse and Bartels, 1965). The contact time in the human placenta is believed to be much longer, mainly because the intervillous, almost capillary-like, channels are in the range of 2 cm., whereas the foetal capillaries in the villi are about 100 times shorter.

The carbonic anhydrase concentration in the foetal blood is much lower than in adult blood and it may even be absent in young foetuses. It can therefore be expected that during carbon dioxide exchange in the foetal blood of the villi, at least in young foetuses, there will be no equilibrium between carbon dioxide tension and bicarbonate concentration. If this is correct, the carbon dioxide tension in the foetal blood of the villi would be lower than its level in the blood of the umbilical vein. After contact of foetal blood with maternal blood, formation of carbon dioxide from H_2CO_3 could still proceed. There is evidence from experiments in goats, rabbits and guinea pigs that such events do take place (Bartels, El Yassin and Reinhardt, 1967).

To obtain quantitative ideas of carbon dioxide exchange and acid base balance during the placental gas exchange, it is convenient to study these processes on the basis of the carbon dioxide dissociation curve. Figure 2 shows such curves for non-pregnant, pregnant and labouring women; and two foetal curves. It is seen that the amount of chemically bound carbon dioxide (bicarbonate and carbaminohaemoglobin, shown in the ordinate) is decreased in pregnant women as the result of the metabolic compensation of the respiratory alkalosis induced by hyperventilation.

The even lower curve of women during labour is obviously the result of muscular activity giving rise to fixed acids, mainly lactic acid, as it is always seen during muscular work. Fixed acids decrease the bicarbonate concentration.

The chemically bound carbon dioxide in the foetal blood at birth is within the same range as in the maternal blood during labour. Demonstration of the carbon dioxide in the blood with the help of carbon dioxide dissociation curves is still rather abstract for the parameter of oxygen transport has to be taken into account.

Figure 3 tries to show the exchange of carbon dioxide from the foetal into the maternal blood in the placenta.

Dissociation curves are presented from 3 maternal (mat. a, b, c) and 3 foetal (foet. a, b, c) blood samples. The transfer of carbon dioxide from foetal into maternal blood will lower the foetal carbon dioxide tension from approximately 60 mm. Hg. to 44 mm. Hg.

The exchange of chemically bound carbon dioxide is determined not only by the change in the carbon dioxide tension, but also by the Christiansen-Douglas-Haldane-effect. In this graph this effect is made evident by the two

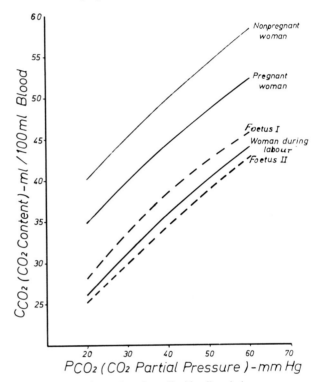

Fig. 2. Sections of carbon dioxide dissociation curves from the blood of non pregnant (Bartels et al. 1955), pregnant women (Rossier and Hotz 1953) and women during labour (Fischer et al. 1965) as well as from foetal blood at term (Beer et al. 1955, Eastman et al. 1933).

carbon dioxide dissociation curves a and c both for maternal and foetal blood. During passage through the placenta, not only is carbon dioxide given off but oxygen is taken up, and thus carbon dioxide binding ability is decreased (curve a); in this way more carbon dioxide can pass from the foetal blood into the maternal blood.

The same effect works in the maternal blood in the opposite direction, which means on the basis of the Christiansen-Douglas-Haldane-effect, that maternal blood can bind more carbon dioxide than without it (curves mat. a and c). The values marked a' and v' would therefore be applicable, were it not that another process, the exchange of fixed acid from the foetal into the maternal blood influences the carbon dioxide exchange. This in turn increases the carbon dioxide combining ability in the foetal blood and decreases it in the maternal blood. In fact, for a given carbon dioxide tension change, less carbon dioxide is exchanged; points a and v respectively represent the final carbon dioxide content and tension in the foetal and maternal blood after exchange in the placenta.

Doubt has been expressed on the diffusion of fixed acids from foetal into maternal blood, because sometimes higher values for lactic acid have been found in maternal arterial blood and in the umbilical vein (Vedra, 1959). It was concluded that the foetus is oxydizing maternal lactic acid. This may happen during labour and with other muscular exercise during pregnancy, but many results suggest that the foetus normally gives off fixed acids into the maternal blood.

yet on the other hand it cannot be considered apart from the questions of oxygen transport.

The uptake of carbon dioxide and fixed acids in maternal blood decreases oxygen combining ability (Bohr effect), on the other hand release of these substances from foetal blood increases the oxygen combining ability of foetal blood so that the Bohr effect comes into action twice. At a given tension difference for oxygen, more oxygen can be transferred than without the Bohr effect in both

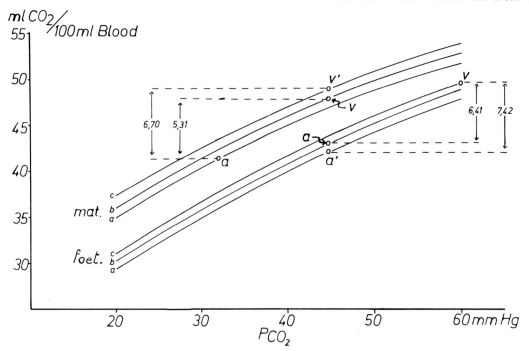

FIG. 3. Carbon dioxide dissociation curves of maternal (mat. a, b, c) and foetal (foet a, b, c) blood, showing the influence of both oxygenation and the level of standard bicarbonate upon the position of the carbon dioxide dissociation curve (after Beer, Bartels and Raczkowski 1955).
mat a Maternal arterial blood (98 % saturated with oxygen) mat b Uterine venous blood (53,5 % saturated with oxygen)
mat c Maternal blood (53,5 % saturated with oxygen, but with the same standard bicarbonate concentration as arterial blood)
foet a Umbilical arterial blood (13,7 % saturated with oxygen)
foet b Umbilical venous blood (47,7 % saturated with oxygen)
foet c Foetal blood (47,7 % saturated with oxygen, but with the same standard bicarbonate concentration as that of umbilical arterial blood).
The vertical distance between curve a and curve c of each group demonstrates the effect of oxygenation upon the affinity of blood for carbon dioxide. The vertical distance between curve c and curve b of each mother and foetus represents the change in carbon dioxide affinity due to the transfer of fixed acids from foetal to maternal blood: in the absence of fixed acid transfer, maternal blood would pick up 6,70 vol% of carbon dioxide during uterine transit while foetal blood would lose 7,42 vol% of carbon dioxide between umbilical artery and umbilical vein. Because of fixed acid transfer these values are reduced to 5,31 vol% for maternal blood (v — a) and 6,41 vol% for foetal blood (v — a).

Results of experiments concerning lactic acid exchange are not in general applicable, for other reasons for Rooth and Nilsson (1964) found that beside lactic acid, glutamic acid, o-oxoglutaric and pyruvic acid are present and exchanged. Recently Štembera and Hodr (1966) showed a fixed acid flow from the foetus to the mother during pregnancy. An indirect indication of the fixed acid transfer from foetal into maternal blood is the decrease of the standard bicarbonate value (carbon dioxide content of 100 ml. plasma at 40 mm. Hg. carbon dioxide tension and full oxygen saturation) of foetal blood after passage through the placenta (Beer, Bartels and Raczkowski, 1955). This mechanism obviously increases the amount of carbon dioxide exchanged at a given difference in tension;

bloods. Thus the mechanism which diminishes carbon dioxide exchange increases oxygen exchange (Fig. 4).

There is no information concerning acid base balance status during pregnancy in the human, and the application of data from sheep and goat foetuses delivered before term appears to be questionable. There are two possible ways of getting information on the foetal acid base status before birth:

1. Measurements in the amniotic fluid.
2. Measurements from capillary blood taken from the foetal scalp during delivery.

Preliminary results on the acid base status of amniotic fluid have been published by Rooth, Sjöstedt and Caligara (1961) and Schreiner, Bühlmann and Held (1961). They conclude that pH and carbon dioxide tensions reflect corresponding values in the umbilical artery and in the foetal subcutaneous tissues. Rooth, Sjöstedt and Caligara (1961), gave results in early pregnancies, from the twelfth to the twentieth week. After this, that is toward the end of pregnancy, there is a significant increase in carbon dioxide tension from 51 to 58 mm. Hg. This method is only applicable for some hours before delivery, and according

There are some measurements and some speculations (Wulf and Manzke, 1964) which give an idea of what happens to the foetus under the influence of changes in the maternal acid base balance. Furthermore, there are some experiments in mammals whose results can be taken into consideration.

It has already been explained that the mother is during almost the whole of pregnancy in a state of respiratory

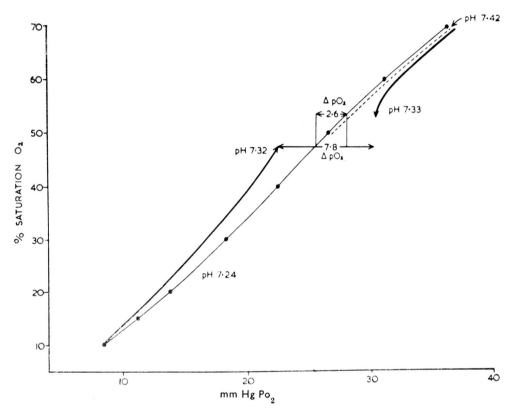

FIG. 4. Maternal (– – – –) and foetal (———) functional dissociation curves during gas exchange in the placenta. It is to be seen that for a given exchange condition there remains a much greater pressure difference for oxygen by the negative (foetus) and positive (mother) Bohr effect (after Bartels 1959).

to later publications, for instance by Rooth and Sjöstedt (1966), is not keeping up to earlier expectations.

Measurements of capillary blood taken from the scalp is a still more recent method (Saling, 1963). There is now agreement that the scalp blood gives values of the carbon dioxide tension similar to those of foetal arterial blood (umbilical artery).

In summary it can be said that information on the acid base status of the foetus depends mainly on information during labour, and this may give us a wrong picture of the acid base status in utero. Presumably foetal acidosis is less pronounced in utero before the onset of labour.

(c) The Effects of the Maternal Acid Base Status on that of the Foetus

It has already been made clear that there is no precise way to judge foetal acid base metabolism except under the extreme condition prevailing at the time of delivery.

alkalosis, partly compensated for by a metabolic acidosis. as shown in Table 1, the main carbon dioxide tension is 32 mm. Hg. instead of about 40 mm. Hg. in the non-pregnant woman.

It may be supposed that this lowered carbon dioxide tension helps the carbon dioxide unloading of the foetus, otherwise foetal carbon dioxide tension would be even higher and the pH lower. Study of Figures 2 and 3 makes it possible to calculate what would happen if the carbon dioxide tension were near 40 mm. Hg. Reduction in the difference of carbon dioxide tension between foetal and maternal blood lessens the amount of exchange carbon dioxide, for two mm. Hg. correspond approximately to about one ml. of carbon dioxide.

The influence of maternal oxygen tension on that of the foetus is determined in quite a different way. Hyperventilation increases the arterial oxygen tension by approximately 8 to 10 mm. Hg., that is to about 105 mm. Hg. for pregnant women living near sea level. As at this tension haemoglobin is almost totally saturated with oxygen the increase in oxygen content will be in the range of only 0·115 ml. O₂ per 100 ml. in maternal blood. Nevertheless, because the oxygen tension, not the oxygen content, governs oxygen transfer into foetal blood, a small increase in foetal oxygen tension should be seen. That as a matter of fact it cannot be observed is explained by the influence of the concomitant alkalosis which occurs during hyperventilation and diminishes placental perfusion, thus opposing the effect of an increase of oxygen transfer to the foetus.

Many authors have shown that the foetal carbon dioxide tension, pH and bicarbonate concentration are in fairly good correlation to the values in maternal blood; this has recently been confirmed by Newman, Braid and Wood (1967), and Newman, Mitchell and Wood (1967). Moya, Morishima, Shnider and James (1965) showed that forced hyperventilation does not facilitate carbon dioxide transport from the foetus to the mother. These authors observed that forced hyperventilation towards the end of pregnancy is accompanied by high carbon dioxide tension and a high degree of base deficit in the foetal blood.

Experiments with guinea pigs (Morishima, Moya, Bossers and Daniel, 1964) with forced hyperventilation with 5 per cent carbon dioxide in the inhaled gas mixture suggest that the mechanics of breathing have a circulatory effect in addition to the hypocapnia caused in the mother. It is assumed that perfusion of the intervillous space is decreased by inhibition of the venous drainage of the placenta.

These results have an important practical application as they show that there is no advantage in lowering the carbon dioxide tension in the maternal blood artificially.

(d) Experimental and Pathological changes of the Acid Base Metabolism in the Mother and its Effects on the Foetus

The influence of forced maternal hyperventilation on the foetal acid base status must be mentioned again in this section. For example the pathological changes of the acid base metabolism in the mother, the acid base status in diabetic mothers and the influence of nitrous oxide inhalation on the foetal acid base status have been used.

1. Kaiser and Goodlin (1958) presented a thorough study of pregnant diabetic women; this disease usually presents as a classic metabolic acidosis. It is likely that diabetic women have a more pronounced metabolic acidosis in labour than normal women. The increase in [H⁺] concentration and carbon dioxide tension is relatively small and cannot be held responsible for the well known neonatal difficulties of infants of diabetic mothers. Extreme changes in the foetal acid base situation might account for foetal death.

2. The use of nitrous oxide as an analgesic agent in labour, increased the amount of metabolic acid in foetal blood, although the carbon dioxide tension in the maternal and the foetal blood is normal (Rooth. 1963). While the cause of this metabolic acid in the foetus is not clear, a

factor may be a brief shortage of oxygen in the mother and consequently in the foetus.

Treatment of foetal acidosis has been attempted by Rooth (1964) by giving sodium bicarbonate intravenously to the mothers during labour.

Conclusions

Maternal hyperventilation, induced by hormone changes, and partially compensated for by a metabolic acidosis, is helpful in carbon dioxide transport from the foetus through the placenta and into the maternal blood. Artificial hyperventilation in the mother does not however increase carbon dioxide transfer, probably because of circulatory effects.

It is very difficult to get information concerning acid base metabolism in the foetus during pregnancy. It is only shortly before delivery that from the amniotic fluid, and after the onset of delivery from the capillaries of the foetal scalp that carbon dioxide tension and content as well as pH can be measured; the results have to be interpreted with great care. An attempt has been made to treat foetal acidosis by giving the mother sodium bicarbonate by the intravenous route during labour.

REFERENCES

Bartels, H. (1959), "Chemical Factors Affecting Oxygen Carriage and Transfer from Maternal to Foetal Blood," in Walker, J. and Turnbull, A. C., *Oxygen Supply to the Human Foetus*, pp. 29–41, Blackwell Scientific Publications.

Bartels, H., Beer, R., Koepchen, H. P., Wenner, J. and Witt, I. (1955), "Messung der alveolär-arteriellen O₂-Druckdifferenz mit verschiedenen Methoden am Menschen bei Ruhe und Arbeit," *Pflügers Arch.*, **261**, 133–151.

Bartels, H., El Yassin, D. and Reinhardt, W. (1967), "Comparative Studies of Placental Gas Exchange in Guinea Pigs, Rabbits and Goats," *Respiration Physiology*, **2**, 149–162.

Bartels, H. and Moll, W. (1964), "Passage of Inert Substances and Oxygen in the Human Placenta," *Pflügers Arch. ges. Physiol.*, **280**, 165–177.

Bartels, H. and Wulf, H. (1965), "Physiologie des Gasaustausches in der Plazenta des Menschen," in Linneweh, F., *Fortschritte der Pädologie*, Band I, pp. 124–146. Springer-Verlag.

Beard, R. W. and Morris, E. D. (1965), "Foetal and Maternal acid-base balance during normal labour," *J. Obstet. Gynaec. Brit. Cwlth.*, **4**, 496–515.

Beer, R., Bartels, H. and Raczkowski, H.-A. (1955), "Die Sauerstoffdissoziationskurve des fetalen Blutes und der Gasaustausch in der menschlichen Plazenta," *Pflügers Arch. ges. Physiol.*, **260**, 306–319.

Cugell, D. W., Frank, N. R., Gaensler, E. A. and Badger, T. L. (1953), "Pulmonary Function in Pregnancy: (1) Serial Observations in Normal Women," *Amer. Rev. Tuberc.*, **67**, 568–597.

Davenport, H. W. (1963), *The ABC of Acid-base-chemistry*. Chicago: University Press.

Döring, G. K. and Loeschcke, H. H. (1947), "Atmung und Säure-Basen-Gleichgewicht in der Schwangerschaft," *Pflügers Arch. ges. Physiol*, **249**, 437–451.

Döring, G. K., Loeschcke, H. H. and Ochwadt, B. (1950), "Weitere Untersuchungen über die Wirkung der Sexualhormone auf die Atmung," *Pflügers Arch. ges. Physiol.*, **252**, 216–230.

Eastman, N. J., Geiling, E. M. K. and De Lawder, A. M. (1933), "Foetal Blood Studies: IV. The Oxygen and Carbon Dioxide Dissociation Curves of Fœtal Blood," *Bull. Johns Hopkins Hosp.*, **53**, 246–254.

Fischer, W. M. (1965), "Untersuchungen zum Säure/Base-Gleichgewicht," *Arch. Gyn.*, **200**, 534–551.

Fischer, W. M., Vogel, H. R. and Thews, G. (1965), "Der Säure-Basen-Status und die CO_2-Transportfunktion des mütterlichen und fetalen Blutes zum Zeitpunkt der Geburt," *Pflügers Arch. ges. Physiol.*, **286**, 220–237.

Goodland, R. L., Reynolds, J. G., McCoord, A. B., and Pommerenke, W. T. (1953), "Respiratory and Electrolyte Effects Induced by Estrogen and Progesterone," *Fertility and Sterility*, **4**, 300–317.

Goodlin, R. C. and Kaiser, I. H. (1957), "The Effect of Ammonium Chloride Induced Maternal Acidosis on the Human Fetus at term. I. pH, Hemoglobin, Blood Gases," *Am. J. M. Sc.*, **233**, 662.

Hasselbalch, K. A. (1912), "Ein Beitrag zur Respirationsphysiologie der Gravidität," *Skand. Arch. Physiol.*, **27**, 1–12.

Hasselbalch, K. A. and Gammeltoft, S. A. (1915), "Die Neutralitätsregulation des graviden Organismus," *Biochem. Z.*, **68**, 206–264.

Hellegers, A., Metcalfe, J., Huckabee, W., Meschia, G., Prystowski, H. and Barron, D. (1959), "The Alveolar pCO_2 and pO_2 in Pregnant and Non-pregnant Women at Altitude," *Proc. Ann. Meeting S. Clin. Invest.*, **38**, 1010.

Kaiser, I. H. and Goodlin, R. C. (1958), "Alterations of pH, Gases and Hemoglobin in Blood and Electrolytes in Plasma of Fetuses of Diabetic Mothers," *Pediatrics*, **22**, 1097–1109.

Loeschcke, H. H. and Sommer, K. H. (1944), "Über Atmungserregbarkeit in der Schwangerschaft," *Pflügers Arch. ges. Physiol.*, **248**, 405–425.

Morishima, H. O., Moya, F., Bossers, A. C. and Daniel, S. S. (1964), "Adverse Effects of Maternal Hypocapnea on the Newborn Guinea Pig," *Amer. J. Obstet. Gynec.*, **88**, 524–529.

Moya, F., Morishima, H. O., Shnider, S. M. and James, L. S. (1965), "Influence of Maternal Hyperventilation on the Newborn Infant," *Amer. J. Obstet. Gynec.*, **91**, 76–84.

Newman, W., Braid, D. and Wood, C. (1967), "Fetal Acid-base Status: I. Relationship between Maternal and Fetal pCO_2," *Amer. J. Obstet. Gynec.*, **97**, 43–51.

Newman, W., Mitchell, P. and Wood, C. (1967), "Fetal Acid-base Status: II. Relationship between Maternal and Fetal Blood Bicarbonate Concentrations," *Amer. J. Obstet. Gynec.*, **97**, 52–57.

Plass, E. D. and Oberst, F. W. (1938), "Respiration and Pulmonary Ventilation in Normal Non-pregnant, Pregnant and Puerperal Women," *Amer. J. Obstet. Gynec.*, **35**, 441–449.

Rooth, G. (1963), "Foetal Respiration," *Acta Pædiatrica*, **52**, 22–35.

Rooth, G. (1964), "Early Detection and Prevention of Fœtal Acidosis," *Lancet*, **I**, 290–293.

Rooth, G. and Nilsson, I. (1964), "Studies on Fœtal and Maternal Metabolic Acidosis," *Clin. Science*, **26**, 121–132.

Rooth, G. and Sjöstedt (1962), "The Placental Transfer of Gases and Fixed Acids," *Arch. of Disease in Childhood*, **37**, 366–370.

Rooth, G., Sjöstedt, S. and Caligara, F. (1961a), "Acid-base Balance of the Amniotic Fluid," *Amer. J. Obstet. Gynec.*, **81**, 4–7.

Rooth, G., Sjöstedt, S. and Caligara, F. (1961b), "Hydrogen Concentration, Carbon Dioxide Tension and Acid Base Balance in Blood of Human Umbilical Cord and Intervillous Space of Placenta," *Arch. Dis. Childh.*, **36**, 278.

Rooth, G. and Sjövall, A. (1966), "Acid-base Status of Amniotic Fluid during Delivery," *Lancet*, **I**, 371–372.

Rossier, P. H. and Hotz, H. (1953), "Respiratorische Funktion und Säurebasengleichgewicht in der Schwangerschaft," *Schweiz. med. Wochenschr.*, **83**, 897–901.

Roughton, F. J. W. (1945), "The Average Time spent by the Blood in the Human Lung Capillary and its Relation to the Rates of CO Uptake and Elimination in Man," *Am. J. Physiol.*, **143**, 621–633.

Saling, E. (1963), "die Blutgasverhältnisse und der Säure/Basen-Haushalt des Fetus bei ungestörtem Geburtsablauf," *Z. Geburtsh. Gynäk.*, **161**, 262–293.

Schlosser, D., Heyse, E. and Bartels, H. (1965), "Flow Rate of Erythrocytes in the Capillaries of the Lung," *J. appl. Physiol.*, **20**, 110–112.

Schreiner, W. E., Bühlmann, A. and Held, E. (1961), "pH- und CO_2-Bestimmung im menschlichen Fruchtwasser," *Gynaec.*, **152**, 66–71.

Schreiner, W. E., Tsakiris, A. and Bühlmann, A. (1962), "Der Einfluß der mütterlichen Atmung auf die fetale Kohlensäurespannung (pCO_2)," *Arch. f. Gynäk.*, **197**, 93–100.

Siggaard-Andersen, O. (1965), *The Acid-base Status of the Blood.* Copenhagen: Munksgaard.

Sjöstedt, S. (1962), "Acid-base Balance of Arterial Blood during Pregnancy, at Delivery and in the Puerperium," *Amer. J. Obstet. Gynec.*, **84**, 775–779.

Štembera, Z. K. and Hodr, I. (1966), "I. The Relationship between the Blood Levels of Glucose, Lactic Acid and Pyruvic Acid in the Mother and in Both Umbilical Vessels of the Healthy Fetus," *Biol. neonat.*, **10**, 227–238.

Vedra, B. (1959), "Acidosis and Anaerobiosis in Full Term Infants," *Acta. pædiat.*, Uppsala, **48**, 60–69.

Wulf, H. (1962), "Der Gasaustausch in der reifen Plazenta des Menschen: I. Teil: Die utero-umbilikalen Sauerstoff- und Kohlensäure-Spannungsdifferenzen," *Z. Geburtsh. u. Gynäk.*, **158**, 117–134.

Wulf, H. and Manzke, H. (1964), "Das Säure-Basen-Gleichgewicht zwischen Mutter und Frucht," *Z. Geburtsh. u. Gynäk.*, **162**, 225–253.

1. BLOOD PRESSURE: ITS MAINTENANCE AND REGULATION

G. W. PICKERING and B. E. JUEL–JENSEN

The flow of blood through the blood vessels follows in a general way hydrodynamic principles. However, blood is not a Newtonian liquid and viscosity depends (apart from variables in the components of the blood such as the cell mass) a good deal on the size of the vessel and the rate of flow. These general principles of relationship between flow in a tube, the viscosity of the fluid, and the radius of the tube are expressed mathematically in Poiseulle's formula:

$$\text{Flow} = \frac{(P_1 - P_2)\pi r^4}{8\eta L}$$

where P_1 and P_2 are the pressures at the two ends of the tube,

    r is the radius of the tube,

    η is the viscosity of the fluid,

    L is the length of the tube.

Figure 1 shows the fall of pressure through the vascular tree as observed by Landis's direct measurement. From the point of view of the economy of the animal as a whole, the important part of the circulation is that through the

capillaries, for it is here that the tissues exchange components with the blood; it is here that the tissues gain their raw materials for metabolism and rid themselves of the waste products. As Landis (1934) showed, the capillary pressure at rest tends to exceed the colloid osmotic pressure of the blood at the arterial end of the capillary and to be smaller at the venous end. From the physiological point of view, arterial pressure is not one of the important constituents in the homeostatis of the body. Its regulation is nothing like so exact as, for example, that of the oxygen or CO_2 tension of the blood or the central body temperature.

Variations during the Day

Until quite recently the extent to which arterial pressure varies during the course of existence was completely unknown. Recent technical innovations are remedying

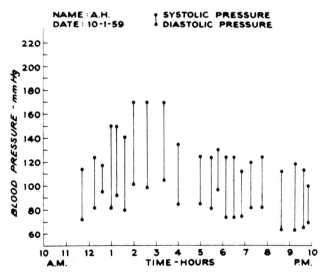

FIG. 2. Levels of blood pressure determined with the portable recorder of Subject A.H. over a ten-hour period. Activities included driving in traffic (1.0 p.m.), speaking at a meeting (2.0 to 3.30 p.m.), and resting at home (9.45 p.m.). (Hinman, Engel and Bickford (1962) *Amer. Heart J.*, 63, 663.)

this defect. Hinman (1962) and his colleagues in San Francisco have developed a portable apparatus. The subject inflates a conventional cuff which is linked via a transducer to a tape-recorder. A microphone over the brachial artery picks up the pulse sounds (Korotkoff sounds). When the cuff is inflated above 50 mm. Hg. a magnetic tape recorder automatically starts recording the blood pressure and the Korotkoff sounds simultaneously. Figures 2 and 3 show two such results and the

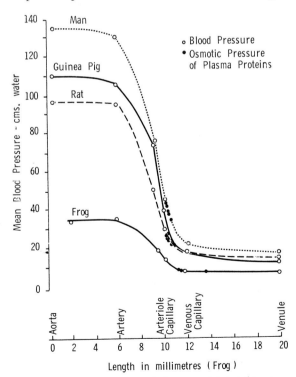

FIG. 1. Chart showing the fall of pressure (circles) in peripheral vessels of man, guinea-pig, rat and frog. Dots indicate the osmotic pressure of the plasma proteins. (Landis (1934) *Physiol. Rev.*, **14**, 404.)

effects on arterial pressure of such things as driving through traffic and a heated argument. Richardson, Honour, Fenton, Stott and Pickering (1964) have developed a more fully automatic machine which, however, is not

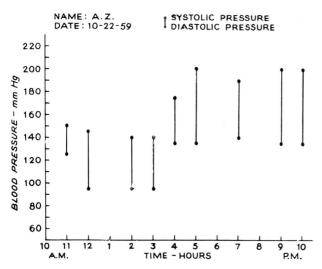

FIG. 3. Levels of blood pressure determined with the portable recorder by Subject A.Z. The first four determinations were made when the subject was alone and reading quietly; the next two were made when he was in a heated discussion about some phase of his work, and the last three were made when he was at home caring for his children. (Hinman, Engel and Bickford (1962) *Amer. Heart J.*, **63**, 663.)

portable. It consists of a Gallavardin double cuff which is inflated automatically at predictable intervals, e.g. 5 min. The pressure in the cuff and the pulsations from the lower cuff are inscribed on a trace. The first increase in pulsation gives the systolic, and the maximum pulsation, the diastolic pressures. The freedom of the subject is

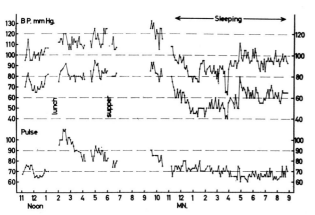

FIG. 4. Blood pressure of a physician during 24 hours. (Richardson, Honour. Fenton, Stott and Pickering (1964) *Clin. Sci.*, **26**, 445.)

limited to the length of tubing connecting the cuff on his arm with the apparatus. Figure 4 shows the recorded pressures in one of the authors. The astonishing new feature in this tracing is the profound fall in arterial pressure during sleep. Figure 5 shows a 24-hour record from

a 34-year-old accountant with elevated arterial pressure, who had episodic forgetfulness and dysphasia but no other complications. The pressor effect of an unpleasant emotional stimulus is illustrated at 3.0 p.m., when he was

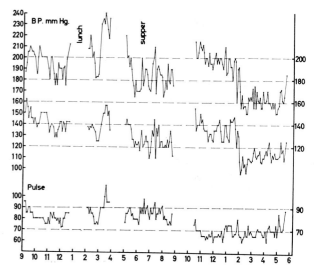

FIG. 5. Blood pressure in a patient with hypertension during 24 hours. (Richardson, Honour, Fenton, Stott and Pickering (1964) *Clin. Sci.*, **26**, 445.)

awakened from a nap by a neurologist who examined his mental function and within the hearing of the patient stated that brain disease was present. Like all the hypertensive subjects we investigated, this patient showed a marked decline in pressure during the early hours of sleep. Figure 6 shows the difference between the maximum and

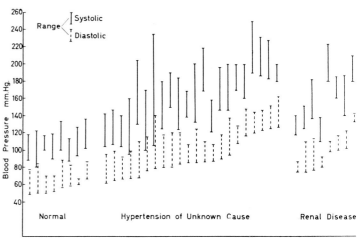

FIG. 6. Ranges of blood pressure in eight normals, 22 patients with essential hypertension and eight subjects with renal disease. Top bar of each range represents average pressure during highest hour of 24-hour record. The bottom bar represents the average during the lowest hour. (Richardson, Honour, Fenton. Stott and Pickering (1964) *Clin. Sci.*, **26**, 445.)

minimum values found with this apparatus in 8 normotensive subjects, 22 subjects with essential hypertension and 8 subjects with renal disease. The range is irregular and has, up to date, not been closely correlated with initial pressure, age or sex.

Richardson, Honour and Goodman (1967) measured the intra-arterial blood pressure by continuous recording during a night of natural sleep in each of 17 healthy subjects. They found an average fall in arterial pressure of 22/12 mm. Hg. during sleep. They recorded EEGs throughout the same period and found that recurrence of alpha rhythm was accompanied by elevation of blood pressure (mean 13/11 mm. Hg.). Dreams were associated

more cumbersome, indirect machines. It has been possible to obtain exclusive continuous records in subjects with the minimum interference with their normal activities throughout the day and night.

The Influence of the Observer

Kapsammer in 1899 was the first to call attention to the elementary and most important fact that the methods

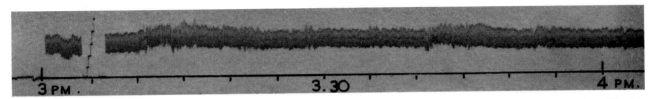

FIG. 7. Part of a 24-hour continuous arterial pressure record. The record represents one hour in time, and shows at the left a stepwise calibration of the trace from 0 to 250 mm. Hg. in 50 mm. steps. (Bevan and Honour (1967). In preparation.)

with little change in the mean arterial pressure and heart rate.

Perhaps the most promising new apparatus is that described by Bevan, Honour and Stott (1966). Here a nylon catheter is inserted into the brachial artery and connected to a transducer which is worn on the chest at heart level and which leads to a galvanometer whose deflections are photographed on slowly moving paper.

used for measurement affect the value we seek to measure. In general, the circumstances of measurement are such that they act as stimuli to two most important reflexes involving the body as a whole including the cardiovascular system, namely the defence reflex and the orienting reflex. It is common experience and an elementary point of method when therapy is being tested that blood pressure tends to fall with repeated measurement. Figure 9 shows the

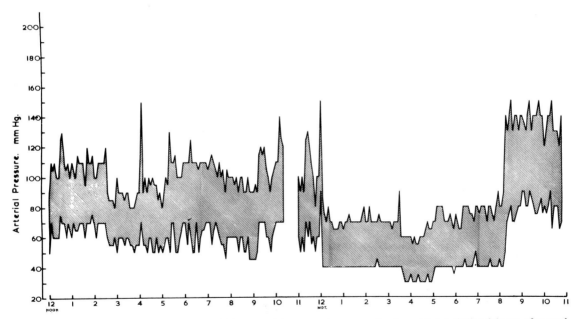

FIG. 8. Plot of 24 hours continuous record of direct arterial pressure in a normotensive subject including 8 hours of natural sleep between 12 midnight and 8 a.m. Readings plotted at five minute intervals. (Bevan and Honour (1967). In preparation.)

The recorder unit can be carried in the pocket. This apparatus is fully portable and fully automatic. Figure 7 shows part of a continuous record from a hypertensive subject during part of a day and night. Figure 8 shows the plot at 5 min. intervals of a continuous record of direct arterial pressure in a normotensive subject. Note the drop in blood pressure during sleep. This instrument has confirmed many of the data which were got with the earlier,

values recorded in a patient treated with a placebo and visiting a clinic at weekly intervals. As the subject becomes more used to the procedure the blood pressure tends to fall. The blood pressure of 100 healthy medical students seated at a table was measured every five minutes for an hour by Diehl and Lees (1929). They found that the blood pressure fell significantly for the first three readings. After that the differences between successive readings were less than the probable error of the differences, until the eighth reading, which was the lowest, the pressure then gradually rising to the twelfth.

Ayman and Goldshine (1940) obtained readings in the home and in the clinic in 34 patients with essential hypertension over long periods. The home readings were made daily by the patient or a member of the family. The home readings were lower in all, the difference

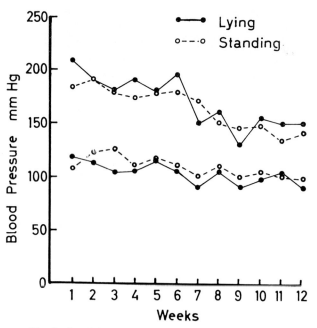

FIG. 9. Arterial pressure, measured at weekly intervals, on a clinic patient receiving inert tablets. (Pickering, Cranston and Pears (1961) *The Treatment of Hypertension*, Charles C. Thomas, Springfield, Illinois.)

amounting to 20 mm. or more in diastolic pressure in 24 per cent of the patients.

We found at St. Mary's that the pressures recorded by the physician at the patient's first visit to out-patients were of the order of 20 mm. higher than those we obtained in the conditions of the St. Mary's survey (Hamilton, Pickering, Roberts and Sowry, 1954a). The reason is obvious. At a patient's first visit he or she is terrified at having to lie naked or semi-naked in front of a crowd of strange people, with the possibility of terrifying news. In the St. Mary's survey, patients only bared their right arm and sat round a table waiting for some 15 minutes while those who had preceded them had their pressures taken.

It is not surprising either that different observers have different pressor effects on their patients. In general, observers of the same sex obtain readings which are lower than those obtained by observers of the other sex (Comstock, 1957).

Position

This has little effect on the blood pressure of a subject despite a fall in right auricular pressure and cardiac output. This is achieved by vascular reflexes initiated by the baro-receptors or the carotid sinus and effected through the sympathetic nerves (Brigden, Howarth and Sharpey Schafer, 1950).

Casual and Basal Arterial Pressure

Addis (1922) was the first to try and obtain readings in which the orienting or defence reflexes had been extinguished. There have been several editions of the so-called basal pressure by Smirk and his colleagues. In their latest method, the patient is admitted to a single room and sleeps with the aid of barbiturates. Early in the morning the patient is wakened by an attractive technician (sex not specified) who talks soothingly to the patient and sits taking readings for approximately half an hour. The end of such a series gives the basal pressure. Readings obtained in this way are probably the most replicable of the pressures that obtain during the waking state. They are not the lowest pressures. They are not, as it were, a floor of arterial pressure but such pressures are much more certain guides of prognosis than the casual pressures obtained in the office, ward, or out-patient department. Unfortunately they require more time and more facilities than most physicians, ourselves included, have at their disposal.

The Mechanism of the Regulation of Blood Pressure

Poiseuille's equation shows the factors on which arterial pressure depends in the physical sense. It is conventional to regard it as the product of the cardiac output and the peripheral resistance. The peripheral resistance in turn depends on viscosity, which depends chiefly on the number of red corpuscles per cu. mm. of blood and on the length and diameter of the arteries, capillaries and veins through which the blood passes. As Figure 1 shows, the fall of pressure is the most rapid in small arteries and arterioles, which are often referred to as the resistance vessels. The cardiac output is dependent on the venous pressure filling the heart. This in turn depends on the relationship between the blood volume and the capacity of the circulation. The capacity of the circulation is chiefly constituted by the capillaries, venules and veins. These then are often referred to as the capacitance vessels.

If blood is removed from the circulation, e.g. from an artery or vein, the blood volume shrinks and cardiac output drops. The arterial pressure is maintained for a time by compensatory vaso-constriction, which affects skin, muscle, gut, kidneys, but not heart or brain. When the arterial pressure drops the cardiac output has already been reduced to about a half. It is thus a sign that the margin of safety in the circulation has been considerably encroached upon. The mechanisms regulating the arterial pressure, as in the example described, are complex. However, one stands out, namely the baroreceptors which are situated in the outer coats of the arterial wall in the arch of the aorta and in the wall of the carotid sinus. When these structures are stretched impulses are sent up the vagus and the carotid sinus nerves with each peak of systolic pressure. The higher the pressure the greater the frequency of impulses. These impulses affect reflexly the heart rate through the vagus and the vasomotor tone through the sympathetic nerves and the adrenal glands. It is these reflexes which account for the maintenance of the arterial pressure when the body is swung from a horizontal to the foot-down position and for the response to haemorrhage.

The blood volume decreases in changing from the recumbent to the upright position (Thompson, Thompson and Dailey, 1928). Cranston and Brown (1963) have shown that the blood volume varies little throughout the day but that it is a little lower in the morning than in the evening in normal subjects. This difference, which is unrelated to posture, becomes much more marked in patients with high blood pressure. This may lead to

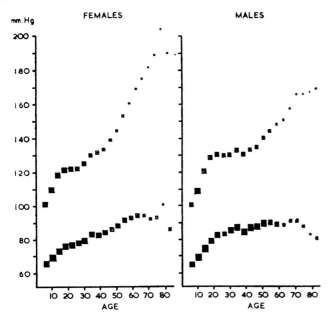

Fig. 10. Mean systolic and diastolic blood pressures in 1261 males and 1305 females living in a mining valley and an agricultural community in South Wales, each subject being measured twice. The area of each square is inversely proportional to the standard error of the mean and so indicates the weight to be attached to each mean. (Miall and Oldham (1963) *Brit. med. J.*, **1**, 75.)

problems in management of such patients when hypotensive agents are employed.

That the arterial pressure falls during sleep, maybe to half its value while awake, is perhaps the outstanding feature of the circulation. Why is there this difference? Recently Smyth, Sleight and Pickering (1967) have attempted to estimate the sensitivity of the baroreceptor reflexes during sleep in man. The baroreceptor reflexes were tested by plotting the pulse interval (as measured by ECG) against the subsequent systolic pressure as measured directly from the brachial artery during the rise of pressure produced by giving a small dose of angiotensin injected intravenously. These observations have shown that the carotid sinus mechanism is active during sleep and indeed its sensitivity greater than when the subject is awake. It is evidence that the striking difference in arterial pressure in the sleeping and waking states reflects the profound difference in the activity of the central nervous system in these two states. It is now held that waking is characterized by activation of the cortex through the reticular formation of the brain. In sleep the cortex is to some extent cut off by the inactivity of the reticular formation.

This is the clearest example of the profound influence of the nervous system on the regulation of arterial pressure.

In an account like this it is not possible to review the other mechanisms regulating arterial pressure. For these reference should be made to *High Blood Pressure* (Pickering, 1968), or to one of the standard textbooks of physiology, such as Best and Taylor.

ARTERIAL PRESSURE IN THE POPULATION

A very large number of surveys of arterial pressure have been made in representative populations all over the globe. These have shown that in every advanced society arterial pressure tends to rise with age. By far the best of these surveys is that by Miall and Oldham (1955, 1958) in South Wales. They selected by true randomization populations in the Rhondda Fach and Vale of Glamorgan, and over 90 per cent of their first degree relatives living within a given radius. Each subject had his or her arterial pressure measured by Miall on two occasions separated by four years. Figure 10 shows the mean values found. It will be seen that the curves are different in men and women, arterial pressure being higher in women from middle age onwards. Figure 11 shows the frequency distribution

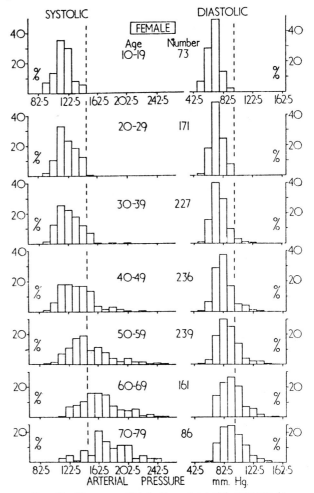

Fig. 11. Frequency distribution of arterial pressures in females of a population sample, arranged by age in decades. (Hamilton, Pickering, Roberts and Sowry (1954) *Clin. Sci.*, **13**, 11.)

of arterial pressures in females in the St. Mary's sample. From this it will be seen that first, the arterial pressure evidently rises more in some subjects than others, indeed there may be some subjects in whom the arterial pressure does not rise at all; second, there is no natural dividing line at any pressure. In fact, to a student of general biology any such dividing line would seem to be nothing more or less than an artefact.

Is there a Dividing Line between Normotension and Hypertension?

Table 1 summarizes some of the suggestions that have been made about whether a dividing line should be drawn.

TABLE 1

SOME SUGGESTED DIVIDING LINES BETWEEN "NORMOTENSION" AND "HYPERTENSION"

Division	Author
120/80	S. C. Robinson and M. Brucer (1939)
130/70	F. J. Browne until 1947
140/80	D. Ayman (1934)
140/90	G. A. Perera (1948)
150/90	C. B. Thomas (1952)
160/100	P. Bechgaard (1946)
180/100	N. M. Burgess (1948)
180/110	W. Evans (1956)

Clearly not all of these suggestions can be right. In fact, not one of these authors produced valid evidence for his suggestion. Table 2 shows the relationship between arterial pressure and expectation of life. There is no dividing line.

TABLE 2

MORTALITY RATIOS* FOR MEN ACCORDING TO GROUPS OF SYSTOLIC AND DIASTOLIC (FIFTH PHASE) BLOOD PRESSURE READINGS, WITHOUT MINOR IMPAIRMENTS. ALL ENTRY AGES TOGETHER
(from Actuarial Society of America and Association of Life Insurance Medical Directors 1941)

Systolic Reading (mm.)	Diastolic Reading (5th Phase) (mm.)				
	64–83%	84–88%	89–93%	94–103%	All %
118–132	90†	91	99	97	92
133–142	99	107	118	134	110
143–152	133	137	141	173	143
153–167	186	178	189	237	210
All	95	100	116	151	106

* Actual to expected deaths (expected = 100)
† This included only systolic readings 128 to 132 mm.

No serious student of arterial pressure now supports the idea of a dividing line between normotension and hypertension though many clinicians continue to use the terms and to employ the concept. Indeed, as always, an old habit dies hard. The fact is that arterial pressure is a quantity and should be treated, as is natural, as a quantity

and not as a quality, good or bad. If this is done then it is found that all the consequences of arterial pressure are related quantitatively to it. In general the higher the worse. This is true for example for foetal salvage as Table 3 shows.

TABLE 3

INFANT MORTALITY IN 27,000 DELIVERIES, BELLEVUE HOSPITAL, NEW YORK
(Wellen (1953), *Amer. J. Obstet. Gynec.*, **66**, 36)

	Infant Mortality	Stillbirths
	%	%
Specific hypertensive disease of pregnancy, mild	7·1	3·1
Specific hypertensive disease of pregnancy, severe	22·0	15·8
Essential hypertension, uncomplicated	10·1	6·5
+ Specific hypertensive disease	27·7	16·8

Factors known to Influence the Arterial Pressure

Age. Arterial pressure rises with age, and more in some subjects than in others. However, the rise is continuous in the individual and is probably related to the changes in properties in elasticity the arterial tree incurs with age.

Sex. The influence of sex is shown in Figure 10.

Weight. The American Actuarial Societies' study of build and blood pressure showed, as others had previously found, the importance of weight. The greater the degree of obesity, the higher the arterial pressure both in males and females. This effect is not entirely due to the error produced by fat arms (see Pickering, Roberts and Sowry, 1954).

Occupation. Miall and Oldham's survey in South Wales showed that the heavier the occupation the lower the arterial pressure.

Smoking. In general smokers have lower arterial pressures than non-smokers. It has been suggested that it may be a reflection of body-weight, as smokers tend to be less obese than non-smokers.

Diet. Apart from obesity, starvation and rigid salt restriction, diet has not been found to influence arterial pressure.

Salt. The influence of salt on arterial pressure is disputed. Dahl (1962) considers that the intake of salt is an important factor determining arterial pressure. Neither Miall and Oldham in South Wales, nor Dawber (1967) and his colleagues in Framingham were able to find any relationship between salt intake and arterial pressure.

Family size. Perhaps the most surprising thing to emerge from the South Wales survey was that the larger the number of children the lower the arterial pressure and this was true both of males and females. Figures 12, 13, 14 and 15 show the relationship.

None of these factors is great enough to account for the variations in arterial pressure observed. Miall and Oldham's survey in particular provided strong evidence for a multifactorial or polygenic inheritance of arterial

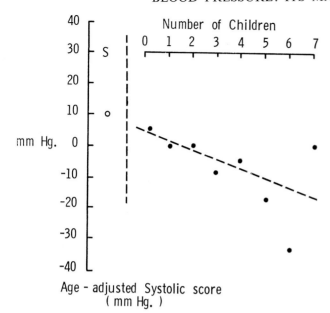

FIG. 12. Age-adjusted systolic scores and family size for females aged 15–45 in the population samples (propositi). (S = single.) (Miall and Oldham (1958) *Clin. Sci.*, **17**, 409.)

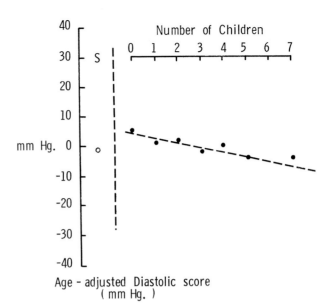

FIG. 13. As Figure 12, but for diastolic scores. (Miall and Oldham (1958) *Clin. Sci.*, **17**, 409.)

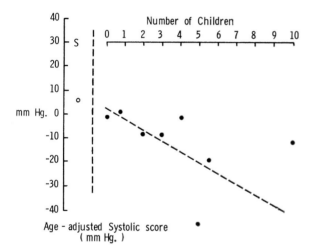

FIG. 14. Age-adjusted systolic scores and family size for males aged 15–50 in the population samples (propositi). (S = single.) (Miall and Oldham (1958) *Clin. Sci.*, **17**, 409.)

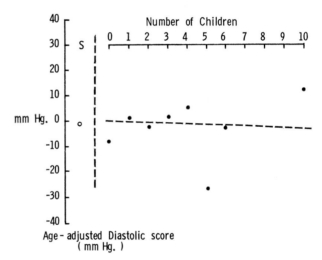

FIG. 15. As Figure 14, but for diastolic scores. (Miall and Oldham (1958) *Clin. Sci.*, **17**, 409.)

pressure. Figures 16 and 17 show the relationship between arterial pressure of first degree relatives and the propositi from which they were derived on the whole population investigated and using the mean of two readings. The age and sex adjusted scores were devised by Hamilton, Pickering, Roberts and Sowry (1954a), to allow for the observed variations between the two sexes and at different ages. These scores were established by a biometrical procedure similar to that used by Francis Galton (1889) in his classic study, *The Inheritance of Stature*. The age and sex adjusted scores express the deviation from the pressures which would be expected at age 60, had the

observed arterial pressure behaved as it has been found to behave in the population at large. It will be noted that the linear relationship is the same for pressures that are below the average (hypotension) or above the average (hypertension). The slope of the line is almost exactly the same as that found by Hamilton and others (1954b) in their relatives of propositi with essential hypertension. This makes it extremely likely that the arterial pressure is inherited in a similar way throughout the ranges commonly called hypotension, normotension and hypertension. It is most unlikely that arterial pressure is inherited by a single gene behaving as a Mendelian dominant or recessive.

Such genes exercise their effects through a specified chemical fault, as implied by the one gene one enzyme hypothesis. No single chemical fault has been discovered in essential hypertension though there are of course disorders associated with hypertension which may be carried through a single gene, as for example, familial phaeochromocytoma.

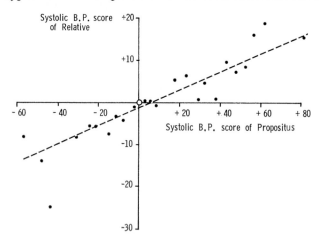

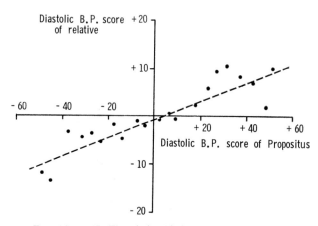

FIGS. 16 AND 17. The relationship between scores of propositi and the mean scores of their relatives in the combined population samples from the Rhondda Fach and Vale of Glamorgan; systolic and diastolic. (Miall and Oldham (1958) *Clin. Sci.*, **17**, 409.)

REFERENCES

Addis, T. (1922), *Arch. intern. Med.*, **30**, 240.

Ayman, D. and Goldshine, A. D. (1940), *Amer. J. med. Sci.*, **200**, 465.

Best, C. H. and Taylor, N. B. (1966), *The Physiological Basis of Medical Practice*, 8th Ed. Baltimore: Williams & Wilkins.

Bevan, A. Honour, A. J. and Stott, F. G. (1966), *J. Physiol.*, **186**, 3P.

Brigden, W., Howarth, S. and Sharpey Schafer, E. P. (1950), *Clin. Sci.*, **9**, 79.

Comstock, G. W. (1957), *Amer. J. Hyg.*, **65**, 271.

Cranston, W. I. and Brown, W. (1963), *Clin. Sci.*, **25**, 107.

Dahl, L. K., Heine, M. and Tassinari, L. (1962), *J. exper. Med.*, **115**, 1173.

Dawber, T. R., Kannel, W. B., Kagan, A., Donabedian, R. K. and McNamara, P. M. and Pearson, G. (1967), "Environmental Factors in Hypertension," in *The Epidemiology of Hypertension*, Ed. J. Stamler and R. Stamler.

Diehl, H. W. and Lees, H. D. (1929), *Arch. intern. Med.*, **44**, 229.

Galton, F. (1889), *Natural Inheritance*. London: Macmillan.

Hamilton, M., Pickering, G. W., Roberts, J. A. F. and Sowry, G. S. C. (1954a), *Clin. Sci.*, **13**, 11.

Hamilton, M., Pickering, G. W., Roberts, J. A. F. and Sowry, G. S. C. (1954b), *Clin. Sci.*, **13**, 273.

Hinman, A. T., Engel, B. T. and Bickford, A. F. (1962), *Amer. Heart J.*, **63**, 663.

Kapsammer, G. (1899), *Wien. klin. Wschr.*, **12**, 1279.

Landis, E. M. (1934), *Physiol. Rev.*, **14**, 404.

Miall, W. E. and Oldham, P. D. (1955), *Clin. Sci.*, **14**, 459.

Miall, W. E. and Oldham, P. D. (1958), *Clin. Sci.*, **17**, 409.

Pickering, G. W., Roberts, J. A. F. and Sowry, G. S. C. (1954), *Clin. Sci.*, **13**, 267.

Pickering, G. W. (1968), *High Blood Pressure*, 2nd Ed. London: Churchill.

Richardson, D. W., Honour, A. J., Fenton, G. W., Stott, F. H. and Pickering, G. W. (1964), *Clin. Sci.*, **26**, 445.

Richardson, D. W., Honour, A. J. and Goodman, A. O. (1967). In preparation.

Smyth, H. S., Sleight, P. and Pickering, G. W. (1967), *J. Physiol.*, **194**, 46P.

Thompson, W. O., Thompson, P. K. and Dailey, M. E. (1928), *J. Clin. Invest.*, **5**, 573.

2. BLOOD PRESSURE IN PREGNANCY

IAN MacGILLIVRAY

Ever since it was recognized that convulsions occurring towards the end of pregnancy, in labour or soon after delivery, were associated with hypertension, obstetricians and others have made intensive studies of the blood pressure in pregnancy. This has been done both with a view to detecting and preventing convulsions or eclampsia and also to see if it might be possible by elucidating the cause of the rise in blood pressure, thereby to determine the cause of eclampsia.

Until quite recently methods of recording the blood pressure have lacked precision and, of course, direct intra-arterial measurements cannot be used in routine practice. It is, therefore, in many ways surprising that there is a fair degree of agreement in published reports about the changes in blood pressure which occur in pregnancy.

Before discussing the changes which have been found it is as well to consider the changes occurring in pregnancy which could influence the blood pressure. There is a marked increase in the blood volume and also in the cardiac output in normal pregnancy which, if not compensated for, would give rise to hypertension.

The cardiac output rises in the early stage of pregnancy from the non-pregnant level of about 4·5 L. up to 5·5 L. and then, more slowly to about 6 L/min. about the twentieth week of pregnancy and remains about this level until term, if the measurements are made with the subjects in the lateral position. It was generally accepted that there was a fall in cardiac output in the later weeks of pregnancy until it was shown by Lees, Taylor, Scott and Kerr (1967a), that the inferior vena caval occlusion associated with the supine position causes a variable fall in cardiac output and all previous measurements of cardiac output in pregnancy had been made with the patients in this position. Lees, *et al.* (1967b), claimed that the rise in the cardiac output is in the order of 30 to 40 per cent. They adduced evidence to show that it is unlikely that placental arterio-venous shunts, increase in plasma volume or foetal demands are relevant to the increase in cardiac output. The increase in plasma volume is more gradual from a starting level of around 2,600 ml. up to a peak of around 3,800 ml. at 34 weeks. Thereafter, there is a decline of about 200 ml. at term (Hytten and Paintin, 1963).

The fall in blood pressure resulting from the supine hypotensive syndrome can be very marked. The incidence of this syndrome is given variously as 11·2 per cent (Howard, Goodson and Mengert, 1953), and 3 per cent (Quilligan and Tyler, 1959). There is very little effect on the blood pressure in the non-pregnant state if a ganglion-blocking agent, tetraethyl ammonium chloride, is injected intravenously, but in pregnant women there is an increasing effect reaching a maximum in the third trimester (Assali, Fergon, Kada and Garber, 1952).

This suggests that the autonomic nervous system in pregnancy is correcting for the effect of an active vaso-dilator substance, the nature of which is unknown.

As many cases of hypertension in the non-pregnant state are of renal origin it might be postulated that the renal changes occurring in pregnancy could predispose to changes in blood pressure. There is a marked rise in plasma renin in normal pregnancy (Brown, Davies, Doak, Lever, Robertson and Trust, 1966). This is an enzyme produced in the renal juxtaglomerular cells and it is found in the kidneys, blood, uterus, placenta, salivary glands and in the amniotic fluid. Renin acts on an α 2 globulin in the plasma, from which it splits off angiotensin 1, a decapeptide. A converting enzyme then removes two amino acids to produce angiotensin 11, an octapeptide, which is the most potent pressor substance known.

The most marked actions of the renin-angiotensin system are the pressor effects, the release of adrenalin and the stimulation of autonomic ganglia, the production of aldosterone and the control of sodium excretion. There is a rise in the output of aldosterone and a retention of some 850 m.eq. sodium in normal pregnancy. Other changes such as the development of the vast vasculature of the placenta occur in pregnancy which might influence the blood pressure regulating mechanisms and it is not surprising that there are blood pressure changes in most women in pregnancy.

Pregnancy is a vascular hyperkinetic state and this adds to the problems of recording the blood pressure. To the usual difficulties of recording the blood pressure, such as the position of the patient, the arm circumference, time of day, and the patient-observer relationship, there is the added difficulty of dealing with a hyperkinetic state in which the blood pressure sounds on auscultation over the brachial artery may persist until zero pressure at the cuff. There has been much controversy about the reliability or otherwise of taking the diastolic pressure at the point of muffling or at disappearance. Most authors are agreed that the systolic pressure is even less reliable than the diastolic pressure. Using direct arterial measurements some workers have found that the indirect technique underestimates the systolic pressure and that phase five of the Korotkoff's sounds (disappearance) correlates best with the direct diastolic pressure, but others have concluded that phase four of the Korotkoff's sounds (muffling) correlated with the direct diastolic pressure better than phase five. While some (Whyte, 1961, and Holland and Hummerfelt, 1964) have found that arm circumference has no influence on indirect readings of blood pressure, others (Pickering, Roberts and Sowry, 1954), suggested that corrections should be applied to allow for arm circumference. A recent study by Raftery and Ward (1968), showed that there was no relationship between arm circumference, skinfold thickness and the direct level of blood pressure. They found good agreement between phase one indirect pressure and the systolic pressure. The phase five (disappearance) indirect pressure agreed better with direct diastolic pressure than phase four (muffling), but they emphasized that the range of variation for all indirect recordings was very wide. The direct intra-arterial pressures were recorded from the upper end of the brachial artery and the indirect pressure was recorded from the same artery using the London School of Hygiene sphygmomanometer (Rose, Holland and Crowley, 1964), which excludes observer bias.

Although there have been many studies of the blood pressure in pregnancy there is still doubt about the normal pattern. This is mainly due to the fact that it has not been possible to standardize the method sufficiently well in the studies which have, so far, been carried out or reported. Most of the difficulties, however, can probably be overcome by studying a sufficiently large number even though there are deficiencies in the standardization of the methods. Such studies have generally agreed that there is a fall in the level of blood pressure in the first trimester of pregnancy which continues in the second trimester and then the level of blood pressure tends to rise again. The level to which it can rise in late pregnancy, however, is uncertain and the border line between normal physiology and pathology has not been clearly established. Probably there is no clear-cut division. Some workers, particularly Browne, have chosen 130/70 as the dividing line, but this would seem to be too low as a very large number of pregnant women would fall into the abnormal category. Even taking a level of 140/90 as suggested by Nelson (1955) and MacGillivray (1961a) means that in some areas a large percentage of primigravidæ are considered abnormal.

On the other hand, a blood pressure rise to 140/90 or more without any associated proteinuria can occur without any deleterious effect on the mother or on the baby. Indeed, it has been shown (Nelson, 1955), that the babies of such women have a lower perinatal death rate than in primigravidæ who were normotensive. Again, it has been shown (MacGillivray, 1967) that women who develop a rise of blood pressure to 140/90 or more without proteinuria have larger babies than the women with normotensive pregnancies. The reason for this appears to be that women who have a high weight gain tend to develop hypertension, but such women who have a high weight gain also have larger babies. A rise of blood pressure at the end of pregnancy, in itself, does not have any effect on the weight of the baby unless there is associated proteinuria, but because women who have a rise of blood pressure also tend to have high weight gains their babies tend to be larger than those of women who are normotensive.

The rise of blood pressure which occurs in some women at the end of pregnancy may represent the temporary unmasking, during pregnancy, of a hypertensive tendency which subsides after delivery, but returns in later life. Many workers have shown that women with hypertensive tendencies are more liable to have a rise of blood pressure during pregnancy and that they would ultimately become hypertensive even if they had never become pregnant.

This view is supported by the finding that nulliparous women as well as women who had pre-eclampsia have a higher mean blood pressure and a greater proportion of higher blood pressures in later life than parous women of comparable age who had not had pre-eclampsia (Adams and MacGillivray, 1961).

TABLE 1

INCIDENCE OF HYPERTENSION IN LATER LIFE
(35–50 YEARS)

	S.B.P. $\geqslant$ 140 mm. %	D.B.P. $\geqslant$ 90 mm. %
Proteinuric Pre-eclampsia	43	40
Late Hypertension	58	60
Normotensive	26	21
Nulliparae	41	35

The level of 140/90 is probably acceptable as a pathological level for Britain, although McClure Browne (1961), concluded from a review of data from all over Britain, that a blood pressure higher than 148/90 must be considered as abnormal.

The diastolic pressure level of 90 mm.Hg. is not necessarily applicable to all the countries in the world. The blood pressure readings in tropical areas are, generally, low, (Doll and Hannington, 1961), and a diastolic pressure of 90 mm.Hg. or more is very unusual. The blood pressure in West African primigravidae is very low in early pregnancy (Lawson, 1961). It is sometimes suggested that blood pressures of less than 90 mm.Hg. should be taken in the tropical areas to indicate pre-eclampsia, but in West African women, just as in British women, proteinuria seldom develops before the diastolic pressure reaches 90 mm.Hg. The diastolic pressure can rise as much as 15 mm.Hg. without the appearance of proteinuria, so long as the diastolic pressure does not reach 90 mm.Hg. and the amount of rise appears to be of less importance than the level reached.

In a survey carried out in 1958–59 the level of blood pressure at the 20th week of pregnancy was recorded in various areas of the British Isles and Eire (MacGillivray, 1961b). This showed that in mid-pregnancy the blood pressure was highest in Eire and Scotland and lowest in London. The blood pressure in late pregnancy was also measured. Again, the highest readings were in Eire and Scotland. This might be due to the methodological differences in taking the blood pressure, but it is probable that this was a true observation as the incidence of proteinuria was, London 2·9 per cent, the rest of England 3·0 per cent, Eire 3·5 per cent and Scotland 4·1 per cent.

The incidence of severe pre-eclampsia, i.e., hypertension and proteinuria in primigravidae in Aberdeen is 9 per cent in those in whom the diastolic pressure was 90 mm.Hg. or more before the 20th week of pregnancy compared to 5 per cent in those in whom the initial pressure was low. It seems probable then that there is a higher initial level of blood pressure in women in Ireland and in Scotland than in those of England. There were also strong indications from Israel, Nigeria and Jamaica that blood pressures there are lower than in Western Europe.

The level of blood pressure is quite clearly influenced by age; or, at least it is true to say that high blood pressure occurs more commonly in older age groups. This also applies in pregnancy, but it is of some interest to note that the diastolic pressure rises steadily with age whereas the systolic pressure shows a change only after the age of thirty. Although it has been stated previously that a rise of blood pressure can be physiological, nevertheless obstetricians cannot afford to consider a blood pressure rise to 140/90 or more as physiological in all cases, even though albuminuria does not appear, because of the risk of eclampsia or other complications occurring.

The triad of hypertension, oedema and albuminuria is usually considered to constitute the condition of pre-eclamptic toxaemia. As a rise to 140/90 or more may be physiological and as oedema occurs with such great frequency in pregnancy that it may also be considered physiological, the only sign which is constantly abnormal is albuminuria. This, however, does not occur without either hypertension or oedema being present. This condition of pre-eclamptic toxaemia is well known to be mostly a disease of primigravidae. Indeed, some maintain that there is no such condition as recurrent toxaemia of pregnancy and that some underlying condition such as a renal lesion must be present in such cases. It is now accepted that pre-eclamptic toxaemia does not cause permanent renal damage. Although pre-eclamptic toxaemia does not tend to recur in second pregnancies about half of the women who have hypertension alone in the first pregnancy will have a recurrence of hypertension in second and subsequent pregnancies. This probably merely indicates that pregnancy reveals a latent tendency to hypertension. There is a well known familial tendency to hypertension and this has also been shown to occur in the hypertension of pregnancy. The incidence of toxaemia in pregnancy approaches 40 per cent in both the sisters and daughters of women who have had eclampsia (Chesley, Cosgrove and Annitto, 1961). A familial tendency to toxaemia does not appear to be related to a hypertensive diathesis.

incidence of pre-eclampsia or hypertension in their first pregnancies than did the sisters of primigravidae who had not had pre-eclampsia or hypertension. Mothers of women who had pre-eclampsia in their first pregnancies had a higher level of blood pressure than those whose daughters did not develop hypertension in their first pregnancies. These findings suggest a strong familial tendency to pre-eclampsia and to hypertension in pregnancy.

Although both a rise of blood pressure and oedema can be considered as physiological there is, nevertheless, no doubt that this combination can herald the onset of pre-eclamptic toxaemia. It is still not clear whether hypertension or oedema is the primary sign of pre-eclamptic toxaemia. It seems fairly clear, however, that pre-eclamptic toxaemia can occur without clinical oedema but also it is clear that women who develop oedema have a greater tendency to develop hypertension and toxaemia. The exact association between oedema and hypertension remains obscure, nor is it even clear whether they have the same basic aetiology. Although it is probable that the excessive weight gain which tends to occur in pre-eclampsia is mostly due to fluid retention it is possible that, at least in some cases, there is also abnormal fat deposition to account for the weight gain.

Most recent studies have shown that the rate of weight gain in itself is of little value in predicting in the individual case which patient will develop pre-eclampsia. When the weight gain is taken in conjunction with the initial blood pressure and with the rise in blood pressure between the 20th and 30th weeks the weight gain was a valuable guide to the subsequent incidence of albuminuria, prematurity and perinatal mortality (MacGillivray, 1961a). Failure to gain weight is at least as important as an excessive gain in terms of perinatal mortality and probably indicates a failure of the foetus to grow.

TABLE 2

PERCENTAGE INCIDENCE IN SISTERS

Sisters (555)	Index Cases (419)		
	Normo-tensive	Late Hyper-tension	Proteinuric Pre-eclampsia
Normotensive	71·8	51·4	51·7
Late Hypertension	23·8	40·2	34·4
Proteinuric Pre-eclampsia	4·5	9·4	13·8

Adams and Finlayson (1961) also showed that sisters of primigravidae who developed pre-eclampsia or some degree of hypertension in pregnancy developed a higher

TABLE 3

DEUTERIUM SPACE RELATED TO HEIGHT IN NORMAL PREGNANCY AND PRE-ECLAMPTIC TOXAEMIA

	Number of Cases	Deuterium Space ml./cm.
Normal pregnancy	15	244
Pregnancy with excess weight gain	5	253
Mild P.E.T. Without oedema	13	251
With oedema	11	267
Severe P.E.T. Without oedema	9	243
With oedema	7	280

Measurements of total body water have shown (MacGillivray, 1961b; Hytten, Thomson and Taggart, 1966) that large amounts of fluid can be retained in women who remain normotensive whilst some women who develop pre-eclampsia have amounts of total body water which are within normal limits. The amount of water in oedematous pre-eclamptic patients is similar to that in high weight gain normotensive women. This could possibly mean that the fluid retained is normal or physiological or that the amount retained is a manifestation of a mild form of pre-eclampsia, or again that the distribution of fluid differs between the normotensives and the pre-eclamptics. In a study of the records of 24,000 pregnant women, Thomson, Hytten and Billewicz, (1967), found that oedema was present in about 40 per cent. Oedema was present in 35 per cent of those who remained normotensive, in 60 per cent of those who developed hypertension and in about 85 per cent of women who had both hypertension and proteinuria. Although this probably means that oedema in pregnancy may be physiological and in itself not an ominous clinical sign, nevertheless some types of fluid retention are probably pathological.

BROMIDE SPACES AND DEUTERIUM SPACES

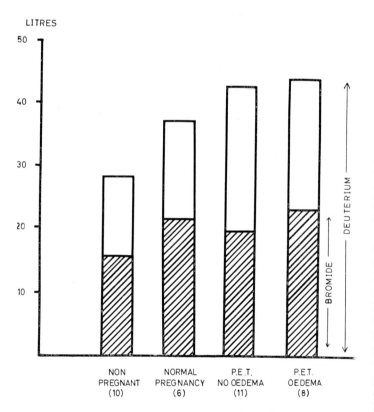

The distribution of fluid between intracellular and extracellular spaces might be a guide to determining which cases are physiological and which are pathological. The extracellular space was measured with bromide and the intra-cellular space was derived by subtracting the bromide space from the total body water space measured with deuterium oxide (MacGillivray, 1967). In the small number of cases in which estimations were done it appears that in normal pregnancy there is relatively more fluid retention outside the cell than in pre-eclamptics without

oedema. The oedematous pre-eclamptic women have more intracellular than extracellular fluid retention. More results will have to be obtained in the various groups before confident conclusions can be drawn, but the findings are suggestive.

When the possible causes of hypertension are being enumerated sodium retention must be considered as a raised blood pressure occurs in such states as aldosteronism in which there is salt retention. In normal pregnancy there is a considerable sodium retention. In normal pregnancy with excess weight gain and probable retention of fluid, the sodium space is similar to mild toxaemia or hypertension with oedema. In severe pre-eclamptic toxaemia, without clinical oedema, the total body water and sodium are similar to those in normal pregnancy, but in severe pre-eclampsia with clinical oedema there is more sodium and more water than in normal pregnancy (MacGillivray, 1967). The conflicting reports reviewed by Chesley (1966) about the amount of sodium retained in pre-eclampsia can probably be explained on the basis that there may be more or less fluid retention in some cases of pre-eclamptic toxaemia than in normal pregnancy. Undoubtedly, however, salt and water retention can occur in pregnancy to a quite marked degree without being associated with hypertension. Conversely, severe pre-eclamptic toxaemia can occur with little salt or water retention. It is unlikely, therefore, that sodium retention is basically involved in the hypertensive process. It is more likely that oedema is physiological in many pregnancies, but in some cases the underlying mechanism of the hypertension also causes changes in the vessels allowing fluid to escape into the interstitial space. This escape of fluid is probably related to the protein shift which occurs in normal pregnancy. The low level of plasma proteins might be due to renal loss of protein, loss into interstitial fluid by capillary leakage, reduced synthesis by the liver or malnutrition.

The percentages of albumin in serum and oedema fluid are directly related (Freeman and Joekes, 1967; Antonaci and Macagnimo, 1957; Hammond and Ross, 1960, and MacGillivray, 1967), and this suggests that the albumin and globulin pass from the plasma into the extracellular fluid by diffusion. The protein pattern in the urine and oedema fluid is very similar in any one individual with toxaemia and the albumin content of the urine and oedema fluid shows a proportionally marked increase compared with the serum. This probably occurs because there is generalized alteration in the systemic and glomerular capillaries allowing an increase in permeability, particularly to albumin. It was also found that there was a significantly smaller amount of sodium per litre of water in the tissue fluid than in the serum of toxaemic patients. The cause of the shift of fluids in pre-eclamptic toxaemia remains obscure.

This is also true of the hypertension occurring in pregnancy. Many substances have been held responsible for the rise in blood pressure but so far no pressor agent has been isolated with certainty. Hunter and Howard (1960), are the most recent authors to have claimed to have isolated a specific pressor substance, but other workers have not been able to confirm this. Brown, *et al.* (1966) have suggested that the substance which Hunter and Howard were estimating was, in fact, renin, and there is good evidence to support their view. The pressor substance liberated from an ischaemic placenta might be analogous to that produced from an ischaemic kidney and the substance which is most likely to cause hypertension in this way is renin.

In women with the most severe forms of pre-eclampsia the renin values were below the mean for normal pregnant women (Brown, *et al.* 1966). Other pressor substances which have been suggested as the cause of pre-eclampsia include vasopressin and noradrenaline, but none has been conclusively shown to be in excess in pre-eclampsia. There is, however, the suggestion that in pre-eclampsia there is an increased sensitivity to normal amounts of a pressor substance. Chesley (1965), has claimed that in four cases of pre-eclampsia he found an increased sensitivity to infused angiotensin. There is, however, evidence that the sensitivity to infused angiotensin varies inversely with the endogenous levels of renin (Kaplan and Silah, 1964). Hocken, Kark and Passovoy (1966), have pointed out that if a potent endogenous hormone is present in excess and is producing an end-organ response, then in order to further stimulate end-organ responses in the patient greater amounts of the hormone will have to be given than that which will produce the same degree of end-organ response in normal subjects. Hence, if there is an increased level of circulating angiotensin present then the patient's tolerance of the effects of exogenous angiotensin ought to be increased. Chesley's findings can, therefore, be interpreted as showing that there are reduced levels of endogenous renin in pre-eclampsia rather than showing that there is a hypersensitivity to angiotensin.

The rise of blood pressure could result from an increase in the blood volume, an increased cardiac output, an increased peripheral vascular resistance, an increased blood viscosity or decreased distensibility of vessel walls. There is no evidence that the last two factors are concerned in the rise of blood pressure which occurs in pre-eclamptic toxaemia. The blood volume instead of increasing is decreased in pre-eclampsia (Cope, 1961; MacGillivray, 1961a). There is, so far, no evidence that the cardiac output is increased in toxaemia more than it is in normal pregnancy. Increased peripheral vascular resistance appears to be the probable cause of the hypertension of pregnancy and this increased peripheral resistance could be the result of renal, endocrine or placental disturbances.

Although there is general agreement that there is reduced renal plasma flow and glomerular filtration rates in pre-eclampsia and that the blood flow through the decidual space is reduced, there is certainly no agreement that either of these changes is primary. The pathological changes in the kidneys are now well-documented from electron microscopic studies; the most important feature is the striking swelling of the endothelial cytoplasm of the glomerular capillaries. The narrowing of the capillary lumen is further added to by the epithelial cytoplasmic swelling and vasculation. The changes in the placental bed vessels have also been studied (Robertson, Brosens and Dixon, 1967). The earliest change is a fibrinoid necrosis of the vessel walls which are later infiltrated by lipophages. Govan (1961), suggested that a common vascular reaction caused the similar lesions in various organs in eclampsia. He considers the hypertension is the underlying cause of the vascular reactions and may produce any degree of change from fibrinoid vasculosis to complete necrosis of the vessel.

Hypertension can then account for both the renal and the placental bed changes but the cause of the hypertension is elusive. When whole blood is taken from patients with severe pre-eclampsia and later reinfused into those patients after delivery there is a transient but significant rise in blood pressure (Tatum and Mulé, 1962). Comparable toxaemic patients who received transfusions of normal bank blood did not have any rise in blood pressure. Page (1938), transfused 400 mls. of blood from patients with eclampsia or severe pre-eclampsia into normal pregnant women without causing any increase in blood pressure. This suggests that a circulating pressor substance causes the rise of blood pressure only in sensitized patients and the pressor substance need not be in abnormal amounts.

It is of interest in this connection that the increased effect of a ganglion blocking agent in pregnant women compared to non-pregnant women is not found in pre-eclamptic women, suggesting that there is a lack of the vasodilator substance presumed to be present in normal pregnancy.

The pressor substance is not known but could be noradrenaline, vasopressin, angiotensin, 5-hydroxy tryptamine or some other pressor substance found circulating in normal pregnancy; probably the more important factor is the one which causes the increased sensitivity. Govan, Mukherjee, Hewitt and Harper (1951), have suggested that this might be chorionic gonadotrophin. Loraine and Matthew (1950), found a significant rise in HCG levels in severe toxaemia, but more recent work (Brody and Carlstrom, 1965), using immunological methods does not support this view as HCG was not found in excess in toxaemia.

An immunological basis for pre-eclampsia producing an increased sensitivity is very attractive but hypotheses which have been postulated by Kalmus (1946) and Platt, Stewart and Emery (1958) do not fully agree with immunological principles and the natural history of toxaemia. Robertson, *et al.* (1967), suggest that there may be an immunological component in the vascular lesions of pre-eclamptic toxaemia because of the morphological similarities of acute atherosis to arterial lesions in other diseases known or suspected to be associated with antigen-antibody reactions. Steblay (1962), has produced evidence that antigens present in the human placenta are very similar to those present in the human kidney. The difficulty of accepting an immune type of mechanism is that the severity of the condition would be expected to increase in subsequent pregnancies and that permanent damage would result. Toxaemia affects mostly first pregnancies and does not cause permanent damage to the kidneys.

Several workers have tried to produce evidence that an antibody is responsible for the production of pre-eclamptic toxaemia (Wagner, Savasal, Kassalova, Maly, Mecl and Prokop, 1959(a), 1959(b) and Hulka, 1963). Brody (1964), claimed that serum from patients with toxaemia of pregnancy contains a factor which agglutinates DNA-sensitized erythrocytes and that the haemagglutination tests strongly suggested that this factor was an antibody. This preliminary finding, however, was not confirmed by Beck and MacGillivray (1968). Although there is no proof from the work that has been done that an antibody is responsible nor has an acceptable theory been presented to explain pre-eclamptic toxaemia on a maternal-foetal incompatability, nevertheless, an immunological basis for the disease cannot yet be discarded.

The role of hormones in the control of blood pressure in pregnancy and in the possible production of pre-eclamptic toxaemia is still debated. Oestrogens may sensitize the vessels, in some way, to a pressor substance but are, themselves, not hypertensive agents. The same applies to progesterone and neither of these substances has been shown to be in excess in pre-eclampsia.

The vascular response to pregnancy is governed by many interrelated factors and thus possibly a disturbance in any one of the many chains of events can produce a rise in the blood pressure. It is probable that the condition known as pre-eclamptic toxaemia can be produced by several mechanisms.

REFERENCES

Adams, E. M. and Finlayson, A. (1961), "Familial Aspects of pre-eclampsia and Hypertension in Pregnancy," *Lancet*, **2**, 1375.

Adams, E. M. and MacGillivray, I. (1961), "Long-term Effects of pre-eclampsia on Blood Pressure," *Lancet*, **2**, 1373.

Antonaci, B. L. and Macagnimo, G. (1957), "Electrophoretic Studies of Serum and Oedema Fluid," *Acta Medica Scandinavica*, **159**, 133.

Assali, N. S., Fergon, J. M., Tada, Y. and Gerber, S. T. (1952), "Studies on Autonomic Blockade," *American Journal of Obstetrics and Gynecology*, **63**, 978.

Beck, J. S. and MacGillivray, I. In preparation.

Brody, S. (1964), "Observations on Toxaemia of Pregnancy," *Lancet*, **1**, 1796.

Brown, J. J., Davis, D. L., Doak, P. B., Lever, A. F., Robertson, J. I. S. and Trust, P. (1966), "Plasma Renin Concentration in the Hypertensive Diseases of Pregnancy," *Journal of Obstetrics and Gynaecology of the British Commonwealth*, **73**, 410.

Browne, F. J. (1947), "Chronic Hypertension and Pregnancy," *British Medical Journal*, **115**, 283.

Browne, J. C. M. (1961), "Survey of Eclampsia—Clinical Aspects, Eclampsia and pre-eclampsia in Pregnancy," Ed. F. C. Roulet, S. Karger, Basle, p. 542.

Brody, S. and Carlstrom, G. (1965), "Human Chorionic Gonadotrophin in Abnormal Pregnancy. Serum and Urinary Findings using Various Immunoassay Techniques," *Acta Obstet. Gynec. Scand.*, **44**, 32.

Chesley, L. C. (1965), "Renal Function in Pregnancy," *Bulletin of the New York Academy of Medicine*, **41**, 811.

Chesley, L. C. (1966), "Sodium Retention and pre-eclampsia," *Amer. J. Obstet. Gynec.*, **95**, 127.

Chesley, L. C., Cosgrove, R. A. and Annitto, J. E. (1962), "A follow-up Study of Eclamptic Women," *American Journal of Obstetrics and Gynecology*, **83**, 1360.

Cope, I. (1961), "Plasma and Blood Volume changes in Pregnancies complicated by pre-eclampsia," *Journal of Obstetrics and Gynaecology of British Commonwealth*, **68**, 413.

De Alvarez, R. R., Bratwold, G. E. and Harding, G. T. (1959), "The Renal Handling of Sodium and Water in Normal and Toxaemic Pregnancy," *American Journal of Obstetrics and Gynecology*, **78**, 375.

Doll, R. and Hannington, E. (1961), "International Survey of Eclampsia and Pre-eclampsia, 1958–59 Epidemiological Aspects in 'Eclampsia and Pre-eclampsia in Pregnancy,'" Editor, F. C. Roulet, S. Karger, Basle, p. 531.

Freeman, T. and Joekes, A. M. (1957), "Nephrotic Proteinuria; a Tubular Lesion," *Acta Medica Scandinavica*, **157**, 43.

Goven, A. D. T. (1961), "The Pathogenesis of Eclamptic Lesions in 'Eclampsia and Pre-eclampsia in Pregnancy'", Editor, F. C. Roulet, S. Karger, Basle, p. 561.

Govan, A. D. T. and Mukherjee, C. L., Hewitt, J. and Harper, W. F. (1951), "Studies of Carbohydrate Metabolism in Pregnancy Hypertension," *Journal of Obstetrics and Gynaecology of the British Empire*, **58**, 788.

Hammond, J. D. S. and Ross, R. S. (1960), "The Proteins of Serum and Oedema Fluid in Heart Failure studied by Paper Electrophoresis," *Clinical Science*, **19**, 119.

Hocken, A. G., Kark, R. M. and Passovy, M. (1966), "The Angiotensin Infusion Test," *Lancet*, **1**, 5.

Holland, W. W. and Hummerfelt, S. (1964), "Measurement of Blood Pressure, Comparison of intra-arterial and Cuff Values," *British Medical Journal*, **2**, 1241.

Howard, B. K., Goodson, J. H. and Mengert, W. (1953), "Supine Hypotensive Syndrome in late Pregnancy," *Obstetrics and Gynaecology*, **11**, 371.

Hunter, C. A. and Howard, W. F. (1960), "A Pressor Substance (hysterotonin) occurring in Toxaemia," *American Journal of Obstetrics and Gynecology*, **79**, 838.

Hulka, J. F. and Brinton, V. (1963), "Antibody to Trophoblast during early Postpartum Period," *American Journal of Obstetrics and Gynecology*, **83**, 130.

Hytten, F. and Paintin, D. B. (1963), "Increase in Plasma volume during Normal Pregnancy," *Journal of Obstetrics and Gynaecology of British Commonwealth*, **70**, 402.

Hytten, F., Taggart, N. and Thomson, A. M., (1966), "Total Body Water in Normal Pregnancy," *Journal of Obstetrics and Gynaecology of the British Commonwealth*, **73**, 533.

Kalmus, H. (1946), "Genetical Antigenic Incorporation as a possible cause of Toxaemias occurring late in Pregnancy. *Annals of Eugenics*. London, **13**, 146.

Kaplan, N. M. and Silah, J. (1964), "The Effect of Angiotensin II on the Blood Pressure in Humans with Hypertensive Disease," *Journal of Clinical Investigation*, **43**, 659.

Lawson, J. B. (1961), "Pre-eclampsia in Nigeria," *Pathology et Microbiology*, Basle, **24**, 478.

Lees, M. M., Taylor, S. H., Scott, D. B. and Kerr, M. G. (1967a), "A Study of Cardiac Output at rest throughout Pregnancy," *The Journal of Obstetrics and Gynaecology of the British Commonwealth*, **74**, 319.

Lees, M. M., Scott, D. B., Kerr, M. G. and Taylor, S. H. (1967), "The Circulatory Effects of Recurrent Postural Change in late Pregnancy," *Clinical Science*, **32**, 453.

Loraine, J. and Matthew, D. (1950), "Chorionic Gonadotrophin in Toxaemias of Pregnancy," *J. Obstet. and Gynaec. Brit. Emp.*, **57**, 542–551.

MacGillivray, I. (1961a), "Hypertension in Pregnancy and its consequences," *Journal of Obstetrics and Gynaecology of the British Commonwealth*, **68**, 577.

MacGillivray, I. (1961b), "Pre-eclampsia in Great Britain and Ireland," in *Eclampsia and Pre-eclampsia in Pregnancy*. Editor, F. C. Roulet, S. Karger, Basle.

MacGillivray, I. (1961c), "Water and Electrolyte Changes in normal and pre-eclamptic Pregnancies," in *Water and Electrolyte Metabolism*, Editors, C. P. Stewart and Th. Strengers, Elsevier, Amsterdam, p. 124.

MacGillivray, I. (1967), "The Significance of Blood Pressure and Body Water Changes in Pregnancy," *Scottish Medical Journal*, **12**, 237.

MacGillivray, I. and Tovey, J. E. (1957), "A Study of the Serum Protein Changes in Pregnancy and Toxaemia using Paper Strip Electrophoresis," *Journal of Obstetrics and Gynaecology of the British Empire*, **64**, 361.

Nelson, T. R. (1955), "A Clinical Study of pre-eclampsia," *Journal of Obstetrics and Gynaecology of the British Empire*, **62**, 48.

Page, E. W. (1938), "The effect of Eclamptic Blood upon the Urinary Output and Blood Pressure of Human Recipients," *Journal of Clinical Investigation*, **17**, 207.

Pickering, G. W., Roberts, J. A. F. and Sowry, G. S. C. (1954), "The Aetiology of Essential Hypertension No. 3, The Effect of correcting for Arm Circumference on the growth rate of Arterial Pressure with age," *Clinical Science*, **13**, 267.

Platt, R., Stewart, A. E. and Emery, E. W. (1958), "The Aetiology Incidence and Heredity of pre-eclamptic Toxaemia of Pregnancy," *Lancet*, **1**, 552.

Quilligan, E. J. and Tyler, C. (1959), "Postural Effects on the cardiovascular status in Pregnancy. A comparison of the lateral and supine postures," *American Journal of Obstetrics and Gynecology*, **78**, 465.

Raftery, E. B. and Ward, A. P. (1968), "The Indirect Method of Recording Blood Pressure," *Journal of Cardiovascular Research*, In Press.

Robertson, H. B., Brosens, I. and Dixon, H. G. (1967), "The Pathological Response of the Vessels of the Placental Bed to Hypertensive Pregnancy," *Journal of Pathology and Bacteriology*, In Press.

Rose, G. Holland, W. W. and Crowley, E. (1964), "A Sphygmomanometer for Epidemiologists," *Lancet*, **1**, 296.

Steblay, R. W. (1962), "Localization in Human Kidneys of Antibodies formed in Sheep against Human Placenta," *Journal of Immunology*, **88**, 434.

Tatum, H. J. and Mule, J. G. (1962), "The Hypertensive Action of Blood from Patients with pre-eclampsia," *American Journal of Obstetrics and Gynecology*, **83**, 1028.

Thomson, A. M., Hytten, F. E. and Billewicz, W. Z. (1967), "The Epidemiology of Oedema during Pregnancy," *Journal of Obstetrics and Gynaecology of the British Commonwealth*, **68**, 577.

Wagner, V., Savazal, V., Kasalova, D., Maly, V., Mecl, A. and Prokop, J. (1959), "Immunology of Toxaemias of Pregnancy (1) Findings of organic specific antibodies," *Experientia*, Basle, **15**, 24.

Wagner *et al.* (1959b), "Immunology of Toxaemia of Pregnancy (II) Immunological reactivity in Eclamptic conditions," *Experientia*, Basle, **15**, 61.

Whyte, H. M. (1959), "Blood Pressure and Obesity," *Circulation*, **19**, 511.

3. CARDIAC FUNCTION

ARTHUR HOLLMAN

The Structure of the Heart

Cardiac anatomy, viewed from the functional aspect, is comparatively simple. The atria are receiving chambers for the venous return, the ventricles are the pumping chambers and the heart valves ensure forward movement of the blood.

The detailed anatomy is however more complex. The thin walled atrial muscle is inserted at its lower edge into the tough fibrous rings of the mitral and tricuspid valves and is thus separated from the ventricles. The aortic and pulmonary valve rings join with the previous two rings to form the "fibrous skeleton of the heart", from which the ventricular muscle mass springs. The ventricles, like the atria, are a *functional syncytium* of muscle fibres, and these are bound together in broad sheets some of which, such as the deep bulbospiral muscle, encircle the left ventricular cavity whilst others wrap themselves round the entire heart. The ventricular septum consists mainly of left ventricular muscle fibres. The aortic and pulmonary valves are fairly simple flap valves, but the mitral and tricuspid valves are complex structures. Briefly they owe much of their function to the restraining action of the papillary muscles, and so disease of the ventricular muscle or chordae tendinae can lead to serious incompetence of these valves. The conventional naming of the chambers as right and left gives rise to confusion, especially when chest radiographs are being analysed. In fact they are much more anterior and posterior than right and left. Whilst the right atrium forms most of the right margin of the cardiac silhouette, the left atrium is a mid-line posterior structure virtually invisible in a normal chest X-ray.

The lateral margins of the normal right ventricle are contained within the cardiac shadow for the left ventricle constitutes the left margin of the heart, but it can be seen in a lateral radiograph where it forms the anterior heart border.

The Mechanism of the Heart Beat

It is interesting to remember that initiation of the heart beat, spread of the excitation wave through the heart, and contraction of the cardiac chambers are all accomplished by one tissue, the striated muscle of the heart—similar in structure to skeletal muscle but functionally closer to smooth muscle.

But these varying tasks require muscle fibres with different properties and this is achieved by variation in size. As Lewis pointed out in his Law of Cardiac Muscle the larger the fibre, the quicker its rate of conduction and the less its rhythmicity. It is a 4 mm. wide collection of small fibres situated at the junction of the superior vena cava and right atrium, possessing a high degree of rhythmicity that forms the sino-atrial node—the *pacemaker* of the heart. The node has a rich nervous connection with nearby parasympathetic ganglia and autonomic nerves and its importance in maintaining normal cardiac rhythm has been clearly demonstrated by Hudson who showed, in abnormal hearts, that a diseased node was nearly always associated with established atrial fibrillation.

The electrical discharge from the sino-atrial node stimulates the atria to contract, the impulse spreading directly through the muscle syncytium itself. It is a rapid movement because atrial systole expels only a third of the stroke volume. The impulse then excites the atrio-ventricular node, another collection of small fibres, with a slow conduction rate. This node is really a delay mechanism (of about 0·11 seconds) which prevents the atria and ventricles from contracting simultaneously. Emerging from the A-V node the impulse enters the large and rapidly conducting Purkinje fibres which transmit the cardiac impulse almost simultaneously, within 0·03 seconds, to all parts of the ventricular muscle mass. These Purkinje fibres form the AV bundle which divides on the ventricular septum into right and left main branches and thence into innumerable tiny branches which spread over the entire endocardial surface of the ventricles.

Control of the Heart Rate

There is a rich autonomic supply to the heart originating in the brain medulla where the cardioregulatory centres receive afferent impulses from all over the body. The parasympathetic nerves are carried in the vagi to the S-A and A-V nodes and atria. Vagal over-activity slows the discharge rate of the S-A node and slows transmission at the A-V node, leading to bradycardia or even ventricular standstill. Depression of S-A nodal activity in this way may result in the A-V node or even the A-V bundle becoming the cardiac pacemaker—situations known respectively as nodal rhythm and ventricular escape.

Stimulation of the cardio-inhibitory centre, causing vagal over-activity, may come from the cerebral cortex (surprise, fear) or from peripheral nerves. Thus the stretch receptors, or baroceptors, in the aortic arch and carotid sinus are stimulated by an increase in arterial pressure leading to bradycardia. Direct digital pressure on the carotid sinus has the same effect, as has pressure on the eyeballs. Stimulation of nerve endings in various viscera may lead to profound vagal slowing of the heart. Examples include the oesophagus (swallowing icy fluids, intubation), the trachea (irritant anaesthetic gases, intubation), the abdominal viscera (mesenteric traction at operation), and deep pain.

The sympathetic fibres, arising in the cardio-accelerator centre, travel to the heart via the sympathetic chain and are distributed, unlike the vagi, to the ventricles as well as the atria. Sympathetic over-activity can thus increase the force of cardiac contraction, in addition to increasing the heart rate by its action on the S-A node. Impulses from the brain (excitement, emotion) and superficial pain from the skin lead to tachycardia. If both types of autonomic nervous activity are blocked in a healthy person by atropine and propranolol the *intrinsic heart rate* is shown to be 110 beats per minute. Since the normal resting rate is 70 this shows that the intact heart is chiefly under parasympathetic control. Stimulation of stretch receptors by distension of the left ventricular wall causes bradycardia but tachycardia due to right atrial distension (Bainbridge reflex) is unproven in man. Fever and hypothermia probably act directly in the nodal tissues causing fast and slow heart rates respectively. The sympathomimetic drugs adrenaline and isoprenaline increase heart rate whilst cholinergic drugs such as acetylcholine and methacholine decrease it.

Regulation of Cardiac Function

Blood is propelled into the atria from the great veins by the residual pressure from the arterial circuits and in varying degrees by inspiration, gravity, and the pumping action of the skeletal muscles. The ventricles receive blood from the atria throughout diastole but the *rapid filling period* immediately after opening of the A-V valves accounts for over half the flow with a later and smaller period of rapid filling due to atrial systole. Ventricular contraction lasts for about 0·3 seconds at a heart rate of 70 and expels about 70 ml. of the 120 ml. diastolic volume giving a normal resting cardiac output of around 5·0 litres per minute in an adult. If the cardiac output is expressed as litres per minutes per square metre body surface, i.e. Cardiac Index, it becomes clear that age has a substantial effect on cardiac performance. Cardiac index starts to fall in adolescence and by the age of 50 it has declined to 75 per cent of the level at age 20. However, the cardiac response to exercise in older subjects has been shown by Julius et al., (1967) to be adequate, with no abnormal arteriovenous oxygen difference appearing in elderly persons on strenuous exertion.

Changes in cardiac output are constantly occurring in a normal person in response to factors such as exercise, posture, emotion, pregnancy and sleep. Since the cardiac output = stroke volume × heart rate it follows that either of these two factors may change output. However, change of heart rate alone has a relatively small effect on output. If for example tachycardia is produced by an electrical pacemaker the stroke volume falls and the output rises only slightly. This is hardly surprising because the prime cause of output changes is the oxygen demand of the tissues. But enormous changes in *stroke volume* can occur and the mechanism of this change is important. The problem was examined many years ago by Frank and also by Starling who epitomized it in his Law of the Heart, "The energy of contraction is a function of the length of the muscle fibres". However this work was done on isolated heart-lung preparations and when attempts were made to confirm it in intact man they appeared to contradict Starling's Law. The reason for this soon became apparent—the contractile properties of the heart are greatly enhanced by sympathetic over-activity or by catecholamines, thus altering the Starling "curve" considerably. It is now clear that there are two fundamental regulatory mechanisms of ventricular function in man and these have been brilliantly investigated by E. Braunwald and his associates. They refer firstly to the Starling Law as the *intrinsic mechanism*. By measuring myocardial segment length and tension at the time of cardiac surgery they have confirmed "that the mechanical activity of heart muscle is determined to a major extent by its length at the onset of ventricular contraction". Now the diastolic length is determined by the end diastolic volume and pressure, in other words by factors occurring during ventricular filling. Hence the *volume* of blood returned to the heart and the venous *pressure*—filling pressure—influence the output by this mechanism. If however a ventricle is diseased its ability to pump blood is impaired and quite large increases in end diastolic pressure result in only a slight increase in stroke work. In heart failure in man it has been shown that a progressive increase in end diastolic pressure may finally result in a decrease in stroke work—the well known descending limb of the Starling curve where further dilatation of the heart becomes ineffective.

The *extrinsic control mechanism* refers to the augmentation of cardiac contraction by catecholamine release at sympathetic nerve endings and from the adrenal gland. This effect is impressively shown by the fact that exercise in the normal human, whilst raising the cardiac output, is accompanied by a decrease in external ventricular dimensions—clearly the ventricles are working more efficiently. This mechanism also protects the circulation from large changes of central blood volume and stroke work when a rapid blood transfusion is given. The relative ineffectiveness of the intrinsic or Starling mechanism in the diseased heart makes the adrenergic nervous system especially important in cardiac patients, who have very high levels of circulating catecholamines under conditions such as exercise or acute myocardial infarction. Blockade of this mechanism by even small doses of propranolol can be extremely dangerous.

The Effects of Sympathomimetic Drugs

Adrenergic responses may be divided into alpha and beta receptor effects. Alpha stimulation leads to vasoconstriction; beta stimulation to (i) vasodilatation, (ii) to increased force and rate of the heart—i.e. positive inotropic and chronotropic effects, and (iii) increased cardiac excitability. The adrenal medullary hormone consists of 20 per cent noradrenaline and 80 per cent adrenaline. The former compound has predominately alpha effects and the stretch receptor response to the hypertension it produces leads to a reflex bradycardia. Adrenaline has both alpha and beta effects: it increases the force and rate of the heart and as a result the systolic blood pressure goes up. Diastolic pressure tends to fall because of the beta effect on arterioles. The synthetic drug isoprenaline has an especially powerful effect in causing tachycardia and it reduces peripheral resistance even more than adrenaline.

SPECIAL CARDIOVASCULAR SITUATIONS

Posture

When a normal person stands up in a relaxed position the venous pressure in the legs increases greatly and nearly one litre of blood is pooled in the lower limbs. As a result the central venous pressure, pulmonary blood volume, and cardiac output all diminish. The vascular resistance in the legs rises, due to reflex vasoconstriction, in order to prevent massive transudation of fluid from the capillary bed.

Syncope

Transient dizziness due to a low arterial pressure is fairly common when normal persons suddenly assume the erect posture but such postural hypotension only rarely causes loss of consciousness. The usual fainting or vasovagal attack is due chiefly to a sudden vasodilatation in muscle mediated by vasomotor nerves—this collapse in peripheral resistance leads to severe hypotension and an inadequate cerebral blood flow. The stimulus for fainting is often psychogenic, but factors such as haemorrhage which cause a critical fall in central venous pressure constitute a separate and important group. An interesting form of postural syncope occurs when pregnant women lie on their backs for too long, compression of the inferior vena cava by the uterus lowering venous pressure and venous return.

Exercise

The increased metabolic need of the muscles during exercise demands an increase in oxygen consumption and this increase is paralleled by a rise in cardiac output. Considerable tachycardia occurs and rates as high as 180 have been recorded even in trained athletes. The peripheral blood flow may increase up to 6 times the resting flow, but blood pressure is only moderately elevated because peripheral resistance falls. Blood flow to the viscera diminishes.

Pregnancy

The haemodynamic changes of pregnancy are dealt with elsewhere whilst the clinical and electrocardiographic features of this high output state with its hyperdynamic circulation are mentioned in this chapter.

The Valsalva Manoeuvre

Forced expiration against a closed glottis leads to a high intrathoracic pressure which cuts off venous return to the heart. This results in a fall of cardiac output with a lowering of the arterial pulse pressure and mean pressure and if the effort is prolonged cerebral ischaemia results in loss of consciousness. This may occur with a sustained bout of coughing. The fall in arterial pressure results in vasoconstriction and the blood flow to the limbs decreases abruptly. When the effort is released the increase of blood flow to a constricted vascular bed causes a sudden overshoot of blood pressure which by baroceptor stimulation leads to bradycardia.

This normal pattern is abolished by conditions such as tabes dorsalis and ganglion blockade which interfere with the baroceptor response. It also occurs when the blood volume is high in cardiac failure, or Conn's syndrome. The abnormal pattern consists solely of a rise in arterial pressure with the strain and is called a "square wave response".

The Coronary Circulation

The heart is supplied with blood by three large vessels, the right coronary artery and the left anterior descending and circumflex arteries but there may be right or left coronary preponderance. Blood flow through the myocardium has two aspects which uniquely separate it from other peripheral vascular beds. Firstly, flow is largely confined to diastole, due to the fact that ventricular contraction squeezes shut the arteriolar and capillary bed, and so diastolic flow accounts for over 70 per cent of the total. Secondly, there is a very high oxygen extraction by the myocardium which results in the coronary venous blood having an oxygen saturation of only about 30 per cent, compared to 70 per cent in the vena cavae. When the oxygen consumption of the heart increases on exercise the coronary A-V oxygen difference hardly alters, blood flow being increased by coronary vasodilation. This high oxygen extraction is mirrored in the heart's metabolism which is *totally* aerobic, unlike skeletal muscle. In fact far from producing lactic acid the heart actually extracts lactate from the blood and converts it to pyruvate. It is only when myocardial ischaemia is present that the heart produces lactate.

There is little evidence that vagal stimulation dilates the coronary arteries, or that sympathetic activity constricts them. The large changes in coronary flow associated with nervous activity are due chiefly to the inotropic and chronotropic effects on the myocardium. However, local coronary spasm, even in apparently normal vessels, does definitely occur.

The Pulmonary Circulation

The outstanding feature of the vascular bed in the lungs is its extremely low resistance compared with the systemic circuit. There is a mean pressure gradient of only about 5 mm. Hg. between the pulmonary artery and the left atrium and the normal pulmonary arterial pressure is 22/8 mm. Hg. Vasomotor control of the pulmonary vessels is of little importance in the normal subject, but anoxia causes vasoconstriction. On exercise the increased cardiac output is easily accommodated and the pulmonary arterial pressure rises very little.

Because the pulmonary resistance is so low the right ventricle has to perform very little pressure work. In fact it has almost a bellows action with the free wall of the ventricle approximating towards the septum—quite unlike the powerful concentric squeezing action of the left ventricle. As a result the right ventricle is ill adapted to meeting a sudden rise in outflow resistance such as occurs with massive pulmonary embolism.

The Electrocardiogram

The electromotive force produced by cardiac contraction may be detected by electrodes placed on the body surface and recorded graphically as the electrocardiogram (ECG). If the instantaneous vectors of electrical activity, referred to the same zero point, are recorded continuously then one obtains a *vectorcardiogram* (VCG). The VCG is not qualitatively different from the ECG and although it has certain academic advantages over the ECG it has been found in practice to yield little or no additional diagnostic information and further it does not record arrhythmias.

Considering the ECG, it is important to remember that it does not record the passage of electrical impulses through the heart (as the EEG does for the brain) although these may be inferred from the sequence of contraction of the atria and ventricles. Atrial contraction gives rise to the P wave and ventricular contraction to the QRST and U waves, A-V conduction time being represented by the PQ or PR interval and intra-ventricular conduction by the QRS duration. The ECG is supreme in its ability to document cardiac rhythm and it is a valuable though less certain way of detecting ventricular abnormalities. For example, ventricular hypertrophy, especially if acquired in adult life, may not alter the QRST deflections. Furthermore the normal range is wide and apparent abnormalities especially of the ST segment and T wave should be interpreted with caution. Racial variations are well known in African and West Indian negroes. A normal ECG

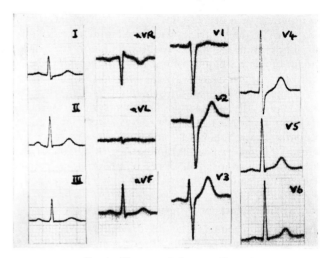

Fig. 1. The normal electrocardiogram.

does not exclude serious heart disease, particularly disease of the coronary arteries.

The spread of the electrical impulse through the heart with its associated cardiac contraction is from the base to the apex and it has been arranged that its projection onto the axes of the standard limb leads in the Einthoven Triangle yields a positive or upward deflection in each lead (Fig. 1). If the direction of activation is abnormal it is therefore represented by an abnormal axis of the P wave or the QRS complex. Consider for example the situation when the pacemaker shifts to the A-V node. The ventricles are normally activated and the QRS complex is upright. The atria however are stimulated from below and yield a negative P wave.

The electrical axis of the *ventricles* is normally in the anatomical axis of the left ventricle since this is the dominant chamber and is at an angle of $+60°$ from the horizontal (range $0°$ to $90°$). If the right ventricle is enlarged the axis shifts to the right, giving right axis deviation. Interruption of the right or left branches of the A-V bundle give respectively right and left axis deviation. The electrical axis is determined by noting the direction of the main QRS deflection in each of the limb leads, and its quantitation using the hexaxial reference system is important but outside the scope of this chapter. Minor degrees of axis deviation are caused by alteration of cardiac position by factors such as pulmonary fibrosis, shape of the chest and position of the diaphragms. It is noteworthy that pregnancy, by causing cardiac rotation from diaphragmatic elevation gives a characteristic ECG pattern with an S wave in lead I and a Q wave and inverted T wave in lead

III—the S1Q3T3 pattern (Fig. 2). A similar pattern may occur in pathological states such as right bundle branch block and pulmonary embolism, but the precordial leads will separate out these conditions.

The precordial or V leads record the anterior projection of the EMF and being relatively close to the ventricular mass they are of especial importance in determining ventricular hypertrophy which is less clearly depicted by the more distant limb leads which are, furthermore, in the frontal plane of the body.

The reference plane for the ST segment is the point where the PR segment joins the ventricular complex and is *not*, as sometimes assumed, the baseline after the T wave. Neglect of this principle leads to erroneous diagnosis of ST depression especially in the presence of tachycardia which lowers the PR segment. The ST segment is elevated when the myocardium is acutely damaged (by infarction, pericarditis or trauma) and is depressed by myocardial ischæmia, hypertrophy, or bundle branch block. Similarly the T wave is inverted by these abnormalities.

Abnormalities of the ventricular complex are often *disease specific*. For example massive pulmonary embolism gives rise to sharp T wave inversion in the "right ventricular" leads V4R to V3, congenital lesions enlarging the right ventricle lead to tall R waves in these leads, whilst acquired right ventricular hypertrophy from lung disease may be manifest only by deep S waves in leads V5 to V7. Left ventricular hypertrophy due to patent ductus arterio-

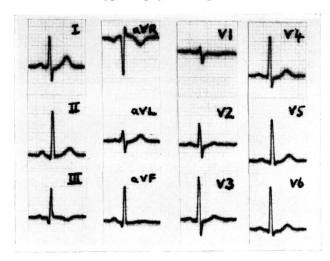

FIG. 2. The electrocardiogram at the 32nd week of pregnancy showing an S wave in lead I and a Q wave and inverted T wave in lead III. The precordial leads are normal.

sus and aortic stenosis both give tall R waves in leads V5 to V7, but the T waves are usually upright in the former condition and often inverted in the latter. Therefore electrocardiographic interpretation should always be related to the clinical problem. "Blind" reading of ECGs is a thoroughly bad procedure which deprives one of the very real help that this investigation can provide. For instance, a normal ventricular complex should not deflect one from diagnosing severe mitral stenosis, but it is incompatible with the diagnosis of Tetralogy of Fallot.

Clinical Evaluation of Cardio-vascular Function

Inspection of the jugular venous pulsations, seen normally above the inner aspect of the clavicles in the jugular bulbs, enable one to determine fairly accurately the form and pressure of the right atrial contractions. The two positive waves *a* and *v* are caused by atrial contraction and atrial diastolic filling, whilst the two negative waves *x* and *y* are due to atrial relaxation plus descent of the tricuspid ring in ventricular systole, and to atrial emptying when the tricuspid valve opens. One can therefore eluci-

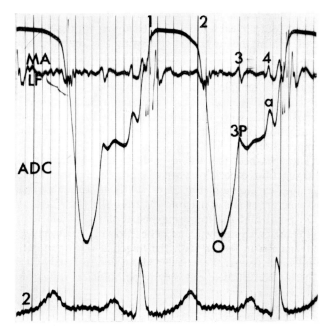

FIG. 3. The normal apex displacement cardiogram (ADC) recorded with the phonocardiogram (mitral area, low frequency, MA LF), and lead 2 of the electrocardiogram. It shows the outward movement of the apex in systole between heart sounds 1 and 2, the rapid filling wave in early diastole (O to 3P) associated with the normal 3rd heart sound, and the clinically undistinguishable features of the *a* wave and 4th heart sound due to atrial systole. In pregnancy the 3rd heart sound is accentuated and occasionally the atrial systolic events may be detected also. (Courtesy of Dr. Peter Nixon).

date abnormalities of right atrial and right ventricular rhythm and function by inspection of the venous pulse. For example A-V nodal rhythm or atrial ectopic beats cause the right atrium to contract against a closed tricuspid valve and lead to a giant *a* wave. The many pathological forms of the venous pulse have been admirably commented on by the late Paul Wood. The pressure of the individual waves may be determined by relating their height to that standard reference point, the sternal angle, and the *mean* pressure in the right atrium is reflected in the height of the *external* jugular vein. In normal subjects this pressure is about 0 cm., subject to respiratory variations but it must always be remembered that atrial pressure is closely related to the cardiac output (Starling). Therefore in healthy young people the venous pressure is higher than in elderly subjects and it may be as high as +5 cms. in high output states such as pregnancy, exercise or fever.

The arterial pulse provides important evidence of the contractile force of the left ventricle and of the cardiac output. The pulse upstroke, or percussion wave, is normally smooth and fairly sharp without being abrupt, whilst the downstroke cannot normally be felt—but mechanical records show it to be interrupted by the dicrotic notch signalling aortic valve closure. The pulse is best examined in the brachial and carotid arteries. High output states lead to an increased pulse volume, and to a more abrupt wave front.

Changes in the cardiac output and blood volume may be usefully detected in the limbs with the patient lying flat. A high output causes warm extremities with well filled veins, whilst the reverse is true with low output states. Experience in the management of patients after heart surgery has taught us that inspection of the dorsal veins of the feet is a reliable guide to blood balance. If these veins are collapsed then it is highly probable that the patient is hypovolemic, with the important proviso that venous contraction is not the result of a low ambient or body temperature.

The apex beat is a useful guide to left ventricular size and function, especially when it is graphically recorded as the apex cardiogram (Fig. 3), which is of particular value in depicting events in diastole. Mitral valve opening at the "O" point and the following phase of rapid ventricular filling are clearly shown, and in healthy young subjects this movement can be felt with the finger at the time of the third heart sound. Ventricular filling due to atrial systole can also be recorded, but only in pathological states such as severe hypertension can it be appreciated clinically. The force and duration of the systolic movement provide good evidence of left ventricular hypertrophy.

Heart Sounds and Murmurs

Vibrations in the heart and great arteries give rise to noises which are conducted to the surface of the chest where they may be detected by palpation or auscultation. These noises have a very wide range of frequency and can only be properly appreciated on auscultation by the use of a stethoscope which has both a bell and a diaphragm. The bell is used for low frequency noises such as the third heart sound whilst the diaphragm accentuates high frequency noises such as the second heart sound or a pericardial friction rub.

The first and second heart sounds signal the beginning and end of ventricular systole and are associated with closure of the atrioventricular and semilunar valves respectively. The first heart sound is caused by closure of the mitral and tricuspid valves and thus has two elements. Due to the lower systolic pressure in the right ventricle the noise of tricuspid closure is softer and later than mitral closure. Therefore the two separate elements of the first sound leading to "splitting" of this sound are normally heard only over the tricuspid valve in the left fourth interspace parasternally. Over the rest of the precordium the first sound is caused exclusively by mitral closure and this loud noise is conducted by the aorta into the neck. Similarly with the second sound there are two elements, due to aortic and pulmonary valve closure,

the latter occurring slightly later and again being a softer noise. Thus splitting of the second sound is normally heard only over the pulmonary valve in the left second space in the pulmonary area. Aortic valve closure is strongly transmitted over the left ventricle and aorta. Mitral and aortic closure are the main determinants of the normal heart sounds and they are heard over the entire precordium.

Significance of Changes in the Heart Sounds

The only ways in which the heart sounds can be altered is by variation in the intensity, or in the timing of closure, of the four heart valves.

The first heart sound is affected chiefly by the interval of time between atrial and ventricular contraction. If this interval is short the valve cusps will still be widely separated by the inrush of blood into the left ventricle when systole occurs and slams them shut, giving a loud first sound. This occurs at irregular intervals in complete heart block when the A-V interval happens to be short ("cannon sounds"). It also occurs with a hyperdynamic circulation and tachycardia although the very rapid onset of ventricular contraction is another factor under these conditions. The A-V interval is long in first degree heart block (long PR interval on the ECG) and the valve cusps having passively floated into apposition before systole make little noise when they finally close, giving a soft or absent first heart sound. Impaired cardiac contractility will cause softening of the first sound but this is an imprecise and usually unnecessary method of diagnosis. Variations in splitting of the first sound are of minor importance.

The second heart sounds at the right and left intercostal spaces are often referred to as the aortic second sound and the pulmonary second sound. This terminology overlooks the dual origin of this sound and leads to confusion especially at the pulmonary area where both aortic and pulmonary closure are heard. It is better to refer to "the second sound at the pulmonary area". When the pulmonary closure can be clearly identified as the second component of a split second sound then its increased intensity in pulmonary hypertension is obvious. However, if aortic and pulmonary closure cannot be separated—and this is frequent in the adult—it is more difficult to diagnose pulmonary hypertension, though a very loud second sound at the pulmonary compared with the aortic area is a useful, but fallible clue. Loud aortic closure occurs with systemic hypertension and with dilatation of the aorta but syphgmomanometry and radiology are better diagnostic methods.

Changes in the interval between aortic and pulmonary closure are of importance. Normally during inspiration an increased volume of blood enters the right ventricle augmenting its stroke volume and prolonging systole. Therefore pulmonary closure is delayed and the second sound becomes more widely split on inspiration. This normal phenomenon is obscured when right ventricular output is higher than the left as in atrial septal defect and the second sound has a "fixed split". Prolongation of right ventricular systole by right bundle branch block or right ventricular hypertension leads to a widely split sound. If left ventricular systole is prolonged because of left bundle branch block or an increased flow or pressure in the left ventricle then aortic closure is delayed. This causes pulmonary closure to precede aortic closure and the second sound is single on inspiration and split on expiration ("reversed split" of the second sound). Detailed texts should be consulted for further explanation of this abbreviated account.

The third heart sound is not due to valve closure. It occurs with the rapid blood flow into the ventricles in early diastole and it is a low pitched noise heard over the apex beat. It is a normal finding when the cardiac output is high and ventricular filling rapid and is thus common in the young and in pregnancy, but rarely heard normally over the age of 40. Pathological third sounds may be heard over the respective chambers when the right or left ventricles are diseased.

The fourth heart sound is never heard in health, though it may be recorded on the phonocardiogram, and like the third sound it is a "filling sound" due to the sudden distension of the ventricles by atrial systole. It becomes audible with pathological states such as systemic or pulmonary hypertension.

Considerable tachycardia can lead to fusion of otherwise inaudible third and fourth sounds to give a "summation gallop" rhythm. This disappears if the heart rate is slowed by carotid sinus pressure.

Heart Murmurs

A high velocity of blood flow through the heart valves gives rise to long continued vibrations which are detected by auscultation (murmurs) or by palpation (thrills). The phemonena of turbulence, and of vortex shedding (Bruns, 1959) are the responsible factors. The pathological aspects of heart murmurs are not within the scope of this chapter, but two normal causes may be mentioned.

"Innocent" murmurs occur when the velocity of blood flow through the aortic and pulmonary valves is high as in children or in high output states such as anaemia and pregnancy. The murmur occurs in early systole and in contrast to pathological murmurs it is short, fairly soft and unaccompanied by a thrill. An interesting murmur which arises in the jugular bulb is the "venous hum". It is a continuous murmur, loudest in systole, which is heard over the base of the neck in normal children, in pregnancy, and in adults with anaemia. Its importance lies in the fact that it may be conducted to the precordium and then erroneously lead to the diagnosis of patent ductus arteriosus.

REFERENCES

Braunwald, E. (1965), "The Control of Ventricular Function in Man," *Brit. Heart J.*, **27**, 1.

Bruns, D. L. (1959), *Amer. J. Med.*, **27**, 360.

Burton, A. C. (1965), *Physiology and Biophysics of the Circulation.* Chicago: Year Book Publishers.

Deuchar, D. C. (1964), *Clinical Phonocardiography.* London: The English Universities Press Ltd.

Friedberg, C. K. (1966), *Diseases of the Heart.* Philadelphia: W. B. Saunders Company.

Hudson, R. E. B. (1960), "The Human Pacemaker and its Pathology," *Brit. Heart J.*, **22**, 153.

Julius, E., Amery, A., Whitlock, L. S. and Conway, J. (1967), *Circulation*, **36**, 222.

Lewis, T. (1925), *The Mechanism and Graphic Registration of the Heart Beat*, 3rd edition. London: Shaw & Sons Ltd.

Marriott, H. J. L. (1962), *Practical Electrocardiography*, 3rd edition. Baltimore: Williams & Wilkins Company.

Rushmer, R. F. (1961), *Cardiovascular Dynamics.* Philadelphia: W. B. Saunders Company.

Wood, P. (1968), *Diseases of the Heart and Circulation.* London: Eyre and Spottiswoode.

4. BLOOD FORMATION AND DEVELOPMENT

LOUIS STEINGOLD

The haemopoietic tissue and the cardiovascular and lymphatic systems develop from the embryonic mesenchyme. Within a few days of implantation of the fertilized ovum angioblastic cells separate from the wall of the blastocyst. This angioblastic tissue develops and spreads, so that when the primitive streak appears, it is present in the body stalk and the wall of the yolk sac. In the wall of the yolk sac it differentiates into solid masses of cells known as blood islands. These hollow out, the peripheral cells forming vascular endothelium while the central cells become the primitive blood cells. Clefts filled with plasma appear between the blood cells. These enlarge and coalesce to form the vascular lumen. Growth and union of these spaces results in a plexus of channels which, along with further channels formed in the mesenchyme, make up the vascular system of the embryo.

At this, the *mesoblastic* stage of blood production, the blood cells are almost entirely large nucleated red cells known as primitive megaloblasts and their continued production is from the cells of the vascular endothelium. However, foci of extravascular haemopoietic tissue soon differentiate from the embryonic mesenchyme, the vascular endothelium loses its haemopoietic capacity and the primitive megaloblasts die out. As the definitive haemopoietic organs appear blood production becomes centred on them, but still remains largely erythropoietic. The red cells are now smaller, with smaller denser nuclei, and are known as definitive megaloblasts. It is from these that the erythrocytes will develop.

When the embryo is 5 to 7 mm. long blood production enters the *hepatic* phase, and by the sixth week of intra-uterine life the liver has become the main haemopoietic organ. This function of the liver diminishes at mid-foetal life and ceases at term. The spleen, thymus and lymph nodes act as supplementary temporary sites of blood formation during this period, but by the eighth month or earlier, even the spleen has ceased to form red cells and granulocytes. The liver and spleen nevertheless retain their haemopoietic potential and may exert it under extreme circumstances such as haemolytic disease of the newborn and myelosclerosis.

By the fourth month of foetal life the bone marrow commences its haemopoietic functions and the *myeloid* phase of blood production is gradually entered. Leucocytes, scanty until now, appear in increasing numbers. By term the bone marrow is the sole source of erythrocytes and granulocytes, while the lymphoid organs and the fixed connective tissue cells other than fibroblasts are the source of monocytes and lymphocytes. The erythrocytes, all nucleated at first, increasingly appear as non-nucleated cells until all are in this form at term.

Throughout infancy and much of childhood the entire bone marrow is haemopoietic. Thereafter the haemopoietic marrow of the small bones and shafts of the long

bones is gradually replaced by fatty tissue, the process being complete by the mid-teens.

There are a number of theories regarding the mode of origin of blood cells. The most important of these are the monophyletic theory and the dualistic form of the polyphyletic theory. The monophyletic theory postulates that the primitive fixed cell of the reticulo-endothelial system gives rise to a totipotential blood-forming cell, the *haemocytoblast*, from which the unipotential stem cells arise, each destined to produce a single type of blood cell; in other words that the stimulus to differentiate is applied to the haemocytoblast. The polyphyletic theory states that this stimulus is applied to the reticulo-endothelial cell itself and that its first generation daughter cell is already destined to produce one type of blood cell only.

Such evidence as there is favours the monophyletic theory although it cannot yet be accepted unreservedly. The identity of the haemocytoblast is certainly not firmly established although there is evidence that it is indistinguishable from the lymphocyte by ordinary microscopy (Cronkite, 1964). As a basis for discussion it is proposed to accept the monophyletic theory, which is illustrated in Fig. 1.

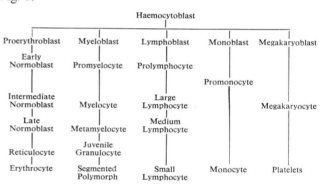

FIG. 1. Development of blood cells.

In the adult the total mass of haemopoietic marrow is about 1500 to 3000 grams, i.e., about that of the liver. There is also an approximately equal mass of fatty marrow. Under normal conditions the proliferative activity of the marrow leaves much in reserve. Under stress the haemopoietic tissue can displace the fatty marrow and increase its proliferative activity to such an extent as to increase haemopoiesis eightfold. In extreme circumstances the haemopoietic potential of the liver and spleen can also be drawn upon.

The Genetic Code
(Crick, Barnett, Brenner and Watts-Tobin, 1961; Davis, 1964.)

It is necessary to understand the nature of the nucleic acids and of the genetic code before considering such subjects as Vitamin B_{12}, folic acid and the abnormal haemoglobins.

Purines and pyrimidines are basic heterocyclic compounds. Their general structure is shown in Fig. 2. The

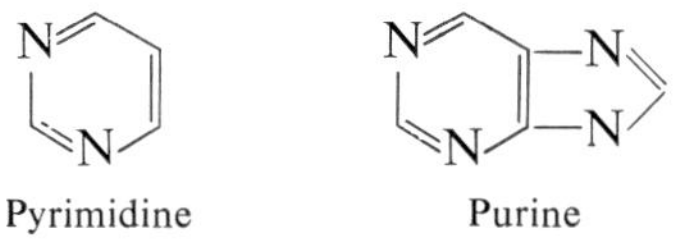

Pyrimidine   Purine

FIG. 2. Basic structure of pyrimidines and purines.

most commonly occurring bases in the nucleic acids are the purines *adenine* and *guanine*, and the pyrimidines *thymine, uracil* and *cytosine*. Thymine occurs in deoxyribonucleic acid (DNA). Its place is taken by uracil in ribonucleic acid (RNA). Thymine is simply methyluracil (Fig. 3). (See also Chap. 1, p. 2.)

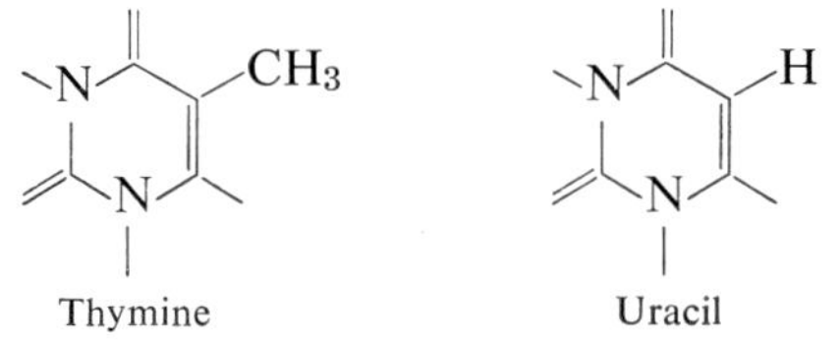

Thymine   Uracil

FIG. 3. Basic structure of thymine and uracil.

When a purine or pyrimidine base combines with the sugars ribose or 2-deoxyribose a *nucleoside* is formed. Thus the nucleoside adenosine consists of the purine adenine combined with ribose.

Nucleotides are monophosphate esters of nucleosides, that is, nucleosides linked to single molecules of phosphoric acid. In these the sugar molecule serves as the link between base and acid. Thus the nucleotide adenylic acid consists of the purine adenine linked to phosphoric acid by means of ribose and is adenosine phosphate. Nucleotides are of two types, ribonucleotides in which the sugar is ribose and which occur in RNA, and 2′-deoxyribonucleotides in which the sugar is 2-deoxyribose and which occur in DNA.

Nucleotides link with one another to form *polynucleotide* chains which, when complete, are the nucleic acids DNA and RNA. The basic structure of the nucleic acids is shown in Fig. 4. DNA consists of two such chains arranged as a double intertwining coil or *helix*, held together by bonds between their bases. Bonding is always between adenine and thymine, or guanine and cytosine. It is apparent therefore that the structure of one chain is intimately related to that of the other. To reduplicate itself DNA unwinds its two chains and each acts as a template for the formation of a new complementary strand. RNA consists of one such chain.

```
Sugar—Phosphate—Sugar—Phosphate—Sugar—Phosphate—etc
  |                |                 |
 Base             Base              Base            etc
```

Fig. 4. Structure of nucleic acids.

Within the cells DNA and RNA occur in the nucleus while the cytoplasm contains RNA only. DNA is the carrier of genetic information. It is the translation of the base composition of an individual's DNA, referred to as the *genetic code*, into protein structure which determines such things as his blood group, his enzymes and the nature of his haemoglobin.

Proteins consist of chains of amino acids (polypeptide chains) held together by "peptide bonds". The amino acid sequence in the polypeptide chain is known as the *primary structure* of the protein. Interaction between the peptide bonds contracts the chain into a loose helix the form of which is the *secondary structure* of the protein. Reactions between the side chains of the amino acids and water cause the helix to fold up into a tangled ball the form of which is the *tertiary structure* of the protein. Many proteins are composed of more than one such chain. Haemoglobin, for example, consists of four. The manner in which these are interwoven is the *quaternary structure* of the protein. It will be noted that, in the absence of outside influences such as excessive heat which causes coagulation by altering the tertiary structure, the primary structure determines the others. The amino acid composition of a protein therefore determines its nature and properties.

The primary structure of proteins is determined by *genes* which, strung together, form the nuclear chromosomes. Each gene controls the synthesis of a single polypeptide chain and a protein composed of more than one chain is controlled by more than one gene. Such related genes generally occur side-by-side in a chromosome.

Genes are segments of DNA. As can be seen from Fig. 4 the "backbone" of DNA is constant. Variation in the sequence of bases attached to this backbone determines the nature of the genetic information residing in the DNA and therefore the nature and properties of the proteins which the cell can synthesize. Four bases only occur in the DNA chain, adenine, cytosine, guanine and thymine. These are usually referred to by their initial letters A, C, G and T. The arrangement of these in consecutive threes (triplets) along the DNA segment constitutes the "code" determining the nature of the genetic information carried, since this determines the sequence of amino acids in the proteins synthesized and therefore their nature and properties.

Twenty different amino acids occur in proteins, while sixty-four (4^3) different triplets can be arranged out of four bases. Many of the amino acids are therefore coded for by more than one triplet, and the code is termed degenerate. Along the DNA strip each triplet is the code word for a specific amino acid, and the linear sequence of the triplets determines the sequence of the amino acids in the protein. Each gene is therefore "programmed" to cause the synthesis of a single specific polypeptide chain.

The DNA code is translated into protein structure by means of RNA. The two DNA strands separate and one induces the formation of a single complementary strand of RNA in much the same way as it induces the formation of the complementary DNA strand during its reduplication. However in the RNA strand ribose replaces 2-deoxyribose and uracil appears in place of thymine. Thus the code letters ACGT on the DNA strand are translated into UGCA on the RNA strand, and each triplet of bases on the DNA strand is represented by a complementary triplet on the RNA strand. As the RNA strand is formed it "peels off" and the double helix of DNA re-forms behind it.

When the RNA strand is complete it is freed and carried into the cytoplasm. This RNA, carrying a translation of the DNA code, is termed messenger-RNA or m-RNA.

Two further RNA's occur in the cytoplasm, soluble-RNA (s-RNA, transfer-RNA) and ribosomal-RNA (r-RNA). Ribosomal-RNA, bound to protein, forms the *ribosomes*. These are minute particles of ribonucleoprotein demonstrable by electron microscopy in the cytoplasm. Each molecule of s-RNA can carry one molecule of a specific amino acid. However since the code is degenerate some amino acids can be carried by different s-RNA's. The s-RNA possesses an exposed triplet base code which determines the nature of the amino acid carried and which is attracted to the correct (complementary) triplet code on the m-RNA strand. The r-RNA then slides along the m-RNA strand binding each s-RNA molecule with its amino acid to its appropriate triplet in a "zipping-up" action. As each amino acid is fixed in position on the m-RNA strand its s-RNA carrier frees itself to become available to carry more amino acid. As the amino acids are deposited they link together by peptide bonds forming a polypeptide chain which peels away from the m-RNA strand. The secondary, tertiary and quaternary structural changes now take place to form the specific protein originally coded for on the DNA tape.

When a triplet on the DNA tape is "wrong" a complementary "wrong" triplet is induced on the m-RNA strand and a "wrong" amino acid occupies this position in the polypeptide chain. An abnormal protein is then produced. Sometimes the change in the biological properties of the protein is considerable. If the change is harmful the subject exhibits disease. If it is beneficial natural selection ensures its continued existence and evolution takes place. It appears that such variations from the normal in the DNA code take place as a change in a single base of a single triplet without alteration of sequence. The protein produced will therefore differ from the normal by a single amino acid, and the code word for this amino acid will differ from that for the normal by a single letter within the triplet.

Very little of a cell's DNA is in action at any one time, and most of it is never put into action at all. This allows the biological differences between, for example, muscle, skin and liver, and for the varying biological activity of the cell at different times. Messenger-RNA disappears when its work is for the moment complete. Its synthesis is again induced when necessary.

The code appears to be universal. In other words it appears to be the same in all living matter.

The Red Cell

In the field of obstetrics much more attention has been paid to the red cell than to the other cells of the blood. It will therefore be considered first and in some detail.

The most immature red cell precursor which can be identified in the bone marrow is the *proerythroblast*. This takes origin from a still unidentified primitive multipotent cell. It is assumed that when this primitive cell undergoes division one of the daughter cells remains in the primitive state while the other differentiates into one of the specific unipotent stem cells, in this case the proerythroblast. In this way depletion of primitive cells does not occur.

The proerythroblast undergoes a series of mitotic divisions which are accompanied by maturation and nuclear condensation, reduction in cell size and increasing haemoglobinization of the cytoplasm. Mitotic division ceases at the stage of the late normoblast. The nucleus, now small and dense, is extruded, and in two or three days the resultant *reticulocyte* enters the circulation. This cell does not contain any DNA since it has lost its nucleus. It does however contain some RNA which it cannot replace (in the absence of DNA) and which will disappear in a few days. Thereafter the cell is a mature *erythrocyte*. The erythrocyte has a life span of about 120 days and the proportion of reticulocytes is normally about one per cent.

Ageing of the red cell is accompanied by loss of stromal lipid. The consequent increase in osmotic fragility is presumed to be the factor determining the removal, mainly by the spleen, of effete red cells from the circulation.

The red cell life span is reduced in women of child-bearing age, particularly in the immediately premenstrual period and during menstruation, and in new-born infants. It is further reduced in eclampsia, in which acute haemolytic episodes may occur, and in pre-eclamptic toxaemia. In the pre-pubertal, post-menopausal and oöphorectomized female it is similar to that in the male.

In conditions of increased red cell production such as haemorrhage, haemolysis and anaemia under appropriate treatment, the proportion of reticulocytes rises.

During normal development a proportion of the nucleated red cells die in the bone marrow. This constitutes "ineffective erythropoiesis". This intramedullary haemolysis is increased in a number of conditions including Addisonian pernicious anaemia.

Under normal conditions regulating mechanisms maintain an accurate balance between the production and destruction of red cells. These mechanisms have now been largely defined. The basic control of erythropoiesis resides in the relationship between oxygen supply to the tissues and their oxygen demands. Thus in persons living at high altitudes and in subjects with chronic bronchitis and emphysema the relative oxygen deficit is compensated for by polycythaemia. Conversely when oxygen supply exceeds demand there is depression of erythropoiesis. Thus the polycythaemia of persons living at high altitudes disappears soon after their return to sea level. It was at first proposed that oxygen acts directly on the bone marrow, a deficit stimulating, and an excess inhibiting red cell proliferation. However studies on bone marrow cultures suggest the reverse; the rate of erythropoiesis and of haemoglobin synthesis increase with increasing oxygen supply. It was also observed that when one only of a pair of parabiotic animals is exposed to hypoxic conditions both show increased erythropoiesis. Such findings directed attention to the possible existence of plasma factors controlling red cell proliferation, and culminated in the discovery of *erythropoietin*.

When tissue demand for oxygen exceeds supply there is increased erythropoietin production. This stimulates erythropoiesis. It will, for example, appear in significant amounts in the plasma of animals rendered anaemic by bleeding. Plasma from such animals, injected into normal animals in sufficient quantity, will induce increased red cell production.

Erythropoietin is a glycoprotein with the electrophoretic mobility of an α_2-globulin. It acts on the most primitive cells of the bone marrow inducing proerythroblast formation. It also stimulates haemoglobin formation in the proerythroblast and early normoblast. These two processes are RNA-dependent and present evidence suggests that erythropoietin acts primarily by stimulating the synthesis of RNA, and particularly of messenger-RNA.

In the hypertransfused experimental animal erythropoietin production is completely inhibited and nucleated red cells are virtually absent from the haemopoietic organs.

Erythropoietin is produced in the renal glomeruli. Its production is diminished, with resulting anaemia, in destructive renal diseases such as nephritis. In renal carcinoma and certain other renal conditions it is increased and there is polycythaemia. Some erythropoietin appears to be produced in other organs and increases have been observed in cases of hepatoma and of uterine fibromyoma.

Linman and Bethell (1960) describe a second erythropoietin in the plasma. This is a lipid produced in the fatty marrow. It appears in the plasma in certain anaemias. Acting alone it causes increased red cell production without any increase in haemoglobin synthesis. The erythrocytes produced are fragile microcytes which are rapidly eliminated from the circulation. It also stimulates the formation of granulocytes and platelets. Its rôle remains uncertain but it presumably functions in conjunction with erythropoietin.

The production of erythropoietin appears to be under the control of the posterior hypothalamus, stimulation of which results in polycythaemia, and of the pituitary, removal of which results in anaemia with hypoplasia of the erythroid marrow. The stimulus to renal erythropoietin production is probably through vasopressin, production of which is increased in haemorrhage and in hypothalamic stimulation.

Increased plasma and urinary erythropoietin levels have been reported in many anaemias including those due to iron deficiency, vitamin B_{12} deficiency and haemolysis. In such cases the anaemia is due to inability on the part of the bone marrow to respond to the stimulus, or to premature destruction of the red cells produced. It is increased in the plasma in pregnancy and in foetal cord blood. There is an unexplained increase, particularly of Linman and Bethell's lipid factor, in polycythaemia vera.

Erythropoietin is metabolized in the liver and excreted in the urine. It is consumed during bone marrow activity, and failure to demonstrate it in normal subjects is due to the balance achieved between production on the one hand, and utilization, catabolism and excretion on the other, under normal circumstances. In animals rendered aplastic by irradiation before being bled, raised erythropoietin levels, which normally subside rapidly after haemorrhage, persist because of the bone marrow inactivity. When the circumstances demanding increased erythropoiesis cease to operate not only does erythropoietin production cease, but an inhibitor appears in the plasma. Thus plasma from humans who have been living at high altitudes and have recently returned to sea level inhibits erythropoiesis in hypoxic animals.

The control of erythropoiesis is therefore mediated through two or possibly three plasma factors; erythropoietin and possibly Linman and Bethell's lipid factor operative when stimulation of erythropoiesis is required, and an erythropoiesis inhibitor operative when it is required that erythropoiesis be depressed. Interplay between these mechanisms maintains the remarkable constancy of the red cell and haemoglobin masses under physiological conditions, while adjusting them to changing circumstances.

It is well known that women of child-bearing age show lower haemoglobin concentrations than men, and that this is due to a considerable extent to minor iron deficiency in the female. The evidence for this has been discussed by the writer in some detail elsewhere (Steingold, 1966). Nevertheless part of the difference is related to the influence of sex hormones on erythropoiesis. Thus testosterone therapy for mammary carcinoma, and some masculinizing ovarian tumours are accompanied by red cell and haemoglobin increases and marrow red cell hyperplasia. Response to testosterone is obtained in some anaemias not responsive to other therapy, such as the anaemias of Hodgkin's disease and leukaemia, and particularly aplastic anaemia of childhood in which complete remission may be obtained. Castrated males and eunuchs show a mild anaemia which responds to testosterone. In contrast, oöphorectomized females show increased erythropoiesis which can be prevented by oestrogens. It is suggested that testosterone acts by causing renal hyperplasia so increasing the amount of erythropoietin produced in response to hypoxia. Oestrogens depress erythropoiesis and this inhibitory effect is abolished by progesterone and testosterone. Of interest in this connection is the observation of Kanaev, Bruk, Kuleshov and Shostka (1966) that in menorrhagia due to excessive oestrogenic stimulation there is a defect in the entry of iron into the cells of the red cell series and in its incorporation into haem. They suggest that this is due to inhibition of erythropoietin by oestrogens.

During lactation the mother shows increased red cell production. This does not occur if lactation is inhibited and the infant is bottle fed. Of the hormones operative at that time, *prolactin* is the only one possessing erythropoietic activity. It appears to act like testosterone, by causing renal hypertrophy.

The administration of cobalt induces polycythaemia in experimental animals. It depresses tissue oxygenation, so increasing erythropoietin production. It is a tissue poison and its use in refractory anaemias is accompanied by disturbing side-effects. Increased erythropoiesis, probably through stimulation of erythropoietin production, has also been reported following the administration of adrenaline and thyro-active substances.

The erythropoietic response may become inadequate because of deficiencies of substances required during the process of maturation or haemoglobinization. Such substances include vitamin B_{12}, folic acid, pyridoxine and iron.

Vitamin B$_{12}$ (Lester Smith, 1965)

Following the discovery that raw liver could be used in the treatment of Addisonian pernicious anaemia, increasingly concentrated liver extracts were prepared, culminating in the isolation of the pure anti-pernicious anaemia factor in 1948. It has been named vitamin B$_{12}$, or cyanocobalamin, although the cyan radicle is a contaminant, the natural vitamin being hydroxycobalamin (vitamin B$_{12a}$). It contains the element cobalt.

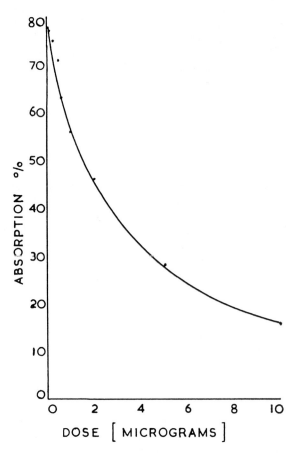

FIG. 5. Effect of dosage on absorption of oral vitamin B$_{12}$ in normal subjects.

Addisonian pernicious anaemia is caused by a deficiency of intrinsic factor, a labile glycoprotein secreted, in man, by the fundus of the stomach. In the absence of intrinsic factor insufficient extrinsic factor is absorbed to maintain optimal erythropoiesis and pernicious anaemia results. Extrinsic factor is now known to be vitamin B$_{12}$ coenzyme, the hydroxyl radicle of the natural vitamin being replaced by a nucleoside in the coenzyme. This is the form in which vitamin B$_{12}$ occurs in the liver, is stored in other tissues and takes part in most if not all of the reactions it mediates. The absence of intrinsic factor is almost invariably accompanied by absolute, histamine-fast achlorhydria. However, children and young adults of families with a history of familial pernicious anaemia can show intrinsic factor deficiency and pernicious anaemia while showing normal gastric secretion of hydrochloric acid.

Intrinsic factor enhances the efficiency of oral vitamin B$_{12}$ about thirty-fold. It combines with the vitamin rendering it unavailable to the bacterial flora of the intestine. The union resists splitting by the usual proteolytic enzymes but not the secretions of the fish tapeworm Diphyllobothrium latum, infestation with which results in megaloblastic anaemia.

Intrinsic factor assists the absorption of vitamin B$_{12}$ more directly also, by binding it to the cells of the intestinal mucosa. A subsequent enzyme mechanism frees the vitamin for absorption as the coenzyme. Absorption by the intrinsic factor mechanism is geared to physiological conditions, when vitamin B$_{12}$ is taken as a constituent of food, and not to its administration in massive oral doses. As the oral dose is increased the total absorbed increases but the proportion falls rapidly. As can be seen from Fig. 5, which refers to normal subjects, when the dose reaches 10 μg only about one-sixth is absorbed (Mollin, 1959).

In man the source of intrinsic factor used in therapy (e.g. man himself, pig, rat) is not important, at least initially. After a time however, foreign intrinsic factors tend to become ineffective because the subject develops inhibitory antibodies. Nevertheless the most commonly used form is a preparation of hog stomach dried at low temperature. The treatment of pernicious anaemia with intrinsic factor and oral vitamin B$_{12}$ is contraindicated in pregnancy, for Adams (1958) has shown that pregnant women on this regime relapse and require parenteral treatment.

Some micro-organisms synthesize large quantities of vitamin B$_{12}$ and this is made use of in its commercial production. Others do not synthesize any and require an external source of the vitamin. Such organisms are used in its microbiological assay. In man some of the normal intestinal bacteria are of this type and their destruction probably explains the success of penicillin and tetracycline therapy in certain megaloblastic anaemias (Foy, Kondi, Hargreaves and Lowry, 1952; Mollin, 1959).

Vitamin B$_{12}$ is essentially an animal product, present in virtually every animal tissue. It is produced by the intestinal flora and stored in the animal's tissues. Its concentration in vegetable matter is negligible. Man depends entirely on his food for the vitamin, for such as is produced in his gut is not released in those areas from which absorption takes place.

In the plasma, vitamin B$_{12}$ is bound to an α_1-globulin. The binding capacity of the plasma is limited and although it is increased by temporary binding of administered vitamin to β-globulin, part of the usual parenteral therapeutic doses remains unbound and is excreted in the urine. With massive doses such as the now popular 1000 μg as much as 75 per cent may be lost in this way. The utilization of 10 μg of vitamin B$_{12}$ in erythropoiesis is sufficient for the production of about 30 million million erythrocytes, or as many as there are in six litres of normal blood, and normal persons do not require to absorb more than 3 μg daily for *all purposes*.

The normal serum vitamin B$_{12}$ level in man is above 200 μμg per ml. In pregnancy increased demands frequently result in a slow fall to levels below this, particularly in anaemic women *regardless of the type of anaemia*. This need not necessarily reflect a tissue deficiency, but may reflect more rapid turnover of the vitamin, including its rapid transfer to the foetus. At term the infant's serum vitamin B_{12} level is often much higher than that of the mother, even when hers is normal.

Vitamin B_{12} is stored, mainly in the liver, as the protein-bound coenzyme. Most of its incorporation into red cells is into the more immature forms. When, in mature circulating erythrocytes, haemoglobin production ceases, vitamin B_{12} activity is almost entirely lost. Incorporation takes place in part by simple diffusion and in part through the intervention of a glycoprotein identical with or closely related to intrinsic factor. As in other tissues, within the red cell the vitamin becomes bound to protein.

Folic Acid

In her studies on the nutritional megaloblastic anaemia of Hindu women, Wills showed that there was a deficiency of a factor other than extrinsic factor. She found it to be present in yeast and crude liver extracts but not in purified liver extracts. The factor was later named vitamin M, and soon accumulated a series of other names. It was finally extracted in the pure state from spinach leaves and named folic acid. It has since been synthesized. Its biological activity depends on its existence in reduced forms related to folinic acid and named folic acid coenzymes. It is widely distributed in foods of animal and vegetable origin. Human requirements are variously estimated but around 0·05 mg. per day for males and rather more than this for females of child-bearing age seems probable. So widely distributed is it that dietary deficiency in normal subjects is almost impossible to imagine. In addition, considerable quantities are produced by the intestinal flora so that excretion usually exceeds dietary intake. In pregnancy however, folic acid requirements are greatly increased and may be as high as 3 to 5 mg. per day. Simple dietary deficiency then becomes distinctly possible.

It is absorbed by passive diffusion across the jejunal mucosa. It is found in all tissues, but particularly in the liver which acts as its main store. It is present in higher concentrations in the more primitive red cell precursors and is not incorporated into mature erythrocytes. Nevertheless folate is present in large amounts in mature red cells, mainly as protein-bound methyl-tetrahydrofolic acid. The transfer of folic acid into cells of the red cell series is vitamin B_{12} dependent and in vitamin B_{12} deficiency red cell folate activity is reduced while serum folate is high.

Folic acid consists of a pteridine-para-aminobenzoic acid complex known as pteroic acid, linked to a molecule of glutamic acid. It is often therefore referred to as pteroyl-glutamic acid or PGA. The natural substance occurs in conjugated forms containing more than one glutamic acid residue. In yeast it is largely present as pteroylhepta-glutamic acid. Another common form is the triglutamic acid.

Conjugates are absorbed from food and converted to folic acid by tissue conjugases (Fig. 6). In the presence of reducing substances such as ascorbic acid this is reduced to tetrahydrofolic acid. It is methylated and the product, N^5-methyl-tetrahydrofolic acid constitutes the form mainly

present in the plasma under normal conditions. In the presence of vitamin B_{12} this transfers its methyl group to homocysteine and is itself reconverted to tetrahydrofolic acid. This rôle of both vitamin B_{12} and folic acid in methionine metabolism is of considerable importance in human protein synthesis. In the presence of iron tetrahydrofolic acid accepts a formimino group from formiminoglutamic acid so playing an essential part in the conversion of histidine to glutamic acid. The N^5-formimino-tetrahydro-

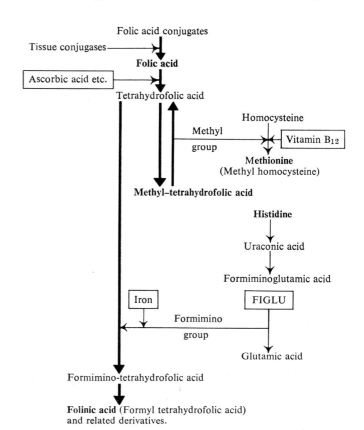

Fig. 6. Metabolism of folic acid and interrelationships with iron and vitamin B_{12}.

folic acid so produced acts as the parent substance from which the labile folic acid coenzymes and the more stable folinic acid are produced. These are the derivatives which play an active part in erythropoiesis.

Folate activity is assayed microbiologically. The most commonly used micro-organisms are Lactobacillus casei, Streptococcus faecalis and Leuconostoc citrovorum (more properly called Pediococcus cerevisiae). Roughly speaking microbiological assays give the following information:

1. *L. casei.* All folates shown in the metabolic table (Fig. 6).
2. *S. faecalis.* Folic acid and folinic acid.
3. *L. citrovorum.* Folinic acid.

Neither S. faecalis nor L. citrovorum determines N^5-methyl-tetrahydrofolic acid, normally the most abundant serum folate.

Four important points arise out of the metabolic table in Fig. 6. The first is that ascorbic acid deficiency may result in inefficient reduction of folic acid and therefore in a form of folic acid deficiency anaemia. Such anaemias are well documented apart from pregnancy. It should be noted that plasma ascorbic acid levels tend to be low in pregnancy and this may contribute to the onset of megaloblastic anaemia (Steingold, Vogel and Suchet, 1966). In megaloblastic anaemias due to ascorbic acid deficiency serum folate and vitamin B_{12} levels may be normal or even high. Administration of ascorbic acid cures the anaemia, this applying particularly to the megaloblastic anaemia of infants fed on dried milk preparations not reinforced with ascorbic acid. These anaemias also respond much better to folinic than to folic acid, verifying that the basis of the anaemia is a defect in folic acid reduction.

The second point to arise is that in vitamin B_{12} deficiency there will be a build-up in serum folate (L. casei) activity, as methyl-tetrahydrofolic acid, resulting in a concomitant metabolic block type of "folic acid" deficiency.

Thirdly, the transfer of the formimino group from FIGLU to tetrahydrofolic acid is iron dependent. Iron deficiency will therefore predispose to "folic acid" deficiency anaemia because of a block in the metabolic pathway of folic acid (Vitale, Streiff and Hellerstein, 1965). This has been observed to occur in pregnancy by Chanarin, Rothman and Berry (1965) who point out that megaloblastic anaemia is most frequent in the most iron deficient women.

The fourth point to arise out of the metabolic table is that FIGLU will accumulate, and appear in significant quantities in the urine, in folic acid deficiency. This will apply whether there is a primary deficiency of the vitamin itself or a block in its metabolic pathway preventing the acceptance of the formimino group by tetrahydrofolic acid. This is the basis of the FIGLU test, usually performed by determining the urinary FIGLU excretion after an oral dose of histidine. It will be apparent that this is not a test for primary folic acid deficiency. It will also be positive in some cases of deficiency of ascorbic acid, vitamin B_{12} or iron.

Mode of Action of Vitamin B_{12} and Folic Acid

Deficiency of vitamin B_{12} or folic acid results in anaemia with megaloblastic erythropoiesis. The erythropoietic marrow becomes hyperplastic and displaces the fatty marrow. Nuclear maturation and division are slowed down and ineffective erythropoiesis is considerably increased. Haemoglobinization is not affected and since there is inhibition of cellular division without interference with growth, the red cells become abnormally large. The result is that megaloblasts appear in the bone marrow. These are large cells with immature nuclei, showing abnormalities in their chromatin structure, while haemoglobinization of their cytoplasm is normal and in advance of their nuclear maturation. In severe cases such cells may appear in significant numbers in the circulation, but usually nuclear extrusion takes place and abnormally large erythrocytes are released into the blood stream. These are referred to as megalocytes or macrocytes.

It is accepted that such abnormalities must be related to abnormalities in nucleic acid metabolism and particularly, since nuclear maturation and division are so obviously implicated, to defects in DNA synthesis. A number of proposals have been put forward on these lines. One such is that of Baldwin and Dalessio (1961), which would explain the precipitate development of spinal cord degeneration in pernicious anaemia treated with folic acid. Their theory is illustrated in Fig. 7. They propose that vitamin B_{12} and folic acid act at different stages of nucleoprotein synthesis. Vitamin B_{12} acts at the stage of uracil formation and is therefore implicated in both DNA and RNA synthesis.

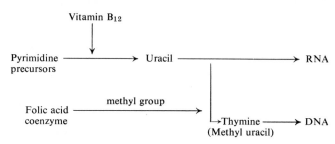

FIG. 7. Suggested rôle of vitamin B_{12} and folic acid in nucleic acid synthesis.

Folate, as methyl-tetrahydrofolic acid, conveys a methyl group to uracil to convert it to thymine and is therefore implicated in DNA synthesis only, and would tend to divert metabolic activity from RNA to DNA synthesis. In pernicious anaemia vitamin B_{12} deficiency results in a deficiency of uracil. Administration of folic acid diverts what little there is away from RNA synthesis to DNA synthesis. The improved DNA synthesis allows mitotic division to proceed and results in improvement in the megaloblastic anaemia. On the other hand, the functioning of axons involves a high turnover of protein and therefore of RNA, and since RNA synthesis is now severely restricted, axon degeneration occurs.

This theory has much in its favour. It explains the folic acid induced spinal cord degeneration in pernicious anaemia and the fall in serum vitamin B_{12} in megaloblastic anaemias treated with folic acid. There is some supporting evidence. Thus a satisfactory haematological response occurs in pernicious anaemia when the presumed block in DNA synthesis is by-passed by the administration of thymine. Subsequent administration of vitamin B_{12} does not elicit any further response.

Both vitamin B_{12} and folic acid are involved in "one-carbon transfers", the transfer from amino acids of small radicles containing single carbon atoms to the synthesis of more complex substances important in tissue metabolism. Examples which have been mentioned are the transfer of formimino groups and the conversion of uracil to thymine by the transfer of a methyl group from the metabolic pathway of folic acid.

One would expect a build-up of uracil and a depletion of thymine in folic acid deficiency. Parry (1966) has shown that this and the corollary, an increase in the ratio of RNA to DNA, both occur in the bone marrow in megaloblastic anaemia. These changes are corrected by treatment of the anaemia. However, observations which appear to be incompatible with this theory remain to be explained, and much of the theory itself remains to be verified.

Many other functions have been ascribed to folic acid and, particularly, to vitamin B₁₂. Some of these are impossible to fit into the processes involved in erythropoiesis. Most of them have been elucidated in work on microorganisms, chick cell preparations or laboratory animals. It remains to be seen which of them are vital or even at all applicable to man. Certainly many of them are not.

Megaloblastic Anaemia of Pregnancy

By this term is meant that megaloblastic anaemia which is specifically related to pregnancy, and not merely the exacerbation by pregnancy of a clinical or subclinical condition present before pregnancy, such as pernicious anaemia or the anaemia of the malabsorption syndrome. While such conditions, and others such as haemolysis and occult blood loss, contribute to the onset of megaloblastic anaemia of pregnancy, the patient is normally healthy before pregnancy. It responds to folic acid and is accepted as being due to a folate deficiency or to a block in its metabolism.

Folic acid is present in a wide variety of foods and dietary deficiency in the absence of pregnancy or disease can only occur in extreme poverty. However, the enormously increased demands for it which occur in pregnancy make such a deficiency possible then. Such increased demands are reflected in the tendency to rather low serum folate levels and increased clearance rates of injected folic acid even in normal pregnancy, and in the frequency with which foetal serum folate levels are considerably higher than those of the mother. Increased demands are greatest in the later stages of pregnancy and in twin pregnancies, and it is then that megaloblastic anaemia most frequently occurs.

While exacerbation of the anaemia of the malabsorption syndrome has been excluded from the definition and earlier workers found no evidence of folic acid malabsorption in megaloblastic anaemia of pregnancy, more recent reports suggest that there is such a disturbance in some cases and that it may be an inherited defect demonstrable apart from pregnancy (Giles, 1966). If this is so then the defect cannot be severe since there is no evidence that these women show megaloblastic anaemia in the non-pregnant state.

True folic acid deficiency, whether due to dietary deficiency or to malabsorption, is now accepted as an important cause of megaloblastic anaemia of pregnancy. Nevertheless, while it is true that serum folate levels are subnormal in most cases, they are not as low as those observed in other folic acid deficiency anaemias of similar severity and a significant proportion of cases show normal levels. Solomons, Lee, Wasserman and Malkin (1962) point out that there is no correlation between the presence or severity of anaemia and the serum folate levels in individual patients, and that there are no haematological differences between patients with high and low serum folate levels.

The discussion so far has referred to folic acid assayed as L. casei factor, in other words to total folate activity including erythropoietically inactive, unreduced and conjugated forms. It is apparent therefore that a block in folic acid metabolism may be an important aetiological factor. Ball and Giles (1964) verified this when they showed that serum "labile folic acid", a reduced coenzyme form related to folinic acid, is low in all patients with megaloblastic anaemia of pregnancy and very rarely so in patients with normoblastic erythropoiesis.

The active forms of folic acid are in the reduced state. Steingold et al. (1966) suggest that ascorbic acid deficiency blocks this reduction and that this is of aetiological significance in the onset of megaloblastic anaemia of pregnancy. Similarly deficiencies of vitamin B₁₂ and of iron will cause a metabolic block type of folic acid deficiency anaemia.

The interrelationships which exist between folic acid metabolism on the one hand, and the metabolism of ascorbic acid, vitamin B₁₂ and iron on the other, and the greatly increased demands for these substances in pregnancy, may well be the answer to the problem of the aetiology of this anaemia.

Red cell folic acid is largely in a functionally inactive, conjugated form, bound to protein. Grzesiukowicz, Jennison and Gowenlock (1965) suggest that this is a folic acid store, released when the cell is destroyed. Its activity is then restored by a plasma factor. They show that such a factor exists and that its concentration is increased in normal pregnancy and reduced in pregnancy with megaloblastic anaemia. If such a factor or factors operate during ordinary folic acid metabolism, as must be accepted to be the case, their theory is not incompatible with that described.

There remains the FIGLU test and its value in pregnancy. It has been shown that a positive test is not diagnostic of primary folic acid deficiency, and that it may also be obtained in deficiencies of iron, ascorbic acid and vitamin B₁₂. Administration of folic acid merely because the test is positive is not necessarily correct therapy. Nor is it correct to withhold it because the test is negative. Thus Chanarin, Rothman and Watson-Williams (1963) found it to be negative in half of their cases of megaloblastic anaemia of pregnancy, and Husain, Rothman and Ellis (1963) obtained variable results with this test throughout pregnancy, results quite unrelated to the patients' haematological status. Berry, Booth, Chanarin and Rothman (1963) go even further and point out that while the incidence of positive FIGLU tests drops considerably in the course of pregnancy, that of megaloblastic anaemia increases. These observations are explained by the slowing of absorption and lowered renal threshold for histidine during pregnancy and the increased demands for histidine during foetal growth.

Finally, there is the association between at any rate severe megaloblastic anaemia of pregnancy and the occurrence of blood group A, suggesting that a genetic factor plays a part in the aetiology of the condition.

Haemoglobin (Ingram, 1963; Rimington, 1959)

The globin fraction of haemoglobin consists of four interwoven polypeptide chains to each of which is attached a haem radicle. The chains are paired, there being, in normal adult haemoglobin, two alpha chains and two beta chains. This is haemoglobin A, and its globin structure is indicated by the formula $\alpha_2 \beta_2$. A considerable part of the haemoglobin of a newborn infant is resistant to denaturation by acid or alkali and is known as foetal haemoglobin or haemoglobin F. Its formula is $\alpha_2 \gamma_2$. This haemoglobin normally disappears more or less completely during the first year of the infant's life. A minor component of normal haemoglobin is haemoglobin A2. Its formula is $\alpha_2 \delta_2$. The gamma and delta polypeptide chains are chemically different from the beta chain.

In the normal haemoglobins of extra-uterine life there are then four different polypeptide chains, alpha, beta, gamma and delta. Their synthesis is controlled by separate genes. All three of the normal haemoglobins contain alpha chains. There occur haemoglobins however which contain no alpha chains. Examples are haemoglobin H (β_4), and haemoglobin Barts (γ_4). These abnormal haemoglobins are associated with disease. It will be observed that in these two cases, while the combination of chains is abnormal, the chains themselves are not.

However abnormal polypeptide chains do occur, in which a single amino acid is replaced by another, the messenger-RNA code of the two differing by a single letter. The haem radicles are unaffected. The synthesis of such abnormal haemoglobins is controlled by genes which are alleles of the genes for haemoglobin A. Only one such abnormal gene can be transmitted from parent to child and the child's genetic pattern will be homozygous or heterozygous depending on whether the parents transmit identical genes or not.

The list of abnormal haemoglobins resulting from the replacement of one amino acid by another is now long and increasing rapidly. Some are accompanied by haemolytic disease. Many are not. They can generally be distinguished from one another by differences in their mobility on electrophoresis. In obstetrics two of them are of considerable importance, haemoglobins S and C. In both of them the glutamic acid in position 6 on the beta chain is replaced. In haemoglobin S it is replaced by valine. In haemoglobin C it is replaced by lysine.

Sickle cell disease occurs in the homozygous inheritance of the gene for haemoglobin S. In other words the individual's genotype is SS. In the heterozygote the normal gene is inherited from one parent and the individual's genotype is AS. His red cells contain both haemoglobins A and S. He shows no clinical disease and is said to exhibit the sickle cell trait. Similarly the homozygous and heterozygous inheritance of the gene for haemoglobin C result in haemoglobin C disease and trait respectively. The inheritance of the genes for both these abnormalities, one from one parent and one from the other, results in haemoglobin SC disease. In these haemoglobinopathies a significant proportion of haemoglobin F usually persists throughout life.

Thalassaemia is an inherited haemolytic disease in which haemoglobin synthesis is defective. No abnormal haemoglobins are produced, the abnormality being an inhibition of normal polypeptide chain synthesis by the presence of an abnormal inhibitor (thalassaemia) gene. Alpha, beta,

gamma and delta chain thalassaemias have been described, depending on which polypeptide chain is inhibited. In alpha chain thalassaemia the haemoglobin produced in the foetus has four gamma chains and is haemoglobin Barts (γ_4). In extra-uterine life the haemoglobin produced has four beta chains and is haemoglobin H (β_4). In beta chain thalassaemia the deficit in beta chains is associated with an increase in gamma and delta chains, so that haemoglobins F and A2 replace haemoglobin A, the former occurring in more severe cases particularly. Thalassaemia major occurs in the homozygote, while the heterozygote has thalassaemia minor.

The thalassaemia genes are not alleles of those controlling the structure of the polypeptide chains. Thalassaemia can therefore occur in association with sickle cell disease, resulting in sickle cell thalassaemia.

Since there is a deficit in haemoglobin synthesis in thalassaemia the red cells are hypochromic. There is, however, no iron deficiency and the serum iron level is high. Iron therapy in this condition and in the haemoglobinopathies is contraindicated unless it is proven that there is concurrent true iron deficiency, such as might be expected if there is ankylostomiasis also.

The gene for thalassaemia occurs in the Mediterranean countries, through the Arab countries and into India and South East Asia. The gene for haemoglobin C occurs in Northern Ghana and has spread into adjacent territories. The gene for haemoglobin S occurs in East Africa and has spread into the countries affected by thalassaemia and across tropical and equatorial Africa. There is considerable overlap of these three genes geographically and the heterozygous haemoglobin diseases are not rare.

A feature of sickle cell disease and, in pregnancy particularly, of sickle cell-haemoglobin C disease is the occurrence of sickling crises. Reduced haemoglobin S is relatively insoluble and tends to precipitate out as long pseudocrystals or *tactoids*. The cells become elongated and distorted, the picture giving the disease its name. The ocurrence of sickling is contributed to by anoxia, circulatory stasis, acidosis, transfusion, and pregnancy itself. Destruction of the sickled cells will result in a haemolytic crisis, or the cells may clump and cause thrombosis, with infarctions. Such infarctions are commonest in the bone marrow and spleen where stasis is most marked. Pulmonary embolism is not rare.

Cases of thalassaemia major seldom survive into adult life, and when they do are usually sexually immature. Successful pregnancy in such women is rare. Thalassaemia minor, normally mild, may become clinically severe in pregnancy.

The presence of the gene for thalassaemia and of that for sickle cell disease protect against malignant tertian malaria. While the homozygote suffers from a lethal disease, the heterozygote does not and is protected against another lethal disease. These are examples of evolution in action, the homozygote being sacrificed for the sake of the much more numerous heterozygote to give protection against the Plasmodium falciparum.

Within the foetal circulation haemoglobin F has a higher affinity for oxygen than haemoglobin A, and this assists in oxygen transfer across the placenta. The infant does not possess two cell populations, both haemoglobins occurring within the one cell. This also applies to the sickle cell trait, in which all the red cells contain both haemoglobins A and S and can be induced to sickle *in vitro*. In contrast with haemoglobin A, the rate of haemoglobin F synthesis is not influenced by erythropoietin so that the polycythaemic effect of hypoxia in the mother is minimized in her infant.

Haemoglobin A first appears at about the thirty-fourth week of foetal life and gradually replaces haemoglobin F. Birth does not accelerate this process which, apart from persistent traces of haemoglobin F, is completed during the first year of life. Since sickle cell anaemia is due to an abnormality of beta chains not present in haemoglobin F, the newborn infant who has inherited the disease does not manifest it at birth.

Haemoglobin synthesis depends on the presence of messenger-RNA and therefore takes place in the less mature red cells. Messenger-RNA is present in the cytoplasm of nucleated red cells where its synthesis is controlled by nuclear DNA. When the nucleus is extruded the residual RNA disappears in two or three days. During this time however, the cell is capable of synthesizing haemoglobin. No haemoglobin synthesis takes place in mature erythrocytes and a haemoglobin-deficient erythrocyte remains so throughout its life.

Attached to each of the four polypeptide chains of haemoglobin is a haem group. This consists of an atom of iron in the ferrous state, linked to protoporphyrin IX (Fig. 8). The iron atom possesses two further coordinate valence bonds in addition to those shown, one attached to the polypeptide chain and the other for oxygen transport. This haem group occurs in other proteins such as myoglobin and the catalase, cytochrome and peroxidase enzymes.

The first step in haem synthesis is the condensation of glycine with succinate. This is dependent on the presence of ferrous ions so that protoporphyrin IX synthesis is inhibited in iron deficiency. It is also dependent on the presence of pyridoxine, a deficiency of which therefore results in hypochromic anaemia with high serum iron levels. There is evidence to suggest that pyridoxine-deficiency anaemia is less uncommon in pregnancy than is generally supposed.

The compound formed by condensation of glycine with succinate converts spontaneously to δ-aminolaevulinic acid, usually referred to as ALA. Two molecules of ALA condense to form porphobilinogen (Fig. 8). Excretion of large amounts of ALA and porphobilinogen occur in the abnormalities of haem synthesis known as the porphyrias. Porphobilinogen is always synthesized in the body. Preformed pyrroles such as occur in chlorophyll, myoglobin and haemoglobin itself are not used.

Four molecules of porphobilinogen combine to form a tetrapyrrolic ring compound. A series of modifying reactions follow, resulting in the formation of protoporphyrin IX. Iron is then inserted into the molecule, by mechanisms to be discussed, and the haem group is complete.

During increased erythropoiesis there is accelerated haem

synthesis. An excess of haem groups operates a feed-back mechanism by inhibiting the enzyme involved in the condensation of glycine with succinate and so inhibiting further haem synthesis, while at the same time stimulating further globin production.

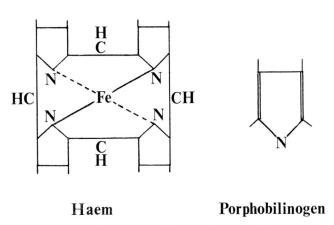

Haem   **Porphobilinogen**

Fig. 8. Basic structure of haem and porphobilinogen.

Iron Metabolism

Iron is conserved in the body. The daily loss is only about 1 mg. in the male and 2 mg. in the female of child-bearing age. This loss is accounted for by the shedding of cells into urine, faeces and bile, from the skin and in sweat. In the female the additional loss is due to menstruation. It is this small daily loss which the diet is required to replace. The average daily intake in a good mixed diet is about 10 to 15 mg. of iron of which the normal person absorbs what he needs. In iron deficiency the proportion absorbed is increased but probably not to levels above 4 mg. per day from such diets.

The total iron in the body of a healthy adult female is about 3·5 g. Its approximate distribution is:

Haemoglobin iron	60–70 per cent
Iron in body stores	20–30 per cent
Tissue iron	5–10 per cent
Plasma iron	0·1 per cent

Iron Absorption. The recommended doses of oral ferrous salts used in the prevention and treatment of anaemia provide 100 to 200 mg. of iron per day. Such doses are unphysiological and conclusions drawn from observations on their absorption are not necessarily applicable to the absorption of iron from food.

In meat diets a high proportion of the iron is in the ferrous form in haem, and appears to be absorbed in this form. It is now known that haemoglobin iron is absorbed at least as well as simpler iron salts in the diet. The mechanism is however different and its absorption is unaffected by the presence of ascorbic acid and increased rather than decreased by dietary phytates and phosphates. The latter form insoluble, unabsorbable compounds with simple iron salts and therefore reduce considerably the absorption of iron from food, and of medicinal iron given with a meal.

The remainder of the dietary iron is largely in the unabsorbable ferric form. In the presence of reducing substances such as ascorbic acid, digestion converts it to the ferrous form. Ascorbic acid increases the absorption of food iron, and by maintaining them in the reduced state, of simple ferrous salts.

Gastric factors in iron absorption. The earlier hypothesis that the hypochlorhydria of pregnancy is a major cause of the iron deficiency so often encountered is not now accepted. In fact the reverse seems to be the case. Iron deficiency causes hypochlorhydria and, unless there are severe irreversible changes in the gastric mucosa, iron therapy will relieve it. The absolute achlorhydria of pernicious anaemia is not usually accompanied by iron deficiency and the administration of hydrochloric acid to achlorhydric subjects has little effect on the absorption of *dietary* iron. However, achlorhydria is accompanied by reduced absorption of inorganic iron (Jacobs, Bothwell and Charlton, 1964), and this is corrected by the administration of hydrochloric acid. However, achlorhydria is not accompanied by deficient absorption of haem iron and it must be accepted, in individuals on an ordinary diet in which much of the iron is in the form of haem compounds, that achlorhydria is unimportant in the pathogenesis of iron deficiency anaemia.

Gastric secretions, other than hydrochloric acid, also play a part in iron absorption. Polya gastrectomy results in the slow development, in a proportion of cases, of a progressive anaemia the incidence of which is less in males than in females of child-bearing age, in whom menstruation is an additional factor (Baird, Blackburn and Wilson, 1959). There is little if any malabsorption of iron given to fasting cases, but considerable malabsorption when the iron is given, either as inorganic iron or as haemoglobin, with a full meal. Development of anaemia in these cases is not accompanied by the expected increase in iron absorption (Baird and Wilson, 1959). Turnberg (1966) was able to correct the deficiency in absorption of iron given with a meal by feeding crude whole hog stomach. He found malabsorption of haemoglobin iron given with food to be the more significant defect, to be present in all Polya gastrectomies and to undergo no correction by giving hog stomach.

Callender (1965) had in fact just previously to Turnberg's paper attracted attention to reports on the existence of two gastric factors influencing iron absorption. One, a "stabiliser", prevents the precipitation of inorganic iron in the alkaline medium of the duodenum and jejunum, and is not increased in iron deficient subjects. The other, demonstrated in dogs and not yet in man, is a muco- or glycoprotein which binds and protects iron and *is* increased in anaemic animals.

That progressive anaemia does not follow Billroth gastrectomies (in which the duodenum is not by-passed), and hog stomach does not correct the malabsorption of haem iron in Polya gastrectomies suggests that by-passing the duodenum rather than a deficiency of gastric factors is the important abnormality in Polya gastrectomy cases. Whether a deficiency of such factors plays any part in the pathogenesis of anaemia in pregnancy remains to be determined.

In man iron is absorbed mainly from the immediately post-pyloric duodenum. In iron deficiency absorption from the rest of the intestine increases but never equals that from the duodenum. Iron absorption is inhibited by the alkaline secretions of the pancreas and over-absorption occurs in the presence of pancreatic damage.

To prevent overloading the body with iron, a mechanism exists which controls its absorption. Such iron as is required is absorbed across the cells of the duodenal mucosa, possibly bound to glycine and serine (Brown and Rother, 1961). Succinic acid, whether given orally or parenterally, enhances its absorption (Brise and Hallberg, 1962) and the possibility that it plays a part in normal iron absorption appears to deserve consideration.

It may be stated at this point that all body iron, apart from that in haem, is in the ferric form except when it is crossing cell membranes when it is in the ferrous form. Reduction is effected by substances such as glutathione and ascorbic acid. Thus mucosal iron, plasma iron and stored iron are all in the ferric form.

The absorption of iron into the bloodstream is enzyme dependent and is controlled by the production of a protein known as *apoferritin* within the cells of the absorptive area. This combines with unwanted iron to form *ferritin* which is returned to the intestinal lumen for excretion when the cells are shed. Iron which enters the mucosal cells and is not bound to apoferritin is absorbed. In iron deficiency little apoferritin appears and iron absorption is maximal (Brown and Rother, 1961; Charlton, Jacobs, Torrance and Bothwell, 1963). In iron repletion apoferritin production is stimulated and iron absorption is minimal. This mechanism effectively controls the absorption of iron from normal diets, adjusting it to the body's needs. The control of absorption is less efficient in the face of massive doses of iron either as medicine, or in food as in the case of the Bantus of South Africa. Thus Smith and Pannacciulli (1959) could demonstrate no limit to the total amount of iron absorbed, even by normal subjects, from increasing doses of ferrous sulphate solution, although the proportion fell as the dose increased. In iron-deficient subjects both the total amount and the proportion absorbed were much higher at all doses (Fig. 9), indicating that even in these circumstances the control mechanism has some effect.

Abnormalities of the intestinal mucosa result in abnormalities of absorption, and the mucosal changes of the malabsorption syndrome are accompanied by reduced iron absorption which is not increased when iron deficiency develops.

Iron transport. Plasma iron is in the ferric form and bound to a β-globulin known as *siderophilin* or *transferrin*. The plasma concentration of siderophilin constitutes the total iron-binding capacity of the plasma (TIBC). That fraction not combined with iron constitutes the unsaturated iron-binding capacity (UIBC). The plasma siderophilin is normally about one-third saturated. One gramme of siderophilin can bind 1·25 mg. of iron. The normal concentration of siderophilin in the plasma is about 250 mg. per 100 ml. The normal TIBC is therefore about 300 μg. of iron per 100 ml. of plasma, and the normal plasma iron about 100 µg. per 100 ml. In iron deficiency, in anaemias responding to therapy and in pregnancy even in the absence of anaemia, the uncombined siderophilin level is high. While there is a total of 3 to 4 mg. of iron in the plasma, some 20 to 26 mg. leave it daily, for conversion to haemoglobin, myoglobin and cell enzymes, and for deposition in body stores. There is therefore a turnover

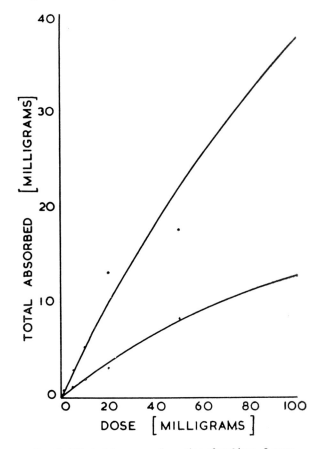

FIG. 9. Effect of dosage on absorption of oral iron. Lower curve—normal subjects. Upper curve—iron deficient subjects.

of plasma iron about 5 to 8 times a day, continuous replenishment being by the absorption of iron from the alimentary canal and the release of iron by haemoglobin breakdown in the reticulo-endothelial system. When these are inadequate, iron is withdrawn from stores.

The mother's plasma iron is also the source of iron for the foetus. The mother's iron is preferentially transferred to the infant even if she is iron deficient, and since the foetus' plasma iron concentration is higher than the mother's the transfer across the placenta is against a concentration gradient and presumably enzyme-dependent. However nothing whatever is known about the mode of transplacental iron transfer.

The determination of the serum iron concentration is frequently used in diagnosing the nature of an anaemia. Occasionally the result can be misleading to the unwary. Low figures, not related to iron deficiency may occur in haemodilution, in infections (in which there is an increase of iron transfer to the tissues) and in megaloblastic

anaemias under appropriate therapy. Unduly high figures may be met with in acute tissue anoxia such as occurs in haemorrhagic shock, iron being liberated rapidly from liver stores under these circumstances. In addition there is a marked diurnal variation in serum iron levels, and random specimens may give misleading results. Waldenström (1946) found, in normal nurses, that the morning serum iron concentration is about 50 per cent greater than the evening level. This situation is reversed in the case of nurses on night duty.

Iron storage. The quantity of iron stored in the body has been variously estimated, but appears to be between 600 and 1500 mg., or about the same as, or a little more than, the excess required in pregnancy over and above what is required over the same period in the non-pregnant state. Absorbed iron and that liberated by the destruction of effete erythrocytes and other cells are preferentially utilised in haem synthesis and there is normally little turnover of stored iron. Such iron as is not used in this way is released from the plasma to the body stores by mechanisms requiring adenosine triphosphate (ATP) and reducing substances. It is stored in the liver, spleen and bone marrow, mainly as water-soluble ferritin, containing about 20 per cent of ferric iron. The remainder is stored as insoluble haemosiderin, containing 35 per cent of iron. When storage is abnormally high the excess is stored as haemosiderin.

The storage of iron is influenced by sex hormones, oestrogens increasing and androgens decreasing it. Thus at sexual maturity the female stores more iron than the male, and removal of the gonads reduces iron storage in the female and increases it in the male. There is, in the female, a marked reduction in serum iron two or three days before the onset of menstruation. This persists for a couple of days after the onset but the serum iron then rises although menstrual blood loss continues. It is believed that this premenstrual fall in serum iron is due to diversion of iron to body stores under the influence of hormones.

However, the most important factor determining the size of the body stores of iron is its availability in the diet, and most women enter pregnancy with inadequate body stores.

Haemochromatosis and haemosiderosis. Haemochromatosis is an uncommon condition in which there is a disturbance of iron metabolism. There is over-absorption of iron, probably due to inefficient synthesis of ferritin within the cells of the duodenal mucosa. Duodenal control of iron absorption is not however eliminated by any means entirely, and venesection in these cases is accompanied by an increase in iron absorption. It usually occurs in males in later life and is rare in females, the ratio between the sexes being about 20 to 1. In women it is almost entirely a disease of the menopause, the few exceptions being women belonging to severely affected families. The protective effect of menstrual blood loss appears to be a sufficient explanation of the sex difference in incidence.

The condition is characterised by grossly excessive deposits of haemosiderin in the organs, particularly the liver, pancreas, skin, spleen and lymph nodes. The total body iron amounts to 20 g. or more, and there is fibrosis of the viscera most involved. Excessive melanin deposition in the skin is usual and reflects the disturbed melanin metabolism associated with fibrosis of the adrenals. The plasma iron level is increased and its iron-binding capacity more or less saturated.

The cause of the visceral fibrosis is not completely understood but it is now widely accepted that it is a direct result of the excessive iron deposits and that similar visceral fibrosis occurs in other forms of siderosis, however caused. Siderosis was once thought to be a benign condition but it is now known that the time factor is important and that if cases are followed up for long enough they will eventually be seen to develop visceral fibrosis.

Siderosis can appear in a number of ways. Haemosiderosis occurs in haemolytic and other non-iron-deficiency anaemias, treated over a long time with transfusions and sometimes, mistakenly, with oral or parenteral iron. The total amount of iron deposited in the tissues in such cases is greater than that administered in the transfusions. The difference is due to the excessive iron absorption which accompanies the anaemia.

A second form is nutritional siderosis which occurs in normal subjects exposed for a long time to grossly excessive dietary iron. The condition leads to hepatic cirrhosis and a high incidence of malignant hepatoma. It is common in the Bantus of South Africa who cook their food in iron pans, and drink Kaffir beer which contains large quantities of iron. Callender (1965) points out that cooking in iron pans increases thirty- to one hundred-fold the iron content of food.

Finally extensive siderosis may occur in cases of portal cirrhosis, usually due to chronic alcoholism, and of postnecrotic cirrhosis.

The deposits of iron in these forms of siderosis may be so large, and the visceral fibrosis so marked as to make them indistinguishable from idiopathic haemochromatosis both clinically and pathologically. MacDonald (1963) goes so far as to say that there is no such condition as idiopathic haemochromatosis. He points out that cases are most frequently reported from France and are readily explained by the large quantities of wine and cider consumed there, these beverages frequently containing large quantities of iron; in other words that these are cases of nutritional or alcoholic siderosis. In this connection it is worth pointing out that alcohol increases the absorption of simultaneously administered iron and that iron absorption is increased in alcoholics even when it is taken without alcohol. MacDonald suggests that this explains even the supposed familial incidence of so-called idiopathic haemochromatosis.

He recommends that a careful search be made for sources of excessive iron intake in every case and states that frequently such sources will be found. Nevertheless it is generally accepted that idiopathic haemochromatosis does exist, although it may be less common than is reported. It is a familial condition exhibiting an intermediate form of inheritance, homozygotes being more severely affected than heterozygotes (Powell, 1965). Examination of relatives of cases will reveal some who show high serum iron levels, excessive tissue iron deposits and increased iron absorption.

Bearing in mind that haemochromatosis is a disease of later life and that presumably the over-absorption of iron is present from an early age, it becomes apparent that the degree of overabsorption need not be very great to explain the total accumulation of iron in the tissues. In fact a number of workers have found the absorption of iron to be within "normal limits" in these cases although at a higher mean level than in normal controls. As MacDonald (1963) points out, over-absorption of as little as 1·8 mg. of iron per day would result in a tissue accumulation of over 20 g. in thirty years.

In chronic pancreatic disease, whether accompanied by hepatic cirrhosis or not, there is over-absorption of iron. Administration of pancreatin reduces iron absorption in these cases and its over-enthusiastic administration may even result in iron deficiency. Pancreatin can also be used successfully to control the over-absorption of iron in hepatic cirrhosis not apparently complicated by pancreatic disease and in haemochromatosis. The nature of the operative constituent in pancreatin is not known but it may be trypsin, which can be shown to have the same effect.

Mobilization of iron from body stores. In addition to reducing substances the release of iron from body stores requires an enzyme made available during the synthesis of uric acid from xanthine and hypoxanthine. Uric acid synthesis does not take place in the liver of the foetus and hepatic iron is therefore not released during intrauterine life. At birth the infant's liver stores of iron are consequently high. Hepatic uric acid synthesis commences within a few days of birth and with it the release of iron for haem synthesis. There is very little iron in milk and, until the infant is weaned, depletion of liver iron takes place. If the infant's iron stores are inadequate or weaning delayed, iron deficiency will ensue. This can be prevented by supplementing the infant's feeds with iron. Iron deficiency in infancy, childhood and adolescence is not a condition to be ignored. It is accompanied by a form of dwarfism. The gain in height and weight when such cases are eventually given iron can be remarkable.

Mobilization of iron from body stores is stimulated by hypoxia (as in haemorrhagic shock). Conversely, high tissue oxygen levels stimulate the storage of iron.

Haem synthesis and haemoglobin breakdown. Haem synthesis takes place in the erythrocyte precursors in the bone marrow, and in tissue cells where it is a component of cell enzymes. None takes place in mature erythrocytes since they contain no RNA and cannot therefore synthesize the necessary enzymes. Within the erythroblast the iron binds to the lipid stroma from which it is released as protoporphyrin becomes available. The union of iron with protoporphyrin is enzyme dependent and, since haem iron is in the ferrous form, requires the presence of reducing substances. When iron incorporation into haem is blocked, as in lead poisoning, the red cell concentration of protoporphyrin is increased and its haemoglobin concentration reduced.

When erythrocytes are destroyed the liberated haemoglobin is broken down by cells of the reticulo-endothelial system. The iron and globin fractions are removed and the iron re-utilized or returned to body stores. The globin fraction appears to be catabolized and not to be used for further haemoglobin synthesis. The porphyrin ring is opened out and converted to bilirubin. This is known as "indirect" bilirubin since it does not react with van den Bergh's reagent without the intervention of some such substance as methanol. It is soluble in lipids and insoluble in water. It cannot therefore be excreted by the kidneys and to be able to circulate in the blood it is bound to plasma albumin. If it is present in considerable excess, as in some cases of haemolytic disease of the newborn, some appears to be attached to plasma lipid and its lipid solubility allows its transfer to the basal ganglia of the brain giving rise to kernicterus. Albumin-bound bilirubin is not transferred in this way and the administration of albumin liberates bilirubin from the basal ganglia.

Salicylates and some sulphonamides have a high albumin-binding capacity and displace albumin-bound bilirubin. Their use in cases of haemolytic disease of the newborn predisposes to kernicterus. Sulphonamides with low affinity for albumin, such as sulphamethizole, sulphadiazine and sulphadimidine, do not predispose to kernicterus (Josephson and Furst, 1966).

Bilirubin is removed from the plasma by the liver which conjugates it with one or two molecules of glucuronic acid, producing mono- and diglucuronides. Conjugation is effected by the enzyme glucuronyl transferase, which is produced in the liver and is responsible for the conjugation of a range of substances excreted in bile. An inherited deficiency of this enzyme occurs in man. The enzyme is also deficient in the newborn and, particularly, premature infant on account of hepatic immaturity, and results in jaundice. It appears within a few days of birth, the accumulated bilirubin is excreted and the jaundice clears. It will be apparent that neonatal glucuronyl transferase deficiency contributes to the hyperbilirubinaemia in haemolytic disease of the newborn.

Certain steroid hormones such as oestriol, pregnanediol, cortisone and prednisolone are also excreted in conjugated form by the liver. Lauritzen and Lehmann (1965, 1966) have shown that the administration of such steroids to the nursing mother or her infant results in an increase in the infant's serum unconjugated bilirubin level. They suggest that this is due to competition between these steroids and bilirubin for glucuronyl transferase. They point out that the infant is required to excrete large quantities of placental and other hormones during the first few days of its life and suggest that this is of importance in the aetiology of kernicterus. In severe haemolytic disease of the newborn there is an increase in bilirubin in the amniotic fluid. The concentration is of considerable prognostic significance (Bower and Swale, 1966).

The conjugated forms of bilirubin are termed "direct" bilirubin since they react with van den Bergh's reagent without the intervention of substances such as methanol. The liver excretes them in bile and they accumulate in the blood by regurgitation in jaundice of an obstructive nature.

They are water soluble and are excreted by the kidneys. In the intestine bacteria convert bilirubin to urobilinogen and urobilin. A significant proportion of these substances in the faeces does not, however, come from haemoglobin breakdown. This proportion is greatly increased in pernicious anaemia. Some bilirubin is eliminated by other, probably metabolic, routes. Thus in infective hepatitis steroid therapy reduces the serum bilirubin without increasing its excretion.

Iron deficiency anaemia. Iron deficiency is the commonest cause of anaemia in pregnancy. The pregnant woman requires twice as much or more iron for herself and her foetus as she does in the same time apart from pregnancy. Approximately 500 to 600 mg. of iron are required for the development of the foetus and placenta, and the increase in maternal tissues associated with pregnancy. A variable loss of blood occurs at parturition and lactation results in a further loss of about 150 mg. of iron. Iron is required for the increase in maternal circulating haemoglobin which accompanies pregnancy. The quantity required is variable but 500 mg. is not at all unusual. These requirements are such that in a normal woman, not given supplementary iron, the body iron stores will be more or less completely used up.

Intercurrent infections and other conditions in which iron is diverted to tissue enzyme formation, infestations such as ankylostomiasis and, in adolescents, the demands for iron occasioned by normal body growth, can be of considerable significance. It is apparent that dietary sources alone will rarely meet these increased demands for iron and, since most women's iron reserves are suboptimal, iron deficiency anaemia will be the rule rather than the exception in pregnancy, unless iron supplements are taken. A common practice therefore, is to give oral iron, usually with ascorbic acid, throughout pregnancy whether or not the patient is anaemic. The major exception is the occasional case of haemolytic anaemia who already has excessive absorption and excessive iron stores.

It does not matter very much which ferrous preparation is used, although ferrous sulphate is to be avoided in out-patient practice since it may accidentally be taken by young children and cause their death. Since intolerance to iron appears to be largely psychological, it seems advisable to withhold from the patient the knowledge that she is on it. The use of hog's stomach, succinic acid and hydrochloric acid remain to be assessed. Parenteral iron offers little advantage over oral iron with ascorbic acid and is really indicated only in the occasional case of the malabsorption syndrome or in patients who cannot or will not take oral iron.

Haemoglobin is a protein. It is to be expected therefore that protein deficiency will result in anaemia. Nevertheless anaemia due entirely, or largely, to protein deficiency is uncommon in man. The almost inevitable concurrent deficiency of other haemopoietic substances is of much greater importance in the production of anaemia. Animal experiments and observations on prisoners in concentration camps have shown that during starvation there is retained a high capacity for haemoglobin synthesis and that this takes priority over the restoration of plasma proteins, when normal diet is resumed.

In terms of haemoglobin synthesis different proteins have different biological efficiencies. Haemoglobin itself has the highest efficiency and vegetable proteins, which often lack essential amino acids, the lowest.

Leucocytes

Unlike red cells, whose life span is spent in the bloodstream, to leucocytes the circulation is merely a means of transport to and from the tissues. Their rate of destruction varies so widely with changing circumstances that, with the exception of lymphocytes, none of them can reasonably be allocated a normal life span. Because of this, such estimates as have been made vary very widely indeed.

Polymorphonuclear leucocytes, or granulocytes, originate in the bone marrow. Lymphocytes and such monocytes as normally appear in the circulation originate in the lymphoid organs. Neutrophile granulocytes are normally the most numerous leucocytes in the blood. They arise from myeloblasts by a series of mitotic divisions and nuclear and cytoplasmic maturation. Mitotic division ceases at the myelocyte stage. These changes take place extravascularly, and the mature cells enter the circulation by diapedesis through the walls of the marrow sinusoids. When the demand for neutrophiles is high the number in the circulation increases and less mature forms appear. This "shift to the left" may be so marked as to cause the blood picture to resemble that of chronic myeloid leukaemia.

Mature neutrophiles exhibit the phenomenon of *taxis*, or directional movement under the influence of physical or chemical stimuli. They are attracted to sites of acute infection and to areas of tissue damage whether bacterial or not, and it has been shown that bacterial products and substances released by damaged tissues exert the necessary chemotactic effect. There is evidence that these substances stimulate the bone marrow to release neutrophiles and to increase their rate of formation (Menkin, 1955). Their production and biological effects are inhibited by ACTH and adrenal cortical steroids, which therefore inhibit the inflammatory reaction.

Menkin's views have not been entirely abandoned but it appears that at least as important are local changes in pH (local acidity attracting leucocytes) and increases in temperature. In addition it appears likely that plasma factors adjust leucopoiesis to meet the body's needs, some factors being stimulatory and some inhibitory. Such work is in its early stages.

Although Menkin found that corticosteroids and ACTH inhibit the factors causing leucocyte production, their administration to man causes leucocytosis. Testosterone also causes leucocytosis, while ovarian hormones appear to have no effect on the production of granulocytes. It has been pointed out that Linman and Bethell's lipid factor causes leucocytosis and thrombocytosis. These workers suggest that this factor makes its appearance along with erythropoietin. Certainly leucocytosis and hrombocythaemia occur in polycythaemia vera.

Considerable attention has been paid to the morpho-logical changes which take place in the circulating neutrophiles and marrow metamyelocytes in megaloblastic anaemia of pregnancy. The changes described are an increase in the proportion of hypersegmented neutrophiles, cells with five or more lobes to their nuclei, and increase in the size of metamyelocytes resulting in giant forms. Some workers have gone so far as to use these changes to diagnose "megaloblastic anaemia" in the absence of megaloblastic changes in the marrow. However Chanarin, Rothman and Berry (1965) found that a significant proportion of cases of megaloblastic anaemia of pregnancy show no hypersegmented neutrophiles and many cases of iron deficiency anaemia do. They also deny the diagnostic significance of giant metamyelocytes, although it is true that large numbers of these are always accompanied by megaloblastic changes. The leucopenia which frequently occurs in megaloblastic anaemias has generally been accepted as resulting from inhibition of leucopoiesis by a deficiency of vitamin B_{12} or folic acid. There is evidence however that it is due to increased turnover of leucocytes (Perillie, Kaplan and Finch, 1967).

Eosinophile polymorphs are generally accepted as originating from the same myeloblast as neutrophiles, differentiation occurring when the specific granules appear in the promyelocyte or myelocyte. However the nucleoproteins of eosinophiles are much more closely related to those of lymphocytes and monocytes than to those of neutrophiles, and it seems likely that eosinophiles have their own stem cell and that this is not identical with that of neutrophiles.

The blood eosinophile count shows pronounced diurnal variation, related to variations in adrenal activity. In females peak counts occur at menstruation. There is a post-ovulatory eosinopenia which precedes the rise in basal temperature by a day or two.

Eosinophilia occurs in allergic conditions but is not induced by histamine. The administration of ACTH and of corticosteroids results in rapid eosinopenia, but deficiencies of these hormones are not accompanied by eosinophilia. Their eosinopenic effect appears to be due to induced migration of eosinophiles into the tissues, particularly of the intestine and lungs, and these hormones appear to have no effect on eosinophile maturation or release.

Other substances such as gonadal hormones, thyroxine, pituitary hormones and adrenaline, which affect the eosinophile count, appear to act by influencing ACTH production or by increasing the susceptibility of eosinophiles to corticosteroids. The eosinopenia of parturition probably arises in this way also.

Senile eosinophiles are phagocytosed by monocytes and tissue histiocytes. It is generally assumed that the majority end up in the gastrointestinal tract, spleen and lungs.

The basophile polymorphs resemble the tissue mast cells and both contain heparin and abundant histamine. Nevertheless they are not identical cells. Blood basophiles originate in the bone marrow. Tissue mast cells arise in the tissues by division of mature mast cells or, in conditions demanding them in large numbers, from fibroblasts and possibly lymphocytes.

Corticosteroids reduce the number of basophiles, but here also there is no evidence of any direct effect on their maturation or release. There is marked reduction in basophiles in pregnancy, and this is probably hormonal in origin.

The mode of origin of blood monocytes has not been entirely elucidated. It is accepted that some at least originate in the lymphoid organs. Some may also originate in the bone marrow. Nevertheless the majority are produced from tissue histiocytes and function in the tissues, using the bloodstream as a means of transport only. Certainly most of the monocytes in inflammatory lesions originate in this way.

Control over the number of monocytes is exerted by the hypothalamus, and severance of its neural connections inhibits monocytosis. The administration of ACTH and of corticosteroids results in a temporary monocytopenia.

The cytoplasm of plasma cells is rich in RNA, this being related to their function of antibody production. They appear during the third month of life, at the same time as antibodies. Their mode of origin has not been defined, but experiments show that antigenic stimuli cause differentiation of plasma cells from reticulum cells of the lymphoid tissues, without concurrent lymphocytosis, and this is probably their tissue and mode of origin.

Of the lymphocytes in the body, no more than two in every ten thousand normally appear in the circulation at any one time. The vast majority are in the bone marrow, the lymphatic tissues and scattered throughout the body. In the adult, lymphocytes are produced in the lymph nodes. The thymus undergoes involution with increasing age and cannot be an important source of lymphocytes except in the young. Lymphocytes in the spleen and lymphoid tissue of the intestine remain in these tissues and do not enter the bloodstream.

The generally accepted mode of development of lymphocytes is shown in Fig. 1. Primitive mesenchyme cells give rise to lymphoblasts from which small mature lymphocytes develop by maturation and a series of mitotic divisions. It has been shown that lymphocytes in areas of inflammation enter such areas from the bloodstream and do not develop locally.

There are two populations of lymphocytes, a smaller population with a short life span and a larger population with a life span of 100 to 200 days or more. They recirculate continuously between blood and lymph nodes and spend only a small part of their life in the bloodstream. The mode and site of their destruction at the end of their life span is not known.

The lymphoid tissues show their maximum development around puberty. Thereafter they undergo gradual involution. Involution is caused by male and female sex hormones, ACTH and corticosteroid hormones. It occurs also in stress situations, including pregnancy and lactation, and is then mediated by ACTH through the adrenal cortex. Such involutions are accompanied by pronounced lymphopenia, and by lymphocytic degeneration and suppression of lymphopoiesis in the lymphoid organs.

Conversely, removal of the gonads or adrenals causes lymphoid hyperplasia. Administration of thyro-active substances induces such hyperplasia also. These findings are reflected in the lymphoid hyperplasia which occurs in Addison's disease and hyperthyroidism.

There remains the question of transformation of cells of the lymphocyte series into other haemopoietic cells. If this occurs in man it is probably rare and takes place only in extreme circumstances. Nevertheless evidence of such transformations is accumulating. It has even been proposed that large or medium lymphocytes are identical with the primitive precursor to the haemocytoblast or the haemocytoblast itself, or at any rate retain such multipotent potential even if it is rarely put into effect. It is suggested that when such transformation takes place the supply of large and medium lymphocytes is maintained by dedifferentiation of small mature lymphocytes.

While such transformations are not entirely proven, and statements on this subject were, at any rate initially, based on observations on cell cultures, there is now strong supporting evidence from *in vivo* experiments, of transformation of lymphocytes into plasma cells and primitive multipotent bone marrow cells. In other words, lymphocytes may form a reserve from which other haemopoietic cells can reconstitute themselves.

Platelets arise in the bone marrow by budding off of fragments of the cytoplasm of megakaryocytes. They have a life span of eight or nine days. Linman and Bethell's lipid factor causes increase in their production. Erythropoietin itself has no such effect and thrombopoiesis is not influenced by hypoxia.

Control over platelet production is exerted by the number of circulating platelets, and platelet transfusions depress thrombopoiesis. Platelets appear to exert this control by modifying the activity of plasma thrombopoietic hormones, and fractionation of normal plasma gives rise to fractions which cause thrombocytosis or thrombocytopenia in animals. This work also is still in its infancy.

REFERENCES

Adams, J. F. (1958), "Pregnancy and Addisonian Pernicious Anaemia," *Scot. med. J.*, **3**, 21.

Baird, I. M., Blackburn, E. K. and Wilson, G. M. (1959), "The Pathogenesis of Anaemia after Partial Gastrectomy. I. Development of Anaemia in Relation to Time After Operation, Blood Loss and Diet," *Quart. J. Med.*, N.S., **28**, 21.

Baird, I. M. and Wilson, G. M. (1959), "The Pathogenesis of Anaemia after Partial Gastrectomy. II. Iron Absorption after Partial Gastrectomy," *Quart. J. Med.*, N.S., **28**, 35.

Baldwin, J. N. and Dalessio, D. J. (1961), "Folic Acid Therapy and Spinal-cord Degeneration in Pernicious Anaemia," *New Eng. J. Med.*, **264**, 1339.

Ball, E. W. and Giles, C. (1964), "Folic Acid and Vitamin B₁₂ Levels in Pregnancy and Their Relation to Megaloblastic Anaemia," *J. Clin. Path.*, **17**, 165.

Berry, V., Booth, M. A., Chanarin, I. and Rothman, D. (1963), "Urinary Formimino-glutamic Acid Excretion in Pregnancy," *Brit. med. J.*, **2**, 1103.

Bower, D. and Swale, J. (1966), "Chemical Test for Bilirubin in Liquor Amnii. For Assessment of Prognosis in Rhesus Immunisation," *Lancet*, **1**, 1009.

Brise, H. and Hallberg, L. (1962), "Effect of Succinic Acid on Iron Absorption," *Acta med. scand.*, **171**, (Suppl. 376), 59.

Brown, E. B. and Rother, M. (1961), "Studies of the Process of Iron Absorption in Rats," *Blood*, **18**, 780.

Callender, S. (1965), "Some Aspects of Iron Metabolism," in *Disorders of the Blood*, p. 84. Edinburgh: Royal College of Physicians.

Chanarin, I., Rothman, D. and Berry, V. (1965), "Iron Deficiency and its Relation to Folic Acid Status in Pregnancy. Results of a Clinical Trial," *Brit. Med. J.*, **1**, 480.

Chanarin, I., Rothman, D. and Watson-Williams, E. J. (1963), "Normal Formiminoglutamic Acid Excretion in Megaloblastic Anaemia in Pregnancy: Studies in Histidine Metabolism in Pregnancy," *Lancet*, **1**, 1068.

Charlton, R. N., Jacobs, P., Torrance, J. D. and Rothwell, T. H. (1963), "The Role of Ferritin in Iron Absorption," *Lancet*, **2**, 762.

Cronkite, E. P. (1964), "Erythropoietic Cell Proliferation in Man," *Medicine*, **43**, 635.

Foy, H., Kondi, A., Hargreaves, A. and Lowry, J. (1952), "Response of Megaloblastic Anaemia in Africans (Kenya) to Oral Crystalline Penicillin," *Lancet*, **1**, 1221.

Giles, C. (1966), "An Account of 335 Cases of Megaloblastic Anaemia in Pregnancy and the Puerperium," *J. Clin. Path.*, **19**, 1.

Grzesiukowicz, H., Jennison, R. F. and Gowenlock, A. H. (1965), "Enzymatic Release of Folate Activity from the Red Cells in Megaloblastic Anaemia of Pregnancy," *J. Clin. Path.*, **18**, 599.

Husain, O. A. N., Rothman, D. and Ellis, L. (1963), "Folic Acid Deficiency in Pregnancy," *J. Obstet. Gynaec. Brit. Cmwlth.*, **70**, 821.

Ingram, V. M. (1963), *The Haemoglobins in Genetics and Evolution*. New York: Columbia University Press.

Jacobs, P., Bothwell, T. H. and Charlton, R. W. (1964), "Role of Hydrochloric Acid in Iron Absorption," *J. Appl. Phys.*, **19**, 187.

Josephson, B. and Furst, P. (1966), "Sulphonamides Competing with Bilirubin for Conjugation to Albumin," *Scand. J. Clin. Lab. Invest.*, **18**, 51.

Kanaev, S. V., Bruk, A. A., Kuleshov, A. V. and Shostka, G. D. (1966), "Inclusion of Fe^{59} into Erythroid Cells during Anaemia Developing as a Result of Uterine Haemorrhage," (Russian), *Meditsinskaya Radiologiya, Moskva*, **11**, 21.

Lauritzen, C. and Lehmann, W. D. (1965), "Die Bedeutung der Steroidhormone fuer Hyperbilirubinaemie und Icterus Neonatorum," *Geburtsh. u. Frauenheilk.*, **25**, 962.

Lauritzen, C. and Lehmann, W. D. (1966), "Die Bedeutung der Steroidhormone fuer die Entstehung von Hyperbilirubinaemie und Icterus Neonatorum," *Z. Kinderheilk.*, **95**, 143.

Lester Smith, E. (1965), *Vitamin B_{12}*, 3rd edition. London: Methuen.

Linman, J. W. and Bethell, F. H. (1960), *Factors Controlling Erythropoiesis*. Springfield, U.S.A: C. C. Thomas.

MacDonald, R. A. (1963), "Idiopathic Haemochromatosis," *Arch. Intern. Med.*, **112**, 184.

Menkin, V. (1955), "Factors Concerned in the Mobilization of Leukocytes in Inflammation," *Ann. N.Y. Acad. Sci.*, **59**, 956.

Mollin, D. L. (1959), "Radioactive Vitamin B_{12} in the Study of Blood Diseases," *Brit. Med. Bull.*, **15**, 8.

Parry, T. E. (1966), "Nucleotide Derangement in the Megaloblast Nucleus," *Nature*, **212**, 148.

Perillie, P. E., Kaplan, S. S. and Finch, S. C. (1967), "Significance of Changes in Serum Muramidase Activity in Megaloblastic Anaemia," *New Engl. J. Med.*, **277**, 10.

Powell, L. W. (1965), "Iron Storage in Relatives of Patients with Haemochromatosis and in Relatives of Patients with Alcoholic Cirrhosis and Haemosiderosis," *Quart. J. Med.* N.S., **34**, 427.

Rimington, C. (1959), "Biosynthesis of Haemoglobin," *Brit. Med. Bull.*, **15**, 19.

Smith, M. D. and Pannacciulli, I. M. (1959), "Absorption of Inorganic Iron from Graded Doses: its Significance in Relation to Iron Absorption Tests and the Mucosal Block Theory," *Brit. J. Haemat.*, **4**, 428.

Solomons, E., Lee, S. L., Wasserman, M. and Malkin, J. (1962), "Association of Anaemia in Pregnancy and Folic Acid Deficiency," *J. Obstet. Gynaec. Brit. Cmwlth.*, **69**, 724.

Steingold, L. (1966), *Anaemia in Pregnancy and the Puerperium*, in *Recent Advances in Obstetrics and Gynaecology*. Ed. by Stallworthy, J. and Bourne, G., p. 96, Ch. 3, 11th edition. London: Churchill.

Steingold, L., Vogel, L. and Suchet, J. (1966), "Ascorbic Acid in the Prevention and Treatment of Anaemia in Pregnancy," *Clin. Trials J.*, **3**, 459.

Turnberg, L. A. (1966), "The Absorption of Iron after Partial Gastrectomy," *Quart. J. Med.*, N.S., **35**, 107.

Vitale, J. J., Streiff, R. R. and Hellerstein, E. E. (1965), "Folate Metabolism and Iron Deficiency," *Lancet*, **2**, 393.

Waldenström, J. (1946), "The Incidence of Iron Deficiency (Sideropenia) in Some Rural and Urban Populations," *Acta Med. Scand.*, *Suppl.* 170, 252.

5. BLOOD COAGULATION AND HAEMOSTASIS

C. R. RIZZA

I. NORMAL HAEMOSTASIS

Thanks to the evolution of a complex and efficient system of haemostasis, damage to all but the largest blood vessels is rarely accompanied by serious haemorrhage in normal people. The mechanism for controlling loss of blood from the body has three main components:

1. Constriction of the injured vessel.
2. Aggregation of platelets at the breach in the vessel wall and formation of platelet plugs.
3. Blood Coagulation.

The exact relationship between these three aspects of haemostasis is not clear but there is no doubt that they are closely linked and inter-dependent.

A short time after a small arteriole or capillary is cut the vessel constricts and platelets are seen to adhere to the injured site to form a plug. In small vessels vaso-constriction and the formation of the platelet plug may be sufficient to staunch the flow of blood, but when larger vessels are breached fibrin formation is also necessary if haemostasis is to be maintained.

The phase of vaso-constriction with platelet adhesion and aggregation may be considered as the phase of primary haemostasis and the phase of fibrin formation and consolidation of the platelet plug the phase of secondary haemostasis. Failure of the primary haemostatic process results in bleeding continuing from the time of the injury, as in thrombocytopenia, whereas failure of the secondary phase is characterized by bleeding which stops initially but recurs some hours later. This is the type of bleeding seen in haemophilia and the related bleeding disorders.

The three components of the haemostatic mechanism will now be considered in detail starting with the vascular component then dealing with platelet function and finally with the coagulation mechanism.

A. The Vascular Function in Haemostasis

As already mentioned the blood vessels play an important part in haemostasis by undergoing constriction in response to injury. Constriction may be complete in which case blood flow through the injured vessels ceases, or may be incomplete, in which case the blood flow tends to be diverted away from the injured vessel and through normal channels. The reaction of vessels to injury depends to some extent on the type and size of vessel involved.

Arterioles have smooth muscle and elastic tissues in their walls and respond to injury by powerful spasm which may last for an hour or more. Capillary vessels also display constriction when injured and although their walls do not contain smooth muscle it is possible that their endothelium possesses contractile elements which are responsible for capillary contraction. The stimulus for vaso-constriction is not yet known but there seem to be several possible mechanisms: a direct response to injury of the vessel wall; the release of vaso-constricting substances from platelets at the site of injury; the appearance of vaso-active kinins in the blood following the initiation of clotting.

B. Platelet Function in Haemostasis

Hayem (1878) studied the occlusive mass formed at the site of incision in a dog's vein and found that it was composed chiefly of "haematoblasts" (platelets). Since then, observations on the mesentery of various animals and the cheek pouch of the hamster have shown that haemostasis in cut arterioles and venules is brought about by the adhesion of platelets to the damaged tissue followed by aggregation of platelets to one another with the build up of a platelet plug. The mechanism of platelet adhesion and aggregation is still not fully understood but recent *in vitro* studies of these phenomena have thrown much light on the problem. The discovery that adenosine diphosphate (A.D.P.) will cause platelets in platelet rich plasma to adhere to one another as well as to glass has aroused great interest. The concentration of A.D.P. required to produce visible clumping is of the order of 0·04 micrograms/ml. although concentrations as low as 0·007 micrograms/ml. will produce microscopical clumping. This reaction of the platelets to A.D.P. requires calcium ions as well as a plasma factor which is so far unidentified.

Other physiologically occurring substances which are known to cause platelet aggregation include adrenaline, noradrenaline, 5-hydroxytryptamine (5 H.T.) and thrombin. Connective tissue suspensions have also been shown to cause platelet clumping. The implications of these *in vitro* studies are obvious and it is possible that the adhesion of platelets and the formation of aggregates at the site of injury in a vessel may be promoted by release of A.D.P. from damaged endothelial cells. Alternatively, A.D.P. may come from the platelets themselves following their contact with connective tissue which has the ability to liberate platelet A.D.P.

The haemostatic plug when first formed is friable especially if the injury is slight and in experimental animal preparations may be seen to break away from the vessel wall, break up and be carried away in the blood stream. For the plug to become more durable strands of reinforcing fibrin must be laid down and this requires the formation of thrombin by the coagulation process with platelets playing yet another important part. The role of platelets in blood coagulation is complex and their importance is evident from the fact that the clotting times of recalcified plasma is prolonged if the plasma is depleted of platelets.

Probably the most important platelet factor involved in the coagulation process is platelet factor 3. This is thought to be a lipo-protein complex contained either within the platelet granules or on the platelet membrane, and probably acts in the clotting process as a catalyst by adsorbing the reacting clotting factors onto the surface of its micelles.

Another activity of platelets which is easily demonstrated *in vitro* is concerned with the retraction or shortening of the threads of fibrin in a clot. Platelets contain a contractile protein like myosin and it is thought that the platelets adhere to fibrin strands and by drawing the strands together reduce the size of the clots and squeeze out red cells and serum. The phenomenon of clot retraction is extremely difficult to study *in vivo* and it is not known how and to what extent it is important in haemostasis.

Besides these functions platelets are thought to be involved in some way in the maintenance of the integrity of the capillary walls since severe thrombocytopenia is usually associated with purpura.

C. Blood Coagulation

One of the most striking properties of normal blood is its ability to remain fluid while circulating in the blood vessels and yet to clot firmly within 10 minutes of coming into contact with a foreign surface. The solidification of the blood is due to the transformation of the soluble protein fibrinogen into a web of insoluble fibrin in which are enmeshed red cells, white cells and platelets.

Fibrinogen is a plasma protein synthesized in the liver and has a molecular weight in the region of 340,000. It is present in plasma in a concentration of 200–400 mg./100 ml. and the level is known to rise during pregnancy. Some of the characteristic properties of fibrinogen along with those of other clotting factors are shown in Tables 1 and 2. The conversion of fibrinogen to fibrin is brought about by the proteolytic enzyme thrombin which splits negatively charged peptides (fibrinopeptides) from the end of the fibrinogen molecules. With the loss of these negatively charged peptides the remaining portions of the fibrinogen

molecules (fibrin-monomer) tend to align themselves side-to-side and end-to-end and polymerize to form strands of fibrin. The fibrin strands so formed are made more durable by the action of a plasma factor, the fibrin stabilizing factor and in the process are rendered insoluble in solvents such as urea or monochloroacetic acid.

Thrombin is not present in the blood in the active form but circulates as an inactive precursor called prothrombin. Prothrombin is synthesized in the liver under the influence of Vitamin K and is present in the plasma in a concentration of 20–30 mg./100 ml. The reactions involved in the conversion of prothrombin to thrombin have been extensively studied during the past 50 years and have been the cause of much confusion in the field of blood coagulation. According to Morawitz's hypothesis, called by later workers The Classical Theory, prothrombin is converted to thrombin by the thrombokinase (tissue thromboplastin) in the presence of calcium ions and the thrombin then converts fibrinogen to fibrin (Fig. 1).

$$\text{Prothrombin} \xrightarrow[\text{Ca}^{++}]{\text{Thrombokinase}} \text{Thrombin}$$

$$\text{Fibrinogen} \xrightarrow{\text{Thrombin}} \text{Fibrin}$$

Fig. 1. The classical theory of blood coagulation.

In 1935 Armand J. Quick introduced his "prothrombin time" test. This test, which was based on the classical theory of blood clotting, was performed by adding tissue thromboplastin (acetone dried rabbit brain) to oxalated plasma and then adding calcium chloride to the mixture and noting the clotting time. Quick argued that since the fibrinogen, thromboplastin and calcium were in excess the clotting time would be related to the prothrombin concentration in the mixture. This test became widely used in

TABLE 1

SOME CHARACTERISTIC PROPERTIES OF BLOOD CLOTTING FACTORS

Factor	Common Synonyms	Site of Production	In vivo $\frac{1}{2}$–life	Normal level in blood	Level required for haemostasis
I*	Fibrinogen	Liver	3–6 days	200–400 mg./100 ml.	50–100 mg./100 ml.
II	Prothrombin	Liver	2–3 days	20 mg./100 ml.	40% of normal
III	Tissue thromboplastin				
IV	Ionized Calcium				
V	Proaccelerin, labile factor	Liver	15–24 hours	100% of normal	10–15% of normal
VII	Proconvertin	Liver	4–6 hours	100% of normal	5–10% of normal
VIII	Antihaemophilic factor (AHF) Antihaemophilic globulin (AHG)	? throughout R.E.S.	12–18 hours	100% of normal	25–30% of normal
IX	Christmas Factor	Liver	18–30 hours	100% of normal	20–25% of normal
X	Stuart Factor	Liver	48–60 hours	100% of normal	15–20% of normal
XI	Plasma thromboplastin antecedent (PTA)	?	60 hours	100% of normal	?
XII	Hageman Factor	?	50–70 hours	100% of normal	
XIII	Fibrin Stabilizing Factor	?	? 3 days	100% of normal	Less than 10% of normal

*Because of the increasing confusion which developed during the 1950s with regard to terminology of blood clotting factors, an International Committee was set up to deal with nomenclature. This Committee laid down the Roman Numeral System of naming coagulation factors which is now generally accepted.

TABLE 2

SOME PHYSICO-CHEMICAL CHARACTERISTICS OF BLOOD CLOTTING FACTORS

Factor	Heat Resistance	Adsorption by $Al(OH)_3$ and $BaSO_4$	Precipitated by $(NH_4)_2SO_4$ (% saturation)	Present in Cohn's Fraction	Electrophoresis
I	Destroyed at 47°C	Not adsorbed	25	I	Fibrinogen
II	Stable at 56°C	Adsorbed	50	III	α_2 globulin
V	Destroyed at 50°C	Not adsorbed	50	III	Albumin
VII	Destroyed at 56°C	Adsorbed	50	III	β globulin
VIII	Partly destroyed at 56°C	Not adsorbed	33	I	β_2 globulin
IX	Destroyed at 56°C	Adsorbed	50	III and IV	β globulin
X	Destroyed at 56°C	Adsorbed	50	III	Albumin
XI	Destroyed at 56°C	Not adsorbed	33	III and IV	Between β and α globulins
XII	Destroyed at 60°C	Not adsorbed	50	III and IV	Between β and α globulins
XIII	Stable at 58°C for 5 mins.	Not adsorbed	33	I	A globulin closely associated with fibrinogen

clinical practice for the study of bleeding in liver disease and for the control of anticoagulant therapy and as a consequence of this widespread use it soon became apparent that other unknown factors were involved in the conversion of prothrombin to thrombin. Quick himself showed that in addition to thromboplastin and calcium a labile plasma factor was required and in 1947 Owren described a young woman with a bleeding disorder and a prolongation of the prothrombin time who had a deficiency of this labile factor. Owren called the factor, Factor V, since it was the fifth factor then known to be concerned in blood coagulation, the others being fibrinogen, prothrombin, tissue thromboplastin and calcium. Subsequently it was found that two more factors were required for the conversion of prothrombin to thrombin in the presence of tissue extracts and these were designated Factors VII and X. The classical theory may now be re-written in a modified form as in Fig. 2. The preoccupation during the

conclusively that normal blood contains all the factors necessary for the generation of a powerful prothrombin converting substance. At that time the factors thought to be essential for the generation of this activity were Factor V, Factor VIII, Factor IX and Calcium, but again, as with the "prothrombin" time test, the widespread use of the thromboplastin generation test in the study of bleeding disorders soon showed the existence of other factors which had previously not been recognized. The factors now thought to take part in prothrombin activation by the intrinsic pathway are shown in Fig. 3. Factors V and X are required for activation of prothrombin by both the extrinsic and intrinsic system.

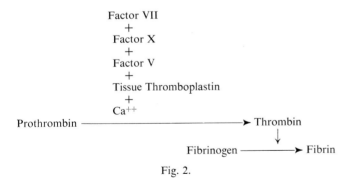

Fig. 2.

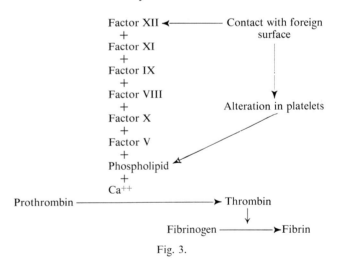

Fig. 3.

earlier part of this century with this extrinsic or tissue system of prothrombin activation drew attention away from the possible existence of a powerful intrinsic or plasma system of prothrombin activation, not requiring tissue extracts for its action. In 1953, Biggs and Douglas devised the thromboplastin generation test and showed

It is unlikely that more than two of these factors react together at any one time and much work has been undertaken to determine the kinetics and sequence of clotting factor reactions in both the intrinsic and extrinsic systems of blood coagulation. A major step in elucidating the sequence of reactions was made by Macfarlane and his colleagues in their study of the venom of the Russell Viper. They showed that the coagulant activity of the venom is due to enzymatic splitting of the Factor X molecule in plasma to form a derivative of lower molecular weight which has esterase activity. This derivative then reacts with Factor V and phospholipid in the presence of calcium ions to form an activator of prothrombin. In the reaction phospholipid probably acts by providing a surface on to which the reacting factors are adsorbed and kept in close proximity to one another. Subsequent work has shown that during coagulation, whether by the intrinsic or extrinsic pathways, there appears in the blood a substance, probably an enzyme, which like Russell's Viper Venom, can split and activate the Factor X molecule. In addition there is evidence now to suggest that most of the blood clotting factors exist in an inactive form in the blood but like Factor X and prothrombin are capable of being activated to yield derivatives which then activate the next factor involved in the clotting reaction. The sequence of events is now thought to be as follows:

Factor XII is activated on coming into contact with a foreign surface; this activation is thought to be associated with a change in its molecular configuration. Activated Factor XII then activates Factor XI which in turn activates Factor IX which activates Factor VIII. Activated Factor VIII is probably the physiological activator of Factor X. The next step, the activation of Factor V by activated X is not so well defined and the evidence for this is not so convincing as that for activation of the other coagulation factors. But it is known that activated Factor X in the presence of Factor V and phospholipid will convert prothrombin to thrombin. The sequence of events outlined above has been depicted by Macfarlane as a cascade of proenzyme-enzyme transformations (Fig. 4) each

enzyme activating the next until thrombin is formed. Calcium and phospholipid are required at various stages of the process. In addition, positive and negative feedback mechanisms probably affect the system. For example, thrombin in trace amounts is known to activate Factor VIII and Factor V but at high concentrations it destroys Factor VIII and Factor V and so may be a means of "switching off" the clotting reaction.

The life span of these very active enzymes is short and they are probably inactivated by a system of natural inhibitors in the blood. In this way the clotting reactions are localized to the site of injury and not permitted to spread into the general circulation with disastrous consequences.

D. Changes in the blood coagulation mechanism during pregnancy and in the neonatal period

Certain important changes take place in the blood coagulation mechanism during pregnancy and the puerperium. The most striking changes involve fibrinogen and Factor VIII both of which show a progressive rise from about the 3rd or 4th month of pregnancy, until term when the fibrinogen level may be twice the normal level and Factor VIII three times the normal level. In addition the stress and exertion of labour may bring about a further increase in the Factor VIII level, which often persists for 7–10 days after delivery. Significant increase in Factors V, VII, IX and X have also been reported, from the 3rd month of pregnancy onwards.

The mechanism of the increase of these blood coagulation factors is not known but in view of the raised level of some of these factors in women taking oral contraceptive preparations the rise is probably related to the hormonal changes in pregnancy. The raised level of blood clotting factors in association with the reduced fibrinolytic activity in the blood late in pregnancy are thought by some to reflect a hypercoagulable state which may predispose to the thrombo-embolic complications of the puerperium. There is no doubt that the relationship between the *in vitro* tests of blood coagulation and *in vivo* coagulation and thrombosis is not simple and although it would seem logical to think that the raised levels of clotting factors predispose to intravascular clotting, much work still has to be done before this simple relationship can be accepted.

In contradistinction to the raised level of coagulation factors found in the mother's blood at term, the blood of the normal newborn infant is usually deficient in Factors II, VII, IX and X. During the first two to three days of life the levels of these factors fall still lower and thereafter there is a gradual rise until the normal adult level is reached within one to two weeks. The deficiency of these Vitamin K dependent clotting factors is in large part due to the immaturity of the newborn child's liver and to poor stores of Vitamin K in the body and if severe enough may result in spontaneous bleeding from the gastro-intestinal tract and umbilical stump. The bleeding state can be eliminated by giving Vitamin K_1 prophylactically to the mother during the week before her confinement if the circumstances warrant it; for example, in prematurity, foetal distress or where a difficult delivery is anticipated. Alternatively,

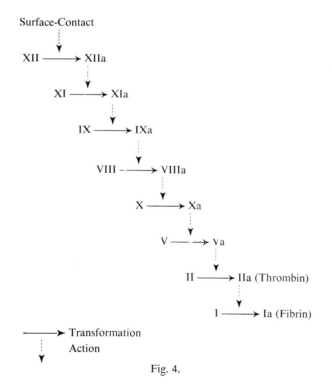

Surface-Contact

XII ⟶ XIIa

XI ⟶ XIa

IX ⟶ IXa

VIII --⟶ VIIIa

X ⟶ Xa

V --⟶ Va

II ⟶ IIa (Thrombin)

I ⟶ Ia (Fibrin)

⟶ Transformation

Action

Fig. 4.

Vitamin K_1 may be given to the child in a dose of 1–2 mg. by intra-muscular injection on the first day of life. Should the full blown haemorrhagic disease appear the child should then be given 1–2 mg. intra-muscularly daily until the laboratory tests have returned to normal. In some cases transfusions of blood or plasma may be required to replace haemoglobin and blood coagulation factors.

Factor VIII, unlike the Vitamin K dependent clotting factors is present in normal amounts in the newborn child's blood and bears a closer relationship to the mother's factor VIII level before pregnancy than to the elevated level at term. It therefore seems that very little factor VIII crosses the placenta from the mother to the child and this is supported by the finding that the cord blood of boys born with haemophilia has very little or no factor VIII activity.

II. DEFECTS OF HAEMOSTASIS

A failure of haemostasis will come if one or more of the three components of haemostasis are defective. Coagulation and platelet defects account for the majority of severe haemorrhagic disorders, vascular defects being an extremely uncommon cause of dangerous bleeding.

The bleeding manifestations seen in the coagulation disorders are usually different from those seen in the platelet disorders (Table 3). Severe coagulation disorders

A. Defects of Blood Vessels and Connective Tissue

Bleeding disorders due to vascular abnormality are ill-defined and difficult to classify. Capillary function is difficult to assess and the classical tests, such as the bleeding time and the tourniquet test, which are used to study this aspect of the haemostatic mechanism are sensitive also to qualitative and quantitative changes in platelets. Von Willebrand's disease has for a long time been thought to be due to a vascular defect because of the findings of a prolonged bleeding time, increased capillary fragility and reports of abnormal nail-bed capillaries, but recent work suggests that the prime defect may not be in the vessels. The bleeding disorder associated with scurvy is thought to be due to a defect of cement substance in the capillary wall but there is now evidence suggesting that platelet thromboplastin function as well as platelet adhesiveness are defective in the condition.

Hereditary Telangiectasia

This is a familial condition characterized by small vascular lesions in the skin and mucous membranes. The characteristic lesion consists of dilated capillaries, arterioles and veins, lined by a single layer of endothelial cells and lacking muscular or elastic coats. Bleeding takes place from the areas of vascular abnormality and the bleeding time in areas of skin not affected is normal. Epistaxis, gastro-

TABLE 3

MAIN CLINICAL FEATURES DISTINGUISHING COAGULATION DEFECTS FROM CAPILLARY AND PLATELET DEFECTS

Clinical Features	Coagulation Defects	Platelet and Capillary Defects
Bleeding from superficial cuts	Usually not excessive	Often profuse
Spontaneous bruises and haematomata	Common, involving deep tissues	Small and usually superficial
Haemarthroses	Common	Rare
Time of onset of bleeding	Usually delayed several hours after injury or operation	Usually immediate
Main bleeding symptom	Bleeding into joints and muscles and following injury	Petechial haemorrhages, ecchymoses epistaxis, menorrhagia and gastro-intestinal bleeding
Effect of pressure on the lesion	Bleeding not controlled	Bleeding usually controlled

are characterized by bleeding into deep tissues such as joints or muscles with consequent crippling and deformity. These haemorrhages may be spontaneous or may follow trauma. Cutaneous bruises following injury are common but petechial haemorrhages are rare. Haematuria and bleeding from the gastro-intestinal tract may also occur. Small cuts and abrasions do not bleed unduly but larger wounds and operation sites after an initial period of haemostasis may bleed persistently and uncontrollably.

Platelet deficiencies are characterized by bleeding from superficial cuts and scratches and bleeding from the mucous membranes of nose and gastro-intestinal tract and uterus. Ecchymoses and petechial haemorrhages in the skin are common. Haemorrhages in muscles are rare and haemarthroses practically never occur.

intestinal bleeding and haemoptysis are the chief haemorrhagic manifestations. In *Ehlers-Danlos syndrome*, a rare hereditary disorder of connective tissue, bleeding may occur from gums, nose or skin. The bleeding is thought to be due to a connective tissue defect in the vessel walls as well as in the supporting tissues about the vessels. The bleeding in *Henoch-Schönlein purpura* is probably due to increased vascular permeability brought about by bacterial toxins or by drugs. Despite the damage to capillaries the bleeding time is usually normal.

B. Bleeding Due to Platelet Deficiencies

Bleeding may come about if the blood platelets are reduced in numbers or defective in function. The type of bleeding, whether due to a quantitative or to a qualitative platelet deficiency is similar, with purpura, ecchymoses and bleeding from mucous membranes being the commonest manifestations. The bleeding is due principally to a defect of primary haemostasis and the failure of platelets to contribute to the coagulation mechanism may be relatively unimportant. Bleeding from wounds starts immediately after the injury and is not delayed as in the coagulation disorders. If haemostasis can be achieved in a wound in a thrombocytopenic patient, as can often be done by gentle local pressure or packing, the wound usually remains dry.

(i) Thrombocytopenia

This is the commonest cause of abnormal bleeding and is with rare exceptions an acquired disorder. There is a rough correlation between the degree of platelet deficiency and bleeding, counts of 60,000 platelets per cu. mm. or less being associated with excessive bleeding.

Thrombocytopenia may be classified broadly into:
1. Primary (idiopathic) thrombocytopenia and
2. Secondary thrombocytopenia.

(a) Primary Idiopathic thrombocytopenic purpura. Idiopathic thrombocytopenia is one of the commonest forms of thrombocytopenia and its aetiology as the name implies is still obscure. There is no doubt the diagnosis embraces more than one entity and that there are several underlying causes including infection and exposure to drugs. A careful search should always be made for such causes before a diagnosis of idiopathic thrombocytopenia is accepted.

The acute form of ITP occurs mainly in children and usually runs a short course from weeks to a few months. The platelet count may be as low as 10–20,000/cu. mm. and the bleeding time is prolonged. If a spontaneous remission does not occur treatment consists of blood and platelet transfusions when required and adrenocortical steroids. If high doses of steroids are required to control serious bleeding then splenectomy becomes the treatment of choice.

(b) Secondary thrombocytopenic purpura. This may be due to a failure of the bone marrow to produce platelets, the thrombocytopenia being only one aspect of a condition in which all of the cellular elements of the marrow are usually involved. Bone marrow failure may be due to drugs or ionizing radiations. Myelofibrosis or infiltration of the marrow by leukaemia, myeloma or carcinoma cells is often associated with thrombocytopenia. The treatment of bleeding in secondary thrombocytopenia consists of giving transfusions of fresh blood and platelet rich plasma and at the same time treating, wherever possible, the underlying cause of the marrow failure.

(ii) Qualitative Platelet Deficiencies

Hereditary Thrombasthenia (Glanzmann's Disease). This is a hereditary bleeding disorder affecting either sex and transmitted as an autosomal dominant disorder. The platelets are normal in number but abnormal in function, and sometimes bizarre in shape. The bleeding time is prolonged and the tourniquet test positive. The platelets fail to adhere to glass and do not form aggregates in the presence of A.D.P. In addition they do not release their platelet factor 3, although it is present in normal amounts. Clot retraction is grossly abnormal. Bleeding may be severe with epistaxis, excessive bruising and prolonged bleeding from cuts being common. Defective platelet function is occasionally found in uraemia, where the platelet factor 3 is either deficient or not "available" for the coagulation reaction.

C. BLOOD COAGULATION DEFECTS

Defects in the blood coagulation process are usually due to the deficiency of one of the essential clotting factors, although very occasionally coagulation may be defective as the result of some inhibitory substance interfering with the reactions between clotting factors. Of the ten clotting factors known to be present in the blood only deficiency of Factor XII (Hageman factor), is not associated with a haemorrhagic disorder. Deficiencies of all the other nine factors have been described either in a congenital or an acquired form. In the congenital bleeding states usually only one coagulation factor is deficient, whereas in the acquired bleeding disorders several clotting factors may be lacking. The treatment of the various coagulation disorders rests on the general principle of raising the blood concentration of the missing clotting factor to a level which will ensure haemostasis. This may be achieved by the intravenous transfusion of materials rich in the appropriate coagulation factor (Table 6). The levels of the different clotting factors required for haemostasis are shown in Table 1.

(i) Congenital Deficiencies of Coagulation Factors

(a) Factor VIII Deficiency (Haemophilia). Classical haemophilia is a sex linked recessive bleeding disorder due to a congenital deficiency of Factor VIII. Males are primarily affected although there are few reports of affected females. It is the most important congenital bleeding disorder, accounting for more than 90 per cent of hereditary bleeding. Deficiency of Factor VIII may be partial or complete and there is good correlation between the level of Factor VIII in the blood and the severity of the bleeding manifestations (Table 4).

TABLE 4

RELATIONSHIP OF BLOOD FACTOR VIII LEVELS TO HAEMORRHAGIC MANIFESTATIONS

Factor VIII level (% average normal)	Haemorrhagic Manifestations
50–100	None
25–50	Excessive bleeding occasionally after serious injury or major surgery
5–25	Excessive bleeding after minor injury and surgery, e.g. dental extractions, tonsillectomy.
1–5	Severe bleeding after minor injury and surgery. Occasional haemarthrosis and "spontaneous" bleeding.
0	Severe haemophilia with "spontaneous" bleeding into joints and muscles and crippling

Because of the absence of Factor VIII there is a failure of formation of the intrinsic activator of prothrombin with delayed and impaired conversion of prothrombin to thrombin and delayed fibrin formation. In the severely affected patient, the disorder manifests itself by seemingly spontaneous haemorrhages into joints, muscles and skin. Repeated bleeding into joints and muscles leads to damage of these tissues with subsequent crippling.

which he is suffering (Table 5). The various therapeutic materials available and the dosages required for different lesions are shown in Table 5. Because of the probable antigenic nature of the animal AHG preparations their use has up until now been reserved for life saving surgery. Local forms of treatment such as the application of pressure to the bleeding site have little to recommend them, and indeed if the pressure is too great and too prolonged it

TABLE 5

THE USE OF VARIOUS THERAPEUTIC MATERIALS IN THE TREATMENT OF HAEMOPHILIA

Lesion	Plasma Factor VIII level to be aimed at in patient (% average normal)	Therapeutic Material	Dose * units/Kg. body wt.
Minor spontaneous bleeding	15–25	Fresh or fresh frozen plasma. Cryoprecipitated Fibrinogen fraction of human plasma	15–20 u/kg.
Dangerous haematomata Multiple Dental Extractions	20–40	Human A.H.G. Cryoprecipitated Fibrinogen fraction of human plasma	20–30 u/kg.
Major Surgery Serious accidents	80–120	Animal A.H.G. Cryoprecipitated Fibrinogen fraction of human plasma	50–100 u/kg.

* A unit of Factor VIII activity is the average amount present in 1 ml. of fresh normal human plasma.

Treatment consists of replacing the missing factor by giving intravenous transfusions of fresh or fresh frozen plasma or potent concentrates of AHG (anti-haemophilic globulin) prepared from human or animal blood. The level of Factor VIII in the patient's blood required for haemostasis will depend on the particular lesion from

may do more harm than good by bringing about sloughing of the tissues.

(b) Factor IX Deficiency (Christmas Disease)

This condition is clinically indistinguishable from haemophilia and like haemophilia is a sex linked recessive congenital bleeding disorder. Treatment consists of giving transfusions of plasma or preferably transfusions of protein concentrates rich in Factor IX (Table 6).

(c) Fibrinogen (Factor I) Deficiency

This is an extremely rare condition and about 30 cases have been described. Because of the absence of fibrinogen the blood is completely incoagulable even on the addition of a strong solution of thrombin. Either sex may be affected and several of the cases reported have been offspring of consanguineous marriages. The bleeding manifestations may be severe and include bleeding from the umbilicus at birth, haemarthroses, bleeding from lacerations and venepunctures and subcutaneous haemorrhages. The bleeding is usually less severe than that found in severe haemophilia and this is surprising in view of the complete absence of fibrinogen from the blood. It is also interesting to note that females suffering from the condition rarely are troubled with menorrhagia. The minimum level of fibrinogen required for haemostasis is thought to be in the region of 50–100 mg./100 ml. and this level can be achieved by transfusions of fresh or stored plasma or concentrated fibrinogen.

TABLE 6

SOURCES OF COAGULATION FACTORS USED FOR THE TREATMENT OF COAGULATION DISORDERS

Factor Deficient	Therapeutic Materials
I	Fresh frozen plasma Fibrinogen concentrate
II	Fresh frozen plasma Plasma concentrates
V	Fresh frozen plasma
VII	Fresh frozen plasma Plasma concentrates
VIII	Fresh frozen plasma Cryoprecipitated fibrinogen fraction of human plasma AHG Concentrates from human plasma AHG Concentrates from animal plasma
IX	Fresh frozen plasma Plasma concentrates
X	Fresh frozen plasma Plasma concentrates
XI	Fresh frozen plasma
XII	Fresh frozen plasma
XIII	Fresh frozen plasma

(d) Deficiencies of Factors II, V, VII and X

Congenital isolated deficiencies of these factors have been described but are very rare. Either sex may be affected and the inheritance seems to be through autosomal recessive genes. Deficiencies of these factors are usually clinically mild and bleeding is rarely as severe as in haemophilia.

Treatment consists of replacement therapy. Menorrhagia may be troublesome in affected females and can often be controlled by one of the oral contraceptive preparations.

(e) Factor XI (P.T.A.) Deficiency

This condition is familial, affects the sexes equally and is thought to be due to an autosomal recessive gene. The majority of patients so far described are of Jewish extraction. Bleeding is not very severe and usually follows surgery or serious injury. Epistaxis and haematuria have occurred and menorrhagia is common. Transfusions of fresh frozen plasma are usually sufficient to maintain haemostasis following surgery.

(f) Factor XII (Hageman Factor) Deficiency

In spite of the fact that their blood may take 1–2 hours to clot in a glass tube, patients with Factor XII deficiency rarely bleed excessively and therefore do not present a clinical problem. From the academic point of view they are of great interest and importance and much work is being done to try to find out why these patients do not bleed.

(g) Factor XIII (Fibrin Stabilizing Factor) Deficiency

In this condition both the blood fibrinogen level and its conversion to fibrin are normal but because of the absence of a factor necessary for fibrin stabilization, the fibrin clots formed are weak and easily broken down. As a consequence there is a tendency for severe bleeding to occur following injury together with delayed healing and abnormal scar formation. Diagnosis is made by testing the solubility of the patient's plasma clots in a solution of 30 per cent urea or 1 per cent monochloroacetic acid. Treatment with fresh frozen plasma usually proves effective in controlling bleeding.

(h) Combined Congenital Coagulation Deficiencies

Congenital combined deficiencies of Factors V and VIII and IX and Factors VII and IX have been described but are rare. The bleeding manifestations are on the whole mild and are usually controlled by transfusion of fresh frozen plasma.

(i) Von Willebrand's Disease

Von Willebrand's disease as originally described by von Willebrand in the Aaland Islanders was defined as a bleeding tendency affecting either sex, transmitted as an autosomal dominant and characterized by a long bleeding time, normal clotting time and normal platelet count. More recently it has been shown that the more severely affected patients have low levels of Factor VIII in their blood and that there is rough correlation between the degree of Factor VIII deficiency and the severity of bleeding. There is also evidence to suggest that the platelets in von Willebrand's disease are abnormal, showing reduced clumping in the presence of A.D.P. and reduced adhesion to glass. How these platelet abnormalities affect the haemostatic defect is not yet clear. There is at present great interest being shown in von Willebrand's disease for several reasons:

1. The Factor VIII deficiency is passed on by an autosomal gene whereas the Factor VIII deficiency in haemophiliacs is a sex-linked recessive characteristic.

2. Since the bleeding time in haemophilia is normal there must be some other defect in von Willebrand's disease to account for the long bleeding time in the latter condition.

3. When a patient with von Willebrand's disease is transfused with normal plasma or serum there may be a progressive rise in Factor VIII activity in the patient's blood over the course of 24–48 hours. The level attained is usually higher than one would expect on the basis of the amount of Factor VIII transfused.

4. But more interesting still when a patient with von Willebrand's disease is transfused with plasma from a severely affected haemophiliac the recipient shows a rise of Factor VIII activity in his blood after several hours similar to that seen after transfusion of normal plasma. This rise of Factor VIII is accompanied by a variable correction of both the bleeding time and the abnormal platelet adhesiveness. There has been a good deal of speculation about the possible explanation of these findings and the following hypothesis seems at present to be the most acceptable:

In von Willebrand's disease there is a deficiency of some substance necessary for the synthesis of Factor VIII. This substance is present in normal blood and also in the blood of haemophiliacs who, for some reason, are unable to make use of it for Factor VIII synthesis. In addition normal plasma contains a factor necessary for normal platelet adhesiveness. This latter factor, which is not Factor VIII, is lacking in von Willebrand's disease and may be identical with the factor necessary for Factor VIII synthesis.

Diagnosis of the severely affected patient is not difficult since there is usually a clear history of bleeding after injury, a prolonged bleeding time and a deficiency of Factor VIII. Diagnosis is more difficult in the mildly affected cases in whom the bleeding time may be near normal.

Clinically the condition is characterized by easy bruising, bleeding from superficial cuts and in particular bleeding from mucous membranes. Epistaxis and gastro-intestinal bleeding may be very difficult to control and in the female, menorrhagia may be severe. Post-partum bleeding is sometimes a problem but may be minimized in some cases by the rise of Factor VIII which is known to take place during pregnancy. In general, treatment of bleeding consists of giving transfusions of fresh frozen plasma or concentrates rich in Factor VIII together with packing of the bleeding site if it is accessible. Menorrhagia may be controlled by one of the oral contraceptive preparations. Curettage of the uterus to control bleeding is not recommended since this rarely helps and may make the bleeding worse.

(ii) Acquired Deficiencies of Coagulation Factors

(a) Factors II, VII, IX and X

The most common cause of acquired coagulation defects is hepatic dysfunction as a consequence either of liver cell damage (e.g. cirrhosis) or of non-availability to the liver of Vitamin K. Fibrinogen, Factors II, VII, IX, X and possibly Factor V are produced in the liver and except for fibrinogen and Factor V, all require Vitamin K for their synthesis. In hepatocellular disease, although Vitamin K may be present in normal amounts there is impaired synthesis of the above clotting factors. The combined deficiencies result in a bleeding disorder which may be severe and may be aggravated by concomitant hypersplenism and thrombocytopaenia. Treatment of the bleeding consists of replacing the missing factors by giving transfusions of fresh frozen plasma or concentrates rich in Factors II, VII, IX and X.

Vitamin K deficiency may come about in several ways: there may be failure of Vitamin K production by the intestinal bacteria, as in haemorrhagic disease of the new born, or when broad spectrum antibiotics are used to sterilize the gut; there may be failure of absorption of Vitamin K from the gut as in steatorrhea and obstructive jaundice. Finally, Vitamin K may be absorbed but its action in the liver inhibited by the use of one of the coumarin type anticoagulant drugs. Bleeding due to Vitamin K deficiency is usually controlled by the administration of Vitamin K.

(b) Defibrination Syndrome

The term "defibrination syndrome" is used for an acquired bleeding disorder usually acute in onset and often clinically severe in which there is depletion of various clotting factors together with thrombocytopenia. The most striking laboratory abnormality is complete incoagulability of the blood even on the addition of strong thrombin solutions. Hence the use of the word "defibrination". During the last 10–15 years the mechanism of the syndrome has been intensively investigated and although the circumstances are complex and not completely understood there are thought to be at least two important mechanisms acting in the production of the syndrome:

1. Intra-vascular clotting is thought to be triggered by the release into the circulation of tissue or tissue juice with consequent generation of thromboplastin in the circulating blood. This converts prothrombin to thrombin which then converts fibrinogen to fibrin as well as attacking Factors V and VIII which are known to be susceptible to thrombin's proteolytic action. The consequences of this chain of reactions are doubly dangerous since the patient not only develops a haemostatic defect but at the same time is forming microemboli which may lodge in the small vessels of liver, kidney and brain.

2. Activation of fibrinolysis (proteolysis) may lead to destruction of certain blood clotting factors. Although the chief substrate for the fibrinolytic enzyme is fibrin the enzyme may attack fibrinogen, Factor VIII and Factor V. The resulting haemostatic defect is further complicated by the fact that certain breakdown products of fibrinogen are potent anticoagulants acting as anti-thrombins or as inhibitors of fibrin polymerization. It is not known for certain how activation of fibrinolysis comes about but it may be caused by tissue entering the circulation or as a response to intra-vascular coagulation.

There are several well recognized clinical situations in which the defibrination syndrome may be seen. In obstetrical and gynaecological practice defibrination has been described in amniotic fluid embolism, septic abortion and hydatidiform mole as well as in the classical situation of premature separation of the placenta. In such cases a process of "auto-extraction" is thought to take place whereby uterine contents rich in clot promoting substances reach the maternal circulation and cause generalized clotting.

In the field of surgery, operations on the lungs, prostate and pancreas may be associated with the defibrination syndrome. Here it is thought that handling of the tissue may squeeze coagulant tissue juices into the circulation and bring about intravascular coagulation. Defibrination may also be seen following mismatched blood transfusion, as a component of the generalized Schwartzman reaction and following the use of the extra-corporeal pump. The haemorrhagic manifestations are usually sudden in onset with generalized bruising and bleeding from venepuncture sites and from surgical wounds. The detailed management which is beyond the scope of this chapter consists of replacing the depleted clotting factors by transfusions of fresh frozen plasma and fibrinogen, and where judged necessary by blocking the intravascular coagulation and fibrinolytic process by giving anti-coagulants (e.g. heparin) and an anti-fibrinolytic agent (e.g. epsilon amino caproic acid or Trasylol).

(c) Circulating Anticoagulants

Occasionally a coagulation disorder may be caused by the appearance in the blood of substances which interfere with coagulation. These materials may disrupt the coagulation process by inactivating or destroying one of the clotting factors or by blocking some reaction between clotting factors. The most commonly seen and most extensively investigated anticoagulants are those which act against Factor VIII. Inhibitors of Factor VIII occasionally develop in haemophiliacs who have received numerous transfusions of Factor VIII containing material and are therefore thought to represent an immune response. Circulating inhibitors of Factor VIII may also develop in women following childbirth or in association with rheumatoid arthritis, regional ileitis, or penicillin allergy. The effect of the inhibitor is to produce a haemophilia-like state which is extremely difficult to treat since transfused Factor VIII is rapidly destroyed. Patients with disseminated lupus erythematosus occasionally develop inhibitors which affect the reaction between Factor VIII and IX or between Factors V and X. The inhibitory substance may be one of the abnormal proteins which are known to be produced in this disease.

REFERENCES

Biggs, R. and Macfarlane, R. G. (1966)., *Treatment of Haemophilia and Other Coagulation Disorders*. Oxford: Blackwell Scientific Publications.

Biggs, R. and Macfarlane, R. G. (1962), *Human Blood Coagulation and Its Disorders*. Third edition. Oxford: Blackwell Scientific Publications.

Hecht, E. R. (1965), *Lipids in Blood Clotting*. Springfield, Illinois, U.S.A.: Charles C. Thomas.

Marcus, A. J. and Zucker, M. B. (1965), *The Physiology of Blood Platelets*. New York and London: Grune and Stratton, Inc.

McKay, D. G., Hoeber Medical Division (1965), *Disseminated Intravascular Coagulation*. New York, Evanston and London: Harper and Row.

6. BLOOD VOLUME AND THE HEMODYNAMICS OF PREGNANCY

JOSEPH J. ROVINSKY

Accurate measurements of the changes in the components of the maternal intravascular space and of the alterations in maternal cardiovascular hemodynamics induced by pregnancy have been attempted by a number of investigators over the past five decades. A variety of methods of increasing sophistication, if perhaps not always of increasing accuracy, have been applied to this problem. The existing medical literature on the subject has been reviewed extensively and critically by Gregerson and Rawson (1959), Overall and Williams (1959), Guyton (1963) and Hytten and Leitch (1964). It is evident that methodologic difficulties in general, and the variability imparted to results by the technical modifications of the individual investigators, have not been completely resolved. Furthermore, the applicability of certain investigative techniques to the pregnant woman, in view of the physical alterations of pregnancy, has been questioned. It is therefore safe to assume only that to date our knowledge of the maternal hemodynamic physiologic adaptations to pregnancy remains at best an approximation.

Plasma Volume

Studies of plasma volume in pregnancy are in almost universal agreement in reporting an increase, whether the studies be serial or cross-sectional and whatever method is employed. Many reports describe changes in plasma volume in pregnancy as a percentage of the non-gravid control volume. Of these, the results presented by Rovinsky and Jaffin (1965) are characteristic: Plasma volume in normal single pregnancy was found to be 34 per cent above non-gravid control levels at 21–24 weeks of gestation, and rose to a peak increment of 49 per cent at 33–36 weeks of gestation, remaining essentially at this level to term. Hytten and Paintin (1963) pointed out that absolute rather than percentage values are more reliable for comparative purposes, and that there was no correlation between the non-pregnant plasma volume and the actual increment during pregnancy. The results reported by Rovinsky and Jaffin (1965) translate into a mean non-gravid plasma volume of 2,768 ml., and a mean peak pregnancy increment of 1,258 ml.

Peak pregnancy plasma volume increments of similar magnitude have been reported by other cross-sectional

studies; Werkö, Bucht, Lagerlöf, and Holmgren (1948) found a mean peak rise of 1,300 ml, and Berlin, Goetsch, Hyde and Parsons (1953), 1,165 ml. In serial studies on the same patients throughout pregnancy, Thomson, Hirsheimer, Gibson and Evans (1938) found a maximal

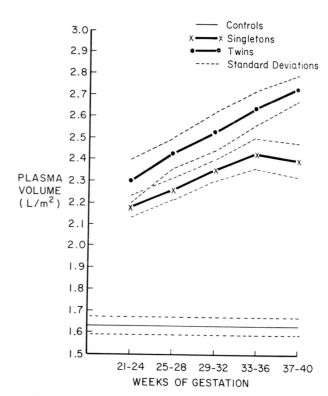

FIG. 1. Plasma Volume Changes in Pregnancy. From Rovinsky and Jaffin, *Amer. J. Obstet. Gynec.*, **93**, 1, 1965, The C. V. Mosby Company, St. Louis, Missouri.

pregnancy plasma volume increment of 1,300 ml. and more recent reports by Caton, Roby, Reid and Gibson (1949), Tysoe and Lowenstein (1950) and Hytten and Paintin (1963) provide results of the same order of magnitude for both non-gravid plasma volume, approximately 2,600 ml. and for peak plasma volume increment in pregnancy, approximately 1,250 ml. These reports further agree that, with marked individual variation, the peak plasma volume increment occurs at about 34 weeks gestation and is followed by a small decrease in plasma volume of about 200 ml. in the last few weeks pre-term. However, Werkö *et al.* (1948), Bucht (1951), Berlin *et al.* (1953), Rovinsky and Jaffin (1965) and Lund and Donovan (1967) question whether this reported decrease is real or significant, and suggest that the peak increment is maintained to term.

A number of questions remain unresolved. The majority of plasma volume studies reported have been carried out in the second half of pregnancy. Lund and Donovan (1967) found the first increase in plasma volume as early as 6 weeks of gestation, with a rapid rise to mid-pregnancy and a slower rise to term; more data are needed on the changes in early gestation.

Few reports have remarked on the significance of a parity difference. Dieckmann and Wegner (1934) noted a mean peak increase in plasma volume of 17·4 per cent in primigravidae and 31·6 per cent in multigravidae; this differential seems to be confirmed by the results of Thomson *et al.* (1938), McLennan and Thouin (1948), Lowenstein, Pick and Philpott (1950), and Cope (1958). On the basis of their critical analysis, Hytten and Leitch (1964) conclude that the peak plasma volume increment is approximately 300 ml. greater in multigravidae than in primigravidae. The reasons for this observed difference are not clear.

In the only report specifically concerned with multiple pregnancy, Rovinsky and Jaffin (1965) described a mean peak plasma volume increment in twin pregnancy of 1,963 ml., or 705 ml. more than in single pregnancy; this peak increment occurred at term. In a few isolated studies in triplet pregnancy, the same report indicates a mean peak plasma volume increment at term of 2,402 ml., or 1,144 ml. more than in single pregnancy. Additional data are necessary in this area as well.

Marked and rapid changes in plasma volume occur immediately postpartum, but these have been best studied and described in relation to total blood volume (q.v.). The major initial factor is blood loss at delivery, measured variously in normal delivery at from 400 ml. of whole blood by Gahres, Albert and Dodek (1962) to around 800 ml. by Osofsky and Williams (1964) and Bhatt (1965). It has been suggested by Osofsky and Williams (1964) that there is a differential loss of plasma in the immediate puerperium; Brown, Sampson, Wheeler, Gundelfinger and Giansiracussa (1947) and Duhring (1962) propose, on the basis of hematocrit changes, the immediate transfer postpartum of a volume of plasma from the intravascular to the extravascular compartment, over and above actual blood loss, and a return of this plasma to the intravascular compartment on the second or subsequent postpartum days. Adams (1954) reported the re-establishment of non-gravid plasma volume levels by the end of the second postpartum week, but the consensus of the other reports cited is closer to four weeks. Additional data, especially as may be obtained from continuous monitoring of plasma volume, are required to clarify this area.

Red Cell Volume

Data on changes in red cell volume in pregnancy show considerable disagreement, since some values are obtained from direct measurement of red cell volume and others derived from measurement of plasma volume and estimation of whole body hematocrit, the latter often without application of an appropriate correction factor for trapping of plasma between red cells and the physiologic alterations of blood flow in pregnancy. Davis (1962), Hytten and Paintin (1963), and Pritchard and Rowland (1964) are in agreement that a correction factor of 0·874 must be applied in pregnancy to venous blood hematocrit values to obtain true whole body hematocrit levels. In addition, marked individual variations may occur, dependent on such factors as supplemental iron intake.

Despite these methodologic difficulties, Thomson *et al.* (1938), Lowenstein *et al.* (1950), Caton, Roby, Reid, Caswell, Maletskos, Fluharty and Gibson (1951), Berlin *et al.* (1953), Verel, Burry and Hope (1956), Pritchard and Adams (1960), and Rovinsky and Jaffin (1965) reported peak mean increments in red cell volume in pregnancy near term averaging about 394 ml. and well concentrated around this value; the same investigators agree on a non-gravid red cell volume of approximately 1,400 ml. These figures represent the best estimate to date of red cell volume increment in pregnancy; the curve of increase is not well established, but is probably linear from beginning to end of gestation. Hytten and Leitch (1964) suggest that in the absence of supplemental iron intake the physiologic increment of red cell volume in pregnancy is probably only 250 ml.

Rovinsky and Jaffin (1965) found a mean peak red cell volume increment in twin pregnancy of 684 ml. and in triplet pregnancy of 947 ml.

A moderate decrease in red cell volume occurs at delivery, and Pritchard, Wiggins and Dickey (1960) have shown that this decrement is directly and securely linked to blood loss alone. From the data of Caton *et al.* (1951) and Paintin (1962), return to non-gravid red cell volume levels occurs within 60 days after delivery.

Whole Blood Volume

Whole blood volume is best estimated when plasma volume and red cell volume are measured simultaneously but independently. The two measurements have seldom been made together, and most reports of whole blood volume are derived from calculations based on measured plasma volume or red cell volume and hematocrit levels. The approximations of plasma volume and red cell volume presented above need only be combined to arrive at an estimate of whole blood volume changes in pregnancy. Thus, the non-gravid whole blood volume approximates 4,168 ml. and the mean peak pregnancy increment in blood volume near term, 1,654 ml. Hytten and Leitch (1964) arrive at a similar estimate in their analysis. As mentioned previously, there is some difference of opinion as to whether there is a significant decrease in whole blood volume in the few weeks prior to term.

In the cases of twin pregnancy reported by Rovinsky and Jaffin (1965), the mean peak whole blood volume increment near term was 2,647 ml.; in the few cases of triplet pregnancy, a value of 3,349 ml. was obtained.

A major change in total blood volume occurs at delivery, the constituents of which have been discussed under plasma volume and red cell volume changes (q.v.). Decrement in total blood volume after normal vaginal delivery has been measured as 505 ml. by Pritchard, Baldwin, Dickey and Wiggins (1962); at delivery by Cesarean section, measured blood loss was 930 ml. Other reports of measured blood loss at normal vaginal delivery have ranged from that of Gahres *et al.* (1962) at 400 ml. to those of Osofsky and Williams (1964) and Bhatt (1965) at slightly more than 800 ml. All are agreed that the non-gravid blood volume is restored by 4–6 weeks postpartum. Donovan, Lund and Hicks (1965) reported no significant difference in plasma volume, red cell volume, and hematocrit in lactating versus non-lactating women 6–8 weeks postpartum.

Cardiac Output

Studies of cardiac output during pregnancy, labor, delivery and the puerperium are subject to a number of significant methodologic problems, and current information cannot be considered definitive.

The values reported by Rovinsky and Jaffin (1966a) for cardiac output in pregnancy are typical of current

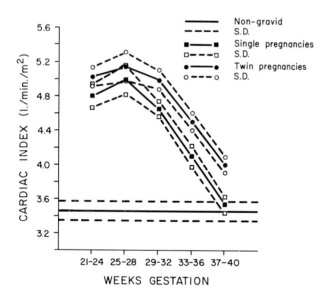

Fig. 2. Cardiac Index Changes in Pregnancy. From Rovinsky and Jaffin, *Amer. J. Obstet. Gynec.*, **95**, 781, 1966, The C. V. Mosby Company, St. Louis, Missouri.

teaching on the subject, which largely is based upon the work of Burwell and Metcalfe (1958). The mean cardiac index (expressed as liters per minute per square meter of body surface area) in single pregnancy rose to a peak of 44·2 per cent above non-gravid control levels in the interval 25–28 weeks of gestation and then fell progressively to normal by term. In twin pregnancy, the cardiac index remained on a relatively stable plateau of 48 per cent above non-pregnant values from the twenty-first through

the thirty-second weeks of gestation, and then fell progressively but was still 15 per cent above control levels at term. In absolute values, non-pregnant cardiac output was 5·87 liters per minute, the mean peak single pregnancy increment in cardiac output, 2·69 liters per minute, and the mean peak twin pregnancy increment, 3·14 liters per minute. Throughout, calculated increments in left ventricular work paralleled increments in cardiac output.

These results tend to confirm the work of Hamilton (1949), Palmer and Walker (1949), Adams (1954), Bader, Bader, Rose and Braunwald (1955), and Roy, Malkham, Virek and Bhatia (1966), but are subject to a number of searching questions. Very few studies have been carried out in early pregnancy, and the shape of the curve of cardiac output before 20 weeks of gestation is not clearly established; the data of Palmer and Walker (1949), Hamilton (1949), Blum de Schwarcz, Aramendia and Taquini (1964), Walters, MacGregor and Hills (1966) and Lees, Taylor, Scott and Kerr (1967) indicate a marked increment in cardiac output at rest as early as the third month of pregnancy. More detailed studies, proceeding from the non-pregnant state into early pregnancy, are needed to define more clearly this phase of alteration of cardiac output.

The reported decrease in cardiac output during the last trimester of pregnancy has been questioned. Hamilton (1949), Adams (1954), Brehm and Kindling (1955), Rovinsky and Jaffin (1966a) and Walters *et al.* (1966) have suggested that cardiac output declines to non-pregnant levels by term. More recently, Lees, Scott, Kerr and Taylor (1967), on the basis of their own work and with support from the study of Pyörälä (1966), have questioned whether the decrease in cardiac output in the weeks prior to term previously described by almost all investigators is not the result solely of methodologic error in performing cardiac output studies on subjects in the supine position. Decrease in cardiac output in late pregnancy when moving from the lateral recumbent to the supine position was demonstrated by Vorys, Ullery and Hanusek (1961) and Lees *et al.* (1967) to be in the range of 12–14 per cent. The causal relationship of compression of the inferior vena cava in the supine position by the near-term gravid uterus, and of the resultant decline in venous return to the heart, to decreased cardiac output and the clinical "supine hypotensive syndrome" has been well documented by Farber, Becker and Eichne (1953), Howard, Goodson and Mengert (1953), Pritchard, Barnes and Bright (1955), Holmes (1960) and Wright (1962), among many others. Quilligan and Tyler (1959) found no significant change in cardiac output near term as estimated by the pulse-pressure method while moving their subjects from the lateral to the supine position; their data may be questioned because of the indirectness of the method. However, Rose, Bader, Bader and Braunwald (1956) studied output by means of cardiac catheterization in pregnant women while exercising, and found a significant decrease in resting cardiac output toward term. Rovinsky and Jaffin (1966a), to eliminate this innate methodologic error, carried out their studies on subjects in the right lateral recumbent rather than supine position, and also found a significant decrease in cardiac output after 28 weeks of gestation; further, the exaggerated decrease in cardiac output because of uterine compression in cases of multiple pregnancy anticipated by Eastman (1958) and described in a few cases by Wright (1962) did not occur—rather, the data in this study indicated the reverse. It therefore seems to be a fair assumption that cardiac output does indeed decline in the last trimester of pregnancy, although additional and more precise studies may be necessary to determine the actual decrement.

Marked changes in cardiac output occur during labor and delivery and in the puerperium, but these have been inadequately investigated. Using the pulse-pressure method for estimating cardiac output, Hendricks and Quilligan (1956) found an increase of cardiac output of 30·9 per cent with each uterine contraction in labor, and a cumulative increase in cardiac output of 35 per cent toward the end of the first stage; uterine contractions and Valsalva maneuvers in the second stage of labor caused even higher and longer lasting increments in cardiac output. Adams and Alexander (1958), using a dye dilution technique, found that cardiac output increased by 20 per cent over the resting state with each uterine contraction in labor, and that calculated left ventricular work increased proportionately; they did not find any cumulative increase in cardiac output as labor progressed. Cunningham (1966), also using a dye-dilution technique, reported similar increases in cardiac output with each uterine contraction in labor, and as labor progressed did find a cumulative increase in cardiac output, which reached a peak late in the first state; in the second stage, cardiac output increased by 50 per cent with each contraction. All are agreed that there is a marked rise in cardiac output immediately after delivery primarily because of markedly increased venous return to the heart secondary to marked diminution in volume of the uteroplacental vascular bed and elimination of uterine pressure on the inferior vena cava, that left ventricular work is greater after delivery than at the end of the first stage, and that this increased cardiac effort is maintained until at least the fourth postpartum day.

Cardiac Rate

Cardiac rate rises progressively through pregnancy, to reach a maximum near term. From the data of Hamilton (1949), Brehm and Kindling (1955), Gemzell, Robbe and Ström (1957) and Ihrman (1960), the cardiac rate is increased by some 15 beats per minute at term after a gradual rise throughout gestation. Rovinsky and Jaffin (1966b) reported a gradual progression to a maximum increase of 21 per cent above non-gravid levels at term in single pregnancy; in twin pregnancy, they found a similar gradual progression to 33–36 weeks of gestation, followed by a sudden upsurge to 40 per cent above non-gravid level at term.

Cunningham (1960) reported marked and very variable tachycardia during labor with many extrasystoles, and a relative bradycardia immediately postpartum. Adams (1954) confirmed the puerperal relative bradycardia which from his data persisted for about 2 weeks.

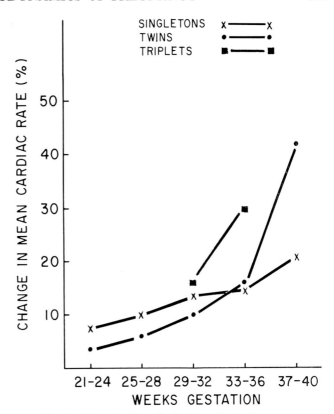

Fig. 3. Changes in Mean Cardiac Rates During Pregnancy. From Rovinsky and Jaffin, *Amer. J. Obstet. Gynec.*, **95**, 787, 1966, The C. V. Mosby Company, St. Louis, Missouri.

Stroke Volume

Increasing stroke volume is the major component responsible for greater cardiac output in pregnancy. Adams and Alexander (1958), Rovinsky and Jaffin (1966b), Roy *et al.* (1966) and Walters *et al.* (1966) are in agreement that increased stroke volume rather than elevated cardiac rate is the primary physiologic adaptation made to raise cardiac output. This increase in stroke volume roughly parallels the curve of cardiac output, and at its peak is approximately 25 per cent above non-gravid control levels in single pregnancy, and 38 per cent higher in twin pregnancy. Adams (1954) and Cunningham (1966) reported a marked increase in stroke volume immediately postpartum, which persisted for 2 weeks.

Total Peripheral Resistance

Total peripheral resistance is a measure of the totality of all factors which affect the blood flow: effective viscosity of the blood, the lengths of the vessels, and their individual and collective cross-sectional areas as determined by intrinsic tone, vasomotor nerve impulses, presence of constrictor or dilator substances, and extravascular pressure provided by tissue tensions. The values of total peripheral resistance are derived mathematically from a formula in which they are directly proportional to mean arterial pressure and inversely proportional to cardiac output. In the calculations of Adams (1954) and Rovinsky and Jaffin (1966b), total peripheral resistance was essentialiy the converse of cardiac output. Adams and Alexander (1958) found a marked decrease in total peripheral resistance in the immediate puerperium which persisted for at least 4 days.

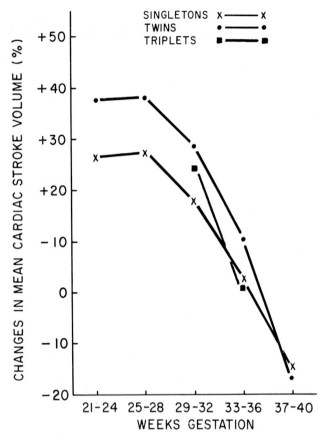

FIG. 4. Changes in Mean Cardiac Stroke Volumes During Pregnancy. From Rovinsky and Jaffin, *Amer. J. Obstet. Gynec.*, **95**, 787, 1966, The C. V. Mosby Company, St. Louis, Missouri.

Circulation Time

Data concerning circulation time in pregnancy are equivocal, but tend toward an increase in velocity of blood flow. Manchester and Loube (1946) reported a decrease in arm-tongue time from 12·4 seconds in the first trimester to 10·2 seconds in the third; the mean arm-lung time fell from 6·6 to 5·0 seconds. Rovinsky and Jaffin (1966b) measured arm-thigh circulation time, and found a decrease of approximately 18 per cent in the interval 21–32 weeks of gestation, and a progressive increase to non-gravid levels at term; there was no significant difference between the results in single and multiple pregnancy. Adams (1954) reported a marked decrease in circulation time postpartum, and a return to non-gravid levels in 2 weeks.

Central Blood Volume and Distribution of Hypervolemia

Central blood volume is a mathematical concept derived from the mean circulation time (arm to thigh) and the cardiac output. In an idealized circulation schema, the calculated central blood volume represents the volume

of blood interposed between the injection site of the indicator dye and the point of sampling; there are obvious difficulties in translating this concept to the human subject. In pregnancy, changes in central blood volume offer an inexact indication of alterations in uterine and placental blood capacity, and may help to delineate the distribution of the pregnancy hypervolemia.

Rovinsky and Jaffin (1966b) found that the central blood volume was elevated approximately 20 per cent over that of the non-gravid state in the interval 21–32 weeks of gestation in both single and multiple pregnancy, and then decreased progressively to term; the values in multiple pregnancy decreased more slowly than those in single pregnancy, and were still elevated significantly at term. The ratio of central blood volume to total blood volume

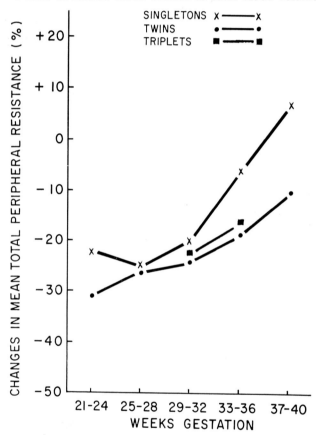

FIG. 5. Changes in Mean Total Peripheral Resistances During Pregnancy. From Rovinsky and Jaffin, *Amer. J. Obstet. Gynec.*, **95**, 787, 1966, The C. V. Mosby Company, St. Louis, Missouri.

was 30 per cent at 21–24 weeks of gestation, and was a progressively diminishing fraction to term. This represents a very crude approximation of the blood volume in the placenta and uterus (assuming little pooling in the pulmonary, gastrointestinal, or renal circulations). That the uteroplacental vascular bed contains about 20 per cent of the total maternal blood volume at term is in agreement with the previous work of White (1950). From this the corollary can be developed that from mid-pregnancy on an ever increasing proportion of total blood

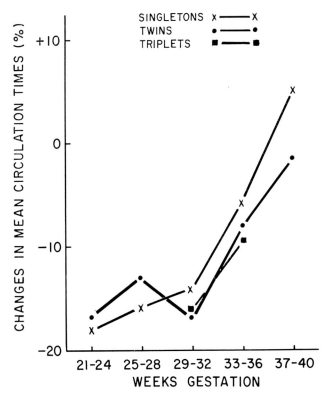

FIG. 6. Changes in Mean Circulation Times During Pregnancy. From Rovinsky and Jaffin, *Amer. J. Obstet. Gynec.*, **95**, 787, 1966, The C. V. Mosby Company, St. Louis, Missouri.

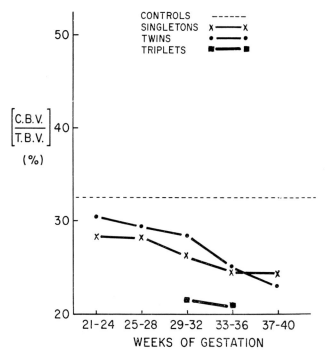

FIG. 7. Relation of Central to Total Blood Volumes During Pregnancy. From Rovinsky and Jaffin, *Amer. J. Obstet. Gynec.*, **95**, 787, 1966, The C. V. Mosby Company, St. Louis, Missouri.

volume comes to lie outside of the central blood volume "space"—an area including, among other things, the lower extremities and the maternal great veins. Hypervolemia and increased venous pressure in the lower extremities have been documented by McLennan (1943) and McCausland, Hyman, Winsor and Trotter (1961), among others, but the extent of hypervolemia of the lower extremities is limited. By far the greater increase in maternal blood volume occurs in the great veins, as evidenced by the fact that diastolic pressures on the right side of the heart have been shown by Rose *et al.* (1956) to be elevated in late pregnancy to an extent ordinarily concomitant with light ventricular failure.

Mechanisms of Physiologic Adaptations in Pregnancy

In summary, maternal cardiovascular adaptation to pregnancy proceeds along fairly well recognized lines. In single pregnancy, blood volume increases progressively to reach a peak increment of about 40 per cent which is maintained through the last 12 weeks of gestation.

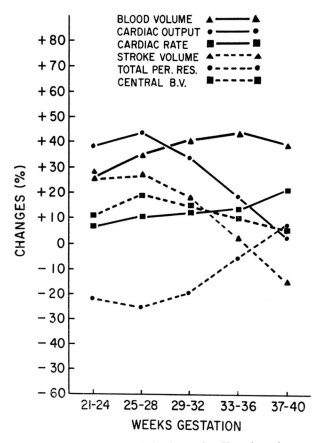

FIG. 8. Parameters of Cardiovascular Hemodynamics During Single Pregnancy. From Rovinsky and Jaffin, *Amer. J. Obstet. Gynec.*, **95**, 787, 1966, The C. V. Mosby Company, St. Louis, Missouri.

Cardiac output rises progressively to a peak increment of about 44 per cent at 25–28 weeks of gestation, and then falls toward non-gravid levels at term. Alterations in cardiac output bear no relation to changes in blood volume, but are inversely related to changes in maternal total peripheral resistance. The major role in raising cardiac output is played by an increasing stroke volume; there is only a small elevation of cardiac rate. The major portion of the maternal hypervolemia is distributed to the lower extremities and the maternal great veins.

In twin pregnancy, the peak increment of blood volume of about 60 per cent occurs at term. Peak cardiac output, some 48 per cent above non-gravid levels, is maintained through the interval 21–32 weeks of gestation, and then falls in the remaining weeks but is still 16 per cent above control levels at term. Increased stroke volume is the major factor maintaining elevated cardiac output until near term, when a markedly increased cardiac rate assumes a more significant role.

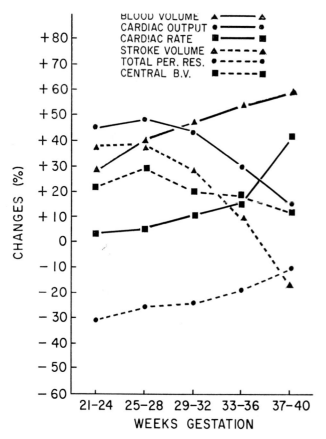

FIG. 9. Parameters of Cardiovascular Hemodynamics During Twin Pregnancy. From Rovinsky and Jaffin, *Amer. J. Obstet. Gynec.*, **95**, 787, 1966, The C. V. Mosby Company, St. Louis, Missouri.

The basis for these physiologic hemodynamic adaptations remains unsettled. Burwell (1938) proposed that the placenta serves as a functional arteriovenous shunt, and that the circulatory adjustments are secondary to this effect. Heckel and Tobin (1956) demonstrated the presence of arteriovenous connections of 200 microns diameter in the uterine vasculature. Attempts at a critical analysis of this thesis and exhaustive reviews of the literature have led Herd, Franklin and Metcalfe (1960), Hytten and Leitch (1964), and Winner (1965) to reject the premise that an arteriovenous shunt mechanism alone is primarily

responsible for all of the described hemodynamic alterations. The concept cannot be completely dismissed, however, and may yet play a significant role in association with other factors. Romney, Reid, Metcalfe and Burwell (1955) referred pregnancy blood volume increments to the oxygen needs of the growing fetus. Hytten and Paintin (1963) found the maximal increase in plasma volume directly related to the weight of the fetus. Rovinsky and Jaffin (1965) described a linear relationship between peak plasma volume increments and placental mass at delivery. In essence, all three reports restated, in different terms, the dependence of blood volume increment on the products of conception. Indeed, Pritchard (1965) suggested from a study of molar pregnancy that a fetus is not necessary for the development of pregnancy-induced hypervolemia. Burchell (1967), using radiologic techniques to visualize uterine and intervillous space blood flow, developed objective evidence which tends to support the presence of a functional arteriovenous shunt; the study suggests that the vascular resistance of this "fistula" is low early in pregnancy, and increases gradually as pregnancy progresses because of syncytial clumping and the proliferation of villi, to reach equilibrium with the resistance of the systemic circulation at about 30 weeks gestation. This correlates well with the time of occurrence of peak blood and plasma volume increments.

Alterations of cardiac output may well be dependent to a large extent upon other factors. Ueland and Parer (1966) and Goodrich and Wood (1966) have demonstrated the marked effect of estrogens on the circulatory system; in many respects, this effect mimics the changes of pregnancy. In essence, estrogens cause a marked reduction in total peripheral resistance, with secondary increase in cardiac output, stroke volume, and cardiac rate. This may be the pre-eminent influence modifying cardiac output early in pregnancy, and may be superimposed to a significant degree on the placental factor in later pregnancy. The influences of sympathetic nervous system activity and of circulating norepinephrine and other hormonal substances suggested by Herd *et al.* (1960) remain undetermined.

Clinical Implications

One must conclude that much remains unsettled in our knowledge of the cardiovascular hemodynamics of pregnancy, and that a large volume of data from many detailed and more critical investigations is needed before definitive answers can be given to some of the questions raised in this chapter. Nevertheless, clinical application of even this incomplete knowledge is effective in reducing maternal morbidity and mortality from heart disease in pregnancy.

The normal heart can compensate with ease, using very efficient mechanisms such as increased stroke volume, for the additional cardiac stress imposed by single pregnancy. In twin pregnancy, the duration of cardiac stress is extended, although not much higher; near term, less efficient compensatory mechanisms such as increased cardiac rate begin to come into play, and cardiac work is considerable even before the onset of labor. Labor and delivery impose transient but severe additional cardiac stress on the mother, and postpartum cardiac stress may be even higher temporarily than in labor itself. Cardiac stress does not return to non-pregnant levels for at least two weeks by many of the parameters investigated.

Application of this information clinically puts the management of the pregnant patient with cardiac disease on a rational base, points out the areas of maximum stress and risk to the diseased heart, and yields more satisfactory therapeutic results.

REFERENCES

Adams, J. Q. (1954), "Cardiovascular Physiology in Normal Pregnancy; Studies with the Dye Dilution Technique," *Amer. J. Obstet. Gynec.*, 67, 741.

Adams, J. Q. and Alexander, A. M. (1958), "Alterations in Cardiovascular Physiology during Labor," *Obstet. Gynec.*, 12, 542.

Bader, R. A., Bader, M. E., Rose, D. J. and Braunwald, E. (1955), "Hemodynamics at Rest and during Exercise in Normal Pregnancy as Studied by Cardiac Catheterization," *J. clin. Invest.*, 34, 1524.

Berlin, N. I., Goetsch, C., Hyde, G. M. and Parsons, R. J. (1953), "The Blood Volume in Pregnancy as Determined by P³²-labelled Red Blood Cells," *Surg., Gynec. Obstet.*, 97, 173.

Bhatt, J. R. (1965), "Blood Volume Variations during Labor and the Early Puerperium," *Obstet. Gynec.*, 26, 243.

Brehm, H. and Kindling, E. (1955), "Das Kreislauf während Schwangerschaft und Wochenbett," *Arch. Gynäk.*, 185, 696.

Brown, E., Sampson, J. J., Wheeler, E. O., Gundelfinger, B. F. and Giansiracussa, J. E. (1947), "Physiologic Changes in the Circulation during and after Obstetric Labor," *Amer. Heart J.*, 34, 311.

Bucht, H. (1951), "Studies on Renal Function in Man with Special Reference to Glomerular Filtration and Renal Plasma Flow in Pregnancy," *Scand. Journal of Laboratory and Clinical Medicine*, 3 (Supplement 3), 1.

Burchell, R. C. (1967), "Arterial Blood Flow into the Human Intervillous Space," *Amer. J. Obstet. Gynec.*, 98, 303.

Burwell, C. S. (1938), "The Placenta as a Modified Arteriovenous Fistula Considered in Relation to the Circulatory Adjustments of Pregnancy," *Amer. J. med. Sci.*, 195, 1.

Burwell, C. S. and Metcalfe, J. (1958), *Heart Disease in Pregnancy. Physiology and Management.* London: J. and A. Churchill.

Caton, W. L., Roby, C. C., Reid, D. E., Caswell, R., Maletskos, C. J., Fluharty, R. G. and Gibson, J. G. (1951), "The Circulating Red Cell Volume and Body Hematocrit in Normal Pregnancy and the Puerperium," *Amer. J. Obstet. Gynec.*, 61, 1207.

Caton, W. L., Roby, C. C., Reid, D. E. and Gibson, J. G. (1949), "Plasma Volume and Extravascular Fluid Volume during Pregnancy and the Puerperium," *Amer. J. Obstet. Gynec.*, 57, 471.

Cope, I. (1956), "Plasma and Blood Volume Changes in Late and Prolonged Pregnancy," *J. Obstet. Gynæc. Brit. Emp.*, 65, 877.

Cunningham, I. (1966), "Cardiovascular Physiology of Labour and Delivery," *J. Obstet. Gynaec. Brit. Commonwealth*, 73, 500.

Davis, H. A. (1962), *Blood Volume Dynamics*, p. 106. Springfield, Ill.: Charles C. Thomas.

Dieckmann, W. J. and Wegner, C. R. (1934), "The Blood in Normal Pregnancy. I. Blood and plasma volumes," *Arch. intern. Med.*, 53, 71.

Donovan, J. C., Lund, C. J. and Hicks, E. L. (1965), "Effect of Lactation on Blood Volume in the Human Female," *Amer. J. Obstet. Gynec.*, 93, 588.

Duhring, J. L. (1962), "Blood Volume in Pregnancy," *Amer. J. med. Sci.*, 243, 808.

Eastman, N. J. (1958), editorial comment, *Obstet. gynec. Surg.*, 13, 48.

Farber, S. J., Becker, W. H. and Eichne, L. W. (1953), "Electrolyte and Water Excretions and Renal Hemodynamics during Induced Congestion of the Superior and Inferior Vena Cava of Man," *J. clin. Invest.*, 32, 1145.

Gahres, E. E., Albert, S. N. and Dodek, S. M. (1962), "Intrapartum Blood Loss Measured with Cr⁵¹-tagged Erythrocytes," *Obstet. Gynec.*, 19, 455.

Gemzell, C. A., Robbe, H. and Ström, G. (1957), "Total Amount of Hemoglobin and Physical Working Capacity in Normal Pregnancy and the Puerperium," *Acta obstet. gynec. scand.*, 36, 93.

Goodrich, S. M. and Wood, J. E. (1966), "Effect of Estradiol-17-β on Peripheral Venous Distensibility and Velocity of Venous Blood Flow," *Amer. J. Obstet. Gynec.*, 96, 407.

Gregersen, M. I. and Rawson, R. A. (1959), "Blood Volume," *Physiol. Rev.*, 39, 307.

Guyton, A. C. (1963), *Circulatory Physiology: Cardiac Output and its Regulation*, pp. 3–124. Philadelphia: W. B. Saunders Co.

Hamilton, H. F. H. (1949), "The Cardiac Output in Normal Pregnancy, as Determined by the Cournand Right Heart Catheterization Technique," *J. Obstet. Gynaec. Brit. Emp.*, 56, 548.

Heckel, G. P. and Tobin, C. E. (1956), "Arteriovenous Shunts in the Myometrium," *Amer. J. Obstet. Gynec.*, 71, 199.

Herd, J. A., Franklin, M. J. and Metcalfe, J. (1960), "Circulatory Adjustments of Pregnancy," *Clin. Obstet. Gynec.*, 3, 364.

Holmes, F. (1960), "Incidence of Supine Hypotensive Syndrome in Late Pregnancy. A clinical study of 500 subjects," *J. Obstet. Gynaec. Brit. Emp.*, 67, 254.

Howard, B. K., Goodson, J. H. and Mengert, W. F. (1953), "Supine Hypotensive Syndrome in Late Pregnancy," *Obstet. Gynec.*, 1, 371.

Hytten, F. E. and Leitch, I. (1964), *The Physiology of Human Pregnancy*, pp. 2–86. Oxford: Blackwell Scientific Publications.

Hytten, F. E. and Paintin, D. B. (1963), "Increase in Plasma Volume during Normal Pregnancy," *J. Obstet. Gynaec. Brit. Commonwealth*, 70, 811.

Ihrman, K. (1960) "A Clinical and Physiological Study of Pregnancy in a Material from Northern Sweden. VI. Arterial blood pressure at rest and in orthostatic test during and after pregnancy," *Acta Soc. Med. upsalien.*, 65, 315.

Lees, M. M., Scott, D. B., Kerr, M. G. and Taylor, S. H. (1967), "The Circulatory Effects of Recumbent Postural Change in Late Pregnancy," *Clin. Sci.*, 32, 453.

Lees, M. M., Taylor, S. H., Scott, D. B. and Kerr, M. G. (1967), "A Study of Cardiac Output at Rest throughout Pregnancy," *J. Obstet. Gynaec. Brit. Commonwealth*, 74, 319.

Lowenstein, L., Pick, C. A. and Philpott, N. W. (1950), "Correlations of Blood Loss with Blood Volume and Other Hematological Studies before, during, and after Childbirth," *Amer. J. Obstet. Gynec.*, 60, 1206.

Lund, C. J. and Donovan, J. C. (1967), "Blood Volume during Pregnancy. Significance of plasma and red cell volume," *Amer. J. Obstet. Gynec.*, 98, 393.

McCausland, A. M., Hyman, C., Winsor, T. and Trotter, A. D. (1961), "Venous Distensibility during Pregnancy," *Amer. J. Obstet. Gynec.*, 81, 472.

McLennan, C. E. (1943), "Antecubital and Femoral Venous Pressure in Normal and Toxemic Pregnancy," *Amer. J. Obstet. Gynec.*, 45, 568.

McLennan, C. E. and Thouin, L. G. (1948), "Blood Volume in Pregnancy. A critical review and preliminary report of results with a new technique," *Amer. J. Obstet. Gynec.*, 55, 189.

Manchester, B. and Loube, S. D. (1946), "The Velocity of Blood Flow in Normal Pregnant Women," *Amer. Heart J.*, 32, 215.

Osofsky, H. J. and Williams, J. A. (1964), "Changes in Blood Volume during Parturition and Early Postpartum Period," *Amer. J. Obstet. Gynaec.*, 88, 396.

Overall, J. E. and Williams, C. M. (1959), "A Note Concerning Sources of Variance in Determinations of Human Plasma Volume," *J. Lab. clin. Med.*, 54, 186.

Paintin, D. B. (1962), "Size of Total Red Cell Volume in Pregnancy," *J. Obstet. Gynaec. Brit. Commonwealth*, 69, 719.

Palmer, A. J. and Walker, A. H. C. (1949), "The Maternal Circulation in Normal Pregnancy," *J. Obstet. Gynaec. Brit. Emp.*, 56, 537.

Pritchard, J. A. (1965), "Blood Volume Changes in Pregnancy and the Puerperium. IV. Anemia associated with hydatidiform mole," *Amer. J. Obstet. Gynec.*, 91, 621.

Pritchard, J. A. and Adams, R. H. (1960), "Erythrocyte Production and Destruction during Pregnancy," *Amer. J. Obstet. Gynec.*, 79, 750.

Pritchard, J. A., Baldwin, R. M., Dickey, J. C. and Wiggins, K. M. (1962), "Blood Volume Changes in Pregnancy and the Puerperium. II. Red blood cell loss and changes in apparent blood volume during and following vaginal delivery, cesarean section, and cesarean section plus total hysterectomy," *Amer. J. Obstet. Gynec.*, **84**, 1271.

Pritchard, J. A., Barnes, A. C. and Bright, R. H. (1955), "Effect of Supine Position on Renal Function in Near-term Pregnant Women," *J. clin. Invest.*, **34**, 777.

Pritchard, J. A. and Rowland, R. C. (1964), "Blood Volume Changes in Pregnancy and the Puerperium. III. Whole body and large vessel hematocrits in pregnant and non-pregnant women," *Amer. J. Obstet. Gynec.*, **88**, 391.

Pritchard, J. A., Wiggins, K. M. and Dickey, J. C. (1960), "Blood Volume Changes in Pregnancy and the Puerperium. I. Does sequestration of red blood cells accompany parturition?" *Amer. J. Obstet. Gynec.*, **80**, 956.

Pyörälä, T. (1966), "Cardiovascular Response to the Upright Position during Pregnancy," *Acta obstet. gynec. scand.*, **45** (Supplement 5), 1.

Quilligan, E. J. and Tyler, C. (1950), "Postural Effects on Cardiovascular Status in Pregnancy," *Amer. J. Obstet. Gynec.*, **78**, 465.

Romney, S. L., Reid, D. E., Metcalfe, J. and Burwell, C. S. (1955), "Oxygen Utilization in the Human Fetus in Utero," *Amer. J. Obstet. Gynec.*, **70**, 791.

Rovinsky, J. J. and Jaffin, H. (1965), "Cardiovascular Hemodynamics in Pregnancy. I. Blood and plasma volumes in multiple pregnancy," *Amer. J. Obstet. Gynec.*, **93**, 1.

Rovinsky, J. J. and Jaffin, H. (1966a), "Cardiovascular Hemodynamics in Pregnancy. II. Cardiac output and left ventricular work in multiple pregnancy," *Amer. J. Obstet. Gynec.*, **95**, 781.

Rovinsky, J. J. and Jaffin, H. (1966b), "Cardiovascular Hemodynamics in Pregnancy. III. Cardiac rate, stroke volume, total peripheral resistance, and central blood volume in multiple pregnancy. Synthesis of results," *J. Obstet. Gynec.*, **95**, 787.

Roy, S. B., Malkain, P. K., Virek, R. and Bhatia, M. L. (1966), "Circulatory Effects of Pregnancy," *Amer. J. Obstet. Gynec.*, **96**, 221.

Thomson, K. J., Hirsheimer, A., Gibson, J. G., 2nd, and Evans, W. A. Jr. (1938), "Studies on the Circulation in Pregnancy. III. Blood volume changes in normal pregnant women," *Amer. J. Obstet. Gynec.*, **36**, 48.

Tysoe, S. W. and Lowenstein, L. (1950), "Blood Volume and Hematologic Studies in Pregnancy and the Puerperium," *Amer. J. Obstet. Gynec.*, **60**, 1187.

Ueland, K. and Parer, J. T. (1966), "Effects of Estrogens on the Cardiovascular System of the Ewe," *Amer. J. Obstet. Gynec.*, **96**, 400.

Verel, D., Bury, J. D. and Hope, A. (1956), "Blood Volume Changes in Pregnancy and the Puerperium," *Clin. Sci.*, **15**, 1.

Vorys, N., Ullery, J. C. and Hanusek, G. E. (1961), "Cardiac Output Changes in Various Positions in Pregnancy," *Amer. J. Obstet. Gynec.*, **82**, 1312.

Walters, W. A. W., MacGregor, W. G. and Hills, M. (1966), "Cardiac Output at Rest during Pregnancy and the Puerperium," *Clin. Sci.*, **30**, 1.

Werkö, L., Bucht, H., Lagerlöf, H. and Holmgren, A. (1948), "Cirkulationen vid graviditet," *Nord. Med.*, **40**, 1868.

White, R. (1950), "Blood Volumes in Pregnancy," *Edinb. med. J.*, **57**, (Transaction 14).

Winner, W. (1965), "The Role of the Placenta in the Systemic Circulation; a re-appraisal," *Obstet. gynec. Surv.*, **20**, 545.

Wright, L. (1962), "Postural Hypotension in Late Pregnancy," *Brit. med. J.*, **1**, 760.

SECTION V

METABOLISM AND NUTRITION

1. CARBOHYDRATE METABOLISM

JEAN GINSBURG

Definition and Function

Of the three primary organic foodstuffs (carbohydrates, proteins and fats), carbohydrates provide the main source of metabolic fuel for the cell. They contain carbon together with oxygen and hydrogen in the proportion found in water; some carbohydrates also contain nitrogen or sulphur. The simplest carbohydrates are the so-called monosaccharides and include 6-carbon compounds or hexoses, of which glucose is the most important example, and 5-carbon sugars or pentoses, such as D-ribose. The more complex carbohydrates—the oligosaccharides and polysaccharides—are made from two or more monosaccharides joined together, a hydroxyl group of one sugar condensing with the reducing group of another, so that the two sugars are linked by a glycosidic bond (C–O–C). Disaccharides contain two sugar molecules joined in this way; lactose, the characteristic sugar of milk, and sucrose, the main sugar of "civilized" diets are both disaccharides. Long chains of monosaccharides, with each sugar unit linked to its neighbours by a glycosidic bond, can also be formed; the polysaccharide macro-molecules such as starch are made up of multiple branched chains containing hundreds of sugar units with glycosidic links present also at the point of branching. The glycosidic bonds of the more complex carbohydrates are thus analogous to the peptide bonds found in proteins.

Carbohydrates, in addition to releasing energy for cellular activity on metabolism, provide essential building blocks for the intricate components of cell structure. Tissue polysaccharides such as glycogen can be considered storage material releasing glucose in accordance with the needs of the organism. Polysaccharides also form part of the organism's structural framework as exemplified by cellulose in plants, chitin in arthropods and the mucopolysaccharides of mammalian cartilage, tendon or subcutaneous intercellular cement.

Metabolism of Glucose

Glucose is the principal energy source for the cell; by its breakdown into smaller molecules and eventually to CO_2, energy, which can be stored as ATP, is made available for cellular function. The two and three carbon fragments produced by glucose metabolism enter the common "metabolic pool" where interconversion takes place between the products of fat, protein and carbohydrate catabolism. The products of glucose metabolism can then take part in the biosynthesis of amino acids, fatty acids and other basic cellular constituents or are further metabolized to CO_2 with the production of additional energy.

An important limiting factor in carbohydrate metabolism is the rate of entry of glucose into the cell. Several substances, including insulin and certain poisons, are known to influence this process *in vitro* but it is not yet clear how variations in rate are normally effected *in vivo*. The entry of glucose into the cell is not purely a function of the concentration gradient, i.e. diffusion of glucose from a region of higher to lower concentration, but requires active cellular intervention in the process.

After glucose has penetrated into the cell, phosphorylation with the formation of glucose-6-phosphate is considered an essential preliminary for the entry of glucose into the majority of metabolic sequences. The phosphorylated sugar can then take part in at least five different metabolic pathways, though the distribution and relative importance of these routes varies in different tissues and may also alter in accordance with physio-pathologic demands. Phosphorylation of glucose is catalysed by the ubiquitous hexokinase enzyme and requires the assistance of a high energy phosphate compound such as ATP. In the liver, a second enzyme, a glucokinase, also catalyses this reaction; the liver also contains glucokinases which specifically catalyse the phosphorylation of galactose and fructose.

(1) Catabolic Routes

(a) Glycolysis and the formation of pyruvate. The major route for glucose catabolism in most mammalian tissues is the glycolytic or Emden–Meyerhof pathway—the series of reactions which start with glucose-6-phosphate and which continue through into the production of pyruvic acid. As a result of the operation of this pathway each hexose molecule is converted into two molecules of pyruvate and four molecules of ATP are produced. But at the same time two molecules of ATP are used for phosphorylation—one in the conversion of glucose to glucose-6-phosphate and one in the conversion of fructose-6-phosphate to fructose-1-6-phosphate. Hence there is a net production of two molecules of ATP for each molecule of glucose which enters the pathway and forms pyruvate. But with glycogen as the starting point, as may occur in contracting muscle, ATP is only required for the reaction fructose-6-phosphate to fructose–1-6-phosphate. The net gain when glycogen is degraded to pyruvate is therefore 3 molecules of ATP.

The sequence of events up to the formation of pyruvate are identical in the presence or absence of oxygen. Thereafter, the products vary with the available oxygen supply and pyruvic acid is either reversibly converted to lactate or decarboxylated to form acetyl-co-enzyme A. The former reaction predominates in anaerobic conditions, but if sufficient oxygen is available, acetyl-co-enzyme A is formed with the evolution of a further 3 molecules of ATP. Acetyl-co-enzyme A can then enter the citric acid cycle (see below) for complete combustion and formation of various essential intermediate metabolites.

Pyruvate is a key substance at the crossroads of fat, protein and carbohydrate metabolism. It is mainly produced by carbohydrate metabolism but can also be derived from other precursors such as amino-acids. As a result of the formation of acetyl-co-enzyme A, the residual molecule enters the citric acid cycle and in so doing provides further energy, as well as vital intermediates for

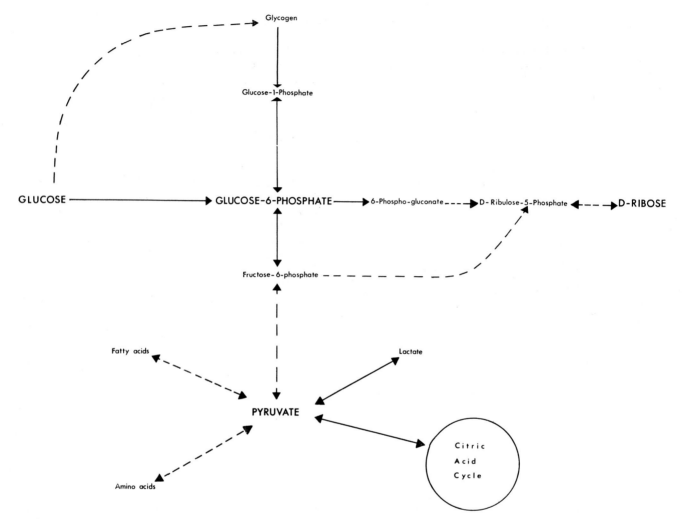

FIG. 1. Schematic outline of main pathways of glucose metabolism (after Beaconsfield, P. and Morris, N. F. (1967) *Europa Medica*, 3, 3).

The rate of tissue glycolysis, conventionally assessed in relation to the rate of lactate production, varies with the oxygen supply and in accordance with cellular demands at the time. Thus in anaerobic conditions energy requirements may be met by increased breakdown of tissue glycogen and glycolysis proceeds more rapidly than in aerobic conditions. A classical example of this is seen in rapidly contracting skeletal muscle; similar considerations apply to uterine muscle, especially in labour. On the other hand when aerobic conditions prevail, the rate of resynthesis of glucose is increased and there is a relative inhibition of glycolysis. This decrease in glucose utilization in the presence of oxygen is frequently referred to as the Pasteur effect.

protein and other biosynthetic processes. Another anabolic process dependent on glucose metabolism to pyruvic acid, and for which acetyl co-enzyme A is also required, is fatty acid synthesis. Pyruvic acid itself can also take part in the resynthesis of glucose, though it should be remembered that anabolic routes consume energy and are not exact reversals of the catabolic process.

Citric Acid Cycle

This cycle, also known as the tricarboxylic acid cycle or Krebs cycle, was originally proposed to account for the complete combustion of pyruvic acid and of the two and three carbon end products of fatty acid oxidation. Its metabolic influence, however, extends beyond a purely catabolic function. By its perpetual activity it forms the hub and central metabolic meeting point for almost all cellular activity. Nearly all the reactions and substrates of this cyclical manoeuvre have a crucial role in the synthesis of a multitude of essential metabolites, e.g. those concerned with amino acid, purine, pyrimidine, long-chain fatty acid and porphyrin synthesis. Additionally the operation of the cycle converts potential chemical energy into metabolic energy in the form of ATP. For each complete operation of the cycle, twelve molecules of ATP are generated. The complete metabolism of one molecule of glucose through the glycolytic pathway and associated citric acid cycle thus releases 32 molecules of ATP (two molecules of ATP generated in the sequence from glucose to pyruvate, three molecules when pyruvate is converted into acetyl co-enzyme A and 12 with each molecule of acetyl co-enzyme A entering and completing the cycle. And since one molecule of glucose produces *two* molecules of pyruvate, the total net production of ATP from the complete oxidation of one molecule of glucose is $2 + 6 + 24$ i.e. 32.) The citric acid cycle is the principal process responsible for harnessing the contained energy in carbohydrates and thereby makes ATP continuously available for cellular activity. It will be remembered that acetyl-co-enzyme A is also formed during the oxidation of long chain fatty acids (see chapter on Lipid Metabolism by N. B. Myant). The citric acid cycle thus also provides for complete combustion of fatty acids.

The continued operation of the cycle requires a continuous supply of oxidized co-enzymes. This is achieved by coupling the reactions in which the co-enzymes are reduced with a sequence of hydrogen carriers—the electron transport sequence—thereby ensuring the complete oxidation of pyruvate or acetyl co-enzyme A and continued formation of ATP.

(b) Pentose-phosphate pathway. Of the alternative pathways of glucose catabolism which start with glucose-6-phosphate, the best known and probably the most important is the pentose-phosphate pathway, variously known as the pentose shunt, the direct oxidative route, the hexose monophosphate pathway or the Warburg-Dickens pathway. As a result of glucose metabolism along this route there is increased formation of reduced NADP (nicotine-adenine dinucleotide phosphate)—an essential co-enzyme for lipid and steroid synthesis and for many detoxification reactions—and production of the pentose sugars essential for nucleic acid biosynthesis.

In most tissues the amount of glucose metabolized by the pentose-phosphate pathway is quantitatively very much less than that which is degraded by glycolysis. The relative activity of the two main pathways for glucose catabolism can be assessed in relation to the relative rates of production of labelled CO_2 after parallel incubation of tissue with glucose labelled in the first carbon atom and with glucose labelled in the sixth carbon atom respectively. The fractional recovery of labelled CO_2 after such incubation provides a qualitative indication of the relative activity of the pentose route in that particular tissue, for when glucose enters the Emden–Meyerhof pathway,* the CO_2 evolved is derived equally from the first and sixth carbon atoms of glucose so that the ratio of labelled CO_2 after incubation ($G_1 : G_6$) is one, whereas when glucose enters the pentose route CO_2 is produced from the first carbon atom only. Since the glycolytic route is generally overwhelmingly the predominant pathway, glycolysis may be the only route of glucose catabolism measurable in normal physiological conditions in some tissues. However, if there is a major increase in pentose shunt activity, the amount of CO_2 produced from glucose labelled in the first carbon atom is increased and the ratio of G_1 to G_6 becomes greater than one.

On this basis an elevated activity of the direct oxidative route for glucose metabolism has been demonstrated in a variety of conditions, for example in the lactating mammary gland, in healing wounds and in the early human placenta. With the use of more complex techniques and the determination of glucose incorporation into various metabolites, a quantitative assessment of the contribution of the pentose route to total glucose catabolism has also been obtained. In this manner it has been found that in certain circumstances the pentose pathway may be responsible for over 40 per cent of the glucose metabolized by that particular tissue.

(c) Other catabolic routes. Glucose-6-phosphate can also be degraded through other catabolic pathways but though these may be of major importance in other species, such as micro-organisms, they are either not present or apparently of only minor significance in mammalian tissues.

(2) Synthetic Processes

Synthetic pathways of glucose metabolism require energy and consume ATP in the process. The most important product of anabolism starting from glucose is glycogen, manufactured mainly in liver and muscle. The synthesis of glycogen does not proceed by a reversal of the phosphorylase reaction which releases glucose from tissue glycogen but by a more complicated process involving the co-enzyme uridine triphosphate. The formation of other glucose polymers, such as oligosaccharides and hexose isomers such as galactose also requires this co-enzyme.

Lactic and pyruvic acids produced by glycolysis and, similarly, intermediates between these acids and glucose can be rebuilt in the liver into glucose. The energy required for these reactions is provided by the ATP formed during energy liberating reactions, such as operation of the citric acid cycle, the ATP produced during complete oxidation of 2 molecules of pyruvate or lactate, for example, being more than sufficient for the resynthesis of 5 molecules of glucose from 10 molecules of pyruvate. The liver can also synthesize glucose from non-carbohydrate residues such as those produced by deamination of amino-acids or by fatty acid metabolism to glycerol and also from any other compound which can be metabolized via pyruvate; a continued supply of glucose for energy purposes is thus ensured. Glucogenesis and gluconeogenesis are the terms used to describe the processes whereby glucose is formed from carbohydrate and non-carbohydrate precursors

---

* For details of individual reactions in the Emden–Meyerhof and other pathways, the interested reader should refer to a textbook of biochemistry as indicated in the references.

respectively. Much of the glucose formed in this way is converted into glycogen, the main sites of glycogen synthesis (glycogenesis) being the liver and muscles. In skeletal muscle, phosphorylated 3 carbon compounds such as α-glycerophosphate can also be converted into glycogen.

Release of Glucose from Glycogen

The mobilization of glucose from glycogen (glycogenolysis) is effected mainly through the medium of a phosphorylase enzyme; the (1–4) glycosidic bonds are broken and a phosphate group introduced from a supply of inorganic phosphate, with the production of glucose-1-phosphate. Intramolecular phosphate transfer, catalysed by a phospho-glucomutase then results in formation of glucose-6-phosphate and free glucose is finally liberated by means of a phosphatase. Free glucose is also released by the action of amylo-glucosidases which rupture the (1–6) glucosidic bonds in branched polysaccharides. In the glycogen storage diseases, where excess glycogen is deposited in the tissues—especially in muscle and liver—there is a deficiency of one or other of the enzymes involved in the sequence between glycogen and free glucose.

Interconversion of Glucose and Fats

Fat and carbohydrate metabolism are intimately linked, with a common meeting point in acetyl-co-enzyme A and links through the citric acid cycle and through the formation of glycerol. Thus, fatty acid and neutral fat synthesis are coupled with oxidation of carbohydrates and conversely, glycerol from fat metabolism can be used in the synthesis of glucose. Changes in glucose metabolism also affect the concentration or release of free fatty acids and a reciprocal relationship has been postulated, whereby increased levels of fatty acids depress tissue glucose utilization (see chapter 2. in this section).

Blood Glucose Homeostasis and Gluco-regulatory Hormones

The complex carbohydrates present in plant and animal foods cannot be used by the cells until they have been broken down in the gut into monosaccharides which are then absorbed into the blood stream and taken to the liver (see chapter on Pancreas by C. W. H. Havard). Here, depending on the particular sugar absorbed and physiological requirements at that time, the monosaccharides are either stored in the form of glycogen, converted into glucose and liberated into the blood stream, metabolized with the production of energy or passed on into the general circulation.

The level of circulating glucose is kept remarkably constant despite vaying rates of tissue glucose metabolism and the irregular influx of sugar absorbed from the gut. The constancy of blood glucose, an essential feature of the "milieu intérieur", is achieved by a complex interplay between intrinsic changes in hepatic carbohydrate metabolism and the effects of the gluco-regulatory hormones—insulin (the only known hormone which lowers blood glucose) and growth hormone, glucagon, the catecholamines and gluco-corticoids (which all raise blood sugar). A balance between glycogenesis and glycolysis on the one hand and glycogenolysis and gluconeogenesis on the other is thereby maintained.

The liver is the principal source of glucose entering the blood stream and ensures an adequate level of blood glucose, even in the fasting state. After hepatectomy in dogs, there is a progressive fall in blood sugar and within a few hours convulsion, coma and finally death. The clinical signs parallel the degree of hypoglycæmia and injection of glucose produces a remarkably rapid—albeit temporary—recovery.

Hepatic glucose output depends on the breakdown of hepatic glycogen or other complex carbohydrate molecules, on de novo synthesis of glucose from smaller units and on glucose transferred from the portal system after absorption from the gut. Glucose outflow from the liver is regulated partly by a homeostatic action of the liver itself and partly by hormonal influences. When the level of circulating glucose falls, the formation of glucose from glycogen or from 2 and 3 carbon fragments is increased, whereas when blood glucose begins to rise, this process ceases and the excess glucose is converted into glycogen or broken down into smaller units. The liver therefore acts as a "glucostat", adjusting its metabolism and hence the rate at which glucose enters the blood stream, so that the level of circulating glucose is maintained within relatively narrow limits.

The gluco-regulatory hormones influence hepatic glucose output directly, in consequence of their effect on hepatic metabolism and also indirectly, as a result of their metabolic action in other tissues. The most studied, probably the most important, yet still perhaps the least understood of these hormones is insulin, secreted by the α-cells of the pancreas. The classic effect of injecting insulin, a fall in blood glucose, results from increased peripheral glucose utilization with increased glycogen deposition in liver and muscle, and increased glucose metabolism to fatty acids, combined with lowered rates of lipolysis, gluconeogenesis and hepatic glycogenolysis. It has not yet been possible to find a single biochemical locus for the action of insulin; the most likely possibilities include increased glucose transfer across the cell membrane and an influence on hexokinase activity or availability of ATP. Insulin secretion is regulated in the first instance, by the glucose concentration in the pancreatic artery and secondly by the action of the other gluco-regulatory hormones, which all raise circulating glucose and can be considered insulin "antagonists".

Thus, growth hormone (HGH) from the anterior pituitary inhibits glucose uptake in fat and muscle, promotes fatty acid release and increases protein catabolism-effects which are the direct opposite of those of insulin. At the same time however it stimulates the secretion of insulin by the pancreas. Blood levels of growth hormone are increased in the fasting state and some hours after a meal.

Glucocorticoids from the adrenal cortex cause hyperglycæmia mainly by their effect on protein metabolism and secondary stimulation of gluco-neogenesis. Their antagonism to insulin is illustrated by the extreme sensitivity to insulin of adrenalectomized animals and patients with Addison's disease.

Adrenaline (from the adrenal medulla) is considered one of the most important factors counteracting the hypoglycaemic effect of insulin. It suppresses the secretion of insulin and induces a rapid rise in blood sugar and lactate through increased glycogenolysis in liver and muscle, an effect dependent on activation of the phosphorylase system. Noradrenaline also raises blood glucose on injection in man but only after relatively high doses. Both amines, additionally, are powerful lipolytic agents. The release of the catecholamines—and particularly of adrenaline—in response to emotion, trauma and a variety of stressful stimuli thus rapidly mobilizes metabolites and energy from carbohydrate and fat stores.

Glucagon (secreted by the α cells of the pancreas) similarly raises blood glucose by a glycogenolytic effect mediated through phosphorylase but its action in this respect is limited to the liver; muscle glycogen is unaffected. Though a peripheral synergistic activity has been suggested between glucagon and insulin, the physiological role of the former and the factors controlling its release are not clear.

The differential release of the glucoregulatory hormones is adjusted to maintain blood glucose constant in the face of ingress from the alimentary tract after a meal and its utilization in accordance with tissue needs. The prime mover is probably the actual level of blood glucose and glucoreceptors in the brain, sensitive to changes in circulating glucose, have been postulated for this purpose. However, the fact that injection of amino acids such as arginine may evoke considerable changes in blood levels of human growth hormone and insulin but with only minor changes in blood glucose, suggests that, at tissue level, the trigger mechanism may involve factors other than changes in the level of blood glucose.

Diabetes Mellitus

The characteristic signs of diabetes mellitus, hyperglycaemia and glycosuria, can be produced experimentally in animals by interference with pancreatic function, either surgically by pancreatectomy or chemically by the injection of substances such as alloxan, streptozotocin, or anterior pituitary extracts. Clinically, however, it is the exception rather than the rule to find a pancreatic lesion, though insulin remedies many of the signs and symptoms of the disease. Hyperglycaemia and other classical accompaniments of the diabetic state may also be found in hyper-adrenocorticalism and hyper-pituitarism.

Changes in blood and urine glucose are the most striking and easily demonstrable diagnostic feature of diabetes but abnormalities can also be demonstrated in other aspects of carbohydrate and also of fat metabolism. Glycogen levels are lowered in liver and muscle, tissue glucose utilization is decreased and gluconeogenesis increased, the latter phenomenon being consequently associated with a negative protein balance; mobilization of fat and ketogenesis are increased. It has not been possible to pinpoint a single biochemical lesion in this condition, any more than it has been possible to define the precise site of action of insulin. There is no simple explanation in terms of insulin lack or antagonistic factors.

The development of the condition has been related, amongst other factors, to obesity, increased parity in women and increased levels of the synalbumin insulin antagonist. The raised levels of insulin found in people with normoglycaemia but with some degree of impaired carbohydrate tolerance has further been suggested as signalling the prelude of a diabetic diathesis, the initial response being an overproduction of insulin so as to maintain glucose homeostasis; eventually, the pancreas becomes exhausted, insulin secretion falls and hyperglycaemia develops.

Relevance to Obstetrics and Gynaecology

With this brief background in mind, certain aspects of carbohydrate metabolism in the foetus and pregnant women and possible clinical applications will now be considered.

Metabolism in pregnancy is essentially anabolic; the increased weight maintained by many women after delivery testifies to the efficiency of this process. Increasing demands by the conceptus for energy and synthetic materials are supplied by the mother across the placenta. Dietary standards in modern sophisticated communities are generally more than adequate for pregnancy and labour and even in the emergent countries the fertility of some of those on the poorest diet shows how little may suffice for a woman to produce a viable infant. Foetal nutrition depends much more on the adequacy of placental function than on the precise composition of maternal diet. Lactation, however, imposes greater demands which are normally met by the fat stored during pregnancy.

1. Foeto-Placental Metabolism

The foetus derives its energy almost exclusively from carbohydrate metabolism and requires a continuous supply of glucose for this purpose and also for manufacture of the basic metabolites essential in biosynthetic processes. Foetal tissues may in fact utilize glucose in preference to other precursors. Thus, cerebral cholesterol synthesis in the early human foetus depends largely on glucose; acetate incorporation into foetal brain cholesterol is apparently negligible.

A discussion of foetal carbohydrate metabolism requires consideration of two factors—firstly that the foetus depends on the mother for its glucose supply and secondly that, in view of the functional immaturity of many foetal organs, especially of the liver and the consequent incomplete development of many metabolic systems, the foetus is unable to carry out all aspects of synthetic function itself and depends on placental and maternal activity in this respect.

The foetus receives its supply of glucose by continuous "transfusion" across the placenta. Glucose crosses the placenta by facilitated diffusion, i.e. the direction of transfer is in accordance with the glucose concentration gradient between maternal and foetal blood, but the rate of glucose transfer from mother to foetus is accelerated beyond that expected on physiochemical grounds alone. Specialized carrier mechanisms have been postulated for the placental transport of glucose and of other sugars.

Our knowledge of human placental and foetal metabolism is based in the main on *in vitro* experiments. Extrapolation on the basis of data derived from *in vitro* studies of tissue metabolism to *in vivo* physiological function in the intact organism has obvious quantitative

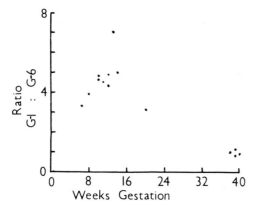

Fig. 2. Ratio of radioactive (^{14}C) carbon dioxide yields from placentae incubated with glucose-1-^{14}-C and glucose-6 ^{14}C at different stages of gestation. (From Beaconsfield, P., Ginsburg, J. and Jeacock, M. K. (1964) *Develop. Med. Child. Neurol.*, **6**, 469.)

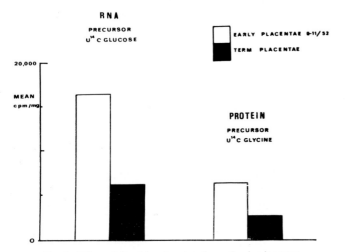

Fig. 3. Ribonucleic acid and protein formation in placentae incubated with U-^{14}C-glucose and U-^{14}C-glycine respectively (data from Beaconsfield, P., Ginsburg, J. and Kosinski, Z. (1965) *Nature*, **205**, 50).

limitations but as shown in tissues such as adult liver or brain, *in vitro* tissue metabolic sequence provides a valid qualitative reflection of physiological processes in the corresponding organ.

Human placental carbohydrate metabolism varies with the stage of gestation. In the early human placenta, the activity of the pentose pathway is considerably increased and, as in other tissues, the rates of nucleic acid and protein synthesis parallel the level of pentose pathway activity. At term, placental glucose metabolism by the pentose route is very much less than in the first trimester;

nucleic acid turnover and protein synthesis are also correspondingly lower. The observed differences in placental glucose metabolism during gestation parallel the relative rates of cell replication and placental growth in the first and third trimesters respectively.

The demonstration of glycogen in the placenta led Claude Bernard to describe this organ as "un veritable organe hépatique" and since that time the placenta has been held to subserve hepatic function for the foetus, pending the development of adequate homeostatic mechanisms in the foetus itself. Placental glycogen has been considered a potential store of glucose for the foetus, providing energy for foetal activity when metabolized; the fact that placental glycogen content is greater early in gestation than at term and that placental lactate production is higher in the early placenta before 14 weeks' gestation, than in term placentae, has been held to support

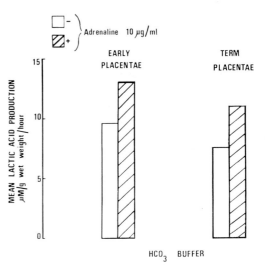

Fig. 4. Mean lactic acid production in early and term placentae incubated in the presence and absence of adrenaline (10 μg/ml.) (from Ginsburg, *J. Proc. Roy. Soc. Med.* (1966) **59**, 16).

this view. However, the observation that adrenaline increases placental lactate output and does not release glucose, even from early placentae, casts doubt on the concept of the placenta as the biochemical equivalent of the foetal liver. In fact, in respect of its metabolic response to adrenaline as to other hormones, the placenta bears a closer resemblance to skeletal muscle than to liver. Human placental carbohydrate metabolism is also affected by other hormones, at least *in vitro*. Insulin increases glucose uptake and glycogen deposition in the placenta and synthetic oxytocin (syntocinon) increases placental glucose uptake and lactate production. The disposal of excess placental lactate could be via the foetus or mother. The metabolite is freely diffusible across the primate placenta in either direction, but the high levels of lactate in amniotic fluid (about ten times that found in arterial blood) suggests that concentration occurs on the foetal side of the barrier.

The relative activity of the two main pathways for glucose metabolism has also been studied in foetal tissues at different stages of gestation. The developing blastocyst has an extremely active pentose shunt, and in foetuses of less than 8–10 weeks, cerebral and cardiac tissue showed elevated pentose phosphate activity. Later in gestation, however, the pattern of carbohydrate metabolism in each organ studied was similar to that of the corresponding adult tissue.

The relative rates of development of specific metabolic pathways and serial studies of enzyme activity during gestation in the human foetus are limited for obvious reasons. But, by analogy with experiments in rodents, where the enzymes concerned with glycogen synthesis increase rapidly towards the end of gestation, in parallel with the rate of glycogen deposition, the marked increase in human foetal hepatic and muscle glycogen observed near term is presumably related to the development of the enzymes required for glycogen synthesis in these tissues.

The foetus and newborn are more resistant to anoxia than the adult organism. The biochemical basis of the foetus' ability to withstand oxygen lack has not yet been related to a particular metabolic change. Altered rates of glycolysis and lipogenesis have been suggested and indeed the rate of glycolysis in foetal tissues, in anaerobic conditions, is generally greater than in adult tissues. But the brain, which is notoriously sensitive to interference with its glucose supply, has little glycogen and has similar rates of glycolysis in aerobic and anaerobic conditions. Recent studies have shown that metabolic protection for the brain during intra-uterine anoxia may be provided by the ability of foetal and neonatal cerebral tissue to metabolize substrates other than glucose, such as pyruvate, lactate and acetate.

The citric acid cycle can proceed in the absence of molecular oxygen provided that an adequate supply of the oxidized co-enzymes are available. It has been postulated that, in foetal tissues, the synthesis of fatty acids—a process which requires the hydrogen contained in reduced co-enzymes—may be increased during anoxia. Oxidized co-enzymes would thus be reformed and enable the pyruvate produced by glycolysis to be completely metabolized with release of further energy. Definitive evidence of a coupling of lipogenesis with glycolysis in foetal tissues during hypoxia has not yet however been provided.

The resistance of the foetus and neonate to hypoxia probably depends on a number of alterations in metabolic pattern in different tissues, each of which provides a small increase in metabolic efficiency and hence, overall, ensures a greater safety margin during oxygen lack.

2. Foetal Blood Glucose Homeostasis

The mechanisms responsible for maintenance of blood glucose homeostasis in the foetus have been surprisingly little studied. Whether maternal insulin crosses the placental barrier and thereby alters foetal blood glucose or whether its action is limited to an influence on maternal tissues and on placental metabolic activity is still disputed. Similarly, the factors determining release of foetal insulin are not known, nor have the effects of foetal and placental steroids on foetal carbohydrate metabolism been investigated.

The level of circulating glucose in the foetus is low *in utero*; glucose levels of under 50 mgm per cent may be found at birth, even in apparently normal babies and similarly, in monkeys before labour, foetal blood glucose is about half that found in maternal blood. The mechanisms responsible for foetal and neonatal hypoglycaemia have still not been fully explained. Possible factors include impaired foetal ability to release glucose from hepatic glycogen stores and limited rates of gluconeogenesis in placental and foetal tissues. The persistence of low levels of blood sugar after birth and the ocurrence of a fall in circulating glucose during the first few hours of life suggest altered mechanisms of glucose production or utilization in the neonate. Increased peripheral utilization has been suggested and supported by the fact that though insulin levels are normal in the newborn, the infant is extremely sensitive to the action of insulin. Against this, however, is the finding of prolonged hyperglycaemia after administration of glucagon and a diminished clearance rate of injected glucose, galactose or fructose. Impaired gluconeogenesis from precursors such as amino acids has also been suggested.

3. Maternal Metabolism

Profound changes occur in maternal carbohydrate and fat metabolism during pregnancy as evidenced by the increased blood levels of lactate, pyruvate and plasma lipid fractions, the rise being particularly marked in respect of phospholipids and non-esterified fatty acids, though little is known of the alteration in tissue metabolic sequence. Fasting blood glucose is not, however, raised in pregnant women.

In considering the mechanism maintaining blood glucose homeostasis during pregnancy, we must take into account, in addition to the factors discussed earlier on (see page 346), the influence on tissue carbohydrate metabolism of steroids produced by the placenta and foetus, and possible effects of foetal insulin and placental lactogen.

It has generally been assumed that carbohydrate tolerance is impaired in pregnancy and that pregnancy itself constitutes a diabetogenic stress for the woman. The increased incidence of diabetes after the menopause, in association with increased parity, the fact that diabetes may first present in pregnancy, that diabetic women frequently require increased amounts of insulin as pregnancy advances, the occurence of glycosuria in pregnancy and the increased resistance to insulin and tolbutamide demonstrated in late pregnancy, are all cited as evidence in support of this view.

However, fasting blood sugar is not increased in normal pregnancy and serial studies of carbohydrate tolerance in standard conditions, have failed to demonstrate impairment of carbohydrate tolerance in healthy women during gestation. Tolerance to intravenous glucose may in fact be improved in early pregnancy, compared with that recorded in the non-pregnant state.

In late pregnancy tolerance to exogenous glucose may be decreased relative to that recorded in the first trimester, but it is not necessarily reduced when compared with the pre-pregnant value or that measured after delivery. In the immediate post-partum period, there may, however, be a definite impairment.

Though carbohydrate tolerance is not reduced in normal pregnancy, peripheral resistance to insulin is increased; the fall in blood glucose after exogenous or endogenous insulin is less despite a greater rise in blood insulin after the injection of tolbutamide. These findings indicate that additional insulin is required in order to maintain normoglycaemia in pregnancy. Blood insulin levels are in fact raised in pregnancy both in the fasting state and after a glucose load. The increase in insulin secretion during pregnancy may strain pancreatic reserve which in turn may relate to the subsequent development of diabetes.

The paradox of increased amounts of circulating insulin in the absence of a hyperglycaemic stimulus, suggests either altered metabolism of insulin in the pregnant organism or the presence of additional "anti-insulin" factors. The former possibility is supported by the reduced half-life of insulin in pregnancy. Increased degradation of insulin by placental and foetal tissues has also been postulated, but insulin degradation by the human placenta has not been demonstrated. Indeed *in vitro* studies have shown that the hormone affects placental glucose metabolism and increases placental glycogen deposition.

As for "anti-insulin" factors, increased levels of the synalbumin antagonist to insulin have been reported in pregnant women and since urinary insulin clearance is reduced, altered protein binding of serum insulin has been suggested. Of the known humoral antagonists, growth hormone is unlikely to be responsible for the increased resistance to insulin, since fasting levels of human growth hormone were similar in pregnant and non-pregnant subjects. Placental lactogen, a polypeptide produced by the placenta has been suggested as the main antagonist to insulin in pregnancy. This hormone cross-reacts immunologically with HGH and shows some of the biological properties of growth hormone. Placental lactogen can be detected in serum at eight weeks' pregnancy; by the third trimester blood levels have increased at least ten times. Immediately after delivery the hormone disappears rapidly from the circulation and is virtually absent from the serum within 24 hours. Glucose tolerance is impaired, despite increased levels of insulin, after prolonged infusion over 8–12 hours of physiological amounts of placental lactogen in men. But whether placental lactogen antagonizes insulin directly in consequence of its own activity or as a result of a synergistic effect on HGH activity, has not been settled.

Alterations in other gluco-regulatory hormones—cortico-steroids, catecholamines and glucagon—in pregnancy, are less well defined. Plasma hydroxycorticosteroids are raised, largely as the result of an increase in binding protein associated with raised level of oestrogen. Whilst much of this bound steroid may be metabolically inactive, the alleviation of rheumatoid arthritis in pregnancy suggests greater availability of biologically active steroid. The half life of free cortisol is also increased in pregnancy. The increased secretion of insulin in pregnancy may therefore partially result from the presence of increased gluco-corticoid activity. Catecholamine and glucagon

levels are apparently unchanged in pregnancy, though the latter hormone induces a greater hyperglycaemic response in pregnancy than normal. We can only speculate on the possible effects of the increased levels of oestrogen and progesterone in pregnancy, for though oestrogens increase endometrial glucose utilization and glycogen formation, their influence on carbohydrate tolerance and tissue metabolism has not been adequately studied.

Increased secretion of both insulin and placental lactogen are thus apparently the main alterations in gluco-regulatory factors, which ensure normoglycaemia during gestation.

The stimulus for the observed metabolic and hormonal adjustments to pregnancy is not clear. Two concepts have been proposed in explanation—"Accelerated starvation" whereby the metabolic demands of the foetus and placenta preferentially divert glucose and gluconeogenic precursors, and induce a shift towards metabolism of fat in the peripheral maternal tissues, thereby ensuring that sufficient endogenous glucose is available for the brain. The increasing amounts of placental lactogen produced during gestation would thus provide an additional means of "sparing" maternal glucose and the raised fasting levels of plasma free fatty acids and insulin in pregnancy would be secondary phenomena. The alternative concept assigns a prime regulatory role to the secretion of placental lactogen and its antagonism to insulin.

Clinical Considerations

Discussion of the clinical consequences of changes in carbohydrate metabolism in pregnancy is limited both by our ignorance of many fundamental mechanisms and by the paucity of metabolic studies in obstetric disorders; the concluding sections deal with a few somewhat unrelated problems.

(1) Methodology

(a) **Blood glucose determinations.** Blood sugar determination by reduction procedures, which measure total reducing substances in the blood, give higher values than those recorded with an enzymic method measuring "true" glucose. Enzymic methods are preferred because of their greater specificity and reproductibility. Differences in the technique of collection and storage of blood samples before analysis also influence the results, particularly in the newborn, where the rate of red cell glycolysis *in vitro* is increased. Separation of the cells and precipitation should be carried out immediately after collection of the blood, or if this is not possible, the sample must be refrigerated with addition of a suitable preservative to the anticoagulant.

(b) **Glucose tolerance tests.** Carbohydrate tolerance can be assessed in response to oral or intravenous glucose. The oral test has been considered more physiological and has certain technical advantages in that relatively few samples are required and the entire test can be carried out by laboratory staff. It has the disadvantage that it may be affected by altered gastro-intestinal function and that pregnant women may vomit after hypertonic glucose, especially in late pregnancy. The intravenous response is more consistent and intravenous glucose is well tolerated by pregnant women; frequent samples and medical supervision are however, required during the test.

Neither test is totally acceptable in all circumstances. In the non-pregnant patient, the fasting blood sugar level will exclude or confirm active diabetes; a sample taken two hours after oral glucose or a full oral tolerance test will detect potential diabetes. If diabetes is suspected in early pregnancy, a fasting sample will similarly be adequate but a glucose tolerance test at this stage may give a misleading normal value. If potential diabetes is therefore suspected on clinical grounds, the tolerance test should be repeated after 30 weeks' gestation; an intravenous test is preferable at this stage. Glucose tolerance has been found impaired in the early puerperium; an abnormal response at this stage may not, therefore, be diagnostic of potential diabetes but requires confirmation by subsequent testing say at about 4 months.

(2) Glycosuria in Pregnancy

Glycosuria is relatively common in pregnant women; in fact, before the days of biological tests for pregnancy, sugar in the urine, especially after a glucose load, was taken as an indication of early pregnancy. The incidence of pregnancy glycosuria varies, in different series, from 5 per cent to over 50 per cent but with the increased use of papers impregnated with glucose oxidase for urine testing, the sensitivity of the procedure has greatly increased and glycosuria is now more frequently detected. Opinions differ, however, as to whether there is any correlation between the occurrence of glycosuria and the response to ingested glucose or foetal size, morbidity and mortality and hence as to whether the occurrence of glycosuria of itself necessitates a glucose tolerance test in a pregnant woman. Glucose is not the only sugar excreted; lactose and, to a lesser extent, ribose, xylose and fructose are also excreted but sensitive chromatographic procedures are required for detection of these sugars.

The mechanism of glycosuria in pregnancy is not clear. Glomerular filtration rate is increased in pregnancy but the rise in glomerular filtration rate is not related to the presence or absence of glycosuria in individual women. The most likely explanation is in terms of the decreased tubular capacity to reabsorb glucose demonstrated in pregnant women with glycosuria.

(3) Diabetes in Pregnancy

Diabetic women have a high incidence of foetal death in utero, both before and during labour. Their babies tend to be large, fat and may be "cushingoid" in appearance, but at the same time they are generally feeble and flabby, behaving like a very premature infant despite their greater size. Hypoglycaemia and feeding difficulties are common. Neonatal morbidity is high and the incidence of neonatal death increased; congenital malformations are more frequent.

The mechanism of altered foetal growth in diabetic pregnancy is not settled. Maternal hyperglycaemia, foetal islet-cell hypertrophy (a post mortem finding in babies born to diabetic women) with consequent foetal hyper-insulinism, excess pituitary growth hormone and glucocorticoids have all been implicated, but their precise role, individually or collectively, has not been determined.

That a primary disturbance in placental metabolism might be responsible is suggested by the raised glycogen content and enhanced placental lactate production, even in women whose diabetes was well controlled by insulin. Many of the foetal accompaniments of maternal diabetes are evident before the clinical onset of the disease;

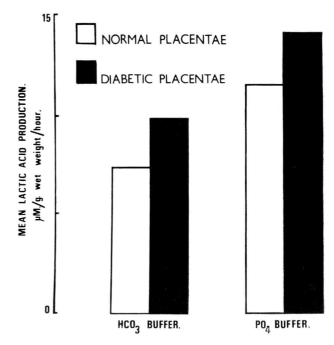

Fig. 5. Mean lactic acid production in normal and diabetic placentae incubated in phosphate or bicarbonate buffer (data from Ginsburg, J. and Jeacock, M. K.) (1966), **73,** 452.

perinatal mortality may, in fact, be higher before active diabetes is diagnosed because of the failure to take adequate precautions. The incidence of hydramnios and hypertension is greater than normal in diabetic women. Their insulin requirements generally increase and hypertensive disease of pregnancy is said to be more frequent.

The obstetric hazards of a diabetic pregnancy are reduced by careful dietary and drug control. The presence of glycosuria in pregnancy invalidates the customary aim of keeping the urine sugar free. Insulin requirements may therefore, have to be adjusted in relation to the level of blood glucose. Intermittent or even continuous supervision in hospital may be advisable from 32–34 weeks onwards. Induction of labour before term is general, with early intervention by caesarean section if delay in labour or foetal distress supervenes. The obstetric complications of latent or of potential diabetes can similarly be minimized by careful antenatal supervision and the clinical management of labour. Hence, the importance of timing and methodology in evaluating glucose tolerance in women whose obstetric or family history indicate the possibility of a diabetogenic trait.

(4) Labour and Caesarean Section

In any form of sustained vigorous exercise, the increased energy requirements are rapidly met by metabolism of glycogen, its contained energy being liberated with the formation of lactate. Similarly the energy demands of labour are met by breakdown of carbohydrates and shortly after each uterine contraction, there is a significant increase in maternal arterial lactate. Maternal metabolic acidosis is common in labour and is related to the onset of strong uterine contractions; foetal acidosis accompanies severe maternal acidosis. Uterine contractions also result in some degree of foetal anoxia, and hence foetal acidosis may increase further. Though, the foetus is relatively resistant to hypoxia, the severe asphyxia which may occur in prolonged labour or in cases of placental inadequacy would cause a rapid fall in cardiac and liver carbohydrate reserves; thus prolonged intra-uterine anoxia might exhaust foetal glycogen stores and hence result in foetal hypoglycaemia.

Experimental studies in animals have shown that the initial carbohydrate concentration in cardiac tissue is among the factors which determine foetal survival time after anoxia and that glucose injections prolong survival time. Studies in monkeys have shown further that the combined administration of glucose and alkali, so as to reduce the degree of metabolic acidosis, lowers the incidence and extent of permanent brain damage. The empirical administration of intravenous glucose to women in prolonged labour with acidosis gains support from these studies and the findings in primate experiments suggest that rational therapy should include the additional administration of base.

The pattern of metabolism in the puerperium has been little studied. Healing of the placental site has an obvious parallelism with wound healing after surgery and a caesarean section presumably evokes an endocrine and metabolic response essentially similar to that described after surgical trauma—namely increased adrenal activity (both cortical and medullary) and increased anterior pituitary activity, with a resultant increase in both glycogenolysis and gluconeogenesis. The impairment of glucose tolerance found in the immediate post-partum period is in accordance with this assumption. The extent to which the metabolic demands imposed by lactation modify this pattern is not however clear.

(5) Severe Hypoglycaemia in the Newborn

Blood sugar levels at birth and for some time thereafter may be significantly lower than normal in the premature and low birth weight infant. These low values have been attributed to two main factors—inadequate liver function with consequent impaired glucose output and the relatively large glucose dependent brain. Transient severe hypoglycaemia may also be found in babies of diabetic mothers, in infants with lesions of the central nervous system, or adrenal haemorrhage and in so-called symptomatic neonatal hypoglycaemia, which may be associated with maternal toxaemia. Treatment with intravenous glucose is recommended immediately on diagnosis, together with

ACTH or hydrocortisone if the hypoglycaemia recurs and persists after further glucose infusion. It has also been suggested that women at risk, i.e. with toxaemia, or premature labour, should be given intravenous glucose during labour, especially when foetal distress supervenes. Foetal blood glucose undoubtedly increases after maternal glucose or fructose infusion but controlled studies are needed to determine the effect of such procedures on foetal metabolism and neonatal function.

Prolonged, severe hypoglycaemia which persists after treatment may be due to a hereditary metabolic disturbance—glycogen storage disease where failure of glycogen degradation results from one of several specific enzyme defects, from impaired glycogen synthesis, or from fructose or galactose intolerance; rarely, an islet cell adenoma may be responsible.

(6) Glucose Tolerance and Hyperglycaemia in the Neonate

Despite the low levels of blood sugar which may be found at birth the new born infant has a relatively poor tolerance to injected glucose during its first month of extra-uterine life; thereafter carbohydrate tolerance improves. The lowered tolerance of the early neonatal period has been attributed, amongst other factors, to hyperadrenocorticalism (for the foetal adrenal gland is extremely active and impaired conjugation of cortisol has been demonstrated in the neonate), to insulin antagonists and to some degree of islet cell failure. Cases have also been reported with hyperglycaemia and glycosuria—so called idiopathic neonatal hyperglycaemia or transient neonatal diabetes mellitus—associated with polyuria, polydypsia and dehydration but in the absence of ketosis. This rare condition characteristically occurs in full term infants of low birth weight; small doses of insulin are sufficient to restore normoglycaemia and the hormone is usually only required for a relatively short period.

(7) Glucose Tolerance during the Menstrual Cycle

It would be reasonable to expect that the phasic changes in steroid production which occur in the normal menstrual cycle, would be accompanied by changes in secretion rate and activity of other hormones and thus influence tissue metabolism. Diabetic control is said to deteriorate and insulin requirements to increase at the time of menstruation, but there are no studies of the secretion rate of glucoregulatory hormones at different stages of the menstrual cycle. The available studies of carbohydrate metabolism during the cycle have provided conflicting data. Fasting blood sugar has been variously reported as raised or lowered premenstrually, compared with levels recorded at mid-cycle; similarly, carbohydrate tolerance is said to be unchanged during a normal ovulatory cycle or improved in the early part of the cycle. Large scale studies are needed to determine whether cyclical changes occur consistently in a significant proportion of women, and hence whether it is necessary to consider the "time of the month" in the performance and interpretation of glucose tolerance tests.

(8) Effects of Oral Contraceptives on Carbohydrate Metabolism

A rise in fasting blood sugar and impaired tolerance to ingested or intravenous carbohydrate have been demonstrated in a proportion of women taking different progestin and oestrogen mixtures, especially in those with a family history of diabetes. Elevated levels of plasma non-esterified fatty acids, pyruvic acid, insulin and HGH have also been reported and established diabetics may require increased amounts of insulin while on oral contraceptives. The oestrogen component has been considered responsible for the impairment in glucose tolerance, but at the time of writing, the available studies have not distinguished between the separate effects on carbohydrate metabolism of the oestrogen and progestogen constituents of current oral contraceptives.

Long term consequences of these metabolic changes and the extent to which they are reversible when progestational agents are discontinued have not yet been established. Short term studies in women taking Enovid over 18 months have shown a partial reversal of the initial decline in glucose tolerance during continued oral contraception. Since, however, this relative improvement may be achieved through increased pancreatic stimulation, as evidenced by the rise in plasma insulin in women taking oral progestogens, pancreatic exhaustion and a diabetic state with the inevitable accompaniments, could eventually result. Impaired carbohydrate tolerance in other circumstances undoubtedly precedes the onset of diabetes in later years.

(9) Carbohydrate Tolerance in Genital Carcinoma, Sterility and Abortion

It is not surprising, in view of the central role of glucose in metabolic processes, that abnormalities of carbohydrate metabolism should have been found in women with gynaecological disease. Altered carbohydrate metabolism with glycosuria, raised fasting levels of blood glucose and impaired tolerance to a glucose load has been demonstrated in women with cervical carcinoma. In endometrial carcinoma, which occurs in an older age group, an association with diabetes and impaired glucose tolerance has long been presumed, but recent studies with carefully matched controls conflict with the earlier findings.

Before the discovery of insulin it was exceptional for the young diabetic to become pregnant and even nowadays the poorly controlled diabetic has difficulty in conceiving. A high incidence of impaired carbohydrate tolerance has been reported in women with sterility and previous abortions; abnormalities of endometrial carbohydrate metabolism have also been described in such cases. Our present tests are, however, too crude and non-specific to provide an adequate guide to therapy in such cases.

Much of the above description will undoubtedly require revision in the light of current and subsequent research, particularly with increasing use of sensitive radio-immunological assay techniques for estimating hormones in biological fluids. It is surprising, however, with all the specialized techniques now available that we are still so ignorant of the factors which make pregnancy possible. Perhaps it is because the clinicians lack the necessary expertise and the basic scientists are not aware of their potential clinical significance. Either way, it is time that a marriage was arranged.

REFERENCES

Baker, D. P., Hutchison, J. R. and Vaughan, D. L. (1968), **31**, 475.

Beaconsfield, P., Ginsburg, J. and Jeacock, M. (1964), *Develop. med. Child. Neurol.*, **6**, 469.

Beaconsfield, P., Ginsburg, J. and Kosinski, Z. (1965), *Nature*, **205**, 50.

Beaconsfield, P. and Morris, N. F. (1967), *Europa Medica*, **3**, 3.

Bleicher, S. J., O'Sullivan, J. B. and Freinkel, N. (1964), *New Eng. J. Med.*, **271**, 866.

Cornblath, M. and Schwartz, R. (1966), *Disorders of Carbohydrate Metabolism in Infancy*. Philadelphia: W. B. Saunders Co.

Dawkins, M. J. R. (1966), *Brit. med. Bull.*, **22**, 27.

Fine, J. (1967), *Brit. med. J.*, **i**, 205.

Freinkel, N. (1964), *Diabetes*, **13**, 260.

Fruton, J. S. and Simmonds, Sofia (1966), *General Biochemistry*. New York: John Wiley & Sons. Inc.

Ginsburg, J. and Jeacock, M. K. (1964), *Bio. Chem. Bio. Phys. Acta.*, **90**, 166.

Ginsburg, J. and Jeacock, M. K. (1968), *Amer. J. Obstet. Gynec.*, **100**, 357.

Kyle, G. K. (1963), *Ann. intern. Med., Supplement*, **3**.

Mahler, H. R. and Cordes, E. H. (1966), *Biological Chemistry*, New York: Harper and Co.

Oakley, W., Pyke, D. A. and Taylor, K. W. (1968), *Clinical Diabetes*, Blackwell Sci.

Pyke, D. A. (edited by), (1962), *Disorders of Carbohydrate Metabolism*. London: Pitman Medical Publishing Co.

Shelley, H. J. and Neligan, G. A. (1966), *Brit. med. Bull.*, **22**, 37.

Spellacy, W. N. and Carlson, K. L. (1966), *Amer. J. Obstet. Gynec.*, **95**, 474.

Trayner, I. M., Welborn, T. A., Rubenstein, A. H. and Russell-Fraser, T. (1967), *J. Endocr.*, **37**, 443.

Villee, C. A. (1962), *Amer. J. Obstet. Gynec.*, **84**, 1684.

Wright, A. D., Dixon, H. G. and Joplin, E. F. (1968), *Brit. med. Bull.*, **24**, 25.

Wynn, V. and Doar, J. W. H. (1966), *Lancet*, **ii**, 715.

2. LIPID METABOLISM

N. B. MYANT

INTRODUCTION

Definition

The lipids are a chemically heterogeneous group of substances characterized by their solubility in chloroform, benzene and other non-aqueous solvents. Strictly speaking, the term includes, in addition to the major energy-providing and structural lipids, many other substances such as fat-soluble vitamins and essential fatty acids. In this chapter we shall be concerned mainly with fatty acids, triglycerides and cholesterol.

Functions of lipids

Lipids carry out a wide variety of functions in the body. The fatty acids and their breakdown products act as sources of oxidative energy in muscle and other tissues. Adipose tissue, whose main constituent is triglyceride, acts as a heat-insulator and as a readily available store of fuel in the form of fatty acids and glycerol. The storage capacity of adipose tissue is remarkably high; in a normal human being the potential chemical energy stored as triglyceride in the whole of the adipose tissue is several hundred times greater than that stored as carbohydrate, including the glycogen of liver and muscle and the glucose in the blood. Brown fat, a specialized form of adipose tissue, plays an important part in the production of heat in response to cold in new-born animals and in adult animals adapted to a cold environment (see Section VI, Ch. 2). Subcutaneous adipose tissue also contributes to sex differences in body contour.

Lipids act as structural components of the cellular and intracellular membranes of all animal tissues. This may be one of the functions of essential fatty acids, since they are present in the phospholipids of cell walls and of mitochondrial membranes. The function of the lipids in membranous structures is far from clear. They may help to determine the selective permeability of the cell wall, so important for the proper functioning of the cell. But they may also act in a more subtle way, perhaps by participating in the many biochemical reactions that are catalyzed by enzymes bound to membranes.

Cholesterol serves as a structural lipid, particularly in the central nervous system. It is also a precursor of bile acids and of most, if not all, of the steroid hormones, including those formed by the gonads.

Relevance to Obstetrics and Gynaecology

A rational approach to the practice of any branch of medicine requires some understanding of what lipids are and of how they are synthesized and metabolized; these questions are dealt with in the first sections of this chapter. Certain aspects of the biochemistry and physiology of lipids, however, are of special importance in Obstetrics and Gynaecology. For example, the growing fœtus must lay down considerable quantities of lipids of all classes, including a store of fat in preparation for neonatal life. Again, during pregnancy and lactation there are marked changes in the output of hormones by the mother, some of which have effects on lipid metabolism. These effects may have a bearing on the changes in body fat that commonly occur in women at various stages in reproductive life. There is also the question of the production of milk fat during lactation. These and other related topics are considered in the later sections of this chapter.

CHEMISTRY

A convenient way of classifying the chief animal lipids is to divide them into the following groups:

1. Fatty acids.
2. Triglycerides (neutral fats).
3. Complex lipids, including phospholipids and glycolipids.
4. Steroids.

Fatty Acids

The commoner fatty acids of animal tissues are unbranched aliphatic acids with one carboxyl group and an even number of carbon atoms. They may be fully saturated or they may have one or more double bonds in the carbon chain. The short-chain fatty acids, such as acetic acid, are soluble in water and are not, therefore, true lipids. Fatty acids with more than six carbon atoms are immiscible with water and are soluble in lipid solvents. Table 1 shows the molecular formula, common name and

TABLE 1

SOME LONG-CHAIN FATTY ACIDS OF ANIMAL TISSUES

Molecular formula	Common name	Abbreviation	Positions of double bonds (carboxyl carbon = 1)
$C_{16}H_{32}O_2$	Palmitic	16:0	—
$C_{16}H_{30}O_2$	Palmitoleic	16:1	9,10
$C_{18}H_{36}O_2$	Stearic	18:0	—
$C_{18}H_{34}O_2$	Oleic	18:1	9,10
$C_{18}H_{32}O_2$	Linoleic	18:2	9,10; 12,13
$C_{18}H_{30}O_2$	Linolenic	18:3	9,10; 12,13; 15,16
$C_{20}H_{32}O_2$	Arachidonic	20:4	5,6; 8,9; 11,12; 14,15

positions of the double bonds of some of the more important long-chain fatty acids. The carbon atoms are numbered from the carboxyl end of the molecule.

A useful system of notation for saturated and unsaturated fatty acids is to write the number of carbon atoms in the molecule, followed by the number of double bonds. Thus, linoleic acid,

$$\overset{13}{CH_3}.(CH_2)_4.\overset{12}{CH}=\overset{11}{CH}.\overset{10}{CH_2}.\overset{9}{CH}=CH.(CH_2)_7.\overset{1}{COOH}$$

is denoted by 18:2, and arachidonic acid is denoted by 20:4.

Triglycerides

The triglycerides, often called "neutral fats", are esters of long-chain fatty acids with glycerol, a trihydroxy alcohol ($CH_2OH.CHOH.CH_2OH$). The general formula of triglycerides is:

$$
\begin{array}{ll}
R.COO.CH_2 & (\alpha) \\
R'.COO.CH & (\beta) \\
R''.COO.CH_2 & (\alpha')
\end{array}
$$

where R.COO, R'.COO and R".COO stand for three molecules of the same or different fatty acids. The three carbon atoms of the glycerol molecule are referred to as α, β and α'. A given triglyceride molecule may contain both saturated and unsaturated long-chain fatty acids. On complete hydrolysis, each molecule of triglyceride yields three molecules of fatty acid and one of glycerol:

$$
\begin{array}{l}
R.COO.CH_2 \\
R'.COO.CH + 3H_2O \rightarrow \\
R''.COO.CH_2
\end{array}
\quad
\begin{array}{l}
R.COOH \\
+ \\
R'.COOH \\
+ \\
R''.COOH
\end{array}
\quad
\begin{array}{l}
CH_2OH \\
CHOH \quad (1) \\
CH_2OH
\end{array}
$$

Triglyceride   Fatty acids   Glycerol

Most of the fat in adipose tissue is in the form of triglyceride. The fatty acid composition of triglyceride in the depot fat varies with the stage of development of the individual and with the proportions of different fatty acids in the diet. In adult human beings on a balanced diet, oleic and palmitic acids together account for more than 65 per cent of the triglyceride fatty acids of adipose tissue, linoleic, palmitoleic, stearic and arachidonic acids accounting for a smaller proportion (Table 2).

TABLE 2

FATTY ACID COMPOSITION OF THE TRIGLYCERIDES OF SUBCUTANEOUS ADIPOSE TISSUE FROM NEW-BORN INFANTS AND FROM NORMAL ADULTS

Fatty acid	Percentage of total fatty acids	
	New-born	Adult
16:0	40·2	19·5
16:1	14·6	6·9
18:0	5·1	4·2
18:1	25·2	46·7
18:2	1·3	11·4
20:4	0·3	0·2

Values taken from Hirsch (1965).

Complex Lipids

(a) Phospholipids

These are lipids with one or more phosphorus atoms in the molecule. The most abundant phospholipid is lecithin, a structural derivative of an α', β-diglyceride in which a choline residue is attached to the α carbon of the glycerol through a phosphate group:

$$
\begin{array}{l}
CH_2.OOC.R \\
R'.COO.CH \quad\quad O \\
CH_2-O-P-\boxed{O-CH_2.CH_2.N(CH_3)_3OH} \\
\quad\quad\quad OH \quad\quad\quad\quad\text{(choline residue)}
\end{array}
$$

Lecithin

In a typical lecithin, R.COO would be 18:0 and R'.COO would be 18:2. In other phospholipids, the choline residue is replaced by ethanolamine, serine or inositol. In sphingomyelin, an important structural phospholipid, the diglyceride residue is replaced by an amino alcohol (sphingosine) linked to a fatty acid.

(b) Glycolipids

The glycolipids are complex lipids containing sphingosine attached to a long-chain fatty acid, and one or more carbohydrate residues per molecule. In the cerebrosides the carbohydrate may be glucose or galactose. In the gangliosides, in addition to one or more hexose residues in each molecule, there are also several molecules of an amino sugar. Both cerebrosides and gangliosides are important constituents of nerve tissue and of cell membranes.

Steroids

The steroids are tetracyclic compounds containing the phenanthrene ring-system (rings A, B and C of cholesterol). By far the most abundant steroid is cholesterol, a steroid alcohol (or sterol) with a 3β-hydroxyl group and a branched side-chain with eight carbon atoms (Fig. 1).

About two thirds of the plasma cholesterol is esterified with long-chain fatty acids through the formation of an ester bond between the carboxyl group of the fatty acid and the hydroxyl group of cholesterol. Most of the cholesterol in the tissues is free, or unesterified. By modification of the ring-system and side-chain, cholesterol is converted in the body into a number of steroids of biological importance (Fig. 1). Of these, the bile acids are quantitatively the most important. The bile acids, of which cholic acid (Fig. 1) is the most abundant in human bile, are conjugated with glycine or taurine to form the bile salts.

REQUIREMENT FOR DIETARY FAT

Provided that the requirements for fat-soluble vitamins and essential fatty acids are satisfied, dietary lipid is not essential for normal growth and maintenance since the body can synthesize adequate amounts of lipids from carbohydrates and other sources. Nevertheless, owing to its high calorie value, a moderate amount of triglyceride fat is desirable in a well-balanced diet.

Essential Fatty Acids

Young animals given a fat-free diet supplemented with the fat-soluble vitamins develop skin lesions and do not grow at the normal rate. The addition to the diet of linoleic acid or arachidonic acid brings about normal growth and cures the skin lesions. Linolenic acid restores

ABSORPTION

Dietary fat is absorbed in the upper part of the small intestine.

At the pH in the lumen of the upper intestine the fatty acids arising from the hydrolysis of triglycerides form soaps. The soaps and bile salts in the intestinal fluid act as detergents, forming molecular aggregates with triglycerides, partial glycerides, cholesterol and other lipids. These mixed molecular aggregates are known as "micelles". The particles of a micellar solution are less than $10 \, m\mu$

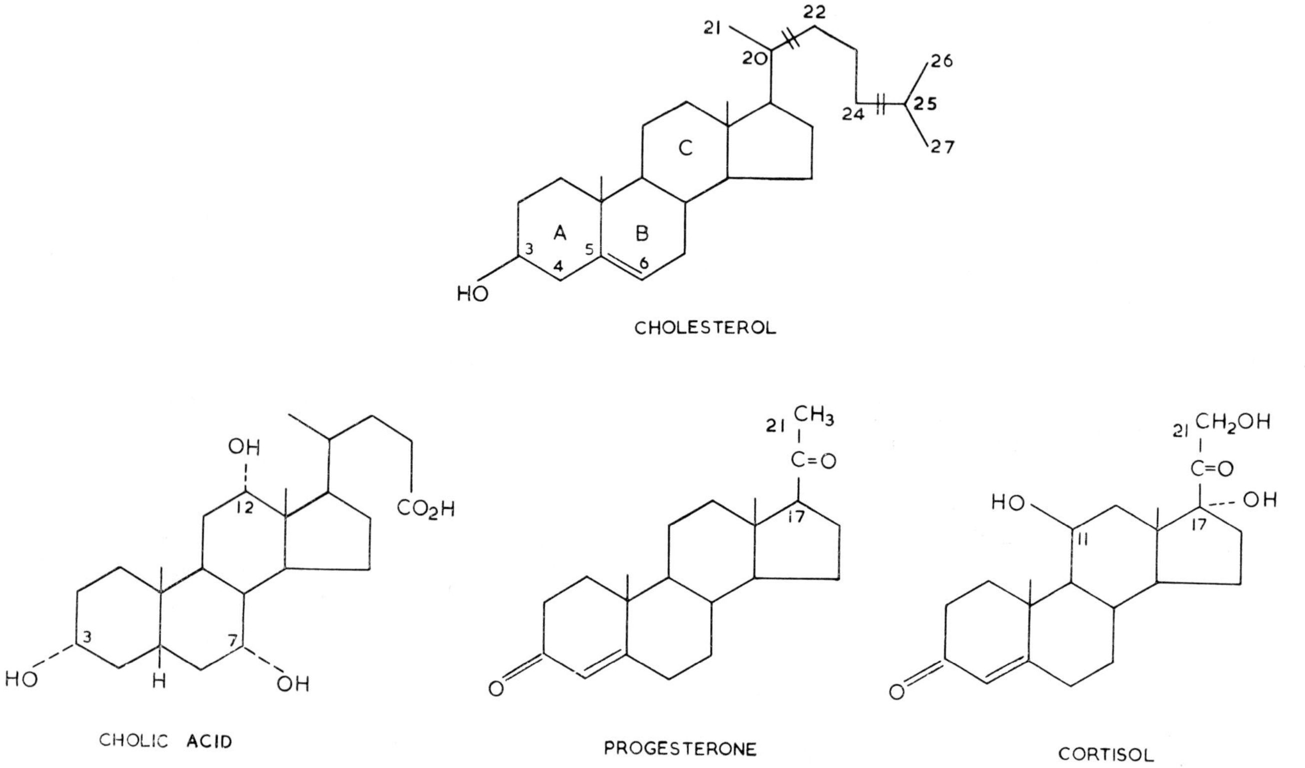

FIG. 1. Cholesterol and three of its biologically active metabolites formed in the animal body.

growth to the normal but does not cure the skin lesions. Linoleic, linolenic and arachidonic acids are usually classed as essential fatty acids, but this is open to criticism because it is not necessary to provide all three fatty acids in the diet. Arachidonic acid can be formed in the animal body from linoleic acid, so that arachidonic acid need not be added to the diet if linoleic acid is present.

There is some evidence that man has the same requirement as animals for unsaturated fatty acids; a syndrome resembling that seen in animals given a diet with no essential fatty acids occurs in infants fed artificial diets lacking fatty acids with two or more double bonds, and the symptoms of this disease are cured by giving linoleic acid. Owing to the wide distribution of unsaturated fatty acids in plant and animal foods, disease due to an absolute dietary deficiency of essential fatty acids probably does not occur in man. It is possible, however, that a partial deficiency of essential fatty acids may contribute to the high plasma cholesterol level seen in people who eat a diet rich in saturated fats and poor in unsaturated fats.

in diameter (far smaller than the particles of a fine emulsion) and readily enter the cells of the intestinal mucosa. According to current ideas, once the lipids have entered the mucosal cells, they are detached from the micelles and recombined, together with protein, to form chylomicra (particles $1–10 \, \mu$ in diameter). The chylomicra enter the intestinal lymphatics and reach the circulation via the thoracic duct. The bile salts do not enter the lymphatics with the chylomicra, but return to the intestinal lumen and pass down to the ileum, from which they are reabsorbed via the portal blood.

The fat-soluble vitamins and some of the steroid hormones, including cortisol, are readily absorbed by the human intestine. The mechanism by which these substances are absorbed is not fully understood, but it is likely that they enter the mucosal cells of the intestine in micellar form and that they then become incorporated into the chylomicra.

Fatty acids with a chain length of less than ten are absorbed in non-esterified form via the portal venous system, appearing only to a small extent in the chylomicra. This is of practical importance since the fats of some milks contain high proportions of short-chain fatty acids (see Table 4).

BREAKDOWN AND SYNTHESIS OF LIPIDS

All the lipids in the animal body are in a state of continuous breakdown and resynthesis. The rate of turnover, however, varies widely among the different lipid fractions. For example, the free fatty acids of the plasma are almost completely replaced every few minutes, whereas renewal of the structural lipids of adult myelin may take months, or even years. Most animal tissues can synthesize lipids of all classes from precursors of low molecular weight throughout life. A notable exception is the central nervous system. Synthesis of cholesterol and other myelin lipids by central nervous tissue is rapid in the foetus and immature animal, but falls to a low level in the adult.

Fatty Acids

(a) Oxidation

Fatty acids are a major source of oxidative energy, not only in starvation, but also under conditions of normal feeding. Under basal conditions, oxidation of fatty acids probably accounts for about half the total oxygen consumed by the whole body. During prolonged moderate exercise the requirement for extra energy is met largely by oxidation of fatty acids. Individual tissues vary considerably in their ability to oxidize fatty acids.

The main pathway for the oxidation of long-chain fatty acids is by β-oxidation. In this pathway, the fatty acid, in the form of its coenzyme-A (CoA) ester (see reaction 2), is degraded by repeated oxidative removal of two-carbon units of acetyl-CoA from the carboxyl end of the molecule. Each step requires an additional molecule of CoA and results in the formation of one molecule of acetyl-CoA and the CoA ester of a new fatty acid with two carbon atoms less than the parent molecule. All the enzymes required for the whole process are present in the mitochondria.

The first two steps in the β-oxidation of a fatty acid may be written:

$$CH_3.(CH_2)_n.\overset{\beta}{C}H_2.\overset{\alpha}{C}H_2.CO.CoA + CoA + O_2 \rightarrow$$
$$CH_3.(CH_2)_n.CO.CoA + CH_3.CO.CoA + H_2O$$
$$\text{Acetyl-CoA} \quad (2)$$

$$CH_3.(CH_2)_{n-2}.\overset{\beta}{C}H_2.\overset{\alpha}{C}H_2.CO.CoA + CoA + O_2 \rightarrow$$
$$CH_3.(CH_2)_{n-2}.CO.CoA + CH_3.CO.CoA + H_2O$$
$$\text{Acetyl-CoA} \quad (3)$$

At each step, one molecule of oxygen is consumed and the β carbon atom of the fatty acid ester becomes the carboxyl carbon of the new acid. Repetition of this sequence results in the conversion of the whole carbon chain into units of acetyl-CoA, which are then oxidized to CO_2 and water by mitochondrial enzymes of the citric acid cycle.

Unsaturated fatty acids are oxidized as rapidly as are the saturated acids, probably by a modification of the β-oxidation pathway.

(b) Synthesis

In animal tissues, long-chain fatty acids are synthesized in two ways. Most fatty acid synthesis takes place by a process which consists essentially in the joining together of two-carbon units derived from acetate. This may be called *de novo* synthesis. In addition to this, some fatty acid is synthesized by another pathway in which preformed fatty acids are elongated by the addition of one or more two-carbon units.

(i) **Synthesis *de novo*.** The first step in *de novo* synthesis of fatty acids is the formation of the CoA ester of malonic acid by the addition of CO_2 to the CoA ester of acetic acid:

$$CH_3.CO.CoA + CO_2 \rightarrow CH_2.CO.CoA \quad (4)$$
$$\underset{COOH}{|}$$
$$\text{Acetyl-CoA} \qquad \text{Malonyl-CoA}$$

This reaction is catalyzed by an enzyme, acetyl-CoA carboxylase, and requires ATP, biotin and manganese. In the next step, one malonyl unit condenses with the carboxyl group of an acetyl unit, with loss of the CO_2 added in reaction 4. There is therefore a net addition of two carbon atoms to the two-carbon acetyl unit. Since this reaction takes place while the reacting molecules are attached to the surface of an enzyme complex (E), it may be written:

$$CH_3.CO.E + CH_2.CO.E \rightarrow$$
$$\underset{COOH}{|} \qquad \overset{\beta}{C}H_3.CO.\overset{\alpha}{C}H_2.CO.E + CO_2$$
$$\underset{\text{enzyme}}{\text{Acetyl}} \quad \underset{\text{enzyme}}{\text{Malonyl}} \quad \underset{\text{enzyme}}{\text{Acetoacetyl}}$$
$$(5)$$

The product of this reaction is an enzyme-bound acid with four carbon atoms and a keto group in the β position. Reduction of the keto acid by a reduced coenzyme (NADPH₂), while the acid is still attached to the enzyme complex, gives rise to a saturated enzyme-bound fatty acid:

$$CH_3.CO.CH_2.CO.E + 2 NADPH_2 \rightarrow$$
$$\text{Acetoacetyl enzyme}$$
$$CH_3.CH_2.CH_2.CO.E + 2 NADP + H_2O \quad (6)$$
$$\text{Butyryl enzyme}$$

By a reaction analogous to reaction 4, another malonyl unit is added to the carboxyl end of the new fatty acid, with loss of CO_2, to give a six-carbon β-keto acid:

$$CH_3.CH_2.CH_2.CO.E + CH_2.CO.E \rightarrow$$
$$\underset{COOH}{|}$$
$$\underset{\text{Butyryl enzyme}}{} \qquad \underset{\text{Malonyl enzyme}}{}$$
$$CH_3.(CH_2)_2.\overset{\beta}{C}O.\overset{\alpha}{C}H_2.CO.E + CO_2 \quad (7)$$
$$\text{β-keto caproyl enzyme}$$

The new keto acid is then reduced to the corresponding saturated fatty acid. Repetition of the whole process results eventually in the formation of a 16- or 18-carbon-atom fatty acid bound to the enzyme complex. The fatty acid is then split off from the enzyme as free palmitic or stearic acid.

The complete sequence may be summarized as the successive addition of two-carbon units to the carboxyl end of a growing fatty acid chain, each addition being followed by a reduction. This method of synthesis explains the preponderance in animal fats of fatty acids with an even number of carbon atoms. The apparently wasteful addition and removal of CO_2 at each step probably serves to activate the carbon atom that condenses with the carboxyl carbon of the growing fatty acid.

From the above description it will be seen that fatty acid synthesis requires, in addition to the necessary enzymes, a supply of carbon in the form of acetyl-CoA and a supply of reductive hydrogen in the form of $NADPH_2$. The acetyl-CoA is derived largely from the breakdown of carbohydrate, and the hydrogen for maintaining $NADPH_2$ in the reduced state is derived partly from glucose oxidation and partly from other reactions.

(ii) **Synthesis by elongation.** An enzyme system catalyzing the elongation of saturated and unsaturated fatty acids with 12 or more carbon atoms is present in the mitochondria and microsomes of most tissues. The fatty acids formed by this pathway have up to 24 carbon atoms.

(c) **Transformations of Fatty Acids**

In addition to their conversion into triglycerides, and into cholesteryl esters and complex lipids, long-chain fatty acids undergo several metabolic transformations in the animal body.

Saturated fatty acids may be desaturated to give fatty acids containing one or more double bonds. In this way, palmitic and stearic acids can be converted, respectively, into palmitoleic and oleic acids (see Table 1). In animal tissues, only certain double bonds can be introduced into the carbon chain of a fatty acid. A double bond cannot, for instance, be introduced into the 12, 13 position of oleic acid to form linoleic acid. If, however, linoleic acid is supplied in the diet, it can be converted into arachidonic acid by chain elongation and the introduction of the two additional double bonds required to give the 20:4 acid.

Arachidonic acid may be converted into prostaglandins. These are a group of substances first isolated from seminal plasma, but since shown to be present in several other tissues. They arise from arachidonic and other essential fatty acids by a series of modifications which include the formation of a bridge between C-8 and C-12. Figure 2 shows the structure of prostaglandin E_1.

Prostaglandins, when injected in very small doses (0·2 μg./kg./min.), lower the blood pressure and inhibit the release of fatty acids from adipose tissue in man. When instilled into the vagina during ovulation, prostaglandins cause an initial increase in the motility of the uterus, followed by relaxation of the cervix. They also inhibit the motility of human uterine muscle *in vitro* at extremely low concentrations. The potent pharmacological effects of prostaglandins suggest that they are necessary for the normal functioning of the body. They may play some part in controlling fat mobilization. It has also been suggested that the effect of prostaglandins on uterine motility is to give the spermatozoa an "assisted passage" to the ovum at a critical stage in fertilization.

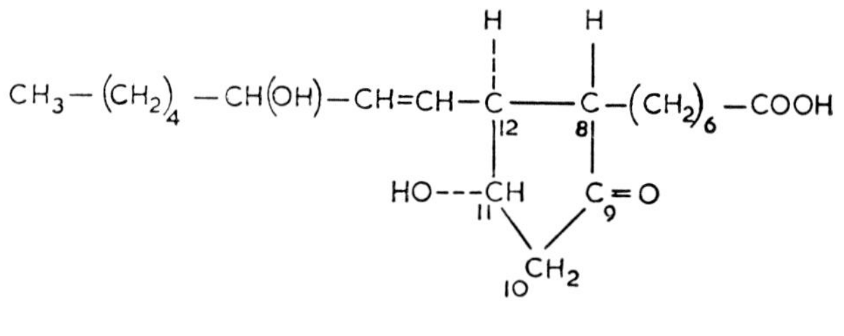

$$CH_3-(CH_2)_4-CH(OH)-CH=CH-\underset{12}{C}-\underset{8}{C}-(CH_2)_6-COOH$$

PROSTAGLANDIN E_1

FIG. 2. Prostaglandin E_1, showing the bridge between C-8 and C-12 of the carbon chain of arachidonic acid.

Triglycerides

The triglycerides of adipose tissue and liver are not, as was once believed, an inert store of fat used only during starvation. On the contrary, triglycerides are constantly broken down and resynthesized, although the total amount of triglyceride fat in the body remains roughly constant from day to day when caloric balance is maintained. Breakdown of tissue triglyceride is catalyzed by intracellular lipases whose action, like that of the pancreatic lipase secreted into the intestine, results in the formation of free fatty acids, partial glycerides and glycerol.

Triglycerides are synthesized from the CoA esters of long-chain fatty acids and the phosphate ester of glycerol (α-glycerophosphate). The overall reaction may be written:

$$3\ R.CO.CoA + \begin{matrix} CH_2OH \\ | \\ CHOH \\ | \\ CH_2OPO_3H_2 \end{matrix} \rightarrow$$

Fatty acid ester α-Glycero-phosphate

$$\rightarrow \begin{matrix} R.COO.CH_2 \\ | \\ R.COO.CH \\ | \\ R.COO.CH_2 \end{matrix} + 3\ CoA + Pi \quad (8)$$

Triglyceride   Phosphate

α-Glycerophosphate is synthesized in liver and in some other tissues by the phosphorylation of glycerol, a reaction which requires ATP and an enzyme, glycerokinase:

$$\begin{matrix} CH_2OH \\ | \\ CHOH \\ | \\ CH_2OH \end{matrix} + ATP \xrightarrow{\text{glycerokinase}} \begin{matrix} CH_2OH \\ | \\ CHOH \\ | \\ CH_2OPO_3H_2 \end{matrix} + ADP \quad (9)$$

Glycerol α-Glycero-phosphate

Adipose tissue has no glycerokinase and therefore cannot synthesize α-glycerophosphate from glycerol. In adipose tissue, α-glycerophosphate is formed by reduction of dihydroxyacetone phosphate, a product of glycolysis. This is important in the regulation of triglyceride synthesis in adipose tissue (see Mobilization of Fat).

Cholesterol

Cholesterol is removed from the body either by excretion in the bile, or by metabolism to other substances. The major route for the metabolism of cholesterol is its conversion into bile acids by oxidative removal of the last

released into the bloodstream. Within the cells of adipose tissue, triglycerides undergo a continual cycle of hydrolysis to free fatty acids and glycerol (reaction 1), followed by resynthesis of triglycerides (reaction 8). At each turn of the cycle, some fatty acid diffuses into the bloodstream and is reversibly adsorbed to the plasma albumin. In this form, fatty acids circulate as the plasma free fatty acids, or "FFA". The plasma FFA are transported to the tissues, where they are oxidized, or metabolized in other ways. As may be seen from Fig. 3, the amount of FFA released into the blood is a function of the relative rates of hydrolysis and resynthesis. A net increase in FFA release could

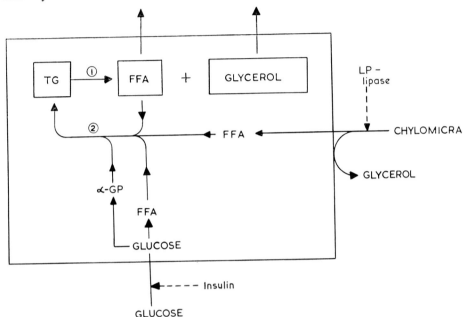

FIG. 3. Diagram representing the inside of an adipose tissue cell, to show the main features of the triglyceride cycle. Intracellular triglycerides are hydrolyzed (1) to FFA and glycerol. Some FFA and all the glycerol diffuse into the bloodstream. Triglycerides are resynthesized (2) from α-glycerophosphate derived from glucose, and from FFA. The FFA used for resynthesis is derived from glucose, from triglyceride hydrolysis and from triglyceride in the chylomicra. Hydrolysis of chylomicra at the surface of the cell is catalyzed by lipoprotein lipase. The FFA from chylomicra enter the fat cell and the glycerol is released into the bloodstream. Transport of glucose from the plasma into the cell requires insulin. *Abbreviations*: α-GP, α-glycerophosphate; FFA, free fatty acids; LP-lipase, lipoprotein lipase; TG, triglycerides.

three carbon atoms of the side-chain and modification of the ring-system (Fig. 1). All the enzymes necessary for these reactions, and for the conjugation of bile acids with taurine and glycine, are present in the liver.

The adrenal cortex and the gonads contain an entirely different set of enzymes which catalyze the cleavage of the side-chain of cholesterol between C-20 and C-22 to give pregnenolone, which is then converted into progesterone (Fig. 1). Progesterone is converted into glucocorticoids in the adrenal cortex and into sex hormones in the gonads.

Cholesterol is synthesized from acetate, synthesis being especially active in liver, intestinal wall and developing nervous system.

MOBILIZATION OF FAT

The Triglyceride Cycle

The triglycerides of adipose tissue act as a labile store of oxidizable substrates which can be rapidly mobilized and

arise as a result either of increased hydrolysis or of decreased resynthesis of adipose tissue triglycerides. Similarly, a net decrease in FFA release could be caused by decreased hydrolysis or increased synthesis.

The Sources of Adipose Tissue Triglyceride

The fatty acids used for resynthesis of adipose tissue triglyceride are derived from several sources.

(a) Intracellular Triglyceride

Some of the fatty acids formed by the hydrolysis of adipose tissue triglyceride are reconverted into triglyceride by combination with α-glycerophosphate derived from glucose (see below).

(b) Chylomicra

The chylomicra present in the bloodstream during the absorption of a fatty meal are taken up by the tissues, particularly by adipose tissue and liver. The triglycerides of chylomicra taken up by adipose tissue are hydrolyzed to fatty acids and glycerol by an enzyme known as "clearing factor lipase" or "lipoprotein lipase" (different from the intracellular lipases). The fatty acids released by lipoprotein lipase at or near the surfaces of adipose tissue cells enter the cells and thus become available for resynthesis of triglyceride.

(c) Glucose

The plasma glucose taken up by adipose tissue cells contributes to triglyceride synthesis in three ways.

In the first place, the pyruvate arising from the glycolysis of glucose is decarboxylated to acetyl-CoA. Glucose therefore supplies the two-carbon units from which long-chain fatty acids are synthesized, either *de novo* through the malonyl-CoA pathway (reactions 4–7), or by chain elongation.

Secondly, a supply of glucose is necessary for the formation of the α-glycerophosphate used in reaction 8, since adipose tissue cannot re-utilize free glycerol by direct phosphorylation (reaction 9). Glycolytic breakdown of glucose leads to the formation of dihydroxyacetone phosphate, which is then reduced to α-glycerophosphate:

$$
\begin{array}{ccc}
\text{CH}_2\text{OH} & & \text{CH}_2\text{OH} \\
| & & | \\
\text{C}=\text{O} & +\,2\text{H} \rightarrow & \text{CHOH} \qquad (10)\\
| & & | \\
\text{CH}_2\text{OPO}_3\text{H}_2 & & \text{CH}_2\text{OPO}_3\text{H}_2 \\
\text{Dihydroxyacetone} & & \alpha\text{-Glycero-} \\
\text{phosphate} & & \text{phosphate}
\end{array}
$$

The glycerol formed during the breakdown of adipose tissue triglyceride is released into the circulation. Increased triglyceride breakdown is therefore accompanied by a rise in the plasma glycerol concentration.

Thirdly, the oxidation of glucose-6-phosphate leads to the formation of the reduced coenzyme, $NADPH_2$, necessary for the reductive step in fatty acid synthesis (reaction 6).

Regulation of FFA Release

(a) The Glucose-Fatty Acid Cycle

The plasma FFA concentration tends to be maintained at a constant level by a homeostatic mechanism which operates through an interaction between glucose metabolism and fatty acid metabolism. The uptake and breakdown of glucose by skeletal and heart muscle is inhibited by FFA. When, therefore, the plasma FFA concentration rises, glucose is diverted from muscle to adipose tissue. This results in increased resynthesis of adipose tissue triglyceride and, hence, in diminished output of FFA. When the plasma FFA concentration falls, glucose is diverted from adipose tissue to muscle, resulting in an increased rate of FFA release. The controlling influence of glucose on triglyceride resynthesis is readily explained by the fact that glucose is necessary for the supply of α-glycerophosphate used in reaction 8 (see Fig. 3).

(b) Hormonal Factors

In addition to this homeostatic mechanism, both the hydrolysis and the resynthesis of adipose tissue triglyceride are controlled by hormones, so that the rate of release of FFA can be adjusted to the changing requirements of the body for oxidizable fuel or, alternatively, for temporary storage of nutrients convertible into fat.

Several hormones stimulate FFA release *in vivo* and *in vitro*. Hormones with an "adipokinetic" action include adrenaline, noradrenaline, growth hormone, glucagon, thyroxine, glucocorticoids, some of the pituitary peptide hormones (including ACTH and vasopressin) and human placental lactogen (see Lipids in Pregnancy). Some of these hormones act by activating intracellular lipase; others may act partly by inhibiting the effect of insulin on adipose tissue (see below). Although some of these effects are undoubtedly of physiological significance, it is by no means certain that all of them are.

The release of FFA from adipose tissue is inhibited by glucose, insulin and prostaglandins. The inhibitory effect of glucose may be seen in the prompt fall in the plasma FFA concentration that follows an intravenous infusion of glucose into a normal person. This effect of glucose requires the presence of insulin and cannot, therefore, be elicited in untreated diabetic patients. The inhibitory effect of insulin on FFA release is due mainly to its stimulatory effect on the transport of plasma glucose into adipose tissue cells, but insulin may also have some direct inhibitory effect on intracellular lipase.

The rate of mobilization of FFA from adipose tissue fluctuates widely under physiological conditions. This is seen in the increased rate of release of FFA caused by fasting, muscular exercise, exposure to cold, or mental stress. Physiological variations in FFA release probably result from the interaction of several factors. For example, the increased rate of release of FFA in fasting seems to be due to the combined effects of a low plasma glucose level, a low plasma insulin level, an increased rate of secretion of growth hormone by the pituitary and, possibly, increased activity of the sympathetic nerves supplying adipose tissue.

In diabetes, the plasma FFA concentration rises to a very high level owing to an abnormally rapid rate of release of FFA from adipose tissue. The increase in FFA release is due mainly to a deficiency of glucose in the cells of adipose tissue, resulting in a decreased rate of resynthesis of triglyceride, but there may also be some increase in the rate of hydrolysis of triglyceride.

STORAGE OF FAT

A net increase in the amount of fat stored in adipose tissue tends to occur whenever caloric intake exceeds caloric output. Indeed, the body's capacity for storing fat is almost unlimited. This seems to have been recognized by Rumanika, a 19th century African king who force-fed his wives with milk until they were so fat that they were unable to rise from the ground. As we have seen, adipose tissue triglycerides can be formed either directly from fatty acids or by lipogenesis from glucose. A diet containing an excess of carbohydrate may, in fact, be more fattening than one containing an excess of trigly-cerides, because the intestine cannot absorb more than a limited amount of fat. This is one reason why carbohy-drate, rather than fat, is used for fattening farm animals.

The amount of adipose tissue that can be laid down in a human being or an animal is certainly remarkable, but equally so is the ability of the normal adult to maintain an almost constant body weight over many years despite wide variations in the day-to-day output of energy. The way in which the body regulates long-term storage of fat is still not fully understood. One possibility is that under normal conditions adipose tissue cells automatically adjust their rate of triglyceride synthesis to the quantity of nutrient with which they are supplied. If this were so, the question of how fat deposition is regulated would resolve itself into the question of how the appetite is regulated in relation to caloric output. There is much to be said for this point of view. It is well known, for instance, that psychological factors can bring about marked changes in the amount of body fat, and that these changes are often attributable to alterations in food intake. It is also possible to produce extreme degrees of obesity in experimental animals by means of hypothalamic lesions which give the animals a voracious appetite.

However, there can be little doubt that hormonal factors also play some part in the regulation of the total amount of fat in the body through their effects on adipose tissue metabolism. A possible example of a hormonal influence on fat deposition is the obesity that often precedes diabetes. Obese people tend to have impaired glucose tolerance and to secrete abnormal amounts of insulin in response to glucose. Vallance-Owen (1965) has suggested that the impaired glucose tolerance of pre-diabetes is due to the presence of a substance which inhibits the action of insulin on glucose uptake by muscle, but which has little effect on the action of insulin on adipose tissue. The presence of this antagonist in the circulation might be expected to evoke an abnormally high rate of insulin secretion after a carbohydrate meal and, hence, to cause excessive uptake of glucose by adipose tissue. Randle, Garland, Hales and Newsholme (1963) have put forward a different explanation for the obesity of pre-diabetes, based on the idea that there is an intrinsic defect in the glucose-fatty acid cycle. On either view, it is assumed that the obesity is caused by an abnormality in the relative sensitivity of muscle and adipose tissue to insulin, leading to increased lipogenesis from glucose in adipose tissue. However, the abnormal carbohydrate metabolism found in some obese people can be restored to the normal by weight reduction (Conn and Fajans, 1961). This suggests that in some cases obesity is a cause, rather than a result, of impaired glucose tolerance and insensitivity to insulin.

Another factor that contributes to changes in fat deposi-tion is an alteration in the activity of enzymes concerned in the various reactions necessary for triglyceride synthesis. A high carbohydrate diet leads to an increase in the activity of lipoprotein lipase and of several adipose-tissue enzymes necessary for converting glucose into fatty acids. Changes in the opposite sense occur during starvation. These changes in enzyme activity are adaptive rather than causa-tive, but they probably enable the body to take full advan-tage of an increase in the amount of nutrients available for fat storage when food intake exceeds caloric require-ments. In mice with hereditary obesity, the adipose tissue does not mobilize fatty acids at the normal rate during prolonged starvation. This seems to be due to a relative insensitivity of the adipose tissue lipase of these animals to adrenaline and other adipokinetic agents. It remains to be seen whether a failure to respond normally to fat-mobil-izing stimuli ever contributes to excessive fat storage in human beings.

The problem of assessing the importance of factors other than changes in caloric balance in causing changes in total body fat is a formidable one. A slight but persistent change in food intake or caloric output could lead eventually to a marked change in body fat. For this reason, measurement of caloric balance may not provide unequivocal answers to the problem of fat deposition until methods have been devised for measuring caloric output (including loss of calories via the excreta) and food intake, more or less continuously, over long periods of time and under the conditions of normal everyday life. It should also be remembered that the mechanism by which hormones and other substances bring about changes in body fat may be quite complex. Part of the effect may be due to a direct action on adipose tissue metabolism, but there may also be an effect on appetite or on muscular activity.

KETOSIS

Ketosis is a condition in which acetoacetic acid, β hydroxybutyric acid and acetone (together known as ketone bodies) accumulate in abnormal amounts in the blood and urine. Ketosis occurs in its severest form in diabetes and starvation, but may also occur in a milder form in many other states. Ketone bodies are formed almost exclusively in the liver, where they arise as normal products of the metabolism of long-chain fatty acids. However, they do not accumulate under normal conditions because they are rapidly oxidized in the muscles and other tissues. According to the current view, ketosis arises when there is excessive production of ketone bodies in the liver and is not due to a failure to oxidize them in the peripheral tissues.

Formation of Ketone Bodies

The liver is capable of oxidizing long-chain fatty acids completely to CO_2 and water, but it also contains an enzyme system that converts acetyl-CoA into acetoacetic acid by a series of steps which may be simplified to:

$$CH_3.CO.CoA + CH_3.CO.CoA \rightarrow$$

Acetyl-CoA   Acetyl-CoA

$$CH_3.CO.CH_2.COOH + 2\,CoA \qquad (11)$$

Acetoacetic acid

Some of the acetyl-CoA formed by the β-oxidation of fatty acids (reaction 2, etc.) is therefore converted into aceto-acetic acid instead of undergoing oxidation in the mito-chondria. Since acetoacetic acid cannot be oxidized in the liver, it is released into the bloodstream, either without further change or after reduction to β-hydroxybutyric acid:

$$CH_3.CO.CH_2.COOH + 2H \rightarrow$$
Acetoacetic acid

$$CH_3.CHOH.CH_2.COOH \quad (12)$$
β-Hydroxybutyric acid

Acetoacetic acid is also converted into acetone by spontaneous decarboxylation:

$$CH_3.CO.CH_2.COOH \rightarrow CH_3.CO.CH_3 + CO_2$$
Acetoacetic acid   Acetone

$$(13)$$

the deficiency of insulin, or the presence of insulin antagonists in the blood, leads to defective transport of glucose from the plasma into the cells of adipose tissue. In diabetes, and in other ketotic states, an increased rate of hydrolysis of adipose tissue triglyceride may also contribute to the high rate of FFA release (see Regulation of FFA release).

(b) Defective Removal of Acetyl-CoA

The acetyl-CoA formed in the liver is removed by several metabolic pathways, of which the most important are oxidation to CO_2 via the citric acid cycle, and conversion

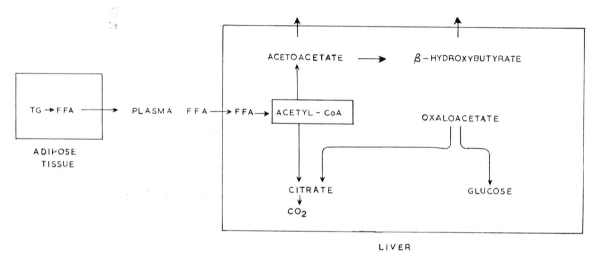

Fig. 4. Diagram to show the main pathways for the formation and removal of acetyl-CoA in the liver. Acetyl-CoA is formed in the liver by the β-oxidation of free fatty acids (FFA) released from adipose tissue triglyceride (TG). Gluconeogenesis removes oxaloacetate, necessary for entry of acetyl-CoA into the citric acid cycle, and thus favours increased formation of acetoacetate.

Causes of Increased Ketone Body Formation

Excessive formation of ketone bodies tends to occur whenever acetyl-CoA accumulates in the liver in abnormal amounts, leading to overproduction of acetoacetic acid by reaction 11. Ketosis, at any rate in its severer forms, is now thought to be due to a combination of two factors, both tending to promote the accumulation of acetyl-CoA in the liver. These factors are increased mobilization of FFA from the adipose tissue and diminished oxidation of acetyl-CoA in the liver.

(a) Increased Mobilization of FFA

In all conditions giving rise to ketosis, the plasma FFA concentration is abnormally high owing to an increased rate of release of FFA from the adipose tissue. This leads to an increased flow of FFA into the liver. Some of the extra load of FFA is converted into triglycerides and returned to the bloodstream, but a large fraction is degraded by β-oxidation, giving rise to acetyl-CoA (reaction 2, etc.).

In most conditions in which ketosis occurs, the increased rate of FFA release from adipose tissue is due mainly to a decrease in the supply of intracellular glucose required for the resynthesis of triglyceride. In diabetes, for example,

into acetoacetic acid. The oxidation of acetyl-CoA requires a supply of oxaloacetate for the formation of citric acid by a condensation reaction:

$$CH_3.CO.CoA + \overset{\displaystyle CO.COOH}{\underset{\displaystyle CH_2.COOH}{|}} + H_2O \rightarrow$$
Acetyl-CoA   Oxaloacetic acid

$$\rightarrow \overset{\displaystyle CH_2.COOH}{\underset{\displaystyle CH_2.COOH}{\overset{|}{\underset{|}{C(OH).COOH}}}} + CoA \quad (14)$$
Citric acid

Oxaloacetic acid, in addition to acting as a condensing partner in the oxidation of acetyl-CoA, also acts as an intermediate in gluconeogenesis (the formation of glucose from non-carbohydrate sources). Since ketosis is almost always accompanied by increased gluconeogenesis, the supply of oxaloacetic acid available for the oxidation of acetyl-CoA through reaction 14 tends to be diminished in the ketotic state.

The Present View on the Mechanism of Ketosis

The biochemical basis of ketosis is still the subject of a good deal of controversy, particularly with regard to the part played by increased gluconeogenesis. However, the following explanation accommodates most of the facts and is now fairly generally accepted (see Fig. 4). Ketosis is caused by overproduction of acetyl-CoA in the liver due to an excessive influx of FFA from the adipose tissue, coupled with defective oxidation of acetyl-CoA in the liver due to increased utilization of oxaloacetate for gluconeogenesis.

PLASMA LIPIDS

The major lipids present in normal plasma are free cholesterol, cholesteryl esters, triglycerides, phospholipids and free fatty acids. All the lipids present in plasma during the fasting state are held in solution by combination with proteins to form lipoproteins, or, in the case of the free fatty acids, by adsorption to the plasma albumin. During the absorption of a fatty meal, chylomicra enter the plasma from the lymphatic duct and may cause the plasma to become turbid. Chylomicra are not normally present in the plasma of a person who has fasted for 12 hours or more, and under these conditions the plasma should be completely translucent.

The Classes of Lipoproteins

The plasma lipoproteins are classified according to their specific gravity or flotation constant (S_f), as determined in the ultracentrifuge, or according to their electrophoretic mobility. Table 3 shows the main classes of

It is generally believed that the FFA present in the plasma in the post-absorptive state are derived almost entirely from the breakdown of adipose tissue triglyceride. The normal concentration of FFA in the plasma of a resting adult human being is about 15 mg./100 ml. (0·5 μEq/ml.). This is only about 2 per cent of the total plasma lipids and is equivalent to less than 400 mg. of FFA in the whole circulation. However, the rate of turnover of the plasma FFA is so rapid that about one quarter of the whole quantity of FFA in the plasma is replaced every minute by uptake into the tissues and release of new FFA from the fat depots. This corresponds to a total flow of about 150 g. of fatty acids through the circulation every 24 hours. If all the fatty acids removed from the plasma were oxidized to CO_2 and water, this would provide the body with at least 60 per cent of the energy required in the basal state. In fact, some of the FFA taken up by the tissues are not burnt, but are metabolized in other ways. In the liver, for example, some FFA taken up from the plasma are incorporated into triglyceride and returned to the plasma as the triglyceride fraction of the very low density lipoproteins (see Table 3). Nevertheless, as we have already seen, FFA probably provide about half the energy required by the whole body under basal conditions.

The plasma FFA concentration is raised in a great many physiological and pathological states which give rise to increased mobilization of FFA from adipose tissue. These

TABLE 3

THE CLASSES OF LIPOPROTEINS IN HUMAN PLASMA, SHOWING THEIR DENSITY, FLOTATION CONSTANT, ELECTROPHORETIC MOBILITY ON FILTER PAPER AND LIPID COMPOSITION

Class of lipoprotein	Density (g./ml.)	S_f	Electro-phoretic fraction	Lipid composition (mg./100 ml. serum)		
				Cholesterol	Triglyceride	Phospholipid
Chylomicra	<1·000	>400	Origin	Variable	Variable	Variable
Very low density	<1·006	20–400	Pre-β or α_2	25	85	30
*Low density	1·006–1·063	0–20	β	125	10	90
High density	>1·063	—	α_1	50	5	100

*The low density plasma lipoproteins are sometimes defined as those having a density between 1·019 and 1·063 (S_f 0–12).
The values for lipid composition are rounded averages.

the plasma lipoproteins, including the chylomicra, together with the contributions made by each lipoprotein fraction to the major lipid components of the plasma. As may be seen from Table 3, the very low density lipoproteins contain most of the triglycerides of the plasma, and the low density lipoproteins (or β-lipoproteins) contain most of the cholesterol.

The Plasma FFA

Free fatty acids have already been mentioned in connection with the mobilization of fat and the production of ketosis, and they will be mentioned again in the sections that follow. However, it may be useful to bring together in one place the main facts about the physiology of the plasma FFA.

states, several of which are mentioned in this chapter, include fasting, prolonged muscular exercise, exposure to cold, mental stress, pregnancy, the early neonatal period, diabetes and thyrotoxicosis.

LIPIDS IN FOETAL AND NEONATAL LIFE

Special Requirements of the Foetus and New-born Animal

Owing to the special conditions of life *in utero* and during the early stages of post-natal life, lipid metabolism in the foetus and new-born animal differs in certain respects from that in the adult.

First, the foetus must deposit substantial quantities of structural lipids at a rapid rate in all its tissues, and it must achieve this with materials brought across a placenta of limited permeability. Second, the foetus as a whole obtains most of its energy from the breakdown of carbohydrate. Within a few hours of birth, however, fat becomes the major source of energy. This change is associated with the release of FFA from adipose tissue and, subsequently, with the ingestion of milk, a diet rich in fat. Finally, adipose tissue plays a much less important part in lipid metabolism in foetal than in post-natal life, but the foetus must nevertheless build up a store of adipose tissue in time to provide the new-born animal with a source of endogenous fuel. These three aspects of lipid metabolism are closely interrelated, but for convenience they are considered separately in this section.

The Origin of the Foetal Lipids

(a) Fatty Acids and Triglycerides

Synthesis of long-chain fatty acids and triglycerides from acetate and glucose takes place in foetal liver, brain and other tissues at an early stage of foetal development (Goldwater and Stetten, 1947; Popják, 1954; Roux, 1966; Myant and Cole, 1966). In general, the rate of synthesis per unit of fresh tissue is considerably higher in the foetus than in the adult.

Long-chain fatty acids also reach the foetus from the mother. This has been demonstrated directly in sheep (Van Duyne, Parker, Havel and Holm, 1960) and in rabbits (Van Duyne, Havel and Felts, 1962) by showing that radioactive fatty acids injected intravenously into the mother appear in the foetal circulation within a few minutes. The passage of fatty acids across the human placenta may be inferred from the fact that essential fatty acids are present in the adipose tissue triglycerides of new-born infants (Bagdade and Hirsch, 1966; and see Table 2).

It is difficult to say what proportion of the foetal fatty acids is synthesized *in situ* and what proportion is supplied by the mother. The fatty acid composition of the adipose tissue triglycerides of the human foetus suggests, however, that synthesis *in situ* becomes increasingly important towards the end of foetal life. As the human foetus grows, the proportion of linoleic acid in its subcutaneous fat decreases and the proportion of palmitic acid increases until, at the time of birth, the foetal fat contains one tenth as much linoleic acid and twice as much palmitic acid as the subcutaneous fat of a normal adult (Table 2). When the new-born infant is breast-fed, the proportion of palmitic acid in its subcutaneous fat falls within a few weeks to that found in human milk (Table 4). These are the changes that would be expected if fatty acid synthesis *in situ* contributes an increasing fraction of the total fatty acids of the adipose tissue of the developing foetus, since linoleic acid is not synthesized in the human body, whereas palmitic acid is the chief fatty acid synthesized from acetate or glucose by the malonyl-CoA pathway. The fatty acid composition of the subcutaneous fat of new-born infants is, in fact, similar to that of animals given a diet rich in carbohydrate and poor in fat. The subsequent changes in the composition of the adipose tissue triglycerides of breast-fed infants is due,

no doubt, to a relative increase in the proportion of their triglyceride fatty acids derived from exogenous fat.

Räihä (1954) has pointed out that synthesis of fat from carbohydrate may provide the human foetus with a means of decreasing its oxygen requirement. This saving of oxygen comes about because the reductive step in fatty acid synthesis (reaction 6) leads to regeneration of oxidized cofactor (NADP) which would otherwise have to be regenerated through oxygen-requiring reactions. Villee (1954) has estimated that the triglyceride synthesized during the last month of foetal life might save the foetus a maximum of one sixth of its total oxygen requirement. However, the actual saving of oxygen is probably smaller than this, because fat synthesis requires energy, and the energy must come ultimately from the oxidation of fuel.

(b) Complex Lipids

Very little is known about the origin of the phospholipids and glycolipids laid down in the tissues of the human foetus, but it is reasonable to assume that they are synthesized entirely from precursors of low molecular weight, since this appears to be the case in animals. In experimental animals, the phospholipids and, presumably, the other complex lipids, cannot pass from the maternal to the foetal circulation. However, liver and brain, as well as other foetal tissues, synthesize phospholipids at a rapid rate *in vivo* (Popják, 1954; Myant and Gamble, 1965) and *in vitro* (Myant and Cole, 1966).

(c) Cholesterol

Most, if not all, foetal tissues can synthesize cholesterol from glucose or acetate. However, experiments in which pregnant animals are fed radioactive cholesterol continuously for long periods of time have shown that a substantial fraction of the cholesterol deposited in the foetal tissues is derived from the mother. The proportion of the total cholesterol derived from synthesis *in situ* varies in different tissues. Synthesis within the foetus accounts for only about 80 per cent of the cholesterol of foetal liver and serum, but for more than 90 per cent of the cholesterol in fœtal brain (Chevallier, 1964; Connor and Lin, 1967).

Undernutrition and the Brain Lipids

Cholesterol and several of the complex lipids are of special importance in the formation of myelin in developing brain. Davison and Dobbing (1966) have pointed out that myelination in brain takes place only during a restricted period, and that once it is completed many of the enzyme systems concerned in the synthesis of myelin lipids cease to be active. They suggest, therefore, that there is a vulnerable stage in the development of a mammal during which brain formation can be permanently retarded by undernutrition sufficient to limit the supply of precursors for the synthesis of lipids and other substances in the brain. Dickerson, Dobbing and McCance (1966) have shown that the brains of pigs severely undernourished during the first year of post-natal life have an abnormally low content of cholesterol and phospholipid, and that this defect cannot be completely repaired by subsequent re-feeding. In man, myelination in the brain is most rapid from the seventh month of foetal life to the first few months of post-natal life. This is therefore the time during which the human brain should be most susceptible to the effects of undernutrition. In view of the extreme degree of undernutrition required to cause brain damage in experimental animals during the post-natal period, it would be surprising if the brain of a human foetus *in utero* could be affected by undernutrition of its mother, except under extreme conditions such as a famine or a siege. However, the brains of premature infants may well be susceptible to minor degrees of undernutrition. The brains of infants born at term may also be susceptible during the early months of life, though perhaps to a smaller extent (see Davison and Dobbing, 1966, for a discussion of this controversial question).

Fat as Energy Source in the Foetus and New-born Animal

(a) The Foetus

It is generally believed that the foetus obtains most of its energy from the breakdown of carbohydrate, and that oxidation of fatty acids contributes little towards its total energy consumption. This is certainly consistent with the changes in lipid and glucose metabolism that take place in the mother during pregnancy. These changes, as we shall see, tend to divert glucose from the mother's tissues to those of the foetus.

The view that glucose, rather than fatty acid, is the predominant fuel used by the foetus is also supported by the finding that the FFA concentration in foetal plasma is low (Van Duyne and Havel, 1959) or very low (Novák and Jirásek, 1966). Reliable measurements of the respiratory quotient (RQ) of the whole human foetus under physiological conditions have not been made, but a value of unity, or slightly higher, has been deduced by Räihä (1954). The RQ of foetal tissues *in vitro* has also been shown to be above unity (Roux, 1966), indicating that synthesis of fatty acids from carbohydrate outweighs oxidation of fatty acids. It should be remembered, however, that a high RQ does not exclude the possibility that oxidation of fat and synthesis of fat from carbohydrate occur simultaneously. Indeed, in view of the ability of the new-born animal to oxidize fatty acids (see below), it is difficult to believe that fatty acid oxidation does not occur to some extent in the foetus.

(b) The New-born Animal

When the foetus is born there is an abrupt change in the contribution of fatty acids and triglycerides to total energy metabolism. As we have seen, carbohydrate derived from the mother is the main source of energy used by the foetus. However, as soon as the foetus is born, the new-born infant must rely on its own stores of fuel until it can get an adequate supply of milk, and this is not usually available from the mother for at least 24 hours. Once the store of glycogen in the infant's liver has been used up, the main source of energy is FFA mobilized from stores of adipose tissue triglyceride built up during the final stages of gestation.

Shortly after the birth of a human infant the RQ falls progressively (Cross, Tizard and Trythall, 1957; Smith,

1959), indicating that an increasing proportion of the total energy consumed is derived from the oxidation of fat. In less than one hour after birth the plasma FFA concentration begins to rise, eventually reaching a level several times that in cord blood (Van Duyne and Havel, 1959; Novák, Melichar, Hahn and Koldovský, 1965). At the same time, the plasma glucose level falls and the plasma glycerol level rises. There is also a slight increase in the level of ketone bodies in the blood, due presumably to an increased flow of FFA to the liver (see Ketosis). The rise in the plasma glycerol level points to the adipose tissue as the source of the increased FFA entering the circulation.

The extreme rapidity with which fat is mobilized in new-born infants suggests that the stimulus to FFA release is an increased activity of the sympathetic nerves supplying the adipose tissue. In agreement with this, Van Duyne, Parker and Holm (1965) have shown that the rise in the plasma FFA level in new-born sheep is prevented by injections of hexamethonium. In the new-born human, other factors may contribute to the maintenance of a high plasma FFA level during the first few days of life. One possible factor is the low plasma glucose level, since Novák, Melichar, Hahn and Koldovský (1961) have shown that the rise in the plasma FFA level of new-born infants can be prevented by infusions of glucose. Another possibility is that FFA release from adipose tissue in the new-born human is kept at a high rate by increased secretion of growth hormone during the first 48 hours of life (Cornblath, Parker, Reisner, Forbes and Daughaday, 1965).

Some practical consequences of the need for a potential store of FFA during the early neonatal period are considered below.

Adipose Tissue

The foetus receives a continuous supply of nutrients from its mother and therefore does not require the labile energy store which becomes necessary in post-natal life, when energy output and food intake are intermittent. Moreover, since the foetus lives in a warm environment at a constant temperature it needs no insulation. It must, however, have a store of adipose tissue in readiness for birth.

In keeping with these changing requirements, the human foetus has little adipose tissue until the last few weeks of its life. At the fifth month, subcutaneous adipose tissue is confined largely to the neck and shoulders and to the region including the buttocks and the upper parts of the thighs. Only later does adipose tissue spread to other subcutaneous areas in substantial amounts. The growth curve of adipose tissue is reflected in the changing fat composition of the developing foetus (Kelly, Sloan, Hoffman and Saunders, 1951; Widdowson and Spray, 1951). Throughout the first 20–25 weeks of foetal life, lipid accounts for only about 1 per cent of the total body weight. Thereafter, the proportion of lipid increases progressively, eventually accounting for 10–15 per cent of the body weight of a full-term new-born infant. The increase is particularly marked from the 34th week.

The ability to release FFA into the plasma in response to the stimulus of birth, and thus to provide the tissues with an emergency ration of oxidizable fuel, may well be an important factor in the survival of the new-born mammal. Van Duyne (1966) has shown that lambs born under conditions leading to suppression of the normal rise in plasma FFA concentration tend to die within a few hours of birth.

(a) The Premature Infant

In the premature new-born infant there is a marked deficiency of subcutaneous fat, particularly if birth occurs before the final spurt in the laying down of adipose tissue. This deficiency not only deprives the infant of its normal insulation. It may also limit the mobilization of FFA at birth, since Melichar, Novák, Hahn and Koldovský (1964) have shown that the plasma FFA concentration in premature infants born before 32 weeks is abnormally low 12 hours after birth. Both these consequences of adipose-tissue deficiency may contribute to the high death rate of premature infants. They also point to the need to provide the premature infant with early and continuous nutrition, in addition to a warm environment (See Section VI, Chap. 2).

(b) The Post-mature Infant

A relative deficiency of adipose tissue may also occur in post-mature new-born infants or in some full-term infants who have been undernourished *in utero*, though it is not at all clear why this should be so. One of the explanations that have been put forward to account for it is based on the idea of placental insufficiency. In the second half of pregnancy the foetus normally grows more quickly than the placenta. But the rate of increase in foetal weight decreases towards the end of pregnancy, suggesting that even in a normal pregnancy the rate-limiting factor in foetal growth at this stage is not the growth potential of the foetus, but the ability of the placenta to transport nutrients from the mother. Failure of the placenta to keep pace with the foetus during an extended period of gestation might give rise to a relative placental insufficiency in post-maturity, which might, in turn, lead to mobilization of the foetal adipose tissue to satisfy the energy requirements of the foetus.

As with the premature infant, the need to supply these infants with early and adequate nutrition should be obvious.

(c) Obesity in the Infants of Diabetic Mothers

The babies of diabetic mothers tend to have an excess of body fat (Pařízková, 1963) and to be abnormally large at birth. The excess of fat, which may be no more than one aspect of a general increase in foetal growth (Driscoll, Benirschke and Curtis, 1960), has not been fully explained. It may be due partly to a high plasma glucose level, causing increased lipogenesis. But it may also be related to over-secretion of insulin by the foetal pancreas. The infants of diabetic mothers usually have hyperplasia of the pancreatic islets, and their glucose tolerance tends to be increased. Farquhar (1962) has suggested that the increased insulin secretion is a response of the foetus to insulin antagonists derived from the mother. If such insulin antagonists did not inhibit the lipogenic and somatotrophic effects of insulin, the foetus would tend to become abnormally large and to lay down an excess of fat. It should be noted, however, that the evidence for the presence of insulin antagonists in the blood of the foetus of a diabetic mother is indirect.

LIPIDS IN PREGNANCY

The Plasma Lipids

In pregnancy there is a rise in the plasma concentration of triglyceride and cholesterol, and there may also be a slight increase in the plasma phospholipid concentration (Dannenberg, Burt and Leake, 1962). The plasma cholesterol level begins to rise during the third month and increases to a value 40–50 per cent above the normal level by the 30th week of pregnancy (Oliver and Boyd, 1955; de Alvarez, Gaiser, Simkins, Smith and Bratvold, 1959). According to Oliver and Boyd (1955), the increase is confined mainly to the cholesterol in the β-lipoprotein fraction. There is also an increase in the plasma FFA concentration (see below).

Mobilization of FFA

During pregnancy, the metabolism of lipids and carbohydrates in the mother tends to change towards that seen in early diabetes or pre-diabetes. Moreover, clinical diabetes often appears for the first time during pregnancy. In pregnancy, as in diabetes, the plasma FFA concentration is abnormally high owing to increased mobilization from adipose tissue. Burt (1960) has shown that the plasma FFA concentration begins to rise at about the 20th week and that it eventually reaches a level 4–5 times that in the post-partum period, the rate of rise being particularly marked during the last month. Within two or three days of delivery the plasma FFA concentration falls to the normal level.

During the last three months of pregnancy, there is a rise in the plasma insulin concentration, while the blood glucose level remains normal or slightly raised. The glucose tolerance may or may not be impaired, but there is decreased sensitivity to insulin, as shown by the relatively small effect of intravenous insulin on the blood glucose level in pregnant women (Burt, 1956). There is also an abnormally large rise in the plasma insulin level in response to intravenous glucose, without any acceleration in the rate at which the injected glucose disappears from the blood (Bleicher, O'Sullivan and Freinkel, 1964).

This combination of metabolic changes points to the presence of an insulin-antagonist in the blood during pregnancy. In particular, inhibition of the effect of insulin on the transport of glucose into adipose tissue cells would enhance FFA release by diminishing the rate of resynthesis of triglyceride (Fig. 3).

It has been suggested that the loss of sensitivity to insulin in pregnancy is due to an increased blood level of growth hormone. This would certainly explain the raised plasma FFA concentration in pregnancy, since growth hormone stimulates FFA release from adipose tissue by inhibiting the insulin-dependent entry of glucose into adipose tissue cells. However, it seems unlikely that the blood level of growth hormone is, in fact, raised in pregnancy (Ehrlich and Randle, 1962; Kaplan and Grumbach, 1965; Yen, Samaan and Pearson, 1967).

Josimovich and MacLaren (1962) have shown that a substance with growth-promoting and lactogenic activity is present in human placenta and in the serum of pregnant women. This substance, which they have called "human placental lactogen" (HPL), is distinct from growth hormone and from prolactin, though it cross-reacts to some extent with anti-serum to human growth hormone. Samaan, Yen, Friesen and Pearson (1966) have shown that HPL is detectable in the serum at the sixth week of pregnancy, its concentration rising progressively until the fifth month, and that it disappears from the serum very rapidly after delivery. Very little of it, if any, crosses the placenta (Kaplan and Grumbach, 1965). HPL produces diabetogenic effects when injected into diabetic patients (Domínguez, Cottini and Fabregat, 1965) or into normal people (Beck and Daughaday, 1967) and stimulates the release of FFA from adipose tissue *in vitro* (Turtle and Kipnis, 1967).

The physiological properties of HPL and the time-course of its appearance in the blood of pregnant women suggest that it is responsible for some, at least, of the diabetogenic effect of pregnancy. It remains possible, however, that other ketogenic hormones, including ACTH, the glucocorticoids and glucagon, also contribute to the increased mobilization of FFA that occurs in pregnancy.

The biological advantage of increased mobilization of FFA in pregnancy is not hard to see. The high plasma FFA concentration, together with the presence of insulin antagonists in the blood, must tend to diminish the utilization of glucose by the mother's skeletal and heart muscle and to substitute FFA for glucose as the main source of energy for these tissues. The net effect is therefore to save glucose for the foetus, which, as we have seen, requires glucose in preference to fat as its energy-providing fuel. A parallel to the saving of maternal glucose for the foetus may be seen during starvation or prolonged exercise. In both cases, the mobilization of FFA, and the substitution of FFA for glucose as the fuel used by muscle, enable the brain to receive an adequate supply of glucose, without which it cannot function.

Body Fat

The weight gained during pregnancy is very variable and is influenced by many factors, particularly by the extent to which food is restricted. Hytten and Leitch (1964), who have sifted the available information with great care, conclude that a normal pregnant woman eating without restriction gains, on the average, 12·5 Kg. (27·5 lb.). Taking into account the probable increase in weight of the uterus and its contents, and of the breasts and the body fluids of the mother, Hytten and Leitch (1964) estimate that about 4 Kg. of the total increase in weight during pregnancy is due to fat storage in the mother's body. In agreement with the conclusion that body fat is

stored during pregnancy, Edwards (1951) and Taggart (1961) have shown that the skin-fold thickness on several skin sites increases in pregnant women. McCartney, Pottinger and Harrod (1959) also found that the percentage of fat in the body, calculated from the volume of body water and the density of the whole body, was higher in pregnant than in non-pregnant women. The measurements of skin-fold thickness and the estimates of Hytten and Leitch (1964) agree in indicating that fat storage begins during the first three months of pregnancy, and that it ceases after about the 30th week. The time-course of fat deposition differs, therefore, from that of fat mobilization, which reaches its peak towards the end of pregnancy (see above).

Very little is known about the stimulus to fat storage during pregnancy. The deposition of fat cannot readily be explained simply as a response to the growth of the foetus and placenta because, as Thomson and Hytten (1961) have pointed out, the greatest increase in the weight of the contents of the uterus occurs in the second half of pregnancy, whereas little or no fat storage occurs during the last ten weeks. The stimulus may well be hormonal. But if so, there remains the question as to how oestrogens, or other hormones formed in increased amounts in pregnancy, enhance fat storage. As we have seen, a net increase in body fat tends to occur when caloric intake exceeds caloric output. Fat storage could, therefore, be due to a combination of the increased food intake and decreased physical activity that so commonly occur in pregnancy. It is not inconceivable that both these changes are the result of hormonal actions on the central nervous system. In this connection, it should be noted that increased appetite is a very early symptom of pregnancy, and that the appetite may increase in women taking oral contraceptives; the effect of sex hormones on the appetite is clearly a subject worth investigating. There is also the possibility that the hormones concerned in the maintenance of pregnancy alter the activities of the enzyme systems necessary for the synthesis and mobilization of fat in adipose tissue, an explanation that has been put forward from time to time to account for the fattening effect of oestrogens on birds. It must be remembered, however, that no amount of change in enzyme activity can lead to a long-term deposition of fat in adipose tissue unless there is a surplus of calories available, either from the breakdown of tissues elsewhere in the body, or from increased food intake in relation to caloric output.

SEX DIFFERENCES IN BODY FAT

Women at all ages tend to have more body fat than men. The absolute amount of fat in the body is difficult to estimate during life, but measurement of skin-fold thickness, combined with other measurements, suggests that the proportion of fat to total body weight is about twice as high in young women as in young men (Kekwick, 1965). There are also sex differences in the distribution of subcutaneous fat. As well as having more fat on the breasts and buttocks, women tend to have more fat on the legs and less on the trunk than men (Edwards, 1951). Sex differences in body fat may be due in part to cultural factors that affect habits of working and eating. However, there can be little doubt that both the high fat content and the characteristic distribution of subcutaneous fat in women are determined largely by biological factors. Full development of the female pattern of fat requires either the presence of oestrogens or, since the body fat of men castrated before puberty tends towards the female pattern, the absence of androgens. There seems also to be an intrinsic difference between the adipose tissue of male and female human beings, since sex differences in the pattern of subcutaneous fat have been demonstrated in new-born infants (Garn, 1958; Pařízková, 1963).

The high proportion of fat in the female body is worth considering from the point of view of human evolution. The female distribution of subcutaneous fat no doubt arose partly through sexual selection. The ideal of female beauty is admittedly influenced by cultural factors. But, to judge from the "Venus of Willendorf" and other palaeolithic statues found throughout Europe, fat on the buttocks and thighs was thought beautiful by Stone Age men. The ability to deposit body fat may also have been advantageous to women in prehistoric communities subject to intermittent shortages of food. Since men are, of course, more expendable biologically than women, increased survival of women would have been more useful to the species than increased survival of men. Whether or not women do, in fact, survive prolonged starvation better than men is a question that might, perhaps, be answered by a study of records available from the recent past.

SEX HORMONES AND PLASMA LIPIDS

Plasma Lipids in Women

Women have a much lower death rate from heart disease than men. A knowledge of this fact, together with the well known correlation between plasma lipid concentrations and disease of the coronary arteries, has led to intensive study of the plasma lipids in women, and to investigation of the effect of sex hormones on the plasma cholesterol and triglycerides. The incentive to much of this work has been the hope that sex hormones might prove useful in the prevention and treatment of heart disease, particularly in people with high plasma lipid concentrations. Though this hope has not been completely fulfilled, the widespread use of oral contraceptives has led to renewed interest in the effects of sex hormones on the blood lipids.

Comparisons between plasma lipid concentrations in men and women have given conflicting answers, perhaps because differences due to sex alone are small, and because the plasma lipids are influenced by many factors besides sex, such as diet, age, economic status, amount of exercise taken and genetic factors other than sex. Nevertheless, it is generally agreed that the plasma lipids of men and women do differ consistently, especially with regard to the distribution of the lipids among the different lipoprotein fractions.

The total plasma triglyceride level in women below the age of about 50 is, on the average, lower than that in men (Schaefer, 1964; Furman, Alaupovic and Howard, 1967),

but in women over 50 it rises above the level in men (Furman et al., 1967). The plasma cholesterol shows a similar trend. In women under 40, the total plasma cholesterol level tends to be lower than that in men of the same age, but in post-menopausal women it is higher (Adlersberg, Schaefer, Steinberg and Wong, 1956; Schaefer, 1964).

Almost all workers agree that the cholesterol concentration in the α-lipoprotein fraction is greater in pre-menopausal women than in men (Havel, Eder and Bragdon, 1955; and see Furman et al., 1967, for other references). There is also fairly general agreement that the cholesterol concentration in the β-lipoprotein fraction is lower in pre-menopausal women than in men. However, Furman et al. (1967) found that the cholesterol concentration in the β-lipoprotein fraction of a group of pre-menopausal women was similar to that in men, but that the women had much less cholesterol than the men in their very low density fraction (defined by Furman et al. (1967) as the fraction of density less than 1·019). After the menopause, the pattern of distribution of the plasma lipids in women changes to one similar to that in men.

To summarize, both the plasma concentration of cholesterol and triglyceride, and the proportion of the total plasma cholesterol carried in the lipoproteins of low or very low density, are lower in women in the reproductive period than in men. This, it may be noted, is the opposite of the pattern seen in patients with disease of the coronary arteries. In these patients, not only does the total plasma cholesterol concentration tend to be raised, but there is an increase in the proportion of the total cholesterol carried in the lipoproteins of low and very low density. If it is assumed that coronary atherosclerosis is caused by the abnormality in the plasma lipids with which it is associated, an assumption that is open to argument, then it follows that the low death rate from heart disease in women may be due to their having a favourable plasma lipid pattern during the reproductive period.

Rôle of Sex Hormones

(a) Endogenous Hormones

The plasma lipid pattern characteristic of pre-menopausal women is generally assumed to be determined by the preponderance of oestrogenic over androgenic hormones. In favour of this, there is a change towards the male pattern after the menopause (see above) and after bilateral removal of the ovaries (Robinson, Higano and Cohen, 1957), and there is a change towards the female pattern in young adult eunuchs (Furman, Howard, Shetlar, Keaty and Imagawa, 1956). Furthermore, in women at about the time of ovulation there is a fall in the plasma cholesterol concentration (Oliver and Boyd, 1953) and an increase in the concentration of α-lipoproteins (Barclay, Barclay, Skipski, Terebus-Kekish, Mueller and Elkins, 1965).

The changes in plasma lipid that occur in pregnancy have already been noted. These changes are presumably caused by many interacting factors, besides a rise in the production of oestrogens.

(b) Exogenous Hormones

The effects of exogenous oestrogens and androgens on the plasma lipids are, for the most part, consistent with the view that the gonadal hormones determine the sex pattern of the plasma lipids. Oestrogens given to men or to post-menopausal women have generally been found to lower the total plasma cholesterol concentration and to cause a shift in cholesterol from the β- to the α-lipoprotein fraction (Barr, Russ and Eder, 1952; Robinson, Higano and Cohen, 1960). Androgens, on the other hand, cause a shift in plasma cholesterol from the α- to the β-lipoproteins (Russ, Eder and Barr, 1955). Despite their effect on the plasma cholesterol, oestrogens appear to have no significant effect on the incidence of myocardial infarctions in survivors of a single previous infarct (Oliver and Boyd, 1961). Nor has it been possible to prevent the feminizing effects of oestrogens by means of androgens without inhibiting the effect of oestrogens on the plasma lipids (Eder, 1959).

Although several groups of workers have confirmed the observation of Barr *et al.* (1952) that oestrogens tend to promote a female pattern of distribution of the plasma lipids, Furman *et al.* (1967) found that oestrogens given to oestrogen-deficient women caused a marked increase in the plasma concentration of triglycerides and of very low density lipoproteins. Wynn, Doar and Mills (1966) have also shown that in women taking oral contraceptives there is an increase in the plasma concentration of triglycerides and cholesterol, and of lipoproteins of low density and very low density. There is thus a change towards the pattern of plasma lipids associated with a high death rate from heart disease.

LIPIDS IN LACTATION

Composition of Milk Fat

Milk provides a diet rich in fat. The lipid component of milk is present almost entirely as the triglycerides of

TABLE 4

FATTY ACID COMPOSITION OF THE TRIGLYCERIDES OF MILK FROM HUMANS, COWS AND GOATS

Fatty acid	Percentage of total in each fraction		
	Human	Jersey cow	Goat
4:0 to 14:0	9	38	33
16:0	27	37	16
16:1	4	1	1
18:0	8	9	14
18:1	38	13	27
18:2	10	0·4	3
20:4	0·8	0	0
22:2, :5, :6	0·7	0	0

Modified from Breckenridge and Kuksis (1967).

long-chain and short-chain fatty acids, but small quantities of cholesterol (about 20 mg./100 ml. in cow's milk), phospholipid, fatty acids and fat-soluble vitamins are also present. Human milk contains about 3·5 per cent of

total lipid. This is about the same as the lipid content of cow's milk. There are, however, important differences between human milk and cow's milk with regard to the fatty acid composition of the triglycerides. Table 4 shows the main fatty acids present in the triglycerides of milk from lactating women, cows and goats. The most striking differences are the relatively large amounts of 4:0 to 14:0 fatty acids in milk from cows and goats, and the relatively high proportion of essential fatty acids (18:2 and 20:4), and of highly unsaturated acids with 2, 5 and 6 double bonds, in human milk. Milk from cows and goats contains no acids with chain length greater than 18 and only small quantities of linoleic acid (18:2).

Origin of Milk Fat

There is no direct evidence on the origin of the fat in human milk, but work on lactating ruminants has shown that the fatty acids in the milk triglycerides arise partly by synthesis in the mammary gland itself (Glascock, 1958) and partly from triglycerides carried in the β-lipoproteins of the plasma (Glascock, Welch, Bishop, Davies, Wright and Noble, 1966). Since dietary fat contributes to the plasma triglycerides, the fatty acids of neutral fat in the food may make a significant contribution to milk fat. Indeed, Glascock (1958) has estimated that nearly one third of the fatty acids in the triglycerides of cow's milk may be derived from dietary fat.

There is no reason to doubt that the fatty acids of human milk triglycerides also arise partly from synthesis in the mammary gland and partly from the plasma triglycerides. It seems unlikely, however, that the precursor from which fatty acids are synthesized in the mammary gland is the same in human beings as in ruminants. Acetate, produced in large quantities in ruminants by the fermentation of intestinal cellulose, is the major precursor of the fatty acids synthesized in the cow's udder. This source of acetate is peculiar to ruminants, and it seems more likely that the human mammary gland synthesizes fatty acids from glucose, as is the case with the mammary gland of rodents. In the lactating mammary gland, acetyl-CoA derived from glucose is converted into long-chain fatty acids by the malonyl-CoA pathway. Immediately after parturition, the capacity of the mammary gland for synthesizing fatty acids rises very markedly, and this increase is accompanied by increased synthesis of the enzymes catalyzing reactions 4, etc., and of the enzymes necessary for the generation of reductive hydrogen (as $NADPH_2$) by the oxidation of glucose. The increased synthesis of enzymes in the lactating mammary gland, which is initiated and maintained by the actions of hormones, provides one of the most striking examples of the reversible induction of new enzyme protein known to occur in animal tissues.

REFERENCES

Adlersberg, D., Schaefer, L. E., Steinberg, A. G. and Wang, C. (1956), "Age, Sex, Serum Lipids, and Coronary Atherosclerosis," *J. Amer. med. Ass.*, **162**, 619.

Bagdade, J. D. and Hirsch, J. (1966), "Gestational and Dietary Influences on the Lipid Content of the Infant Buccal Fat Pad," *Proc. Soc. exp. Biol.*, **122**, 616

Barclay, M., Barclay, R. K., Skipski, V. P., Terebus-Kekish, O., Mueller, C. H., Shah, E. and Elkins, W. L. (1965), "Fluctuations in Human Serum Lipoproteins during the Normal Menstrual Cycle," *Biochem. J.*, **96**, 205.

Barr, D. P., Russ, E. M. and Eder, H. A. (1952), "Influence of Estrogens on Lipoproteins in Atherosclerosis," *Trans. Ass. Amer. Phys.*, **65**, 102.

Beck, P. and Daughaday, W. H. (1967), "Human Placental Lactogen: Studies of its Acute Metabolic Effects and Disposition in Normal Man," *J. clin. Invest.*, **46**, 103.

Bleicher, S. J., O'Sullivan, J. B. and Freinkel, N. (1964), "Carbohydrate Metabolism in Pregnancy. V. The interrelations of glucose, insulin and free fatty acids in late pregnancy and post partum," *New Engl. J. Med.*, **271**, 866.

Breckenridge, W. C. and Kuksis, A. (1967), "Molecular Weight Distributions of Milk Fat Triglycerides from Seven Species," *J. Lipid Res.*, **8**, 473.

Burt, R. L. (1956), "Peripheral Utilization of Glucose in Pregnancy. III. Insulin tolerance," *Obstetrics and Gynecology*, **7**, 658.

Burt, R. L. (1960), "Plasma Nonesterified Fatty Acids in Normal Pregnancy and Puerperium," *Obstetrics and Gynecology*, **15**, 460.

Chevallier, F. (1964), "Transferts et synthèse du cholestérol chez le rat au cours de sa croissance," *Biochim. biophys. Acta*, **84**, 316.

Conn, J. W. and Fajans, S. S. (1961), "The Prediabetic State. A Concept of Dynamic Resistance to a Genetic Diabetogenic Influence," *Amer. J. Med.*, **31**, 839.

Connor, W. E. and Lin, D. S. (1967), "Placental Transfer of Cholesterol-4-^{14}C into Rabbit and Guinea-pig Fetus," *J. Lipid Res.*, **8**, 558.

Cornblath, M., Parker, M. L., Reisner, S. H., Forbes, A. E. and Daughaday, W. H. (1965), "Secretion and Metabolism of Growth Hormone in Premature and Full-term Infants," *J. clin. Endocrin.*, **25**, 209.

Cross, K. W., Tizard, J. P. M. and Trythall, D. A. H. (1957), "The Gaseous Metabolism of the Newborn Infant," *Acta paediat.*, **46**, 265.

Dannenburg, W. N., Burt, R. L. and Leake, N. H. (1962), "Plasma Lipids in the Early Puerperium," *Amer. J. Obstet. Gynec.*, **84**, 1091.

Davison, A. N. and Dobbing, J. (1966), "Myelination as a Vulnerable Period in Brain Development," *Brit. med. Bull.*, **22**, 40.

De Alvarez, R. R., Gaiser, D. F., Simkins, D. M., Smith, E. K. and Bratvold, G. E. (1959), "Serial Studies of Serum Lipids in Normal Human Pregnancy," *Amer. J. Obstet. Gynec.*, **77**, 743.

Dickerson, J. W. T., Dobbing, J. and McCance, R. A. (1966), "The Effect of Undernutrition on the Postnatal Development of the Brain and Cord in Pigs," *Proc. roy. Soc. B*, **166**, 396.

Domínguez, J. M., Cottini, E. P. and Fabregat, A. N. (1965), "Diabetogenic Effect of a Placental Factor in Man." In *Excerpta Medica International Congress Series*, 99, *VIth Pan American Congress of Endocrinology*, 1965, edited by A. S. Mason and A. Moragas Redecilla, p. E72. Amsterdam: Excerpta Medica Foundation.

Driscoll, S., Benirschke, K. and Curtis, G. W. (1960), "Neonatal Deaths among Infants of Diabetic Mothers," *Amer. J. Dis. Child.*, **100**, 818.

Eder, H. A. (1959), "The Effects of Sex Hormones on Serum Lipids and Lipoproteins." In *Hormones and Atherosclerosis, Proceedings of the Conference held in Brighton, Utah, March 11–14, 1958*, edited by G. Pincus, pp. 335–348. New York: Academic Press.

Edwards, D. A. W. (1951), "Differences in the Distribution of Subcutaneous Fat with Sex and Maturity," *Clin. Sci.*, **10**, 305.

Ehrlich, R. M. and Randle, P. J. (1962), "Immunoassay of Serum Growth Hormone in Diabetes Mellitus." In *Ciba Foundation Colloquia on Endocrinology*, 14, *Immunoassay of Hormones*, edited by G. E. W. Wolstenholme and M. P. Cameron, pp. 117–132. London: J. and A. Churchill.

Farquhar, J. W. (1962), "Maternal Hyperglycæmia and Fœtal Hyperinsulinism in Diabetic Pregnancy," *Postgrad. Med. J.*, **38**, 612.

Furman, R. H., Alaupovic, P. and Howard, R. P. (1967), "Effects of Androgens and Estrogens on Serum Lipids and the Composition and Concentration of Serum Lipoproteins in Normolipemic and Hyperlipidemic States." In *Progress in Biochemical Pharmacology*, Vol. 2, *Drugs Affecting Lipid Metabolism*, Part I, edited by D. Kritchevsky, R. Paoletti and D. Steinberg, pp. 215–249. Basel: S. Karger.

Furman, R. H., Howard, R. P., Shetlar, M. R., Keaty, E. C. and Imagawa, R. (1958), "A Comparison of the Serum Lipids, Lipoproteins, Glycoproteins, Urinary 17-ketosteroids, and Gonadotropins in Eunuchs and Control Male Subjects," *Circulation*, **17**, 1076.

Garn, S. M. (1958), "Fat, Body Size and Growth in the Newborn," *Hum. Biol.*, **30**, 265.

Glascock, R. F. (1958), "Recent Research on the Origin of Milk Fat," *Proc. roy. Soc. B*, **149**, 402.

Glascock, R. F., Welch, V. A., Bishop, C., Davies, T., Wright, E. W. and Noble, R. C. (1966), "An Investigation of Serum Lipoproteins and of Their Contribution to Milk Fat in the Dairy Cow," *Biochem. J.*, **98**, 149.

Goldwater, W. H. and Stetten, D. (1947), "Studies in Fetal Metabolism," *J. biol. Chem.*, **169**, 723.

Havel, R. J., Eder, H. A. and Bragdon, J. H. (1955), "The Distribution and Chemical Composition of Ultracentrifugally Separated Lipoproteins in Human Serum," *J. clin. Invest.*, **34**, 1345.

Hirsch, J. (1965), "Fatty Acid Patterns in Human Adipose Tissue." In *Handbook of Physiology, Section 5, Adipose Tissue*, edited by A. E. Renold and G. F. Cahill, Jr., pp. 181–189. Washington, D.C.: American Physiological Society.

Hytten, F. E. and Leitch, I. (1964), *The Physiology of Human Pregnancy*. Oxford: Blackwell Scientific Publications.

Josimovich, J. B. and MacLaren, J. A. (1962), "Presence in Human Placenta and Term Serum of Highly Lactogenic Substance Immunologically Related to Pituitary Growth Hormone," *Endocrinology*, **71**, 209.

Kaplan, S. L. and Grumbach, M. M. (1965), "Serum Chorionic 'Growth Hormone-prolactin' and Serum Pituitary Growth Hormone in Mother and Fetus at Term," *J. clin. Endocrin.*, **25**, 1370.

Kekwick, A. (1965), "Adiposity." In *Handbook of Physiology, Section 5, Adipose Tissue*, edited by A. E. Renold and G. F. Cahill, Jr., pp. 617–624. Washington, D.C.: American Physiological Society.

Kelly, H. J., Sloan, R. E., Hoffman, W. and Saunders, C. (1951), "Accumulation of Nitrogen and Six Minerals in the Human Fetus during Gestation," *Hum. Biol.*, **23**, 61.

McCartney, C. P., Pottinger, R. E. and Harrod, J. P. (1959), "Alterations in Body Composition During Pregnancy," *Amer. J. Obstet. Gynec.*, **77**, 1038.

Melichar, V., Novák, M., Hahn, P. and Koldovský, O. (1964), "Free Fatty Acid and Glucose in the Blood of Various Groups of Newborns." Preliminary report. *Acta pædiat.*, **53**, 343.

Myant, N. B. and Cole, L. A. (1966), "Effect of Thyroxine on the Deposition of Phospholipids in the Brain *in vivo* and on the Synthesis of Phospholipids by Brain Slices," *J. Neurochem.*, **13**, 1299.

Myant, N. B. and Gamble, J. (1965), "The Accumulation of Maternal Phosphate in the Brain, Liver and Bone of Fœtal and Newborn Rabbits from Normal and Thyroid-deficient Mothers," *J. Endocr.*, **33**, 405.

Novák, M. and Jirásek (1966), Unpublished work quoted in Novák, M., Melichar, V. and Hahn, P., *Biologia Neonatorum*, 1966, **9**, 105.

Novák, M., Melichar, V., Hahn, P. and Koldovský, O. (1961), "Levels of Lipids in the Blood of Newborn Infants and the Effect of Glucose Administration," *Physiol. Bohemoslovenica*, **10**, 488.

Novák, M., Melichar, V., Hahn, P. and Koldovský, O. (1965), "Release of Free Fatty Acids from Adipose Tissue Obtained from Newborn Infants," *J. Lipid Res.*, **6**, 91.

Oliver, M. F. and Boyd, G. S. (1953), "Changes in the Plasma Lipids during the Menstrual Cycle," *Clin. Sci.*, **12**, 217.

Oliver, M. F. and Boyd, G. S. (1955), "Plasma Lipid and Serum Lipoprotein Patterns during Pregnancy and Puerperium," *Clin. Sci.*, **14**, 15.

Oliver, M. F. and Boyd, G. S. (1961), "Influence of Reduction of Serum Lipids on Prognosis of Coronary Heart-disease," *Lancet*, **1**, 499.

Pařízková, J. (1963), "Impact of Age, Diet, and Exercise on Man's Body Composition," *Ann. N.Y. Acad. Sci.*, **110**, 661.

Popják, G. (1954), "The Origin of Fetal Lipids," *Cold Spr. Harb. Symp. quant. Biol.*, **19**, 200.

Räihä, C. E. (1954), "Tissue Metabolism in the Human Fetus," *Cold Spr. Harb. Symp. quant. Biol.*, **19**, 143.

Randle, P. J., Garland, P. R., Hales, C. N. and Newsholme, E. A. (1963), "The Glucose Fatty-Acid Cycle. Its Rôle in Insulin Sensitivity and the Metabolic Disturbances of Diabetes Mellitus," *Lancet*, **i**, 785.

Robinson, R. W., Higano, N. and Cohen, W. D. (1957), "The Effects of Estrogens on Serum Lipids in Women," *Arch. intern. Med.*, **100**, 739.

Robinson, R. W., Higano, N. and Cohen, W. D. (1960), "Effects of Long-term Administration of Estrogens on Serum Lipids of Postmenopausal Women," *New Engl. J. Med.*, **263**, 828.

Roux, J. F. (1966), "Lipid Metabolism in the Fetal and Neonatal Rabbit," *Metabolism*, **15**, 856.

Russ, E. M., Eder, H. A. and Barr, D. P. (1955), "Influence of Gonadal Hormones on Protein-Lipid Relationships in Human Plasma," *Amer. J. Med.*, **19**, 4.

Samaan, N., Yen, S. C. C., Friesen, H. and Pearson, O. H. (1966), "Serum Placental Lactogen Levels during Pregnancy and in Trophoblastic Disease." *J. clin. Endocrin.*, **26**, 1303.

Schaefer, L. E. (1964), "Serum Cholesterol-Triglyceride Distribution in a 'Normal' New York City Population," *Amer. J. Med.*, **36**, 262.

Smith, C.A. (1959), *The Physiology of the Newborn Infant*, Third Edition, p. 210. Oxford: Blackwell Scientific Publications.

Taggart, N. (1961), "Skinfold Measurements during Human Pregnancy," *Proc. Nutr. Soc.*, **20**, xxx.

Thomson, A. M. and Hytten, F. E. (1961), "Calorie Requirements in Human Pregnancy," *Proc. Nutr. Soc.*, **20**, 76.

Turtle, J. R. and Kipnis, D. M. (1967), "The Lipolytic Action of Human Placental Lactogen on Isolated Fat Cells," *Biochim. biophys. Acta*, **144**, 583.

Vallance-Owen, J. (1965), "Synalbumin Antagonism in Obesity and Maturity Onset Diabetes Mellitus," *Ann. N.Y. Acad. Sci.*, **131**, 315.

Van Duyne, C. M. (1966), "Free Fatty Acid Metabolism during Perinatal Life," *Biol. Neonatorum*, **9**, 115.

Van Duyne, C. M. and Havel, R. J. (1959), "Plasma Unesterified Fatty Acid Concentration in Fetal and Neonatal Life," *Proc. Soc. exp. Biol.*, **102**, 599.

Van Duyne, C. M., Havel, R. J. and Felts, J. M. (1962), "Placental Transfer of Palmitic Acid-1-C14 in Rabbits," *Amer. J. Obstet. Gynec.*, **84**, 1069.

Van Duyne, C. M., Parker, H. R., Havel, R. J. and Holm, L. W. (1960), "Free Fatty Acid Metabolism in Fetal and Newborn Sheep," *Amer. J. Physiol.*, **199**, 987.

Van Duyne, C., Parker, H. R. and Holm, L. W. (1965): "Metabolism of Free Fatty Acids during Perinatal Life of Lambs," *Amer. J. Obstet. Gynec.*, **91**, 277.

Villee, C. A. (1954), "The Intermediary Metabolism of Human Fetal Tissues," *Cold Spr. Harb. Symp. Quant. Biol.*, **19**, 186.

Widdowson, E. M. and Spray, C. M. (1951), "Chemical Development *in utero*," *Arch. Dis. Childh.*, **26**, 205.

Wynn, V., Doar, J. W. H. and Mills, G. L. (1966), "Some Effects of Oral Contraceptives on Serum-lipid and Lipoprotein Levels," *Lancet*, **2**, 720.

Yen, S. S. C., Samaan, N. and Pearson, O. H. (1967), "Growth Hormone Levels in Pregnancy," *J. clin. Endocrin.*, **27**, 1341.

3. PROTEIN METABOLISM

R. W. CARRELL

The human body is thought to contain about 100,000 different proteins. Each protein is composed of polypeptide subunits which themselves are polymers formed by the peptide linkage of combinations of the twenty or more different amino acids. Each polypeptide usually contains up to several hundred of these amino acids which are arranged in a unique sequence giving each protein its own characteristic primary structure. As a consequence of this sequence each polypeptide spontaneously takes up a particular three dimensional conformation with the formation of an ordered structure along the amino acid chain, the secondary structure, and then bending and interaction of this in turn to give the tertiary structure. The final order of structure, the quaternary structure, describes the form taken up by the associated polypeptide subunits of the protein. Each protein then has a precise shape or configuration which arises directly from the sequence of amino acids contained in its polypeptide chains. It is this three dimensional conformation that confers on natural or native proteins their biological properties and loss of this conformation will result in loss of biological function and the rendering of the protein susceptible to enzymic digestion. In order then to maintain the integrity of body proteins they must be constantly renewed by a continuous or dynamic process of protein synthesis and degradation.

DIGESTION OF FOOD PROTEINS

The proteins of foodstuffs are broken down in the digestive tract to progressively smaller fragments. The initial cleavage occurs due to endopeptidases, enzymes such as trypsin, chymotrypsin, and pepsin, that produce hydrolysis at specific amino acids resulting in the formation of small peptides. These small peptides are broken down in turn by the diverse enzyme group, the exopeptidases which are potentially capable of the complete splitting of such peptides to free amino acids.

In order for the initial cleavage by the endopeptidases to occur all the amino acid side chains of the protein must be made available to the action of the enzymes. In the native protein many of the amino acid side chains are obscured in the interior of the molecule and the protein only becomes susceptible to digestion after the occurrence of the process of denaturation in which there is an unfolding of the polypeptide chain. Initial denaturation of protein usually occurs in the course of the cooking and preparation of food. The process is furthered in the stomach both by the gastric acid and the action of the enzyme pepsin which will give some partial peptide cleavage. The other important role of the stomach in protein digestion is the control it exercises over the release of proteins into the intestine—it is probably the impairment of this function that is responsible for the decreased protein assimilation that may be observed following gastrectomy.

On leaving the stomach the protein encounters the alkaline secretion of the pancreas. This contains a number of proteolytic enzymes the most important of which is trypsin. This as well as being a powerful digestive enzyme, is also responsible for the activation of other digestive enzymes. The pancreatic enzymes are capable of splitting proteins to very small peptides but the subsequent breakdown of these peptides to free amino acids is still conjectural. Inferentially it seems likely that this takes place due to the action of the exopeptidases of the intestinal villi, probably as the peptides come into contact with the epithelial border.

The absorption of 80–90 per cent of the dietary nitrogen takes place in the distal duodenum and proximal half of the jejunum. By this stage almost all proteins will be appreciably digested although, as is shown by food allergies, small amounts of whole protein may be absorbed, perhaps by the process of pinocytosis but more likely by absorption through the lymphatic system. The absorption of whole protein is of particular physiological importance to the newborn infant who utilizes the immunoglobulins of the colostrum by this process. It is possible that the absorption of the immunoglobulins by the intestinal epithelium occurs by a similar mechanism to that involved in placental transport. Here the major immunoglobulin fraction, IgG, is uniquely transported across the trophoblastic cells to the foetal circulation by a process whose specificity depends on the presence of certain "transmission sites" on the heavy chain of the IgG. The survival of these proteins in the gut of the newborn infant is attributed to the absence of gastric acid secretion in the first few days of life and to the presence in the colostrum of potent enzyme inhibitors. It will also be assisted by the inherent resistance to trypsin of the colostrum immunoglobulin, IgA. For the most part the absorption of the products of protein digestion is confined to that of the isolated amino acids though there is evidence that absorption of dipeptides can also occur, probably as a passive process. The absorption of free amino acids has been shown to involve active transport mechanisms.

Curiously, the amino acids absorbed by the gut are often only to a lesser extent derived from foodstuffs since there is a considerable secretion into the gut of endogenous protein. This is formed by the secreted digestive enzymes, abraded cells of the intestinal mucosa, and exuded serum proteins and mucoproteins. These are all digested and absorbed by the same mechanisms as are the proteins of foodstuffs, although, because of their native state, the digestive process is slower. The endogenous protein secretion provides, as a short term effect, some balance to the intake of protein. However, it also makes the interpretation of protein uptake studies particularly difficult and has led to the misinterpretation of numbers of protein labelling experiments.

AMINO ACID METABOLISM

Although the majority of absorbed amino acids pass via the portal circulation to the liver, from the moment of their absorption they are available for protein synthesis. Thus a small proportion of the absorbed amino acids will be utilized for the synthesis of protein in the cells of the villi, at the same time some of the protein of these cells break down with the release of amino acids for general metabolism. This continuous interchange between amino acids and proteins is the general pattern for almost all the body proteins. There are no true stores of protein in the body but the liver, muscle, and plasma proteins all undergo a rapid turnover (liver protein has a half-life of seven days) and are able to be drawn on in times of protein depletion. In the period of recovery from protein depletion there is evidence that some of the body proteins take precedence over others in utilizing the amino acids that become available. A practical application of this follows from the observation that haemoglobin synthesis takes priority over the formation of plasma proteins. For this reason the first step in the treatment of malnutrition should be the correction, by transfusion, of any anaemia present.

Amino acids as well as being directly utilized for the synthesis of protein may also be converted to other amino acids, converted to carbohydrate, or utilized for energy production. The pathways involved are often quite complex and for details of them reference should be made to standard biochemical texts. There is however one major pathway of amino acid metabolism of general importance. This is available for both the synthesis and breakdown of amino acids and is based on two enzymically controlled reactions.

(i) **Transamination.** Here there is effectively a transfer of the amine of an amino acid to a keto acid resulting in the formation of a new amino acid, and leaving a new keto acid which is available for further degradation or metabolic use.

$$
\begin{array}{cc}
\begin{array}{c} R \\ | \\ CHNH_2 \\ | \\ COOH \end{array}
+
\begin{array}{c} COOH \\ | \\ CH_2 \\ | \\ CH_2 \\ | \\ CO \\ | \\ COOH \end{array}
\rightleftharpoons
\begin{array}{c} R \\ | \\ CO \\ | \\ COOH \end{array}
+
\begin{array}{c} COOH \\ | \\ CH_2 \\ | \\ CH_2 \\ | \\ CHNH_2 \\ | \\ COOH \end{array}
\end{array}
$$

amino acid   α-keto glutaric acid   new keto acid   glutamic acid

Use of this reaction in the forward direction will give the breakdown of an amino acid with acceptance of its amine group by α-ketoglutarate. The reverse reaction can be used for the synthesis of new amino acids with the acceptance by a keto acid of an amine group from glutamic acid. The enzymes that catalyse these reactions are the aminotransferases which are perhaps better known by their former name, the transaminases. These enzymes are widely distributed in the tissues, the two most important being glutamic-oxaloacetic transaminase (GOT) and glutamic-pyruvic transaminase (GPT). The occurrence of rapid tissue breakdown results in the raising in the serum levels of these enzymes, the level of GOT being particularly raised in muscle necrosis (as in myocardial infarction), a raised GPT level being more indicative of liver damage.

(ii) **Deamination.** The breakdown of amino acids by the process of transamination would soon result in an accumulation of glutamic acid since α-ketoglutarate is the major amine group acceptor in this reaction. There is however another widely distributed enzyme, glutamic dehydrogenase, which catalyses the direct deamination of glutamic acid with the release of ammonia.

$$
\begin{array}{ccc}
\text{COOH} & & \text{COOH} \\
| & & | \\
\text{CH}_2 & & \text{CH}_2 \\
| & & | \\
\text{CH}_2 + \text{NAD} + \text{H}_2\text{O} \rightleftharpoons & \text{CH}_2 + \text{NADH}_2 + \text{NH}_3 \\
| & & | \\
\text{CHNH}_2 & & \text{CO} \\
| & & | \\
\text{COOH} & & \text{COOH} \\
\text{glutamic} & & \text{α-ketoglutaric} \\
\text{acid} & & \text{acid}
\end{array}
$$

It can be seen then that the coupling of transamination and deamination will provide a versatile pathway for both the synthesis and degradation of amino acids. The coupled process has been termed *Transdeamination*.

Metabolism of Ammonia

The ammonia formed by deamination may alternatively be utilized in the reverse reaction, used to give amidation of glutamic acid with the formation of glutamine, or metabolized to urea in the liver. The liver is the major site of ammonia removal and it is especially responsible for the detoxication of the appreciable amounts of ammonia formed in the intestines by bacterial action and absorbed into the portal circulation. It is the presence of abnormal concentrations of ammonia in the circulation that is responsible for the most acute manifestations of liver failure. The toxic effect of ammonia on the brain causes the tremor, delusions and eventual coma, seen in hepatic failure. This has provided the rationale for the treatment of a hepatic crisis with antibiotics in order to suppress the intestinal bacterial flora thus reducing ammonia production from this source.

Essential Amino Acids

It has been shown that the adult must be supplied, in the diet, with the essential amino acids; lysine, tryptophan, phenylalanine, threonine, valine, methionine, leucine, and isoleucine. These amino acids are dietary essentials because their corresponding keto acids cannot be synthesized in the human or because the amino acids cannot be formed by one of the limited number of special pathways for the interconversion of one amino acid to another.

Glycogenesis and Ketogenesis

It was pointed out that the chief pathway of amino acid breakdown was that of transamination, with the formation from the amino acid of a corresponding keto acid. For the most part the deaminated products of the amino acids can be utilized, via the citric acid and glyolytic pathways, for the formation of carbohydrate. These amino acids are therefore glycogenic whereas the minority of amino acids whose terminal products are ketone bodies are said to be ketogenic.

Specific Dynamic Action of Proteins

It has long been observed that, in animals, an increase in heat production by the body occurred after the ingestion of food. Explanations that have been advanced in the past for this increased heat production have been sufficient to explain the small increase in heat noted after the ingestion of fats and carbohydrate but have not satisfactorily explained the very large increase in heat production (20–40 per cent) noted after the ingestion of protein, an effect that has been termed the specific dynamic action of protein. Krebs, in the text edited by Munro and Allison (1964), has proposed an acceptable reason for this effect. He points out that in order for the chemical energy of food to be utilized by the body it must ultimately be converted to the high energy nucleotide ATP. He demonstrated that, by comparison with fat and carbohydrate, additional calories of protein were required for the production of a given amount of ATP. Thus more calories of protein than of carbohydrate are required to produce the same amount of ATP, the difference representing the heat produced by the specific dynamic action of protein.

The reason for this difference is that urea synthesis, the end-point of protein catabolism, is an energy requiring process and also that by comparison with carbohydrate or lipid catabolism, amino acid breakdown is an incomplete and wasteful process. The end effect then is that the protein provides less useful energy per calorie than do fats and carbohydrate, the energy loss being dissipated in body heat production.

Inborn Errors of Metabolism

There are now a number of well documented hereditary diseases which arise from defects in the pathway of amino acid metabolism. A full account of these diseases is given in Stanbury, Wyngaarden and Fredrickson (1966). Of particular relevance to this discussion is the disease phenylketonuria which presents in the newborn due to a defect in the pathway for the conversion of phenylalanine to tyrosine. This defect results in the accumulation in the serum, and excretion in the urine of phenylalanine, phenylpyruvate and their degradation products.

In surveys for the disease it has been found to occur as frequently as 1:10,000 births. The abnormality becomes detectable about six days after birth when the serum phenylalanine levels rise and the excretion of phenylpyruvate appears in the urine. Routine testing usually consists of a simple urine/ferric chloride colour test but this may give false negative results and there is a strong case for the routine screening of serum levels of phenylalanine or its products. The disease generally results in brain damage but this can be prevented by early enough treatment of the condition by use of a diet restricted in phenylalanine content. It is now realized, however, that the disease may be expressed in several manners and that brain damage is not necessarily an inherent feature of the disease. This has been advanced as a reason for caution in the institution of the radical dietary treatment.

PROTEIN SYNTHESIS

One of the most remarkable scientific developments of the past decade has been the advance in our knowledge of the molecular processes involved in protein synthesis. The advances in the next decade are likely to be even more considerable and will be of increasing relevance to the obstetrician whose responsibility covers the most critical period of protein development, that of foetal growth. Our knowledge is already sufficient for some general understanding of the processes involved in mutation and genetic variation, in the mode of action of hormones, and of the action of some of the drugs affecting protein synthesis.

The relationship of the chromosome to the genetic material DNA (deoxyribonucleic acid) and RNA (ribonucleic acid) has been described in section 1. Briefly, DNA is a polymer formed by combinations of the four bases, adenine (A), guanine (G), cytosine (C), and thymine (T), linked together by a sugar (deoxyribose) and phosphate groups. It is the arrangement of these bases in the DNA that provides the code determining the sequence of amino acids in the polypeptide whose synthesis the DNA ultimately controls. The success of DNA as a genetic material is dependent on the occurrence of the phenomenon of base pairing. The bases of DNA project from the molecule and will spontaneously form weak bonds with other bases which have a complementary physical structure to give, in DNA, the base pairs T–A and C–G. As the result of this pairing each DNA molecule can act as a template for the formation of another molecule that lies parallel to it and has a completely complementary base composition. In this way the two form a double stranded molecule, the two strands being bridged by the base pairs and for reasons of stability taking up a helical conformation. This occurrence of spontaneous base pairing means that the molecule can always be readily duplicated. Thus in the passage of genetic material, as in the dividing cell, the process of replication occurs with each strand of the DNA undergoing duplication, by base pairing, to give rise to two daughter double stranded molecules.

The process of protein synthesis can best be described in conjunction with the diagrammatic representation shown in Fig. 1. In order for the code of the DNA to become available for the determination of amino acid sequence, transcription of the code into RNA must first occur. The only difference between RNA and DNA is that in RNA the sugar present is ribose, not deoxyribose, and the base thymine (T) is replaced by uracil (U). Thus a molecule of RNA is built up with complementary structure to that of the DNA strand on which it is based, in this way the RNA retaining the coded sequence of the DNA. This RNA, because it passes from the nucleus to the cytoplasm, is termed the messenger or m–RNA. During active protein synthesis the portion of DNA coding for each polypeptide will produce many m–RNA molecules each of which acts as a template for synthesis of the polypeptide. The actual formation, or translation, of the polypeptide is brought about by a particulate body, the ribosome. This passes along the length of the m–RNA successively adding amino acids according to the coded message of the RNA to give at the end the complete polypeptide. The process occurs rapidly with several ribosomes moving in succession on the one m–RNA molecule, the compound structure so formed being called the polysome.

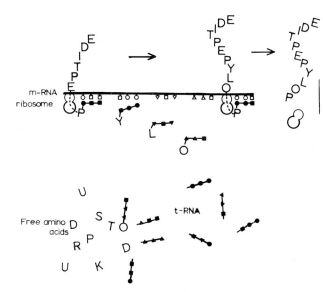

Fig. 1. Protein Synthesis. The free amino acids (capital letters), on activation combine with their appropriate transfer RNA (t-RNA) and are taken to the messenger (m-RNA) seen in the upper part of the diagram. Here the t-RNA is matched with its triplet code and the amino acid added by the ribosome to the growing polypeptide. The ribosomes move along the m-RNA to the right, being released after the addition of the final (COOH-terminal) amino acid.

There are several requirements before an amino acid can be utilized by the ribosome for peptide linkage. Each amino acid has first to undergo activation in the presence of ATP and an enzyme to form a compound with another smaller RNA molecule, the transfer or t-RNA. Each amino acid has its own specific t-RNA which is able to recognize the code on the m-RNA for its particular amino acid. In this way the transfer RNA molecules bring the activated amino acids to their appropriate positions on the m-RNA template, the ribosome incorporating the amino acid into the forming polypeptide as it moves along the m-RNA molecule.

Protein Genetics and Variation

Our knowledge of molecular genetics in the human rests largely on studies that have been made of the abnormal haemoglobins, variant forms of haemoglobin which have usually been detected as the result of population surveys. These have confirmed that the mechanisms of molecular genetics in man are the same as those in all other living organisms. The abnormal haemoglobins have also indicated the existence in the population of a good deal of variation in protein structure which seems only occasionally to cause dysfunction of the protein and therefore to give rise to hereditary disease.

Each amino acid is coded in the DNA molecule by a group of three bases. The four bases of DNA provide 64 possible triplet combinations, giving ample allowance for the coding of the twenty amino acids and also for the provision of punctuation, i.e. instructions for the commencement or termination of a polypeptide. There is then, at least one and usually more, triplet codes for each amino acid. The codes for valine and isoleucine are illustrated below, there being four triplets that code for valine and three for isoleucine.

Valine GUU	Isoleucine AUU
GUC	AUC
GUA	AUA
GUG	

Protein variants resulting from a mutation usually have a change confined to one position in their amino acid sequence with the replacement of one amino acid by another. By studying the nature of these amino acid replacements it has been possible to show that the underlying change occurring in a natural mutation is almost always the replacement of just one of the bases of DNA by another. It is clear then that numbers of undetectable mutations must be occurring since the change in one base of a triplet may result in another triplet coding for the same amino acid and hence have no affect on the amino acid sequence of the protein. For example:

$$GUU \xrightarrow{\text{mutation}} GUC$$
$$\text{valine} \qquad\qquad \text{valine}$$

Again, even when a mutation does affect the amino acid sequence of the protein it is probable that it will not cause any gross change in the function of the protein. For instance, five every thousand of a European population are thought to have a haemoglobin of variant structure yet very few of these have any noticeable handicap as a result. There are several reasons for this. Firstly the genetic code is so arranged that a change in one base is most likely to produce an alteration in coding from one amino acid to another of similar physical characteristics. It is unlikely, for instance, that the mutation

$$GUU \longrightarrow AUU$$
$$\text{valine} \qquad \text{isoleucine}$$

would result in protein dysfunction as the amino acids valine and isoleucine are of very similar structure. Secondly, even when the change produced is from one amino acid to another of very different structure, it does not necessarily result in an alteration in the function of the protein. This is because there are a number of positions in the amino acid sequence of a protein which make a minimal contribution to the overall function of the molecule.

In this way then considerable variation in protein structure can occur within a population, the variation only giving rise to a hereditary disease when there is a replacement of an amino acid in an important portion of the molecule by one of differing physical properties.

Hormonal Control of Protein Synthesis

Many hormones produce a stimulation of protein synthesis. Some of these, such as growth hormone and insulin, cause a generalized increase in protein synthesis, whilst others, such as luteinising hormone and ACTH, stimulate the synthesis of specific proteins. It was an attractive thought that the mode of action of all hormones could be explained by the one mechanism and an immediate proposition was that hormones acted by freeing the production of the m-RNA which coded the required proteins. It is possible that this mechanism might be involved in the action of some hormones but increasingly, evidence seems to point to the controlling mechanism being at the ribosomal level, i.e. at the translational stage of protein synthesis. It has been found for example, that in preparations from the tissues of growth hormone deficient animals the rate of protein synthesis is still depressed even after the addition of excess m-RNA. More recent experiments with preparations from diabetic animals suggests that insulin may stimulate protein synthesis by causing ribosomal activation. How this occurs is not clear but on other grounds it is evident that there is a, as yet ill-understood, mechanism controlling the rate of protein synthesis at the translational level and it is likely that the action of some hormones will be involved at this stage.

Drugs and Protein Synthesis

A number of drugs effect protein synthesis and amongst the best studied of these are certain of the antibiotics. A number of antibiotics, of which penicillin is the outstanding example, achieve their effect by their action on the bacterial cell wall and for this reason function as specific antibacterial agents. However, other of the antibiotics have a general action on protein synthesis, their antibacterial effect depending only on the greater specificity of this action on the bacterial rather than on the mammalian cell. A number such as streptomycin, chloramphenicol, and the tetracyclines are bound by the ribosome and cause an inhibition of the translational process in which formation of polypeptide occurs. Another mode of action is that of actinomycin which becomes associated with the double helix of DNA causing it to distort. A last example is puromycin which functions as a structural analogue of t-RNA and can be added on the ribosome to the growing polypeptide resulting in its termination.

From these examples it can be seen that it is now becoming possible to assess the effects of drugs, at the molecular level, on protein synthesis. It is to be hoped that further work of this type will allow a more reasoned approach in the choice of drugs for administration to the pregnant woman.

FURTHER READING

Altschul, A. M. (1965), *Proteins. Their Chemistry and Politics.* London: Chapman and Hall.

Korner, A. (1967), Ribonucleic Acid and Hormonal Control of Protein Synthesis," *Progress in Biophysical and Molecular Biology,* **17,** 63.

Munro, H. N. and Allison, J. B. (1964), *Mammalian Protein Metabolism,* Vol. i and ii, New York: Academic Press.

Newton, B. A. and Reynolds, P. E., (1966), *Biochemical Studies of Antimicrobial Drugs,* London: Cambridge University Press.

Stanbury, J. B., Wyngaarden, J. B. and Fredrickson, D. S. (1966), *The Metabolic Basis of Inherited Disease.* 2nd Edition. New York: McGraw-Hill.

Watson, J. D. (1965), *Molecular Biology of the Gene,* New York: Benjamin.

4. NUTRITION

C. GOPALAN

Introduction

The physiological stress of pregnancy imposes some specific and additional nutritional requirements. There is strong evidence that if these requirements are not adequately met, not only would the nutritional status of the mother be affected, but also the course of her pregnancy and the condition of her offspring at birth. There is a great deal of evidence gathered from work on experimental animals pointing to the role of nutrition in pregnancy. However, the question arises how far these experimental results are applicable to human subjects. As far as human subjects are concerned, the evidence for the role of nutrition in pregnancy rests largely on epidemiological evidences. The unfortunate nutritional situation prevalent in many developing countries affords opportunities for the study of the effects of maternal nutrition on the course of pregnancy and the condition of the offspring at birth.

Nutritional requirements in pregnancy are quite often computed as the requirement of the mother in the non-pregnant state plus the nutritional requirement of the foetus. This approach, however, obviously ignores the possible effects of the profound maternal hormonal and metabolic changes which are bound to condition nutritional requirements in pregnancy. The full significance and implications of the metabolic changes in pregnancy have, however, not been fully elucidated.

It would appear that the alterations in hormonal balance during pregnancy are such as generally to favour anabolic processes. A growth hormone like substance has been isolated from human placenta. This has been partially characterized and has been shown to be very similar to human growth hormone of pituitary origin. The efficiency of absorption of iron, vitamin B-12 and of calcium have been shown to increase during pregnancy.

On the other hand, basal metabolism increases significantly during pregnancy and this increase may be as high as 20 per cent towards the end of pregnancy. The glomerular filtration rate and the clearance of substances like creatinine, urea and uric acid are also considerably increased during pregnancy. There is a quantitative as well as qualitative increase in the pattern of excretion of amino acids in the urine. Glycosuria is not an uncommon feature.

There is a marked increase in plasma volume, on an average, by about 50 per cent. This is accompanied by an increase in red cell mass by about 20 per cent. Haemoglobin concentration and the packed cell volume, therefore, drop in spite of an absolute increase in the total circulating haemoglobin. There is a fall in serum proteins; however, all the fractions of serum proteins are not affected proportionately. There are also definite changes in the concentration of various nutrients in the plasma, but not all of this can be attributed to the changes in plasma volume. Thus, while there is a decrease in the concentration of haemoglobin, serum proteins, serum vitamin A and ascorbic acid, the concentration of carotene, tocopherols, cholesterol and N-methyl nicotinamide, increases.

There is also an increase in the total body water from a normal value of over 50 per cent in the first few weeks of gestation to about 70 per cent or more, in the last trimester. The manner in which water is distributed in different compartments may vary and this is probably determined to a certain extent by the nutritional status of the subject.

In the assessment of the nutritional status of subjects, concentrations of various nutrients in serum and urine are often used as indices. It is essential to appreciate physiological variations in these constituents during pregnancy in order to avoid misleading conclusions with regard to nutritional status during pregnancy.

Nutritional Requirements in Pregnancy

Calorie requirement. During pregnancy, extra energy is needed for the growth of the foetus, the placenta and the associated maternal tissues. The caloric requirements during pregnancy are conditioned by the following factors:

1. Extra energy needed for the growth of the foetus, placenta and the associated maternal tissues.
2. Increase in B.M.R. of the mother by about 20 per cent above usual rate, towards the end of pregnancy.
3. Increased energy expenditure involved in the movements of the mother whose bodyweight is increased during pregnancy.

The FAO committee on Calorie Requirements computed that the increased total calorie requirements would be of the order of 80,000 KCalories for the entire duration of the pregnancy. In women of the well-to-do groups who gain, on an average, nearly 12 kg. during the entire course of pregnancy, it has been estimated that nearly 40,000 calories are accounted for by increased fat storage. Since fat accumulation in maternal tissues in pregnancy may not be considered as an essential part of the reproductive process, the increased caloric requirements in pregnancy would be of the order of 40,000 calories or around 150 calories, daily. However, an allowance has also to be made for the fact that during pregnancy in the great majority of cases, there is reduced physical activity. In most cases, energy balance during pregnancy is achieved partly by increased food intake and partly by reduced physical activity. The precise increase in calorie requirement in a given case of pregnancy will depend upon the extent to which physical activity is reduced. It is reasonable to expect that in the great majority of well-to-do women with few domestic responsibilities, energy balance may be achieved purely by restricted physical activity and, in these cases, no additional calories would be required during pregnancy.

Protein requirement. An estimate of the additional protein requirement during pregnancy may be attempted by various methods. Nitrogen balance studies, extent of protein retention with different dietary levels of protein and increase in body-weight during pregnancy may be used as indicators. Protein requirement may also be assessed indirectly by determining the basal energy expenditure in pregnancy.

During pregnancy, additional protein is required for the growth of the products of conception and the enlargement of organs of reproduction. The quantity of protein laid down during the course of pregnancy has been computed by Thomson and Hytten. According to these authors, the growth of the products of conception and the increase in the weight of maternal organs account for only 60 per cent of the actual maternal weight gain during pregnancy. However, nitrogen balance studies in pregnant women indicate that the nitrogen retention which occurs in pregnancy is considerably in excess of the actual requirements of the foetus and the accessory organs.

Long-term nitrogen balance studies by Macy and co-workers have indicated a nitrogen retention of 200 to 400 g. in excess of retention in foetus and reproductive organs, during the entire course of pregnancy. It has been estimated that in the successive quarters of pregnancy the daily amount of protein laid down would be around 0·5, 3·0, 4·5 and 5·7 g. giving a cumulative total of 950 g. as the additional need for protein during pregnancy. The precise significance of the increased deposition of protein in maternal tissues other than the reproductive organs, is not clear. It has been claimed that this may represent a reserve which may be called upon during the post-partum period. However, it is well-known that nitrogen balance studies are subject to several cumulative errors. Hytten and Leitch have questioned the validity of the assessment of nitrogen retention based on nitrogen balance studies.

On the basis of available data, the FAO/WHO Expert Group on Protein Requirements recommended that the increased requirement of protein during the last two trimesters of pregnancy may be considered to be 5 g. to which figure 20 per cent may be added as allowance for individual variation. It is, therefore, recommended that the increased demand for protein in pregnancy may be met by providing an additional 6 g. of good quality protein daily, during the 2nd and 3rd trimesters of pregnancy.

Calcium requirement. It has been estimated that about 30 g. of calcium is deposited in the foetus. This takes place mostly during the third trimester. On this basis, a daily intake of additional 350 mg. of calcium would be needed during the third trimester. However, there is evidence now that during pregnancy certain metabolic adaptations resulting in better absorption and conservation of calcium, are brought into play. Sufficient data are, however, not available to indicate the extent to which such adaptation modifies calcium requirement. On the basis of available evidence, it may be, therefore, accepted that an additional allowance of about 300 mg. of calcium during the latter half of pregnancy would be adequate. The FAO/WHO Expert Group have suggested a total intake of 1000 to 1200 mg. calcium daily, during pregnancy.

Iron requirement. A full-term foetus is known to contain about 300 mg. of iron and the placenta, about 70 mg. The increase in red cell mass in the mother during pregnancy would represent an increment of nearly 290 mg. of iron, while the blood loss during parturition would represent an additional 50 mg. of iron. On the other hand, the cessation of menstruation during pregnancy would result in an over-all reduction in iron requirement equivalent to 150 mg. during the entire course of pregnancy. The net physiological cost of iron in pregnancy would, therefore, work out to around 550 to 600 mg. Of this amount, the iron needed for expansion of haemoglobin mass will be met from the tissue stores and will return to the stores after pregnancy. The real extra need which has to be supplemented through diet will consist of the amount needed for transfer to the foetus and the loss during parturition. This amounts to about 300 mg. This would imply that an additional amount of 2 to 3 mg. of iron daily would be needed by the mother during her pregnancy. Generally, about 10 per cent of dietary iron is believed to be absorbed. There is evidence that efficiency of absorption of dietary iron is considerably increased during pregnancy. Recent studies have shown that this can be as high as 20 per cent. An additional 10 mg. of dietary iron may, therefore, have to be provided daily, during pregnancy.

In many developing countries, women start their pregnancy with poor iron stores. The intake of available iron in the dietaries of these women is relatively low. For this reason, the incidence of anaemia in pregnancy is very high in such countries and accounts for a high proportion of maternal mortality. Under these circumstances, it is essential to ensure that in addition to improvement of diets, additional iron supplements are provided during pregnancy.

Iodine requirement. A precise estimate of the physiological cost of pregnancy in terms of iodine is not possible. That there is an increased requirement for iodine during pregnancy is, however, clear from the increased incidence of goitre during pregnancy. Special attention should, therefore, be given to iodine needs of pregnant women particularly in areas where endemic goitre is a problem.

Vitamin A requirement. The additional need for vitamin A during pregnancy is largely due to the transfer of the vitamin from the mother to the foetus. The data obtained from autopsy studies indicate that the liver of the newborn infant may contain about 45 μg. of vitamin-A/g. of tissue. Since the liver of a newborn infant weighs around 150 g., the whole liver may be expected to contain around 7000 μg. of vitamin A. This implies that there will be withdrawal from the maternal stores, to the extent of about 50 μg. of vitamin A per day during the last half of pregnancy to provide for the foetal stores. Information as to the efficiency of transfer of vitamin A across the placenta is still very scanty. Moreover, we do not as yet have any precise indication as to how the needs for vitamin A of the maternal tissues are modified during pregnancy. There is now some evidence that vitamin A is concerned with progesterone metabolism; and, it is possible that the hormonal changes in pregnancy may necessitate increased maternal requirement of vitamin A.

Among malnourished women in developing countries, clinical signs of vitamin A deficiency are frequently seen. Further, while a fall in serum vitamin A levels in the last trimester of pregnancy may be considered to be a physiological event in pregnancy, the extent of this fall in malnourished women would appear to be much greater. It is also found that, unlike in well-to-do mothers, among undernourished women supplementation of vitamin A to the mother during the last weeks of pregnancy has been found to produce a significant increase in the vitamin A level of cord blood.

The FAO/WHO Expert Committee concluded that since the additional amount of vitamin A required during pregnancy was an insignificant fraction of the total normal daily requirement, no special additional allowance over and above the normal daily requirement of 750 μg. of vitamin A need be recommended during pregnancy.

Thiamine, Riboflavin and Niacin requirements. It is the customary practice to express the requirement of thiamine, riboflavin and niacin in terms of caloric value of the diet. On the basis of available evidence, it is not possible to give any precise indication of the physiological cost of pregnancy in terms of these vitamins. There is some evidence of changes in the urinary excretion of thiamine and riboflavin in pregnancy. There is also an indication that the conversion of tryptophan to niacin is probably more efficient in pregnancy. Some national nutrition bodies have recommended increased allowance of these nutrients during pregnancy. However, the available data would suggest that the requirement of these vitamins in relation to calories is no greater in pregnancy than in the non-pregnant state. The FAO/WHO Expert Group have in fact concurred with this view. There is no evidence that there is an increase in thiamin, riboflavin and niacin requirements in pregnancy over and above what is dictated by increased caloric intake. An intake of 0·4 mg./1000 calories of thiamine, 0·55 mg./1000 calories of riboflavin and 6·6 niacin equivalents/1000 calories (for the calculation of the niacin equivalent, 60 mg. of tryptophan may be considered equivalent to 1 mg. of niacin) in pregnancy may be considered adequate.

Pyridoxine requirement. Pregnant women excrete abnormally large amounts of xanthurenic acid following a tryptophan load. This can be corrected in a number of pregnant subjects by the administration of pyridoxine. It has, therefore, been suggested that the requirement for pyridoxine increases during pregnancy.

On the other hand, there is evidence that functional pyridoxine deficiency may not be the total explanation for the abnormal xanthurenic acid excretion in pregnancy. Apparently, abnormal tryptophan metabolism induced by endocrine factors may also be partly concerned. The demonstration of direct effect of estrogens on the kinurenine transaminase system in the tryptophan metabolic pathway is in support of this possibility.

Vitamin C requirement. It is of course well-known that a nursing mother will furnish to her nursing infant nearly 20 mg. of ascorbic acid daily. While, thus, the need for increased vitamin C in lactation is clear, there is no evidence pointing to the need for extra allowance of vitamin C during pregnancy. The normal vitamin C allowance which ranges from 50 to 100 mg. according to various national bodies, may be considered to include a safety margin covering the possible needs of vitamin C in pregnancy.

Vitamin D requirement. It is essential that the diet contains adequate supply of vitamin D in order to ensure proper calcium absorption and utilization. This is specially the case in communities where, for cultural or religious reasons, or as a result of climatic factors, the subjects may be insufficiently exposed to light. In any case, it is desirable that the diet in pregnancy provides 400 I.U. of vitamin D.

Vitamin K. The practice of administration of vitamin K to the pregnant woman a few hours before delivery to prevent neonatal haemorrhage, which was once widely in use has now been abandoned. It has been demonstrated that vitamin K and analogues, especially in high doses, can produce definite toxic manifestations in the newborn.

Folic acid and vitamin B-12 requirements. Deficiencies of folic acid and probably, of vitamin B-12 are apparently common during pregnancy. Serum folate levels decline significantly especially in the last trimester of pregnancy. Folic acid requirement in pregnancy is not known with certainty. Some studies have indicated that the minimum intake of folic acid in diet needed to maintain serum folate levels would be as high as 300 μg. daily.

It has been computed that during pregnancy, foetal storage of vitamin B-12 may be around 50 to 100 μg. To provide for this, additional 0·1 to 0·2 μg. of absorbed vitamin B-12 would be necessary. To ensure this, an additional intake of 1 μg. daily of vitamin B-12 over and above the normal requirement may be needed, bringing the total desirable vitamin B-12 intake in pregnancy to 2 μg. daily. Serum vitamin B-12 levels are known to decline in pregnancy and to revert to normal values after parturition without additional vitamin B-12 supplementation. The fall in serum vitamin B-12 levels in pregnancy cannot be totally averted by vitamin B-12 supplementation. It is necessary to ensure that especially in areas of the world where megaloblastic anaemias are common, adequate levels of folic acid and vitamin B-12 in the diets are provided.

Effect of Nutrition on the Course of Pregnancy

From the foregoing discussion of the nutritional requirements in pregnancy, it will be obvious that expectant women constitute a highly vulnerable group from the nutritional standpoint. In any public health programme concerned with the improvement of the nutritional status of populations, pregnant women, along with nursing mothers, infants and children, require special consideration. The current situation with regard to dietary patterns in pregnancy in different parts of the world may now be briefly reviewed and the epidemiological and experimental data pointing to the possible effects of nutritional factors on the course of pregnancy may be discussed.

Dietary pattern in pregnancy. The diets of pregnant women in different parts of the world generally reflect the habitual diets of the rest of the population in these areas. In most of the technologically advanced countries of the world, diets of pregnant women generally provide on an average, more than 2500 calories, except where on the advice of physicians calories in diets are reduced to 2000–2200 calories. In these diets, proteins provide more than 12 per cent of the calories. On the other hand, among the poorer segments of populations in developing countries, the calorie intake is well below 2000 calories and only about 8 per cent of calories are derived from protein. In some areas, the intakes are as low as 1500 calories. The intake of calcium is generally more than 1 g. daily among well-nourished population groups, but it rarely exceeds 500 mg. daily in many countries of Asia and Africa. Vitamin A intake of the mothers in pregnancy in poor undernourished segments is 300 μg. of vitamin A or less, as against 800 μg. in well-to-do communities. The intake of iron in the dietaries among undernourished communities subsisting on cereals is above 20 mg. daily—a level which is seemingly adequate. Since, however, these diets are generally predominantly based on cereals rich in phytin, absorption of dietary iron is poor and the diets are, therefore, in fact deficient in iron.

Apart from such poor diets, pregnant and lactating women in large areas of the world are also subjected to other stresses, in the nature of chronic infections and parasitic infestations which tend further to aggravate the nutritional inadequacy. Social, cultural and family environment and specific customs and taboos also greatly influence dietary habits during pregnancy. In the actual application of scientific knowledge with regard to the nutritional requirements in pregnancy and in the translation of the nutrient requirements into practical recommendations under field conditions, an appreciation of all these factors is essential.

Pregnancy wastage. A great deal of information is available pointing to the effect of nutrition on the course of pregnancy in experimental animals. When the dietary protein levels are reduced to less than 5 per cent in rats, the incidence of foetal resorptions is found to be as high as 70 per cent to 100 per cent. The critical need for protein

in these experimental studies is apparent only during the early stages of placental and foetal development. The practical significance of these experimental observations from the point of view of human subjects requires cautious appraisal.

In a survey carried out in South India among poor women whose dietaries during pregnancy provided barely 1500 calories and about 40 g. of protein daily, nearly 20 per cent of the pregnancies were found to terminate in abortions, miscarriages and still-births. Even this figure may be an underestimate and may not include abortions in early stages of pregnancy. Such high incidence of pregnancy wastage seems to be a usual finding among undernourished population groups in other parts of the world. It must, however, be pointed out that the standard of obstetric care among the underprivileged population groups is also low. To what extent the high pregnancy wastage is a reflection of poor obstetric care is a moot question.

Gain in bodyweight during pregnancy. A relatively low gain in bodyweight in pregnancy has been observed among undernourished women. While the usual weight gain during pregnancy among well-to-do women is around 12 kg., in Indian women of the poor socioeconomic groups weighing on an average 42 kg., the gain in body weight during pregnancy is only of the order of 6 kg. Similar observations have been made among undernourished populations in other parts of the world also. The significance of this comparatively small gain in bodyweight requires consideration specially in the context of the profound changes in body composition which are known to occur during pregnancy. Lower weight gain may be a reflection of smaller gain of body protein or of smaller accretion of body fat. Body composition studies among poorly nourished pregnant women indicate that unlike in well-to-do groups, there is actually a loss of body fat in these women during pregnancy.

Hyperemesis gravidarum. It was earlier pointed out that the abnormal xanthurenic acid excretion observed in pregnancy may be a manifestation of functional pyridoxine deficiency. It has been demonstrated that in cases of hyperemesis gravidarum the increase in blood urea following the ingestion of alanine is of a much higher order than in normal pregnancy, and such higher levels are maintained over a longer period of time. It has also been found that this abnormal response could be corrected by pyridoxine. It would thus appear there is some biochemical support for the role of pyridoxine deficiency in the development of hyperemesis gravidarum.

Toxaemias of pregnancy. A high incidence of eclampsia is reported in pregnant women of the low socioeconomic group in certain parts of the world where malnutrition is widespread. On this basis, it has been claimed from time to time that malnutrition may play a contributory role in the development of toxaemias of pregnancy. While a possible effect of dietary status on toxaemias of pregnancy may not be ruled out, it would seem more probable on the basis of available epidemiological evidence that the higher incidence of eclampsia in poor communities is largely a result of poor obstetric care.

Effect of Maternal Nutrition on the Condition of the Infant

Apart from affecting the course of pregnancy, there is evidence that maternal nutritional status may considerably influence the condition of the offspring at birth. The evidence for the role of malnutrition in this regard is provided by several experimental and epidemiological observations.

Birthweight and incidence of immaturity. There is now ample evidence pointing to the effect of maternal nutritional status on the birthweight of the infant. In a survey carried out in South India, birthweights of infants of the low socioeconomic group was found to be 2·8 kg. while that of the infants of high socioeconomic group was around 3·1 kg.—a difference which was found to be statistically significant. If all infants including those who were not born full term had been included in the study, the difference between the two groups would have been even wider.

Using a birthweight of 2·5 kg. as the criterion, it was found that incidence of immaturity among infants of the low socioeconomic group was nearly 30 per cent while the corresponding figure for the high socioeconomic groups was about 14 per cent. If a birthweight of 2·0 kg. was used as criterion, the incidence of immaturity was less than 2 per cent among the high socioeconomic group as compared to 10 per cent in the poor socioeconomic group.

Among malnourished communities, a birthweight of less than 2·5 kg. or even 2·0 kg. need not necessarily indicate functional inadequacy in all cases. In fact, it has been observed that several infants with such low birthweights thrive normally. Birthweights may be a useful yardstick in assessing the maternal nutritional status of population groups. Low birthweights in poor communities are also associated with high neonatal mortality rates. Thus, in South India nearly 73 per cent of neonatal deaths occur in infants whose birthweights are less than 2 kg. It would thus appear that birthweight in a community may be an index of neonatal viability and that maternal nutritional factors which result in low birthweight could contribute to the high infant mortality observed in developing countries of the world.

The possibility that low birthweights in malnutrition are mediated through impaired placental function can only be speculated upon, at present. Urinary excretion of estrogens in pregnancy of undernourished women has been found to be significantly lower than in well-to-do women. Dietary supplementation to undernourished women has been shown to result in an increase of urinary excretion of estrogen. A direct correlation between urinary estrogen excretion and the birthweight of infants has also been demonstrated in these studies. The possibility of the effect of undernutrition on birthweight being mediated through changes in placental function would thus seem to merit consideration.

Congenital malformations. It is well-known that congenital malformations can be induced in the offspring of mammals by maternal dietary deficiencies. But congenital anomalies due to spontaneously occurring maternal nutritional deficiency have not been recognized in the human being. The available literature does not lend support to the view that the incidence of congenital malformations in infants of malnourished mothers is significantly different from that in infants of well-to-do mothers. Obviously, the rigid conditions and devices necessary to induce congenital anomalies in experimental animals find no counterpart in human reproduction. In contrast to the rat, in relation to the total period of gestation, the organogenetic period in which most malformations are determined, is relatively short in the human subject, and it is followed by a long period of foetal growth in which malformed foetuses can be eliminated. It may be argued that the increased incidence of pregnancy wastages among malnourished mothers may in fact be a reflection of such elimination of damaged foetuses.

The syndrome of endemic cretinism may be justifiably looked upon as an effect of the maternal deficiency of iodine, on the offspring. In fact, the results achieved in Switzerland with regard to the incidence of endemic cretinism by iodization of salt very convincingly demonstrate this. It is, however, possible that other factors may also contribute to the etiology of this syndrome. Congenital anomalies following ingestion of aminopterin by the mother during early pregnancy have been reported. This observation would highlight the dangers of inducing congenital anomalies by use of potent antimetabolites during pregnancy.

Effect of maternal nutrition on foetal storage of nutrients. Among the major nutritional deficiency disorders in infancy and early childhood encountered in many of the developing countries of the world today, are hypovitaminosis-A and anaemia. The extent to which maternal malnutrition during pregnancy may contribute to the development of these important deficiency syndromes, may be briefly considered.

Available literature with regard to placental transfer of vitamin A and carotene reveals considerable differences in the behaviour of different species. In the rat, the amount of vitamin A which passes into the foetal livers appears small and independent of the vitamin A fed to the mothers. In calves, the vitamin A content of the maternal diet has been found to determine the amount of vitamin A transferred to the foetal liver. In pups, kittens, lambs, goats and pigs also it has been demonstrated that foetal storage of vitamin A can be greatly improved by dosing the pregnant mother with vitamin A.

It is well known that the vitamin A concentration in serum steadily declines during pregnancy. In pregnant women drawn from undernourished populations, this decline is very striking. Thus, among poor pregnant women in South India it was found that the vitamin A concentration declined from 32 μg. in the first trimester to 21 μg. in the third trimester. The vitamin A content of the cord blood from the infants of these mothers was around 15 μg./100 ml. On the other hand, cord blood obtained from a group of infants whose mothers had received vitamin A supplements orally during the last trimester of pregnancy showed an average value of about 26 μg./100 ml. It would appear that especially in areas of the world where vitamin A deficiency in infants and children is a serious problem, correction of vitamin A deficiency in the mother during pregnancy might significantly improve the nutritional status of the infant with regard to vitamin A.

Data with regard to the vitamin A content of livers of newborn infants are few. Among infants of undernourished communities, values for hepatic vitamin A, as low as 3 μg./g. have been reported, while among infants in well-fed groups this value is nearly 45 μg./g. It seems reasonable to expect that maternal malnutrition with regard to vitamin A because of poor foetal liver storage, may predispose to vitamin A deficiency in late infancy and early childhood.

The possible effect of anaemias in pregnancy on the haematological status of the infant at birth and neonatal period also deserves consideration. This problem acquires particular significance and importance in regions of the world where anaemias of pregnancy as well as of infancy and childhood are common. It has been stated that the foetal iron stores are largely deposited in the last trimester of pregnancy and that they are influenced by the mother's intake of iron. The normal full-term infant born of a non-anaemic mother is believed to possess adequate iron stores at birth, so that dietary supplementation is not required for several months. However, conclusions with regard to foetal storage of iron and its adequacy for the formation of new haemoglobin in full-term infants are not in complete agreement. Early studies had indicated that these foetal iron stores fully compensated for the meagre iron content of milk. Later studies, however, seem to indicate that stores of non-haemoglobin iron in newborn infant's liver are not as much as had been assumed. Chemical and microscopic studies have shown no deposition of iron in the liver in the last four months of gestation. Progressive siderosis of liver and spleen apparently starts only three days after birth and reaches a maximum after a week of life. The recession in extramedullary haemopoiesis and red blood cell haemolysis are believed to be factors which increase the neonatal iron stores. If, therefore, neonatal iron stores are derived to a great extent from haemoglobin iron, the question arises whether the content of haemoglobin iron in the newborn infants of undernourished mothers is inadequate. Studies on the newborn infants of the poor socioeconomic group do not reveal low haemoglobin concentration in these infants in spite of the poor haematological status of the mothers; but, in the absence of data regarding blood volume of these infants, no precise information as to the total circulating haemoglobin is available. Clinical experience would, however, clearly indicate that infants born of undernourished mothers who receive no iron supplements tend to develop anaemia in the neonatal period much more readily than infants born of well-fed mothers. This would suggest poor iron storage resulting from poor maternal nutrition with regard to iron as being responsible.

Nutritional Factors in some Gynaecological States

In several gynaecological disorders, nutritional deficiencies may arise secondarily. There is, however, no convincing evidence for a primary role of nutritional deficiencies in such conditions.

There are several reports pointing to the occurrence of amenorrhoea in women and of delayed onset of menstruation in adolescent girls subjected to privation and suffering from hunger or war oedema. However, in such situations, the possible role of anxiety and other emotional factors has to be borne in mind. The role of emotional factors would particularly seem to merit attention since in a number of such cases, the onset of amenorrhoea actually precedes food shortage. The role of nutrition, however, cannot be entirely discounted. The effect of inanition on estrous cycles of young experimental animals is well established. Chronic inanition in experimental animals leads to a state of "pseudohypophysectomy" characterized by marked gonadal atrophy. Apart from general inanition, numerous studies have also shown that diets chronically deficient in vitamins of the B-group bring about atrophic changes in the genital tract.

It has also been demonstrated that animals maintained on folic acid deficient diets exhibit diminished response to estrogen administration. Reports of the Ukranian famine refer to extreme atrophy of the ovaries and uterus in undernourished women. Obviously, these changes represent advanced stages of continued inanition.

It has also been shown that vitamins of the B-group are concerned in the inactivation of estrogens by the liver. There is evidence that excess of estrogen may be involved in certain forms of pathological uterine bleeding and of chronic cystic mastitis. It has been claimed that associated deficiency of vitamins of the B-group may aggravate such clinical states in view of the need of these vitamins for the proper inactivation of estrogens. Menorrhagia and metrorrhagia associated with cirrhosis of the liver and pellagra have been attributed to deficiency of vitamins of the B-group.

These considerations may be of particular importance in women subsisting on diets which are already on the borderline of deficiency.

It has been found that women using a combination of progesterone and estrogen for ovulation control have abnormal levels of xanthurenic acid excretion and show abnormal urinary metabolites of tryptophan after a loading dose of tryptophan. Pyridoxine supplementation was found to correct this phenomenon completely. It would, therefore, appear that there is an increased requirement of pyridoxine in women using steroid hormones for ovulation control. Excretion of abnormal metabolites of tryptophan in the urine has been associated with carcinoma of the bladder. The routine administration of pyridoxine supplements to women receiving such steroid hormones for ovulation control over prolonged periods would, therefore, seem desirable.

REFERENCES

Gopalan, C. (1962), *Bull. Wld. Hlth. Org.*, **26**, 203.

Hytten, F. E. and Leitch, I. (1964), in *The Physiology of Human Pregnancy*. Blackwell.

Venkatachalam, P. S. (1962), *Bull. Wld. Hlth. Org.*, **26**, 193.

Nutrition in Pregnancy and Lactation, (1965), W. H. O. Tech. Rept. Ser. No. 302, Pub: W. H. O. 1965.

5. CALCIUM AND PHOSPHORUS METABOLISM, INCLUDING RENAL CALCULI, PARATHYROID DISEASE, OSTEOPOROSIS, AND OSTEOMALACIA

MARY G. McGEOWN

In normal human subjects the serum calcium is maintained at a fairly constant level of 10 mg. per 100 ml. (range 9·0 to 10·5 or 9·5 to 10·9 mg. per 100 ml. according. to the method used).

The serum inorganic phosphorus is also fairly constant under normal conditions, within a range of 2·5 to 4·0 mg. per 100 ml. In childhood it is higher, between 4·0 and 6·0 mg. per 100 ml. The serum phosphorus has a diurnal rhythm, the lowest values being present in the morning.

The very precise regulation of the serum calcium and phosphorus is most probably related to the conditions which favour proper mineralization of bone without production of calcification of soft tissues.

The serum calcium is divided into fractions (in mg. per 100 ml.) as follows:

Uitrafiltrable		6·0 (5·9–6·5)
Ionized	5·5	
Bound to citrate	0·5	
Non-filtrable		4·0
Total		10·0 (9·5–10·9)

The ionized fraction is the most important biologically. It is important for the maintenance of normal neuro-muscular transmission. When it is reduced the excitability of nerve fibres is increased so that they respond to stimuli below the response threshold of normal nerve fibres, or respond abnormally by sending off several impulses in response to a single stimulus of normal strength. There is also increased excitability of autonomic ganglion cells. At very high levels of serum calcium the excitability of nerve fibres is reduced. These changes do not occur until there are quite large deviations from the usual level of serum calcium and the susceptibility to these changes varies from individual to individual, so that there is no precise level which is always associated with abnormal excitability.

The ionized fraction of the serum calcium takes part in blood clotting, where it is necessary for the formation of active thromboplastin, and for the formation of thrombin from prothrombin. All levels of calcium which are compatable with life are adequate for clotting of shed blood.

Calcium accounts for about 25 per cent of the weight of dry fat free bone and this is the major store of this ion within the body. It is relatively poorly absorbed from the gut and losses of endogenous calcium occur into the gut. It is excreted in urine and sweat, but in temperate climates the loss in sweat is small and insignificant.

Phosphate forms part of adenosine triphosphate and diphosphate systems which provide energy for many important enzyme systems, including glycolysis; it is a major source of buffer in the body.

Both calcium and phosphate are present within cells as well as extracellularly. Calcium is present in mito chondria. Mitochondria release calcium and also uncouple oxidate phosphorylation. This does not happen in vitamin D deficient cells.

Calcium Homeostasis

The ionized fraction of the serum calcium appears to be controlled mainly by changes in the level of secretion of parathyroid hormone. Vitamin D is necessary for satisfactory homeostasis of calcium in most species, but, as it is exogenous in origin, it cannot correct acute changes in the calcium concentration of the internal environment. The recently discovered calcitonin reduces elevated levels of serum calcium, but there is still doubt as to its role in normal physiological control of calcium.

The thyroid and adrenal glands are known to affect calcium metabolism in disease states, but it is doubtful whether they are at all concerned with the physiological control of calcium.

The level of the protein-bound calcium reflects the level of the plasma proteins. It has been claimed that the parathyroid hormone affects the proportion of the plasma calcium bound by protein, but this has not been confirmed.

The Parathyroid Hormone

There are usually four parathyroids which are situated on either side of the upper and lower poles of the thyroid gland. They may lie close to the pole of the thyroid or may even be so closely applied as to appear to be continuous with it, or may be some distance away in loose areolar tissue. In rare instances they are situated in the thyroid lobe. Occasionally five or even six glands may be present. The ectopic glands can lie at a considerable distance from the thyroid. The lower glands may lie at any level from the level of the inferior thyroid artery to the arch of the aorta. They may be related to the upper pole of the thymus, and occasionally may be embedded within it.

The normal gland measures up to 5 × 4 × 1 mm. and weighs about 40–50 mg. It is typically pale fawn in colour and often lies in a little pad of fat, through which run the blood vessels to the hilum of the gland.

Histologically the normal gland consists of a fine stroma of anastomosing sinusoids which supports islands of secretory cells interspersed with fat cells. Fat is absent from the glands of very young subjects and appears in increasing amount from puberty onwards. The majority of the active cells in the normal gland are "chief" or "principal" cells, which are small cells with a poorly staining cytoplasm containing vacuoles and a small vesicular nucleus. There are also less numerous oxyphil cells which are larger with an oxyphilic granular cytoplasm and deeply staining nuclei. The "chief" or "principal" cells appear to be those which produce the parathyroid hormone.

The parathyroid hormone is a relatively small polypeptide with a molecular weight of 9,000.

Purified parathyroid hormone has both calcium mobilizing and phosphaturic activity, and acts mainly on bone and kidney.

When the parathyroids are removed there is a rapid fall in the serum calcium to about 6 mg. per 100 ml. which is manifested by the development of increased neuromuscular excitability (tetany). The administration of parathyroid hormone raises the serum calcium of the parathyroid deficient subject or elevates it above normal in the euparathyroid subject. It appears to do this mainly by solution of the mineral content of bone crystal. Fragments of parathyroid tissue when implanted in bone erode it with the formation of lacunae, associated with the appearance of large numbers of osteoclasts.

The parathyroid hormone decreases the urinary excretion of calcium by increasing tubular reabsorption of this ion, but in conditions where there is excess circulating hormone this effect is often overshadowed by the increase in filtered calcium due to the elevation of the serum calcium. This helps to conserve the body stores of calcium.

A reduction in the serum calcium stimulates secretion of parathyroid hormone which then raises the serum calcium at the expense of bone, but at the same time decreases urinary excretion of calcium. It has been shown in cows that an infusion of ethylene diamine tetra-acetic acid is rapidly followed by an increase in circulating parathyroid hormone, and that elevation of the serum calcium is equally rapidly followed by a reduction in circulating parathyroid hormone, within about 20 minutes. There is an inverse relationship between the level of parathyroid hormone and the serum calcium which holds good from 4–14 mg. per 100 ml.

The parathyroid hormone increases absorption of calcium from the gut and it appears to influence the excretion of calcium by the breast, at any rate, in rats. After parathyroidectomy it has been shown that the concentration of calcium in milk is increased despite a considerable fall in the serum calcium. It has been suggested that this is due to a reduction in the volume of milk, but the concentration of calcium is increased even when expressed as mg. per g. solids.

There seems to be some relationship between the parathyroids and magnesium metabolism, though this has not been as clearly defined as that of calcium. Buckle and Care (1968) report that parathyroid hormone, measured directly by radioimmunoassay in the effluent blood from surgically isolated parathyroid glands, was reduced by perfusion with high magnesium blood, and increased when low magnesium blood was perfused. In patients with hyperparathyroidism there is often, but not invariably, hypermagnesuria pre-operatively and hypomagnesaemia may develop following removal of the tumour.

In the parathyroid deficient animal the serum phosphorus is raised above the normal adult level of 3–4·5 mg. per 100 ml. The administration of parathyroid hormone will reduce the serum phosphorus towards normality, though usually less effectively than it raises the serum calcium. Administration of parathyroid hormone increases urinary excretion of phosphorus and is usually followed by reduction of the serum phosphorus, by reducing the re-absorption of phosphate by the renal tubules. It was suggested by Albright many years ago that this is the main action of the hormone and that the changes in the serum calcium are secondary to the increased resorption of phosphate by the renal tubules. However, the evidence that parathyroid hormone will increase the serum calcium in nephrectomized animals, with absorption of bone, is against this hypothesis. After removal of a parathyroid adenoma the serum calcium falls without a preceding rise in the serum phosphorus, and indeed the serum phosphorus may become lower.

There is some evidence that increase in the serum phosphorus stimulates the parathyroids but the evidence for this is not convincing and it is probable that it does so only indirectly by inducing hypocalcaemia.

In the presence of excess parathyroid hormone, the urinary excretion of hydroxyproline is increased, which is a reflection of the increased breakdown of bone.

It has recently been reported that there is an increase in serum glucagon levels in the hyperparathyroid state.

A radioimmunoassay for parathyroid hormone has been developed, using an antibody to bovine parathyroid. This has been useful for physiological experiments in cows related to the control of parathyroid hormone secretion. It is not yet sufficiently sensitive reliably to detect changes in parathyroid function in the human, probably due to a species difference in the hormone. The recent isolation of human parathyroid hormone may lead to improvement in the assay.

Action of Vitamin D

Vitamin D affects calcium metabolism at gut, bone and kidney levels.

Vitamin D increases the absorption of calcium from the intestine, which apparently occurs principally from the upper jejunum. It may do this by increasing cellular permeability to calcium or by releasing citrate. It is also possible that the release of calcium bound to mitochondria by vitamin D is involved in the absorption of calcium.

Vitamin D appears to promote resorption of bone in a similar way to the parathyroid hormone. In the vitamin D deficient animal it increases the resorption of bone, even in doses too small to increase absorption of calcium from the intestine. It has been shown to mobilize calcium[45] *in vivo* from labelled bones in rats. In the vitamin D deficient state, wide unmineralized borders of osteoid appear along bone trabeculae. These rapidly become mineralized when vitamin D is given. Vitamin D, can, therefore, promote both resorption and deposition of bone mineral.

In vitamin D deficiency in man the serum calcium is normal or low, while the serum phosphorus is low. This is reversed by vitamin D. It is thought that the lowered serum calcium stimulates excretion of parathyroid hormone and that this is the main explanation of the low serum phosphorus which often accompanies vitamin D deficiency.

It may also explain why the reduction in the serum calcium is usually minimal.

Vitamin D differs from parathyroid hormone in causing an increase in the serum phosphorus, presumably mostly due to mobilization of bone. There is no increase in urinary phosphate. Vitamin D increases urinary excretion of calcium and this occurs before any increase in the serum calcium, so that it is not due to increase in filtered load.

Calcitonin

In 1962 Copp (Copp & Cheney, 1962) perfused the thyroparathyroid glands of dogs with blood high in calcium, and found a more rapid fall in systemic calcium than could be accounted for by inhibition of parathyroid hormone secretion by the elevated serum calcium. Perfusion of the parathyroid glands in isolation from the thyroid is not possible in the dog, but has been done in the goat (Foster, Baghdiantz, Kumar, Slack, Soloman & MacIntyre, 1964) to show that the presence of the thyroid is essential for the calcium lowering effect. Perfusion of the parathyroid alone has no calcium lowering effect. Copp named his calcium-lowering hormone calcitonin. It was later renamed thyrocalcitonin when it was shown to be of thyroid origin. The source of calcitonin in the thyroid gland is the parafollicular cells, which are granular cells, parafollicular in location, now known as C cells. It has recently been shown that the parafollicular cells are derived from ultimobranchial tissue from the fifth pharyngeal pouch. In mammals the ultimobranchial body becomes incorporated in the thyroid gland, but in fish, reptiles and birds, remains separate and has been shown to contain large quantities of calcium-lowering substance. In view of the ultimobrarchial origin of the new hormone, the term thyrocalcitonin has been dropped and the original name of calcitonin resumed. Porcine calcitonin has recently been purified and it is a small polypeptide with a molecular weight of 3,600. It has been shown to produce significant hypocalcaemia and hypophosphatemia when injected into animals in the absence of the gastrointestinal tract, kidney, and parathyroid glands.

Calcitonin lowers plasma calcium by inhibiting bone breakdown and causing retention of calcium in bone. The hypophosphatemia appears to be accompanied by increased urinary excretion of phosphate. It reduces hydroxyproline excretion. Its efficacy in reducing serum calcium appears to depend on the prevaling rate of bone resorption.

The stimulus to the release of calcitonin appears to be an increase in the serum calcium.

Copp (Copp, Cockcroft, Kueh and Melville, 1968) has suggested that calcitonin plays an important part in calcium homeostasis by counteracting the effects of the parathyroid hormone, preventing calcium overshoot and hence adding greatly to the stability of the serum calcium. In support of this concept is the fact that there is impaired control of hypocalcaemia in thyroparathyroidectomized dogs and totally thyroidectomized human subjects. However, the part it plays in normal physiology is less clearly defined as protection against hypocalcaemia may be of little or no importance in normal circumstances.

It does not appear to be effective in controlling hyper calcaemia arising in the course of spontaneous hyperparathyroidism. Munsen (1968) has suggested that its main importance in normal physiology may be related to the development and maintenance of the healthy skeleton rather than to calcium homeostasis.

Evidence has been produced by Gaillard (1968) that in addition to inhibiting bone resorption there may be an increased formation of bone with increase in osteoblasts.

A state of chronic calcitonin deficiency has been induced in thyroidectomized rats. The plasma calcium was maintained at the normal level and the animals grew normally and appeared quite healthy. However, recent work has shown that C cells (derived from ultimobranchial tissue) are present in many other tissues in the thorax, and even in the liver and the parathyroids in the human, as well as in thyroid. In patients who have been totally thyroidectomized an intravenous infusion of calcium has produced a prolonged hypercalcaemia as compared with control subjects. This difference was considered to be due to lack of calcitonin in the thyroidectomized subjects.

A short intravenous infusion of calcitonin in three patients with hypercalcaemia secondary to malignant disease produced an eight to ten per cent reduction in the serum calcium level without affecting either serum sodium or magnesium. It is possible that the small response obtained may have been related to the fact that the calcitonin used was of porcine origin and there may be a species difference.

The only indication so far that calcitonin may play a part in any human disease is the observation that thyroid tissue from two patients with longstanding pseudo-hypoparathyroidism contained 100 times more calcitonin than that of normal man (Munson, 1968). It is, however, uncertain whether the high concentration of calcitonin in the thyroid gland in these patients caused the persistent hypocalcaemia, or whether the long-term hypocalcaemia was in some way responsible for the observed excessive storage of calcitonin.

Calcitonin is at present assayed by its hypocalcaemic effect in starved weanling rats. Attempts to produce an immunoassay have not yet been successful due to difficulty in producing an anti-body, but very recently Potts (1968) has obtained one by the use of relatively enormous quantities of calcitonin.

Thyroxine

Hypercalcaemia occurs occasionally in thyrotoxicosis, while hypercalciuria is almost invariably present. There is an increase in glomerular filtration rate in thyrotoxicosis, which may contribute to the hypercalciuria. However, there is also an increased turnover of bone and this may be severe enough to lead to osteoporosis. In normal circumstances thyroxine probably does not take part in calcium homeostasis.

Adrenals

The serum calcium is sometimes raised in Addison's disease, and in one series of 62 cases, 8 had hypercalcaemia. Adrenalectomy in dogs results in hypercalcaemia, and this hypercalcaemia occurs in the absence of the parathyroids, and without an increase in absorption of calcium. It is accompanied by an increase in plasma citrate, which suggests that there is increased resorption of bone.

Osteoporosis may develop in Cushing's syndrome, and it is not uncommon as a complication of prolonged steroid treatment. Cortisone induces a negative calcium balance by increasing both faecal and urinary excretion of calcium. In sarcoidosis and in vitamin D poisoning cortisone reduces an elevated serum calcium to normal, while increasing faecal excretion of calcium.

It is doubtful whether the adrenal hormones take part in normal calcium homeostasis.

Calcium Absorption

The absorption of calcium from the diet is incomplete, and the proportion absorbed varies with the adjustment of the subject to the calcium content of his diet. If an individual is adjusted to a high calcium intake, change to a low intake at first results in a negative calcium balance because a large percentage of the dietary calcium is unabsorbed. When the low intake is prolonged the efficiency of absorption increases, and the faecal loss is reduced. The power to adapt in this way may differ in different individuals. A greater proportion of ingested calcium is absorbed in the young, and during pregnancy and lactation. Man can thus remain in calcium balance over a wide range of intake levels. It is, therefore, very difficult to define minimum requirements for dietary calcium.

Calcium absorption is in part conditioned by the other contents of the diet. High phosphate diets, and those containing excessive amounts of phytate reduce absorption of calcium. This is made use of in the treatment of idiopathic hypercalciuria by sodium phytate or cellulose phosphate. Since calcium and magnesium share a common absorptive pathway in the intestinal mucosa, high magnesium diets will depress calcium absorption. Fatty acids in the diet form insoluble soaps, and failure of fat absorption leads to decreased calcium absorption. It has been found that calcium absorption is impaired from diets deficient in protein. The calcium in milk is better absorbed than any inorganic or available organic salt of calcium (82 per cent of milk calcium absorbed compared with 32 per cent from calcium chloride). Milk calcium is thought to be better absorbed because it is in the form of calcium caeseinophosphate, but in calves lactose has been shown to increase calcium absorption.

Vitamin D is essential for absorption of calcium, and the parathyroid hormone also influences it: this has already been considered under "Calcium Homeostasis."

The faecal calcium is made up mainly of calcium not absorbed from the diet, but a small amount is actively secreted into the intestine. Work with Ca^{45} suggests that the secreted calcium reaching faeces amounts to about 70–100 mg. daily. It is independent of the level of dietary calcium. Large intravenous injections of calcium do not appreciably increase faecal excretion of calcium, suggesting that this is not an important route for calcium excretion. It can, however, lead to increase in negative balance as faecal calcium excretion continues even in starvation, and in severe vitamin D deficiency.

Decreased absorption of calcium

Calcium absorption is decreased in many clinical conditions which are grouped together under the term "malabsorption syndrome." It is theoretically possible that an increase in secreted calcium contributes to the increase in faecal excretion of calcium, but available evidence suggests that this is not so. The conditions leading to the malabsorption syndrome can be classified under the following headings:

1. Gluten sensitivity: coeliac disease, idiopathic steatorrhoea.
2. Inflammatory conditions: jejunitis, regional ileitis, chronic pancreatitis.
3. Following surgery; post-gastrectomy steatorrhoea, resection of massive lengths of small intestine.
4. Infiltrating conditions: Whipple's disease, amyloidosis, scleroderma, Hodgkin's disease, lymphosarcoma.
5. Chronic infective diarrhoeas, including sprue.
6. Miscellaneous causes: stagnant loop syndrome, stricture, fistula between small and large intestine.

In these malabsorption conditions, there is also deficiency of vitamin D which must contribute to the poor absorption of calcium.

The malabsorption of calcium may manifest itself clinically by tetany, (see "hypocalcaemia"), by bone pain, bone deformity or pathological fractures (see "Osteoporosis," "Osteomalacia").

The malabsorption of calcium is associated with other deficiencies leading to the development of macrocytic anaemia. The diagnosis rests on the finding of a negative calcium balance mainly due to large faecal losses of calcium, usually together with a macrocytic anaemia. Helpful tests include barium meal, faecal excretion of fat, D-xylose absorption test, serum carotene level, absorption of radio-active vitamin B_{12}, and intestinal biopsy.

Increased calcium absorption

Vitamin D intoxication is associated with increased absorption of dietary calcium. Severe vitamin D intoxication is associated with hypercalcaemia but this is probably only partly due to increased absorption of calcium, increased turnover of bone being thought to be more important. It is difficult to give any precise definition of what constitutes over-absorption of calcium, but Dent (Dent and Watson, 1965) appears to consider 50 per cent absorption of dietary calcium to be excessive.

The absorption of calcium is also increased in sarcoidosis, and may fairly rarely be associated with hypercalcaemia. In both sarcoidosis and vitamin D intoxication the faecal calcium is decreased and hypercalcaemia, if present, is abolished by administration of cortisone for five to ten days. This suggests that there is an increased sensitivity to vitamin D in sarcoidosis. It has also been found that the toxic effects of vitamin D overdosage can be produced in patients with sarcoid by relatively tiny doses of the vitamin.

There is evidence to suggest that increased calcium absorption may be the cause of idiopathic hypercalciuria (*see* "Calcium Excretion").

Calcium Excretion

Knapp (1947) studied the urinary excretion of calcium in a large number of normal individuals of all ages on different levels of calcium intake. She found that urinary calcium increased with increasing age, which appeared to be related to increase in skeletal weight, roughly represented by total body weight. At any given age, the mean excretion of a group of subjects increased with increased intake, being greater in adults than in children. Dietary factors other than the calcium content had relatively minor effects on the urinary calcium. Ingestion of acids, a ketogenic (high protein) diet, or a high ratio of calcium to phosphorus in the diet, all increased the urinary calcium. She found that for individuals of the same weight and eating the same diet, there is a wide range of values for urinary calcium.

It is, therefore, difficult to define the normal range of urinary calcium.

Hodgkinson and Pryah (1958) measured the urinary calcium in sixty men convalescing after minor surgery, on an intake of 800 ± 200 mg. per day, and were able to find values in the literature for another 72 men and 126 women. They concluded that normal men on a normal diet excrete 100–300 mg. calcium per day, and normal women excrete 100–250 mg per day. They consider that calcium excretion in excess of this represents hypercalciuria.

While this definition of hypercalciuria has been fairly generally accepted, it should be realised that 10 per cent of normal men and 6 per cent of normal women excrete more calcium than this. There is considerably less variation in the urinary excretion of calcium on a low calcium intake, and the author has always preferred to estimate the urinary calcium while the patient is receiving a standard diet containing 150 mg. calcium, on the assumption that it is more likely to reflect true metabolism. The author has found, in normal ambulatory laboratory staff eating this diet, that the upper limit of urinary calcium is 154 mg. per 24 hours (mean plus 2 S.D.; mean 83, S.D. 32 mg.). She considers that true hypercalciuria is excretion of calcium in excess of 150 mg. on a diet containing 150 mg. calcium. There are, however, some patients whose urinary calcium rises more steeply than normal with increase in calcium in the diet.

Recently, Peacock, Hodgkinson and Nordin (1968) have re-investigated hypercalciuric stone formers, normocalciuric stone formers, hypercalciuric "controls" and normocalciuric controls. Using calcium infusions they have not found any consistent difference in tubular absorption between these groups, and have concluded that hypercalciuria should be defined in relation to the dietary calcium at the time of observation.

Causes of increased urinary excretion of calcium:

1. Hormonal:

   (i) Hyperparathyroidism
   (ii) Thyrotoxicosis
   (iii) Cushing's syndrome
   (iv) Acromegaly
   (v) Steroid therapy.

2. Immobilization of the skeleton:

   (i) Following fractures ⎫
   (ii) Poliomyelitis   ⎬ associated with acute
   (iii) For tuberculosis   ⎭ osteoporosis
   (iv) Paraplegia

3. Vitamin D intoxication.

4. Sarcoidosis.

5. Renal tubular acidosis.

6. Tumours destroying bone:

   (i) Multiple myeloma

   (ii) Tumours metastazing to bone: breast, thyroid, oat cell carcinoma of lung, prostate, hypernephroma.

   (iii) Tumours with parathormone-like activity: oat cell tumour of lung, some ovarian tumours.

7. Idiopathic (generally detected in patients with urinary stones).

The hormonal causes of hypercalciuria have already been considered, with the exception of acromegaly, under "Calcium Homeostasis." Hypercalciuria is often present in the active stage of acromegaly. This may be mediated via the parathyroids as growth hormone has some parathyropic activity, and the parathyroid glands are often enlarged. More rarely parathyroid adenomas occur.

The acute osteoporosis which follows immobilization of the body for any reason is often associated with hypercalciuria. Before the importance of early mobilization was realised urinary calculi frequently complicated such situations.

Vitamin D used for the treatment of post-operative and idiopathic hypoparathyroidism or for the treatment of metabolic bone disease, can lead to elevated excretion of calcium, even before hypercalcaemia appears. This is rapidly abolished by cortisone.

The close resemblance of sarcoidosis to vitamin D intoxication, as regards calcium metabolism, has already been pointed out.

In renal tubular acidosis there is a failure of the tubules to excrete hydrogen ion, with the production of a systemic acidosis with a relatively alkaline urine. There may be increased excretion of cations, including calcium. The condition may lead to either urinary stones, nephrocalcinosis or osteomalacia (cf.).

Idiopathic hypercalciuria is the presence of increased excretion of calcium without any obvious cause. It occurs in association with renal stones, but as already pointed out, the older definition of hypercalciuria also included some normal healthy individuals. It has been shown that it is associated with increased absorption of calcium from the intestine, but it has also been suggested that the primary lesion is an inability of the kidney tubules to reabsorb calcium, and that increased absorption of calcium by the intestine is compensatory. In support of this is the fact that in some patients there is but little reduction in the urinary excretion of calcium even when the calcium intake is greatly reduced for a long period, e.g. Dent and Watson

(1965) has reported a patient who excreted 220 mg. calcium daily on an intake of 200 mg. after one year's equilibration. However, there is also evidence to support primary over-absorption of calcium as the cause of hypercalciuria—the calcium infusion studies of Peacock, *et al.* (1968) already mentioned, and their evidence that a standard load of calcium citrate orally is, in hypercalciuric subjects, followed by a greater rise in serum and urinary calcium than in normal individuals.

Idiopathic hypercalciuria is sometimes accompanied by increased urinary excretion of phosphate and a low serum phosphorus. This syndrome resembles hyperparathyroidism except for the absence of a raised serum calcium, but it does not appear to be a variant of hyperparathyroidism, as exploration of the neck in a number of these patients has not shown overactive parathyroids. Hyperphosphaturia and a low serum phosphorus can occur in patients with stones, but without hypercalciuria. The most likely explanation of the increased excretion of phosphate is an inherent tubular defect, but these patients can acidify their urine and do not have glycosuria or aminoaciduria.

Renal Calculi

Calculi may co-exist with pregnancy, and are now discovered with increasing frequency due to recent interest in urinary infections occurring in pregnancy. In the past such infections were treated and then forgotten. In modern obstetric practice women who develop urinary tract infection, or even asymptomatic bacteriuria, should be investigated after the pregnancy and should usually have an intravenous pyelogram, which may reveal a hitherto unsuspected calculus. The author has seen ten women with calculi which were discovered in this way, over the past two years. Calculi can present during pregnancy as an attack of severe renal pain, often but not always radiating downwards towards the groin. The author has twice had to treat anuria due to bilateral calculi during pregnancy.

Causes of Renal Calculi

Certain types of stones appear to be due simply to precipitation from a supersaturated urine. Uric acid, cystine and the very rare xanthine calculi are of this type.

The pH of the urine may in some cases favour precipitation of the stone-forming substance, for example, both cystine and uric acid are less soluble at low pH. These types of stones are all rare, and the majority are composed of various compounds of calcium, phosphate, oxalate, carbonate and magnesium. Recently Lonsdale (1968) has reported x-ray diffraction analysis of a large number of urinary stones, and has found 7 calcium compounds and 2 magnesium compounds. The pathogenesis of these common types of stones is much less well understood, but certain conditions are commonly associated with them.

Associated conditions:

(a) Increased excretion of calcium in the urine.
(b) Dehydration.
(c) Urinary infection.
(d) Urinary stasis.

(e) Hydrogen ion concentration of the urine.
(f) Hyperphosphaturia.

(a) Many, but not all of the causes of increased urinary excretion of calcium, are associated with renal stones.

(b) The sparingly soluble salts which form calculi can be more readily excreted without precipitation if the urine volume is high. It therefore is reasonable to expect that conditions which favour dehydration will increase the prevalence of stone disease.

(c) Urinary infections, especially with urea-splitting organisms, are commonly associated with mixed stones.

(d) Urinary stasis could take part in the formation of stones by providing time for crystallization of salts to take place, and by favouring retention of minute fragments of organic or inorganic material which might form a nidus for crystallization.

(e) The influence of pH of the urine in providing conditions suitable for the precipitation of the stone-forming salts is clearly of importance.

(f) It has already been mentioned that patients who form stones and have idiopathic hypercalciuria, may also have hyperphosphaturia.

It is evident that none of the above factors can provide any complete explanation of the formation of stones. All stones, no matter what their crystalline constituents, contain a matrix of a mucopolysaccharide material.

Many of the observed facts about calculus formation suggest that urine of normal individuals may contain some substance, or substances, which prevents the precipitation of calcium salts. A deficiency of this, or its destruction by bacteria, might then lead to calculus formation. This is in keeping with the known association of high urinary calcium with stones.

Diseases of the Parathyroid Glands

Hyperparathyroidism: (a) Primary.
                           (b) Secondary.
Hypoparathyroidism: (a) Following operations on the thyroid gland (or radiotherapy).
                           (b) Idiopathic.

Primary Hyperparathyroidism

(a) Over-action of the parathyroid glands usually develops insidiously, and it may lead to signs and symptoms related to many different systems.

Eighty to ninety per cent of patients with hyperparathyroidism suffer from renal calculi. It is rarer to find nephrocalcinosis. The calculi are often bilateral before the diagnosis is made. Even if calculi are not formed, the hypercalcaemia if allowed to persist, may lead to serious impairment of kidney function. The kidneys of patients dying from hyperparathyroidism without calculi contain microscopic deposits of calcium, and are contracted and fibrotic.

In the second commonest form of hyperparathyroidism the skeleton is predominently affected. It was once thought that stones are formed early in the disease or in mild cases, and that the bone form represents an advanced form of the disease. This is not so, as occasionally very severe bone changes occur without involvement of the kidneys. Stones, or nephrocalcinosis may occur along with the bone changes.

The bone changes associated with hyperparathyroidism (osteitis fibrosa) lead to aching pain in long bones, ribs, spine and joints, but sometimes despite marked radiological changes pain may be remarkably little. When the disease is of long standing, deformities may occur due to softening of the skeleton, especially deformity of the chest and spine. Pathological fractures may occur—one of the author's patients, a woman of 30 years, developed bilateral fractures of neck of femur. Bone cysts or giant cell pseudo-tumours (osteoclastoma) are fairly common.

Often the earliest, as well as the most typical radiological changes are seen in the hands and skull, and in the distal ends of the clavicles. The cortical layer of the affected bones becomes progressively decalcified until it is no longer clearly demarcated. In addition tiny areas of bone resorption appear beneath the periosteum (subperiosteal erosions). The whole skull develops a mottled appearance, which can be described as moth-eaten. The loss of bone trabeculae can be seen in the long bones and pelvis as a coarsening of the pattern. The cortex of the long bones becomes thin and cystic enlargements, or osteoclastomata, may appear, especially common in the lower ends of tibia and fibula and in the jaws. Large clear areas are occasionally seen in the tables of the skull, which heal to become very dense areas.

These changes do not occur in diseases other than hyperparathyroidism, but occur in the secondary form of the disease as well as the primary. The cystic changes, however, are rare, if they occur at all, in the secondary disease.

A few patients with hyperparathyroidism suffer from very severe and intractable symptoms of peptic ulceration. The presence of stones or of bone changes may give a clue to the underlying hyperparathyroidism.

Nearly all patients with hyperparathyroidism have vague symptoms which are due to hypercalcaemia; they are also seen in patients with hypercalcaemia from other causes. Lack of energy, lack of appetite and constipation are very frequent complaints, and the patients may not fully appreciate the extent of these troubles until they disappear following recovery. Thirst and polyuria are classical symptoms, but are not very common, although many patients do excrete somewhat larger than normal amounts of urine. The higher the serum calcium, the more marked are these general symptoms. Very high levels of serum calcium lead to nausea and vomiting, and dehydration; oliguria and renal failure may develop. These severe symptoms associated with very high levels of serum calcium (16–20 mg. per 100 ml.) constitute acute hyperparathyroidism. Hypotonia and tachycardia may be the only signs of the condition, apart from dehydration. This very serious condition, which may rapidly lead to death unless adequately treated, has presented in the guise of hyperemesis gravidarum. It may be difficult to recognise unless a history of renal stones, or bone symptoms, or a chance x-ray showing typical bone lesions give a clue to the true condition.

Pancreatitis may complicate hyperparathyroidism, usually in patients with very high levels of serum calcium.

Occasional cases of hyperparathyroidism present in more bizarre ways. A few have mental symptoms, or depression (one of ours had hallucinations during an episode of acute hyperparathyroidism). A tumour may be felt in the neck, or may even be found accidentally during thyroid surgery. A very few patients have been detected, including one of the author's, because a new-born infant developed tetany, the infant's parathyroid glands having been depressed *in utero* by the mother's over-active glands. Anaemia is common, and rarely it may be the prominent feature of the disease.

Physical signs of hyperparathyroidism are usually few. It is unusual to be able to feel the enlarged gland in the neck, as it is seldom above 2 cm. in diameter, and it is soft.

Calcium deposits occur in the superficial layers of the periphery of the cornea in advanced cases. Calcium deposits in the conjunctiva may be present and are associated with a remarkable increase in vascularity.

Biochemical changes: In the cases without radiological bone changes, the diagnosis can only be made from the biochemical abnormalities.

The most important abnormality is the raised calcium. This is present in almost all cases, although it may be present only intermittently. It is usually greatest in the patients with bone changes. In the less obvious cases without radiological bone changes, the elevation may be less than 1 mg. above the normal upper level, and it may be present only intermittently, so that repeated and very accurate measurements of the serum calcium are necessary in patients in whom the disease is suspected. In the author's experience it is most helpful to repeat the serum calcium at fairly long intervals, over a year or more, in suspect cases. Care must be taken to obtain the blood sample without stasis.

A low serum phosphorus occurs in most patients with primary hyperparathyroidism but again may occur only intermittently, and is no longer present in advanced cases with renal failure. The existence of the low serum phosphorus-hyperphosphaturia syndrome in association with renal stones, already described, may also lead to confusion.

The urinary excretion of calcium is often high in hyperparathyroidism, but is normal or low when renal function becomes impaired. The hypercalciuria of hyperparathyroidism must be distinguished from the idiopathic hypercalciuria associated with renal stones.

The serum alkaline phosphatase is raised only in the patients with radiological evidence of bone disease.

More exotic tests of parathyroid function have been used, including various methods of measurement of phosphate excretion, the response to calcium infusion, measurement of ionized calcium, and renal tubular functions, but have been of little practical value. Attempts to measure plasma levels of parathyroid hormone have been successful in only a few laboratories. Scanning of the parathyroids using selenomethionine—Se[75] has proved disappointing (McGeown, Bell, Soyannwo and Fenton, 1968).

Differential diagnosis: When the serum calcium is found to be raised it is convenient to consider the causes of hypercalcaemia according to whether or not there are radiological changes in the bones.

1. With radiological changes:

    (i) Hyperparathyroidism.

    (ii) Secondary carcinomatosis (from breast, bronchus, thyroid, kidney, cervix).

    (iii) Multiple myelomatosis.

    (iv) Sarcoidosis.

    (v) Acute osteoporosis.

2. Without radiological changes:

    (i) Hyperparathyroidism.

    (ii) Vitamin D intoxication.

    (iii) Sarcoidosis.

    (iv) Secondary to certain tumours without bone metastases (hypernephroma, bronchus, ovary).

    (v) Multiple myelomatosis.

    (vi) Thyrotoxicosis.

    (vii) Milk alkali syndrome.

    (viii) Infantile hypercalcaemia.

    (ix) Addison's disease.

The radiological changes of hyperparathyroidism are quite characteristic and once seen are easily distinguished from the changes which occur in the other conditions mentioned. Examination of the sites of tumours which commonly produce secondary deposits in bone is important in any patient known to have hypercalcaemia.

There are characteristic changes in the electrophoretic pattern of the plasma proteins, in both sarcoidosis and myelomatosis, which separate these conditions from other types of hypercalcaemia.

In patients suffering from vitamin D intoxication, there may be a history of taking large doses of some form of the vitamin. The diagnosis is obvious in patients who are receiving treatment for osteomalacia or as replacement therapy in hypoparathyroidism, but vitamin D is still occasionally used in pregnancy and the treatment of certain skin diseases and in arthritis, and the patient may be unaware of the nature of the treatment. This type of hypercalcaemia is rapidly reduced to normal by five to ten days' treatment with cortisone acetate, in a dosage of 150 mg. daily.

The hypercalcaemia of hyperparathyroidism differs from that of vitamin D intoxication, and of sarcoidosis, in almost always persisting during treatment with cortisone. There are no characteristic changes in the plasma proteins in hyperparathyroidism.

Certain tumours seem able to produce hypercalcaemia without directly involving bone, and it is thought that they secrete a substance with an action similar to that of the parathyroid hormone.

Milk alkali syndrome occurs in patients with peptic ulcers who have been taking very large amounts of milk and alkali. It is probably very rare and is more likely in patients who already have impaired renal function. The hypercalcaemia slowly subsides when the intake of milk ceases, but it may take a very long time to do so, possibly even as long as a year.

Infantile hypercalcaemia was first described by Lightwood in 1952, and was followed by numerous reports of other cases. It occurred in babies being artificially fed, who fed poorly, failed to thrive, began to vomit and were constipated. There was considerable elevation of the serum calcium and the blood urea, and anaemia. It was considered to be due to excessive intake of vitamin D. The serum calcium fell to normal on reducing the intake of calcium. Cortisone also appeared to be beneficial, though less dramatically so than in vitamin D intoxication in adults. The blood urea took longer to fall and in some babies remained permanently elevated. As a result of investigations by the British Paediatric Association in 1957 the vitamin D addition to proprietary baby foods was approximately halved. In the 1960's, the disease seems to have become rare again, though it appears to have remained fairly frequent for some years after the reduction in vitamin D content of infant foods.

Treatment of Primary Hyperparathyroidism: The only treatment is removal of the overactive parathyroid gland or glands. It is important to try to identify all four glands because in about 20 per cent of cases more than one gland is enlarged. There may be multiple adenomata, or primary hyperplasia may affect all 4 glands. It is essential to carry out a careful dissection in a blood-free field as otherwise normal glands, and even enlarged ones, may not be seen.

The normal parathyroid gland is usually not larger than 5 mm. in diameter, and is of a yellowish colour. Over-active glands are both larger and darker in colour, becoming more definitely brownish or reddish brown. The upper glands are usually found above the point of entry of the upper branches of the inferior thyroid artery into the thyroid gland, often well posterior to this plane.

The lower pair are usually situated at the lower pole of the thyroid, antero-lateral to the trachea, and in front of the inferior thyroid artery and recurrent laryngeal nerve. The lower glands are much more variable in position than the upper ones, and may be within the upper mediastinum, the thymus, the thyroid itself, or even as low in the mediastinum as the arch of the aorta. Those in the upper mediastinum are usually visible from the neck. In our experience, 1 to 2 per cent of tumours are situated so low in the mediastinum as to be inaccessible from the neck, and about 10 per cent are in one or other of the ectopic situations mentioned above.

Pathology: Parathyroid tumours vary greatly in size, ranging from the size of a normal gland (0.5 cm. diameter) up to 5 cm. diameter or more. In primary hyperplasia all the glands are enlarged, though the enlargement may be unequal. In one of our cases 29 g. of parathyroid was removed from a patient with primary hyperplasia, leaving behind a sizeable portion of one gland.

A typical adenoma has a compressed rim of normal parathyroid tissue at the periphery of the tumour, but this may be impossible to identify without serial section of the gland. There are no other specific features by which an adenoma may be distinguished from hyperplasia.

The predominant cell type is frequently a variant of the normal cell, which has a copious vacuolated cytoplasm, and is known as the "water-clear cell". In some tumours chief cells predominate, or are mixed with water-clear cells. There may be islands of oxyphil cells, which may sometimes occur in large sheets, but it is doubtful whether true oxyphil adenomata occur.

Post-operative course: This is usually uneventful in the patients suffering only from stones. Tetany is unusual unless there is radiological evidence of bone disease or injudicious biopsies have been taken from the remaining normal glands. The treatment of post-operative tetany will be described (see "Hypocalcaemia"). In advanced cases renal failure may occur post-operatively and dialysis may be required to maintain the patient temporarily. Pancreatitis is a rare but very serious complication of the post-operative period.

In patients with bone disease, the skeleton heals over a period of months, with reformation of bone leading to healing of the subperiosteal erosions, and appearance of new trebuculae. Cysts persist for long periods although their walls become thicker. Deformities persist and continue to cause disability.

A survey of the post-operative five years in the author's patients has shown an almost complete cessation from the formation of stones. The only patients in whom stones recurred or increased in size had already had enormous staghorn calculi removed repeatedly and the kidneys were greatly damaged structurally and the site of intractable infection.

In addition to the above benefits, the patient experiences a great increase in general well-being, with increase in energy, appetite and weight.

b. *Secondary hyperparathyroidism:*

Chronic hypocalcaemia stimulates increase in parathyroid hormone secretion. This has been demonstrated in the cow by the immunoassay method already mentioned, and it has been claimed to occur also in patients with hypocalcaemia due to chronic renal failure by Sherwood (1968). The cause of the hypocalcaemia in renal failure is not fully understood. It is not due to excessive urinary loss of calcium, as urinary calcium becomes very low in renal failure, and there is evidence that there is no defect of calcium absorption. It is tempting to try to fit calcitonin into a hypothesis to account for the hypocalcaemia occurring in chronic renal failure. Increased secretion of calcitonin, if chronic, would be expected to lead to bone sclerosis, and this occurs commonly in patients with chronic renal failure, although its distribution is usually patchy. If excess calcitonin contributes to the hypocalcaemia in chronic renal failure, the stimulus to its production remains unexplained but could be hyperphosphataemia, acidosis or some abnormal component of uraemic plasma.

Patients suffering from renal failure develop a bone disease which closely resembles the radiological and microscopical changes seen in primary hyperparathyroidism. Often there are no symptoms until a pathological fracture occurs. While the changes are similar to those already described in primary hyperparathyroidism, cysts rarely, if ever, are present. In long-standing cases the vertebral bodies may show transverse stripes of sclerotic bone alternating with bands of decreased density, the so-called "rugger jersey" spine.

Vitamin D, in large doses to the tolerance of the individual patient, is used for the treatment of patients with hyperparathyroid bone disease and a low serum calcium. However, if the condition has become autonomous, and the serum calcium is normal or elevated, this cannot safely be used because of the danger of calcification of soft tissues, since the serum phosphorus is also high. The only treatment is total parathyroidectomy followed by long-term replacement of parathyroid function with vitamin D (see Treatment of Hypoparathyroidism). It is interesting that bone healing can occur even though both serum calcium and phosphorus remain at their previous level.

The hypocalcaemia produced by malabsorption can also lead to parathyroid stimulation and the production of radiological lesions of hyperparathyroid bone disease. It is treated with vitamin D and calcium, as well as correction of the cause of malabsorption, if possible. This type of secondary hyperparathyroidism can also become autonomous and parathyroidectomy may become necessary.

Hypoparathyroidism:

(a) Following damage to the parathyroid glands during operation on the thyroid.

(b) Idiopathic hypoparathyroidism.

The symptoms, signs and biochemical findings of both types of hypoparathyroidism are related to the low serum calcium due to lack of parathyroid hormone. The serum phosphorus is raised but this is of little practical importance.

The level at which reduction of the serum calcium produces symptoms varies in different individuals, some having symptoms at about 8.0 mg. per 100 ml., others tolerating much lower levels without complaining. The symptoms are known as tetany. In mild cases the patient experiences pins and needles in the extremities and perhaps twitching of the facial muscles. There may be muscle spasm which begins with a feeling of stiffness and goes on to a tonic and painful contraction often described as cramp. The spasm may follow a voluntary action such as writing or walking. The fingers are flexed at the metacarpal-phalangeal joints, and are held tightly bunched together, with the thumb adducted. The palm is hollowed and the wrist is flexed. When the feet are affected, the toes are flexed under the feet, pressed together with the big toe underneath the others. The posterior muscles of the leg contract and draw the heel upwards. These spasms are known as carpo-pedal spasms. Spasm of the glottis may cause stridor, and spasm of the diaphragm, back and chest muscles may also occur.

When spasms are not present at the time of examination, latent tetany may sometimes be demonstrated by the following tests:

1. Chvostek's sign is elicited by tapping on the facial nerve in front of the ear. A positive sign is twitching of the facial muscles, especially of the upper lip, though occasionally the alae of the nose and the eyelids may also twitch.

2. Trousseau's sign is elicited by raising the blood pressure cuff on the upper arm above the systolic pressure. When positive the hand assumes the position of carpo-pedal spasm.

3. Erb's sign is the demonstration of hyperexcitability of the muscles to electrical stimulation.

In idiopathic hypoparathyroidism, which is very rare, tetany in infancy or early childhood may be manifest as fits of epileptiform type, and be mistaken for idiopathic epilepsy. If not recognized and treated, both mental and physical development are retarded, and stunted growth and mental deficiency may result. In adequately treated cases development is normal, and the author has one patient who is an undergraduate in an honours school, although treatment was not commenced until after the appearance of a cataract at the age of 5.

Cataracts are a common complication of hypoparathyroidism, but may occur in any condition in which there is long continued hypocalcaemia.

Atrophic changes may occur in hair, nails, teeth and skin. Monilial infections of the nails are relatively common. Dent and Garretts (1960) have drawn attention to the association of exfoliative dermatitis with hypocalcaemia.

Calcification of the basal ganglia on the x-ray of skull is a classical sign of idiopathic hypoparathyroidism.

Differential diagnosis of hypoparathyroidism· Hypoparathyroidism must be separated from other conditions in which hypocalcaemia occurs:

Causes of hypocalcaemia:

    (a) Renal Failure.
    (b) Malabsorption syndrome.
    (c) Following operation on the thyroid.
    (d) Idiopathic hypoparathyroidism.

Treatment of hypoparathyroidism: Parathyroid hormone is not used in the treatment of hypoparathyroidism because it is expensive and other effective treatment is available. Vitamin D is used instead, the dose being tailored to the needs of the individual patient. The maximum effect does not appear for some time, and as it is stored in the liver, the effect is cumulative. A loading dose of 400,000 units (10 mg.) is followed by doses up to 200,000 units (5 mg.) daily. The dosage must be controlled by twice weekly estimations of the serum calcium until a dose is found which keeps the serum calcium at about 9·0 mg. per 100 ml. The urinary excretion of calcium may be increased at a dose which does not maintain the serum calcium satisfactorily, so occasional estimations of the urinary excretion of calcium are necessary. After a suitable dose has been found, it is usually possible to manage the patient with serum calcium estimations once a month or less frequently. If hypercalcaemia is inadvertently produced, it is rapidly abolished by a short course of cortisone in a dose of 150 mg. daily.

Occasional patients do not respond to Vitamin D, or later cease to respond. In these cases dihydrotachysterol (A.T. 10) can be tried. Three ml. A.T. 10 are given daily until calcium appears in the urine, after which a maintenance dose of 1 ml. three to seven times weekly is enough. Such patients may later again become responsive to vitamin D.

During the acute phase of post-operative hypoparathyroidism it may be necessary to give calcium intravenously to control tetany, while waiting for the action of vitamin D to build up. Twenty ml. of 10 per cent calcium gluconate can be given intravenously four-hourly, or as necessary to keep the patient comfortable. In addition, effervescent tablets of calcium lactate gluconate (Sandocal) are given orally, one tablet four times daily, each tablet containing 400 mg. of calcium.

Osteoporosis

Osteoporosis has been defined as an absolute loss of bone substance. The bone trebeculae are reduced in number and in thickness, but each one is normal in appearance and is fully calcified. The condition may be confined to the spine or it may also involve the peripheral skeleton. Radiologically the vetebral bodies appear less dense, but only after about 30 per cent of bone has been lost. Later the vertebral bodies may appear to be little more dense than the intervertebral discs, and the discs expand to occupy the space lost as the rarefied bones collapse. Peripheral osteoporosis is shown only by increased radiolucency.

Osteoporotic bones are brittle and tend to fracture rather than to deform, but deformities eventually occur as a result of fractures, especially spinal deformity from collapse of vertebral bodies.

The patient may complain of acute back pain, when collapse of a vertebra has occurred, but there may be no pain at other times. Bone tenderness is not usually present.

The serum calcium, phosphorus and alkaline phosphatase are usually normal in osteoporosis. In the acute osteoporosis associated with immobilization of the skeleton, the serum calcium may (rarely) become elevated.

The pathogenesis of osteoporosis is not clear. It was formerly considered to be a disease related to deficiency of bone matrix, and that the matrix formed was fully calcified. More recently evidence has been produced, notably by Nordin (1961), that it may be a disease of calcium deficiency. It is obvious that the end result of too little bone could be produced either by deficient formation of bone or increased bone destruction.

There is a gradual and steady decline in bone mass, beginning in the fourth decade and continuing throughout life. There is radiographic osteoporosis in about 25 per cent of women and 5 per cent of men over the age of 60, and it would appear that osteoporosis would be inevitable if one lived long enough. It has been suggested by Wachman and Bernstein (1968) that bone mineral represents a store of buffer base as phosphate, which is gradually used up. It has long been known that an acid load leads to dissolution of bone, and conditions which tend to produce acidaemia would accelerate this dissolution. They suggest that the predominantly "acid-ash" diet of meat-eating civilized man may thus favour the production of osteoporosis.

Osteoporosis is associated with the following conditions:

(a) Hormonal, including Cushing's syndrome, steroid therapy, thyrotoxicosis and post-menopausal osteoporosis.

(b) Nutritional, including simple dietary lack of calcium, protein deficiency and malabsorption syndromes.

(c) Immobilization of skeleton, possibly including that associated with rheumatoid arthritis.

(d) Idiopathic: juvenile, adult and senile.

The commonest variety of osteoporosis is the idiopathic form in which no cause can be found. The juvenile form is rare but is self-limiting. The form which occurs in relatively young adults is a serious disease which tends to progress inexorably to severe loss of stature and other deformities and ends fatally. Senile osteoporosis is protracted in course.

Treatment: There is no satisfactory treatment. If any associated condition can be found it should be treated but in the majority there is none. Calcium supplements are used by those who believe that it is a disease of calcium deficiency, and cannot be harmful. There is little evidence that they produce any increase in bone mass, although calcium balance becomes positive for a time. A generous diet and vitamin intake are reasonable measures.

Oestrogens have long been used for the treatment of senile and post-menopausal osteoporosis. They seem often to be effective in reducing symptoms, but again there is little evidence that there is increase in bone mass. The dose is 1–3 mg. stilboestrol daily. In women it must be interrupted by one week out of 4, to avoid metropathia. Androgens are equally good, but in women increase facial hair, and produce baldness.

Osteomalacia

In this condition the trabeculae are also reduced in number, but the characteristic feature is that they are not fully calcified, and their periphery is formed of uncalcified osteoid. The condition is widespread throughout the skeleton. The bones are soft rather than brittle and tend to deform rather than to fracture. Deformity of the pelvis and legs is often striking and leads to considerable disability.

Rickets is the childhood form of osteomalacia and is similar in all respects.

Radiologically osteomalacia resembles osteoporosis in that in both conditions there is increased radiolucency, with fewer trabeculae. In osteomalacia, however, there may be characteristic breaks in the cortex of bone, especially in the pelvis, femora, scapulae, and other long bones. These are known as Looser's zones, or Milkman's fractures. They may easily escape notice unless looked for carefully, but become more obvious during healing as callus forms around them.

The patient may complain of aching pain in the bones, or in childhood a deformity of the legs such as bow legs may drawn attention to the condition. Fractures are uncommon. When the disease occurs in childhood there is considerable dwarfing. Looser zones are absent in the childhood form, but the epiphyseal lines are broadened, less distinct, irregular and broken. The end of the metaphysis may become goblet shaped.

Apart from the presence of deformities, there may be striking tenderness on deep palpation of the bones.

The biochemical findings are very different from those of osteoporosis. The serum alkaline phosphatase is raised, usually only moderately in adults, but may reach high levels in children. The serum calcium is reduced or almost normal. The serum phosphorus is usually reduced though it may occasionally be normal.

The causes of osteomalacia are:

1. Vitamin D lack (nutritional, malabsorption syndrome, vitamin D resistant rickets).

2. Renal tubular defects.

3. Chronic renal failure.

Nutritional osteomalacia is sometimes unmasked by the demands of the foetus during pregnancy, and bone pain appears for the first time. The author has seen this occur in an Indian woman living in this country, who ate a very poor diet because she disliked European food.

Treatment: Vitamin D is used in the treatment of all types of osteomalacia. In simple vitamin D lack and malabsorption, it is rarely necessary to give more than 40,000 units (1 mg.) daily for a short time but in malabsorption a maintenance dose may need to be given once or twice weekly.

Much larger doses of vitamin D are necessary in vitamin D resistant rickets, which is a familial condition characterized by hypophosphataemia. Almost all patients, even if treated, are somewhat dwarfed. The dose is worked out for the individual patient, the maximum being given that will not produce hypercalcaemia, the aim being to raise the serum phosphorus.

The treatment of renal tubular defects, and of chronic renal failure, have already been described.

Calcium Metabolism in Pregnancy and Lactation

Surprisingly little is known about calcium metabolism in pregnancy. About 30 g. of calcium is deposited in the foetal skeleton, mainly during the second half of pregnancy, and approximately 250 mg. of calcium are required by the foetus per day during the last quarter. This amounts to about 2·5 per cent of the maternal store of calcium. Even if all of it came from the mother, rather than from diet, a single pregnancy should not cause significant depletion, unless she was suffering for example, from malabsorption syndrome, or prolonged dietary deficiency. On the other hand, absorption of 250 mg. calcium daily from the diet would require a dietary intake considerably higher than this as calcium absorption is inefficient (*see* Calcium Absorption), and repeated pregnancies, especially if the dietary intake is inadequate, would be expected to deplete the mother. The author has seen both osteomalacia and osteoporosis produce symptoms for the first time during late pregnancy, but this appears to be rare in Great Britain.

In farm animals calcium is stored in maternal tissues during pregnancy, to be later mobilized for the production of milk, but there is no information about whether this occurs in humans. Urinary excretion of calcium falls during pregnancy and there is a further fall after parturition.

Approximately 300 mg. of calcium is excreted daily when lactation is fully established, and the excretion remains unchanged when the maternal diet is deficient in calcium. The parathyroid glands influence the excretion of calcium in milk (*see* Parathyroids).

REFERENCES

Buckle, R. M. and Care, A. D., (1968), *Medical Research Association*.
Copp, D. H. and Cheney, B. (1962), *Nature, Lond.*, 193, 381.
Copp, D. H., Cockcroft, D. W., Kueh, Y. and Melville, M. (1968), *Calcitonin* (in press).
Dent, C. E. and Garretts, M. (1960), *Lancet*, i, 1011.
Dent, C. E. and Watson, L. (1965), *Brit. med. J.*, ii, 449.
Foster, G. V., Baghdiantz, A., Kumar, M. A., Slack, E., Soliman, H. A. and MacIntyre, I. (1964), *Nature, Lond.*, 202, 1303.
Gaillard, P. J. (1968), *Calcitonin* (in press).
Hodgkinson, A. and Pyrah, L. N. (1958), *Brit. J. Surg.*, 46, 10.
Knapp, E. L. (1947), *J. clin. Investig.*, 26, 182.
Lonsdale, K. (1968), *Science*, 159, 1199.
McGeown, Mary G. (1960), *Clin. Sci.*, 19, 465.
McGeown, Mary G., Bell, T. K., Soyannwo, M. A. O. and Fenton, S. S. A. (1968), *Brit. J. Radiol.*, 41, 300.
Munson, P. L. (1968), *Calcitonin* (in press).
Nordin, B. E. C. (1961), *Lancet*, i, 1011.
Peacock, M., Hodgkinson, A. and Nordin, B. E. C. (1968), *Brit. med. J.*, iii, 469.
Potts, J. (1968) (in press).
Sherwood, L. M. (1968), *New Engl. J. Med.*, 278, 663.
Wachman, A. and Bernstein, A. (1968), *Lancet*, i, 958.

6. FOLATE METABOLISM IN PREGNANCY

BRYAN M. HIBBARD

and

ELIZABETH D. HIBBARD

Folates are essential for normal cellular reproduction and growth, and the demand for these substances during pregnancy is considerable.

Deficiency of folates in the diet, or failure to convert them to appropriate active forms in the body, results in impaired cellular metabolism. This may have far-reaching effects on the mother, the most commonly recognised manifestation being megaloblastic anaemia, and on the conceptus.

THE NATURE AND FUNCTION OF FOLATES

Folates are a group of chemically related compounds which owe their metabolic activity to the possession of pteroylglutamic radicals. (Fig. 1)

The term "folic acid," formerly applied to pteroylglutamates collectively, is best reserved for the simplest form, pteroylmonoglutamic acid (Folacin, PGA) which is found in liver and yeast. It can be prepared synthetically and is used for therapeutic purposes.

The majority of naturally occurring folates are polyglutamates with three or seven acid radicals. In the body these polyglutamates are converted to PGA conjugates, usually in the form of 5, 6, 7, 8, tetrahydrofolic acid (THFA) with attached methyl, formyl, hydroxymethyl or formimino groups at N_5 or N_{10} (Fig. 2). These groups provide the means of transfer of single carbon units.

Such transfers play an important part in the synthesis of amino-acids, purines and pyrimidines, and in the formation of RNA and DNA.

The suggested inter-relationships of the various PGA derivatives and other substances are shown in Figure 3.

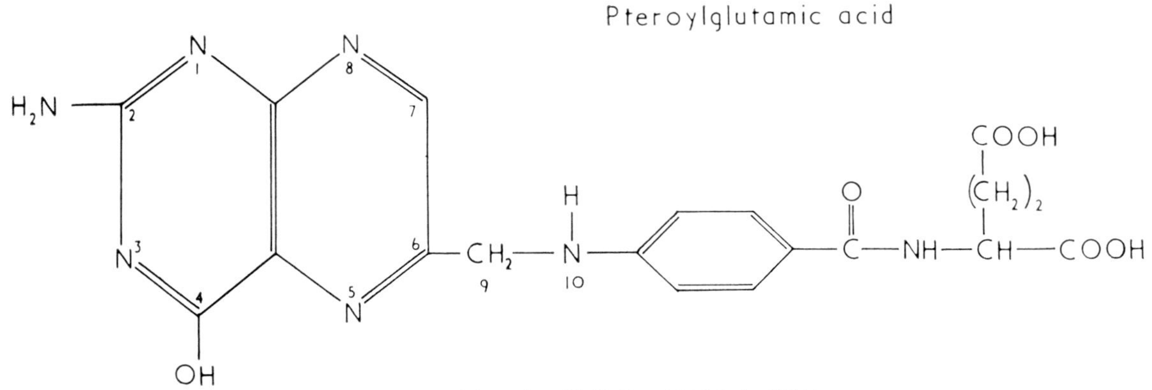

Fig. 1. Pteroylglutamic acid (Folic acid, Folacin, PGA).

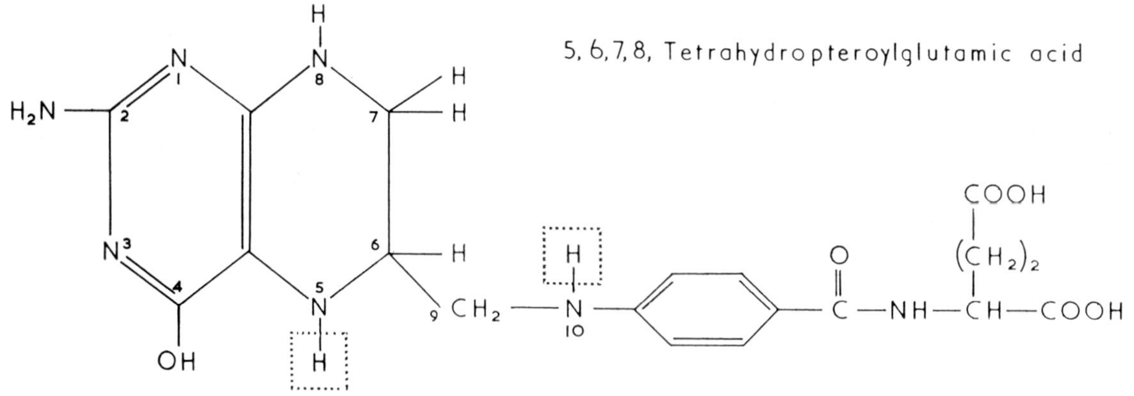

5, 6, 7, 8, Tetrahydropteroylglutamic acid

FIG. 2.   5,6,7,8-Tetrahydropteroylglutamic acid (Tetrahydrofolic acid, THFA).   Transfer of single carbon units is mediated at N_5 and N_{10}, indicated by broken squares.

Cyanocobalamin (Vitamin B_{12}) plays an important part in some of the metabolic processes with which folates are associated. Ascorbic acid (Vitamin C) may also be involved but its exact role has not yet been fully evaluated. There is also a relationship between the metabolism of iron and folates, and a severe iron deficiency can induce a secondary defect in folate utilization (Chanarin, Rothman and Berry, 1965). This is probably mediated through the iron-containing cytochromes, and it has been shown experimentally that in iron-deficient animals the activity of the enzyme formimino transferase is significantly reduced (Vitale, Restrepo, Velez, Riker and Hellerstein, 1966).

There is evidence that folates influence the metabolism and biological activity of steroid hormones. A deficiency of PGA results in severe limitation of growth response of the chick oviduct to oestrogen (Klein and Dorfman, 1951), but this may be to some degree a reflection of the overall growth impairment resulting from folate deficiency. In humans, Martin, Davis and Hahnel (1964) showed reduced urinary oestrogen excretion in patients with low serum folate levels. In vitro studies suggest that THFA enhances enzymatic hydroxylation of progesterone (Hagerman, 1964). The exact significance and biochemical basis of these relationships has not been evaluated but clinical evidence suggests that they may be of relevance in the progress of pregnancy.

REQUIREMENTS AND SOURCES OF FOLATES

A non-pregnant adult requires an intake of approximately 50 micrograms of PGA daily to maintain health (Herbert, 1964). Indirect evidence from the administration of folic acid supplements indicates that requirements in pregnancy may be increased to the order of 300 to 500 micrograms daily. The needs at different stages of gestation are unknown but changes in folate metabolism can be demonstrated even in the early weeks (Hansen 1964; Hibbard and Hibbard, 1966).

The important dietary sources of folates in most communities are green vegetables and liver. From any particular item of food the amount of folate ingested shows wide variation depending on farming and marketing methods, storage and cooking. Naturally occurring folates vary in their metabolic value and their utilisation is influenced by the overall nature of the diet of which they form a part; also, a measurement of microbiological activity may not necessarily be an index of nutritional availability to man. Therefore precise figures cannot be given but Hurdle (1967), investigating diets in London, found that after cooking, "poor" diets often contained as

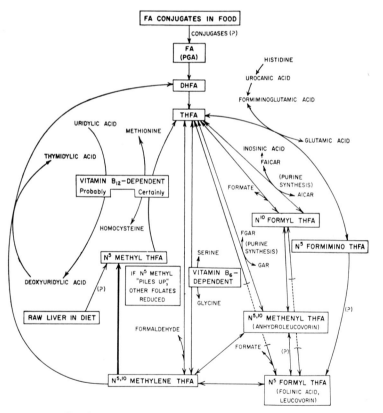

FIG. 3.   Interrelations of vitamin B_{12} and folate metabolism. FA = Folic acid (pteroylglutamic acid); DHFA = dihydrofolic acid; THFA = tetrahydrofolic acid; AICAR = aminoimidazolecarbozamide ribotide; FAICAR = formyl-AICAR; GAR = glycinamide ribonucleotide; FGAR = formyl-GAR. (Reproduced by kind permission from Herbert, V., in *The Pharmacological Basis of Therapeutics*, edited by Goodman and Gilman, page 1412, Collier-Macmillan Limited, London, 1965.)

little as 50 micrograms, whereas good diets contain about 250 micrograms folate daily.

FACTORS LEADING TO DEFECTIVE FOLATE METABOLISM

Defective folate metabolism commonly results from a dietary intake which is inadequate to meet the increased demands of pregnancy. However, many factors may contribute to a negative folate balance and disturb the normal metabolic processes.

1. Supply and Demand

Many women who are apparently well early in pregnancy have a sub-optimal folate intake resulting from poverty, ignorance, customs or fads. Their limited reserves may become rapidly exhausted and may not be adequately replenished between pregnancies, especially if these occur in rapid succession. Thus folate deficiency is found more than three times as often among women of high parity as in nulliparae (Hibbard, Hibbard and Jeffcoate, 1965). Moreover 3 out of 4 patients with defective folate metabolism during pregnancy show a recurrence of the defect in subsequent pregnancies (Hibbard and Hibbard, 1966).

The result of exceptional demands is also illustrated by the fact that there is a fivefold increase in the incidence of folate depletion in women carrying twins (Hibbard *et al.*, 1965).

2. Defective absorption

The detection of defective folate metabolism early in pregnancy, before the foetal demands are great, suggests that in some cases absorption or utilisation of folates is impaired. Even in normal pregnancy, intestinal absorption may be less efficient than in the non-pregnant state. Whitfield (1967) demonstrated intestinal villous flattening in patients with folate deficiency. It is possible that such atrophic changes result in a vicious circle of depletion and malabsorption.

3. Defective utilisation

Deficiencies of dietary factors, enumerated previously, which are closely associated with folate metabolism may result in defective utilisation of ingested folates. Folate metabolism is also impaired by certain drugs, such as phenytoin. In a recent study, eight out of ten patients receiving such therapy showed evidence of defective folate metabolism. (Hibbard and Hibbard, 1968).

Girdwood (1960) postulated a metabolic impairment related to hormonal changes and this might explain the alterations in folate metabolism which can sometimes be demonstrated in the very early weeks of pregnancy. It is also possible that genetically determined but, as yet unidentified, enzymatic defects may be involved.

4. Other Contributory Factors

Several pathological states may increase the overall demands for folates and contribute to a negative folate balance. These include:

(a) Nausea and vomiting in early pregnancy;
(b) Helminthic infestation;
(c) Disorders of intestinal absorption, such as sprue;
(d) Haemolytic anæmias and haemoglobinopathies;
(e) Chronic blood loss from the alimentary tract;
(f) Preceding menorrhagia.

INCIDENCE OF FOLATE DEFICIENCY

Wide variations in the incidence of folate deficiency are reported, depending principally on socio-economic factors as well as methods of assessment and completeness of sampling. In Great Britain there is general agreement that in poorer communities, such as the conurbations of the North, anaemia associated with megaloblastic erythropoiesis occurs in approximately 5 per cent pregnant women, whereas in the South the incidence may be 1 per cent or less (Chisholm, 1966). In addition, megaloblastic bone marrow changes are frequently found in patients who have not reached a state of clinical anaemia. Defective folate metabolism, as judged by biochemical tests, is found at least twice as frequently as megaloblastic erythropoiesis (Hibbard *et al.*, 1965).

Studies from other parts of the world also indicate varying incidences of folate deficiency, resulting principally from differences in dietary habits and nutritional status. In Scandinavia generally folate deficiency is uncommon, but in certain areas where raw fish is eaten megaloblastic anaemia occurs secondary to infestation with Diphyllo-o thriu m latum. In mixed Eastern communities, such as are found in Malaysia, Singapore and Fiji the incidence among Indians is much higher than in other racial groups. Other regions where folate deficiency is known to occur commonly include West Africa, where haemoglobinopathies and malaria are associated factors, and in Bantu tribes, whose diet is exceptionally poor in folates.

LABORATORY ASSESSMENT OF FOLATE STATUS

Full assessment of folate status depends on the summation of results of investigations concerned with various parameters, but it should be emphasised that variations in folate metabolism demonstrated by laboratory tests may not always be of obvious clinical relevance. Investigations can be considered in three groups:

(1) Haematological changes in the blood and bone marrow, which reflect the role played by folates in cell maturation.
(2) Microbiological assay of folate activity in serum and erythrocytes.
(3) Metabolic studies of certain biochemical interactions and of the intestinal absorption and plasma clearance of folates.

The choice of investigations undertaken depends on the nature of the population and available laboratory facilities.

1. Haematological investigations

The haematological changes resulting from folate depletion are characterised by disordered maturation of both erythroid and myeloid cells, leading ultimately to anaemia and leucopenia. Thrombocytopenia may also be observed.

The most obvious changes in the bone marrow morphology are the appearance of giant metamyelocytes and megaloblasts. The degree of megaloblastosis may vary considerably, depending on the severity and duration of folate depletion. The haemopoietic changes are reflected in the peripheral blood by the presence of polylobed neutrophils and macrocytes. Occasionally megaloblasts can be identified, particularly if the "buffy layer" is examined. These typical morphological appearances are often modified or obscured by the effects of a co-existent iron deficiency.

Deficiencies of folate and cyanocobalamin produce identical cellular changes, so that the two conditions cannot be differentiated by morphological studies. Although in some communities dietary Vitamin B_{12} deficiency is common, untreated Addisonian anaemia due to lack of intrinsic factor is rarely, if ever, seen in pregnancy.

Whole blood folate levels are influenced considerably by variations in haematocrit and therefore in pregnancy can be misleading, if considered in isolation. Erythrocyte folate levels show little diurnal variation and closely reflect tissue levels. They are calculated from the haematocrit and serum and whole blood activities (Hansen, 1964; Hoffbrand, Newcombe and Mollin, 1966). The normal range of erythrocyte folate levels in non-pregnant subjects is 166–640 ng/ml. (Hoffbrand *et al.*, 1966). No detailed observations are so far available of erythrocyte folate levels through pregnancy.

3. Metabolic Studies

(a) **Assay of urinary formiminoglutamic acid (FIGLU)** provides an assessment of folate metabolism. FIGLU is a normal intermediary in histidine metabolism (Fig. 4). Degradation of FIGLU to glutamic acid takes place in the presence of formiminotransferase, with THFA acting as coenzyme. If THFA is not available FIGLU accumulates, and is excreted in the urine in excessive amounts. This

TABLE 1

GROWTH PROMOTING ACTIVITY OF PTEROYLGLUTAMIC ACID AND RELATED COMPOUNDS

	PGA (Folic acid Folacin)	THFA	N_5 Methyl THFA	N_5 Formyl THFA (folinic acid)	N_{10} Formyl THFA	Dietary Polyglutamates of PGA and THFA
L. casei	+	+	+	+	+	+
Strep. faecalis	+	+	−	+	+	−
P. cerevisiae	−	+	−	+	+	−

2. Folate assays

Folate activity of human blood is due predominantly to conjugated derivatives of N_5 methyl THFA. The fact that these conjugates support the growth of certain microorganisms forms the basis of almost all methods of assay. The original technique of Toennies and Gallant (1949) has been adapted by several groups of workers (Waters and Mollin, 1961; Herbert, 1961; Hansen, 1964).

Differential assay using a range of organisms (e.g. Lactobacillus casei, Streptococcus faecalis, Pediococcus cervisiae) facilitates the identification of the various pteroylglutamates. Lactobacillus casei is the most sensitive organism and has the widest range of response. Assays using this organism therefore provide the most useful information for clinical purposes.

Less than 10 per cent of the folate activity of the blood is found in the serum. Serum levels are liable to transitory fluctuations which result mainly from dietary variations. Nevertheless, because of technical considerations, they have been widely adopted and give a reasonable indication of folate status. Serum folate levels tend to fall progressively during pregnancy, the mean values being 6–8 nanograms/ml. in the first trimester, and 3·5–4·5 nanograms/ml. in the third trimester (Hansen, 1964; Hibbard—unpublished observations). Foetal levels are usually 5–8 times those found in the mother.

defect can be accentuated by the administration of a loading dose of 1–histidine.

Assay of urinary FIGLU is readily performed spectrophotometrically (Chanarin and Bennett, 1962) or by high voltage electrophoresis (Knowles, Prankerd and Westall, 1960). Its value has been confirmed in large scale studies (Hibbard *et al.*, 1965; Stone, Luhby, Feldman, Gordon and Cooperman, 1967) but Berry, Booth, Chanarin and

BIOCHEMICAL BASIS OF FIGLU EXCRETION TESTS

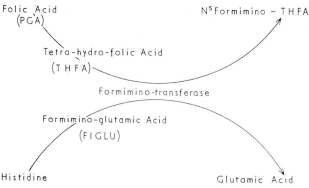

FIG. 4. Biochemical basis of FIGLU excretion tests.

Rothman (1963) have suggested that false negative results may be obtained in the last trimester of pregnancy because of delayed intestinal absorption, lowered renal threshold for histidine and increased passage of histidine to the foetus.

Excessive FIGLU excretion normally indicates that folate metabolism is impaired. This is commonly due to a lack of folates, but can be caused by an enzymatic defect; it may also result from deficiency of cyanocobalamin. Other histidine degradation products such as urocanic acid can be assayed by similar techniques, but such measurements are not of great practical value.

(b) **Folic acid absorption** may be judged by measuring plasma levels following the administration of folic acid orally and intravenously (Girdwood, 1960; Chanarin, MacGibbon, O'Sullivan and Mollin, 1959). The amount subsequently excreted in the urine provides an index of tissue saturation. Similar tests using orally administered tritiated folic acid are also described. Assay of faecal radioactivity after oral administration of radioactive folate gives a measure of the unabsorbed folic acid (Anderson, Belcher, Chanarin and Mollin, 1960).

(c) **Associated studies.** Assays of serum iron, iron combining power, vitamin B_{12} and possibly ascorbic acid all provide useful information relating to the metabolism of folates.

CLINICAL MANIFESTATIONS

1. Maternal

The most important manifestation of folate depletion is megaloblastic anaemia but, even in the absence of anaemia, certain general effects may be evident. These include anorexia, lassitude and fatigue. The hair lacks lustre and muscle tone is poor. Treatment with folic acid alone usually produces dramatic improvement in the physical and mental well-being of affected patients.

Megaloblastic anaemia of pregnancy shows certain characteristic clinical features. It is commonly diagnosed in the last trimester of pregnancy or early in the puerperium but, with increased awareness and improved antenatal care, it is now detected with increasing frequency earlier in pregnancy. Spontaneous remission invariably occurs post partum, but may be delayed as a result of lactation. Although the condition usually develops insidiously, rapidly fulminating cases are sometimes seen. Megaloblastic anaemia is almost invariably associated with excessive urinary FIGLU excretion. Serum and erythrocyte folate levels are generally depressed but there is some overlap with the values found in patients with normal erythropoiesis.

2. Foetal

Folate depletion may affect the development of the foetus directly or by impairment of placental and decidual growth. Animal experiments show that total folate deprivation can give rise to foetal malformation or death, the end result being influenced by the stage of gestation at which the deprivation is inflicted (Nelson, 1960). Folic acid antagonist drugs have been administered to a few pregnant women, either for therapeutic purposes or to induce abortion (e.g. Thiersch, 1960). In the majority of such cases abortion ensued and in the remainder the foetus showed major malformations.

The less severe degrees of folate deprivation encountered in clinical practice are also associated with an increased risk to pregnancy, the principle manifestations being abortion, foetal malformation and abruptio placentae. However, the aetiology of these conditions is usually multifactorial and factors other than folate depletion are important in many cases. Also, the demonstrable folate deficiency in such cases often reflects a more general nutritional inadequacy which may contribute to the overall picture.

Abortion. A significant correlation between threatened abortion and low serum folate levels was observed by Martin and Davis (1964). They subsequently suggested that oestrogen metabolism is adversely affected by folate deficiency and this may be an important factor in relation to the growth of the foetus and the occurrence of abortion (Martin et al., 1964).

A study of over 700 patients suffering abortion (Hibbard, 1967) showed an association with defective folate metabolism, as judged by serum and erythrocyte folate levels and by FIGLU excretion. There was a particularly high incidence of deficiency in patients with recurrent (3 or more consecutive) abortions. In this series and in that reported by Martin, Harper and Kelso (1965) low serum folate levels were found in approximately 50 per cent of patients with non-recurrent abortion. Erythrocyte folate levels, which are uninfluenced by diurnal effects and are more indicative of recent folate status in the tissues, showed the same general trend but to a lesser degree. Abnormally low levels were found in 16 per cent of all abortions and 36 per cent of recurrent abortions, as compared with 6 per cent in clinically normal pregnancies.

Foetal Malformation. Malformations are twice as common in the infants of women with defective folate metabolism as compared with normal women. The commonly occuring defects are those involving errors in fusion, such as anencephaly and cleft palate. In an investigation of mothers with anencephalic foetuses, abnormal folate metabolism was found in nearly 60 per cent of cases, about four times the incidence found in a control series of patients matched for age, parity and gestation period. (Hibbard and Smithells, 1965). However, the investigations were usually carried out late in pregnancy and it would be desirable to have more knowledge of the folate status obtaining at the period of organogenesis.

Abruptio Placentae. Hibbard and Jeffcoate (1966) have suggested that if folate depletion is present at the time of implantation, both placental and decidual cells may be adversely affected. It is postulated that a cellular defect, once produced, results in an insecure implantation which persists through pregnancy. Such a placenta is more liable to premature separation and disruption as a result of any strain imposed in pregnancy, such as the onset of uterine contractions.

Placental abruption was noted to be associated with megaloblastic erythropoiesis in a large proportion of cases by Coyle and Geoghegan (1962). Similar findings were reported from Liverpool, where two thirds of women with unequivocal evidence of abruptio placentae showed megaloblastic erythropoiesis and nearly all had excessive FIGLU excretion (Hibbard, 1964). Similar correlations have been shown by Streiff and Little (1967) and Stone et al (1967). In addition Streiff and Little showed erythrocyte folate levels to be consistently low, suggesting a long-standing pre-existing deficiency.

Investigators in some other centres, especially in the Far East (Menon, Sengupta and Ramaswamy, 1966; Thambu and Llewellyn-Jones, 1966), failed to find an association between placental abruption and abnormal folate metabolism. However, their clinical and laboratory criteria differ from those in the studies reported above. Also in such communities, other nutritional deficiencies may be relevant.

TREATMENT OF FOLATE DEPLETION

Folate depletion can be prevented in the majority of patients if they can be persuaded to improve their dietary and cooking habits and, if possible, to space and limit childbearing. For patients at known increased risk prophylactic therapy should be started early in pregnancy.

Local circumstances influence the need for and desirability of prophylactic therapy. If facilities for clinical and laboratory supervision are limited the routine administration of supplements to all pregnant women may be advisable, at least in high risk populations. This does not obviate the need for continued vigilance, for many women fail to take the therapy prescribed and up to 10 per cent fail to respond to oral therapy.

It is suggested that because of the likelihood of folate depletion, certain patients, irrespective of their socio-economic status, should be given folic acid supplements:

(i) Those pregnant for the 5th or subsequent time;
(ii) Those carrying a multiple pregnancy;
(iii) Those giving a history of folate deficiency, megaloblastic or severe anaemia in a previous pregnancy;
(iv) Those with a history of abruptio placentae in a previous pregnancy;
(v) Those who have suffered recurrent abortion associated with folate deficiency or with no obvious aetiology;
(vi) Those receiving anti-convulsant therapy during pregnancy.

In some patients, such as those suffering from recurrent abortion and those with a past history of abruptio placentae, folic acid should be administered as early as possible in pregnancy, or even before conception. Pursuing this policy, Martin et al (1965) reported favourable results in patients with a history of abortion associated with low serum folate levels, but this awaits confirmation. Personal observations (unpublished data) indicate that administration of folic acid and general dietary advice reduces the risk of recurrence of abruptio placentæ in women who have had a previous pregnancy complicated by this condition.

Once folate deficiency is recognised treatment with folic acid should be commenced and continued until several weeks after delivery, or until the cessation of lactation. Oral therapy is usually preferred, but sometimes failure to respond adequately necessitates parenteral therapy.

The dosage of oral folic acid most commonly used has been 5 mgms. twice or three times daily. Such amounts are far in excess of physiological or therapeutic needs and recent surveys suggest that a reasonable dose lies in the microgram range (Hansen, 1964; Willoughby and Jewell, 1966). 500 μgm daily is adequate for prophylactic therapy, even in poorly nourished, poorly motivated communities (Hibbard and Hibbard, 1969a). A larger dose may be necessary for treatment of established deficiency and for this purpose 500 μgm thrice daily is adequate (Hibbard and Hibbard, 1969b).

Folinic acid, which is one of the physiologically active derivatives of folic acid, is also effective in correcting folate depletion, but is more costly and can only be given by injection. The exact indications for this type of therapy are uncertain but it may be essential if there is an intrinsic defect in the metabolism of folates.

It is important to correct any other co-existent deficiency and also to treat any intercurrent infection or infestation which may interfere with response to therapy. If iron deficiency is not already present, it may be induced as a result of the haemopoietic response to folic acid. In practice, therefore, it is wise always to administer iron in addition to folic acid.

CONCLUSIONS

Increased metabolic demands and limited body reserves coupled with poor dietary intake can readily lead to the development of folate deficiency during pregnancy, often with serious results to both mother and foetus. Biochemical, morphological and clinical evidence of folate depletion appear in succession as pregnancy progresses.

The most commonly recognised clinical manifestation is megaloblastic anaemia, but there is a predisposition to abortion, foetal malformation and abruptio placentae, all of which occur more commonly in patients with defective folate metabolism. Although additional aetiological factors operate in many cases, prevention or correction of folate depletion may result in improved prognosis for the foetus.

The recurrent nature of defective folate metabolism and its frequent demonstration early in pregnancy suggest that in many cases there is an underlying metabolic disorder. The exact relationship with enzymatic deficiencies and steroid metabolism is uncertain at present.

The widespread administration of folic acid supplements during pregnancy is often considered desirable because of the high incidence of deficiency and inadequate facilities for detailed investigation in some areas. Such a policy may be of individual benefit but hampers epidemiological research and may delay full understanding of the nature and results of defective folate metabolism in pregnancy.

REFERENCES

Anderson, B., Belcher, E. H., Chanarin, I. and Mollin, D. L. (1960), "Urinary and Faecal Excretion of Radioactivity after Oral Doses of ³H Folic Acid," *Brit. J. Haematology*, **6**, 439.

Berry, V., Booth, M. A., Chanarin, I., and Rothman, D. (1963), "Urinary Formimino Glutamic Acid Excretion in Pregnancy," *Brit. med. J.*, **ii**, 1103.

Chanarin, I. and Bennett, M. C. (1962), "A Spectrophotometric Method for Estimating Formiminoglutamic and Urocanic Acid," *Lancet*, **i**, 27.

Chanarin, I., MacGibbon, B. M., O'Sullivan, W. J. and Mollin, D. L. (1959), "The Pathogenesis of Megaloblastic Anaemia of Pregnancy," *Lancet*, **ii**, 634.

Chanarin, I., Rothman, D., and Berry V. (1965), "Iron Deficiency and Its Relation to Folic Acid Status in Pregnancy: Results of a Clinical Trial," *Brit. med. J.*, **i**, 480.

Chisholm, M. (1966), "A Controlled Clinical Trial of Prophylactic Folic Acid and Iron in Pregnancy," *J. Obstet. Gynaec. Brit. Cwlth*, **73**, 191.

Coyle, C. V. and Geoghegan, F. (1962), "The Problem of Anaemia in a Dublin Maternity Hospital," *Proc. roy. Soc. Med.*, **55**, 764.

Girdwood, R. W. (1960), "Folic Acid, its Analogs and Antagonists," in *Advances in Clinical Chemistry*, Vol. 3 Ed. Sobotka, H. and Stewart, C. P., Academic Press, New York.

Hagerman, D. D. (1964), "Pteridine Cofactors in Enzymatic Hydroxylation of Steroids," *Fed. Proc.*, **23**, 480.

Hansen, H. A. (1964), *On the Diagnosis of Folic Acid Deficiency*, Alquist and Wiksell, Stockholm.

Herbert, V. (1961), "The Assay and Nature of Folic Acid Activity in Human Serum," *J. clin. Invest.*, **40**, 81.

Herbert, V. (1964), "Studies of Folate Deficiency in Man," *Proc. roy. Soc. Med.*, **57**, 377.

Herbert, V. and Zalusky, R. (1962), "Interrelations of Vitamin B12 and Folic acid Metabolism: Folic acid clearance studies," *J. Clin. Invest.*, **41**, 1263.

Hibbard, B. M. (1964), "The Role of Folic Acid in Pregnancy," *J. Obstet. Gynaec. Brit. Cwlth.*, **71**, 529.

Hibbard, B. M. (1967), "Abortion and Defective Folate Metabolism," *Fifth World Congress of Gynaecology and Obstetrics Supplement*, p. 40. Butterworths, Australia.

Hibbard, B. M. and Hibbard, E. D. (1966), "Recurrence of Defective Folate Metabolism in Successive Pregnancies," *J. Obstet. Gynaec. Brit. Cwlth.*, **73**, 428.

Hibbard, B. M. and Hibbard, E. D. (1968), "Folate Metabolism and Reproduction," *Brit. med. Bull.*, **24**, 10.

Hibbard, B. M. and Hibbard, E. D. (1969a), "The Prophylaxis of Folate Deficiency in Pregnancy," *Acta Obstet. Gynec. Scand.*, **48**, in press.

Hibbard, B. M. and Hibbard, E. D., (1969b), "The Treatment of Folate Deficiency in Pregnancy," *Acta Obstet. Gynec. Scand.*, **48**, in press.

Hibbard, B. M., Hibbard, E. D., and Jeffcoate, T. N. A. (1965), "Folic Acid and Reproduction," *Acta obstet. gynec. scand.*, **44**, 375.

Hibbard, B. M. and Jeffcoate, T. N. A. (1966), "Abruptio placentae," *Obstet. Gynec.*, **27**, 155.

Hibbard, E. D. and Smithells, R. W. (1965), "Folic Acid Metabolism and Human Embryopathy," *Lancet*, **i**, 1254.

Hoffbrand, A. V., Newcombe, B. F. A. and Mollin, D. L. (1966), "Method of Assay of Red Cell Folate Activity and the Value of the Assay as a Test for Folate Deficiency," *J. clin. Path.*, **19**, 17.

Hurdle, A. (1967), Unpublished Observations quoted in *British Medical Journal*, **i**, 415.

Klein, I. T. and Dorfman, R. I. (1951), "Estrogen Stimulation of the Oviduct in Vitamin Deficient Chicks," *Endocrinology*, **48**, 345.

Knowles, J. P., Prankerd, T. A. J. and Westall, R. G. (1960), "Simplified Method for Detecting Formiminoglutamic Acid in Urine as a Test of Folic Acid Deficiency," *Lancet*, **ii**, 347.

Martin, J. D. and Davis, R. E. (1964), "Serum Folic Acid Activity and Vaginal Bleeding in Early Pregnancy," *J. Obstet. Gynaec. Brit. Cwlth.*, **71**, 400.

Martin, J. D., Davis, R. E. and Hahnel, R. (1964), "Reduced Urinary Oestrogen Excretion Associated with Low Serum Folic Acid Activity in Pregnancy," *Lancet*, **i**, 1075.

Martin, R. H., Harper, T. A. and Kelso, W. (1965), "Serum Folic Acid in Recurrent Abortion," *Lancet*, **i**, 670.

Menon, M. K., Sengupta, M. and Ramaswamy, N. (1966), "Accidental Haemorrhage and Folic Acid Deficiency," *J. Obstet. Gynaec. Brit. Cwlth.*, **73**, 49.

Nelson, M. M. (1960), "Teratogenic Effects of PGA Deficiency in the Rat", *Ciba Symposium on Congenital Malformations*, J. & A. Churchill, London, p. 134.

Stone, M. L., Luhby, A. L., Feldman, R., Gordon, M. and Cooperman, J. M. (1967) "Folic Acid Metabolism in Pregnancy," *Amer. J. Obstet. Gynec.*, **99**, 638.

Streiff, R. R. and Little, A. B. (1967), "Folic Acid Deficiency in Pregnancy," *New Engl. J. Med.*, **276**, 776.

Thambu, J. and Llewellyn-Jones, D. (1966), "Bone Marrow Studies in Abruptio Placentae," *J. Obstet. Gynaec. Brit. Cwlth.*, **73**, 930.

Thiersch, J. B. (1960), Discussion in *Ciba Symposium on Congenital Malformations*, J. & A. Churchill, London, p. 152.

Toennies, G. and Gallant, D. L. (1949), "Bacterimetric Studies III: Blood Level Studies on Teropterin Metabolism," *J. Lab. Clin. Med.*, **34**, 501.

Vitale, J. J., Restrepo, A., Velez, H., Riker, J. B., and Hellerstein, E. E. (1966), "Secondary Folate Deficiency Induced in the Rat by Dietary Iron Deficiency," *J. Nutr.*, **88**, 315.

Waters, A. H. and Mollin, D. L. (1961), "Studies on the Folic Acid Activity of Human Serum," *J. clin. Path.*, **14**, 335.

Whitfield, C. R. (1967) "Sprue Complicating Pregnancy in Singapore," *J. Obstet. Gynaec. Brit. Cwlth.*, **74**, 537.

Willoughby, M. L. N. and Jewell, F. J. (1966), "Investigation of Folic Acid Requirements in Pregnancy," *Brit. med. J.*, **ii**, 1568.

SECTION VI

THE NEWBORN

1. THE FIRST BREATH AND DEVELOPMENT OF LUNG TISSUE

JOHN A. DAVIS

Knowledge of the development of the foetal lung is of importance to the obstetrician for three main reasons; the first, that it makes it possible to determine the gestational age at which independent viability is conceiveable, since this largely depends on efficient respiration; the second, that it makes it possible to define the vulnerability of the lung to insults suffered at particular stages of gestation (Landing 1957): the third, that it may help the pathologist to estimate the gestational age in abortions and still-born babies (Parmentier 1962). From the first point of view, which is the most important, the lungs cannot be considered in isolation since their proper functioning depends upon that of the respiratory musculature with its innervation and upon that of the pulmonary circulation: that is, on the circulatory and central nervous systems. In this chapter the various factors on which respiratory function depends will be considered in turn, the reader being referred to the separate chapter on the perinatal pulmonary circulation for further details.

Embryology

The first rudiments of the lungs appear at about 24 days gestation as a ventral outgrowth from the endoderm of the foregut which soon divides into two main branches, the anlagen of the main bronchi (Schulz 1959). These in turn divide again—the right into three divisions, the left into two—to form the bronchi to the principal lobes of the lungs (Fauré-Fremiet and Dragoiu 1923). Further growth takes place by sequential dichotomous branching until at about 16 weeks a maximum of some 24 generations has been achieved. (Bucher and Reid 1961.) Growth and differentiation appear to depend upon glycolysis; the large stores of glycogen present in the lung at this time presumably serving as the source of energy (Sorokin 1960); and they are to some extent inhibited by compression, as may occur in cases of congenital diaphragmatic hernia. (Areechon and Reid 1963.) The bronchi are initially solid (stade bronchique), but somewhere between 16 and 24 weeks they become patent (stade canalaire) and develop a lining of ciliated epithelium (Bucher and Reid 1961). At 24 weeks the terminal branches develop into respiratory bronchioles: these are initially lined with cuboidal epithelium which is partly shed (Plank 1967) at about 27 weeks when there is a breakdown of the walls of the terminal air-spaces to form larger units. Finally, *true* alveoli are formed at sometime after the 37th week (stade alveolaire) (Dubreuil *et al.* 1936). Dunnill (1962) has calculated that there are some 20 million alveoli at birth as opposed to 300 million in the adult, but the studies of Boyden, quoted by Reid (1966) suggest that Dunnill's

figures refer to terminal air spaces rather than to true alveoli with limiting elastic tissue which probably do not form until after birth.

At 90–120 days mucous and serous glands first become apparent in the bronchial walls; mucous glands at first predominate and the adult ratio is not attained until the age of three. There is evidence that the nature of the mucus secreted by the foetus and young infant is also different from that in older children, with a higher proportion of sulphate to sialate; and this may affect its physical properties (Lamb 1968).

TABLE 1

Gestational age	Appearance and maturation of tissue elements
Stade bronchique	
3–4 weeks	Bronchial "buds"
3–4 weeks	Pulmonary blood vessels
9–13 weeks	Pulmonary lymphatics
9–13 weeks	Pleural sacs: lung develops lobar structure
9–13 weeks	Elastic fibres of bronchial walls
10–17 weeks	Bronchial cartilage
Stade canalaire	
10–17 weeks	Mucus glands appear
10–17 weeks	Ciliated bronchial epithelium differentiates
10–17 weeks	Alveolar ducts demonstrable
17–20 weeks	Serous glands appear
24–37 weeks	Terminal air spaces form
26–30 weeks	Proliferation of pulmonary capillary network Increasing muscularity of pulmonary arterioles
22–27 weeks	Type II alveolar cells
Stade alveolaire	
37–42 weeks	True alveoli with elastic tissue in lining membrane and flattened epithelium

Two types of "pneumocyte" become distinguishable at this time in the lining of the terminal "air spaces" (Bertalanffy and Leblond 1953); cuboidal cells, which elongate and flatten during development between six and nine months of gestation to become the alveolar epithelium (Palmer 1935; Barnard and Day 1937; L'Aumonier 1952), and less numerous cells which contain osmophilic inclusions and may be responsible for the secretion or re-absorption of the alveolar lining layer—the so-called pulmonary surfactant (Pattle 1958). The function of this important substance is considered later.

Alongside the development of the pulmonary endoderm, the mesenchyme of the thoracic cavity differentiates into a dense layer around the bronchi and a looser tissue into which they ramify (Ham and Baldwin 1941). From the denser layer are formed the cartilage and muscle of the bronchial walls; the looser tissue forms the pulmonary interstitium comprising elastic and connective tissue and arterial, venous, capillary and lymphatic vessels. The pulmonary capillaries come into close relation with the future air spaces at about 20 weeks and proliferate over

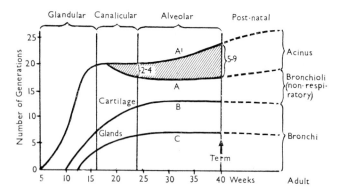

FIG. 1. Intra-uterine development of the bronchial tree. Line A represents the number of bronchial generations, and A^1 the respiratory bronchioles and alveolar ducts. B is the extension of cartilage along the bronchial tree and C the extension of mucous glands. (From Bucher, U. and Reid, L. *Thorax*, **16**: 207, 1961.)

the succeeding 3 months until the lung is more or less completely vascularized as pregnancy approaches term. (Loosli and Potter, 1958). The development of supernumerary in addition to conventional branches results in the establishment of an effective collateral blood supply to the terminal air spaces, which thereafter are no longer discrete units in this respect (Reid 1966). The anatomical basis of the ventilation/perfusion ratio that underlies adequate respiratory gas exchange is probably not reached until relatively late in gestation; and this may be responsible for some of the respiratory difficulties of the premature infant (Klemola 1937). In the human foetus the walls of the pulmonary arterioles are more muscular than in the child or adult, providing the basis for the high pulmonary arterial resistance which is a feature of the unborn fetus as it approaches term. However it is noteworthy also that at this stage of development muscular arteries are not usually found within the alveolar wall as in the adult (Hislop 1968). This marked muscularity of the foetal pulmonary vessels regresses after birth, except in certain disease states (Heath and Edwards 1958) but its persistence in the immediate neonatal period results in a tendency for the infant to revert to foetal circulatory pattern in conditions of partial asphyxia (Naeye 1961; O'Neal, Ahlvin, Bauer and Thomas, 1957). The adult ratio between the area of lung capable of effecting gas exchange and the body surface area as an index of metabolic needs appears on the evidence available to be reached fairly early in gestation and is therefore unlikely to be a factor in the viability of the premature baby (Karlberg, 1957; Dunnill, 1962). The time-table of this essentially anatomical phase of development is set out in Table 1.

Functional Development

The second phase of development renders the lungs capable of carrying out their respiratory function as the site of gas exchange between the blood and the atmosphere. For this to be fully effective, the essential developments are—(i) the formation of stable alveoli in close relation to the pulmonary capillaries and with a large enough total surface area to allow adequate oxygen uptake and CO_2 elimination, and (ii) the establishment of rhythmic respiration. The work of breathing consists in overcoming the frictional, elastic and surface tension components of the resistance to inflation of the lungs. At birth an important component is that due to surface forces, which resist both the initial expansion of the lungs and the establishment of an adequate functional residual capacity (that is, the volume of air remaining in the lungs after expiration). In this context the alveoli can be compared to minute bubbles blown on the ends of the terminal bronchioles (Fig. 2). The alveoli would tend to collapse in expiration, and to fill unevenly in inspiration, were surface tension at the high values (20 dynes per cm.) characteristic of body fluids (Avery and Mead, 1959), but in healthy term babies the surface tension at the alveolar interface is lowered by the presence of a surface tension reducing substance, known as pulmonary surfactant, which is a lipo-protein containing dipalmitoyl-lecithin (Tierney, Clements and Trahan, 1965) (Abrams, 1966). The reduction in surface forces brought about by surfactant is almost certainly due to its

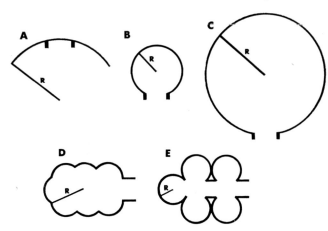

FIG. 2. Diagram to illustrate the effect of surface tension forces, unmodified by surfactant, on alveoli. Since the constricting force in a sphere $= 2T/R$ (where T is the surface tension of the lining and R the radius) it will be relatively low in case (A), representing an uninflated alveolus, in case (D), representing an alveolar duct without fully formed alveoli in a very premature infant, and in case (C), representing a fully expanded alveolus, relatively high in case (B) representing a partially expanded alveolus.

forming a coherent layer at the interface between gas and water with lower intermolecular attraction than is the case with water molecules. As a consequence, stretching the film so that it becomes functionally discontinuous will greatly reduce its activity. When at its minimum radius during late expiration, an alveolus lined with surfactant will be protected from progressive collapse; while during inspiration the lining may be broken up and surface tension forces will then act to prevent its expansion at the expense of alveoli with smaller radii and therefore greater resistance to stretch (Clements, Brown and Johnson, 1958). For this mechanism to function efficiently, the total amount of surfactant available at one time must be limited; but since its half-life is comparatively brief—less than 18 hours (Clements, 1967)—and it is readily denatured (Abrams, 1966) the capacity of the lung to produce and

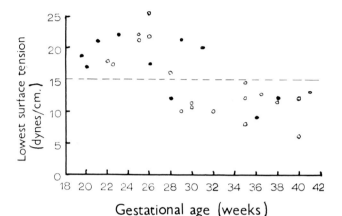

Gestational age (weeks)
● still-born infants   o live-born infants

FIG. 3. Graph to illustrate the relation between gestational age and the concentration of surfactant (as measured by the compression in lung extracts from human infants dying of other causes than respiratory distress). Figures below the dashed line indicate a sufficiency. (From the data of Reynolds, Orzalesi, Motoyama, Craig and Cook (1965) *Brit. Med. Bull.*, 1966.)

release it needs to be relatively large. Some surfactant can be shown to be present in human foetal lungs from about 23–24 weeks gestation onwards (Reynolds, Orzalesi, Motoyama, Craig and Cook, 1965), and pressure volume curves may be normal in the lungs of new-born infants dying in the first week of life at this gestational age; but most truly premature infants are probably relatively deficient, and this probably accounts for their high mortality and morbidity from the so-called respiratory distress syndrome (Wigglesworth, Reynolds and Roberton, 1968) (Fig. 3). This deficiency may be less important for very immature infants with relatively larger terminal air-spaces than for babies nearer term with "alveoli" of smaller diameter—according with a generally held impression that clinical respiratory distress is commoner in babies born at 30–37 weeks gestation than in those born before 30 weeks (though the mortality is of course much higher in the latter group).

Oxygen uptake and CO_2 elimination depend not only on the ventilatory capacity, but on pulmonary perfusion, haemoglobin concentration, the oxygen dissociation curve, circulation time, oxygen diffusion capacity and carbonic anhydrase activity. The factors which result in the huge increase in pulmonary perfusion brought about by the first breath are considered in Section III, Ch. II; animal studies indicate that they include expansion of the lungs, a decrease in alveolar CO_2 tension, and an increase in alveolar oxygen tension (Cassin, Dawes, Mott, Ross and Strang, 1964). There is little evidence that there is

any gross abnormality of diffusion capacity at birth; haemoglobin levels and oxygen capacities (Bartels, 1966) are on the high side by adult standards; and the presence of foetal haemoglobin does not affect the dissociation curve in such a way as to make a significant difference to oxygen uptake at "normal" alveolar oxygen tensions (Bartels, 1966); but it is conceivable that the very low levels of carbonic anhydrase activity in the blood of very immature fetuses may impose a limit on CO_2 elimination since in the absence of this enzyme CO_2 equilibration between capillary blood and alveolar air may be slower than the circulation time (Kleinman *et al.*, 1968).

It appears then that the respiratory apparatus with its circulation and CNS connections is capable of supporting independent existence, given the best possible circumstances, from about 24 weeks gestation; and newborn infants of this gestation do in fact sometimes survive although the mortality up to 28 weeks (B.W. 1,000 grs.) is for various reasons very high (Perinatal Mortality Survey, 1958).

The Initiation of Pulmonary Respiration

Given a respiratory apparatus capable of functioning, it remains to consider how it is set in motion. During fetal life the lung occupies the same volume of the thorax as after birth, the difference being that the lungs of the fetus in utero are filled with liquid whereas after birth they are of course filled with gas. This liquid is quite different in composition from amniotic fluid, perhaps as a result of physical separation due to closure of the glottis (Smith, 1959 and Adams, Desilets and Towers, 1966). During birth the lung liquid is partly expelled from the air passages, perhaps by pressure in the birth canal, and is partly absorbed by the pulmonary lymphatics, which at any rate in the foetal lamb are capable of draining large volumes of liquid at term (Adams, Fujiwara and Rowsham, 1963) (Humphrey, Normand, Reynolds, Strang, 1967) as expansion of the lungs and rhythmic breathing are established.

That respiratory movements occur in utero is well established (Snyder and Rosenfeld, 1937; Davis and Potter, 1946; Shaffer, 1956) but whether these represent normal rhythmic respiration is doubtful; it is perhaps more likely that in most of the instances reported they were of the nature of asphyxial or post asphyxial gasping.

The actual cause of the first extra-uterine breath is still not established. It cannot be asphyxia, though all babies are to some extent asphyxiated at birth (Oliver, Dennis and Bates, 1961) because blood gas tensions in the fetus of the same order as those that result from being born do not as a rule initiate breathing in utero except when anoxia is so severe as to induce gasping (Harned, Rowsham, MacKinney and Sugioka, 1964). The most reasonable explanation would seem to lie in an activation of the chemoreceptors at birth by sympathetic stimulation caused by clamping the cord—possibly as a result of a fall in carotid body perfusion—with a consequent increase in input to the respiratory "centre"; certainly in the human infant tying the cord accelerates the onset of respiration (Purves, 1967; Dunn, 1967).

Another important component of sensory input at birth, at any rate in certain species, is cold, which stimulates inspiration just as warmth appears to inhibit it (Tchobroutski, 1967). It has also been shown that in the newborn human infant Head's so-called paradoxical reflex will result in augmented respiratory effort as the lungs are inflated (Cross, Klaus, Tooley and Weisser, 1960); and this presumably contributes to their initial expansion.*

In the totally asphyxiated baby the course of events is somewhat different. If any mammal is rendered anoxic, it goes through a "crisis" characterized by bradycardia, hypotension, voiding and apnoea. Subsequently, after a variable interval, apnoea is succeeded by regular gasping; and finally, after the last gasp, the circulation fails and death follows (Davis, 1961; Mott, J., 1961) (Fig. 4). The total duration of life in these circumstances varies with age, being much longer in the new-born of most species, and seems to depend on the initial cardiac glycogen reserves (Stafford and Weatherall, 1960) and the rate of build up of potassium and hydrogen ions in the blood (Klionski, 1968). From the respiratory point of view, what it is important to stress is that apnoea in the new-born baby may be the consequence of previous asphyxia and that in these circumstances it may be primary—before the first spontaneous gasp—or terminal—after the last gasp—with quite a different prognosis in the two situations. The period of primary apnoea is in most species prolonged very greatly by the prior administration of narcotics or hypnotics which can reach a foetus across the placenta, after administration to the mother (Moore and Davis, 1967) and can be shortened by stimulation, which may bring forward the first gasp; but animals in terminal apnoea can only be induced to breathe again by reoxygenation (Cross, 1966). Brain damage begins at the last gasp but is unlikely to be extensive before the heart fails (Dawes, Hibbard and Windle, 1964). Thus in asphyxiated babies the first breath is likely to be a gasp which in practice is often induced by artificial inflation of the lung and the induction of Head's reflex. One significant implication of the occurrence of this pattern of reaction in total asphyxia is that gasping may indicate a more serious situation than primary apnoea; which the prognosis and treatment of terminal apnoea would be quite different from that of primary apnoea could they always be distinguished in the clinical setting.

In the normal term infant, even if asphyxiated just before or after birth, the first cry, breath or gasp will establish a functional residual capacity (Hey and Kelly, 1968; Klaus, Tooley, Weaver and Clements, 1962; Fawcitt, Lind and Wegelius, 1960) as has been shown by both radiological and plethysmographic methods. If

* It might appear that the evidence cited lends scientific support to old fashioned remedies for apnoea at birth such as slapping, plunging into cold water, the giving of CO_2 etc., but it must be stressed that the inevitable sensory stimulation consequent on being born is enough to start most babies breathing and that those who remain apnoeic are abnormal and for that reason unlikely to respond to extra stimulation—for reasons discussed later in the chapter. There is no evidence to suggest that premature infants lack the CNS connections necessary for the initiation of breathing, albeit there are often problems in its maintenance.

animal studies are any guide, this will in turn bring about a big increase in pulmonary perfusion and initiate a return to normal breathing (Cross, 1966). The first breaths in healthy infants are characterized by a short inspiration followed by prolonged expiration, i.e. are sighing in character; and a higher negative pressure is usually

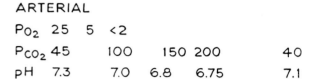

ARTERIAL

P_{O_2}	25	5	<2		
P_{CO_2}	45	100	150	200	40
pH	7.3	7.0	6.8	6.75	7.1

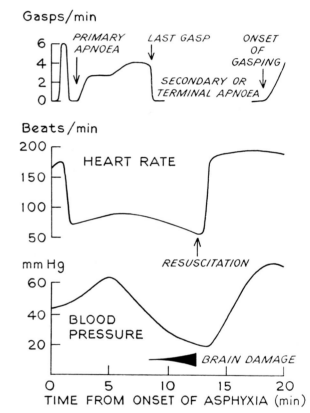

Fig. 4. Figure to illustrate the pattern of events immediately following acute asphyxia and subsequent resuscitation in the foetal rhesus monkey. (From the data of Dawes, 1968.)

needed to establish than to maintain regular respiration (Karlberg, Cherry, Escardo and Koch, 1962). Within an hour or two of birth respiratory performance in the baby reaches its full capacity, with no further improvement over the first week. In the rat it has been shown that alveolar surface area increases sharply in the first five days before returning to its normal rate of growth (Weibel, 1967), and this accords with the abrupt increase in oxygen consumption seen in the first few days of age in human infants who initially exhibit a limited capacity to increase their metabolic rate in response to cold and exhibit lower than normal oxygen tensions (Scopes, 1966; Tizard, Roberton, Gupta, Dahlenburg, (1968).

Finally, there are certain secondary consequences of the first breath that are of importance. The creation of a high negative pressure in the thorax will inevitably influence the distribution of the foetal blood volume between baby and placenta so that the size of the so-called "placental transfusion" may be affected considerably by whether the cord is tied early or late and before or after a breath or uterine contraction (Redmond, Isana and Ingall, 1965). The size of the placental transfusion has certain effects on the baby which have been investigated in some detail, but it does not seem to be critical for survival (Buckels and Usher, 1965). Another possibly important accompaniment of the first breath, at any rate in the lamb, is a great increase in cerebral blood flow (Purves, 1968) that could have clinical implications: for instance, intraventricular haemorrhage, a common cause of death in very immature infants (Grontoft, 1954) is very seldom found in still-born infants. A third likely effect is an alteration in the distribution of blood inside the baby as a result of the decrease in intra-thoracic and the increase in intra-abdominal pressure consequent on inspiration, an effect that may be concerned with other factors in the establishment of pulmonary perfusion. This aspect of the subject is dealt with more extensively in other chapters (Section III, Chs. 11 & 12; Section VI, Ch. 3.)

To sum up, independent pulmonary respiration demands clear airways, an adequate alveolar area, stably expanded alveoli, sufficient pulmonary perfusion, adequate oxygen carrying capacity, satisfactory lymphatic drainage, minimal carbonic anhydrase activity and rhythmic respiration. A number of these desiderata are not fulfilled until relatively late in gestation; and premature birth is therefore associated with a high incidence of respiratory problems in the new-born period.

ACKNOWLEDGMENTS

The author takes pleasure in acknowledging the help of Professor Lynne Reid and her co-workers in the preparation of this chapter, for the content of which however they are in no way responsible; thanks are also due to Dr. W. W. Payne for helpful criticism; to Professor Reid, Dr. Plank and the editor of Ciba Foundation Symposium on Development of the Lung, and to Dr. Reynolds and the editor of the British Medical Bulletin, for permission to reproduce diagrams for Figures 1 and 3 respectively; to Dr. R. G. W. Ollerenshaw of the Department of Medical Illustration, Manchester Royal Infirmary, for the preparation of Figure 2 and to Dr. Geoffrey Dawes of the Nuffield Institute of Medical Research for Figure 4, and to Miss Nina Burns for the preparation of the manuscript.

BIBLIOGRAPHY

Avery (1964), "The Lung and its Disorders in the New-born Infant," *Major Problems in Clinical Paediatrics.* Vol. 1. W. B. Saunders.

Engels (1966), *The Prenatal Lung.* Pergamon Press.

Dawes (1968), *Foetal and Neonatal Physiology.* Year Book Medical Publishers.

Symposium (1967), "Development of the Lung," *Ciba Foundation,* eds. de Reuck and Potter. Churchill.

"The Foetus and the New-born—Recent Research," (1966), eds. Cross and Dawes. *Brit. med. Bull.* The British Council.

REFERENCES

Abrams, E. (1966), "Isolation and Quantitative Estimation of Pulmonary Surface—Active Lipo-protein, *J. appl. Physiol.,* **21,** 718–20.

Adams, F., Fujiwara, T. and Rowshan, G. (1963), "The Nature and Origin of the Fluid in the Fetal Lamb Lung," *J. Pediat.,* **63,** 5, 881.

Adams, F. H., Desilets, D. T. and Towers, B. (1966), "Control of Flow of Fetal Lung Fluid at the Laryngeal Outlet," *J. Pediat.,* **69,** 63.

Areechon, W. and Reid, L. (1963), "Hypoplasia of Lung with Congenital Diaphragmatic Hernia," *Brit. med. J.,* **1,** 230–3.

Avery, M. E. and Mead, J. (1959), "Surface Properties in Relation to Atelectasis and Hyaline Membrane Disease," *Amer. J. Dis. Child.,* **97,** 517–23.

Barnard, W. and Day, T. D. (1937), "The Development of the Terminal Air passages of the Human Lung," *J. Path. Bact.,* **45,** 67–73.

Bartels, H. (1966), "Carriage of Oxygen in the Blood of the Foetus," *CIBA Symposium on Development of the Lung,* eds. de Reuck and Ponter, p. 276–96, J. & A. Churchill.

Bertalanffy, F. D. and Leblond, C. P. (1953), "The Continuous Renewal of the Two types of Alveolar Cell in the Lung of the Rat," *Anat. Rec.,* **115,** 515–46.

Bucher, U. and Reid, L. (1961), "Development of the Intrasegmental Bronchial Tree," *Thorax,* **16,** 207.

Buckels, L. J. and Usher, R. (1965), "Cardio-pulmonary Effects of Placental Transfusion," *J. Pediat.,* **67,** p. 239.

Cassin, S., Dawes, G. S., Mott, J. C., Ross, B. B. and Strang, L. B. (1964), "The Vascular Resistance of the Foetal and Newly Ventilated Lung of the Lamb," *J. Physiol. (Lond.),* **171,** 61.

Clements, J. A., Brown, E. S. and Johnson, R. F. (1958), "Pulmonary Surface Tension and the Mucus Lining of the Lung—some Theoretical considerations," *J. appl. Physiol.,* **12,** 262–8.

Clements, J. A. (1967), "The Alveolar Lining Layer," *CIBA Symposium on Development of the Lung,* eds. de Reuck and Ponter, p. 223, J. & A. Churchill.

Cross, K., Klaus, M., Tooley, W. H., Weisser, K. H. and Clements, J. A. (1960), "The Response of the New-born Baby to Inflation of the Lungs," *J. Physiol.,* **151,** 551.

Cross, K. W. (1966), "Resuscitation of the Asphyxiated Infant," *The Foetus and the Newborn—Recent Research, Brit. med. Bull.,* eds. Cross & Dawes, p. 74.

Davis, M. and Potter, E. (1946), "Intra-uterine Respiration of the Human Fetus," *J. Amer. med. Ass.,* **131,** 1194–1200.

Davis, J. A. (1961), "The Effect of Anoxia in Newborn Rabbits," *J. Physiol.,* **155,** 56.

Dawes, G. W., Hibbard, E. and Windle, W. F. (1964), "The Effect of Alkali and Glucose Infusion on Permanent Brain Damage in Rhesus Monkeys Asphyxiated at Birth," *J. Pediat.,* **65,** 801.

Ditchburn, R. K., Hull, D. and Segall, M. M. (1956), "Oxygen Uptake during and after Positive Pressure Ventilation for the Resuscitation of Asphyxiated New-born Infants," *Lancet,* **II,** 1096.

Dunn, P. (1967), "Cord Occlusion and the Onset of Respiration," *Society for Paed. Res.*—Programme and Abstracts—37th Annual Meeting, Atlanta City, 160.

Dunnill (1962), "Postnatal Growth of the Lung," *Thorax.,* **17,** 329.

Fauré-Fremiet, E. and Dragoiu, J. (1923), "Le developpement du poumon fetal chez le mouton," *Archives d'anatomie microscopique.* Tome XIX. Fasc., **IV,** 413.

Fawcitt, J., Lind, J. and Wegelius, C. (1960), "The First Breath. A Preliminary Communication Describing Some Methods of Investigation of the First Breath of a Baby and the Results Obtained from Them," *Acta Paediat.,* **49,** supp. 123, 5–17.

Grontoft, O. (1954), "Intracranial Haemorrhage and Blood Brain Barrier Problems in the New-born," *Acta path. microbiol. scand.,* **34,** Supp. 100.

Ham, A. W. and Baldwin, K. W. (1941), "Histological Study of Development of Lung with Particular Reference to Nature of Alveoli," *Anat. record,* **8,** 363–79.

Harned, H., Rowsham, G., Mackinney, L. and Sugioka, K. (1964), *Trans. Soc. paediat. Res.*, "Relationship of PO₂, PCO₂ and PH to the Onset of Breathing," *Amer. J. Dis. Child.*, **10**, 517.

Heath, D. and Edwards, J. E. (1958), "The Pathology of Hypertensive Vascular Disease," *Circulation*, **18**, 533–47.

Hey, E. and Kelly, J. (1968), "Gaseous Exchange during Endotracheal Ventilation for Asphyxia at Birth," *J. Obstet. Gynaec. Brit. Commonwealth*, **75**, No. 4.

Hislop Alison, (1968), Communication to Brompton Hosp. Symposium on Resp. Problems in the new-born.

Humphreys, P. W., Normand, I. C. S., Reynolds, E. O. R. and Strang, L. B. (1967), "Pulmonary Lymph Flow and the Uptake of Liquid from the Lungs of the Lamb at the Start of Breathing," *J. Physiol.*, **193**, 1.

Karlberg, P. (1957), "Breathing and its Control in Premature Infants," *Trans. Second Confer. on the Physiology of Prematurity, Jos. Macy Foundation*, ed. Lanman.

Karlberg, P., Cherry, R. B., Escardo, F. and Koch, G. (1962), "Respiratory Studies in New-born Infants. II. Pulmonary vent. and Mechanics of Breathing in the First Minutes of Life, including onset of Respiration," *Acta Pediat.*, **51**, 121–36.

Kleitman, L., Petering, H. and Sutherland, J. (1967), "Blood Carbonic Anhydrase Activity and Zinc Concentration in Infants with Respiratory Distress Syndrome," *N.E.J.M.*, **277**, 1157.

Klemola, E. (1937), "Ueber den lungenbau der fruhgeburt," *Acta Pediat.*, **21**, 236.

Klionski, B. (1968), "The Role of Hyperkalaemia in Experimental Foetal Asphyxia," *Proc. Brit. Pediat. Assoc.* meeting, Dublin.

Kluas, M., Tooley, W. H., Weaver, R. and Clements, J. A. (1962), "Lung Volume in the New-born Infant," *J. Pediat.*, **30**, 111–16.

Lamb, D. (1968), Communication to: Colloqu. internat. de pathologie thoracique: Lille. (September.) To be published in proceedings.

Landing, B. H. (1957), "Symposium on Respiratory Disorders—Anomalies of the Respiratory Tract," *Pediat. Clinics. N. Amer.* (February.)

L'Aumonier, R. (1952), "Recherches sur la Structure Pulmonaire des Prématures," *Semaines des Hopitaux de Paris*, 28.

Loosli, C. G. and Potter, L. (1958), "Symposium on Emphysema and the Chronic Bronchitis Syndrome, 80, part II, p. 5. Pre- and Post-natal Development of the Respiratory Portion of the Human Lung," *Amer. Rev. Resp. Dis.*

Moore, M. and Davis, J. A. (1967), "Simultaneous Administration of Narcotic and Narcotic Anatagonist Drugs in the Newborn Rabbit," *J. Pediat.*, **71**, 420.

Mott, J. C. (1961), "The Ability of Young mammals to Withstand Oxygen Lack," *Brit. med. Bull.*, **17**, 144.

Naeye, R. L. (1961), "Arterial Changes During the Prenatal Period," *Arch. Path.*, **71**, 121–28.

Oliver, T. K., Demis, J. A. and Bates, G. D. (1961), "Serial Blood Gas Tensions and Acid-base Balance during the First Hour of Life in Human Infants," *Acta. Pediat.*, **50**, 346–60.

O'Neil, R. M., Ahlvin, R. C., Bauer, W. C. and Thomas, W. A. (1957), "Development of Fetal Pulmonary Arterioles," *A.M.A. Arch. Path.*, **63**, p. 309.

Palmer, D. M. (1935), "The Lung of a Human Fetus at 170 mm," *Amer. J. Anat.*, **158**, 59–72.

Parmentier, R. (1962), "L'aeration néonatale du poumon," *Rev. Belge de Pathologie et de Medicine Experimentale*, **XXIX**, Fasc. 3–4, 123–33.

Pattle, R. E. (1958), "Properties, Function and Origin of the Alveolar Lining Layer," *Proc. roy. Soc. (Lond.)*, 148 Series V.

Perinatal Mortality Survey (1963), ed. Butler, N. and Bonham, D. Table 43, 135.

Plank, J. (1967), "A Morphological Contribution to the Development of the Human Lung: Observations in the Non-retracted Lung," *Development of the Lung, CIBA Foundation Symposium*, eds. de Reuck and Potter, p. 156–65. J. & A. Churchill.

Purves, M. (1967), "Initiation of Respiration," *Development of the Lung—CIBA Foundation Symposium*, eds. de Reuck and Potter. J. & A. Churchill.

Purves, M. (1968), Accepted by Circulation Research. Title not yet available.

Redmond, A., Isana, S. and Ingall, D. (1965), "Relation of Onset of Respiration to Placental Transfusion," *Lancet*, **i**, 283.

Reid, L. (1966), "The Embryology of the Lung," *Development of the Lung—CIBA Foundation Symposium*, eds. de Reuck and Potter, pp. 109–23. J. & A. Churchill.

Reid, L. (1966), *Development of the Lung—CIBA Foundation Symposium*, eds. de Reuck and Potter, p. 114. J. & A. Churchill.

Reynolds, E. O. R., Orgalesi, M. M., Motoyama, E. K., Craig, J. M. and Cook, C. D. (1965), "Surface Properties of Saline Extracts from Lungs of New-born Infants," *Acta paediat. Stockh.*, **54**, 511.

Reynolds, E. O. R., Roberton, N. R. C. and Wigglesworth, J. S. (1968), "Hyaline Membrane Disease, Respiratory Distress and Surfactant Deficiency," *Pediatrics*. In press.

Schaffer, A. J. (1956), "The Pathogenesis of Intra-uterine Pneumonia: Evidence Concerning Intra-uterine Respiratory Movements," *Pediatrics (N.Y.)*, **17**, 747–56.

Schulz, H. (1959), *Die submikroskopische anatomie und pathologie der lunge*, Springer-Verlag.

Scopes, J. (1966), "Metabolic Rate and Temperature Control in the Human Body," *The Foetus and the New-born—Recent Research*, eds. K. W. Cross and G. S. Dawes, p. 90, *Brit. med. Bull.*

Smith, A. (1959), "Obstruction of Respiratory Tract in the Flexed Foetus," *Brit. med. J.*, **1**, 1344.

Snyder, F. F. and Rosenfeld, M. (1937), "Intra-uterine Respiratory Movements of the Human Foetus," *J. Amer. med. Ass.*, **108**, 1946–8.

Sorokin, S. (1960), "Histochemical Events in Developing Human Lungs," p. 19, *Act. anat.*, **40**, 105.

Stafford, A. and Weatherall, J. A. C. (1960), "The Survival of Young Rats in Nitrogen," *J. Physiol.*, **153**, 457–72.

Taylor, F. B. and Abrams, E. (1966), "Effect of Surface Active Lipo-protein on Clotting and Fibrinolysis and of Fibrinogen on Surface Tension of Surface-active Lipo-protein," *Amer. J. Med.*, **40**, 346.

Tchobroutski, Catherine (1967), "Respiratory Movements Induced in the Foetal Lamb near Term by Cold Stimulus Applied to the Face." Communication to the Neonatal Society.

Tierney, D. F., Clements, J. A. and Trahan, H. J. (1965), "The Metabolic Activity of Pulmonary Lecithens," *The Physiologist, Washington (abstract)*, **8**, 288.

Tizard, Peter (1964), "Intracranial Haemorrhage of the Newborn," *Acta Pædiatrica Latina*. Vol. XVII. Supp. al fasc 6.

Tizard, J. P. M., Gupta, J., Dahlenburg, G. and Roberton, J. (1968), "Oxygen Therapy in the Newborn," *Lancet*, **1**, 1323.

Weibel, E. R. (1967), "Post-natal Growth of the Lung and Pulmonary Gas Exchange Capacity," *Development of the Lung—CIBA Foundation Symposium*, eds. Reuck and Potter, p. 137.

2. BROWN ADIPOSE TISSUE IN THE NEW BORN

DAVID HULL

The physiological mechanisms of thermoregulation are some of the many biological processes which become active at birth. In the uterus the developing mammal enjoys all the benefits of homoeothermy without effort. After birth, newborn mammals achieve thermal stability despite their dependence on untried physiological mechanisms but the energy necessary for the extra heat production is often an important drain on their limited reserves. Because of their poor thermal insulation and relatively large exposed surface, a small fall in the surrounding temperature below body temperature leads to rapid heat loss and thus high rates of heat production are often necessary to keep the body temperature constant. The physiological awakening which occurs at birth in many ways resembles the arousal of the hibernating mammal from its winter sleep. Here, also, thermoregulatory mechanisms suddenly become active and large rates of heat production are required, in this instance, to warm the dormant animal. It is interesting to find that in both situations the thermoregulatory responses are dependent on a special heat producing tissue, brown adipose tissue.

Because brown adipose tissue is especially prominent in hibernating mammals, it has been called the hibernating gland. However, it is found in many non-hibernating adult mammals including man. In 1902 Hatai first described the "hibernating gland" in a human infant and Bonnot (1908) extended these findings and described its anatomical distribution in foetal, new born and adult humans. His illustration (shown in Fig. 1) suggests a more defined gland than is present, but certainly brown adipose tissue can be found at this site in the neck as well as in the axillae, between the shoulder blades, and around the vessels and organs in the thorax and posterior abdominal wall (Fig. 2) (Dawkins and Hull, 1965). Bonnot thought that the tissue formed part of the lympho-haemopoietic system. There is, in fact, very little evidence of physiological or clinical curiosity about the function of brown adipose tissue in man. This is largely due to the misconception, which is still helb by many, that the brown adipose tissue found in young mammals is merely a stage in the development of white adipose tissue. In pathological texts brown adipose tissue is often called embryonal fat. The factors leading to this view and the evidence against it have recently been reviewed (Hull and Segall, 1966).

Although the hibernating gland provoked very little medical interest it fascinated biologists. Over the years many facts came to light. Microscopically brown adipose tissue resembles an endocrine gland and many attempts were made to extract an active principle and observe its biological effects, all without success (for refs. see Johansson, 1958). A little surprisingly brown adipose tissue of the woodchuck was subsequently found to contain more androgens, per unit tissue weight than the bull's testis (Sweet and Hoskins, 1940). Impressive though this may

sound, it is only fair to point out that the bull's testis produces androgens and it does not necessarily store them, and the high content in brown adipose tissue may reflect only the holding capacity of its stored fat. Other workers investigated the effects of excising brown adipose tissue (Trusler, McBirnie, Pearson, Gornal and Bigelow, 1953).

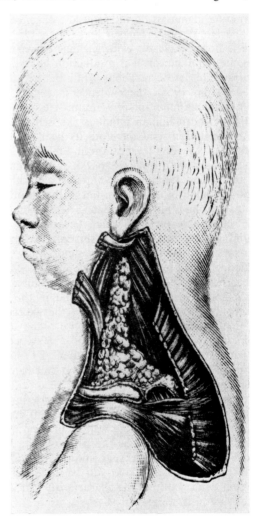

FIG. 1. A foetus of 4½ months dissected to show the hibernating gland, from E. Bonnot: The interscapular gland. *J. Anat. Physiol.*, 1908, 43.

The only positive finding was that animals after "hibernectomy" were less able to withstand prolonged cold exposure. Trusler *et al.* (1953) quoted two interesting observations. Firstly, that ground squirrels can be induced to hibernate at any time of the year except during the mating season. At this time the amount of brown adipose tissue is at its lowest and its fat content is small. Secondly, that old marmots die at the onset of cold weather. The brown adipose tissue of these animals is shrunken and fibrotic. Physiologists studying the effects of prolonged cold exposure on experimental animals found that whereas the total amount of white adipose tissue decreased, the amount of brown adipose tissue increased. During cold adaptation adult mammals develop the ability to produce heat without shivering. Although they can hardly be considered to be cold-adapted, newborn mammals including man have a similar ability to produce heat without shivering. It was whilst studying this phenomenon in newborn rabbits that Michael Dawkins and I demonstrated that brown adipose tissue was an organ of heat production (Dawkins and Hull, 1963). At the same time other workers demonstrated that it played a similar role in hibernating mammals during arousal from hibernation (Smith and Hock, 1963; Smalley and Dryer, 1963).

There is now conclusive evidence that brown adipose tissue is the main site of heat production in response to cold exposure in newborn rabbits (Hull and Segall, 1965; Heim and Hull, 1966), the evidence that it is equally important in the human infant is impressive but indirect. When the newborn human infant is exposed to cold its oxygen consumption, and therefore its heat production, increases from a resting level of about 5 ml./kg. body wt. min. to a maximum around 15 ml./kg. min. (Adamsons, Gandy and James, 1965). This compares favourably with the response found in adult man, but in the infant unlike the adult shivering is not prominent. There is some doubt whether the muscle twitches which occasionally can be seen in infants exposed to cold is shivering or not; it is hard to imagine that it contributes significantly to heat production. It is more difficult to discount the possibility, which has been raised, that heat production in response to cold exposure occurs in the liver and in the muscle without contraction. On the basis of the experimental finding that 1·5–2·0 g. of brown adipose tissue supports a rise in the oxygen consumption of a 60 g. newborn rabbit, from a resting level of about 20 ml./kg. min. to a maximum of 60 ml./kg. min. it can be calculated that a human infant, weight 3·5 kg., would require 20–30 g. of brown adipose to produce the observed rise in oxygen consumption of 10 ml./kg. min. Anatomical dissection suggests that this amount could well be present and thus brown adipose tissue could be the principle site of heat production. Other evidence suggesting its participation in the infant's response to cold will be discussed in the next section which outlines the characteristics of nature's system of central heating.

The Heating System

Anatomically brown adipose tissue has many features which are relevant to its function as an organ of heat production. For example most of the lobes of brown adipose tissue are situated deep in the body which reduces to a minimum the heat wastage by loss from the surface. Many lobes surround major arteries and veins and thus the blood supplying the metabolically active tissues and organs will provide not only oxygen and nutrients but also tend to keep the cells at an optimal temperature. Brown adipose tissue, itself, has a very rich capillary bed (Hausberger and Widelitz, 1963), in fact, when stimulated

to produce heat, its blood supply per gram tissue is higher than that of the other major organs and tissues of the body (Heim and Hull, 1966a). In this instance the rich blood supply will disperse the heat and prevent the tissue becoming overheated.

At one site, on the back between the scapulae, brown adipose tissue lies immediately under the subcutaneous white adipose tissue and it is not close to any major

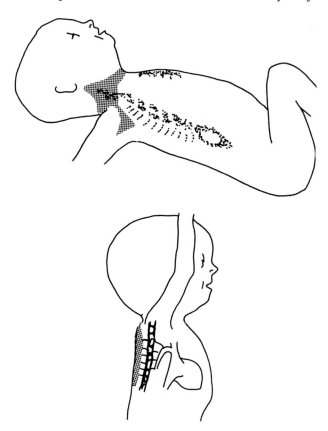

FIG. 2. Anatomical distribution of brown adipose tissue. The uniformly shaded area indicates the sites where brown adipose tissue may be found underneath the covering layer of white adipose tissue. The lower drawing illustrates the venous drainage from the interscapular pads of brown adipose tissue to the vertebral venous sinuses.

arteries. However it does have an unusual and interesting venous drainage which may be important in relation to its function (Smith and Roberts, 1964). The blood from these pads drains via the external and internal vertebral venous plexuses before it reaches the azygos veins and the heart (Fig. 2). The warmed blood would therefore protect the vital nerve centres during cold exposure. Heat production in these lobes of brown adipose tissue in infants is suggested by the observations of Silverman, Zamelis, Sinclair and Agate (1964) who showed that the skin on the nape of the neck of infants exposed to cold is relatively warmer than elsewhere.

The unit of the heating element is the subcellular organelle of oxidation, the mitochondria. Figure 3, is a schematic diagram based on electron micrographs of brown adipose tissue of newborn rabbits (Hull, 1966).

The large complex mitochondria can be seen lying adjacent to the fat vacuoles. White adipose tissue stores fat in the most economical way, as a single spherical vacuole. In contrast the cell of brown adipose tissue usually contains many vacuoles of fat and therefore there is a larger area of cytoplasm-fat interface relative to the volume of fat store. There is some evidence to suggest that as the fat content falls the number of vacuoles per cell increases

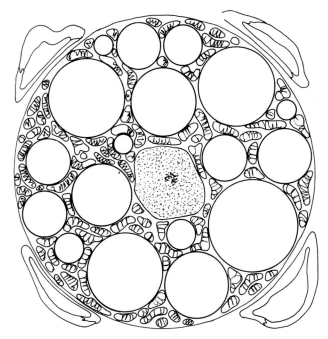

FIG. 3. Diagrammatic representation of a cell of brown adipose tissue taken from electron micrographs. The cell contains many vacuoles of fat, the remaining cytoplasm is filled with large mitochondria and a central nucleus. In each corner is a capillary which illustrates the rich capillary bed of brown adipose tissue.

thus maintaining the large area of interface. Apart from a round nucleus, the cell contains little evidence of any structure other than fat vacuoles and mitochondria and therefore it is difficult, on the grounds of structure alone, to postulate that the cell has any function apart from the storage and oxidation of fat.

The Fuel

The burners may be described as "oil-fired" for they convert the chemical energy of fat to heat. The stored fat is largely triglyceride and this must first be hydrolyzed to free fatty acids and glycerol. In white adipose tissue the free fatty acids released after hydrolysis enter the circulation along with the glycerol, but in brown adipose tissue the free fatty acids are metabolized within the cell. Some are oxidized to carbon dioxide and water which provides energy in the form of adenosinetriphosphate and some are re-esterified to trigylceride which requires energy. The breakdown and resynthesis of triglyceride is an apparently purposeless cycle, the net effect is the oxidation of fatty acid to produce heat (Ball and Jungas, 1961). The process can be demonstrated *in vitro*. If a hormone, i.e.

noradrenaline, which stimulates hydrolysis of triglyceride, is added to slices of brown adipose tissue there is a rise in the rate of the tissue's oxygen consumption and a large increase in the release of glycerol but not free fatty acids into the surrounding medium. Brown adipose tissue from newborn rabbits like white adipose tissue lacks the enzyme glycerol-kinase which is necessary for the intracellular conversion of glycerol back to glucose. Thus the rate of release of glycerol is a measure of the rate of hydrolysis of triglyceride. This finding formed the basis of the demonstration of hydrolysis of triglyceride in brown adipose tissue *in vivo* for it seems reasonable to assume that it occurs if a rise in plasma glycerol level occurs without an equivalent rise in free fatty acids. Experimentally, noradrenaline infusion and cold exposure in newborn rabbits cause a large rise in plasma glycerol relative to the rise in free fatty acids (Dawkins and Hull, 1964). In newborn human infants a small fall in environmental temperature also stimulates a rise in plasma glycerol but not free fatty acid (Dawkins and Scopes, 1965).

Control of the Heating System

Heat production in brown adipose tissue can be caused by stimulation of the sympathetic nervous system (Hull and Segall, 1965b) and by infusion of various hormones including noradrenaline, adrenaline, isoprenaline, glucagon and corticotrophin (Heim and Hull, 1966b). In physiological conditions the principle controlling mechanism is probably the sympathetic nervous system for after section of the nerves the tissue is no longer able to produce heat on cold exposure (Hull and Segall, 1965b). It remains to establish what role, if any, is played by the catecholamines and the other lipolytic hormones. There is some evidence

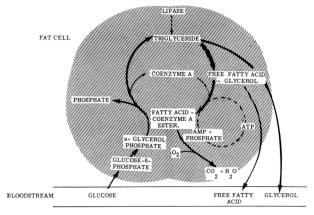

FIG. 4. A schematic representation of the triglyceride cycle which may be the basic biochemical process which leads to the conversion of chemical energy to heat.

to suggest that thyroxin and the corticosteroids have a permissive action. Brown adipose tissue like white adipose tissue is very sensitive to insulin which influences the rate of glucose uptake and lipogenesis but insulin itself is not calorigenic (Joel, 1966; and Hull, unpublished).

Noradrenaline is probably the mediator at the sympathetic nerve endings, for brown adipose tissue has been shown to have a high content of noradrenaline some of which is located outside the cells and close to the nerve endings. *In vitro* noradrenaline has many effects on adipose tissue; it is possible that it influences the rate of heat production by first releasing 3–5 cyclic adenosine monophosphate which in turn activates tissue lipases (Rizack, 1961). The lipases control the rate of hydrolysis of triglyceride and thus the intracellular supply of free fatty acids. It may be that the supply of fuel is the rate limiting step.

Clinical Implications of this Heating System

In clinical practice biological systems require attention if they are involved in disease processes or cease to work. With respect to brown adipose tissue the first possibility has not received much attention. Swellings of brown adipose tissue occur in cretins and occasionally benign (hibernomas) and malignant tumours have been described but these are all rare. Of more importance is the finding that viruses grow well in brown adipose tissue and they may be harboured there. Rabies virus, for example, may be carried from country to country in the brown adipose tissue of hibernating bats (Sulkin, Krutzsh, Wallis and Allen, 1957). There is no evidence to my knowledge that brown adipose tissue plays any part in virus disease in man.

The failure of brown adipose tissue to function, however, may be responsible for a fall in body temperature. Hypothermia most commonly occurs in the young and the elderly. In some instances it is due to failure of the controlling mechanisms secondary to diseases of the central nervous system but in others it is due to the exhaustion of the fuel supply. Experimentally it has been shown that the fat content of brown adipose tissue falls during prolonged cold exposure (Hull and Segall, 1965c). After severe cold exposure it may be totally depleted of fat, even though fat is present in white adipose tissue and elsewhere (Hull and Segall, 1966). In animals it has been shown that when the fat content of the tissue falls below a certain level the ability of the tissue to produce heat falls and hypothermia ensues. The clinical parallel to this observation is found in infants with the cold syndrome. In all the six infants admitted to the Radcliffe Infirmary, Oxford, who died with this condition, the brown adipose tissue was found to be grossly depleted of fat (Aherne and Hull, 1964). The brown adipose tissue of some, though not all elderly patients with hypothermia was also found to be depleted. In a histological survey of brown adipose tissue from over 200 infants dying in the newborn period Aherne and Hull (1966), found that the fat content of brown adipose tissue was high at birth and then gradually fell over the next few days. In extremely premature infants, in infants undernourished at birth dying in the first week of life and in infants with severe disease (e.g. inoperable intestinal obstruction or congenital heart disease) dying in the second week of life, the brown adipose tissue was often totally depleted of fat. In the first two groups it is probable that the brown adipose tissue was poorly filled at birth but in the second group it is hard to avoid the conclusion that they experienced considerable cold exposure. It is still not generally appreciated that a warm environment to an adult is often cold to an infant. For example a naked man is comfortable at an environmental temperature of 28°C (82°F) which is a considerable cold stress to an infant, on the other hand a naked infant is comfortable at an environmental temperature of 35°C (95°F) which would be intolerably warm to his attendant nurse.

The newborn infant is most likely to experience rapid heat loss during and immediately after delivery. At this time evaporative heat loss is considerable. Unfortunately during this period the infant is changing from placental to lung respiration and perforce there is a varying period when the infant is hypoxic and therefore dependent on anaerobic metabolism. During hypoxia the blood flow to brown adipose tissue remains high but the fall in oxygen content of arterial blood leads immediately to a fall in the rate of heat production. Brown adipose tissue appears unable to produce heat to any significant degree anaerobically (Heim and Hull, 1966a). Therefore the asphyxiated infant at birth is unable to compensate for the rapid heat loss by extra heat production. This further emphasizes the need for drying and gently swaddling of newly born infants especially if the onset of spontaneous breathing is delayed.

Conclusion

The human infant, like many newborn mammals has a sophisticated, efficient and economic organ of heat production. In this respect the physiological mechanisms in the newborn compare favourably with those in the adult where shivering is considered to be the principle means of heat production and where the role of brown adipose tissue, although as yet undefined, would appear to be of less importance. The heat organ of newborn mammals demonstrates again that physiological mechanisms in the newborn are not necessarily immature but are frequently different from those present in the adult.

REFERENCES

Adamsons, K., Gandy, G. M. and James, L. S. (1965), "The Influence of Thermal Factors upon Oxygen Consumption of the New-born Human Infant," *Journal of Pediatrics*, **66**, 495.

Aherne, W. and Hull, D. (1966), "Brown Adipose Tissue and Heat Production in the Newborn Infant," *The Journal of Pathology and Bacteriology*, **91**, 223.

Aherne, W. and Hull, D. (1964), "The Site of Heat Production in the Newborn Infant," *Proceedings of the Royal Society of Medicine*, **57**, 1172.

Ball, E. G. and Jungas, R. L. (1961), "On the Action of Hormones which Accelerate the Rate of Oxygen Consumption and Fatty Acid Release in Rat Adipose Tissue (*in vitro*)," *Proceedings of the National Academy of Sciences, Washington*, **47**, 932.

Bonnot, E. (1908), "The Interscapular Gland," *Journal of Anatomy and Physiology*, **43**, 43.

Cox, R. W. (1954), "Hibernoma: The Lipoma of Immature Adipose Tissue," *Journal of Pathology and Bacteriology*, **2**, 511.

Dawkins, M. J. R. and Hull, D. (1963), "Brown Fat and the Response of the New-born Rabbit to Cold," *Journal of Physiology*, **169**, 101.

Dawkins, M. J. R. and Hull, D. (1964), "Brown Adipose Tissue and the Response of New-born Rabbits to Cold," *Journal of Physiology*, **172**, 216.

Dawkins, M. J. R. and Hull, D. (1965), "The Production of Heat from Fat," *Scientific American*, **213**, 62.

Dawkins, M. J. R. and Scopes, J. W. (1965), "Non-shivering Thermogenesis and Brown Adipose Tissue in the Human Newborn Infant," *Nature*, **206**, 201.

Hatai, S. (1902), "On the Presence in Human Embryos of an Inter-scapular Gland Corresponding to the so-called Hibernating Gland in the Lower Animals," *Anatomischer Anzeiger*, **21**, 369.

Hausberger, F. X. and Widelitz, M. M. (1963), "Distribution of Labelled Erythrocytes in Adipose Tissue and Muscle in the Rat," *American Journal of Physiology*, **204**, 649.

Heim, T. and Hull, D. (1966a), "The Blood Flow and Oxygen Consumption of Brown Adipose Tissue in the New-born Rabbit," *Journal of Physiology*, **186**, 42.

Heim, T. and Hull, D. (1966b), "The Effect of Propranalol on the Calorigenic Response in Brown Adipose Tissue of New-born Rabbits to Catecholomines, Glucagon, Corticotrophin and Cold Exposure," *Journal of Physiology*, **187**, 271.

Hull, D. (1966), "Brown Adipose Tissue, Structure and Function," *British Medical Bulletin*, **22**, 92.

Hull, D. and Segall, M. M. (1965a), "The Contribution of Brown Adipose Tissue to Heat Production in the Newborn Rabbit," *Journal of Physiology*, **181**, 449.

Hull, D. and Segall, M. M. (1965b), "Sympathetic Nervous Control of Brown Adipose Tissue and Heat Production in the Newborn Rabbit," *Journal of Physiology*, **181**, 458.

Hull, D. and Segall, M. M. (1965c), "Heat Production in the New-born Rabbit and the Fat Content of the Brown Adipose Tissue," *Journal of Physiology*, **181**, 468.

Hull, D. and Segall, M. M. (1966), "Distinction of Brown from White Adipose Tissue," *Nature*, **212**, 469.

Joel, C. D. (1965), in *Handbook of Physiology—Section 5, Adipose Tissue* (A. E. Renold and G. F. Cahill, eds.), pp. 59–85. Washington: American Physiological Society.

Johansson, B. (1959), "Brown Adipose Tissue: A Review," *Metabolism*, **8**, 221.

Rizack, M. A. (1961), "An Epinephrine-sensitive Lipolytic Activity in Adipose Tissue," *Journal of Biological Chemistry*, **236**, 657.

Silverman, W. A., Zamelis, A., Sinclair, J. C. and Agate, F. J., Jr. (1964), "Warm Nape of the Newborn," *Pediatrics*, **33**, 984.

Smalley, R. and Dryer, R. (1963), "Brown Fat: Thermogenic Effect during Arousal from Hibernation in the Bat," *Science*, **140**, 1333.

Smith, R. E. and Hock, R. J. (1963), "Brown Fat: Thermogenic Effect of Arousal in Hibernators," *Science*, **140**, 199.

Smith, R. E. and Roberts, J. C. (1964), "Thermogenesis of Brown Adipose Tissue in Cold-acclimated Rats," *American Journal of Physiology*, **206**, 143.

Sulkin, S. E., Krutzsch, P. H., Wallis, C. and Allen, R. (1957), "Role of Brown Fat in the Pathogenesis of Rabies in Insectivorous Bats," *Proceedings of the Society of Experimental Biology and Medicine*, **96**, 461.

Sweet, J. E. and Hoskins, W. H. (1940), "Androgen in the Wood-chuck Hibernating Gland," *Proceedings of the Society of Experimental Biology and Medicine*, **45**, 60.

Trusler, G. A., McBirnie, J. E., Pearson, F. G., Gornall, A. G. and Bigelow, W. F. (1953), "A Study of Hibernation in Relation to the Technique of Hypothermia for Intracardiac Surgery," *Surgical Forum*, **4**, 72.

3. THE RESPIRATORY DISTRESS SYNDROME

SHIELA G. HAWORTH and L. STANLEY JAMES

Introduction

During the first half of the twentieth century the perinatal mortality rate in most western countries has gradually and consistently declined. Improved standards of living and nutrition, improved obstetric and perinatal care and the advent of antibiotics have probably all contributed to a varying degree. While this rate has continued to decline to levels as low as 12·6/1,000 in Sweden, the rate in the U.S.A. is almost 22·8/1,000 in 1967 and has remained relatively stationary since 1955. The rate for the U.S.A. is probably a reflection of population shifts and an inability of medical and social standards to keep up with the movement of lower income groups into the cities.

Immaturity, congenital malformations and respiratory malfunction all contribute to this high mortality. Of the numerous causes of respiratory insufficiency, the idiopathic respiratory distress syndrome or hyaline membrane disease is by far the most common. Formerly it was believed that the syndrome could be diagnosed only at autopsy, but after many years of controversy it is now generally agreed that there is a distinct clinical picture and diagnosis may be made during life. Appreciation of the fact that between 30 and 50 per cent of infants with this condition will die has been a most potent stimulus for the current intensive investigation into etiology, pathogenesis and treatment.

Progress has been slow, primarily because all forms of respiratory insufficiency in the neonate have been regarded as a manifestation of immaturity. The natural history of the syndrome has been poorly understood due to lack of early observations and understanding of pathogenesis impeded by the prerequisite of hyaline membranes at autopsy.

Incidence and Predisposing Factors

The syndrome is of widespread occurrence. No environmental or racial factors can be incriminated since the incidence is similar in many areas including Europe, North America, Singapore, Hawaii, Lebanon and India (Cohen, Weintraub and Lilienfeld, 1960; Neligan, 1961; Sivanesan, 1961; Chuang, 1962; Younozai, 1962; Webb, John, Jadhar, Graham and Walter, 1962). There is a 2:1 sex ratio for both morbidity and mortality, males being twice as susceptible.

Immaturity appears to be the most important predisposing factor although the condition is occasionally seen in term infants. The clinical incidence in babies weighing less than 2·5 kg. has been estimated as being between 10 and 14 per cent (Miller and Jennison, 1950; Usher, 1961; Gairdner, 1965). Both incidence and mortality are higher in the more immature (Silverman and Silverman, 1958; Cohen et al., 1960; Driscoll and Smith, 1962). When the diagnosis is based on the demonstration of hyaline membranes at necropsy the incidence varies from 4–7 per cent of live births in infants weighing less than 2·5 kg., to 0·2 per cent in those weighing over 2·5 kg. (Miller, 1950; Latham, Nesbitt and Anderson, 1955;

Cohen *et al.*, 1960; Neligan, 1961). These figures are probably too low since hyaline membranes are rarely present in the lungs of infants dying within 4 hours of birth (Briggs and Hogg, 1958). In evaluating the degree of immaturity, gestational age rather than weight should be considered. An overall mortality rate of about 40 per cent is found when autopsy diagnosis of RDS depends on the demonstration of hyaline membranes (Gairdner, 1965). This figure corresponds well with clinical observations made on untreated infants (Usher, 1963; Gairdner, 1965).

Birth asphyxia is frequently associated. There is a significant correlation between the condition at birth and subsequent respiratory distress. The majority of infants who develop the syndrome have an Apgar score of 6 or less (James, 1959; Rudolph, Desmond and Pineda, 1966) and difficulty or delay in the onset of respiration (Miller, 1962, 1963). Over a third of mothers whose infants are severely affected suffer from such conditions as dystocic labor or intrauterine bleeding which are likely to produce a degree of intrauterine anoxia. (Cohen *et al.*, 1960; Miller, 1962; Gairdner, 1965).

Infants of diabetic mothers are particularly susceptible to RDS. This is surprising because they are usually more mature and have a higher birth weight than the majority of affected babies. One series reported an incidence of 57 per cent, over three quarters of the infants weighing more than 2·5 kg. Hyaline membranes were present in half of those who died (Driscoll, Benirschke and Curtis, 1960). Other series report that smaller infants are more susceptible to the syndrome (Farquhar, 1962).

Cesarean section alone does not appear to increase the incidence when indications for the operative procedure are taken into account (Craig and Fraser, 1957; Strang, Anderson and Platt, 1957; Cohen *et al.*, 1960). It has been alleged that the procedure itself predisposes to the development of RDS if the infant is delivered before 270 days gestation (Usher, 1964) but clarification of the separate effects of prematurity and cesarean section has yet to be made.

Clinical Features

The respiratory distress syndrome has a rather characteristic clinical course. As noted above, the majority of infants are in poor condition at birth, have an Apgar score of less than 7, and difficulty in initiating respiration. In those who initially appear normal, signs of distress develop in the first hour or two of life (Miller, 1955; Auld, 1961). On the other hand, any baby who remains well until the 6th to 8th hour of life will not develop the syndrome (Avery, 1964). Mild and transitory respiratory distress probably occurs more frequently than is generally realized, respirations being somewhat labored and increasing in frequency for the first 3 to 6 hours of life (Rudolph, Desmond and Pineda, 1966). Whether or not this is a manifestation of idiopathic respiratory distress is not known.

The syndrome is usually fully developed by 4 to 6 hours of age. The infants are hypotonic, inactive and lie in a frog-like position. Breathing is labored with retraction of the subcostal and intercostal spaces on inspiration, later

accompanied by an expiratory grunt. Air entry is poor. Frequency of respiration may be as high as 100/min., but is less in severely ill infants who have respiratory depression. The lower sternum becomes deeply and permanently indrawn, while the upper chest appears hyper-inflated. Respiration becomes almost entirely diaphragmatic and "see-saw" in nature. Rales are occasionally present, but are indicative of intrauterine pneumonia. The severity of retraction may be assessed numerically (Silverman and Anderson, 1956).

Most infants are cyanotic early if breathing room air. This sign is less evident when the ambient oxygen is increased to 40 per cent or higher but persists in the most severe cases. Heart rate does not have the lability so characteristic of healthy infants; persistent fixation is associated with a poor prognosis (Rudolph, 1965). Bradycardia is a preterminal feature.

Systemic hypotension is present, infants with RDS having a lower blood pressure than asymptomatic infants of the same gestational age (Neligan and Smith, 1960). Poor peripheral circulation is manifested by dusky, pale extremities which become edematous. Poor visceral circulation is manifested by oliguria which may be followed by anuria; bowel sounds are diminished and later the abdomen may become distended, resembling an impending ileus (Dunn, 1963). Thermal control is impaired, body temperature initially falls precipitously and the infants remain cold unless a special effort is made to conserve heat. Sclerema may develop, particularly in those exposed to cold. Apneic spells occur with increasing frequency and duration. Death from uncomplicated RDS usually takes place before 72 hours of age, the highest mortality being during the first 24 hours.

The first sign of recovery is an increase in air entry, followed by reduction in cyanosis, and initiation of spontaneous movements accompanied by improved muscle tone. Respiratory effort gradually becomes less labored but the rate remains elevated for some time. Lability of the heart rate returns, and with improved peripheral circulation, urine flow increases.

Residual pulmonary damage has recently been proposed as a sequel (Sheperd, Gray and Stahlman, 1964), and evidence of pulmonary insufficiency has been reported in babies maintained by artificial ventilation for considerable periods of time (Northway, Rosan and Porter, 1967).

Differential Diagnosis

A number of different conditions may present in a similar fashion.

Congenital anomalies	Choanal atresia
	Laryngeal web
	Cysts and tumors in the neck, thorax or abdomen
	Tracheo-esophageal fistula
	Diaphragmatic hernia
	Congenital heart disease with failure
Intrauterine and Intrapartum	Meconium aspiration
	Congenital pneumonia
	Aspiration of amniotic fluid

Trauma | Vocal cord paralysis
Phrenic nerve paralysis
Pneumothorax and pneumome-
diastinum

Anemia (very rare) due | Placenta previa
to blood loss | Abruptio placentae

Some of these require prompt surgical intervention and others specific medical treatment. It is therefore essential to establish a definitive diagnosis as soon as possible.

A chest x-ray is an important ancillary aid in differential diagnosis. The classical findings consist of a diffuse reticular granularity throughout both lung fields, and against this opacification the air filled bronchial tree is seen extending out to the periphery. The granularity has been interpreted as being due to atelectic areas, and increases as the condition progresses; the air bronchogram is probably due to dilated alveolar ducts. Films taken during the first hour of life may show fine granularity with abnormal prominence of hilar and perihilar bronchial and vascular strands, and thus enable a preclinical diagnosis to be made (Feinberg and Goldberg, 1957). However, the radiological signs are not pathognomonic and therefore of limited value in diagnosis (Bauman and Nadelhaft, 1958). They are most useful in excluding conditions which may present in a similar fashion, particularly those requiring specific treatment such as pneumothorax, diaphragmatic hernia, congenital pneumonia and meconium aspiration.

Pathology

Hyaline membranes are not found invariably at necropsy, but atelectasis is always present and widespread (Gruenwald, 1953, 1958; Ranstrom, 1953; Briggs and Hogg, 1958; Bauman, 1958). A period of air breathing is apparently necessary for their formation since they are not seen in stillborn infants nor in those dying during the first few hours of life. The lungs are airless, provided expansion has not been maintained by artificial ventilation or as a terminal resuscitative procedure. The pattern of atelectasis is determined by the degree of maturation (Gruenwald, 1963). When the gestational age is less than 37 weeks, respiratory bronchioles are distended with air and the alveoli so collapsed as to render their outlines difficult to determine. If membranes are present they will line the respiratory bronchioles. Beyond 37 weeks distribution of air is random and membranes are found more peripherally. They contain fibrin (Gitlin and Craig, 1956; Van Breeman, Neustein and Bruns, 1957; Wade-Evans, 1962), which is present as regular masses by about approximately the 12th hour, increasing in thickness as the condition progresses.

The earliest lesion, consisting of a marked constriction of small arterioles with edema and loss of definition of the smooth muscle coat, has been demonstrated in a lamb dying with experimental respiratory distress at 15 minutes of age (Stahlman, LeQuire, Young, Birmingham, Payne and Gray, 1964). There is also a loss of glycogen from epithelial cells and sloughing of cells into the lumen. Recovery, on the 4th or 5th day, is accompanied by

phagocytosis of the fragmented masses lying free in the alveolar air spaces. Lung biopsies of the surviving infants reveal thickened alveolar walls with an increase in the number of fibroblasts and excess reticular and collagen fibers (Robertson, 1964).

Infants who die following prolonged treatment with artificial ventilation and high oxygen mixtures show chronic lung lesions (Northway et al., 1967). This picture has been called bronchopulmonary dysplasia and appears to be an extension of the healing phase of the respiratory distress syndrome combined with certain features seen in oxygen poisoning (Bruns and Shields, 1964; De and Anderson, 1964; Berfenstam, Edlung and Zettergren, 1958; Nash, 1967; Lancet, 1967). Mucosal, alveolar and vascular tissues are involved and there is bronchiolar metaplasia. At present it is not possible to relate these lesions specifically to oxygen therapy, but a cause and effect relationship has to be borne in mind.

Pathogenesis

Abnormal Capillary Permeability. The membranes were at one time thought to originate from aspirated amniotic fluid (Ahvenainen, 1948). This theory was largely abandoned when they were stained with a fibrin antibody tagged with fluorescein (Gitlin and Craig, 1956). Later a hemoglobin-like compound was also demonstrated (Lynch and Mellor, 1956), so there was little doubt that the membranes were produced endogenously, probably by a process of transudation.

Abnormal permeability of pulmonary capillary endothelium is suggested by the concomitant presence of dilated lymphatics (Wade-Evans, 1962; Boston, Humphreys, Reynolds and Strang, 1965), but this may be only one aspect of a more generalized process which is manifested by peripheral edema and the presence of dilated lymphatics in many organs of the body (James, 1959). Studies of lymph flow and rate of protein clearance suggest that permeability of pulmonary capillaries to protein is higher in the fetal lamb than in the newborn of more than 6 hours of age, and that this may be due to different permeability properties rather than to hypodynamic factors (Boston et al., 1965; Humphreys, Normand, Reynolds and Strang, 1967). Electron microscopic studies showing swollen capillary endothelium, with an unchanged alveolar epithelium, also support such a concept (Campiche, Prod'hom and Gautier, 1961).

Pulmonary Surfactant. A substance is present in normal lungs which alters surface tension as the alveolus changes in size (Pattle, 1955, 1963). Using autofluorescent (Bolande and Klaus, 1964; Bernstein, Wittner and Scarpelli, 1965; Desai, 1965), and immunofluorescent techniques (Craig, 1964), the surfactant has been shown to reside in a liquid layer covering the alveolar epithelium. It has been identified as a complex phospholipid containing dipalmitoylecithin as an active component (Pattle and Thomas, 1961; Klaus, Clements and Havel, 1961) and is synthesized and stored in lamellar inclusions of the large type II alveolar cells (Buckingham, 1964). The exact time at which these lamellar inclusions appear in the human fetus has not been determined, but it appears to be about 20 weeks (Campiche *et al.*, 1963). Surface activity has been demonstrated in previable fetuses of 200 to 500 grams (Gruenwald, 1960). In the lamb the increase in number of the type II alveolar cells with maturation precedes the development of surface activity (Kikkawa, Motoyama and Cook, 1965).

Surfactant is present in lesser amounts in the lungs of distressed infants and not found in lung washings of babies below 1·2 kg. birth weight (Avery and Mead, 1959).

The early lesions described by Stahlman in both the newborn lamb and human infant dying from RDS (see Pathology) reflect the severity of this vasoconstriction. If the integrity of the alveolar cells is to be maintained an adequate pulmonary circulation is necessary both before and after birth (Gardner, Finley and Tooley, 1962; Finley, Tooley, Swenson, Gardner and Clements, 1964; Chu, Clements, Cotton, Klaus, Sweet and Tooley, 1967). This sequence of events could therefore account for the

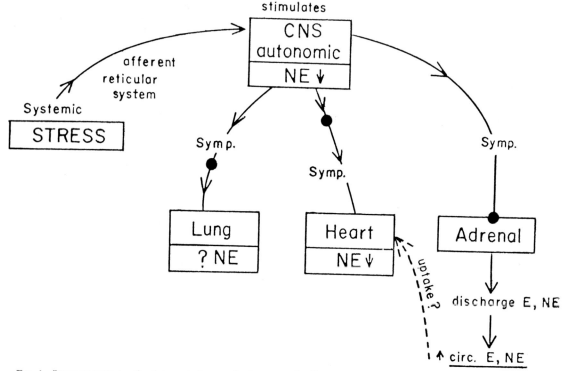

FIG. 1. Stress appears to stimulate central sympathetic centers, leading to excess utilization and eventual loss of brainstem NE[6]. Efferent nerve discharges to peripheral organs may contribute to subsequent losses of myocardial and adrenal catecholamines, and to increased circulating catecholamines. From Buckingham, S. (1967): *57th Ross Conference on Pediatric Research*, 104, and Buckingham, S., Sommers, S. C., McNary, W. F. (1968): *Biologica Neonatorum, 12*, May, 1969. (In press.)

This finding suggested that immaturity alone was the cause of RDS.

However, this is unlikely since activity of pulmonary surfactant may be demonstrated in previable fetuses. Damage to the alveolar cells before, during or after birth could interfere with the production of surfactant (Gruenwald, 1960).

Asphyxia. As noted above, asphyxia during labor and delivery is an important predisposing factor. Furthermore, hyaline membranes have been produced experimentally in rhesus monkeys following intrauterine or immediate postnatal asphyxiation (Windle, 1964; Adamsons, Behrman, Dawes, James and Ross, 1963). The pulmonary arterioles of the fetus constrict in response to asphyxia (Dawes and Mott, 1962) the vessels responding independently to hypoxia, hypercarbia and acidosis (Cook, Drinker, Jacobson, Levine and Strang, 1963; Cassin, Dawes, Mott, Ross and Strang, 1964; Rudolph and Yuan, 1966). In the fetal lamb asphyxia results in an intense arteriolar constriction which reduces blood flow to an almost immeasurable level (Cassin, Dawes and Ross, 1964).

diminution or absence of pulmonary surfactant. However, pulmonary hypoperfusion does not explain the pulmonary congestion and it is possible that there is also a post-capillary venular constriction (see below).

Disturbances of the Central Nervous System. RDS has several features suggesting autonomic nervous system derangement—hypotonia, hypotension, hypothermia and a fixed heart rate. Demonstrations of lesions in the dorsal vagal nuclei (Buckingham, Sommers, Sherwin, 1967) and the experimental production of RDS by bilateral vagotomy (Farber, 1937; Miller, Behrle and Gibson, 1951) provide strong circumstantial evidence for the involvement of the autonomic nervous system. Furthermore the manifestations of respiratory distress have been produced in newborn piglets by injecting epinephrine and norepinephrine (Cheek and Rowe, 1966). The pulmonary vascular bed is under autonomic control (Dawes and Mott, 1964; Colebatch, Dawes, Goodwin and Nadeau, 1965) and in the fetus and neonate is extremely reactive.

A tentative scheme correlating observed central nervous system and pulmonary events with norepinephrine release has been suggested (Buckingham, 1967) (Fig. 1). Catecholamines released both centrally and peripherally in response to asphyxial stress could damage the pulmonary venular endothelium and permit fibrin to leak into the alveolar space.

Cardiac Failure or Circulatory Insufficiency. Infants with left ventricular failure in the neonatal period may present a clinical picture indistinguishable from that of the respiratory distress syndrome (Rudolph, 1965). In the infant with RDS the ductus is widely patent. Large left to right and right to left shunts have been demonstrated at both the foramen ovale and the ductus level (Stahlman, 1966). Recovery in both lamb and baby is accompanied by a rise in systemic pressure and predominantly left to right shunts which diminish as the ductus closes (Stahlman, 1966). Deterioration is accompanied by a fall in systemic pressure and large bidirectional shunting.

Because left atrial pressure is not elevated, left ventricular failure has been considered unlikely. This argument is not tenable if there is circulatory collapse. Under such circumstances pulmonary edema may occur in the presence of a normal left atrial pressure. Constriction of the post-capillary venule in response to an autonomic disturbance (Buckingham, Sommers and McNary, 1966) could also lead to pulmonary edema in the absence of raised left ventricular pressure.

Although the heart may be enlarged and intracardiac shunts are invariably present, the precise role of circulatory insufficiency has not been defined. In our opinion, intracardiac shunts result in a diminution of effective tissue perfusion which is exemplified by the low oxygen consumption (Levison, Delivoria-Papadoupoulos and Swyer, 1964). There is an acute loss of blood volume due to leakage of edema fluid through anoxic capillaries. One would not expect to find the classical signs of failure under these conditions.

Placental Transfusion. The possibility that early clamping of the cord is related to the development of RDS remains unproven (Bound, 1962; Moss, 1963; James, 1966). Additional blood, far from being beneficial to the infant may, in some instances, even be dangerous (Burnard and James, 1963). It can lead to abnormally high blood viscosity particularly at a low pH, the increase being as much as 6 fold at a pH of 7 and a hematocrit of 70 (Burnard, 1966).

Serum Plasma Proteins and Fibrinolytic Activity. Low serum proteins may be a contributing factor by predisposing to transudation from the vascular bed. Total serum proteins are lower in babies with RDS than in healthy premature infants and there is an increased rate of fall in concentration between $1\frac{1}{2}$ and 6 hours of age (Markarian, Jackson and Bannon, 1966). While the concentration of albumin is somewhat depressed the concentration of gamma globulin is abnormally low and these changes become more pronounced as the illness progresses (Hardie, 1965). It is of interest that mothers of infants with RDS have significantly lower levels of gamma globulin, but not of albumin or total protein, than do controls, even at 16 to 20 weeks of pregnancy. This defect persists until 6 weeks postpartum (Hardie, 1967). The significance of this finding remains to be elucidated.

Plasminogen levels are also low and because of this a defect in fibrinolysis has been suspected (Phillips and Skrodelis, 1958). Absent fibrinolytic activity in lung tissue was demonstrated and an inhibitor of plasminogen activator identified in the placenta. High levels of the inhibitor were also found in the placentas of infants of diabetic mothers (Lieberman, 1959, 1961, 1963). Pulmonary surfactant and fibrinogen may interact in such a manner as to establish a vicious cycle. Fibrinogen can inhibit the surface activity of lipo-proteins obtained from lung extracts and at the same time lipo-proteins can inhibit the activation of the fibrinolytic system and activate the coagulation system by accelerating generation of thromboplastin (Taylor and Abrams, 1966).

Disturbances in Pulmonary and Cardiovascular Function

Labored respiration with soft tissue retraction on inspiration reflects a marked decrease in lung compliance. Minute volume is larger than in normal infants early in the disease, due primarily to the rapid respiratory rate. Physiological dead space and the ratio of physiological dead space to tidal volume is increased (Karlberg, Cook, O'Brien, Cherry, Smith, 1954; Strang, 1961; Nelson, Prod'hom, Cherry, Lipsitz, Smith, 1962; Chu et al., 1967). Effective pulmonary blood flow is significantly less than in normal infants (Chu et al., 1967). Lung volume is also reduced (Berglund, Karlberg, 1956; Auld, Nelson, Cherry, Rudolph, Smith, 1963; Chu et al., 1967), but the distribution of ventilation appears to be as uniform as in normal infants.

Those who die become progressively more acidotic as alveolar ventilation and pulmonary blood flow become further reduced. In surviving infants acid-base derangement is corrected as alveolar ventilation and effective pulmonary blood flow increase; lung compliance increases more gradually over the next 5–10 days. The deranged pulmonary mechanics can be explained on the basis of diminished or absent pulmonary surfactant activity but pulmonary congestion may also play a role.

Cyanosis is present early and is due to large right to left shunts which are both intracardiac and intrapulmonary. Intrapulmonary shunts occur through atelectatic areas and the intracardiac shunts through both foramen ovale and ductus arteriosus (Rudolph, 1961; Stahlman, 1966). Because cyanosis persists even in 100 per cent oxygen, the volume of blood shunted can amount to as much as 80 per cent of the right ventricular output (Prod'hom, Levison, Cherry and Smith, 1965; Strang and MacLeish, 1961). The volume of blood shunted appears to increase as the alveolar ventilation decreases (Strang and MacLeish, 1961). The volume of blood flowing through the foramen ovale is to a certain extent dependent upon the volume and direction of the ductus shunt. The direction of shunting through the ductus arteriosus in turn depends upon the relative resistances in the systemic and pulmonary circuits and the relative pressures in the pulmonary artery and aorta (James and Rowe, 1957; Stahlman, LeQuire, Young, Merrill, Birmingham, Payne and Gray, 1964). Deterioration is accompanied by a fall in systemic pressure and large bidirectional shunting, while recovery is accompanied by a rising systemic pressure and a predominantly left to right shunt that diminishes as the ductus closes (Stahlman *et al.*, 1964; Stahlman, 1966).

There is some evidence that the heart is enlarged and decreases in size with recovery (Burnard, 1959). ECG abnormalities are present in a high proportion of the infants, particularly in the most severely ill and those who have been hypothermic. They consists chiefly of conduction defects with prolongation of the PR and QRS intervals. T wave changes also occur (Keith, Rose, Braudo and Rowe, 1961). In some infants the only changes may be a marked reduction in voltage. ECG changes have been correlated with high potassium levels (Usher, 1959) although the derangements are nonspecific and rarely present the characteristics of potassium intoxication.

The presence of the foramen ovale and ductus arteriosus, together with a reactive pulmonary vasculature, provide conditions for marked circulatory instability. Bidirectional shunts at both foramen ovale and ductus arteriosus will, if large, markedly reduce effective cardiac output. Increasing right to left shunting combined with progressive atelectasis and diminution in pulmonary flow make oxygenation increasingly difficult.

Metabolic Sequelae

Healthy infants achieve a normal acid-base state after delivery principally by prompt establishment of effective pulmonary ventilation and the pulmonary excretion of carbon dioxide (Weisbrot, James, Prince, Holaday and Apgar, 1958; Reardon, Baumann and Haddad, 1960). In those with RDS respiratory acidosis is variably reduced. A few infants achieve normal values of pCO_2 for a few hours, but this is unusual, the pCO_2 in the majority being about 45 mm. Hg. Progressive anoxemia is associated with a progressive metabolic acidosis, lactic acid levels rising (Stahlman, Young and Payne, 1962) and pH falling. Oxygen consumption is low (Levison *et al.*, 1964). While this is probably a reflection of circulatory insufficiency a direct depression of metabolism as a consequence of anoxemia cannot be ruled out. High lactic acid levels are associated with a poor prognosis (Stahlman, 1962, 1967).

Other manifestations of disordered function frequently found in immature infants are present in a more exaggerated form in RDS. These include elevated potassium levels with evidence of increased tissue catabolism, shift of water from the intracellular to the extracellular compartment, with increase in sodium excretion during the first 48 hours of life (Nicolopoulos and Smith, 1961). Peripheral edema which develops quite rapidly has been considered in part as a reflection of the metabolic derangement. Its degree and rate of development would argue against this being the sole explanation (Sutherland, Oppé, Lucy and Smith, 1959).

Hyperbilirubinemia occurs more frequently at 5 to 7 days of life in infants recovering from RDS. This suggests an association between anoxia and hyperbilirubinemia, but a cause and effect relationship has not been demonstrated (Miller, Reed, 1958; Odell, Reed, 1964).

Prognosis

Outcome has been difficult to predict except in those infants who are severely ill from the moment of birth.

A scoring system to calculate probability of survival has been proposed (Stahlman, Battersby, Shepard and Blankenship, 1967). It employs the principle of linear discriminants involving arterial oxygen tension, pH, birth weight, respiratory rate and serum potassium, the measurements being made during the first 12 hours of life. The Stahlman technique should be valuable in assessing new forms of therapy, since infants at greater risk will be more readily identified.

Treatment

Since etiology and pathogenesis are incompletely understood, treatment at present is more supportive than specific. Several therapeutic measures are currently employed in most centers but it is difficult to evaluate their relative efficacy; diagnosis is imprecise, severity varies, approximately half of the infants will survive irrespective of the treatment given, outcome is difficult to predict, and the infants are in a precariously unsteady state which may deteriorate suddenly as a result of only small changes in ambient oxygen concentration. Although there is a sound physiological basis for many of the measures employed, they do not always achieve the desired effect. This may be due to harmful side effects, to their incorrect application or to additional and unsuspected complications.

For these reasons control observations are essential. These must be made on the same type of patient at the same time (Sinclair, 1966). Because of the large number of variables, such studies require large numbers of patients; groups of even 20 or 30 may be too small.

Temperature and Humidity

Body temperature should be maintained at 37·5°C and exposure to the mild cold stress of normal room temperature (25°C) should be as brief as possible. Placing the incubator near a window or an air conditioning jet should also be avoided at all times, since this permits excessive heat loss by radiation to cold incubator walls.

Newborn infants have a limited ability to maintain body temperature when exposed to cold (Brück, 1961). The surface area is large and energy stores are limited. This is more pronounced in the immature (Silverman and Agate, 1964), particularly those with RDS probably because the metabolic response to cold is impaired under conditions of hypoxia (Adamsons, 1959; Hill, 1959). In the human newborn it appears to be abolished at a pO_2 of 30 mm. Hg. (Scopes and Ahmed, 1966). Several investigators have demonstrated an increased mortality in association with only mild cold exposure (Silverman, Fertig and Berger, 1957; Buetow and Klein, 1964; Day, Caliguiri, Kamenski and Erhlich, 1964). While the exact cause for this mortality has not been determined it is likely that the increased metabolic demands in response to cold play a major role.

Because the infant's ability to lose heat is also impaired, they are easily overheated. A poorly controlled incubator temperature will result in wide swings in the infant's body temperature. Stability is best achieved through a servo-control mechanism. It has been found satisfactory to keep the skin temperature between 36° and 37° (Silverman, Sinclair and Agate, 1966). This may be achieved by the incubator air temperature or by the use of an infra red source of heat.

High humidity does not seem to be more beneficial than moderate relative humidity (Silverman, Agate and Fertig, 1963). Increased survival in high humidity is apparently due to a thermal effect, heat loss being less in the more humid environment. Nebulized water mist also offers no particular advantage (Silverman and Anderson, 1956). However if high concentrations of oxygen are administered (the gas is cold and dry as it emerges from the cylinder), and an endotracheal tube is in use, inspired gas will bypass the moist nasal mucosa. Under these circumstances it is necessary to use a nebulizer to prevent drying of secretions in the trachea.

Oxygen

Oxygen administration presents many problems. Mild degrees of hypoxemia lead to depression of the respiratory center (Miller and Behrle, 1954; Brady and Ceruti, 1966; Ceruti, 1966) pulmonary vasoconstriction and dilatation of the ductus. On the other hand, hyperoxia may cause retrolental fibroplasia and is toxic to the lungs (Pichotka, 1940; Bean, 1945, 1965; Buckingham et al., 1966; Northway et al., 1967). These difficulties are aggravated by the fact that cyanosis is a late sign of hypoxia in RDS. Even arterial pO_2 measurements are of limited value since they do not indicate whether tissue requirements for oxygen are being met.

40 per cent oxygen in the inspired gas mixture has been recommended as a safe concentration which will not lead to retrolental fibroplasia. The risk of this complication appears to be a function of arterial oxygen tension rather than the ambient concentration (Ashton, 1964). Using 40 per cent oxygen the arterial pO_2 will not rise above 150 mm. Hg. in normal premature and full term infants (Klaus and Meyer, 1966). However, this pO_2 is not attained in infants with severe RDS even with 100 per cent oxygen. Thus we are faced with the dilemma that alveolar concentration of oxygen necessary to maintain arterial pO_2 above 50 mm. Hg. in the very sick infant may also damage the lung parenchyma.

Acid-base Correction

The recognition of a mixed metabolic and respiratory acidemia (James, 1959) led to a clinical trial of acid-base correction using intravenously infused glucose and sodium bicarbonate (Usher, 1961). This resulted in a reduction of mortality. Since that time the principle of correcting at least the metabolic component of acidemia has gained widespread acceptance. THAM (trihydroxy-methylaminomethane) has also been used (Hutchison, 1962; Troelstra, Jonxis, Visser, Van der Vlugt, 1964; Gupta, Dahlenburg and Davis, 1967) and appears to offer theoretical advantages if there is CO_2 accumulation. Correction of pH would seem desirable from several points of view. It should increase pulmonary blood flow by reducing pulmonary vasoconstriction (Rudolph, 1966) and diminish right to left intracardiac shunting by raising

systemic blood pressure (Stahlman, 1966). Correction of pH has other indirect but important effects on metabolic processes: binding of bilirubin to albumin is increased and intracellular diffusion reduced (Odell, 1960, Cole, 1964).

Exchange Transfusion

Kernicterus has been observed in infants suffering from RDS in whom peak levels of bilirubin have remained below 20 mgm. per cent (Stern, Paton, 1965). Our own experience confirms this finding, kernicterus being present in some infants with peak levels as low as 14 mgm. per cent. In consequence when there has been severe acidosis or a history of birth asphyxia, exchange transfusion is recommended at a lower serum bilirubin concentration than for hyperbilirubinemia of prematurity.

Respirator Therapy

Artificial or assisted ventilation becomes the logical form of treatment with progressive impairment of alveolar ventilation and the onset of respiratory failure. Nevertheless, the introduction of this therapy has brought with it additional hazards and complications which must be weighed against the beneficial effects of improved oxygenation and CO_2 elimination. It is difficult to treat an adult for prolonged periods of time by artificial ventilation. These difficulties are compounded in a small infant and are almost inversely proportional to size. Of all the therapeutic regimes introduced, this is the hardest to evaluate. While physicians caring for infants in ventilators will be convinced that individual cases would not have survived without the use of artificial ventilation, a controlled clinical trial failed to indicate that artificial ventilation resulted in an improved outcome (Silverman, Sinclair, Gandy, Finster, Bauman and Agate, 1967).

Feeding

The provision of adequate calories is an added problem. Although various feeding policies have not been shown to be important in determining the immediate outcome (Hsia, Peterson and Gellis, 1957; Bauman, 1960; Butterfield, O'Brien and Lubchenco, 1962; Hubbell et al., 1961; Lethin and Eisner, 1965) certain biochemical derangements may be influenced by early feeding. There is evidence of excessive catabolism (Nicolopoulos and Smith, 1961; Auld, Mehta and Bhangananda, 1965) and hyperkalemia is sometimes present (Usher, 1959). Initially calories can be supplied in part by the use of intravenous 10 per cent glucose. Because this solution is hypertonic it acts as an osmotic diuretic. Once renal function begins to improve there may be a rather prompt diuresis accompanied by loss of sodium. It is essential that the infant's electrolytes be monitored daily and maintenance requirements supplied.

Conclusion

Probably more information has accumulated about the respiratory distress syndrome in the last few years, than about any other condition. Despite this unprecedented research activity many unanswered questions remain. We are still trying to treat a condition for which the cause is far from understood. Until our knowledge of the development of the fetus and its adaptation to extrauterine life is more complete, and until differences between the immature and mature infant are more fully appreciated our therapeutic efforts are likely to be a fumbling procession of errors.

The challenge of the respiratory distress syndrome is the challenge of prematurity and it will not be fully met until we understand and can control the mechanisms involved in the onset of labor.

REFERENCES

Adamsons, K. (1959), "Breathing and The Thermal Environment of Young Rabbits," *J. Physiol. (Lond.)*, **149**, 144.

Adamsons, K., Behrman, R., Dawes, G. S., Dawkins, M. J. R., James, L. S. and Ross, B. (1963), "Treatment of Acidosis with Alkali and Glucose during Asphyxia in Foetal Rhesus Monkeys, *J. Physiol.*, **169**, 679.

Adamsons, K., Behrman, R., Dawes, G. S. and James, L. S. (1964), "Resuscitation of Rhesus Monkeys Asphyxiated at Birth by Positive Pressure Ventilation and Tris-hydroxymethylaminomethane," *J. Pediat.*, **65**, 807.

Ahvenainen, E. K. (1948), "On Changes in Dilatation and Signs of Aspiration in Fetal and Neonatal Lungs," *Academic dissertation* (paperback) Helsinki.

Andrews, B. F. (1965), "Epsom Salts for Hyaline Membrane Disease" (Letter), *Lancet*, **1**, 215.

Ashton, N. (1964), "Retrolental Fibroplasia in Kittens," Personal communication to J. P. M. Tizard, *Pediatrics*, **34**, 771.

Auld, P. A. M., Nelson, N. M., Cherry, R. B., Rudolph, A. J. and Smith, C. A. (1963), "Measurement of Thoracic Gas Volume in the Newborn Infant, *J. clin. Invest.*, **42**, 476.

Auld, P. A. M., Mehta, S. and Bhangananda, P. (1965), "Effect of Glucose on Catabolism in the Premature Infant" (Abstract), *J. Pediat.*, **67**, 950.

Avery, M. E. and Mead, J. (1959), "Surface Properties in Relation to Atelectasis and Hyaline Membrane Disease," *Amer. J. Dis. Child.*, **97**, 517.

Avery, M. E. (1964), *The Lung and its Disorders in the Newborn Infant.* Philadelphia and London: W. B. Saunders Company, **1**, 111.

Bauman, W. A. (1958), "The Respiratory Distress Syndrome and its Relationship to Hyaline Membrane Formation," *Bulletin Sloane Hospital for Women, New York*, **4**, 113.

Bauman, W. A. and Nadelhaft, J. (1958), "Chest Radiography of Prematures. A Planned Study of 104 Patients including Clinicopathologic Correlation of the Respiratory Distress Syndrome," *Pediatrics*, **21**, 813.

Bauman, W. A. (1960), "Early Feeding of Dextrose and Saline Solution to Premature Infants," *Pediatrics*, **26**, 756.

Bean, J. W. (1945), "Effects of Oxygen at Increased Pressures," *Physiol. Rev.*, **25**, 1.

Bean, J. W. (1965), "Factors Influencing Clinical O_2 Toxicity," *Ann. N.Y. Acad. Sci.*, **117**, 745.

Berfenstam, R., Edlund, T. and Zettergren, L. (1958), "The Hyaline Membrane Disease. A Review of Earlier Clinical and Experimental Findings and some Studies on Pathogenesis of Hyaline Membranes in O_2 Intoxicated Rabbits," *Acta paediat.*, **47**, 82.

Berglund, G. and Karlberg, P. (1956), "Determination of the Functional Residual Capacity in Newborn Infants," Preliminary report, *Acta paediat., scand.*, **45**, 541.

Bernstein, J., Wittner, M. and Scarpelli, I. M. (1965), "Morphologic Changes in the Alveolar Lining Film as Related to the Surface Tension Properties and Structure of the Lung in the Respiratory Distress Syndrome," *Amer. J. Path.*, **46**, 270.

Blystad, W. (1956), "Blood Gas Determinations on Premature Infants: II. Investigations of Premature Infants with Early Neonatal Dyspnea," *Acta Paediat.*, **45**, 103.

Bolande, R. P. and Klaus, M. H. (1964), "The Morphologic Demonstration of an Alveolar Lining Layer and its Relationship to Pulmonary Surfactant," *Amer. J. Path.*, **45**, 449.

Boston, R. W., Humphreys, P. W., Reynolds, E. O. R. and Strang, L. (1965), "Lymph Flow and Clearance of Liquid from the Lungs of the Foetal Lamb," *Lancet*, **2**, 473.

Bound, J. P., Harvey, P. W. and Bagshaw, H. B. (1962), "Prevention of the Pulmonary Syndrome of the Newborn," *Lancet*, **1**, 1200.

Brady, J. P. and Ceruti, E. (1966), "Chemoreceptor Reflexes in the Newborn Infant. Effects of Varying Degrees of Hypoxia on Heart Rate and Ventilation in a Warm Environment," *J. Physiol. (Lond.)*, **184**, 631.

Briggs, J. N. and Hogg, G. (1958), "Perinatal Pulmonary Pathology," *Pediatrics*, **22**, 41.

Brück, K. (1961), "Temperature Regulation in the Newborn Infant," *Biologica Neonatorum*, **3**, 65.

Bruns, P. D. and Shields, L. V. (1954), "High Oxygen and Hyaline-like Membranes," *Amer. J. Obstet. Gynec.*, **67**, 1224.

Buckingham, S., McNary, W. F. and Sommers, S. C. (1964), "Pulmonary Alveolar Cell Inclusions: Their Development in the Rat," *Science*, **145**, 1192.

Buckingham, S., Sommers, S. C. and McNary, W. F. (1966), "Sympathetic Activation and Serotonin Release as Factors in Pulmonary Edema after Hyperbaric Oxygen," *Fed. Proc.*, **25**, 566 (Abstract).

Buckingham, S., Heineman, H. O., Sommers, S. C. and McNary, W. F. (1966), "Phospholipid Synthesis in the Large Alveolar Cell," *Amer. J. Path.*, **48**, 1027.

Buckingham, S., Sommers, S. C. and Sherwin, R. P. (1967), "Lesions of the Dorsal Vagal Nucleus in the Respiratory Distress Syndrome," *Amer. J. clin. Path.*, **48**, 269.

Buckingham, S. (1967), "Sympathetic and Parasympathetic Nervous System," *57th Ross Conference on Pediatric Research*, 104.

Buckingham, S., Sommers, S. C., McNary, W. F. (1968), "Experimental Respiratory Distress Syndrome. I. Central, Autonomic and Humoral Pathogenetic Factors in Pulmonary Injury of Rats induced with Hyperbaric Oxygen and the Protective Effects of Barbiturates and Trasylol," *Biologica Neonatorum*, **12**, 261.

Buetow, K. C. and Klein, S. W. (1964), "Effects of Maintenance of Neonatal Skin Temperature on Survival of Infants with Low Birth Weight," *Pediatrics*, **34**, 163.

Burnard, E. D. (1959), "Changes in Heart Size in the Dyspnoeic Newborn Baby," *Brit. med. J.*, **2**, 134.

Burnard, E. D. and James, L. S. (1963), "Atrial Pressures and Cardiac Size in the Newborn Infant," *J. Pediat.*, **62**, 815.

Burnard, E. D. (1966), "Influence of Delivery on the Circulation," *The Heart and Circulation in the Newborn and Infant.* Edited by Cassells, D. E. New York and London: Grune and Stratton.

Butterfield, J., O'Brien, D. and Lubchenco, L. O. (1962), "Respiratory Distress Syndrome in Premature Infants: An Evaluation of the Early Feeding of Glucose Water," *Amer. J. Dis. Child.*, **104**, 230.

Campiche, M., Prod'hom, S. and Gautier, A. (1961), "Étude au microscope électronique du poumon des prématurés morts en detresse respiratoire," *Annals of Pediatrics*, **196**, 81.

Cassin, S., Dawes, G. S., Mott, J. C., Ross, B. and Strang, L. (1964), "The Vascular Resistance of the Foetal and Newly Ventilated Lung of the Lamb," *J. Physiol.*, **171**, 61.

Cassin, S., Dawes, G. S. and Ross, B. (1964), "Pulmonary Blood Flow and Vascular Resistance in Immature Foetal Lambs," *J. Physiol.*, **171**, 80.

Ceruti, E. (1966), "Chemoreceptor Reflexes in the Newborn Infant: Effect of Cooling on the Response to Hypoxia," *Pediatrics*, **37**, 556.

Cheek, D. B. and Rowe, R. D. (1966), "Aspect of Sympathetic Activity in the Newborn including the Respiratory Distress Syndrome," *Pediatric Clinics of North America, The Newborn I,* Edited by James, L. S., p. 863. Philadelphia and London: W. B. Saunders, Company.

Chu, J. and others (1965), "Preliminary Report: The Pulmonary Hypoperfusion Syndrome," *Pediatrics*, **35**, 733.

Chu, J., Clements, J. A., Cotten, E. K., Klaus, M. H., Sweet, A. Y. and Tooley, W. H. (1967), "Neonatal Pulmonary Ischemia. I. Clinical and Physiological Studies," *Pediatrics*, **40**, 709.

Chuang, K. A. (1962), "Pulmonary Hyaline Membrane Disease in Hawaii," *Amer. J. Dis. Child.*, **103**, 718.

Cook, C. D., Drinker, P. A., Jacobson, H. N., Levison, H. and Strang, L. (1963), "Control of Pulmonary Blood Flow in the Foetal and Newly Born Lamb," *J. Physiol.*, **169**, 10.

Cohen, M. M., Weintraub, D. H. and Lilienfeld, A. M. (1960), "The Relationship of Pulmonary Hyaline Membrane to Certain Factors in Pregnancy and Delivery," *Pediatrics*, **26**, 42.

Colebatch, H. J. H., Dawes, G. S., Goodwin, J. W. and Nadeau, R. A. (1965), "The Nervous Control of the Circulation in the Fetal and Newly Expanded Lungs of the Lamb," *J. Physiol.*, **178**, 544.

Craig, J. and Fraser, M. S. (1967), "The Respiratory Difficulties of Cesarean Babies," *Annals Paediatrics*, Fenn. **13**, 143.

Craig, J. (1964), "The Distribution of Surface Active Material in the Lungs of Infants with and without Respiratory Distress," *Biologica Neonatorum*, **7**, 185.

Cropp, G. J. (1967), *Effect of Magnesium in Pulmonary Vasomotor Response to Hypoxia*. Abstract. Society for Paediatric Research, Atlantic City, New Jersey, April, 28, 29.

Dawes, G. S. and Mott, J. C. (1962), "Vascular Tone of Foetal Lung," *J. Physiol.*, **164**, 465.

Dawes, G. S. and Mott, J. C. (1964), "Changes in Oxygen Distribution and Consumption in Fetal Lambs with Variations in Umbilical Blood Flow," *J. Physiol.*, **170**, 524.

Day, R. L., Caliguiri, L., Kamenski, C. and Ehrlich, F. (1964), "Body Temperature and Survival of Premature Infants," *Pediatrics*, **34**, 171.

De, T. D. and Anderson, G. W. (1954), "The Experimental Production of Pulmonary Hyaline-like Membranes with Atelectasis," *Amer. J. Obstet. Gynec.*, **68**, 1557.

DeSa', D. J. (1965), "Microscopy of the Alveolar Lining Layer in Newborn Infants," *Lancet*, **1**, 1369.

Driscoll, S. A., Benirschke, K. and Curtis, G. W. (1960), "Neonatal Deaths among Infants of Diabetic Mothers," *Amer. J. Dis. Child.*, **100**, 818.

Driscoll, S. G. and Smith, C. A. (1962), "Neonatal Pulmonary Disorders." *Pediatric Clinics of North America*, **9**, 325. Philadelphia and London: W. B. Saunders Co.

Dunn, P. M. (1963), "Intestinal Obstruction in the Newborn with Special Reference to Transient Functional Ileus Associated with Respiratory Distress Syndrome." *Arch. Dis. Child*, **38**, 459.

Farber, S. (1937), "Studies on Pulmonary Oedema: I. The Consequence of Bilateral Cervical Vagotomy in the Rabbit," *J. exp. Med.*, **66**, 397.

Farquhar, J. W. (1962), "Birth Weight and the Survival of Babies of Diabetic Women," *Arch. Dis. Child.*, **37**, 321.

Feinberg, S. B. and Goldberg, M. E. (1957), "Hyaline Membrane Disease: Preclinical Roentgen Diagnosis; a Planned Study," *Radiology*, **68**, 185.

Finberg, L. (1967), "Dangers of Change in Osmolal Concentration, *Pediatrics*, **40**, 1031.

Finley, T. N., Tooley, W. H., Swenson, E. W., Gardner, R. E. and Clements, J. A. (1964), "Pulmonary Surface Tension in Experimental Atelectasis," *Amer. Rev. res. Dis.*, **89**, 372.

Gairdner, D. (1965), *Recent Advances in Paediatrics*, Third Edition, p. 57. London: J. A. Churchill Ltd.

Gardner, R. E., Finley, T. N. and Tooley, W. H. (1962), "Effect of Cardiopulmonary Bypass on Surface Activity of Lung Extracts," *Bull. Soc. Internat. de Chir.*, **21**, 542.

Gitlin, D. and Craig, J. M. (1956), "The Nature of the Hyaline Membrane in Asphyxia of the Newborn," *Pediatrics*, **17**, 64.

Gruenwald, P. (1953), in "Pulmonary Hyaline Membranes. *Report of the 5th Ross Conference on Pediatric Research*, p. 71.

Gruenwald, P. (1958), "The Significance of Pulmonary Hyaline Membranes in Newborn Infants," *J. Amer. med. Ass.*, **166**, 621.

Gruenwald, P. (1963), "Normal and Abnormal Expansion of the Lungs of Newborn Infants obtained at Autopsy: III. The Pattern of Aeration as affected by Gestational and Postnatal Age," *Anat. Rec.*, **146**, 337.

Gruenwald, P. (1960), "Prenatal Origin of Respiratory Distress (Hyaline Membrane) Syndrome of Premature Infants," *Lancet*, *1* 230.

Gruenwald, P. (1966), "Pulmonary Pathology in the Respiratory Distress Syndrome," *Pediatric Clinics of North America*. The Newborn: I., edited by James, L. S., **13**, No. 3, 703. Philadelphia and London: W. B. Saunders, Company.

Gupta, J. M., Dahlenberg, G. W. and Davis, J. A. (1967), "Changes in Blood Gas Tension following Administration of Amine Buffer THAM in Infants with Respiratory Distress Syndrome," *Archi. Dis. Child.*, **42**, 416.

Hardie, G., Hesse, H. deV. and Kench, J. E. (1966), "Serum Porteins in the Idiopathic Respiratory Distress Syndrome of the Newborn," *Lancet*, **2**, 876.

Hardie, G. (1967), "Maternal Serum Proteins in Idiopathic Respiratory Distress Syndrome of the Newborn," *Lancet*, **1**, 809.

Hill, J. R. (1959), "The Oxygen Consumption of Newborn and Adult Mammals. Its Dependence on the Oxygen Tension in the Inspired Air and on the Environmental Temperature," *J. Physiol.*, (*Lond.*), **149**, 346.

Hubbell, J. P., *et al.* (1961), "'Early' versus 'Late' Feeding of Infants of Diabetic Mothers," *New Eng. J. Med.*, **265**, 835.

Humphreys, P. W., Normand, I. C. S., Reynolds, E. O. R. and Strang, L. B. (1967), "Pulmonary Lymph Flow and the Uptake of Liquid from the Lungs of the Lamb at the Start of Breathing," *J. Physiol.*, **193**, 1.

Hutchinson, J. H., *et al.* (1962), "Studies in the Treatment of the Pulmonary Syndrome of the Newborn," *Lancet*, **2**, 465.

James, L. S. and Rowe, R. D. (1957), "The Influence of Short Induced Periods of Hypoxia on the Pulmonary and Systemic Arterial Pressures," *J. Pediat.*, **51**, 5.

James, L. S., Weisbrot, I. M., Prince, C. E., Holaday, D. A. and Apgar, V. (1958), "The Acid-base Status of Human Infants in Relation to Birth Asphyxia and the Onset of Respiration," *J. Pediat.*, **52**, 379.

James, L. S. (1959), "Physiology of Respiration in Newborn Infants and in the Respiratory Distress Syndrome," *Pediatrics*, **24**, 1069.

James, L. S. and Burnard, E. D. (1961), "Biochemical Changes Occurring during Asphyxia at Birth and Some Effects on the Heart." In Wolstenholme, G. E. W. and Connor, M. O., eds., Ciba Foundation Symposium on *Somatic Stability in the Newly Born*, p. 75. London: J. A. Churchill, Ltd.

James, L. S. (1966), "Onset of Breathing and Resuscitation," *Pediatric Clinics of North America*, **13**, No. 3, 621, James, L. S., ed. Philadelphia and London: W. B. Saunders Co.

Karlberg, P., Cook, C. D., O'Brien, D., Cherry, R. B. and Smith, C. A. (1954), "Studies of Respiratory Physiology in the Newborn Infant: II. Observations during and after Respiratory Distress" (Suppl. 100), *Acta Paediat., scand.*, **43**, 397.

Keith, J. D., Rose, V., Braudo, M. and Rowe, R. D. (1961), "Electrocardiogram in the Respiratory Distress Syndrome and Related Cardiovascular Dynamics," *J. Pediat.*, **59**, 167.

Kincaid-Smith, P. and Bullem, M. (1965), "Bacteriuria in Pregnancy," *Lancet*, **1**, 395.

Klaus, M. H., Clements, J. A. and Havel, R. J. (1961), "Composition of Surface-active Material Isolated from Beef Lung," *Proc. nat. Acad. Sci.*, **47**, 1858.

Klaus, M. and Meyer, B. P. (1966), "Oxygen Therapy for the Newborn," *Pediatric Clinics of North America*, **13**, 731, No. 1. Philadelphia and London: W. B. Saunders Company.

Latham, E. F., Nesbitt, R. E. L. and Anderson, G. W. (1955), "A Clinical Pathological Study of the Newborn Lung with Hyaline-like Membranes," *Bull. Johns Hopk. Hosp.*, **96**, 173.

Lethin, A. and Eisner, V. (1965), "Glucose Therapy in Neonatal Respiratory Distress," *Amer. J. Dis. Child.*, **110**, 140.

Levison, H., Delivoria-Papadopoulos, M. and Swyer, P. (1964), "Oxygen Consumption of Newly Born Infants, with Respiratory Distress Syndrome," *Biologica Neonatorum*, **7**, 255.

Lieberman, J. (1959), "Clinical Syndromes Associated with Deficient Lung Fibrinolytic Activity: I. New Concept of Hyaline Membrane Disease," *New Eng. J. Med.*, **260**, 619.

Lieberman, J. (1961), "The Nature of the Fibrinolytic Enzyme Defect in Hyaline Membrane Disease," *New Eng. J. Med.*, **265**, 363.

Lieberman, J. (1963), "Unified Concept and Critical Review of Pulmonary Hyaline Membrane Formation" (Editorial), *J. Amer. med. Ass.*, **35**, 443.

Low, F. N. (1954), "Electron Microscopy of Sectioned Lung Tissue after Varied Duration of Fixation in Buffered Osmium Tetroxide," *Anat. Rec.*, **120**, 827.

Lynch, M. J. D. and Mellor, L. D. (1956), "Hyaline Membrane Disease of the Lungs," *J. Pediat.*, **48**, 168.

Markarian, M., Jackson, J. J. and Bannon, A. E. (1966), "Serial Serum Plasma Protein Values in Premature Infants with and Without Respiratory Distress Syndrome," *J. Pediat.*, **69**, 1046.

Miller, C. A. and Reed, H. R. (1958), "The Relation of Serum Concentration of Bilirubin to Respiratory Function of Premature Infants," *Pediatrics*, **21**, 362.

Miller, H. C. and Jennison, M. A. (1950), "Study of Pulmonary Hyaline-like Material in 4,117 Consecutive Births," *Pediatrics*, **5**, 7.

Miller, H. C., Behrle, F. C. and Gibson, D. M. (1951), "Comparison of Pulmonary Hyaline Membranes in Vagotomized Rabbits with those in Newborn Infants," *Pediatrics*, **7**, 611.

Miller, H. C. and Behrle, F. C. (1954), "Effects of Hypoxia on Respiration of Newborn Infants," *Pediatrics*, **14**, 93.

Miller, H. C. (1962), "Respiratory Distress Syndrome of Newborn Infants: I. Diagnosis and Incidence: II. Pathogenesis," *J. Pediat.*, **61**, 2.

Miller, H. C. and Conklin, E. V. (1955), "Clinical Evaluation of Respiratory Insufficiency in Newborn Infants," *Pediatrics*, **16**, 427.

Miller, H. C., Behrl, F. C., Smull, N. W. and Blim, R. D. (1957), "Studies of Respiratory Insufficiency in Newborn Infants: II. Correlation of Hydrogen Ion Concentration, Carbon Dioxide Tension, Carbon Dioxide Content and Oxygen Saturation of Blood with trend of Respiratory Rates," *Pediatrics*, **19**, 387.

Miller, H. C. (1963), "Respiratory Distress Syndrome of Newborn Infants: III. Statistical Evaluation of Factors possibly affecting Survival of Premature Infants," *Pediatrics*, **31**, 573.

Moss, A. J., Duffie, E. R. and Fagan, L. (1963), "Respiratory Distress Syndrome in the Newborn," *J. Amer. med. Ass.*, **184**, 48.

Nash, G., Blennerhassett, J. B. and Pontoppidon, H. (1967), "Pulmonary Lesions Associated with Oxygen Therapy and Artificial Ventilation," *New Engl. J. Med.*, **276**, 368.

Nelson, N. M., Prod'hom, L. S., Cherry, R. B., Lipsitz, P. J. and Smith, C. A. (1962), "Pulmonary Function in the Newborn Infant: II. Perfusion-estimation by Analysis of the Arterial Alveolar Carbon Dioxide Difference," *Pediatrics*, **30**, 975.

Neligan, G. A., Smith, C. A. and Oxon, O. M. (1960), "The Blood Pressure of Newborn Infants in Asphyxial States, and in Hyaline Membrane Disease," *Pediatrics*, **26**, 735.

Neligan, G. A. (1961), quoted by Webb, *et al.*, 1962.

Nicolopoulos, D. A. and Smith, C. A. (1961), "Metabolic Aspects of Idiopathic Respiratory Distress (Hyaline Membrane Syndrome) in Newborn Infants," *Pediatrics*, **28**, 206.

Northway, W. H., Rosan, R. C. and Porter, D. Y. (1967), "Pulmonary Disease following Respirator Therapy of Hyaline Membrane Disease," *New Eng. J. Med.*, **276**, 357.

Odell, G. B. and Cohen, S. (1960), "The Effect of pH on the Protein Binding of Bilirubin (Abstract)," *Amer. J. Dis. Child.*, **100**, 525.

Odell, G. B. (1964), "The Influence of pH on the Distribution of Bilirubin between Albumin and Mitochondria," *J. Pediat.*, **65**, 1108.

Pattle, R. E. (1955), "Properties, Function and Origin of the Alveolar Lining Layer," *Nature* (*Lond.*), **175**, 1125.

Pattle, R. E. and Thomas, L. R. (1961), "Lipoprotein Composition of film Lining Lung," *Nature* (*Lond.*), **189**, 844.

Pattle, R. E. (1963), "The Lining Layer of the Lung Alveoli," *Brit. med. Bull.*, **19**, 41.

Phillips, E. L. and Skrodelis, V. (1958), "A comparison of the Fibrinolytic Enzyme Systems in Maternal and Umbilical Cord Blood," *Pediatrics*, **22**, 715.

Pichotka, J. (1940), "On the Histologic Change of the Lungs after Breathing High Concentrations of Oxygen Experimentally," *Beitr. path. Anat.*, **105**, 381.

Prod'hom, L. S., Levison H., Cherry, R. B. and Smith, C. A. (1965), "Adjustment of Ventilation, Intrapulmonary Gas Exchange and Acid-base Balance during the Frist Day of Life: Infants with Respiratory Distress," *Pediatrics*, **35**, 662.

Ranstrom, S. (1953), "On the Effect of the Hyaline Membrane in the Lungs of Newborn Infants," *Acta Paediat.*, **42**, 323.

Reardon, H. (1958), "Adaptation to Extrauterine Life; Infants of Diabetic Mothers, Bio-Chemical Studies and Management," in the *Report of the 31st Ross Pediatric Research Conference*, Columbus, Ohio, Ross Laboratories, p. 72.

Reardon, H. S., Baumann, M. L. and Haddad, E. J. (1960), "Chemical Stimuli of Respiration in the Early Neonatal Period," *J. Pediat.*, **57**, 151.

Robertson, B., Tunell, R. and Rudhe, U. (1964), "Late Stages of Pulmonary Hyaline Membrane of the Newborn," *Acta Paediat. scand.*, **53**, 433.

Rudolph, A. M., Auld, P. A. M., Golinko, R. J. and Paul, M. H. (1961), "Pulmonary Vascular Adjustment in the Neonatal Period," *Pediatrics*, **28**, 28.

Rudolph, A. M., Drorbaugh, J. E., Auld, P. A. M., Rudolph, A. J., Nadas, A. S., Smith, C. A. and Hubbell, J. P. (1961), "Studies on the Circulation in the Neonatal Period: The Circulation in the Respiratory Distress Syndrome," *Pediatrics*, **27**, 551.

Rudolph, A. M. (1965), "Diagnosis and Treatment: Respiratory Distress and Cardiac Disease in Infancy," *Pediatrics*, **35**, 999.

Rudolph, A. J., Vallbona, C. and Desmond, M. M. (1965), "Cardiodynamic Studies in the Newborn: III. Heart Rate in Infants with Idiopathic Respiratory Distress Syndrome," *Pediatrics*, **36**, 551.

Rudolph, A. J., Desmond, M. M. and Pineda, R. G. (1966), "Clinical Diagnosis of Respiratory Difficulty in the Newborn," *Pediatric Clinics of North America*, **13**, No. 3, 669. The Newborn: I., ed. James, L. S. Philadelphia and London: W. B. Saunders Co.

Rudolph, A. M. and Yuan, S. (1966), "Response of the Pulmonary Vasculature to Hypoxia and H^+ Ion Concentration Changes," *J. clin. Invest.*, **45**, 399.

Scopes, J. W. and Ahmed, I. (1965), "Indirect Assessment of Oxygen Requirements in Newborn Babies by Monitoring Deep Body Temperature," *Arch. Dis. Childh.*, **41**, 25.

Shepherd, F., Gray, J. and Stahlman, M. (1964), "The Occurrence of Pulmonary Fibrosis in Children who had Idiopathic Respiratory Distress Syndrome," presented at the Annual Meeting of the Society for Pediatric Research, Washington, June 14–19.

Shirodkar, V. N. (1955), "Surgical Treatment of Habitual Abortion. Tendances actuel les en gynecologie et obstetrique," Librairie de l'Universite, S.A. Geneve, George, 0, CIE.

Silverman, W. A. and Anderson, D. H. (1956), "A Controlled Clinical Trial of Effects of Water Mist on Destructive Clinical Signs, Death Rate and Necropsy Findings among Premature Infants," *Pediatrics*, **17**, 1.

Silverman, W. A., Fertig, J. W. and Berger, A. P. (1958), "The Influence of the Thermal Environment upon the Survival of Newly Born Premature Infants," *Pediatrics*, **22**, 876.

Silverman, W. A. and Silverman, R. (1958), "Incidence of Hyaline Membrane in Premature Infants," *Lancet*, **2**, 588.

Silverman, W. A., Agate, F. J. Jr., and Fertig, J. W. (1963), "A Sequential Trial of the Nonthermal Effect of Atmospheric Humidity on Survival of Newborn Infants of Low Birth Weight," *Pediatrics*, **31**, 719.

Silverman, W. A. and Agate, F. J. (1964), "Variation in Cold Resistance Among Small Newborn Infants," *Biologica Neonatorum*, **6**, 113.

Silverman, W. A., Sinclair, J. C. and Agate, F. L., Jr. (1966), "The Oxygen Cost of Minor Changes in Small Newborn Infants," *Acta Paediat.*, **55**, 294.

Silverman, W. A., Sinclair, J. C., Gandy, G. M., Finster, M., Bauman, W. A. and Agate, F. J. (1967), "A Controlled Trial of Management of Respiratory Distress Syndrome in a Body Enclosing Respirator: I. Evaluation of Safety," *Pediatrics*, **39**, 740.

Sinclair, J. C. (1966), "Prevention and Treatment of the Respiratory Distress Syndrome," *Pediatric Clinics of North America*, **13**, No. 3, 711. The Newborn: I., ed. James, L. S. Philadelphia and London: W. B. Saunders Co.

Sivanesan, S. (1961), "Neonatal Pulmonary Pathology in Singapore," *J. Pediat.*, **59**, 600.

Stern, L. and Denton, R. L. (1965), "Kernicterus in Small Premature Infants," *Pediatrics*, **35**, 483.

Stahlman, M. T., Young, W. C. and Payne, G. (1962), "Prognostic Significance of Blood Lactic Acid Levels in Hyaline Membrane Disease (Abstract)," *Sth. med. J.*, **55**, 1320.

Stahlman, M., LeQuire, V. S., Young, W. C., Merrill, R. E., Birmingham, R. T., Payne, G. A. and Gray, J. (1964), "Pathophysiology of Respiratory Distress in Newborn Lambs," *Amer. J. Dis. Child.*, **108**, 375.

Stahlman, M. T., Battersby, E. J., Shepard, F. M. and Blankenship, W. J. (1967), "Prognosis in Hyaline Membrane Disease: Use of a Linear Discriminant," *New Engl. J. Med.*, **276**, 303.

Stahlman, M. (1966), *The Heart and Circulation in the Newborn and Infant*, Cassels, D. E., ed., p. 121, New York and London: Grune and Stratton.

Strang, L. B., Anderson, G. S. and Platt, J. W. (1957), "Neonatal Death and Elective Caesarian Section," *Lancet*, **1**, 954.

Strang, L. B. (1961), "Alveolar Gas and Anatomical Dead-space Measurements in Normal Newborn Infants," *Clin. Sci.*, **21**, 107.

Strang, L. B. and MacLeish, M. H. (1961), "Ventilatory Failure, and Right-to-left Shunt in Newborn Infants with Respiratory Distress," *Pediatrics*, **28**, 17.

Sutherland, J. M., Oppe, T. E., Lucy, J. F. and Smith, C. A. (1959), "Leg Volume Observed in Hyaline Membrane Disease," *Amer. J. Dis. Child.*, **98**, 24.

Taylor, F. B. and Abrams, M. E. (1966), "Effect of Surface Active Lipoprotein on Clotting and Fibrinolysis, and of Fibrinogen on Surface Tension of Surface Active Lipoprotein with a Hypothesis on the Pathogenesis of Pulmonary Atelectasis and Hyaline Membrane in Respiratory Distress Syndrome of the Newborn," *Amer. J. med.*, **40**, 346.

Thomsen, A. (1964), "Arterial Blood Sampling in Small Infants," *Acta Paediat.*, **53**, 237.

Troelstra, J. A., Jonxis, J. H. P., Visser, H. K. A. and Van der Vlugt, J. J. (1964), "Metabolism and Acid-base Regulation in the Respiratory Distress Syndrome: Treatment with Tris-hydroxymethylaminomethane (THAM)," *Maandschr. Kindergeneesk*, **32**, 569.

Usher, R. H. (1959), "The Respiratory Distress Syndrome of Prematurity: I. Changes in Potassium and the Electrocardiogram and the Effects of Therapy," *Pediatrics*, **24**, 562.

Usher, R. H. (1961), "Clinical Investigation of the Respiratory Distress Syndrome of Prematurity—Interim Report," *N.Y. St. J. Med.*, **61**, 1677.

Usher, R. H. (1963), "Reduction of Mortality from Respiratory Distress Syndrome of Prematurity with Early Administration of Administration of Intravenous Glucose and Sodium Bicarbonate," *Pediatrics*, **32**, 966.

Usher, R. H., McLean, F. and Maughan, G. B. (1964), "The Respiratory Distress Syndrome in Infants Delivered by Caesarean Section," *Amer. J. Obstet. Gynec.*, **88**, 806.

van Breeman, V. L., Neustein, H. B. and Bruns, P. D., (1957), "Pulmonary Hyaline Membrane Studied with the Electron Microscope," *Amer. J. Path.*, **33**, 769.

Wade-Evans, T. (1962), "The Formation of Pulmonary Hyaline Membranes in the Newborn Baby," *Arch. Dis. Child.*, **37**, 470.

Webb, G. K. G., John, T. J., Jadhar, M., Graham, M. D. and Walter, A. (1962), "The Incidence of Hyaline Membrane Syndrome in South India," *J. Indian Paediat. Soc.*, **1**, 193.

Weisbrot, I. M., James, J. S., Prince, C. E., Holaday, D. A. and Apgar, V. (1958), "Acid-base Homeostasis of the Newborn Infant during the first 24 Hours of Life," *J. Pediat.*, **52**, 395.

Windle, W. F. (1964), "Respiratory Distress: Relation to Prematurity and Other Factors in Newborn Monkeys," *Science*, **143**, 1345.

Younozai, M. K. (1962), "Hyaline Membranes in Lebanon," *Pediatrics*, **29**, 332.

SECTION VII

LACTATION

1. THE MAMMARY GLAND AND LACTATION

A. T. COWIE and S. J. FOLLEY

Lactation, the production of milk for the nourishing of the young, is the last phase of the reproductive cycle of mammals. In almost all species the maternal milk is necessary for the sustenance of the young during their neonatal period and adequate lactation is essential for survival of the species, although the human infant has for long had the benefit of substitute mothers or substitute milks.

MAMMARY GROWTH

The physiology of lactation is concerned not only with the functioning of the mammary gland but also with the processes of its growth through the foetal to adult stages. Interference at any stage with its normal growth may reduce or even abolish the future functional capacity of the mammary gland. An understanding of the processes of mammary growth may therefore be of some importance.

Mammary Growth in the Foetus

The various stages in the embryonic and foetal growth of the mammary gland have been described in a number of species including man (see review by Raynaud, 1961). The *mammary band*, the first sign of the future mammary glands, appears as a raised band of ectoderm on either side of the mid line of the very young embryo (in the human embryo when it attains a length of 4–6 mm.); along the band then appears a narrower ribbon of raised epithelium known as the *milk line*. The mammary band generally disappears but the fate of the milk line depends on the number and distribution of the mammary glands in the species in question. In man the line diminishes in length from its caudal end, while its cranial extremity thickens and becomes a small nodule of ectodermal cells (human embryo length 13–15 mm.). This nodule sinks into the dermis becoming lenticular, hemispherical and then spherical in shape—the *primitive mammary bud* (human embryo length 20–30 mm.). In those species with multiple mammary glands the milk line becomes fragmented along its length giving rise to small separate nodules (the number depending on the species) which sink into the dermis and become mammary buds. The mammary buds give rise, according to the species, to one or more secondary buds which lengthen into epithelial cords; these branch at their distal ends forming the anlagen of the adult duct system. At this stage a pause occurs in the development of the mammary anlagen; in the human embryo this pause lasts from the 3rd to the 5th months of foetal life. During the fifth month (embryo length 120 to 150 mm.) the deep layer of the bud proliferates, producing 15–25 secondary epithelial buds which lengthen into solid cords and these traverse the underlying mesenchymal tissue into sub-cutaneous cellular tissue. In embryos of 180–200 mm. these cords branch at their ends and develop a lumen, further growth and branching continuing to term.

Only in the mouse and rat is there any substantial information about how the growth of the mammary anlage is controlled. In these species the initial stages of mammary growth are apparently independent of the influence of any hormones of the foetal gonads and are the same in both male and female foetuses up to the 14th day. However, on the 15th day in the female the mammary bud sinks into the underlying mesenchyme but remains connected to the epidermis by a long neck of ectodermal cells; the mammary bud then lengthens into a cord which, near term, begins to branch at its distal end. In the male foetus on the 15th day the mammary bud also sinks into the mesenchyme but becomes disconnected from the epidermis; the isolated bud grows into a small cord which near term becomes slightly branched; as a result in the adult male mouse and rat the mammary glands are without nipples and do not open to the exterior. The above pattern of mammary growth in the male foetus is controlled by hormones from the foetal testis; on the other hand, the female pattern is not due to the presence of foetal gonadal hormones. Castration of the male foetus (see Raynaud, 1961) or inhibition of the hormonal activity of its testes by suitable drugs (see Neumann and Elger, 1966 and Fig. 1) induces the female pattern of mammary growth, while injection of androgens into female foetuses induces the male pattern of growth. The injection of oestrogens into mouse or rat foetuses may cause exaggerated nipple growth but may also partially or totally arrest the growth of the mammary anlagen. Thus in the mouse and rat the male pattern of mammary growth is a specialized type due to a process of inhibition of the normal female type of growth by a hormone or hormones from the foetal testis (see review by Raynaud, 1961; also Jean and Delost, 1965). It may be noted that this type of differentiation, the diversion of the neutral (female) type under the influence of foetal androgens is characteristic also of the early differentiation of the reproductive tract and of the sexual differentiation of the central nervous system.

Whether similar hormonally controlled mammary differentiation occurs in other species is not so far known. The question may be of some clinical importance as it is conceivable that hormones administered during pregnancy could cause congenital malformations of the mammary gland.

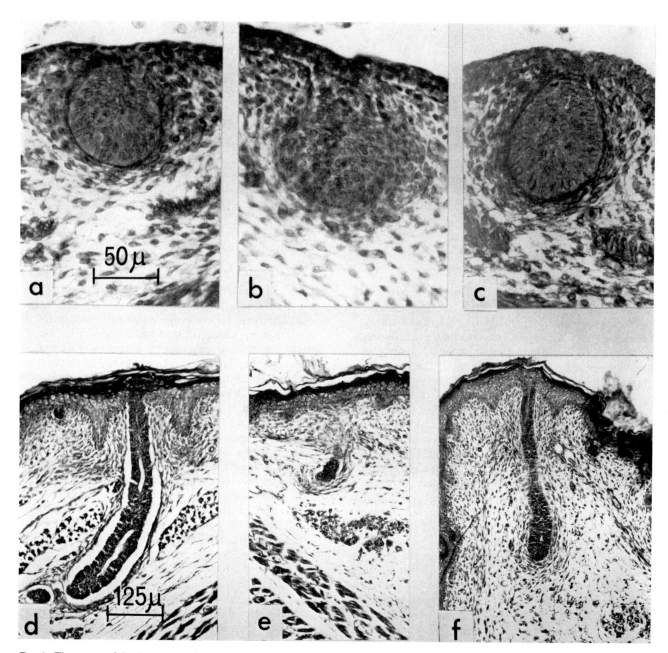

FIG. 1. The pattern of development of the mammary anlagen in the foetal mouse. (a) Mammary bud of the normal 14-day-old female foetus. (b) Mammary bud of the normal 14-day-old male foetus. Note that the outline of the bud is less clearly defined as mesenchyme condenses prior to rupture of the connexion between the bud and the epidermis. (c) Mammary bud of the 14-day-old male foetus whose mother has been treated with an antiandrogen (cyproterone acetate, 3 mg./day) from day 12 of pregnancy. Note the similarity with the normal female bud (a). (d) Mammary cord of the normal 18-day-old female foetus. Note that the cord is attached to the epidermis and that around the base of the cord there is an invagination of the epidermis representing the anlagen of the nipple. (e) Mammary rudiment of the normal 18-day-old male foetus. Note that the connexion with the epidermis has disappeared and that invagination of the epidermis is virtually absent. (f) Mammary cord of the 18-day-old male foetus whose mother has been treated with an antiandrogen (cyproterone acetate, 3 mg./day) from day 12 of pregnancy. Observe the similarity with the normal female (d); the mammary cord is attached to the epidermis and there is clear evidence of nipple formation. (Photographs by courtesy of Dr. F. Neumann, Schering AG, Berlin.)

Postnatal Mammary Growth

The postnatal growth pattern of the mammary gland depends mainly on the type of sex cycle of the species in question. In species exhibiting short cycles (e.g. rat and mouse) growth is limited to extensions of the duct system until pregnancy occurs. In species in which there is a long luteal phase of the cycle (e.g. dog) then considerable lobulo-alveolar growth may occur before pregnancy ensues (see reviews by Folley, 1952, 1956; Jacobsohn, 1961). In women some degree of proliferation and regression of alveolar tissues occurs during the menstrual cycle; a detailed description of the development of the human breast has been given by Dabelow (1957) and Bonser, Dossett and Jull (1961). In most species, however, it is only during pregnancy that extensive lobulo-alveolar growth occurs although growth may not be completed until the early stages of lactation (see Munford, 1964).

The postnatal phases of mammary growth are hormonally controlled but only in the rat and mouse have detailed analyses of the hormones concerned been made. In both these species a phase of rapid duct growth sets in some days before the onset of the first oestrus and continues until the ducts have reached their full adult extension. This phase of rapid growth is evoked by oestrogenic hormones from the ovaries. Studies on the stimulation of mammary growth in hypophysectomized-gonadectomized-adrenalectomized rats and mice have revealed that proliferation of the mammary duct system is dependent on the presence of pituitary growth hormone, oestrogen and adrenal corticoids while the stimulation of lobulo-alveolar growth requires the presence of two further hormones, progesterone and prolactin. Thus in the rat and mouse after the surgical removal of the pituitary, gonads and adrenals it is experimentally possible to induce full mammary growth similar to that observed in late pregnancy by administering prolactin, growth hormone, oestrogen, progesterone and adrenal corticoids. In these species hormones from the placenta probably participate in normal mammary growth during pregnancy as hormonal factors allied to prolactin and growth hormone have been detected in the placentae (see reviews by Lyons, 1958; Cowie and Folley, 1961 and Forsyth, 1967).

In the species so far studied the ovarian hormones have no mammogenic activity if the anterior pituitary and its hormones are absent and it is probable that the ovarian hormones exert their main mammogenic effects by causing the release of anterior-pituitary hormones. In some species (e.g. guinea-pig and rhesus monkey) the administration of oestrogen alone will induce considerable growth of normal lobulo-alveolar tissue while in others (e.g. goat) the alveoli tend to be abnormal in structure. In general both ovarian hormones seem necessary for full lobulo-alveolar growth to occur (see Folley, 1956).

Prolactin free from growth hormone activity has not yet been isolated from primate pituitaries and it is still uncertain whether such a hormone exists in primates. However, highly purified preparations of human and monkey pituitary growth hormone exhibit prolactin-like activity when tested in laboratory animals and this activity seems to be intrinsic to the growth hormone molecule. There has,

moreover, been isolated from the human placenta a substance, termed human placental lactogen, which also exhibits marked prolactin-like activities in test animals. It is thus probable that in primates pituitary growth hormones and endocrine substances from the placenta play an important role in mammary growth during pregnancy (see review by Forsyth, 1967).

Advances in our knowledge of the phases of mammary growth and of its regulatory hormonal mechanism have been slow because of the difficulties of accurately assessing mammary growth and of assaying the levels of the various mammogenic hormones in the blood. The overall size of the mamma or udder in the adolescent animal may provide no reliable indication of the amount of glandular tissue within it. As the parenchyma grows, however, it extends into an already existing pad (consisting mainly of fatty tissue in ruminants and of connective tissue in man) so that by late pregnancy and in lactation the fatty and connective tissues are largely replaced by mammary parenchyma; there is then a more satisfactory correlation between the volume of the mamma or udder and the parenchymatous tissue it contains. Measurements of the volume of the mamma or udder may therefore be useful in functional studies in the fully lactating gland (see Hytten, 1954; Linzell, 1966). Other clinical methods of assessing the degree of development of the mammary parenchyma include the assessing of the dimensions of the parenchyma by palpation, or by specialized radiographic techniques. As yet no clinical method is wholly satisfactory for detailed investigations of mammary growth (see review by Munford, 1964).

In the case of material obtained by biopsy or at autopsy a number of histometric methods exist which permit an accurate evaluation of the extent and morphological characteristics of mammary growth; unfortunately these tend to be tedious. In species such as the mouse, rat and rabbit, in which for part of its development the mammary gland is virtually a flat sheet of tissue, whole-mounts of the gland can be prepared and the area of the duct system measured. This area provides a useful index of growth especially if it is supplemented by studies on the complexity of the duct arborescence (based on counts of duct junctions) within the area. However, as soon as the ducts begin to grow in three dimensions, as occurs in these species during pregnancy and in other species before pregnancy, the above procedures are no longer applicable and other histometric methods must then be used whereby such parameters as the ratio of glandular non-glandular tissue, surface area of secretory tissue, or volume of glandular tissue can be obtained (see Munford, 1964).

Recently, certain biochemical procedures which are much less laborious have been introduced for assessing the numbers of the cells in the mammary gland and for indicating the functional state of the cells of the gland. The commonest of these is the determination of the deoxyribonucleic acid (DNA) content of the mammary gland as an index of the cell numbers. The DNA is concentrated mainly in the nucleus of the cell and it is widely believed that the amount of DNA in a nucleus is constant for the somatic tissues of a given species; thus changes in the total

DNA of an organ give an indication of changes in the total number of cells, i.e. an increase indicates true growth and a decrease reveals involution. Unfortunately it is still uncertain whether the DNA concentration in the nucleus is constant under all circumstances (see Munford, 1964, also Sod-Moriah and Schmidt, 1968) and so conclusions drawn from DNA estimations must be treated with some caution. Ribonucleic acid (RNA) which occurs in several forms mainly in the cytoplasm of cells is concerned with the synthesis of proteins including cellular enzymes, and the level of RNA: DNA may be used as an index of the secretory activity of the mammary cells.

While studies based on DNA and RNA estimations are in a number of species providing considerable information on the growth processes of the mammary gland far too few of these studies have included detailed comparisons of biochemical and structural changes and we would reaffirm the admonition given by Munford (1964) "It should perhaps be stressed that indices of structure and measures of biochemical changes are to be regarded not as alternatives, but rather as complementary methods of assessing the state of the gland in studies on mammary development".

Regarding the assay of mammogenic hormones in the blood it may be noted that methods of determining oestrogen and progesterone by techniques based on gas-liquid chromatography are becoming available (see Lipsett, 1965; Grant, 1967). Assays for prolactin, growth hormone and placental lactogen are at present the subject of much research activity (see review by Forsyth, 1967) and so the dearth of information about the blood levels of these hormones in relation to mammogenesis may soon be remedied.

While the post-natal phases of growth of the mammary gland during the sex cycles and pregnancy are essentially controlled by the hormonal changes associated with the phase of reproduction, mammogenesis may be influenced by external stimuli acting via the central nervous system on the secretory activity of the anterior pituitary (see also p. 430). There exist numerous reports on the induction of mammary growth and lactation in non-pregnant women arising from the repeated application of the suckling stimulus (see review by Foss and Short, 1950), while heifers and even ovariectomized virgin goats may be brought into milk production by regular milking (see Cowie, Knaggs, Tindal and Turvey, 1968). In some species external nervous stimuli may play an integral role in mammogenesis for it has been demonstrated that if pregnant rats are prevented from licking their nipples during pregnancy then full mammary development is not attained (Roth and Rosenblatt, 1968).

LACTATION

Lactation comprises two main phases: first the milk has to be secreted and stored within the mammary gland—the phase of *milk secretion*; secondly, the stored milk must be made available to the suckling as required—the phase of *milk removal*. The recognition of these phases is necessary for the proper understanding of the physiological processes involved in lactation.

Milk Secretion

Milk secretion comprises the processes by which the alveolar cells synthesize milk constituents from precursor substances derived from the blood and then pass or excrete these constituents into the lumen of the alveolus. The milk thus formed is stored within the alveoli and fine ducts and a portion of it may pass into the larger ducts, storage sinuses or cisterns depending on the architecture of the gland of the species under consideration. The composition of the milk can alter during its storage period since the milk remains in osmotic equilibrium with the blood flowing through the gland and exchanges of water and water-soluble constituents between the blood and milk may occur (see review by Rook and Wheelock, 1967).

Studies with the electron microscope have considerably clarified the mechanism of how the secretory products of the alveolar cells are excreted into the alveolus. The milk fat appears at the base of the cell as small droplets associated with the ergastoplasm, these droplets migrate towards the apex of the cell, increasing in size, until they lie under the cell membrane. The membrane becomes pushed out and envelops the droplet. As the protrusion proceeds, the membrane constricts behind the droplet and finally becomes pinched off; the droplet enveloped in cell membrane then falls free into the alveolar lumen.

The protein is synthesized in the ergastoplasm and appears as small granules within the Golgi vacuoles. The vacuoles move towards the apex of the cell and finally open into the alveolar lumen (see reviews by Mayer and Klein, 1961; Bargmann, 1964; also Hollmann, 1966).

Hormonal Control of Milk Secretion

There is no evidence that the activity of the mammary alveolar cells is in any way controlled by secretory nerves; indeed the mammary gland can be transplanted to another part of the body and will secrete milk normally as long as satisfactory vascular connexions with the general circulation are achieved (Linzell, 1963). The secretory activity of the mammary gland is regulated by the endocrine system and in particular by the hormones of the anterior pituitary. The first evidence of the active participation of anterior-pituitary hormones in the initiation of milk secretion or lactogenesis was obtained by Stricker and Grueter in 1928 when they observed that injections of anterior-pituitary extract induced copious milk secretion in the mammary glands of pseudopregnant rabbits (see review by Stricker, 1951, and also Fig. 2). In 1933 Riddle and his colleagues showed that the lactogenic effects of pituitary extracts were associated with the principle present in the extracts which induced growth of the crop gland when injected into pigeons and doves. This response, the now classical "pigeon-crop" test for prolactin, greatly facilitated the preparation of prolactin in a highly purified form—the first of the anterior-pituitary hormones to be so obtained. While prolactin gave dramatic lactogenic responses in pseudopregnant rabbits it soon became evident that in some other species its lactogenic effects were less marked and attempts to use it clinically for lactational failures in women were not successful. From experimental studies, such as those of Azimov and Krouze and of Folley and Young on cows, it became clear that the ability of prolactin to induce and maintain milk secretion was dependent on the presence of other anterior-pituitary hormones and Folley and Young in 1941 put forward the concept of an anterior-pituitary lactogenic complex of hormones of which prolactin and adrenocorticotrophin were important components. Evidence soon accrued that another component of the complex was growth hormone (see reviews by Folley, 1952, 1956; Cowie, 1966). As in studies on mammary growth the analysis of the hormones concerned in lactogenesis and the maintenance of lactation are best conducted in hypophysectomized animals to avoid the complicating factor of the endogenous anterior-pituitary hormones. Lyons and his colleagues (see Lyons, 1958) using hypophysectomized-adrenalectomized-ovariectomized rats demonstrated that lactogenesis in the rat required the presence of prolactin and adrenal corticoids. Similar observations have been made on mice (Nandi, 1959). Subsequent studies on the maintenance of milk secretion in rats hypophysectomized during lactation showed that prolactin and adrenal corticoids maintained milk secretion although at a sub-normal level (see review by Cowie, 1966). In hypophysectomized goats, prolactin + growth hormone + adrenal corticoids + thyroid hormone are necessary to maintain full lactation, prolactin alone giving a negligible response (see review by Cowie, 1966). Recent studies in this laboratory (Cowie *et al.* 1969) indicate that prolactin alone will restore milk yields in rabbits hypophysectomized during lactation. Similar studies on other species are desirable but the observations to date suggest that considerable differences may occur in the constitution of the anterior-pituitary hormone complexes concerned in the maintenance of milk secretion, or perhaps rather that the relative importance of the various components differs in different species. Although we have just noted that prolactin alone will restore lactation in the hypophysectomized rabbit it is most probable that in the rabbit other anterior pituitary hormones normally participate in the regulation of mammary function. Thus, while prolactin alone will induce lactogenesis in the adrenalectomized pseudopregnant rabbit, adrenal corticoids or adrenocorticotrophin can, in the absence of exogenous prolactin, induce lactogenesis in the pregnant or pseudopregnant rabbit with intact pituitary (Talwalker, Nicoll and Meites, 1961; Chadwick and Folley, 1962).

As noted above (p. 425) pure prolactin has not so far been isolated from primate pituitaries but primate growth hormone is highly lactogenic in animals and it seems that this activity is intrinsic to the growth hormone molecule. The pigeon-crop assay is not a wholly reliable method of assessing the lactogenic potency of primate material since many samples of primate growth hormone may exhibit low activity in the pigeon assay but be highly lactogenic when tested in rabbits (see Fig. 2) and monkeys and *in vitro* in mouse mammary-gland organ cultures (non-primate growth hormone is inactive both in the pigeon-crop assay and in the pseudopregnant rabbit assays although it has prolactin-like effects in some strains of mice) (see review by Forsyth, 1967). Growth hormone in man may therefore play an important role in the initiation and maintenance of milk secretion. Since it is now clear that the growth hormones and prolactins of different species may exhibit biological species specificities and even chemical differences the lack of response in lactating women to prolactin of animal origin as observed in early clinical studies is now explicable. Moreover, in view of immunity reactions such clinical use of prolactins of animal origin could well be dangerous.

In view of the complexities of the hormonal control of milk secretion in the various species it is understandable that the hormonal mechanism responsible for the initiation of milk secretion at parturition remains obscure but reductions in the levels in the blood of oestrogens and progesterone, particularly the latter, associated with adequate or increased levels of prolactin and adrenal corticoids may favour the onset of milk secretion. Whether identical hormone combinations are concerned in the maintenance of milk secretion as in its initiation is still uncertain. The hormonal stimulation of milk secretion—galactopoiesis (although some workers use this term to include the maintenance of milk secretion)—has been studied mainly in the cow in which bovine growth hormone and the thyroid hormones are galactopoietic agents, prolactin being ineffective—observations which suggest that the decline in lactation in the cow is associated with lowered levels of growth hormone and thyroid hormones in the blood and not with a deficiency of prolactin (see Folley, 1956; Meites, 1961).

Oestrogen and combinations of oestrogen and progesterone have been used clinically for many years for the suppression of unwanted lactation in women. Since in such cases the suckling stimulus (see page 430) is also removed, the mode of action of the hormones is uncertain, and may in part be a local action on the breast depressing secretory activity (see review by Barnes, 1947; also papers by Toaff and Jewelewicz, 1963; MacDonald and O'Driscoll, 1965; Hodge, 1967). A possible relationship between such therapy and puerperal thromboembolism requires further study (Daniel, Campbell and Turnbull, 1967).

Oral contraceptives currently available contain oestrogenic and progestogenic substances and there is evidence that their use by nursing women may impair lactation. This effect, however, appears to be dose-dependent and with the lower dosage rates now in use may not present much of a problem particularly if the use of the oral contraceptives is postponed until lactation is established (see Kaern, 1967).

Milk Removal

Milk having been secreted is stored in the alveoli, ducts and cisterns or sinuses. Only the portion in the large ducts, sinuses or cisterns (depending on the species) is immediately available to the suckling; the milk in the alveoli and smaller ducts, which may represent the greater portion, is retained there by physical forces and to become available it must be transferred or ejected from the alveoli into the larger ducts or sinuses. To effect this ejection of milk from the alveoli a complex reflex must occur whereby the alveoli are squeezed by the contraction of a network of

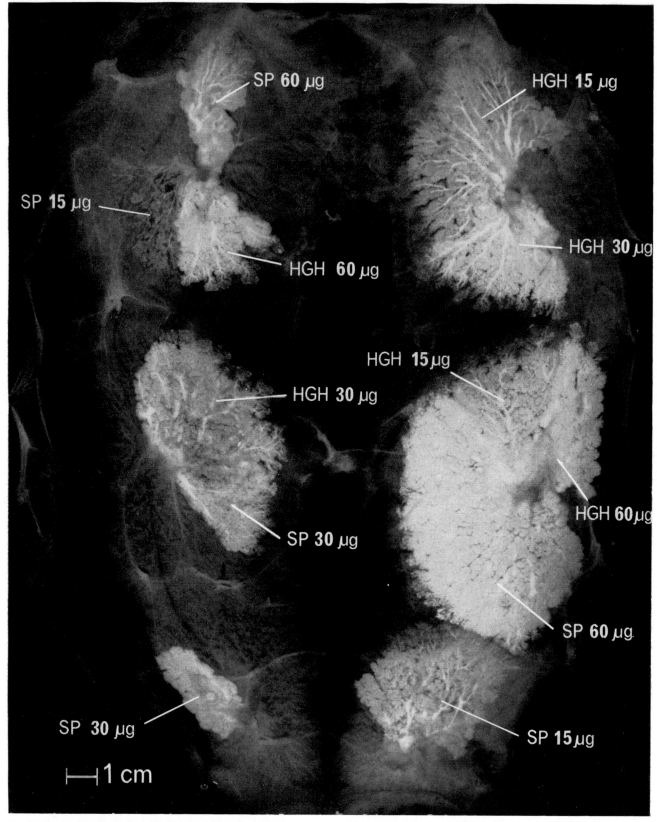

Fig. 2. The freshly dissected mammary glands of a pseudopregnant rabbit showing the lactational responses in the sectors which 7 days previously had received injections of sheep prolactin (SP), assaying 21 i.u. per mg., or human growth hormone (HGH) in doses of 15, 30 or 60 μg (in 0·3 ml. saline) into the mammary duct draining the respective sector. The milk is clearly visible in the injected sectors and both hormones have similar lactogenic potencies. The non-injected sectors contain no milk and their lobulo-alveolar tissue shows only faintly. (Photograph by courtesy of Dr. Isabel A. Forsyth.)

cells—the myoepithelial cells—which overlie them; the milk within the alveoli is thus forced into the duct system and sinuses causing a considerable rise in the pressure of milk within them so that in some instances a stream of milk may be forced through the nipple or teat. This reflex rise in intramammary pressure, now generally termed the milk-ejection reflex, has long been recognized in lactating women and known as the "draught"—this reflex is described in great detail by Waller (1938)—but only within the last few decades has its physiological importance been appreciated and an understanding of its underlying mechanism been achieved. The sudden increase in the tenseness

discussed here (see reviews by Cowie and Folley, 1961; Cross, 1961; Benson and Fitzpatrick, 1966). Only recently, however, has a reliable method of assaying oxytocin in blood become available and studies have been carried out in the cow, goat and sow (Folley and Knaggs, 1966).

There have been numerous clinical studies on the pressure changes within the breast during suckling and the pressure changes in response to injections, inhalations and sublingual administration of oxytocin (see Fig. 3)—reference to these will be found in the reviews by Denamur (1965) and Folley and Knaggs (1970).

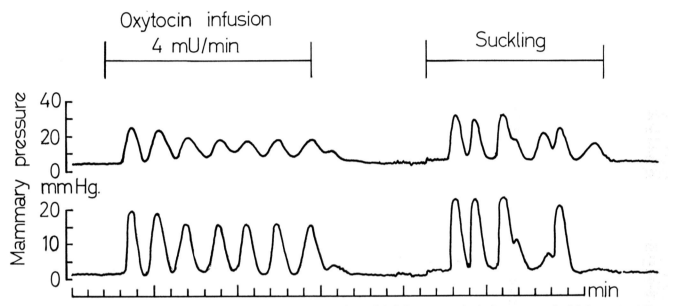

FIG. 3. Intramammary pressure changes recorded simultaneously from two ducts of the left mammary gland of a woman at the 6th day postpartum. The intravenous infusion of oxytocin (4 mu per minute) produced rhythmical increases in pressure which were similar to those recorded when the baby suckled the right breast. These rhythmical increases are characteristic of certain species. (From Y. Sica-Blanco, C. Mendez-Bauer, N. Sala, H. M. Cabot and R. Caldeyro-Barcia (1959), *Archivos de Ginicologia y Obstetricia*, **17**, 63.)

of the gland resulting from the increased milk pressure within the gland was until the mid-twenties erroneously believed to be due to a very active secretion of milk in response to the stimulus of suckling. The secretion of milk, however, progresses steadily between the acts of suckling or milking and the sudden increase in milk pressure is due, not to rapid secretion of milk but, as stated above, to the ejection of the milk stored in the alveoli and fine ducts. In response to the suckling or milking stimulus, or to stimuli the mother has come to associate with these acts, oxytocin is released from the posterior lobe of the pituitary into the blood stream and on reaching the mammary gland it causes the myoepithelial cells to contract. The afferent pathway of the milk-ejection reflex is neural, the efferent is hormonal. The delay involved in the transport of oxytocin in the blood is responsible for the long latent period of the reflex—about half a minute.

The classical experiments of Gaines in 1915, Turner and Slaughter in 1930, Ely and Petersen in 1941 which first suggested the true nature of the physiological mechanism and the role of the posterior-pituitary gland in milk ejection have been frequently reviewed and need not be

In some species reflex alterations in the tonus of the mammary ducts which facilitate the transfer of milk along the duct system are said to occur. These alterations in tonus may arise from stimulation of baroceptors within the ducts or from the suckling stimulus. These are considered to be purely neural segmental reflexes with short latent periods (see Zaks, 1962).

In the majority of species so far investigated, including man, unless the milk-ejection reflex occurs the suckling, or milker, will obtain only a fraction of the milk stored within the gland, exceptions being the goat and sheep in which the udder may be milked out in the complete absence of the milk-ejection reflex. This peculiarity of goats and sheep may be associated with the architecture of the gland in these species which possibly permits more ready drainage of the milk from the alveoli into the cisterns.

The continued ineffective removal of the milk from an actively secreting gland because of the repeated failure of the milk-ejection reflex may lead eventually to an inhibition of the secretory process bringing lactation to an end with the ensuing involution of the mammary parenchyma.

The importance of a quiet regular routine at milking

times in the cow-shed has long been recognized as essential for the efficient milking of cows, but the necessity for ensuring as far as possible for the human mother freedom from pain, fear and embarrassment at the time when she is nursing her baby has not always been widely understood. Thanks, however, to the studies of Waller, Isbister, Gunther and the Newtons the importance of the milk-ejection reflex in human lactation has been demonstrated and proper consideration can now be given to factors, such as emotional stress and pain, which by inhibiting the establishment of the reflex may well cause a failure of the lactation (see reviews by Newton, 1961; Newton and Newton, 1962). The implication, by some writers, that the "draught" reflex in women was only recognized, and so termed, some thirty years ago is quite incorrect. An excellent description of the "draught" was given by Sir Astley Cooper (1840) over a century ago, and he recognized, moreover, that the reflex (in terms introduced by Pavlov some 60 years later) could become "conditioned" although he erred in assuming that a rapid *secretion* of milk was involved: "The secretion of milk may be said to be constant or occasional; by the first, the milk tubes and reservoirs are *constantly* supplied by means of a slow and continued production of fluid, so that the milk is thus, in some degree, prepared for the child. By the *occasional* is to be understood that secretion which is called by mothers and nurses, the *draught* of the breast, by which is meant a sudden rush of blood to the gland, during which the milk is so abundantly secreted, that if the nipple be not immediately caught by the child, the milk escapes from it, and the child when it receives the nipple is almost choked by the rapid and abundant flow of the fluid; if it lets go its hold, the milk spirts into the infant's eyes.

— Even the sight of the child will produce this draught . . . as the thought or sight of food occasions an abundant secretion of the saliva. The draught is also greatly increased by the child pressing the breast with its little hands, by its drawing out the nipples by its tongue, lips and gums, and by the pressure of its head against the breast".

Suckling Stimulus

The suckling stimulus controls mammary function in two main ways: first by regulating, via the hypothalamus, the secretory activity of the anterior pituitary with regard to the hormones concerned in milk secretion; secondly by bringing about the release from the posterior pituitary of the oxytocin required for milk ejection.

It is probable, although there is little or no evidence for or against the view, that the afferent nervous pathway for both these controls is common for the greater part of its length. Studies have indicated that in the spinal cord the path is ipselateral but only in the guinea-pig has the pathway in the brain been studied. In this species it appears to ascend by the spinothalamic system and continues rostrally to relay with the medial and ventral thalamus, the dorsal longitudinal fasciculus and the medial forebrain bundle (see Tindal, Knaggs and Turvey, 1967). Control of the hormonal activity of the anterior pituitary is effected by the release of neurohumoral transmitter substances from the hypothalamus (see review by

Guillemin, 1967; also Schally *et al.*, 1967). These substances are transmitted to the anterior pituitary by a specialized vascular system in the pituitary stalk—the hypophysial portal system—where they stimulate the secretion of the trophic hormones into the blood, with the exception of prolactin whose release is inhibited by its hypothalamic factor. Thus to bring about the secretion of prolactin it is necessary to depress the prolactin inhibitory activity of the hypothalamus. It has, moreover, been shown that the suckling stimulus depresses the prolactin-inhibiting activity in the hypothalamus. Oestrogen and certain derivatives of phenothiazine (e.g. chlorpromazine) and rauwolfia alkaloids (e.g. reserpine) will also depress the prolactin-inhibiting activity of the hypothalamus, an action that may well explain the occasional occurrence of milk secretion in patients being given such drugs for psychotherapeutic reasons (see review by Meites, 1966; also Lampe II, 1967). While the suckling stimulus is normally the principal factor controlling the maintenance of lactation there may in some species be secondary control mechanisms of a wholly humoral nature which can maintain production of the necessary hormone complexes from the anterior pituitary since it is known that lactation will continue in the goat in the complete absence of any nervous connexions between the mammary gland and the CNS (see review by Cowie and Tindal, 1965).

The control of posterior-pituitary function by the suckling stimulus is effected via the supraoptic and paraventricular nuclei of the hypothalamus where oxytocin is synthesized. From these nuclei the hormone—attached to a "carrier protein"—passes down the axons of the cells as a neurosecretion to be stored in the posterior lobe of the pituitary (see review by Denamur, 1965). The regular application of the suckling stimulus is thus, in most species, of prime importance in the maintenance of lactation, since it controls and integrates the functioning of the anterior and posterior lobes of the pituitary.

In conclusion, readers may well question the relevancy of animal studies to the problem of lactation in man and one must indeed be cautious in assuming precise identity of physiological mechanisms even between closely related species. We would, however, give two brief but relevant quotations from a recent World Health Organization Technical Report (1965) on the physiology of lactation:

". . . human lactation cannot be considered in isolation, partly because the evolutionary and comparative aspects are illuminating as well as fascinating and partly because the neural and endocrinological background has necessarily been analysed mainly by experiments on laboratory and farm animals".

"The chain of events leading to milk secretion and milk ejection has been less intensively studied in man than in other animals, but what evidence there is suggests no important difference. As in the animals, both milk secretion and ejection are in part controlled by the hypothalamus and are, through it, subject to influences from higher centres; but in man higher centres of nervous activity play a much larger role and, as a result, psychological influences on lactation are conspicuous".

Peculiar to the human species is the problem of the decline of breast feeding particularly in affluent societies. The rapidity of this decline over the last few decades strongly suggests that sociological factors are concerned. This problem is discussed in the above W.H.O. Technical Report which urges that studies be carried out on the effects of socio-economic conditions on breast-feeding patterns of different population groups and on the psychophysiological mechanisms involved (see also Newton and Newton, 1967).

REFERENCES

Bargmann, W. (1964), "Secretion and 'let-down' of Milk," *German Medical Monthly*, **9**, 309.

Barnes, J. (1947), "Hormonal Inhibition of Lactation with Special Reference to Man," *British Medical Bulletin*, **5**, 167.

Benson, G. K. and Fitzpatrick, R. J. (1966), "The Neurohypophysis and the Mammary Gland," in *The Pituitary Gland*, Vol. 3, p. 414. Eds. G. W. Harris and B. T. Donovan. London: Butterworths.

Bonser, G. M., Dossett, J. A. and Jull, J. W. (1961), *Human and Experimental Breast Cancer*, p. 96. London: Pitman Medical Publishing Co.

Chadwick, A. and Folley, S. J. (1962), "Lactogenesis in Pseudopregnant Rabbits treated with ACTH," *Journal of Endocrinology*, **24**, xi.

Cooper, Sir Astley (1840), *On the Anatomy of the Breast*, p. 129. London: Longman, Orme, Green, Brown and Longmans.

Cowie, A. T. (1966), "Anterior Pituitary Function in Lactation," in *The Pituitary Gland*, Vol. 2, p. 412. Eds. G. W. Harris and B. T. Donovan. London: Butterworths.

Cowie, A. T. and Folley, S. J. (1961), "The Mammary Gland and Lactation," in *Sex and Internal Secretions*, 3rd edition, Vol. 1, p. 590. Ed. W. C. Young. Baltimore: Williams and Wilkins Co.

Cowie, A. T., Hartmann, P. E. and Turvey, A. (1969): The Maintenance of Lactation in the Rabbit after Hypophysectomy. *Journal of Endocrinology*, **43**, 651.

Cowie, A. T., Knaggs, G. S., Tindal, J. S. and Turvey, A. (1968), "The Milking Stimulus and Mammary Growth in the Goat," *Journal of Endocrinology*, **40**, 243.

Cowie, A. T. and Tindal, J. S. (1965), "Some Aspects of the Neuroendocrine Control of Lactation," *Proceedings of the Second International Congress of Endocrinology*, part 1, p. 646. Amsterdam: Excerpta Medica Foundation.

Cross, B. A. (1961), "Neural Control of Lactation," in *Milk: the Mammary Gland and its Secretion*, Vol. 1, p. 229. Eds. S. K. Kon and A. T. Cowie. New York and London: Academic Press.

Dabelow, A. (1957), "Die Milchdrüse," in *Handbuch der mikroskopischen Anatomie des Menschen*, Vol. 3, part 3, p. 277. Eds. W. von Möllendorf and W. Bargmann. Berlin, Göttingen and Heidelberg: Springer Verlag.

Daniel, D. G., Campbell, H. and Turnbull, A. C. (1967), "Puerperal Thromboembolism and Suppression of Lactation," *Lancet*, **ii**, 287.

Denamur, R. (1965), "The Hypothalamo-neurohypophysial System and the Milk-ejection Reflex," *Dairy Science Abstracts*, **27**, 193 and 263.

Folley, S. J. (1952), "Lactation," in Marshall's *Physiology of Reproduction*, 3rd edition, Vol. 2, p. 525. Ed. A. S. Parkes. London: Longmans, Green and Co.

Folley, S. J. (1956), *The Physiology and Biochemistry of Lactation*. Edinburgh and London: Oliver and Boyd.

Folley, S. J. and Knaggs, G. S. (1966), "Milk-ejection Activity (oxytocin) in the External Jugular Vein Blood of the Cow, Goat and Sow, in Relation to the Stimulus of Milking or Suckling," *Journal of Endocrinology*, **34**, 197.

Folley, S. J. and Knaggs, G. S. (1970), "Physiological and Pharmacological Effects of Neurohypophysial Hormones. (c) Mammary Action," in the *International Encyclopedia of Pharmacology and Therapeutics*, Section 41, Chap. 8, p. 295. Ed. H. Heller. Oxford: Pergamon Press.

Forsyth, I. A. (1967), "Prolactin and Placental Lactogens," in *Hormones in Blood*, 2nd edition, Vol. 1, p. 233. Eds. C. H. Gray and A. L. Bacharach. New York and London: Academic Press.

Foss, G. F. and Short, D. (1950), "Abnormal Lactation," *Journal of Obstetrics and Gynæcology of the British Commonwealth*, **58**, 35.

Grant, J. K., editor (1967), "Gas Liquid Chromatography of Steroids," *Memoirs of the Society for Endocrinology, No. 16*, Cambridge University Press.

Guillemin, R. (1967), "The Adenohypophysis and its Hypothalamic Control," *Annual Review of Physiology*, **29**, 313.

Hodge, C. (1967), "Suppression of Lactation by Stilboestrol," *Lancet*, **ii**, 286.

Hollmann, K. H. (1966), "Sur des aspects particuliers des protéines élaborées dans la glande mammaire. Etude au microscope électronique chez la lapine en lactation," *Zeitschrift für Zellforschung*, **69**, 395.

Hytten, F. E. (1954), "Clinical and Chemical Studies in Human Lactation. VI. The Functional Capacity of the Breast," *British Medical Journal*, **i**, 912.

Jacobsohn, D. (1961), "Hormonal Regulation of Mammary Gland Growth," in *Milk: the Mammary Gland and its Secretion*, Vol. 1, p. 127. Eds. S. K. Kon and A. T. Cowie. New York and London: Academic Press.

Jean, Ch. and Delost, P. (1965), "Oestrogènes et malformations congénitales experimentales de la morphogenèse mammaire," *Comptes rendus des séances de la Société de Biologie, Paris*, **159**, 2357.

Kaern, T. (1967), "Effect of an Oral Contraceptive immediately Post Partum on Initiation of Lactation," *British Medical Journal*, **ii**, 644.

Lampe II, W. T. (1967), "Lactation following Psychotropic Agents," *Metabolism: Clinical and Experimental*, **16**, 257.

Lipsett, M. B., editor (1965), *Gas Chromatography of Steroids in Biological Fluids*. New York: Plenum Press.

Linzell, J. L. (1963), "Some effects of Denervating and Transplanting Mammary Glands," *Quarterly Journal of Experimental Physiology*, **48**, 34.

Linzell, J. L. (1966), "Measurement of Udder Volume in Live Goats as an Index of Mammary Growth and Function," *Journal of Dairy Science*, **49**, 307.

Lyons, W. R. (1958), "Hormonal Synergism in Mammary Growth," *Proceedings of the Royal Society*, B, **149**, 303.

MacDonald, D. and O'Driscoll, K. (1965), "Suppression of Lactation: a Double-blind Trial," *Lancet*, **ii**, 623.

Mayer, G. and Klein, M. (1961), "Histology and Cytology of the Mammary Glands," in *Milk: the Mammary Gland and its Secretion*, Vol. 1, p. 47. Eds. S. K. Kon and A. T. Cowie. New York and London: Academic Press.

Meites, J. (1961), "Farm Animals: Hormonal Induction of Lactation and Galactopoiesis," in *Milk: the Mammary Gland and its Secretion*, Vol. 1, p. 321. Eds. S. K. Kon and A. T. Cowie. New York and London: Academic Press.

Meites, J. (1966), "Control of Mammary Growth and Lactation," in *Neuroendocrinology*, Vol. 1, p. 669. Eds. L. Martini and W. F. Ganong. New York and London: Academic Press.

Munford, R. E. (1964), "A Review of Anatomical and Biochemical Changes in the Mammary Gland with particular reference to Quantitative Methods of Assessing Mammary Development," *Dairy Science Abstracts*, **26**, 293.

Nandi, S. (1959), "Hormonal Control of Mammogenesis and Lactogenesis in the C3H/HeCrgl Mouse," *University of California Publications in Zoology*, **65**, 1.

Neumann, F. and Elger, W. (1966), "The Effect of the Anti-androgen 1, 2α-methylene-6-chloro-$\Delta^{4,6}$-pregnadiene-17α-ol-3,20-dione-17α-acetate (Cyproterone acetate) on the Development of the Mammary Glands of Male Fœtal Rats," *Journal of Endocrinology*, **36**, 347.

Newton, M. (1961), "Human Lactation," in *Milk: the Mammary Gland and its Secretion*, Vol. 1, p. 281. Eds. S. K. Kon and A. T. Cowie. New York and London: Academic Press.

Newton, M. and Newton, N. (1962), "The Normal Course and Management of Lactation," *Clinical Obstetrics and Gynecology*, **5**, 44.

Newton, N. and Newton, M. (1967), "Psychologic Aspects of Lactation," *New England Journal of Medicine*, **277**, 1179.

Raynaud, A. (1961), "Morphogenesis of the Mammary Gland," in *Milk: the Mammary Gland and its Secretion*, Vol. 1, p. 3. Eds. S. K. Kon and A. T. Cowie. New York and London: Academic Press.

Rook, J. A. F. and Wheelock, J. V. (1967), "The Secretion of Water and of Water-soluble Constituents in Milk," *Journal of Dairy Research*, **34**, 273.

Roth, L. L. and Rosenblatt, J. S. (1968), "Self-licking and Mammary development during pregnancy in the rat," *Journal of Endocrinology*, **42**, 263.

Schally, A. V., Müller, E. E., Arimura, A., Bowers, C. Y., Saito, T., Redding, T. W., Sawano, S. and Pizzolato, P. (1967), "Releasing Factors in Human Hypothalamic and Neurohypophysial Extracts," *Journal of Clinical Endocrinology and Metabolism*, **27**, 755.

Sod-Moriah, U. A. and Schmidt, G. H. (1968), "Deoxyribonucleic Acid Content and Proliferative Activity of Rabbit Mammary Gland Epithelial Cells," *Experimental Cell Research*, **49**, 584.

Stricker, P. (1951), "Comment fut découverte l'existence d'une hormone lactogène dans le lobe antérieur de l'hypophyse," *Colloques Internationaux du Centre National de la Recherche Scientifique*, No. 32, "*Méchanismes Physiologiques de la Sécrétion Lactée*," p. 15.

Talwalker, P. K., Nicoll, C. S. and Meites, J. (1961), "Induction of Mammary Secretion in Pregnant Rats and Rabbits by Hydrocortisone Acetate," *Endocrinology*, **69**, 802.

Tindal, J. S., Knaggs, G. S. and Turvey, A. (1967), "The Afferent Path of the Milk-ejection Reflex in the Brain of the Guinea-pig," *Journal of Endocrinology*, **38**, 337.

Toaff, R. and Jewelewicz, R. (1963), "Inhibition of Lactogenesis by Combined Oral Progestogens and Oestrogens," *Lancet*, **ii**, 322.

Waller, H. (1938), *Clinical Studies in Lactation*. London and Toronto: Heinemann Ltd.

World Health Organization Technical Report Series (1965) no. 305. *Physiology of Lactation*. Geneva: W.H.O.

Zaks, M. G. (1962), *The Motor Apparatus of the Mammary Gland*. Edinburgh and London: Oliver and Boyd.

SECTION VIII

ORGAN FUNCTION

1. RENAL FUNCTION

G. M. BERLYNE

In this chapter renal function will be discussed so that the reader will be able to understand more readily the changes in renal physiology in normal and pathological states in pregnancy and the puerperium, and in the common renal tract diseases affecting women particularly. This chapter will be divided into the four functional divisions of the nephron—the functional circulation, the glomerulus, the proximal tubule and the distal tubule.

FUNCTIONAL CIRCULATION

Renal Blood Flow

In the normal adult the renal blood flow (RBF) is 1·0–1·2 litres/min., about 90 per cent of the flow going to the cortex and only 10 per cent to the medulla where it circulates through the vasa recta. The relative low blood supply of the medulla compared with the cortex is still fifteen times greater per gm. of tissue than that of resting muscle. RBF is controlled by "autoregulation" so that RBF remains constant in spite of changes in blood pressure above 90 mm. Hg. RBF is increased in normal pregnancy.

Filtration Fraction

(FF) is the ratio $\dfrac{GFR}{RPF}$ where RPF is renal plasma flow and GFR is glomerular filtration rate. Normally this is 15–20 per cent in man, but it varies in many abnormal conditions, and is reduced in hæmorrhagic shock due to the fall in GFR being proportionately greater than the fall in RBF. This may be due to intense vasoconstriction of the afferent arterioles. Blood urea level is a useful clinical measurement of renal function, provided the patient is on a normal protein intake i.e. 80–100 G./day; the blood urea will rise above the upper limit of normal (45 mg./100 ml.) (equivalent to blood urea nitrogen of 20 mg./100 ml.) when GFR falls to 25–30 ml./minute. If protein intake is reduced to very low figures (i.e. 18G./day as on the Giordano-Giovannetti diet), then the blood urea level will remain normal with GFR as low as 3 ml./min. (Shaw *et al.*, 1965).

GLOMERULUS

The normal human glomerular capillaries act as a semipermeable membrane which ultra-filters the plasma circulating through them, leaving a virtually protein-free ultrafiltrate in Bowman's space. The amount of plasma filtered through the glomeruli per minute is termed the glomerular filtration rate or GFR. The normal GFR in women is lower than that in men, when expressed per 1·73 sq. metres of body surface area, being about 120 ml./min./1·73 sq. metres in women compared to 125 ml./min./1·73 sq. metres in men.

Glomerular filtration rate (GFR) can be measured by any substance which has ideally the following attributes:

1. Completely filtered through the glomerular capillaries. This limits the molecular size of the substance to considerably less than that of hæmoglobin, and in practice molecular weights of 5,000 or less are used. Recent measurement has shown the pore size in the capillaries to be 75–100 Ångstrom units.

2. The substance should not be protein-bound as the filterable plasma concentration of the substance cannot then be readily determined.

3. The substance must not be reabsorbed or secreted by the renal tubules.

4. It should be easy to estimate accurately either chemically or physically.

5. Its renal clearance should be unaffected by the plasma level of the substance. It is necessary to define renal clearance of any substance, which is the amount of any substance completely cleared from the plasma by the kidneys in one minute. It is expressed as

$$Cx = \frac{UxV}{Px} \text{ where } \begin{cases} Cx = \text{clearance of X in ml./minute.} \\ Ux = \text{urine concentration in mg./} \\ \quad\ \ 100 \text{ ml.} \\ V \ \ = \text{urine volume ml./min.} \\ Px = \text{plasma concentration of X} \\ \quad\ \ \text{in mg./100 ml.} \end{cases}$$

When a substance is neither reabsorbed nor secreted by the renal tubules its clearance is equivalent to the glomerular filtration rate, (GFR) so

$$GFR = \frac{UV}{P} \text{ where } \begin{cases} U \ = \text{urine concentration in mg./} \\ \quad\ 100 \text{ ml.} \\ V \ = \text{urine volume in ml./min.} \end{cases}$$

6. It should not require constant rate infusion intravenously. In common practice endogenous creatinine is a very useful index of glomerular function and in many patients creatinine clearance is identical with GFR; nevertheless in some patients creatinine is secreted by the tubules, so it should be used with reservation. Urea clearance is less than GFR except in advanced renal failure, because of reabsorption of urea by the renal tubules. The usual exogenous substances used in determination of glomerular filtration are (1) inulin (or its synthetic equivalent "Inutest" a polymer of fructose). Its disadvantage is that it is tedious to estimate chemically,

but nevertheless it is the most reliable method of G.F.R. measurement. (2) ^{57}Co labelled cyanocobalamine (Nelp *et al.*, 1964) can be readily measured accurately but cyanocobalamine is protein-bound in part and estimation of protein binding is tedious. (3) ^{131}I or ^{127}I labelled hyapaque is a convenient method of measuring GFR (Blaufox *et al.*, 1963): measurement is simple and accurate as in all radioactive methods. (4) ^{51}Cr labelled ethylene diamine tetracetate (EDTA). This method was recently introduced by Garnett *et al.* (1967). It is easy to measure accurately and is not protein bound.

The driving force of glomerular filtration is the hydrodynamic force of blood pressure on the glomerular capillaries. When the blood pressure falls to below 60 mm. Hg. the hydrostatic pressure in the glomerular capillaries is unable to overcome the oncotic pressure of the plasma* proteins and the hydrostatic pressure in Bowman's space, so that filtration ceases. The patient becomes anuric. If the patient has had a massive haemorrhage (such as a post-partum haemorrhage) causing the fall in blood pressure, there may be a reduction in renal blood flow due to splanchnic vasoconstriction, which may be associated with a further fall of renal blood flow resulting in renal anoxia with acute tubular necrosis, or cortical necrosis if the anoxia is more severe.

The control of GFR is maintained by the relative tone of the afferent and efferent glomerular arterioles. Efferent arteriolar constriction causes an increase in mean glomerular pressure; afferent arteriolar constriction causes a fall in mean glomerular pressure. GFR increases up to 50 per cent from the second month of pregnancy until two weeks before term. RBF increases by 25 per cent in the middle trimester and falls to normal values in the last trimester. FF is increased throughout the pregnancy. In pre-eclamptic toxaemia there is a fall in GFR, RBF and FF.

Serum creatinine levels are unaffected by the amount of dietary protein, and so are useful as an indication of reduction in GFR. In general serum creatinine remains below 2·0 mg./100 ml. until GFR has fallen to 25–30 ml./minute, rising slowly after this to values of 20–30 mg./100 ml. with a GFR of 3·0–1·5 ml./min. respectively. The drawback to relying on serum creatinine values is caused by the increasing degree of overall tubular secretion of creatinine as renal failure progresses; in many patients with nephrotic syndrome or massive proteinuria, the serum creatinine value likewise is lower than would be expected with the corresponding level of GFR due to overall tubular secretion of creatinine (Berlyne *et al.*, 1964). Thus serum creatinine levels are of limited use in estimating the GFR clinically.

Renal plasma flow is measured biochemically by estimating the renal clearance of paraminohippurate (PAH) at low concentrations (2 mg./100 ml.). This is a simple biochemical test and is dependent on the renal clearance of PAH in the renal venous effluent blood in the normal, so that C_{PAH} equals RPF. RPF is more readily estimated by clearance of ^{127}I or ^{131}I hippuran, which is readily counted accurately. When the PAH concentration is

elevated to about 80 mg./100 ml. clearance of PAH is a method of measuring TmPAH, providing the filtered load of PAH is known by estimation of GFR.

$$TmPAH = UV_{PAH} - \text{Filtered load of PAH}$$

$$TmPAH = \text{Tubular maximum of PAH secretion (mg./min.).}$$

$$UVPAH = \text{excretion of PAH (mg./min.)}$$

where

$$\text{Filtered load} = GFR \times \text{Plasma PAH concentration.}$$

Tubular Function

Tubular function is roughly divisible into proximal and distal tubular function, although many tubular functions take place in both proximal and distal tubules. Nevertheless many functions are best dealt with by separating proximal distal tubular functions, including the loop of Henle in the distal tubule.

PROXIMAL TUBULE

The main functions of the proximal tubule are:

1. Iso-osmotic Reabsorption of Sodium and Water.

Over 80 per cent of the filtered sodium and water are reabsorbed proximally. Four fifths of the oxygen consumption of the mammalian kidney is attributed to the process of reabsorption of sodium, a process of major importance in the maintenance of a constant volume and composition of extracellular fluid. Sodium ions have been shown to be absorbed against an electrochemical gradient; this reabsorption is an active, energy consuming process and the energy is supplied by aerobic oxidation involving high energy phosphate bonds. Proximal tubular sodium reabsorption can be partially inhibited by frusemide and possibly by other diuretics. Water reabsorption is a passive process in the proximal tubule, the fluid at the end of the proximal tubule being iso-osmotic with plasma. Water accompanies the sodium and chloride ions out of the tubular lumen. The proximal tubular walls are freely permeable to the passage of water into and out of the tubular lumen.

2. Potassium Reabsorption.

likewise occurs in the proximal tubule, about 80 per cent of the filtered potassium being removed in this way. Like sodium reabsorption, proximal tubular reabsorption of potassium is an active process, against an electrochemical gradient.

3. Bicarbonate Reabsorption.

The mechanism of proximal tubular handling of bicarbonate is carried out in a complex manner. Hydrogen ions, produced from carbonic acid in the proximal tubular cells under the influence of carbonic anhydrase, diffuse into the lumen of the proximal tubule and combine with

---

* Plasma protein oncotic pressure is the osmotic pressure exerted by Colloids.

bicarbonate ions in the glomerular filtrate to produce carbonic acid which dissociates into carbon dioxide

$$H^+ + HCO_3^- \leftrightarrows H_2CO_3 \rightleftarrows CO_2 + H_2O$$

and water. The CO_2 freely diffuses back into the tubular cells and recombines with water to form hydrogen ions and bicarbonate ions *inside* the cells. The hydrogen ions are exchanged for sodium coming into the cell from the tubular lumen, and the bicarbonate ions pass through the basal region of the cell with sodium ion and enter the peritubular capillaries. The overall net effect is therefore a transfer of sodium, potassium, bicarbonate and chloride ion from tubular lumen to blood stream.

4. Glucose Reabsorption.

There is active proximal tubular reabsorption of glucose which is virtually complete in normal man. In the presence of an increase in blood glucose levels, the filtered load of glucose, i.e. the amount of glucose being filtered per minute is increased, and this results in a point being reached at which the maximum reabsorptive capacity of the tubule for glucose is exceeded, so that some glucose remains unabsorbed at the end of the proximal tubular lumen and eventually appears in the urine as glucose, i.e. glycosuria. The most frequently found reducing sugar in pregnancy is lactose, often misinterpreted as glucose when reducing substances are detected in urine. Clinistix, a glucose oxidase dependent test, is specific for glucose in the urine and should be used to confirm the identity of apparent glycosuria in pregnancy. The maximum amount of glucose which the proximal tubules are able to reabsorb per minute is known as the tubular maximal reabsorption of glucose, or TmG. The term Tm can be used to express tubular maximal reabsorptive or secretory capacity of any substance secreted or reabsorbed by the renal tubules.

5. Amino-Acid Reabsorption.

Most of the filtered amino-acids are reabsorbed in the proximal tubule, but small amounts of some amino-acids escape reabsorption and appear in the urine. There are three major groups of amino-acids which share, within each group, a common method of reabsorption: Group (1) lysine, ornithine, arginine, histidine and cystine. Group (2) contains glutamine and aspartic acids. Group (3) contains alanine and creatinine. Within each group there is competition between the amino-acids for reabsorption. Some amino-acids (i.e. lysine and glycine) have a measurable Tm for reabsorption.

6. Phosphate reabsorption

is influenced by several factors —filtered load of phosphate, parathyroid hormone, thyrocalcitonin, dietary intake of phosphate, hydrocortisone secretion and acidosis. There is a Tm phosphate in the proximal tubule, but this is set at a lower level than TmG, phosphate reabsorption being incomplete so that phosphate appears in the bladder urine under normal circumstances. If there is a moderate *decrease* in filtered phosphate due to a lowering of plasma phosphate levels, then the Tm phosphate is greater than the filtered load of phosphate: the urine becomes phosphate free. Parathyroid

hormone causes a decrease in phosphate reabsorption, thyrocalcitonin causing an increase in phosphate reabsorption.

7. Urate

is absorbed proximally and this reabsorption may go to completion resulting in a urate-free fluid at the end of the proximal tubule, with distal secretion of urate responsible for the urate found in urine. Lactate infusion reduces urate excretion by inhibition of urate secretion distally, and so causes an elevation of the plasma urate level. This is thought to be a possible mechanism of the elevated plasma urate levels in pre-eclamptic toxaemia, in which there is frequently a raised lactate level, i.e. a hyperlactataemia producing similar effects to intravenous infusion of lactate on urate excretion.

Some ammonia secretion occurs proximally in the proximal tubule. This is discussed in the section on ammonia secretion in the distal tubule.

DISTAL TUBULE

Counter Current System of Urine Concentration

The ability to concentrate the urine in patients with pyelonephritis is frequently impaired. The method of concentrating the urine is thought to be one of counter-current *exchange* in the vasa recta, and counter-current *multiplication* in the loop of Henle. Counter-current exchange is a purely passive process by which the medullary hypertonicity is preserved. The counter-current multiplier, in contrast, is an active process whereby a high medullary osmolality is set up. This is an energy-consuming activity, and is mediated through the pumping of sodium from the ascending part of the loop of Henle into the medullary interstitium. The high interstitial osmolality of the medulla causes the content of the collecting ducts to equilibrate at a similar high level of osmolality by abstraction of water, so forming a concentrated urine. The sodium pump can probably be activated by antidiuretic hormone (ADH), so that secretion of ADH results in a higher medullary osmolality and an increase in urine concentration. For further details of the counter-current system readers are referred to Berliner (1962).

A 12–14 hour deprivation of water in the normal person results in a urine osmolality of 600–800 mOsm./Kg. In renal failure, in pyelonephritis, in hydronephrosis, and in diabetes insipidus of various origins, there is an inability to reach these levels of urine osmolality; in pyelonephritis and in hydronephrosis particularly there is a greater reduction in the urinary concentrating ability than would be expected from the reduction in GFR. In advanced renal failure (GFR <10 ml./minute), urine osmolality approaches above that of plasma: this is known as isosthenuria. In patients in whom it is difficult to rely upon voluntary abstinence from fluids it is convenient to use a more convenient test by giving an intramuscular injection of vasopressin tannate, 5 units. The normal response is a urine osmolality of at least 600 mOsm./Kg. after 3 hours.

The two most important substances responsible for producing a high medullary osmolality are sodium and urea. If a low protein diet is fed there is a reduction in urea in the medulla and in the urine, and maximal urinary concentrating ability is diminished, being restored by oral or parenteral urea. It has been shown that the role of urea is complex, for the fall in urinary osmolality on low protein diets cannot be solely accounted for by the reduction in urinary urea. There is some evidence in certain animals, but none in man that is convincing, that urea is actively transported in the medulla. In diabetes insipidus the medullary osmotic gradients are diminished but still present. The urine osmolality is always below that of plasma. Renal diabetes insipidus can be differentiated from that of pituitary-hypothalamic disease by the response to vasopressin, the latter group yielding a normal urine osmolality response while the former group is resistant to the action of vasopressin.

Urinary Dilution

The ability to form a dilute urine is maintained for a long time, well into advanced renal failure. In several patients with GFR below 3 ml./min. urine osmolality of 150–160 mOsm./kg. has been found (Berlyne, unpublished observations). The dilution test is principally of historical interest and should not be carried out as a routine test of renal function. It is, however, most useful as a test of adrenocortical and anterior pituitary function.

Free Water Clearance

When solutes such as sodium, urea, chloride or phosphate are reabsorbed the water left behind is known as free water, i.e. water that is not osmotically obligated. This can be measured conveniently by determining the urine volume, and the urine and plasma osmolality so that we can calculate the osmolar clearance, this being defined as

$$C_{osm} = \frac{Uosm \ V}{Posm}$$

$Cosm$ = osmolar clearance
$Uosm$ = urine osmolality
$Posm$ = plasma osmolality
V = urine volume ml./minute.

Free water clearance is expressed as

$C_{H_2O} = V - Cosm$ where C_{H_2O} is free water clearance. This is a mathematical way of saying: "let us find the volume of urine that would be passed per minute if urine osmolality were equal to that of plasma; thus the difference between this volume and that actually passed per minute is a measure of osmotically unobligated or free water and is known as 'free water clearance'". It is not a true renal clearance as shown elsewhere, and it is used as a sophisticated test of dilutional ability. It is unimpaired in pyelonephritis, whereas concentrating ability is impaired early and specifically. Because of the convenience of measuring tubular maxima (Tm) in proximal and distal tubules the concept of maximal reabsorption of free water was developed to define mathematically the process of water reabsorption in the production of a concentrated urine. This may be shown as a negative free water clearance, but is more conveniently expressed as

$T^c_{H_2O} = V - C_{osm}$ where $T^c_{H_2O}$ = free water reabsorbed ml./min. and $T^c_{H_2O} = - C_{H_2O}$.

Under conditions of osmotic diuresis with mannitol and in the presence of excess ADH in circulation it is possible to measure a Tm for free water, i.e. Tm^cH_2O. This may well be artifactual for no Tm is determinable if hypertonic saline is used to produce an osmotic diuresis. Tm^cH_2O is about 5 ml./min. in normal man, and is early reduced in pyelonephritis and hydronephrosis, the reduction in Tm^cH_2O being greater than that of GFR. A specific reduction in free water reabsorption is found in pyelonephritis when GFR is still greater than 30 ml./min. at a level of GFR when no similar reduction can be found in glomerulonephritis. This may well prove to be useful in the investigation of dubious cases of urinary tract infection in females. The ratio of GFR/TmPAH gives an index of the glomerular : proximal tubular relationship. Similarly in the distal tubule, the GFR/Tm^cH_2O ratio gives an indication of glomerular : distal tubular relationship. In several renal diseases there is no change in the GFR/TmPAH or GFR/Tm^cH_2O ratios, but in pyelonephritis and hydronephrosis GFR/Tm^cH_2O ratio is increased due to a specific decrease in Tm^cH_2O caused by distal tubular damage.

Acidification of the Urine

The process of urinary acidification is an essential distal tubular function which, in association with the respiratory system and body buffers, results in the maintenance of the normal acid-base balance of the extracellular fluid. Acidification of urine in normal man on normal diets can yield urine pH as low as 4·6. With intravenous administration of non-reabsorbed anions such as sulphate, the urinary pH can drop as low as 4·1. In health the urine can be as alkaline as 8·3, so that the urine has a pH range in health of just under 4 pH units. In the process of acidification of the urine, the hydrogen ion concentration in the distal tubular lumen has its concentration increased 800 fold over that in the blood. This passage of hydrogen ion against a large concentration gradient is an active process. In healthy man on a normal North American or West European diet about 50–70 mEq. of hydrogen ion are excreted in the urine daily. Very little of this is in the form of free hydrogen ion—at a pH of 4·6 there are only 0·025 mEq. of free hydrogen per litre. Most of the hydrogen ion is excreted in combination with ammonia as ammonium ion, or with the urinary buffer, principally phosphate, creatinine and the organic acids. Ammonium excretion is important because the ammonium ion is unable to diffuse back into the lipid coated tubular cell, so that ammonia traps hydrogen ion in the tubular lumen and the lower the pH the greater the ammonium content of the urine. The urinary buffers are measured as titratable acidity (TA) defined as the amount of alkali required to titrate the urine up to a pH of 7·4. Total hydrion excretion/day can be expressed as follows:

$$\Sigma H^+ = NH_4^+ + TA - HCO_3^-$$

where ΣH^+ = total hydrion excretion in mEq./day.
NH_4^+ = Ammonium excretion mEq./day
TA = Titratable acidity mEq./day.
HCO_3^- = Bicarbonate mM/day.

In urinary tract infections, hydronephrosis, hypokalaemia, hypercalcaemia and inherited renal tubular acidosis there is an impairment of the ability to acidify the urine. The ability to excrete hydrogen becomes progressively reduced as renal failure increases, with a reduction in ammonium excretion, so that when the GFR has fallen bellow 3 ml./min. the total hydrogen ion excretion is approximately 10 mEq./day, in spite of a severe systemic acidosis, i.e. a maximal stimulus to urinary acidification. The ability to acidify the urine is tested clinically by a modification of the test of Wrong and Davies (1959) in which ammonium chloride (0·1 g./Kg. body weight) is given orally and the urine pH measured hourly, together with ammonia and TA excretion, for 6 hours. The normal response is acidification of the urine giving a pH of 5·1 or less within six hours of oral administration. In renal tubular acidosis (RTA) the urine pH is greater than 5·3, and often greater than 6·0.

Distal ion-exchange mechanism. In the distal tubule 10–20 per cent of the sodium reabsorption occurs. It is here that the final variation of sodium reabsorption takes place so determining urinary sodium composition; this is of major importance in the maintenance of electrolyte homeostasis. The mechanism appears to be partly an ion-exchange mechanism, involving the exchange of sodium ion for potassium and hydrogen ion, and partly an active reabsorption of sodium ion more distally in the collecting tubule. Sodium reabsorption is often impaired in pyelonephritis, sometimes leading to salt-losing nephritis where the sodium loss may be 200 mEq. or more per day. It can be differentiated from Addison's disease by its lack of response to 9αfluorohydrocortisone, a potent mineralocorticoid which stimulates the virtually complete reabsorption of sodium from the distal tubular fluid in normal man. The administration of 1 mg. daily of 9α fluorohydrocortisone for 3 days is a useful clinical test of sodium reabsorption; alternatively 20 mEq. of sodium in the diet for 5 days should result in a fall in urinary sodium excretion to below 20 mEq. of sodium per day by the fifth day. The mechanism of virtually complete sodium reabsorption from the distal tubule in conditions of low salt intake or sodium depletion is by one of the following methods. Lower GFR results in a reduction in filtered sodium and so more complete sodium reabsorption in the proximal tubule. In the distal tubule therefore the tubular sodium concentration, already low, is readily reduced to very low levels. This is one of the mechanisms operative in pre-eclampsia, so that sodium retention occurs leading to oedema and hypertension. Other mechanisms of sodium reabsorption are the action of aldosterone and that of corticosteroids with stimulation of sodium reabsorption and potassium secretion. Aldosterone secretion is probably increased in various severely ill patients as well as in renal failure (Wrong, 1967) in heart failure, in nephrotic syndrome and in cirrhosis. A natriuretic hormone or "third factor" is known to occur in man and is responsible for the ability to excrete sodium. It is remarkable that in heart failure either natriuretic hormone release is diminished or the hormone is unable to cause sodium excretion despite its presence. Potassium secretion occurs as part of the distal tubular $Na^+/H^+/K^+$ exchange mechanism. In the presence of aldosterone secretion potassium secretion is increased: this is one of the major mechanisms of potassium depletion resulting from the administration of diuretics, particularly of the thiazide group. In advanced renal failure potassium secretion is such that potassium clearance may be twice the GFR.

Final bicarbonate reabsorption occurs distally, so that if the urine pH is below 6·0 the urine is virtually free of bicarbonate, i.e. bicarbonate reabsorption is complete. In advanced renal failure bicarbonate may appear in the urine at a pH less than 6·0; this is termed a "bicarbonate leak". In normal man when the plasma bicarbonate is above 28 mEq./L. the urine contains bicarbonate; with a plasma level below 28 mEq./L. the Tm bicarbonate is not exceeded so that the urine is bicarbonate free.

BIBLIOGRAPHY

Berliner, R. W. (1962), In *Diseases of the Kidney*, by Strauss, M. A. and Welt, L. G. Boston: Little Brown.

Berlyne, G. M., Varley, H., Nilwarangkur, S. and Hoerni, M. (1964), "Endogenous Creatinine Clearance and Glomerular Filtration Rate," *Lancet*, 2, 874.

Blaufox, M. D., Sanderson, D. R., Tauxe, W. N., Wakim, K. G., Orvis, A. L. and Owen, C. A. (1963), "Plasma diatrizoate—I^{131} Disappearance and Glomerular Filtration in the Dog," *Amer. J. Physiol.*, 204, 536.

Garnett, E. S., Parson, V. and Veall, N. (1967), "Measurement of G.F.R. in Man Using ^{51}Cr/Edetic-Acid Complex," *Lancet*, 1, 818.

Nelp, W. B., Wagner, H. W. and Reba, R. C. (1964), "Renal Excretion of Vitamin B_{12} and Its Use in the Measurement of Glomerular Filtration Rate in Man," *J. Lab. Clin. Med.*, 63, 480.

Shaw, A. B., Bazzard, F. J., Booth, E. M., Nilwarangkur, S. and Berlyne, G. M. (1965), "The Treatment of Chronic Renal Failure by a Modified Giovannetti Diet," *Quart. J. Med.*, 34, 237.

2. FLUID BALANCES

PHILIP RHODES

Life began in the sea and the first living things were probably unicellular. Each cell used the aquatic environment for its supplies of oxygen and nutrients and for the excretion of waste products. These are activities of the cell membrane. In order to colonize the land, multicellular creatures had to carry their aquatic environment with them for the cells of which they were made still had to use water surrounding them for respiration, nutrition and excretion.

The vastness of the oceans makes for relative constancy of composition of the sea, but when each creature has to carry its own water with it, methods of control become essential to preserve relative constancy of composition, since even quite small additions of chemical compounds to a small volume of water might greatly alter the physical and chemical properties of the medium which could make the life of cells impossible.

The Compartments of Body Water

The water of the body is partly within the cells, partly surrounding the cells in the tissue fluid, and partly within the blood. These are the intracellular fluid (ICF) and the extra-cellular fluid (ECF) which includes the tissue fluid and the plasma. The three "pools" are not rigidly divided from one another and there is constant interchange between them. Some idea of the magnitude of these changes may be gleaned from the fact that about eight litres of fluid is poured into the alimentary tract each day and the total glomerular filtrate per day is of the order of 170 litres. The molecules of water cross and re-cross membranes and cell surfaces. At membranes the water might pass through the cells themselves or through the intercellular spaces.

The methods of measurement of the various compartments of body water will not be detailed here. They depend upon the injection of an indicator whose degree of dilution can later be measured. It is obvious that to measure the total body water (TBW) the indicator must diffuse evenly through all three compartments. To measure the ECF, which includes the vascular and tissue fluids, the indicator must not penetrate into the cells, and to measure the vascular fluid the indicator must stay within the vascular tree. Direct measurements can thus be made of TBW, ECF, and plasma volumes. From these ICF can be calculated since ICF = TBW − ECF and tissue fluid is ECF − plasma volume.

None of the indicators is ideal for its purpose since they obstinately refuse to stay entirely within the compartment which is being measured but examples of each group are as follows:

Total body water	Antipyrine, Urea, Deuterium, Tritium.
Extra-cellular fluid	Inulin, Thiocyanate, Radio-sodium.
Plasma	Evan's blue, Protein-bound radio-iodine.

The Volumes of the various Compartments

In apparently comparable individuals as regards height, weight and general appearance the range of the volumes of the compartments of body water is wide. To make the data obtained from difficult experimentation clinically useable it has been usual to express the amounts of water in the body as percentages of body weight. The following table shows reasonably acceptable rough figures for women. The figures are not transposable to men.

TABLE 1

		Per cent body weight
Total body weight	60.0 kg.	
Total body water	33·0 litres	55
(i) Intracellular water	24·0 litres	40
(ii) Extracellular water	9·0 litres	15
(a) Tissue fluid	6·5 litres	11
(b) Plasma	2·5 litres	4

The problem of using body weight as a standard is the variability of body composition. Body weight can be looked upon as consisting of lean body mass (LBM) and fat. The LBM consists of all tissues other than fat and is an index of the actively functioning tissue of the body. Fat contains almost no water whilst the water content of the LBM is almost constant at about 72 per cent of its weight. Fat is one of the largest variables in body weight and may range from 11 to about 50 per cent. This variability, which is not easily measurable in individual patients, vitiates estimates of body water based on crude body weight. At present there seems to be no half-way house between inspired wild guesses about body water in patients and careful prolonged experimental procedures designed to measure water content with some accuracy. Nevertheless, the above crude figures give a first basis for discussion and understanding.

Control Mechanisms

These will first be dealt with in the non-pregnant woman.

The volumes of the various compartments of body water are maintained within reasonably narrow limits. The volumes could be disturbed by intake of fluid or its excretion and also by variations of distribution of the water between the three compartments.

The intake of fluid is normally by mouth and is controlled by thirst and by habit. Therapeutically fluid may be given parenterally and then control must be by the doctor. Intake is obviously very variable but averages about three litres per day, two litres being actual fluid drunk and one litre coming from the water in food and from the oxidation of food. Replacement therapy in sick patients with normal renal function and no abnormal losses should aim at delivering about three litres of fluid per day.

The output of fluid normally balances the intake. Obligatory loss is that from the lungs and skin, the so-called *insensible loss*. It amounts to about one litre per day or a little more. The remainder of the loss is in the urine and a very little, which can be ignored for clinical purposes, in the faeces.

Thirst is ill-understood but seems to be an expression of intracellular dehydration. Such dehydration must be signalled in some way to the brain, perhaps the hypothalamus, so that the sensation of thirst is aroused. A dry mouth may also be a stimulus for the arousal of the sensation.

The distribution of water between compartments is very complex but is best understood in the first instance by consideration of events at the tissue level. The diagram

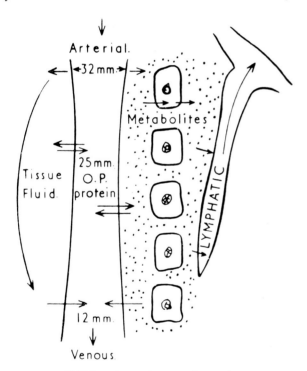

Fig. 1. Fluid interchanges between plasma, tissue spaces, and lymphatics. (*Wright, Proc. roy. Soc. Med., 1939.*)

makes matters clearer. At the arterial end of the capillary the hydrostatic pressure tending to drive fluid out of the vessel is 32 mm. Hg. Tending to hold fluid in the capillary is the osmotic pressure of the plasma proteins estimated at 25 mm. Hg. At the venous end of the capillary the hydrostatic pressure has fallen to 12 mm. Hg. The net force driving fluid into the capillary at the venous end is 13 mm. Hg. The cells are producing metabolites all the time so that the presence of these osmotically active ions and molecules has some effect upon the simplified scheme just outlined.

Factors affecting distribution between the three compartments include (i) the plasma proteins since they remain within the blood stream and (ii) the osmotically active particles in the tissue fluid and in the intra-cellular fluid. In addition the membranes separating the compartments, the capillary walls and the cell membranes, also play a part. The activity of the cell walls is shown by the differences of electrolyte concentrations in the cells and the tissue fluid surrounding them. The following table shows this:

TABLE 2

From Black, D.A.K. (1957) Essentials of Fluid Balance, Blackwell

	Intracellular Fluid (mEq./litre)		Extracellular Fluid (mEq./litre)
Na⁺	8		143
K⁺	151		5
Ca⁺⁺	2	Cell	5
Mg⁺⁺	28	wall	2
Cl′	—		103
HCO₃′	10		27
PO₄″	100		2
SO₄″	10		1
Organic acid	4		6
Protein	65		16

A glance shows significant differences between the two sides of the cell wall. Especially to be noted is that almost all the potassium of the body is within the cells and almost all the sodium in the extracellular fluid. It is probably the specialized activity of the cell membrane which keeps these two major cations relatively separated. The mechanisms controlling the cell walls are little known, but it is likely that some hormones act here and among them may well be the sex steroids, and adrenal steroids. Also, as mentioned previously, the activities both within and outside the cell must alter the distribution of substances which normally pass easily through membranes.

It is now possible to consider the volumes and changes within the three compartments in the light of what is known to be happening at the tissue level just discussed. Virtually all that is known is based on analysis of plasma because this is so easily accessible to observation whilst the other two compartments are not. However, except for the presence of the plasma proteins in the vascular compartment plasma is the same as the tissue fluid. The physiological mechanisms are best understood when an attempt is made to alter the volume of the plasma by either loading it with water or relatively depriving it of water.

Water Load

If a large quantity of water is drunk it is absorbed into the blood, where it causes dilution of all the plasma constituents so lowering the osmotic pressure. Water therefore escapes from the blood into the tissue fluid where it is temporarily stored. Some of the water must also pass into the cells because the osmotic pressure of the tissue fluid is lowered too. It is probable that there are cells in the region of the hypothalamus which are especially sensitive to changes of osmotic pressure within them, for perfusion of the hypothalamic area with relatively dilute plasma causes a diminution in the output of anti-diuretic hormone (ADH) from the posterior lobe of the pituitary gland. ADH, like vasopressin the other secretion of the posterior lobe of the pituitary gland, is an octapeptide whose major action is on the kidney. When it reaches the kidney its effect is to cause conservation of water. Of the water delivered in the glomerular filtrate to the renal tubule a certain amount is reabsorbed into the blood stream as a solvent for such substances as glucose, urea and electrolytes. This is an obligatory reabsorption. The final adjustment of the amount of water to be reabsorbed is made by ADH which affects the function of the distal convoluted tubule and the collecting tubule of the nephron.

This draws attention to the major role of the kidney in getting rid of the excess of water so restoring the volumes of the three compartments to normal and adjusting the osmotic pressures within them. Apart from the special cells in the brain which are responsive to osmotic pressure changes, there are also "volume receptors" within the thorax probably in association with the great veins which are responsive to pressures within them. When the plasma volume is expanded by the large water load the pressure in the great veins increases and reflexly these call into play the ADH mechanisms which will adjust the blood volume.

The excess water can only be excreted through the kidney. The first factors controlling the renal function are the renal blood flow and the glomerular filtration rate (GFR). There is probably little change in blood flow but the GFR depends upon the filtering head of pressure in the glomeruli, i.e. the diastolic pressure of about 70 to 80 mm. Hg. less the osmotic pressure of the plasma proteins. The dilution of the blood has lowered this osmotic pressure so that glomerular filtration is increased. Tubular reabsorption is changed because the filtrate delivered to the tubules is relatively dilute. Since the concentration of sodium ions in the blood is diminished aldosterone secretion from the adrenal gland is increased to help in sodium reabsorption from the tubules whilst at the same time the diminished output of ADH allows more water to escape in the urine so that its specific gravity decreases.

Aldosterone is the secretion of the zona glomerulosa of the adrenal gland. Its secretion is not under the control of ACTH from the anterior pituitary as other steroid secretions of the adrenal gland are. It is the hormone most powerfully affecting the excretion of sodium and potassium by the kidney. Its action is to cause reabsorption of sodium from the renal tubular fluid and to allow the escape of potassium.

It is the lack of aldosterone in Addison's disease which is responsible for the major electrolyte changes, there being gross loss of sodium and a relative retention of potassium. Although ACTH does not control the secretion of aldosterone it is probable that the brain is involved through a diencephalic centre perhaps secreting a hormone called glomerulotrophin in response to the level of circulating electrolyte levels and perhaps in response to the volume receptors in the thorax.

These receptors are responsive to tension which is dependent on blood volume so that appropriate adjustments may be made to maintain homeostasis. Such adjustments necessarily involve ADH and aldosterone among other factors. As the blood has its normal osmotic relationships restored by these renal mechanisms water which has been temporarily stored is withdrawn from the tissue fluid into the plasma and the cycle just described is repeated. As the tissue fluid is restored to normal the ICF also become adjusted by water being passed from the cells into the tissue fluid.

The whole process of dealing with an excessive water load may take something of the order of two to four hours though most of the excess water is excreted in the shorter time.

Water Deprivation

Water deprivation leads to increased concentration of the blood which raises its osmotic pressure. Water is then withdrawn from the tissue fluid and since tissue fluid and plasma must have the same electrolyte content water is withdrawn from the cells too. Cellular dehydration results and with this goes intense thirst. ADH is secreted in increased amount to prevent undue loss of water by the kidney, and because of the higher osmotic pressure of the plasma proteins the GFR is reduced. Aldosterone secretion diminishes to allow for loss of sodium ions so that osmotic equilibrium can be restored.

Sodium excess is rare but because sodium cannot enter the cells in appreciable quantities the osmotic pressure outside the cells increases, water passes out and there is intracellular dehydration. Aldosterone secretion diminishes to allow the kidneys to excrete the excess of sodium whilst ADH secretion is increased so that water may be retained.

Salt deprivation is much more common since it is likely to occur whenever there are undue losses from the alimentary tract as may occur with vomiting or gastric aspiration. Such deprivation is worsened if water is drunk or administered freely. ADH secretion is diminished to attempt to get rid of the apparent excess of water whilst aldosterone production may rise greatly to conserve sodium. Because the osmotic pressure of the ECF is low water passes into the cells which now suffer from overhydration, so there is no thirst. To a small extent potassium may replace sodium in the ECF and so potassium tends to pass out of the cells where there is a large store, and this leads to potassium deprivation in the cells even though the level of potassium in the serum may be very high. Therefore measurement of the serum potassium is only a very indirect measure of its metabolism and may be very misleading if interpreted too simply.

A high serum potassium with a low sodium may indeed be an indication for giving potassium since it may be high in the serum because of a low intracellular content. One very rough guide to changes in intracellular potassium may be an alteration in the electrocardiogram, especially an inversion of the T wave.

In summary the control of fluid balance depends among other things on the following:

1. The "normal" volumes and osmotic pressures in the three main compartments, namely intracellular fluid, tissue fluid, plasma.
2. Intake and out-put of fluid.
   Oral intake. Fluid and food.
   Output. Insensible loss through lungs and skin.
      Urine.
3. Physico-chemical factors in the tissues. ? endocrine factors.
4. Osmotic receptors in the hypothalamus.
5. Volume receptors in the thorax.
6. Renal mechanisms.
   Renal blood flow. Glomerular filtration rate.
   Endocrine factors affecting tubular reabsorption.
      Anti-diuretic hormone.
      Aldosterone.
      Others.

Menstruation

Menstrual losses of water and electrolytes are so small that they can be ignored in a clinical context. Total water loss may be about 50 to 100 ml. sodium loss about 5 mEq. and potassium loss about 2·5 mEq. with each period.

Pregnancy

Pregnancy changes fluid balance appreciably. The weight gain of pregnancy is made up of eight factors which are foetus, placenta, liquor amnii, uterine growth, breast growth, increased blood volume, increased tissue fluid and fat. All of these, with the exception of fat, involve the retention of water and of electrolytes among a host of other things. Hytten and Leitch (1964) produce the following table which epitomizes most of what is known of water retention in pregnancy.

It should be noted that the total body water in normal pregnancy was measured by the deuterium method and the figures obtained are in the bottom line of the table.

The table above these figures is an estimate of where it can be calculated that the measured increment of water may be in the different parts of the weight increase of pregnancy. Looking at the bottom two figures of the last column it will be seen that there is a discrepancy between the measured volume of water and that which can be accounted for in the various components of pregnancy. The difference between these two is accounted for by the tissue fluid, which therefore harbours an increase of about 1·2 litres at term.

The fluid balances of the foetus, placenta, liquor, breasts and red cells are of great interest in their own right, but for present purposes the major interest is concentrated in the increased blood volume and interstitial or tissue fluid.

The blood volume of a non-pregnant woman weighing about 55 to 60 kg. is about 4 litres of which 2,600 ml. is plasma. The plasma volume increases in pregnancy over this volume by about 50 ml. at 10 weeks, 550 ml. at 20 weeks, 1,150 ml. at 30 weeks, 1,300 ml. at 34 weeks and then it declines to 1,000 ml. at 40 weeks. (Hytten and Leitch, 1964). The tissue fluid volumes at these times in pregnancy are not known and there is only the estimate of 1,200 ml. at term. The interest of these estimates is in explaining how they are brought about. Perhaps one of the major determining factors in the increased blood volume is the growth of the vascular tree in the uterus, in the placenta on the maternal side, and in the breasts. The size of the placental blood lake has been estimated at 140 ml. and possibly 250 ml. (Aherne and Dunnill, 1966) but the sizes of the vascular trees of the uterus and breasts are not known. The vascular bed of the skin in pregnancy is also increased in order to dissipate the heat generated by the growing products of conception. If the blood volume increases, the tissue fluid volume must increase as well since both are parts of the ECF. The blood is more dilute during pregnancy as shown by the lower hæmatocrit reading (34 per cent—Hytten and Leitch, 1964) and this lowers the osmotic pressure of the plasma proteins which are also reduced in pregnancy. This presumably allows of a greater escape of fluid from the capillaries. There is

TABLE 3

	Weeks of Pregnancy								
	20			30			40		
	Weight	Water	Water	Weight	Water	Water	Weight	Water	Water
	g.	%	g.	g.	%	g.	g.	%	g.
Foetus	300	88	264	1,500	79	1,185	3,300	71	2,343
Placenta	170	90	153	430	85	366	650	83	540
Liquor amnii	250	99	247	600	99	594	800	99	792
Blood-free uterus	585	82·5	483	810	82·5	668	900	82·5	743
Blood and fat-free mammary gland	180	75	135	360	75	270	405	75	304
Plasma	550	92	506	1,150	92	1,058	1,000	92	920
Red cells	50	65	32	150	65	98	250	65	163
			1,820			4,239			5,805
Measured increment of water			1,500			3,750			7,000

no evidence of alteration of the hydrostatic pressure at the arterial end of the capillary and no direct measurement of the pressure at the venous end. In the legs at least, however, the venous pressure is raised from a normal value of about 9 cms. of water to one of 27 cms. of water (McLennan, 1943). This must help to increase the amount of tissue fluid in the legs and this often shows itself clinically as oedema. Thus the physico-chemical factors in fluid balance in the tissues are altered during pregnancy.

Because of the relatively dilute blood of pregnancy one might expect a fall in the secretion of ADH but so far it has not been found possible to measure its presence in the blood. However, it would seem likely that the osmoreceptors are set at a different level in pregnancy from that which obtains in the non-pregnant. Similarly it would seem that the volume receptors have a different threshold in pregnancy from the non-pregnant.

Renal function is undoubtedly changed in pregnancy. Renal blood flow is about 885 ml. per minute per 1·73 square metres in the non-pregnant. (It is the convention to correct all measurements of renal blood flow to a standard surface area.) By the middle trimester the flow has increased to about 1,200 ml. but thereafter it falls to about 1,100 ml. at 34 weeks and is only about 100 ml. per minute above the non-pregnant values, at term (Hytten and Leitch, 1964).

The significance of this high renal blood flow in early pregnancy followed by a diminishing blood flow to term is quite unknown. Nor is it known if it has any effect on the changed fluid balance of pregnancy. By contrast the GFR is raised from the beginning of pregnancy and stays at the raised level throughout.

In the non-pregnant the GFR is about 90 ml. per minute and in pregnancy it is about 140 ml. per minute. At the least this increase of 60 per cent in the GFR would suggest that the kidneys are quite able to deal with any increase in the water load presented to them. But Hytten and Klopper (1963) showed that pregnant women given a water load of one litre have greater difficulty in getting rid of it the nearer they are to term. Rather than failure in renal function this difficulty would appear to be due to pooling of the water somewhere in the tissue fluids or because of changes in hormone secretion in pregnancy. The role of ADH is uncertain.

It is known that the cortisol of the blood is raised about two and a half times over its non-pregnant level (Cope and Black, 1959) but this is probably because more of it is bound to protein which is an effect of the raised level of œstrogen in the plasma. The hormone bound to protein may not be physiologically active but may be a store perhaps ready for emergency when it may be rapidly drawn upon. In like fashion it is known that the aldosterone excretion is greatly raised in pregnancy. The normal amounts in the urine are of the order of 2–10 μg. in 24 hours. In pregnancy this is raised to 119·2 $\pm$ 27·3 μg. (Rinsler and Rigby, 1957). It should be noted that only about 4 per cent of any injected dose of aldosterone appears in the urine so that this excretion demonstrates a vastly increased production of the hormone. The significance of this rise in aldosterone is not fully known but

sodium has to be retained in large quantities in pregnancy both for growth of the products of conception and for the maintenance of isotonicity in all the body fluids.

The water retention of pregnancy is fairly rapidly reversed in the puerperium. At birth the foetus, placenta, secundines and liquor are lost together with a certain amount of blood. For the first few days after birth it is probable though not proven that there is a relative retention of fluid such as is seen after a major operation (Le Quesne, 1957). This might be mediated by an increased output of ADH. Thereafter the water is lost quite quickly especially if the woman breast feeds her baby, since by the tenth day or so of the puerperium the breasts may be delivering about 500 ml. of milk every 24 hours. The small lochial loss, as well as urine also contributes to the fluid balance. However direct measurements suggest that the excess of water taken on in pregnancy may not be fully excreted until about the sixth week of the puerperium though the greater part is excreted in the first two weeks.

PROBLEMS OF FLUID BALANCE IN GYNAECOLOGICAL PRACTICE

The problems of fluid balance in gynaecology are nearly all concentrated in the post-operative period and are exemplified by paralytic ileus. Here there is a large outflow of fluid and electrolytes into the alimentary canal. When diagnosed the treatment is by gastric suction and replacement of fluid and electrolytes by intravenous drip. The loss of water and ions into the gut inevitably depletes the plasma and the blood volume is diminished. This shows itself by a rise in pulse rate especially and also in a fall in blood pressure. The haematocrit ratio rises and serum electrolytes may be raised too if the loss of water is relatively in excess of that of ions. Thus the serum electrolytes alone may be a poor guide to therapy. Provided that the shock (raised pulse rate and low blood pressure) are not due to blood loss the blood volume depletion must be due to water and salt loss. This will be confirmed when the patient vomits copiously and when a gastric tube withdraws large amounts of intestinal fluids.

The clinical state is the indication for starting an intravenous drip of sodium chloride together with gastric suction. Depending on progress and the amounts of fluid withdrawn estimates of requirements of water and salt must be made 12 hourly or 24 hourly. Carefully kept balance charts are an essential of management. The wellbeing of the patient together with her pulse chart, the passing of flatus or the return of bowel sounds are the best indices of improvement.

The calculations to be done are simple but require ten minutes or so with pencil and paper and written instructions to the nursing staff when the policy for the next 12 or 24 hours has been worked out. The intake for a normal healthy person is about 3 litres of water. The intake of sodium chloride is about 5 gms. in 24 hours. Approximately this amount of sodium chloride is present in 0·5 litre of normal saline. Water has to be given intravenously as 5 per cent dextrose to maintain osmotic relationships. Therefore the daily minimum must be 3 litres of fluid of which 0·5 litre must be given as normal saline. On the output side of the balance are (i) insensible loss, (ii) urine, (iii) the amount of fluid withdrawn from the stomach. One litre is allowed for the insensible loss. The urine volume and the volume of the gastric aspirate will have been measured. Comparing intake with output will soon show whether the coming day's intravenous fluids should be increased or decreased over the basic 3 litres.

The amount of saline to be given has to be calculated separately. At least half a litre of normal saline is always required. In addition, for every 0·5 litre of gastric aspirate, 0·5 litre of normal saline should be administered. This would appear to mean that gastric aspirate is the equivalent of normal saline, but in fact it is not and contains rather less sodium chloride than normal saline. However, it is important to give enough saline and enough water *provided that renal function is not impaired*. It is well to realize that the patient's homeostatic mechanisms are much better at maintaining fluid and electrolyte balance than the most erudite doctor. All the mechanisms require is enough material with which to work. In general the tendency is to give too little rather than too much, though care is needed not to overload the patient. If renal function is impaired then great care is needed in management, but is beyond the scope of this present chapter.

In the first 48 hours after operation there is a relative retention of water which may be caused by an increased output of ADH (Le Quesne, 1957). Therefore, not more than 2 litres of fluid should be given in the 24 hours for the first day, that is the day of operation.

The administration of potassium intravenously can be very dangerous. It is not usually required in the first two or three days of intravenous therapy, and provided that water and sodium chloride losses are quickly dealt with drips can be stopped and potassium given by mouth as potassium citrate and in fruit drinks and in ordinary food. However, potassium may have to be given, and it has already been pointed out that serum potassium levels may be no good guide to the amounts needed since a high serum potassium may be an expression of low serum sodium when the potassium is withdrawn from the cells. In these circumstances the giving of potassium may actually lower the serum potassium since some is sent back into the ICF. This shows that the serum potassium levels are of value when the sodium levels are nearly normal and so it is advised that the sodium balance be quickly restored to normal first. With these provisos the administration of potassium can be undertaken and the following rules should be observed.

1. There must be a good urine output.
2. The kidneys must be normal.
3. The intravenous fluid must not contain more than 40 mEq. potassium per litre.
4. Not more than 20 mEq. of potassium must be given in 1 hour.
5. Not more than 100 mEq. of potassium must be given in 24 hours.

6. The serum potassium must be estimated daily. It must not be allowed to rise above 7 mEq. per litre.

The most convenient solution to use is potassium chloride in a strength 3 gm. per litre. It contains 40 mEq. potassium per litre. Better than intravenous potassium is oral potassium whenever this is possible.

Acid-base problems only very rarely arise with the regime recommended. The kidneys take care of this problem. If serum chloride rises greatly bicarbonate diminishes since the numbers of negatively charged ions in the blood must balance exactly the number of positively charged ones. If there is an excess of chloride then instead of normal saline one-sixth molar sodium lactate should be given. This contains 165 mEq. of sodium per litre.

If there is delay in treating a patient with paralytic ileus it should be realized that the losses of water and electrolytes may amount to about 4 litres before the intravenous therapy is started. It may therefore be necessary to give as much as 5 to 6 litres of fluid per day for two days to such a patient. The best guides to adequacy of intake are the urine output, the pulse rate and the haematocrit reading which will be high with gross dehydration. In addition of course all serum constituents will tend to be high when the plasma is short of water.

OBSTETRIC PROBLEMS OF FLUID BALANCE

Posture

Posture affects the distribution of fluid markedly. This is seen when oedema of the legs disappears with rest in bed. Also posture affects renal blood flow and cardiac output (Lees, Taylor, Scott and Kerr, 1967). In sleep RBF is reduced but recumbency may increase it and this explains the diuresis often seen when a patient with oedema is put to bed. In pregnancy the uterus may occlude the inferior vena cava when the patient is supine (Kerr, Scott and Samuel, 1964) and the excretion of a water load is slower with the patient supine than when she is on her side (Browse, 1965). As pregnancy progresses there is increasing difficulty in getting rid of a water load (Hytten and Klopper, 1963). Also to be taken into account is the fact that aldosterone excretion is greater in the upright posture than when recumbent. In the orthostatic albuminuria of pregnancy it is probable that lordosis raises the venous pressure in the kidneys. The role of the effects of posture on fluid balance mechanisms is only just being appreciated but may turn out to be very important both in gauging the results of experiments done in the past and in understanding oedema in pregnancy.

Hyperemesis Gravidarum

The objective diagnosis of this condition rests on the demonstration of ketones in the urine. Such ketonuria is an expression of depletion of carbohydrate reserves and not of water and salt loss from the stomach. However, depletion of carbohydrates will only occur if the patient is taking little by mouth and so ketonuria is an indirect index of water and salt depletion. Once in hospital the patient's therapy as regards fluid balance is exactly the same as that outlined for paralytic ileus.

Anuria

Obstetric anuria is mainly due to accidental haemorrhage and eclampsia. In accidental haemorrhage the cause is pre-renal in that it is probably caused by prolonged hypotension. In eclampsia the cause is renal and probably due to the renal lesion itself. The important thing to recognize is that both conditions are preventable and therefore obstetric anuria ought to be very rare. Especially is it important to restore the blood volume in accidental haemorrhage by rapid massive early blood transfusion even when the pulse rate and blood pressure seem to show that transfusion may not be needed. In one sense blood losses are part of the problems of fluid balance but they are dealt with elsewhere in this book (p. 333).

Once oliguria or anuria is established the problems of fluid balance are essentially the same as have already been dealt with, except that one channel of output is blocked. The only factor on the output side is the insensible loss. Since the major regulator of fluid, the kidneys, cannot cope, the intake must be reduced to accord with the only output. The object is to maintain biochemical equilibrium so that the patient is not killed, whilst the kidneys are given time in which to recover. They may or may not be able to do this but they must be given the opportunity.

Previously the insensible loss was given as 1 litre per day. This is a generous estimate which is valuable in dealing with water losses since this figure will make the doctor give a slight excess of fluid to his patient. Such amounts are to be avoided in oliguria and anuria and an estimate of 500 to 750 ml. of insensible loss per day is enough. The intake must be reduced to this level. Daily weighing of the patient will give an indication of whether the intake is too much. The other major problem of anuria is the continuing breakdown of tissues the products of which cannot be excreted. Especially is potassium important since a high level in the blood will kill the patient. Therefore tissue breakdown must be kept to minimum and this can be done by a caloric intake of about 2,000 per day. In most patients the intake of fluid and food can be given by mouth but it must be very strictly regulated. In those who have to have their nutrients administered intravenously a very concentrated solution of glucose (20 per cent) has to be given and therefore must be administered through a polythene catheter introduced into the inferior vena cava where the blood flow is fast enough to carry the concentrated solution.

The rise of the blood urea and potassium in anuria gives a guide to progress. Serum potassium can be lowered by ion exchange resins, and by the giving of insulin. Tissue breakdown can be slowed by the administration of an anabolic steroid.

Pre-eclamptic Toxaemia

The fluid balance problems of this disorder have long had a fascination. Oedema is one of its facets and is due to an excess of fluid in the tissue spaces. Such excess can be local as in the legs or it can be general. The causes are probably different. In the legs the excess is mainly due to a rise in venous pressure. In generalized oedema the causes are not fully known.

At the tissue level they could be due to a rise in pressure at the arterial end of the capillary, to a fall in osmotic pressure of the plasma proteins or to altered osmotic relationships between the cells and the tissue fluid. The rise in blood pressure of pre-eclamptic toxaemia is probably due to arteriolar spasm which is proximal to the capillaries so there is no direct evidence of a rise in pressure at the capillary. The osmotic pressure of the proteins is lowered in pregnancy but if anything shows a rise in the severer grades of toxaemia. Nothing is known of the general venous pressure in toxaemia. Few now believe that there is a "toxin" damaging capillary walls. A possibility is that there is a change in cellular metabolism that alters the ionic balance between ICF and ECF. Such a change would involve cell membranes whose permeability is affected by steroid hormones which are much raised in pregnancy.

Nothing is known of the osmoreceptors in the hypothalamic area in pregnancy, nor of the volume receptors in the thorax. Results for ADH are equivocal. Aldosterone excretion is decreased in toxaemia as compared with normal pregnancy (Rinsler and Rigby, 1957); therefore on a simple basis it might be expected that sodium would be excreted and help diminish the oedema. But this leaves out of account the role of the kidneys, and in toxaemia the renal blood flow and the glomerular filtration rate are reduced. These must have their effects on sodium and on aldosterone excretion, and the changes in renal physiology may be due in large measure to the arteriolar spasm.

The fact of oedema in pre-eclamptic toxaemia has led to the assumption that more water must be retained by the subjects of this disorder than the normal pregnant woman. This assumption has been called into question (Rhodes, 1960, 1962). Hytten and Thompson (1966) measured accurately the total body water in 6 women throughout pregnancy who subsequently developed toxaemia. Their conclusions are "Up to 30 weeks of pregnancy the rate of gain of body water was within the limits found for normal pregnancy. Between 30 and 38 weeks the gain in body water was a little more rapid than that found for normal pregnant women with generalized oedema, but total water gained was within normal limits." It would seem that generalized oedema can occur without there being toxaemia and that an increase in total body water is not a necessary concomitant of toxaemia.

The relationship of weight gain in pregnancy to oedema has been investigated by Thomson, Hytten and Billewicz (1967). Of 24,000 patients 40 per cent had oedema, and in 25 per cent it was present in the legs only. Of women with a normal blood pressure throughout pregnancy the incidence of oedema was 35 per cent, in women with a raised blood pressure it was 60 per cent and if proteinuria was added to the hypertension the incidence of oedema was 85 per cent. There would thus seem to be a definite relationship between toxaemia and oedema, but the oedema is not certainly an indication of excess total body water.

Perhaps there may be a different ratio between ECF and ICF in normal pregnancy which is accentuated for reasons unknown in pre-eclamptic toxaemia. Further observations by Thomson *et al.* (1967) which are of importance are that the incidence of leg oedema increased with increasing maternal age and that generalized oedema was more likely in those who were overweight as judged by the weight for height ratio. The relationship of obesity to hypertension and to toxaemia and to oedema is a complex one not yet fully evaluated.

The plasma volume in toxaemia is not greatly if at all in excess of that found in normal pregnancy. In severe toxaemia when the patient is rapidly becoming oedematous the plasma volume is in fact decreased as water moves from the blood into the tissue spaces. Such water could not be held there unless there were some change in osmotic relationships there, and if these are present the changes are probably due to a shift of osmotically active particles from the cells into the ECF. Such changes could only be due to changes in cellular metabolism and especially at the cell membranes (Rhodes, 1960).

As with water the sodium balances of toxaemia are far from clear. It used to be thought that there was an excess of sodium ions present in the body in toxaemia, but several investigations of the total exchangeable sodium by radio-isotopic methods, notably that of MacGillivray and Buchanan (1958) show that this sodium may be less in toxaemia than in normotensive patients. These authors give a figure of 48·3 mEq. Na$^+$ per Kg. in normal pregnancy, and ones of 44·0 and 43·8 mEq. per Kg. in mild and severe toxaemia respectively.

Liquor Amnii

This is dealt with elsewhere, as is the fluid balance of the foetus and placenta (p. 254 and p. 181).

Labour

During normal labour there tends to be little intake of fluid whilst fluid is being lost through urine, lungs and skin. In most labours there is a fall in urine output. This dehydration is quickly put right almost as soon as labour is over and fluid is once more taken in. In labours lasting longer than 24 hours it is inevitable that there will be dehydration. Salt losses are negligible unless the patient vomits. Ketonuria is a measure of starvation and indirectly therefore of dehydration. Correction of fluid balance problems in labour is by glucose and water, given as 5 per cent glucose solution. Because of decreased gastric motility and poor absorption of fluids the therapy must be intravenous. When labour is prolonged there is a rise of serum potassium levels and there are other electrolyte changes too, (Hawkins and Nixon, 1957) but these are seldom of importance at the present day since few women are allowed to be in labour for more than 48 hours (nor should they be) and fluid balance problems have no time to become severe.

Caesarean Section

Post-operatively patients who have had a Caesarean section are no different from other patients who have had surgical operations.

REFERENCES

Aherne, W. and Dunnill, M. S. (1966), *Brit. med. Bull.*, **22**, 5.
Browse, N. L. (1965), *The Physiology and Pathology of Bed Rest*. Springfield, Illinois: Chas. C. Thomas.
Cope, C. L. and Black, E. (1959), *J. Obstet. Gynaec. Br. Emp.*, **66**, 404.
Hawkins, D. F. and Nixon, W. C. W. (1957), *J. Obstet. Gynaec. Br. Emp.*, **64**, 641.
Hytten, F. E. and Leitch, I. (1964), *The Physiology of Human Pregnancy*. Oxford: Blackwell Scientific Publications.
Hytten, F. E. and Klopper, A. I. (1963), *J. Obstet. Gynaec. Br. Commonw.*, **70**, 811.
Hytten, F. E. and Thomson, A. M. (1966), *J. Obstet. Gynaec. Br. Commonw.*, **73**, 714.
Kerr, M. G., Scott, D. B. and Samuel, E. (1964), *Brit. med. J.*, **1**, 532.
Lees, M. M., Taylor, S. H., Scott, D. B. and Kerr, M. G. (1967), *J. Obstet. Gynaec. Br. Commonw.*, **74**, 319.
Le Quesne, L. P. (1957), *Fluid Balance in Surgical Practice*, 2nd Ed. London: Lloyd-Luke Ltd.
MacGillivray, I. and Buchanan, T. J. (1958), *Lancet*, **II**, 1090.
McLennan, C. E. (1943), *Amer. J. Obstet. Gynec.*, **45**, 568.
Rinsler, M. G. and Rigby, B. (1957), *Brit. med. J.*, **2**, 966.
Rhodes, P. (1960), *Fluid Balance in Obstetrics*. London: Lloyd-Luke Ltd.
Rhodes, P. (1962), *Lancet*, **I**, 663.
Thomson, A. M., Hytten, F. E. and Billewicz, W. Z. (1967), *J. Obstet. Gynaec. Br. Commonw.*, **74**, 1.

3. THE LIVER IN PREGNANCY

SHEILA SHERLOCK

LIVER FUNCTION DURING PREGNANCY

In normal pregnancy hepatic function is not significantly impaired although little is known about the detailed functions of the liver (Hytten and Leitch, 1964). The development of vascular spiders and palmar erythema may be due to the physiological increase of circulating oestrogens. These disappear with the termination of pregnancy.

Biochemical tests show a slight rise in the serum alkaline phosphatase level in the ninth month. Serum total cholesterol is raised but esterification normal. Serum albumin is reduced and globulins rise prior to delivery. Serum choline esterase values are reduced (Wetsone and Lamotta; Mildbrook, Pennart and White, 1958). Transaminase values are normal just prior to delivery and post partum (Fote, 1960).

The dye bromsulphalein (BSP) can be used to study hepatic function in more detail. This dye is rapidly removed by the liver and excreted in the bile. In the liver it is conjugated largely with glutathione for transfer from blood to bile. The standard BSP test, using a five mg. per kg. dose and taking one blood sample 45 minutes later, shows occasional slight impairment in the last trimester of pregnancy. If BSP is infused at two different rates and the plasma level analysed at intervals then subsequent calculations allow the measurement of the two independent processes of storage by the liver cells (S) and active secretion into the bile (Tm) (Wheeler, Meltzer and Bradley, 1960). Storage (S) rises 122 per cent during the last half of pregnancy returning towards normal during the first week post partum. In contrast, the Tm decreases 27 per cent in the last half of pregnancy and rapidly increases to normal levels after delivery (Combes; Shibata, Adams, Mitchell and Trammell, 1963). The quantity of BSP in the blood, liver and bile at any time following a single injection can be calculated reliably from knowledge of the plasma content of the dye alone (Richards, Tindall and Young, 1959). During pregnancy the essential changes are a slight increase in the uptake of BSP from the plasma, a twofold increase in the return of dye to the plasma, a reduction by one half to two thirds in the elimination of dye into the bile and an alteration in the proportion of dye lost from the liver cells per minute through the plasma and bile respectively (Tindall and Beazley, 1965). BSP is not transferred across the placenta and its fate after injection is qualitatively the same in the pregnant as in the non-pregnant subject.

Needle liver biopsy in normal pregnancy gives histological appearances that differ very little from the normal (Ingerslev and Teilum, 1951; Nixon, Egeli, Lacqueur and Yahya, 1947). Minor nonspecific changes include difference in size of liver cells, an increase in nuclear size, some increase in binucleate cells and occasionally very mild lymphocytic infiltration in the portal zones.

Liver blood flow is within the normal range (Munnell and Taylor, 1947). This is important because in pregnancy blood volume and cardiac output increase. The liver blood flow comprises 35 per cent of the cardiac output in non-pregnant females and only 28 per cent of the cardiac output in pregnancy. The excess blood volume is shunted through the placenta.

JAUNDICE IN PREGNANCY

TABLE 1 JAUNDICE IN PREGNANCY

Peculiar to pregnancy	Notes
Acute fatty liver.	Poor prognosis. Note relation to tetracycline therapy.
Recurrent cholestasis.	Good prognosis. Develop jaundice and pruritus if given oral contraceptives.
Toxaemias.	Rare cause of jaundice. Rupture of liver may occur.
Hyperemesis gravidarum.	Rare cause of jaundice.

INTERCURRENT JAUNDICE

Viral hepatitis.	Prognosis same as in non-pregnant. High incidence of stillbirths.
Gall stones.	Surprisingly rare as a cause of jaundice in pregnancy.
Hepatotoxic drugs.	Chlorpromazine may cause prolonged cholestasis. Prognosis otherwise as for non-pregnant.
Underlying liver disease.	Rare to become pregnant. No indication for premature termination. Prognosis variable.

Three aetiological types can be distinguished. The jaundice may be peculiar to pregnancy such as acute fatty liver of pregnancy, cholestatic jaundice in pregnancy or jaundice complicating the toxaemias. The jaundice may be an intercurrent one affecting the pregnant woman such as virus hepatitis or gall stones. Finally, the effect of pregnancy on underlying liver disease such as cirrhosis must be considered.

Jaundice occurs in about one out of every 1,500 gestations, an incidence of 0·067 per cent (Haemmerli, 1966). At least 41 per cent of all cases with jaundice are due to viral hepatitis and about 21 per cent to intrahepatic cholestasis of pregnancy. Common bile duct obstruction accounts for less than 6 per cent of all cases. These results are reported from Switzerland and different statistics can be expected from other parts of the world.

JAUNDICE PECULIAR TO PREGNANCY

Acute Fatty Liver

Sheehan (1940) was the first to suggest that there is a specific type of severe jaundice in pregnancy which he

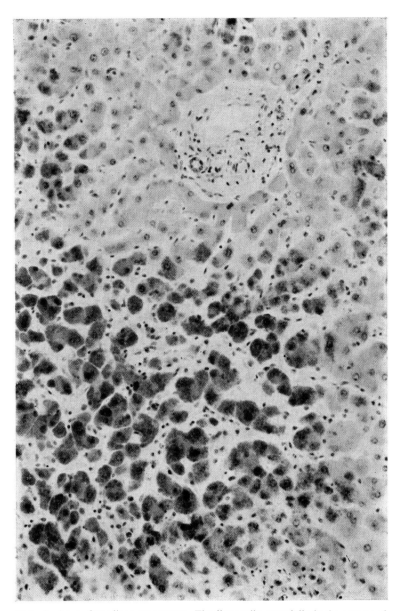

FIG. 1. Acute fatty liver pregnancy. The liver cells, especially in the centres of the lobules and in the mid zones, contain large quantities of fat. The portal area is spared. Necrosis is minimal. Stained Oil Red × 130.

called "obstetric acute yellow atrophy of the liver" but others have termed it "acute fatty liver of pregnancy" (Ober and Le Compte, 1955; Moore, 1956). During the last trimester of pregnancy, these mothers develop jaundice, severe nausea and vomiting, hæmatemesis, abdominal pain, headaches and stupor. Death is the usual outcome, several days after delivery. Survivals are reported (Woolf, Johnston, Stokes and Roberton, 1964; Duma, Dowling, Alexander, Sibrens and Dempsey, 1965). In many ways the course is similar to acute fulminant hepatitis, histology of the liver however is quite different. There is little or no hepatocellular necrosis or inflammatory reaction but many small intracytoplasmic lipid-laden vacuoles arranged around a centrally placed, normal nucleus (Fig. 1).

Recently this rare and severe jaundice of pregnancy has been related to protein malnutrition and in particular to the depression of protein synthesis caused by certain drugs particularly the tetracyclines. Ober and Le Compte (1955) noted that, in addition to acute fatty metamorphosis in the liver, there was fatty change in the renal tubular epithelium. This suggested a diffuse, metabolic disturbance. They postulated that ethionine acted as a competitive metabolite to methionine to produce these changes. Tetracycline is known to be a general inhibitor of cell metabolism and this is particularly apparent in the liver. More specifically, tetracycline apparently interferes with the incorporation of glutamate into protein, inhibits acetate metabolism and impairs oxidative phosphorylation. This depression of cell anabolism is so clear cut that in the 1950s tetracycline was even used in cancer chemotherapy. Bateman and co-workers (1952) gave 1–2 g. of tetracycline daily by the arterial route to 23 patients with cancer; but in several patients, jaundice and renal damage developed and this treatment of malignant disease was abandoned. When the tetracyclines were introduced for the chemotherapy of infections, liver damage was also noted. Lepper and his group (1951) gave 2 g. Chlortetracycline daily by mouth or intravenously to seven patients and, in every one enlargement of the liver and jaundice developed and the five of these who died (chiefly of the disease for which antibiotic therapy was being given) had fatty livers. This association of hepatic dysfunction and tetracycline therapy was largely forgotten until 1963 when Schultz and co-workers reported the deaths of six women who had had acute pyelonephritis associated with pregnancy and who had received tetracycline intravenously. They suffered nausea, vomiting, wide fluctuations in temperature, jaundice, haematemesis, melaena and azotaemia. The dose of tetracycline had been greater than that usually recommended, the maximum daily dose varying from 3·5 to 6 grams intravenously. The chief necropsy finding in each case was fine drops of fat in liver cells throughout the lobules. In addition, acute pyelonephritis was found in four patients, three of whom also had small abscesses in the kidneys. Two others had fatty deposits in the renal tubular epithelium. In 1964 Waller, Adams and Combes reported four cases of fatty liver of pregnancy following tetracycline therapy for acute pyelonephritis. Three of these four patients survived.

Kahil and colleagues (1964) also reported two pregnant patients who died with acute fatty liver, both of whom had received tetracycline, one for pyelonephritis and the other for broncho-pneumonia.

In a review of the subject, Kunelis, Peters and Edmondson (1965) have described sixteen patients with fatty liver of pregnancy. Twelve had acute pyelonephritis and were being treated with large doses of tetracycline intravenously. Four, who had not received tetracycline, had hepatic lesions that were indistinguishable from those seen in fatty liver of pregnancy. Six non-pregnant women who were treated with tetracycline intravenously, had similar fatty changes of the liver. There was a high incidence of pathological and functional involvement of the pancreas, kidneys, and brain. The central nervous system changes were so severe that they could have been responsible for the stupor and coma. The liver in pregnancy, with its increased demands for protein anabolism, may be more sensitive than the non-pregnant one to agents which depress this function, such as the tetracyclines. The similarity between the fatty liver of pregnancy and that seen in experimental lesions produced by other substances which depress protein anabolism such as ethionine or diets deficient in essential amino-acids, is striking. Co-existing pyelonephritis could also predispose to fatty liver of pregnancy.

The acute fatty liver of pregnancy is not found only in those who have received large doses of tetracycline. A patient with this condition, who was studied by serial light and electron microscopy of liver biopsy specimens, had never received tetracycline (Duma, Dowling, Alexander, Sibrans and Dempsey, 1965). She was in a very poor nutritional state and this is believed to have been the prime factor. Nevertheless it is advisable to avoid the use of the tetracyclines, especially intravenously, during the last trimester of pregnancy. The risk of liver damage may be greatest when the patient has pyelonephritis or is undernourished. The differential diagnosis of this condition from virus hepatitis can be difficult. The serum biochemical pattern is of increased serum bilirubin levels, reduced prothrombin time, azotaemia, hyperuricaemia and acidosis. Serum transaminase and alkaline phosphatase values are only moderately raised, a point of distinction from virus hepatitis. Needle liver biopsy may be required to make the diagnosis certain although, if blood coagulation is impaired, this procedure must be postponed until the recovery stage (Woolf et al., 1964). Hepatic histology shows multiple intracellular fat droplets without significant necrosis or cellular infiltrate. The picture is quite unlike the changes of fulminant virus hepatitis or other types of fatty liver. Electron microscopy shows a striking honey comb appearance in the smooth endoplasmic reticulum compatible with nutritional or toxic liver injury (Duma et al., 1965).

The prognosis is very poor, only six of forty cases surviving (Haemmerli, 1966). If survival does transpire however the ultimate prognosis is good (Woolf et al., 1964). The baby is usually stillborn, only five of forty children surviving.

Treatment is symptomatic for hepatic and renal failure.

Recurrent Intrahepatic Cholestatic Jaundice

This type of obstructive (cholestatic) jaundice appears in the last trimester of pregnancy. It has had many names including idiopathic hepatopathy of pregnancy (Ljünggren, 1956), hépatite benigne de la grossesse (Caroli, Puyo and Rampon, 1954) and idiopathic jaundice of pregnancy (King and Kerrins, 1963). The term recurrent intrahepatic cholestatic jaundice of pregnancy seems the most appropriate (Haemmerli, 1966; Sherlock, 1968).

In the mildest form jaundice is absent and the only abnormality is pruritus. Many patients experiencing generalized itching in the last weeks of pregnancy may be suffering from this condition. Jaundice is rarely deep, the urine is dark and the stools pale. General health is preserved and there is no pain. The liver and spleen are impalpable. After delivery jaundice disappears and within one to two weeks the pruritus has ceased, (Thörling, 1955). The condition recurs with subsequent pregnancies. It is a benign condition and prognoses for mother and child are excellent. Mild increases are found in these with itching (Fast and Roulston, 1964).

Serum shows an increase in conjugated bilirubin and alkaline phosphatase values. Serum transaminases are normal or slightly increased although occasionally very high values are found. A prolonged prothrombin time may lead to post partum haemorrhage and should be promptly dealt with by vitamin K_1.

Hepatic histology, obtained by needle biopsy, shows mild focal and irregular bile stasis. Hepatocellular necrosis and cellular reaction are absent. Electron microscopy shows the dilatation, blunting and swelling of the microvilli which is constantly found in all forms of cholestasis (Eliakim, Sadovsky, Stein and Shenkar, 1966).

The aetiology of this condition is unknown. It probably represents an unusual cholestatic reaction to a steroid produced in pregnancy. Whether this is an abnormal response to a natural steroid or due to the production of an unknown, cholestatic one remains uncertain. It has already been mentioned that normal women, in the last trimester, show increased difficulty in transfer of BSP into the biliary canaliculi. Bilirubin is in many ways analogous to bromsulphalein and the response in recurrent cholestatic jaundice of pregnancy may be an exaggeration of the normal one. Moreover natural oestrogens, in large doses, also cause abnormalities in the handling of BSP (Mueller and Kappas, 1964). There is also an association between jaundice following the administration of oral contraceptives and the intrahepatic cholestasis of pregnancy. Jaundice following "the pill" is extremely unusual, only some 100 cases having been reported. In the largest series of 50 patients, reported from Chile, the clinical, biochemical and microscopical findings bore a strong resemblance to those of cholestatic jaundice of pregnancy (Orellana-Alcalde and Dominguez, 1966). Forty of these fifty patients had had previous pregnancies, during which seventeen had suffered jaundice and pruritus and ten late pruritus only. The constituents of "the pill" are known to cause a fall in bromsulphalein transport when given to normal non-pregnant women (Kleiner, Krish and Arias, 1965). A family incidence was shown in one patient who was affected by recurrent intrahepatic cholestasis of pregnancy and who developed cholestasis when given an oral contraceptive (Holzbach and Sanders, 1965). Her mother and her sister also suffered pruritus and jaundice in pregnancy. It is interesting that reports of jaundice following oral contraceptives come from countries where recurrent intrahepatic cholestasis of pregnancy is frequent, such as Chile and Scandinavia (Orellana-Alcalde and Dominguez, 1966; Thulin and Jerker-Nermark, 1966). Oral contraceptives should not be given to patients who have previously suffered pruritus in pregnancy. Care should be taken before applying this method of population control to a country where intrahepatic cholestatic jaundice of pregnancy is frequent and icteric reactions to "the pill" can be anticipated.

In a first pregnancy the diagnosis of idiopathic, cholestatic jaundice from viral hepatitis and other conditions causing jaundice may be difficult. It might be possible to perform a diagnostic test after delivery. Serial serum bilirubin, alkaline phosphatase and bromsulphalein tests are done before, during and at the end of a one cycle course of an oral contraceptive drug in standard dosage. Increasing cholestasis would confirm the diagnosis of idiopathic cholestatic jaundice of pregnancy, contraindicate further use of this method of contraception and warn that subsequent pregnancies would be complicated by idiopathic cholestatic jaundice.

Toxaemias

Although abnormal tests of liver function, such as serum alkaline phosphatase and transaminase are common in pregnancy (Crisp, Miesfeld and Frajola, 1959; Kubli, 1961) jaundice is infrequent. In Sheehan's (1961) autopsy series of ninety cases of toxaemia only ten were jaundiced. The jaundice is mostly haemolytic. It is a grave sign, often being terminal.

Hepatic histology shows periportal fibrin deposition in the sinusoids with haemorrhages. Centrizonal necrosis and haemorrhage represent shock. An inflammatory reaction is characteristically absent. The liver lesions of eclampsia are terminal events. Toxaemia cannot be regarded as primarily involving the liver. Jaundice in the toxaemias rarely enters into the differential diagnosis of icterus in pregnancy.

Rupture of the Liver

Subcapsular liver haematomata with or without rupture and laceration of the liver parenchyma is a rare and grave complication of pregnancy (Barry and Meagher, 1964; Call and Lorentzen, 1965; Panaysis, Garcia-Bunuel and Calalang, 1965). Twenty cases have been reported. Severe eclampsia and pre-eclampsia was also present in nineteen.

The characteristic symptoms and signs are severe epigastric pain usually radiating to the back and right shoulder, vomiting and circulatory collapse (shock).

Treatment consists of early recognition and prompt surgical and supportive measures. Operative procedures include packing and suture of the laceration. Evacuation of the uterus is essential.

Hyperemesis Gravidarum

Jaundice in hyperemesis is rare and mild and does not carry a bad prognosis. Hepatic needle biopsy has not been performed. At autopsy mild fatty and other nonspecific changes are seen (Sheehan, 1961). These are probably nutritional in origin.

INTERCURRENT JAUNDICE IN PREGNANCY

Viral Hepatitis

The agent causing this common type of jaundice remains to be identified. The common experimental animals are not susceptible and there is no specific diagnostic test. Numerous needle punctures during the antenatal period provide a means of transmission of the serum hepatitis virus. Disposable syringes and needles eliminate this hazard. However, women of the child-bearing age are in close contact with the excreta of their children. Hepatitis is most frequent between the ages of three and ten. This family contact exposes them to the risk of infective hepatitis. Pregnant women are not more susceptible to hepatitis, whether infective or serum, than the general population. The incidence in epidemics is the same in the pregnant and non-pregnant (Martini, Von Harnack and Napp, 1953; Ellegast, Gumpesberger, Rissel and Wewalka, 1954). The incidence is equal in all trimesters of pregnancy. The clinical course, liver function tests and hepatic histology, as shown by needle biopsy, are the same as in the disease in the general population. A favourable outcome may usually be anticipated for the mother with hepatitis (Adams and Combes, 1965). It is often stated that virus hepatitis is particularly lethal to the pregnant woman. In Europe and the United States this is certainly not so (Martini et al., 1953; Cahill, 1962; Adams and Combes, 1965; Haemmerli, 1966). High mortality rates are reported from areas where undernutrition is frequent. A high mortality rate has for instance been reported from undernourished women in Israel (Zondek and Bromberg, 1947) and in the Delhi epidemic (Niadu and Viswanathan, 1957; Malkani and Grewal, 1957). Such reports have led the World Health Authority to recommend that, when supplies of prophylactic gamma globulin are limited, these should be used preferentially for pregnant women exposed to the disease (W.H.O., 1963).

In general the disease is managed in a similar fashion in the pregnant and the non-pregnant. Where it is considered necessary to confirm the diagnosis needle biopsy, using the Menghini technique (Sherlock, 1968), can safely be performed. The course of severe hepatitis is not influenced by termination of pregnancy and this should be avoided because it adds the strain of operation upon an already failing liver.

There are variable reports concerning the effects on foetus. Hepatitis is said to induce a tendency towards abortion or premature delivery (Martini, 1953), the survival depending on the stage of maturity at birth and not on the mother's disease (Haemmerli, 1966). Others have not observed an increased foetal wastage in pregnancies complicated by hepatitis (Cahill, 1962; Adams and Combes, 1965).

It might be questioned whether foetal damage, similar to that complicating other virus infections such as rubella, may result from the intra-uterine virus infection. The virus has a widely disseminated septicaemic stage in the mother and it is difficult to believe that the foetus is unscathed. However, there is no positive evidence to incriminate the pregnancy hepatitis as a cause of foetal abnormalities. In fact, infants born of mothers with virus hepatitis do not show evidence of neonatal hepatitis (Aterman, 1963).

In summary, virus hepatitis is the commonest cause of jaundice in pregnancy. It runs the same course as in the non-pregnant. There is no increased hazard. Termination of pregnancy is not recommended and the infant is not at additional risk except from premature birth.

Gall Stones

At all ages gall stones are more frequent in women than men and especially so below the age of 50 (Friedman, Kannell and Dawber, 1966). Gall stones are also associated with obesity and parity but not with the number of pregnancies (Van Der Linden, 1961). Stones in the common bile duct may therefore coincide with pregnancy and cause jaundice. The association is however surprisingly rare. In one combined series it comprised only 27 of 456 patients with jaundice in pregnancy (Haemmerli, 1966). The clinical picture does not differ from that in the non-pregnant and the management should be the same. If necessary needle biopsy of the liver may be used to help in diagnosis.

HEPATOTOXIC DRUGS AND THE PREGNANT WOMAN

The pregnant woman can react to drugs causing jaundice in similar fashion to the non-pregnant. Increased sensitivity to tetracycline has already been discussed and this would apply to any drug which decreases synthetic processes in the liver. Sensitivity to chlorpromazine with consequent cholestatic jaundice is infrequent. When it does affect the pregnant however it may be particularly prolonged, lasting for up to three and a half years (Read, Harrison and Sherlock, 1961).

Jaundice following multiple exposures to the anaesthetic halothane is rare (Davidson, Babior and Popper, 1966). It is however very lethal and note should be taken of any slight fever or jaundice in a pregnant woman following halothane. In these circumstances the anaesthetic should not be repeated.

The effect of drugs in potentiation of jaundice or kernicterus in the newborn must be considered (Sherlock, 1966). In particular, drugs such as sulphonamides which displace bilirubin from its binding site to serum bilirubin or novobiocin which inhibits conjugation of bilirubin in the liver should be avoided. Drugs such as Phenacetin, given to the mother, may precipitate jaundice in an infant with glucose 6-phosphate dehydrogenase deficiency.

EFFECT OF PREGNANCY ON PRE-EXISTING LIVER DISEASE

The mild jaundice associated with the benign, familial hyperbilirubinaemias with conjugated bilirubin in the liver (Dubin-Johnson, Rotor types) are reported both to increase and decrease with pregnancy. In the Gilbert type, where the hyperbilirubinaemia is unconjugated, the effect of pregnancy has not been studied.

The full time parturition of a woman suffering from hepatic cirrhosis is unusual. In one such instance the mother, suffering from cirrhosis, showed no deterioration of hepatic function during the pregnancy. The infant became jaundiced in the first twenty-four hours and this lasted for thirteen days, when recovery was complete and the infant progressed normally (Slater, 1964). It is very rare for such a patient to conceive. The liver disease is not an indication for termination.

The condition of active chronic hepatitis (lupoid hepatitis, juvenile cirrhosis) affects predominantly young women. Amenorrhoea is usual at the onset but occasionally the disease becomes less active and menses return. Jaundice is usually mild. Such patients may become pregnant and one conceived on three occasions and bore two living children (Joske, Pawsey and Martin, 1963). This patient deteriorated during each pregnancy. Another deeply jaundiced patient with active chronic hepatitis became pregnant and delivered normally (Seedat and Raine, 1965). The baby was deeply jaundiced.

The concidence of liver disease and pregnancy should not *per se* indicate termination. Special care must be taken during the pregnancy. Specialist maternity care is essential. Spontaneous delivery should be anticipated.

Oesophageal varices may bleed during pregnancy (Gordon and Johnston, 1963) and portacaval shunt has been successfully performed during the pregnancy (Johnston, Gordon and Rodgers, 1965).

Primary biliary cirrhosis may present as a cholestatic jaundice in or shortly after pregnancy (Sherlock, 1959).

REFERENCES

Adams, R. H. and Combes, B. (1965), "Viral Hepatitis during Pregnancy," *J. Amer. med. Ass.*, **192**, 195.

Adlercreutz, H., Svanborg, A. and Anberg, A. (1967), "Recurrent Jaundice in Pregnancy: II. A Study of the Estrogens and their Conjugation in Late Pregnancy," *Amer. J. Med.*, **42**, 341.

Aterman, K. (1963), "Neonatal Hepatitis and its Relation to Viral Hepatitis of Mother," *Amer. J. Dis. Child.*, **105**, 113.

Barry, A. P. and Meagher, D. J. (1964), "Rupture of the Liver Complicating Pregnancy," *Obstet. Gynaec.*, **23**, 381.

Bateman, J. C., Barberio, J. R., Grice, P., Klopp, C. T. and Pierpoint, H. (1952), "Fatal Complications of Intensive Antibiotic Therapy in Patients with Neoplastic Disease," *Arch. intern. Med.*, **90**, 763.

Cahill, K. M. (1962), "Hepatitis in Pregnancy," *Surg. Gynaec. Obstet.*, **114**, 545.

Call, M. and Lorentzen, D. (1965), "Rupture of the Liver in Pregnancy: Report of a Case," *Obstet. Gynaec.*, **25**, 466.

Caroli, J., Puyo, G. and Rampon (1954), "Remarques sur les hépatites ictérigènes de la grossesse," *Sem. Hop. Paris*, **30**, 1692.

Combes, B., Shibata, H., Adams, R., Mitchell, B. D. and Trammell, V. (1963), "Alterations in Sulfobromophthalein Sodium Removal Mechanisms from Blood during Normal Pregnancy," *J. clin. Invest.*, **42**, 1431.

Cook, G. C. and Sherlock, S. (1965), "Jaundice and its Relation to Therapeutic Agents," *Lancet*, **i**, 3378.

Crisp, W. C., Miesfeld, R. L. and Frajola, W. J. (1959), "Serum Glutamic Oxalacetic Transaminase Levels in the Toxaemias of Pregnancy," *Obstet. Gynaec.*, **13**, 487.

Davidson, C. S., Babior, B. and Popper, H. (1966), "Concerning Hepatotoxicity of Halothane," *New Engl. J. Med.*, **275**, 1497.

Duma, R. J., Dowling, E. A., Alexander, H. C., Sibrans, D. and Dempsey, H. (1965), "Acute Fatty Liver of Pregnancy: Report of a Surviving Patient Studied with Serial Liver Biopsies," *Ann. intern. Med.*, **63**, 851.

Eliakim, M., Sadovsky, E., Stein, O. and Shenkar, Y. G. (1966), "Recurrent Cholestatic Jaundice of Pregnancy: Report of Five Cases and Electron Microscopic Observations," *Arch. intern. Med.*, **117**, 696.

Ellegast, H., Gumpeserger, G., Rissel, E. and Wewalka, F. (1954), "Virus hepatitis und Graviditat; haufigkeit und schwere der hepatitis," *Wien. klin. Wschr.*, **66**, 42.

Fast, B. B. and Roulston, T. M. (1964), "Idiopathic Jaundice of Pregnancy," *Amer. J. Obstet. Gynec.*, **88**, 314.

Fote, F. A. (1960), "Hepatic Effects of Chloroform Anaesthesia in Obstetrics," *Amer. J. Obstet. Gynec.*, **79**, 1142.

Friedman, G. D., Kannell, W. B. and Dawber, T. R. (1966), "The Epidemiology of Gallbladder Disease: Observations in the Framingham Study," *J. Chr. Dis.*, **19**, 273.

Gordon, A. G. and Johnston, G. W. (1963), "Portal Hypertension in Pregnancy," *J. Obstet. Gynæc. Brit. Cwlth.*. **70**, 1056.

Griner, P. F. (1966), "Hepatitis after Repeated Exposure to Halothane: Case Report and Brief Review," *Ann. int. Med.*, **65**, 753.

Haemmerli, U. R. (1966), "Jaundice during Pregnancy with Special Emphasis on Recurrent Jaundice during Pregnancy and its Differential Diagnosis, *Acta med. scand.*, **197** (suppl.), 444.

Holzbach, R. T. and Sanders, J. H. (1965), "Recurrent Intrahepatic Cholestasis of Pregnancy: Observations on Pathogenesis," *J. Amer. med. Ass.*, **193**, 542.

Hytten, F. E. and Leitch, I. (1964), "Physiology of Human Pregnancy." Oxford: Blackwell Scientific Publications.

Ingerslev, M. and Teilum, G. (1951), "Jaundice during Pregnancy," *Acta obstet. gynaec. scand.*, **31**, 74.

Joske, R. A., Pawsey, H. K. and Martin, J. D. (1963), "Chronic Active Liver Disease and Successful Pregnancy," *Lancet*, **ii**, 712.

Johnston, G. W., Gordon, A. G. and Rodgers, H. W. (1965), "Portacaval Shunt Performed during Pregnancy," *J. Obstet. Gynaec. Brit. Cwlth.*, **72**, 292.

Kahil, M. E., Fred, H. L., Brown, H. and Davis, J. S. (1964), "Acute Fatty Liver of Pregnancy." Report of two Cases. *Arch. Intern. Med. (Chicago)*, **113**, 63.

King, M. J. and Kerrins, J. F. (1963), "Recurrent Idiopathic Jaundice of Pregnancy," *New Engl. J. Med.*, **268**, 1180.

Klein, N. C. and Jeffries, G. H. (1966), "Hepatotoxicity after Methoxyflurane Administration," *J. Amer. med. Ass.*, **197**, 1037.

Kleiner, G. J., Kresch, L. and Arias, I. M. (1965), "Studies of Hepatic Excretory Function: II. The Effect of Norethynodrel and Mestranol on Bromsulphalein Sodium Metabolism in Women of Child Bearing Age," *New Engl. J. Med.*, **273**, 420.

Koff, R. S., Grady, G. F., Chalmers, T. C., Mosley, J. W., Swartz, B. L. and the Boston Inter-Hospital Liver Group (1967), "Viral Hepatitis from Shellfish," *New Engl. J. Med.*, **376**, 703.

Kubli, F. (1961), "Transaminase, Lactic Dehydrogenase and Alkaline Phosphatase in Late Pregnancy, during Labour and in Toxicosis," *Gynaecologia*, **151**, 72.

Kunelis, C. T., Peters, J. L. and Edmondson, H. A. (1965), "Fatty Liver of Pregnancy and Its Relationship to Tetracycline Therapy," *Amer. J. Med.*, **38**, 359.

Larsson-Cohn, U. and Stenram, U. (1967), "Liver Ultrastructure and Function in Icteric and Non-icteric Women using Oral Contraceptive Agents," *Acta. med. scand.*, **181**, 257.

Lepper, M. H., Wolfe, C. K., Zimmerman, H. A., Cladwell, E. R., Spies, H. W. and Dowling, H. F. (1951), "Effect of Aureomycin on Human Liver," *Arch. intern. Med.*, **88**, 271.

Ljunggren, G. (1956), "Clinical Aspects of Icterus in Pregnancy," *Nord. med.*, **55**, 373.

Malkani, P. K. and Grewal, A. K. (1957), "Observations on Infectious Hepatitis in Pregnancy," *Indian J. med. Res.*, **45** (suppl.), 77.

Martini, G. A. (1953), "Hepatitis und Schwangerschaft," *Schweiz. Z. allg. Path.*, **16**, 479.

Martini, G. A., von Harnack, G. A. and Napp, J. H. (1953), "Hepatitis und Schwangerschaft; die Auswicking der heparitis auf die Mütter," *Duetsch. Med. Wschr.*, **78**, 661.

Mueller, N. M. and Kappas, A. (1964), "Estrogen Pharmacology: I. The Influence of Estradiol and Estriol on Hepatic Disposal of Sulfobromophthalein (B.S.P.) in Man," *J. clin. Invest.*, **43**, 1905.

Munnell, E. W. and Taylor, H. C. Jr. (1947), "Liver Blood Flow in Pregnancy—Hepatic Vein Catheterisation," *J. clin. Invest.*, **26**, 952.

Naidu, S. S. and Viswanathan, R. (1957), "Infectious Hepatitis in Pregnancy during Delhi Epidemic," *Indian J. med. Res.*, **45** (suppl.), 71.

Nixon, W. C. W., Edeli, E. S., Laqueur, W. and Yahya, O. (1947), "Icterus in Pregnancy: A Clinicopathological Study Including Liver Biopsy," *J. Obstet. Gynaec. Brit. Emp.*, **54**, 641.

Ober, W. and Le Compte, P. M. (1955), "Acute Fatty Metamorphosis of the Liver Associated with Pregnancy: a Distinctive Lesion," *Amer. J. Med.*, **19**, 743.

Orellana-Alcalde, J. M. and Dominguez, J. P. (1966), "Jaundice and Oral Contraceptive Drugs," *Lancet*, **ii**, 1278.

Panayis, A. H., Garcia-Bunuel, R. and Calalang, S. (1965), "Subcapsular Hæmatoma of the Liver Complicating Pregnancy: Report of a Case and Review of the Literature," *Obstet. Gynæc.*, **26**, 115.

Read, A. E., Harrison, C. V. and Sherlock, S. (1961), "Chronic Chlorpromazine Jaundice with Particular Reference to its Relationship to Primary Biliary Cirrhosis," *Amer. J. Med.*, **31**, 249.

Richards, T. G., Tindall, V. R. and Young, A. (1959), "A Modification of the Bromsulphthalein Liver Function Test to Predict the Dye Content of the Liver and Bile," *Clin. Sci.*, **18**, 499.

Schultz, J. C., Adamson, J. S. Jr., Workman, W. W. and Norman, T. D. (1963), "Fatal Liver Disease after Intravenous Administration of Tetracycline in High Dosage," *New Eng. J. Med.*, **269**, 999.

Seedat, Y. K. and Raine, E. R. (1965), "Active Chronic Hepatitis Associated with Renal Tubular Acidosis and Successful Pregnancy," *S. Afr. med. J.*, **39**, 595.

Sheehan, H. L. (1940), "The Pathology of Acute Yellow Atrophy and Delayed Chloroform Poisoning," *J. Obstet. Gynaec. Brit. Emp.*, **47**, 49.

Sheehan, H. L. (1961), "Jaundice in Pregnancy," *Amer. J. Obstet. Gynec.*, **81**, 427.

Sherlock, S. (1959), "Primary Biliary Cirrhosis (Chronic Intrahepatic Obstructive Jaundice)," *Gastroenterol.*, **37**, 574.

Sherlock, S. (1968), *Diseases of the Liver and Biliary System*, 4th edition. Oxford: Blackwell.

Sherlock, S. (1966), "Prediction of Hepatotoxicity Due to Therapeutic Agents in Man," *Medicine (Balt.)*, **45**, 453.

Slater, R. J. (1954), "Investigation of an Infant Born to a Mother Suffering from Cirrhosis of the Liver," *Pediatrics*, **13**, 308.

Thorling, L. (1955), "Jaundice in Pregnancy: A Clinical Study," *Acta med. scand.*, **151** (suppl.), 302.

Thulin, K. E. and Nermark, J. (1966), "Seven Cases of Jaundice in Women Taking an Oral Contraceptive, Anovlar," *Brit. med. J.*, **i**, 584.

Tindall, V. R. and Beazley, J. M. (1965), "An Assessment of Changes in Liver Function during Normal Pregnancy using a Modified Bromsulphthalein Test," *J. Obstet. Gynaec. Brit. Cwlth.*, **72**, 717.

Van der Linden W. (1961), "Some Biological Traits in Female Gallstone-disease Patients," *Acta chir. scand. suppl.*, 269.

Wetstone, H. J., Lamotta, R. V., Middlebrook, L., Tennant, R. and White, B. V. (1958), "Studies of Cholinesterase Activity: IV. Liver Function in Pregnancy: Value of Certain Standard Liver Function Tests in Normal Pregnancy," *Amer. J. Obstet. Gynec.*, **76**, 480.

Whalley, P. J., Adams, R. H. and Coombes, B. (1964), "Tetracycline Toxicity in Pregnancy," *J. Amer. med. Ass.*, **189**, 357.

Wheeler, H. O., Meltzer, J. I. and Bradley, S. E. (1960), "Biliary Transport and Hepatic Storage of Sulfobromophthalein Sodium in the Unanaesthetised Dog, in Normal Man, and in Patients with Hepatic Disease," *J. clin. Invest.*, **39**, 1131.

Woolf, A. J., Johnston, A. W., Stokes, J. F. and Robertson, N. R. C. (1964), "Acute Liver Failure in Pregnancy: Case Report with Survival of Mother and Child," *J. Obstet. Gynaec. Brit. Cwlth.*, **71**, 914.

World Health Organisation (1964), "W.H.O. Expert Committee on Hepatitis," *Tech. Rep. Ser. Wld. Hlth. Org.*, No. 285.

Zondek, B. and Bromberg, Y. M. (1947), "Infectious Hepatitis in Pregnancy," *J. Mt. Sinai Hosp.*, **14**, 222.

1. CENTRAL NERVOUS MECHANISMS OF UTERINE SENSATION

DAVID BOWSHER

The nervous system probably originated as a conducting linkage between a receptor on the one hand and an effector on the other. Phylogenetic studies show that neurones become progressively specialised to conduct more and more rapidly. These considerations have two implications for the study of advanced organisms. First, as animal life started in an aquatic environment, chemoreceptors were the first to develop, and may still be said to hold a certain primacy; the dominating forebrain of higher vertebrates evolved, in the first instance, in response to the importance of the input from the olfactory nerves. The internal environment of even the highest land vertebrates is still, of course, essentially in aqueous solution, and therefore that part of the brain, the hypothalamus, which regulates the internal environment not only has a very ancient phylogenetic history, but retains its pride of functional place among more obtrusive newcomers.

The second point is that the afferent nerve fibres leading from phylogenetically ancient chemoreceptors will themselves be of an "old" type, and will not show the morphological advances which enable more recently evolved neurone systems to conduct impulses so much more rapidly.

All receptors are transducers, which convert some specific form of energy (chemical, mechanical, photic) into the electro-chemical force which we call the nervous impulse. The receptor may be a specialised non-nervous element, such as the acoustic hair cell or the Pacini corpuscle, which in some way activates (i.e. depolarises) the nerve fibre with which it is in contact. But in the case of the more primitive chemoreceptors, the neurone is itself the transducer; olfactory nerve endings are directly depolarised by solutions of the chemical substance to which they are specifically sensitive; hypothalamic neurones are directly sensitive to the concentrations of various substances in the plasma circulating through this part of the brain. Nerve endings in the tegument are sensitive to histamine-like substances released by damaged tissue—for the primitive organism needs a signalling system which will help it to withdraw from noxious situations as much as it needs an olfactory system to draw it towards potential food or mates.

Because the external membranes of neurones, like those of all living cells, are selectively semipermeable, they are electrically charged by the balance of various ions on either side. The special property of nerve fibres consists in the fact that when chemical forces temporarily "dissolve" the membrane, allowing the charges on the two sides to be reversed by ionic flux, the depolarised segment acts as the positive pole of a battery with respect to the next (polarised)

segment, which is the negative pole; a current is thereby set up, the effect of which is to depolarise the formerly resting segment, and so on throughout the length of the axon. The active segments are subsequently restored to resting potential by the metabolic sodium-potassium pump mechanism, which is classically exemplified in the red blood corpuscle. The impulse in nerve fibres is carried not by electrons, as in the case of electricity, but by charged ions. It is therefore several million times slower than electric current—in the primitive, so called unmyelinated (non-noded) axons discussed above, conduction velocity varies from 0·5 to 2 metres per second ($1\frac{1}{2}$ to 6 m.p.h.) according to the diameter of the fibre. In larger axons with classical myelin sheaths, interrupted by nodes of Ranvier, the depolarising process jumps from node to node (saltatory conduction) and so travels much more rapidly—up to 120 metres per second (about 300 m.p.h.) in the largest human fibres. For a full review of nerve conduction, see Hodgkin (1964).

It is interesting that the initiation of the nervous impulse at the receptor sites discussed above is a depolarisation brought about by chemical means, for the transmission of an impulse from one neurone to another at a synapse, and the transmission of an impulse from a neurone to a muscle, is also brought about by secretion of a chemical transmitter substance. When considering impulses passing along chains of neurones, in addition to conduction time, synaptic delay, caused by chemical transmission, must also be taken into account. This is roughly of the order of 1/2000 sec. for each synapse.

Two further basic interlinked concepts must be considered before describing neural pathways and global mechanisms. These are (i) threshold, and (ii) convergence. A certain threshold intensity of stimulation must be achieved to activate a receptor. If, as in the cases discussed above, the receptor is the nerve ending itself, then an adequate stimulus will fire the first neurone. But when the impulse arrives at a synapse, it may not be adequate to initiate a discharge in the next neurone; that is, it may not, of itself, liberate a sufficient quantity of transmitter substance to bring about threshold depolarisation of the second neurone. Adequate depolarisation may, however, be brought about either by the simultaneous arrival of afferent impulses along a number of convergent fibres (spatial summation) or by the arrival of a number of impulses along the same fibre, following one another so closely that their depolarising effects are additive (temporal summation).

Non-myelinated chemosensitive fibres of the type described above may well be responsible for pain casued by mechanical damage to skin and viscera, though clinical experience of the relative insensitivity of viscera to crushing would suggest that the density of distribution of such fibres in hollow viscera is much less than in skin. Non-myelinated axons activated by stretch-compression have also been observed in populations of visceral afferent fibres; whether impulses in such nerves are consciously interpreted as painful or not is as yet unknown.

Recent research directed towards the elucidation of pelvic pain has established that (i) uterine pain can be brought about by electrical stimulation of the uterus (which will, of course, activate all types of afferent fibre); (ii) the (electrical) threshold of such pain is lowered in cases of dysmenorrhoea, and (iii) the pain threshold can be raised by local anaesthesia of the (somatic) ilio-inguinal and ilio-hypogastric nerves. (Theobald *et al.*, 1966). Thus the classical theory of referred pain can be confirmed, for the pelvic viscera are supplied by the same spinal cord segments as the ilio-inguinal and ilio-hypogastric nerves.

Furthermore, the opposite threshold changes caused by uterine irritation on the one hand, and somatic sensory anaesthesia on the other, suggest that conscious pelvic pain depends upon a threshold quantity of summated peripheral afferent activity reaching the spinal cord.

The mechanisms and pathways by which impulses generated by noxious stimuli reach conscious levels are complex, and may be best explained with reference to a diagram (Fig.1). It will be seen immediately that we are essentially dealing with two distinct systems within the C.N.S. which are called specific or lemniscal and non-specific or extralemniscal respectively (Bowsher and Albe-Fessard, 1965). It is therefore most important to realise at the outset that these separate central systems are supplied, by collateral branching, from a single set of peripheral afferent fibres (Fig. 4).

It will be simpler first to deal with the well-known classical lemniscal (specific) systems, which consist of small numbers of long neurones, organised both spatially and in respect to modality, leading eventually through the thalamus to the specific sensory cortex. Although these are probably of less importance in the appreciation of pelvic pain, they are largely responsible for localizing signs, and so must be considered here. Within the spinal cord, two groups of fibres may conveniently be described (Fig. 2). In the first group all large and most medium-sized medullated primary afferent fibres from mechanoreceptors (only) pass directly, without synapse, into the ipsilateral dorsal columns of the spinal cord. Since the arrangement is orderly both for place and for sub-modality (i.e. touch-pressure, hair movement, vibration, joint-movement) as the fibres travel up the dorsal columns to the gracile and cuneate (dorsal column) nuclei at the caudal end of the medulla oblongata, this means that in the upper part of the spinal cord, fibres originating from lower (lumbar and sacral) dorsal roots will go into the most medial part of the dorsal columns (gracile funiculus).

These fibres relay by forming synapses with the neurones of the dorsal column nuclei, and at this point the impulses are subjected to modification both by descending influences from higher (cortical) centres and by the activity of inter-

neurones within the nuclei. Long efferent axons from neurones of the dorsal column nuclei decussate under the central canal (internal arcuate fibres), thereby helping to bring it to the surface to form the floor of the fourth ventricle, and then turn rostrally as the medial lemniscus. This large fibre bundle ascends through the brain stem,

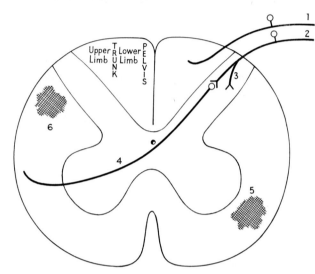

FIG. 2. Diagrammatic cross-section of spinal cord to show location of various pathways. Large mechanoreceptor fibres (1) enter dorsal columns to run up without synapse to the gracile and cuneate nuclei, in the orderly fashion indicated in the left dorsal column. Smaller primary afferent fibres (2) enter dorsal horn of spinal cord to synapse both with specific lemniscal neospinothalamic neurones (4), whose axons cross and ascend in the opposite anterolateral columns and with extralemniscal (non-specific) systems (3) (see Fig. 4). After various synaptic transfers at segmental level in the spinal cord, non-specific spino-reticular fibres ascend in the anterolateral columns, in the position indicated by 5. Descending control system fibres occupy the area marked 6.

without giving off any noteworthy collateral branches, until it reaches the thalamus, where its axons terminate in the lateral part of the ventroposterior nucleus. Both in the medial lemniscus and thalamus, the orderly topographical arrangement is maintained. As the fibres have decussated after leaving the dorsal column nuclei, the lower segments of the body are now represented in the lateral part of the medial lemniscus and thalamus. Again at thalamic level, the impulses are subject to modification at synaptic transfer. The final thalamo-cortical neurone is projected again in an orderly fashion, to the primary sensory areas of the cerebral cortex, mainly in the postcentral gyrus; though there is some evidence that impulses originating in the viscera may reach the cortex of the insula, underlying the Rolandic area.

The second group of lemniscal fibres are represented by smaller medullated primary afferents, coming from some mechanoreceptors, from thermal receptors, and from "fast pain" (pinprick) receptors. These primary afferents relay in the grey matter of the dorsal horn of the spinal cord, whence a second neurone crosses over in the anterior commissure (taking up to 5 segments to do so) and then runs rostrally (cranially) in the anterolateral spinal white matter

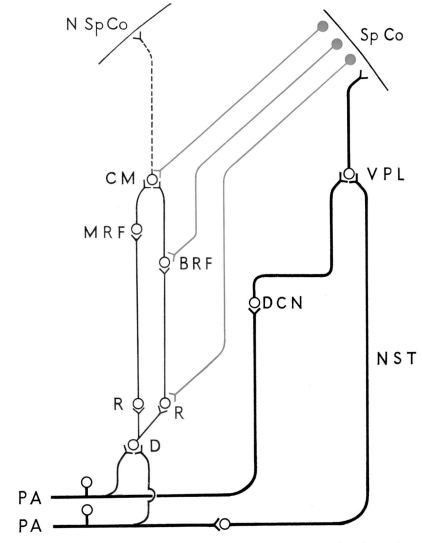

Fig. 1. Specific (lemniscal) systems are shown in black; non-specific (extralemniscal or ascending reticular) in red. Note that primary afferent fibres (PA) give off collaterals on entry into the cord which synapse with neurones of the non-specific system. D and R are segmental common carrier and relay cells respectively, as shown in Fig. 4. BRF: Bulbar (medullary) reticular formation; MRF: midbrain reticular formation; CM: intralaminar thalamic nuclei; N Sp Co: non-specific (non-primary or "associational") cortex. NST: Neospinothalamic fibres: DCN: Dorsal column nuclei; VPL: specific (lemniscal) thalamic relay; Sp Co: Specific (primary) somatosensory cortex. Shown in blue are the descending central neurones which arise in the specific cortex, but exert their influence on the non-specific system.

on the opposite side of the cord (Fig. 2). The lemniscal component of this fibre system (the neospinothalamic fibres) joins the medial lemniscus in the rostral part of the medulla oblongata and is distributed with it to the thalamus (Fig. 1); and thence follows a common pathway to the cortex. It should be emphasised that in comparison with the total numbers of fibres in the anterolateral quadrant of the cord and in the medial lemniscus, the number of neospinothalamic fibres is very small.

Two groups of cells in the grey matter of the spinal cord are concerned with the first relay of the extralemniscal ascending reticular system (Fig. 2), which may be roughly defined as the central grey core of the spinal cord and brain stem (Fig. 3). One group lies fairly deep in the dorsal horn, and receives collaterals from the smaller myelinated primary afferents whose stem axon goes on to feed into the specific lemniscal systems (dorsal column or neospino-thalamic). Note that the two systems, lemniscal and extra-lemniscal, share a common primary peripheral afferent fibre, but that beyond its terminal collateral branching at the segmental entry level, they are completely independent of each other.

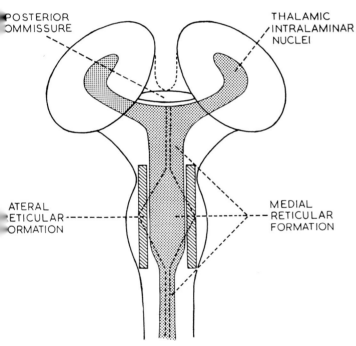

FIG. 3. The central reticular core of the neuraxis is represented by a continuous column of grey matter extending up from the spinal cord through the medial reticular formation of the lower brain stem right up to and including the intralaminar nuclei of the thalamus (reproduced, by permission, from Bowsher, *Brit. J. Anaesth.*, 1961).

In addition to these collaterals, this group of cells (known as common carrier cells) also receives small mye-linated fibres coming from muscle and other deep tissues. In sharp contrast to the relay cells of the dorsal column nuclei or neospinothalamic system, these extralemniscal dorsal horn neurones are supplied by convergent afferents coming from many types of receptor; thus modality

distinction, in the strict sense, is lost at the first synapse (Fig. 4).

The second group of first-order extralemniscal neurones is formed by the cells of the substantia gelatinosa, at the external tip of the dorsal grey horn; non-myelinated primary peripheral afferents converge onto these cells,

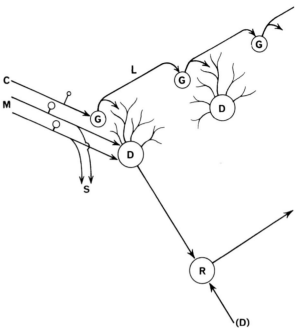

FIG. 4. Myelinated primary afferents (M) of different modalities converge on common carrier cells (D), after giving off long collaterals (S) which feed into specific lemniscal system. Non-myelinated primary afferents (C) make synaptic contact with cells of substantia gela-tinosa (G), whose axons interconnect with one another as the tract of Lissauer (L); collaterals from these axons establish contact with dendrites of common carrier cells, thereby modulating their level of excitability. Common carrier cell axons converge on spino-reticular relay cells (R) which convey impulses upwards to brain stem reticular formation and intralaminar thalamus. For descending control, see Fig. 1 (reproduced by permission from Bowsher, Introduction to the Anatomy and Physiology of the Nervous System, Blackwell Scientific Publications, Oxford and Edinburgh).

which are interconnected with each other, up and down the length of the cord, by their axons which form the tract of Lissauer. Collaterals from the gelatinosal cell axons make synaptic contact with outwardly-reaching dendrites from the extralemniscal dorsal horn cells described in the preceding paragraphs, and are thus able to modulate their level of excitability. Essentially, then, unmyelinated peripheral afferents eventually act, by way of the substantia gelatinosa, on extralemniscal neurones deeper in the grey matter of the dorsal horn (Melzack and Wall, 1965). The fact that gelatinosal cells are themselves interconnected up and down several segments of the cord by the tract of Lissauer already implies that even the first-order extra-lemniscal neurones (D) in the dorsal horn proper are exposed to influences coming from a variety of sites in the body. These common carrier neurones themselves have short axons, which further converge on other spinal neurones (marked R in Fig. 4). The number of inter-neurones at spinal level is not known, but may well be larger than shown in the simplified diagram of Figure 4. Certainly it is known that some R neurones receive, via interneurones, an input from both sides of the body so that at this level, place as well as modality specificity is to some extent lost. That it is not completely lost is due to the frequently overlooked fact that the inter-connections and convergences displayed by these neurones, though multitudinous, are not infinite.

The R neurones of Figure 4 have long axons which project upwards in the anterolateral quandrant of the spinal cord (Fig. 1). Most of them are spinoreticular—i.e. they end in association with neurones of the lower brain stem reticular formation. A small number of them (palæospinothalamic fibres) carry right on up to the intra-laminar nuclei of the thalamus, to which the lower levels of the reticular formation also project. The intralaminar thalamic nuclei also have an input from the limbic system of the forebrain (Fig. 5), the significance of which will be discussed below.

The cells of the intralaminar group of thalamic nuclei are known to send their axons to the corpus striatum, and can thus influence muscle tone through the extrapyramidal motor system, of which the corpus striatum has been described as the "head ganglion". Because of the eventual convergence of both extralemniscal impulses, initiated in somatic and visceral receptors, and limbic influences coming from those parts of the forebrain concerned with affect, it is evident that both somato-visceral stimulation and emotional state can, and do, express themselves in terms of changes in muscle tone (Fig. 5).

There is no anatomically proven direct projection from the intralaminar thalamic nuclei to the cerebral cortex, but nevertheless this nuclear group has long been known to have an important effect on the non-primary areas of the cerebral cortex, i.e. those areas to which lemniscal systems do not project—sometimes known as "association cortex". Because of the ability to produce fast asynchronous EEG activity, the intralaminar nuclei are often said to be the final (or penultimate) link in an "ascending reticular activating system".

It remains to describe the descending influences on the extralemniscal ascending reticular system; it is only by taking these carefully into account that one can hope to elucidate its function.

So-called "second pain" is defined as that which comes relatively slowly to consciousness, is poorly localised, and the sensation of which outlasts the application of the provoking stimulus. It may be reasonably assumed to be mediated within the C.N.S., by the ascending extra-lemniscal reticular system, which should now be considered with particular reference to afferent input from the pelvic viscera.

Although the common carrier cells (D of Fig. 4) receive, as has been shown, a convergent input which is complete so far as modality is concerned, there is evidence suggesting that their output pattern bears some relation-ship to the type of stimulus which provokes their activation. This is only to be expected when it is remembered that a

considerable degree of spatial summation of peripheral input is necessary to raise their level of excitability to firing threshold; and in this respect the input from C fibres through the substantia gelatinosa is of considerable significance. It may be noted in parenthesis that in a case of congenital absence of pain it has been shown that the tract of Lissauer and the substantia gelatinosa were severely affected.

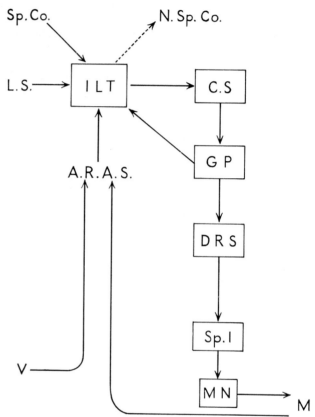

Fig. 5. Intralaminar thalamus (ILT) receives inputs from specific cortex (Sp. Co), ascending reticular activating system (A.R.A.S.), globus pallidus (GP) and limbic system (LS) via fornix. Outputs go in directly to non-specific cortex (N. Sp. Co.) and directly to corpus stria-tum (C.S.). Thence influences pass via globus pallidus (GP) through descending reticular system (DRS) to spinal interneurones (Sp. I) and finally to motor-neurones (MN) whose axons influence muscular activity (M). Afferents from muscles and viscera (V) are among the many influencing the activity of the ascending reticular activating system.

It is in quantitative convergence on common carrier cells that the explanation of Theobald et al's findings may be sought. Thus local anaesthesia of the ilio-inguinal and ilio-hypogastric nerves reduce the total quantity of afferent bombardment of the common carrier cells to which uterine nerves also project.

It is probable that the uterine nerves, being all of the small myelinated or unmyelinated categories, establish central contacts only with the extralemniscal system. However, the somatic ilio-hypogastric and ilio-inguinal nerves, as well as establishing collateral extralemniscal synapses with the same common carrier neurones as the uterine nerves, also take part in a specific lemniscal system; and this could account for many forms of uterine pain being referred to the distribution of these somatic nerves.

Similarly the lowered pain threshold of the diseased uterus may be explained by the assumption that in these cases the level of chronic afferent bombardment is raised, though it may still be sub-threshold so far as conscious experience of pain is concerned; however, very little extra input is required to bring about pain sensation.

In this type of case, it is important to realise that one is dealing not only with temporal summation, but also with spatial summation, such that the extra excitatory impulses necessary to bring about a "pain pattern" of common carrier cell firing may come from a wide receptive field area.

Various spinal extralemniscal interneurones, as well as longer spino-reticular relay neurones, are subjected to descending inhibitory influences from higher levels of the C.N.S. (Fig. 1). Evidence is accumulating to show that (a) this descending inhibition, the pathway for which lies in the dorsolateral part of the spinal white matter (Fig. 2), is tonic in nature; that is to say, the extralemniscal system shows a degree of spontaneous activity which is normally damped down by descending inhibitory impulses, and (b) that the highest centres of inhibitory influences acting on the extralemniscal system lie in the primary (lemniscal) cortex, and not in the association cortex with which ascending extralemniscal activity is associated.

These inhibitory cortical projections do not pass directly to the spinal cord, but to brainstem reticular neurones with descending axons. Other inhibitory cortical efferents are distributed to the intralaminar thalamic nuclei; but these influences are probably phasic in nature, and do not exert a permanent inhibitory influence at this level.

It is probably *partly* because of the tonic nature of descending inhibition that there is some degree of rather poor localisation (e.g. low back pain) in certain forms of pelvic disease. In these cases it must be assumed that only the common carrier cells in a localised region of the lumbar spinal cord receive a sufficient quantity of afferent bombardment to "break through" the tonic descending suppression to an extent sufficient to produce an efferent firing pattern which will be interpreted as painful at conscious (i.e. cortical) level.

Quantitative considerations can also go far to explain the degree of pain experienced in parturition. Thus relaxation of the somatic musculature, brought about by inhibitory processes starting in the cerebral cortex (whether by "will" or conditioned reflex) considerably reduce the afferent bombardment of spinal extralemniscal neurones. Conversely, a state of emotional tension, causing excitatory activity in the circuit: limbic system—intralaminar thalamic nuclei—corpus striatum—extrapyramidal motor system, will cause increased activity to be sent back to the extralemniscal reticular system from muscle receptors connected to small myelinated and unmyelinated fibres; this activity will sum with that already engendered by uterine contraction, and thus increase the upgoing impulses which will be interpreted as increased pain (Fig. 5). However, it is evident from what has been stated earlier that these same impulses originating in the limbic lobe and passing to the intralaminar thalamic nuclei will also affect activity in the association cortex as well as, or even before, affecting the extrapyramidal motor system. In this way, emotional tension may lead to increased apprehensiveness before so-called "physical" pain is increased—if indeed it is either neurologically or philosophically possible to differentiate between organic and non-organic pain.

The sensation which we call pain is an extremely primitive one and is obviously of great value to the organism in maintaining its integrity. When it occurs as the result of noxious stimulation of internal organs, it is equally of great value to the physician both as a symptom and as a sign. What is remarkable is not that pain exists, but that it can be suppressed, by the neurological mechanisms of which an elementary description is given in this chapter. Suppression of pain, particularly chronic ("slow") pain, is a property which is indubitably better developed in the female of our species than in the male; and this is probably why the gynaecologist is, rightly, so struck when encountered by it.

REFERENCES

Bowsher, D., and Albe-Fessard, D. (1965), "The Anatomo-physiological Basis of Somatosensory Discrimination," *Internat. Rev. Neurobiol*, **8**, 35–75.

Hodgkin, A. L. (1964), *The Conduction of the Nervous Impulse*, p.108. Liverpool University Press.

Melzack, R., and Wall, P. D.(1965), "Pain Mechanisms: A New Theory," *Science*, **150**, 971–979.

Theobald, G. W., Menzies, D. N. and Bryant, G. H. (1966), *Critical Electrical Stimulus which causes Uterine pain*, *Brit. med. J.*, **1**, 716–718.

2. NEUROPHYSIOLOGICAL ASPECTS OF GYNAECOLOGY AND OBSTETRICS

H. J. CAMPBELL and J. W. URSCHEL

I. BASIC MECHANISMS

1. Introduction

It is well known that neuroendocrine mechanisms (inter-action of the nervous and endocrine systems) regulate a wide variety of body functions. The best known neuro-endocrine mechanism is that which controls the release of pituitary hormones. Through hypothalamic control of anterior pituitary secretion, the brain regulates thyroidal, adrenocortical and gonadal activity. The oxytocic and vasopressor principles of the posterior pituitary are also controlled by the hypothalamus via a neuroendocrine reflex arc. Hormones in turn exert regulatory influences on the nervous system by means of a feedback mechanism which involves both the anterior pituitary and the hypo-thalamus.

It has been well established that hormones act on neurons in the brain to control some forms of behaviour. In animal studies oestrogens and androgens affect sexual interest and behaviour while luteotrophic hormone (LTH) appears to stimulate maternal behaviour.

Finally, neuroendocrine interrelations have also been found to be important during development and maturation.

2. Neural Control of Endocrine Secretions

The idea that the central nervous system, or more specifically, the hypothalamus plays a key role in the control of the hypophysis has now been well substantiated by experimental evidence. Control is exerted by two possible pathways—a neurosecretory one involving the posterior pituitary and a neurohumoral one involving the anterior pituitary.

It is not surprising that two different pathways exist when one recalls the embryological development of the pituitary gland. This is formed from two elements, a neural downgrowth from the floor of the diencephalon forms the neurohypophysis while an epithelial upgrowth from Rathke's pouch forms the adenohypophysis.

(a) The Hypothalamo-adenohypophysial Pathway

Popa and Fielding described a specialized system of vessels, which connect capillaries located in the median eminence of the tuber cinereum with sinusoids of the pars distalis. In 1949 Green and Harris made direct micro-scopic observation of these portal vessels in living mammals and confirmed that the blood flow was from the median eminence to the pituitary gland.

Early experiments on separation of the pituitary from this connection with the brain by pituitary stalk section or transplantation produced conflicting and puzzling results. Pituitary transplants resulted in a loss of cyclic anterior pituitary gonadotrophic function and atrophy of the reproductive organs while simple pituitary stalk section

did not produce reproductive organ atrophy or discon-tinuation of oestrous cycles. Harris (1955) drew attention to the fact that the portal vessels regenerate quickly after pituitary stalk section. If such regeneration is prevented by the placement of a barrier between the cut ends of the stalk, then the animals remain anoestrous and their reproductive organs undergo atrophy.

The importance of the portal vessels was finally proven when pituitary tissue was placed in the subarachnoid space of hypophysectomized rats, firstly under the median eminence of the tuber cinereum where it became vas-cularized by the portal vessels, and secondly under the temporal lobe of the brain where it became vascularized by cerebral cortical and dural vessels. Hypophysectomized female rats with hypothalamic transplants showed regular oestrous cycles, mated, became pregnant, delivered living young and showed normal milk formation. On the other hand the control animals with temporal lobe transplants remained anoestrous after operation and developed atrophy of their reproductive organs.

Anatomists now agree that the pars distalis receives very few, if any, nerve fibres. Thus making it highly improbable that hypothalamic control over the anterior pituitary is transmitted via a neural pathway.

There is abundant indirect evidence for the existence of humoral hypothalamic control of the secretion of adreno-corticotrophic hormone (ACTH), thyrotrophic hormone (TSH), gonadotrophins and to a less extent growth hormone. The hypothalamus appears to inhibit the secretion of prolactin through a neurohumoral mechanism. Direct evidence has been obtained by extractions from hypothalamic tissue of six factors, corticotrophin-releasing factor (CRF), thyrotrophin-releasing factor (TRF), growth hormone-releasing factor (GHRF), follicle-stimulating hormone-releasing factor (FSHRF), lutein-izing hormone-releasing factor (LRF) and prolactin inhibitory factor (PIF).

The exact nature of these factors is not yet known but they are probably secreted by the nerve fibres which terminate on the capillary loops in the median eminence from which the portal-hypophysial vessels arise. These fibres resemble neurons from the supraoptic and para-ventricular nuclei but unlike them, do not contain demon-strable granules of "neurosecretory material".

The hypothalamus-portal vessel-anterior pituitary unit thus represents a final common pathway from the brain to the pituitary; a path on which many neural inputs converge to influence anterior pituitary secretions.

(b) Hypothalamo-neurohypophysial Pathway

In marked contrast to the adenohypophysis, the neurohypophysis has direct neural connections with the central nervous system. Thus as one would expect, there is total lack of posterior pituitary regeneration following pituitary stalk section. The main nerve supply originates in the supraoptic and paraventricular nuclei of the hypothalamus and consists of the supraoptico-hypophysial tract and the tubero-hypophysial tract. The fibres of these tracts reach the infundibular process through the neural stalk.

Unlike other unmyelinated nerve fibres in the central and peripheral nervous system, the supraoptic-hypophysial nerve fibres showed irregularities in their calibre and swellings or bulb-shaped nerve endings. These swellings

constitutes the final common pathway of posterior pituitary gland function.

3. Feedback Mechanisms to the Pituitary Gland and Brain

The regulatory influence that hormones exert on the nervous system by means of a feedback mechanism is an important aspect of neuroendocrine function. Thyroidal, adrenocortical, and gonadal hormones inhibit, in a negative feedback fashion, the secretion from the anterior

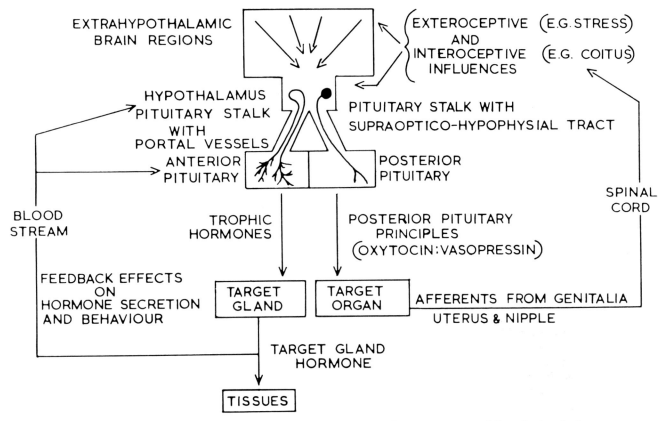

FIG. 1. Schematic diagram of interrelations between the environment, the nervous system and the endocrine glands.

are caused by the presence of vesicles which contain neurosecretory granules. Special staining techniques and electron microscopy have advanced the study of neurosecretion greatly. It was primarily the Scharrers (1940, 1954) who pioneered the concept that neurosecretory cells are specialized neurons in which the ability to secrete has become extensively developed and of primary importance. It is now generally accepted that the cells and axons of the paraventricular and supraoptic nuclei manufacture oxytocin and vasopressin or antidiuretic hormone (ADH) which pass to the posterior pituitary for storage and release. There appears to be simultaneous release of oxytocin and ADH under some conditions but more generally the two hormones are largely under separate control. Their release from the nerve endings in the neural lobe results from a wide range of stimuli which generate impulses in the unmyelinated fibres of the hypothalamico-neurohypophysial tract. This tract therefore

pituitary of TSH, ACTH and the gonadotrophins. It is now accepted that this feedback mechanism acts in part on the anterior pituitary and in part on the hypothalamus by means of neuroendocrine reflexes.

At one time it was thought that sexual cyclicity in females was entirely due to a reciprocal relationship between the ovaries and the anterior pituitary gland. Current studies, however, substantiate the view that gonadal hormones also modify the secretion of gonadotrophin through an action on the brain. A direct and localized action of gonadal hormones upon the hypothalamus has been demonstrated in many animals. For example, implantation of oestradiol into the posterior median eminence-basal tuberal region of the hypothalamus in rabbits abolishes the usual mating-induced ovulation and produces ovarian atrophy, thus illustrating the negative feedback action of oestrogen upon the neural control of gonadotrophin secretion.

Other studies suggest that progesterone also acts primarily on a neural site in its feedback action, since the induction of ovulation by progesterone in domestic fowl is regularly prevented by lesions placed in the anterior region of the ventromedian hypothalamus.

II. ACTION OF THE HYPOTHALAMUS ON THE PITUITARY GLAND

1. Adenohypophysis

(a) Factors Influencing Gonadotrophin Secretion

Reproductive processes in the female are characterized by cyclic alterations in the genital tract which depend upon the rhythmic secretion of hormones by the adenohypophysis and ovary. This rhythm is not intrinsic to these glands however, but is imposed upon them by the central nervous system.

There appear to be two mechanisms in the CNS which control the secretion of gonadotrophic hormones. One mechanism involves the hypothalamus and its hypophysiotrophic influence on the anterior pituitary gland. This system is necessary for the maintenance of normal anterior pituitary histology and function.

The other mechanism is the so-called "release regulating mechanism", which includes all the brain structures that can modify the activity of the hypophysiotrophic cells of the hypothalamus. The influence of the neural structures belonging to this system will be discussed more fully later in this chapter.

(b) Hypothalamic Control of Gonadotrophin Secretion

The effects of electrical stimulation of the tuber cinereum or adjacent hypothalamic areas (Harris, 1937, 1948) and other studies already referred to contradict the theory that the adenohypophysis and ovary are linked together in a self-contained system of purely hormonal interaction. Furthermore, assuming that the number of nerve fibres entering the anterior pituitary would be inadequate for secretomotor function and that the flow of blood in the hypothalamo-hypophysial portal vessels is towards the adenohyophysis, the chemotransmitter hypothesis of Harris (1955) is the most plausible explanation of gonadotrophin regulation.

The first good evidence for this hypothesis was that hypothalamic extracts stimulated ACTH secretion. In 1960 Harris and his colleagues produced evidence which indicated the existence of a hypothalamic luteinizing hormone-releasing factor (LRF) in the hypothalamus. These findings were later extensively confirmed by various workers and LRF has now been isolated chromatographically. Various tests suggest that it is a small polypeptide with a molecular weight of about 1,200–1,400 and that its action is to promote the proteosynthetic reactions involved in the manufacture of LH.

Proof for the existence of FSH–RF is hindered by the lack of a sensitive assay of FSH. However, there is indirect evidence that the hypothalamus influences both the synthesis and release of FSH by means of FSH–RF. Attempts to purify FSH–RF have been made and it is likely that it has slightly greater molecular size than LRF.

Results of both *in vitro* and *in vivo* studies point to the existence of a prolactin-inhibiting factor (PIF) in hypothalamic extracts. Accumulated evidence suggests that the hypothalamus exercises a tonic inhibitory effect on the release of prolactin. It has been observed that suckling induces an acute decrease in the lactating rat. This decrease in the concentration of pituitary prolactin can be prevented if just prior to suckling the lactating rat is given an intraperitoneal injection of rat or bovine median eminence extract. PIF has not yet been purified but it is probably a distinct polypeptide.

It would appear therefore that these hypothalamic releasing factors constitute a new family of polypeptide hormones differing from the known neurohypophysial hormones vasopressin and oxytocin. There is some evidence that the target gland steroids may feed back to the hypothalamus and cause inhibition of secretion of these releasing factors.

The neurosecretory cells in the hypothalamus or "hypophysiotrophic" cells which synthesize the various releasing factors have yet to be identified. These cells may lie in the stalk-median eminence (SME) region or even some distance from there. It seems evident that LRF is concentrated in the SME region.

2. NEUROHYPOPHYSIS

As stated earlier, it is generally accepted that the cells and axons of the paraventricular and supraoptic nuclei constitute the final nervous link in the release of oxytocin and vasopressin into the blood stream. It is likely that both nuclei contain cells in varying proportions which are specialized to secrete either oxytocin or vasopressin. Most of the evidence indicates that the two hormones are largely under separate control. The natural stimuli for release of the two hormones are quite different, i.e. suckling or reproductive processes for oxytocin and increased blood osmotic pressure for ADH.

Knowledge of the role of oxytocin in reproduction and lactation dates from 1906 when Dale published the first account of the uterine contraction induced by extracts of the posterior lobe of the pituitary. There is extensive evidence now that oxytocin has a role in natural milk ejection and during parturition it evokes uterine contractions thus promoting the evacuation of the foetus. It has not been shown to influence any of the mechanisms concerned with the preparation for labour. Chemical studies show that it is an octapeptide.

Complete knowledge of the sensory pathways in the spinal cord subserving reflex release of oxytocin in response to genital and mammary stimuli is lacking. Electrical stimulation of the medial lemniscus in the medulla and stimulation of the brainstem reticular formation, and subthalamus elicit milk ejection responses. It also appears as though excitation of widely scattered points in the limbic forebrain can result in the release of oxytocin from the neurohypophysis.

The feedback mechanisms controlling neurohypophysial secretion of oxytocin have not been studied extensively at the present time. There is fairly good evidence for a positive feedback mechanism, however, in the process of parturition. Positive feedbacks are rare in physiology since they are essentially nonhomeostatic. However, they are well adapted to expulsive processes, such as parturition, since the feedback excitation is removed when the foetus is delivered. In 1941, Ferguson showed that mechanical distension of one cervix or uterus, in the bicornuate uterus of the rabbit, induced contractions of the other uterus. The long latency of the response and its persistence after the stimulus was removed suggested a humoral mechanism. Electrolytic cautery of the pituitary stalk eliminated the uterine effect. Ferguson postulated that cervical dilation by the foetus in labour initiates a neurohumoral reflex, the "Ferguson reflex", whereby the expulsive efforts of the uterus are intensified through increased concentration of circulating oxytocin.

III. ACTION OF HORMONES ON BRAIN

1. The Immature Organism

In addition to their integrative functions throughout life, neuroendocrine mechanisms play key roles in patterning and timing developmental processes. Neural control of the onset of puberty is an example of such a process.

Another example of the operation of neuroendocrine mechanisms during development is the action of steroid hormones on the brain early in life to induce the pattern of sex behaviour and pituitary secretion that develops in adulthood.

(a) The Hypothalamus and Development of Puberty

The inactivity of the gonads that characterizes the prepubertal period of growth cannot be explained by unresponsiveness of the gonads to the gonadotrophic hormones, by a lack of gonadotrophic hormone production or by an inability of the pituitary to secrete these hormones when properly stimulated.

Prior to Foa's work in 1900 it was thought that the onset of puberty was due to an ageing or maturation process in the endocrine glands concerned. Foa showed that this was not the case, since the ovaries of immature animals transplanted to mature animals exhibited cyclic changes typical of the adult organ. Later it was found that the anterior pituitary gland played a key role in ovarian activity and that it contained active gonadotrophic hormone even before the onset of maturity. In 1952 Harris and Jacobsohn found that pituitary tissue obtained from new-born rats grafted under the hypothalamus of hypophysectomized adult female rats became vascularized by the hypophysial portal vessels, and was capable of supporting full adult reproductive functions. Thus the functional activity of the ovary and pituitary gland in the immature animal does not depend on an intrinsic property of the tissue but on the "environment" in which it is situated.

Other studies have shown that a feed-back action of gonadal hormones on pituitary function is present in the immature form. This implies the existence of some control mechanism regulating gonadal activity at this immature age. Hypothalamic disturbance (especially hamartomata)

in clinical cases and experimental hypothalamic lesions in animal studies result in pubertas praecox and an accelerated onset of puberty. This suggests that the essential control mechanism involves the hypothalamus. The detailed physiology of such a control mechanism of the time of onset of puberty is not as yet understood, but it seems clear that during immaturity, the hypothalamus exerts an inhibitory influence upon the pituitary (see Donovan and van der Werff ten Bosch, 1967).

(b) Gonadal Hormones and Sexual Development of the Brain

The cyclic release of LH which occurs in the females of many species, and which results in ovulation and the onset of the luteal phase of the menstrual cycle, has no counterpart in males.

It has been known for some time that the "gonadotrophic mechanism" is undifferentiated (i.e. is neither male nor female) at birth in species such as the rat. It soon became apparent that the cyclic type of release of LH in the female and the acyclic type of release in the male was attributable to some mechanism in the CNS, rather than in the pituitary gland itself. It has now been proven that sexual differentiation of the pituitary gland does not occur. Harris and Jacobsohn (1952) found that male pituitary tissue transplanted beneath the median eminence of hypophysectomized female rats was capable of supporting normal oestrous cycles, mating, pregnancy and milk formation in the female host. Conversely, female pituitaries did not produce cycling in males. Thus pituitary tissue is seen to be pluripotential in nature.

Studies have been made which show that a single injection of about 5–10 μg. testosterone into female rats at 0–5 days of age results in permanent lack of oestrous cycles, lack of ovulation and loss of female sexual behaviour when the rats become adult. Treatment at later ages, e.g. at 10 days, is without this effect. Other evidence suggests that these results are not due to any intrinsic abnormality of ovarian or anterior pituitary tissue brought about by the treatment with testosterone. The site of action of testosterone on the gonadotrophin control mechanism in the neonatal animal appears to be at the CNS level, perhaps at the suprachiasmatic-preoptic area of the hypothalamus.

Recent studies show that ovarian tissue transplanted into adult *male* rats that have been castrated at the first day of life exhibits rhythmic ovulation and formation of corpora lutea with the periodicity characteristic of the normal female.

These findings suggest that in the rat the neural mechanism concerned with the control of LH secretion by the anterior pituitary, is at birth, in an undifferentiated state. If testosterone is lacking in the circulation, then hypothalamic mechanisms develop in the tissue which regulates LH release in a cyclic female fashion. If, on the other hand, testosterone (endogenous or exogenous) is present in the circulation during the early neonatal period, then the neural control mechanism for LH secretion becomes that of the normal male-regulating LH release in a steady-state pattern. Thus sexual differentiation of the brain may be under the control of testicular secretion in the early neonatal period of the rat.

In some other species, in which the young are born at a more advanced stage of development, it is likely that the "critical period" at which the hypothalamus is sensitive to testosterone occurs some time *before* birth. This is almost certainly the case in the rabbit (Campbell, 1966) and is very probably true in the human. Since, in suitable doses, other hormones also have this effect, great caution

of oestradiol into the posterior median eminence is followed by failure of ovulation with mating and later by ovarian atrophy. Implants made into the anterior pituitary and other parts of the brain give negative results in this respect.

Cytological changes have been observed in the cells of the anterior hypothalamus of rats treated with either an increase or decrease of the blood oestrogen level. There is a consistent decrease in nuclear size whenever the blood oestrogen level is altered.

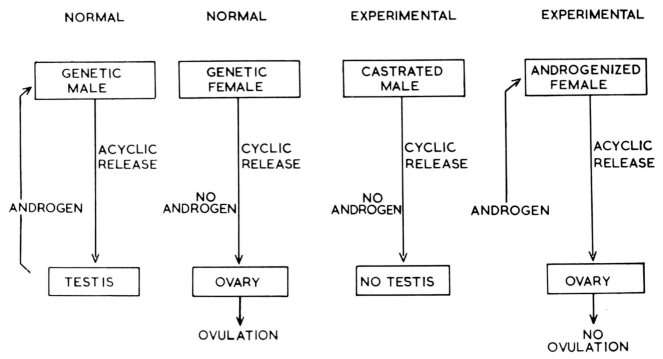

FIG. 2. Schematic diagram of neuroendocrine interrelationships in the immature animal.

should be employed in the therapeutic use of hormones during pregnancy in the human. For a review of this important topic, see Jacobsohn (1965).

2. The Mature Organism

It has been known for many years that interplay occurs between the secretion of the gonadal hormones and the release of gonadotrophic hormone from the anterior pituitary. The first indication that the feedback effect of gonadal steroids involved in ovulation was at a central nervous system level came in 1949 when Sawyer *et al.*, showed that oestrogen-induced ovulation in pregnant rats, and progesterone-advanced ovulation in 5-day cyclic rats, was blocked by administration of drugs (Dibenamine or Atropine) known to have potent effects on the nervous system.

Current studies verify the view that physiological doses of gonadal hormone modify the secretion of gonadotrophin through an action on the brain. The direct, localized action of gonadal hormones upon the hypothalamus is illustrated by intrahypothalamic injections of oestrogen in rats. Such injections result in a fall of gonadotrophin concentration in the pituitary gland. In rabbits an implant

Studies with isotopically labelled oestrogen reveal that the hormone concentrates in an anatomically definable system which involves the septal area and hypothalamus.

The feedback action of progesterone on the hypothalamus is likewise important in the complex physiology of ovulation. It is known that progesterone facilitates LH release and ovulation in rats which have been made persistently oestrous, by say continuous illumination. This effect of progesterone can be blocked by lesions involving the medial pre-optic area of the hypothalamus. Other studies show that ovulation in the hen can be advanced by the injection of progesterone into the hypothalamus.

Apparently the hypothalamus exerts a dual control over the release of adenohypophysial gonadotrophin. The first level of hypothalamic control involves the tonic discharge of gonadotrophin (mainly FSH) in sufficient quantity to maintain oestrogen production in response to the oestrogen feedback mechanism. This steady secretion of gonadotrophin maintains oestrogen levels suitable for the well-being of the secondary sexual apparatus and for the ripening of ovarian follicles. The second higher level of control is responsible for the cyclic increased discharge of gonadotrophin (mainly LH) to cause ovulation. This region of "ovulation-control", or, neural timing mechanism in the hypothalamus is likely dependent on exteroceptive stimuli (see more detail below) such as light, interoceptive stimuli such as oestrogen and progesterone, and other neural controlling influences.

IV. EXTEROCEPTIVE FACTORS

1. Auditory Stimuli

The effect of auditory stimulation upon reproductive organs and functions has been ably presented in detail by Zondek and Tamari (1967). In female rats and rabbits continuous intense sound (100 dB, 4 Kc/s) from an alarm bell does not noticeably affect the general behaviour of the animals. However, after about 14 days rats show prolonged or persistent oestrus and after longer periods (up to 60 days) both species show marked hypertrophy of the ovaries and uterus with histological signs of abnormally elevated LH secretion together with lactation in the rabbits. (No changes were found in the sexual organs of male rats so treated.) Thus the effect of continuous sound on the reproductive apparatus is to simulate the reactions of pregnancy.

Fertility, on the other hand, is very considerably reduced in *both* male and female rats exposed to this same treatment. Sexual behaviour appears to be quite normal but the usual rate of conception is reduced from 80 per cent to 5 per cent. This is partly due to loss of fertilizing capacity in the sperm (which, as well as the testes, appear anatomically normal) and partly to the fact that sound stimulation during pregnancy results in cessation of the gestation processes. But it seems clear that the latter effect is only produced when the stimulus is applied prior to the conceptus becoming well-established in the endometrium for sound applied at later stages was without effect.

None of the above responses is obtained when continuous sound is applied to rats which have been deafened by long treatment with kanamycin indicating that the integrity of the organ of Corti is required. This makes even more remarkable the finding that the effects upon fertility and pregnancy are duplicated in rats exposed to continuous sound well above their range of hearing.

In view of these basic findings, some useful knowledge might accrue from a study of menstrual, fertility and pregnancy conditions among people working in noisy environments or under conditions of supersonic sounds even though the individuals appear to be unperturbed. Should a correlation be found, the only therapeutic measure available would seem to be removal of the individual from the environment, for the effects of continuous sound could not be inhibited by hormone treatment in experiments with that aim in mind.

The effect of intense sound is not limited to the maternal structures and processes. In a long series of investigations on the effects of intense stimulation, including sound, Arvay (for review, see Arvay, 1967) found that rats exposed to these conditions before and during pregnancy produced offspring with a high incidence, 11·4 per cent experimental,

0·75 per cent untreated, of malformations such as absence of crystalline lens, defective atrial development, double ureter, syndactyly, hiatus hernia and cleft palate. The last condition represented 25 per cent of the observed abnormalities. It has also been reported that malformed human infants occurred in higher numbers after a period of bombardment in Hungary during World War II. Two possible causes, perhaps occurring concurrently, have been suggested. The first is that intense sound has been shown to induce degenerative changes in ovarian germinal tissue and the second is that the same stimuli are known to elevate blood levels of adrenal hormones, both cortical and medullary. It is perhaps a synergism between the genetic and phenotypic factors which facilitates teratogeny.

Less intense and discontinuous sounds have not been greatly studied experimentally for it is difficult to establish rigid controls for this kind of stimulus—though it has been suggested that rabbits may ovulate if the animal room door is slammed! Non-experimentally, of course, it is clear that some sounds have a specific relation to sexual behaviour and reproduction, the so-termed mating calls. Sows will make a sexual response to manual pressure upon the back if they are exposed to a recording of the sounds made by a boar during mating. The main constituent of popular music comes to mind when it is remembered that the sow will also respond in this way to the imitated rhythm of the boar's mating sounds.

2. Olfactory Stimuli

The study of the effects of olfactory stimuli upon reproductive processes in mammals has gained considerable impetus only in the last decade or so. Examination of the literature shows, as Bruce (1967) has pointed out in his recent review, that odours may produce three kinds of effects, (i) immediate, non-hormonal, transient, (ii) delayed, neurohormonal, transient, and (iii) non-hormonal, permanent.

It has been shown in rats and mice that purely neural analysis of solely odorous stimuli enables males to differentiate between males and females on the one hand, and between oestrous and anoestrous females on the other hand. Destruction of the olfactory brain regions is followed by deranged sexual selectivity—a situation seen normally in anosmic creatures such as the goat. Under these conditions, choice of an appropriate sexual partner is determined by chance, copulation occurring when a male's repetitive free-lance mounting in the colony or herd brings him in contact with a receptive female. Hence, in fully osmic species, odours may serve as the initial trigger for the chain of responses that together constitute the sexual act, the effect disappearing at the end of consummatory activity. The extent to which this type of stimulus-response pattern is involved in other mammals is not known with scientific rigour. Even so, it is common observation that the sense of smell is employed extensively in social contact among dogs and cats, and it could be that the lucrative perfume industry has some basis in neurophysiological mechanisms that have shifted by social conditioning from the natural animal odours to the synthetic aromas of the botanical kingdom.

Delayed responses to olfactory stimuli occur when the endocrine system becomes involved. Among farm animals the evidence for a specific role for olfaction is not precise, but experiments have shown that, at least in some cases, visual and tactile stimuli are not responsible for the changes observed. These changes have to do with such phenomena as the appearance of synchronous sexual cycles in hitherto non-cyclic ewes some time after a male has been introduced into the herd. More rigorous are the findings in mice. Females of this species, if kept isolated from males, show irregular or absent ovulatory cycles. They become cyclic (i.e. exhibit normal periodicity in pituitary secretion of LH) under three conditions, all of which indicate the role of olfaction—(i) introduction of a male into the colony, (ii) introduction of bedding (e.g. sawdust) soiled by a male, (iii) application of male urine to the nostrils of the females. Further, the stimulation of cyclicity by these procedures does not occur in female mice whose olfactory regions have been destroyed.

In contrast to the stimulatory effects of male odours upon ovulatory cycles, they have an inhibitory action upon conception. Pregnancy after a successful coitus is blocked by the introduction of a strange male, by placing the female on bedding soiled by strange males or by applying strange male urine to the female's nostrils. (Note that the father's odours do not have this effect, but others; see below.) Neither of these treatments is effective after the olfactory apparatus has been destroyed. Interaction of the nervous apparatus with endocrine mechanisms is shown by the facts that neither of the above treatments is effective in intact mice treated with luteotrophic hormone (which aids implantation) or if the mouse bears an ectopic pituitary graft (i.e. free from neural influences) or if the pregnancy is postpartum (i.e. during the lactational period of increased release of luteotrophic hormone).

The overall view, then, is that the release of FSH and LH in female mice is inhibited by female odours and stimulated by male odours, and that the latter inhibit the release of LTH. In this apparent reciprocity of male and female odours, it appears that the odour from one male is able to negate the effect of odour from at least 30 females. More details of these studies are available in the recent review by the principle investigator (Whitten, 1966).

The permanent type of effect produced by olfactory stimuli is perhaps the most remarkable of all. There is clear cut evidence that in female mice, the male odour they are exposed to in infancy (i.e. normally, the father's odour) determines their sexual selectivity throughout the whole of adult life (Mainardi, 1965). Close study of the preferential acceptance of certain males has shown that female mice which have been reared normally will much more readily mate with males of a different strain from themselves. Such behavioural selectivity is absent in females which have been reared with no male present or in females which have grown up with parents who were sprayed daily with a masking perfume. As with the effect of androgen on the developing female, there is a "critical period" during which odours have this imprinting effect, roughly, the period of suckling. Unfortunately, no experimental studies of this phenomenon have been made

in higher animals but it is well known that in several species, especially canine, the oestrous female is not available to all-comers but steadfastly refuses some and actively seeks out others. The role of infantile olfactory imprinting in the human female must, for the moment, remain cogitative.

3. Visual Stimuli

The response of the gonads to changes in visual stimuli has been known for nearly half a century, since Rowan (1925) showed that the periodical fluctuation in size of male gonads in birds was closely coupled with natural or artificial variation in hours of light. It was indeed one of the first pieces of evidence which suggested that the pituitary-gonad system is under neural control. Later observations involved a wide range of species and included studies on ovarian function. These demonstrated that in all cases, light was a factor which influenced the secretion of gonadotrophic hormones, but that its role was greater in some species than in others; its importance decreases with ascent through the phyla. More recently it has become apparent that light may play a part in human reproductive endocrinology, though possibly in a converse manner to that in lower groups.

In subprimate groups such as rodents, the effect of light is clearly positive. Exposure of prepubertal rats or ferrets to more illumination than they would normally receive induces precocious puberty, exhibited by significantly earlier vaginal opening and earlier onset of oestrus. On the other hand, maintenance of constant darkness results in delayed sexual maturation and delayed onset of oestrus in these lower forms. However, in a most carefully controlled study on the human, Zacharias and Wurtman (1964) found a negative effect of light. They determined the age of onset of menstruation in 235 girls who were blind at birth or who became blind within the first year (20/200 or less in both eyes), from causes strictly limited to pathology of the orbit. In comparison with 335 girls with normal vision the visually defective group had an earlier menarche, the earliest of all being found in a group of 80 girls who had no perception of light whatever.

These contrary effects of light upon sexual maturation in humans and lower forms might be related to different organization of the nervous system in day-active and night-active species. On the other hand, the crucial factor may be whether light falls on the eye or on the head. It has been shown quite conclusively that under normal lighting conditions, light can penetrate through the skull to considerable depths in the brain (Ganong et al., 1963) in lower species. Coupled with the fact that removal of the eyes in the female rat is associated with only temporary disturbance of oestrous cycles, the ability of light to penetrate the brain raises the possibility that the control of reproductive rhythms by light is not exerted via the traditional visual system, but is perhaps mediated by activation of the pineal body. Support for this concept comes from a wealth of biochemical studies which have conclusively demonstrated that lighting rhythms control the rhythmic production of enzymes by the pineal body, via a pathway which normally includes the optic tract but is not dependent upon it. Evidence has also been adduced that the pineal organ exerts an influence upon ovarian function, though this is not yet a widely-held belief. Several workers have postulated or claim to have demonstrated the existence of neural pathways direct from the retina to hypothalamic neurones, and suggest that these are responsible for the effects of light upon pituitary gonadotrophic function.

The extent to which light penetrates the human skull and the functions of the human pineal body appear not to have been investigated. Nor, it seems, have studies been made of any relation between environmental lighting (duration, intensity) and menstrual irregularities in women.

A detailed bibliography of the effect of light on endocrine function is available (Wurtman, 1967). Pineal matters are reviewed by Kitay (1966).

4. Stress

To the neuroendocrinologist a stress is defined by its action upon the pituitary-target gland axes, not by a subjective state of mind. Stresses are non-specific; they all produce the same results of inhibition of TSH secretion and increased ACTH secretion. Their effects upon gonadotrophic function are not so well understood. Stresses fall broadly into two categories, (a) those which involve observable damage to the body (laceration, burns toxins, haemorrhage) and which are called systemic stresses, and (b) those which do not damage the body directly (fear, anxiety, anger) and which are called emotional stresses. It is unlikely that systemic stresses occur frequently in the absence of emotional stress, but the converse probably has a high incidence in human society. It should be particularly noted that, from this neuroendocrine point of view, a stress need not necessarily be harmful or distasteful. Birth is a stress and so is coitus.

The hey-day of experimentation upon stress has passed, but during that period about a decade ago many thousands of experiments were carried out with enthusiasm and ingenuity, so that in a very short time a large number of stresses were studied and the mechanism of action clearly established.

Several lines of enquiry led to the concept that systemic stresses act directly upon the pituitary gland by virtue of changes in blood composition such as increased histamine or serotonin due to trauma or foreign proteins and poisons due to infections and intoxications. Emotional stresses, such as restraint, loud noises, brilliant light, required the integrity of the portal vessel system to be effective and therefore exerted their action by nervous pathways to the hypothalamus. This distinction is not so clear now as it seemed then, for the line of demarcation has been clouded by the discovery that various compounds in the blood stream have an action also upon hypothalamic endocrine mechanisms. It is likely that many systemic stresses produce their effects by a dual action—on both pituitary gland and hypothalamus—but most of them are still effective when the hypothalamic influence on the pituitary has been removed by stalk-section, transplantation or lesion.

Systemic stresses, though important with regard to the secretion of ACTH and TSH probably have little influence upon gonadotrophic secretion because of their acute nature. A systemic stress that would affect the long-term rhythms of reproductive processes is probably not compatible with life. Emotional stresses, however, are very clearly related to several disturbances of reproductive mechanisms.

Anorexia nervosa is routinely accompanied by amenorrhoea and is in almost all cases associated with a history of psychic involvement of a particular kind—loss of familial ties in a person highly dependant upon interpersonal relations. Appropriate psychotherapy, with supporting nutritional attention, results in many cures. Disturbances of menstruation, absence, excessive or irregular flow, can result from many different emotional stresses. Similarly, emotional shock may precipitate lactation and various psychic processes may terminate menstruation in the condition of pseudocyesis. Rather interesting for its possible extrapolation to the human is the finding that rats showing spontaneous cessation of cycles, commence to ovulate regularly again after coitus with a selected male.

V. PERIPHERAL NERVE ACTION

1. The Uterus

(i) **Anterior pituitary.** There can be no doubt at all that impulses travelling in afferent fibres from the uterus play a role in reproductive processes. Nor can it be doubted that such impulses do *not* have a decisive influence upon gonadotrophic secretion. Routinely, physical manipulation of the uterine cervix in the rabbit and cat is followed by ovulation. This is perhaps not surprising in these species of reflex ovulators, in which the ovulatory surge of LH normally occurs only after coitus. However, denervation of the uterus or even its total removal does not prevent coitally-induced ovulation. Thus the uterine afferents must have a supporting rather than initiating influence upon the release of gonadotrophins.

Similar mechanical (or electrical) stimulation of the uterine cervix in spontaneous ovulators is followed by a condition somewhat similar to that in reflex ovulators. Cervical stimulation in various rodent species results in prolongation of the life of the corpora lutea, with enlargement of the uterus and mammary glands—pseudopregnancy. During this period, the uterine endometrium reacts to slight mechanical trauma by the formation of a deciduoma, tissue which will later be sloughed off and rejected. Pseudopregnancy is also induced by sterile mating. When the uterus of the spontaneous ovulator is completely denervated, pseudopregnancy still follows sterile mating—indicating the effectiveness of psychic and perhaps genital stimuli—but no longer results from stimulation of the cervix—indicating (a) that under normal conditions impulses in uterine afferents play a role in activation of the pituitary, and (b) that these impulses are not essential for progestational reactions.

The precise pathways by which cervical stimulation affects hypothalamic mechanisms is not known, but unit recordings from neurones in the lateral area of the hypo-thalamus have shown them to be responsive to such stimulation. Interestingly, the threshold of excitation of the lateral hypothalamic neurones to cervical stimulation was shown to be raised within a short time of progesterone administration (Cross and Silver, 1965), correlating with the post-coital EEG reactions in the rabbit (Sawyer and Kawakami, 1961) and the responses of the progesterone-treated rabbit to self-stimulation of the limbic system (Campbell, 1968). It is likely that this general field of study will produce findings of very great importance over the next decade.

A field of greater complexity and less clarity involves the effects produced by distention of the uterus or more accurately perhaps, the presence of objects in the uterine cavity. A simple example is seen in the common hen. The presence of an object (which under normal circum-stances is its own egg) in the large section of the oviduct inhibits subsequent ovulation—an automatic feedback device for, so to speak, keeping the conveyor belt clear. Similar effects are produced in mammals such as sheep, cows and guinea-pigs but there is enormous species variation which makes physiological interpretation diffi-cult. Introduction into the uterus of plastic or glass beads of appropriate size in these forms results in shortened oestrous cycles. The time of the cycle at which the beads are introduced determines the exact nature of the response. When they are small (2 mm. dia. as against 8 mm. dia.) the effect is not produced at all, suggesting that actual distention is the primary cause. With the large beads, denervation of the uterus inhibited the response, indicating that impulses in uterine afferents converge upon the hypothalamus to influence pituitary function.

Beads in one horn of the uterus also cause earlier regres-sion of corpora lutea on that side, in cyclic species such as the guinea-pig, when inserted at an appropriate phase of the cycle and some workers believe that the effect is produced by a luteolytic substance released, apparently unilaterally, by the uterus (Bland and Donovan, 1966), but such a substance has not yet been demonstrated in uterine extracts.

The physiological significance of these various findings is not immediately apparent and it is not yet possible to extrapolate to the human condition. Use of intrauterine devices as a contraceptive measure is not yet fully evaluated, but the evidence so far indicates that pregnancy may be prevented without interference with the menstrual cycle and that the devices do not act by causing distention. Nor, from observations on the human endometrium, do neuro-endocrine factors seem involved. Attachment of a gener-alized physiological role to the uterus in the life of the corpus luteum, either neurally or humorally, does not seem warranted in view of the fact that total hysterectomy in several species, including monkeys and women, does not alter ovarian function.

(ii) **Posterior pituitary.** An excellent detailed review of the relations between the posterior pituitary gland and the female reproductive tract has been prepared by Fitz-patrick (1966). As this author and others have pointed out, the most reliable index of release of posterior pituitary principles is not the uterus itself, for several factors may be responsible for uterine contraction. On the other hand the release of milk from the mammary gland is a highly specific response to oxytocin, and antidiuresis is a good guide to increased blood levels of antidiuretic hormone.

The release of these two hormones by impulses in afferent fibres from the uterus and genitalia is now well established in a range of lower species. Uterine contrac-tions have been observed during orgasm in the human female (Beck, 1874) and mating in women is also accom-panied by antidiuresis (Friberg, 1953) and the milk-ejection response (Pickles, 1953). Although there is no doubt that the release of posterior pituitary principles during coitus is due to a convergence upon the hypo-thalamus of afferent impulses from the whole genitalia region—including vagina and vulva—direct experiments upon the uterus itself have shown that distention of this organ results in the secretion of oxytocin. Absence of the response after spinal section and increased activity of hypothalamic neurones with distention of the uterus testify to the neural nature of the response. That the events of parturition in the human are associated with release of oxytocin is demonstrated by the observation that labour is accompanied by the milk-ejection reflex in women who are lactating from a previous pregnancy (Gunther, 1948) and by a large increase in oxytocic activity of blood withdrawn from the jugular vein during the second stage of labour (Coch et al., 1965). However, it would be naive to consider that these processes are operative only at parturition. Rather, this event must be looked upon as the peak of a progression which begins at the end of the first third of pregnancy. Determination of intra-uterine pressure in the human has shown that con-tractions are present but weak at 12 weeks and progres-sively increase in size and frequency up to term (Caldeyro-Barcia and Sereno, 1961), though there is some disagreement about intermittent periods of quiescence (Theobald, 1961).

Release of oxytocin by uterine distention at parturition has advantages too obvious to dwell upon. Similar oxytocin activity during coitus is not so easily understood. Its postulated role in sperm transport would appear to be tenable only in a few species for the observed rate of migration of sperms in other species, including the human (Egli and Newton, 1961), is well within the capacity of unaided sperm motility.

2. The Nipple

(i) **Anterior pituitary.** There is good evidence that *in some species* mechanical stimulation of the nipple, as at suckling, induces the release of prolactin for use in milk-formation. That this happens by virtue of afferent nerve impulses from the nipples is shown by absence of the effect after denervation of the nipple or spinal section. This response is seen in the rat and rabbit. On the other hand, milk-formation in the sheep and goat appears to be quite independent of nervous connections to the nipples. Studies on women with denervated nipples do not seem to have been made yet; pending such remarkable observa-tions the role of nipple manipulation with regard to prolactin secretion in the human must remain undecided. The common observation that delayed weaning is associated with prolonged lactation in women, suggests that nipple afferents may play a part in the human.

(ii) **Posterior pituitary.** In contrast with the processes of milk-formation the role of mechanical stimulation of the nipple in milk-secretion is well established. Abundant evidence exists to indicate that impulses in nipple afferents cause the release of oxytocin from the posterior pituitary gland. The oxytocin then acts upon the myoepithelium of the mammary gland, causing expulsion of the milk into the ducts. This neurohumoral reflex does not occur after denervation of the nipples, after spinal cord section or after complete posterior lobectomy. Further, direct recording from the hypothalamus demonstrates increased activity of neurones when the nipples are stimulated. Similar release of oxytocin and milk-ejection can be elicited by electrical stimulation of the supraoptico-hypophysial tract and can be abolished by electrolytic lesions in this region. Attempts to delineate the spinal and brain-stem pathways involved in the milk-ejection reflex have so far not met with success, such studies indicating a diffuse pattern which converges only at hypothalamic levels.

An important corollary of the role of nervous excitation in milk-ejection is that the response is therefore conditionable. This fact is known to farmers, who sometimes cannot get the rattling buckets under quickly enough, and to recent mothers whose blouses require laundering after their husbands have smiled in a certain fashion. For those in whom neither this emotional sensitivity nor the natural stimulation of the nipple is effective, the neural loop of the reflex can be therapeutically by-passed by nasal administration of oxytocin.

Detailed reviews of experimental (Meites, 1966) and clinical (Newton, 1961) studies of this whole topic are available.

VI. EXTRAHYPOTHALAMIC REGIONS

The above account has emphasized the role of the hypothalamus in the control of endocrine function. This is partly because by far the greater amount of research in neuroendocrinology has been concerned with diencephalic mechanisms and partly because the hypothalamus must represent the final common path for neural effects upon pituitary secretion. However, despite considerable evidence for a measure of hypothalamic autonomy, especially with regard to the cyclic release of gonadotrophins in the female, it is clear that with ascending phylogeny more recent parts of the brain have become involved in endocrine reactions. While many data have accrued from studies involving several pituitary hormones it is perhaps appropriate to restrict the present account to hormones involved in female reproductive processes. Useful bibliographies are available in this field (Schreiber, 1963; Flerko, 1966).

The extrahypothalamic regions which appear to form the next higher level of endocrine integration are those which are collectively known as the limbic system. Electrical stimulation of the septum pellucidum induces ovulation, as does similar excitation of the amygdalar complex. However, lesions in these regions do not inhibit ovulation or reproduction, hence their role is modulatory rather than generative. Indeed, lesions of the amygdala in immature animals have been followed by precocious ovarian development, while in the adult this procedure somewhat reduces the synthesis of gonadotrophins. Similarly, the release of oxytocin seems also to be influenced by limbic structures, for the milk-ejection reflex (specific indicator of oxytocin release) has been obtained upon electrical stimulation of the septum, hippocampus, fornix, amygdala and pre-piriform cortex. It seems reasonable to suppose that interoceptive influences (e.g. from genitalia and nipples) may travel more or less directly to the hypothalamus via the brain-stem, but that exteroceptive factors, especially those generating emotion (e.g. stress, sexual excitement) involve diffuse activation of the limbic system where some degree of integration occurs before modulating information is relayed to the hypothalamus.

The neocortex would seem to have no direct effect upon endocrine processes (with the exception of the adrenal medulla), for large amounts of it may be removed with no apparent untoward effect upon reproduction, and stimulation of the cortex is without remarkable influence upon ovarian activity. Bilateral temporal lobectomy in the rhesus monkey was associated with somewhat lengthened menstrual cycles, but after this operation the animals are severely defective in many non-endocrine directions and this finding has yet to be properly confirmed and shown to be specific. Nevertheless, it does seem likely that endocrine responses which involve emotion and conditioning must be at least initially triggered by some event in the neocortex, but even this must remain an assumption until considerably more research has been directed at extra-hypothalamic regions.

SUMMARY

The brain controls the activity of the anterior pituitary gland by means of neurohumours formed in the hypothalamus and passed along short portal blood vessels to the gland. Control of the posterior gland is by substances formed by and travelling along nerve fibres which arise in the hypothalamus and pass to the gland via the pituitary stalk. The hypothalamus is the focus of influences reaching it from other parts of the brain by pathways that at the moment are ill-understood.

Pituitary hormones themselves may have a direct effect upon brain activity and their control of target gland (thyroid, ovary etc.) secretion involves an indirect action upon neural regions. Target gland hormones have both excitatory and inhibitory actions upon various parts of the brain, producing (a) feedback control of pituitary secretion, and (b) influences upon behaviour including mental states.

This interaction of the nervous system and endocrine system is continuously operative in the adult organism, guiding the glandular and behavioural responses to changing conditions in the environment and maintaining endogenous hormonal rhythms. Neuroendocrine mechanisms are also of considerable importance during the perinatal period, at which time the action of hormones upon the brain produces changes which are permanent and irreversible.

REFERENCES

Arvay, A. (1967), in *The Effects of External Stimuli on Reproduction* (Eds. G. E. W. Wolstenholme and M. O'Connor). Ciba Found. Study Group No. 6. Churchill, London.

Beck, J. T. (1874), *Amer. J. Obstet. Dis. Wom.*, **7**, 353–391.

Bland, K. P. and Donovan, B. T. (1966), *J. Physiol.*, **186**, 503–515.

Bruce, H. M. (1967), in *The Effects of External Stimuli on Reproduction* (Eds. G. E. W. Wolstenholme and M. O'Connor), Ciba Found. Study Group No. 6, Churchill, London.

Caldeyro-Barcia, R. and Sereno, J. A. (1961), in *Oxytocin*. (eds. R. Caldeyro-Barcia and H. Heller). Oxford: Pergamon Press.

Campbell, H. J. (1966), *J. Anat.*, **100**, 381–387.

Campbell, H. J. (1968), *J. Physiol.*, **196**, 134–135P.

Coch, J. A., Brovetto, J., Cabot, H. M., Fielitz, C. A. and Caldeyro-Barcia, R. (1965), *Amer. J. Obstet. Gynec.*, **91**, 10–17.

Cross, B. A. and Silver, I. A. (1965), *J. Endocr.*, **31**, 251–263.

Dale, H. H. (1906), *J. Physiol.*, **34**, 163–206.

Donovan, B. T. and Van Der Werff Ten Bosch (1966), *The Physiology of Puberty*. London: Edward Arnold.

Egli, G. E. and Newton, M. (1961), *Fertil. & Steril.*, **12**, 151–155.

Ferguson, J. K. W. (1941), *Surg. Gynec. Obstet.*, **73**, 359–366.

Fitzpatrick, R. J. (1966), in *The Pituitary Gland*. (eds. G. W. Harris and B. T. Donovan). London: Butterworth.

Flerko, B. (1966), in *Neuroendocrinology* (eds. L. Martini and W. F. Ganong). London: Academic Press.

Foa, C. (1900), *Arch. ital. biol.* Quoted from Parkes, A. S. *The Internal Secretions of the Ovary*. London: Longmans Green, 1929.

Friberg, O. (1953), *Acta Endocr. (Kbh)*, **12**, 193–196.

Ganong, W. F., Shepherd, M. D., Wall, J. R., Van Brunt, E. E. and Clegg, M. T. (1963), *Endocrinology*, **72**, 962.

Green, J. D. and Harris, G. W. (1949), *J. Physiol.*, **108**, 359–361.

Gunther, M. (1948), *Brit. med. J.*, **i**, 567.

Harris, G. W. (1939), *Proc. roy. Soc. B.*, **122**, 374–394.

Harris, G. W. (1948), *Brit. med. J.*, **i**, 567.

Harris, G. W. (1955), in *Neural Control of the Pituitary Gland*. London: Edward Arnold.

Harris, G. W. and Jacobsohn, D. (1952), *Proc. roy. Soc. B.*, **139**, 263–276.

Jacobsohn, D. (1965), *Acta Univ. Lund.*, Section II, No. 17, 1–19.

Kitay, J. I. (1966), in *Neuroendocrinology* (eds. L. Martini and W. F. Ganong). London: Academic Press.

Mainardi, D. (1965), *Boll. Zool.*, **32**, 1–6.

Meites, J. (1966), in *Neuroendocrinology* (eds. L. Martini and W. F. Ganong). London: Academic Press.

Newton, M. (1961), in *Milk: the Mammary Gland and Its Secretions* (eds. S. K. Kon and A. T. Cowie). London: Academic Press.

Pickles, V. R. (1953), *J. Obstet. Gynaec. Brit. Cmwlth.*, **60**, 301–311.

Popa, G. T. and Fielding, U. (1930), *J. Anat.*, **65**, 88–91.

Popa, G. T. and Fielding, U. (1933), *J. Anat.*, **67**, 227–232.

Rowan, W. (1925), *Nature*, **115**, 494–495.

Sawyer, C. H. and Kawakami, M. (1961), in *Control of Ovulation* (ed. C. A. Villee). New York: Pergamon Press.

Scharrer, E. and Scharrer, B. (1940), *Ass. Res. Publ. nerv. ment. Dis.*, **20**, 170–194.

Scharrer, E. and Scharrer, B. (1954), *Rec. Progr. Horm. Res.*, **10**, 183–240.

Schreiber, V. (1963), in *The Hypothalamo-hypophysial System*. Prague: Czech. Academy of Science.

Theobald, G. W. (1961), in *Oxytocin* (eds. R. Caldeyro-Barcia and H. Heller). Oxford: Pergamon Press.

Wurtman, J. (1967), in *Neuroendocrinology* (eds. L. Martini and W. F. Ganong). London: Academic Press.

Zacharias, L. and Wurtman, R. J. (1964), *Science*, **144**, 1154–1155.

Zondek, B. and Tamari, I. (1967), in *The Effects of External Stimuli on Reproduction* (eds. G. E. W. Wolstenholme and M. O'Connor). Ciba Found. Study Group No. 6. London: Churchill.

3. THE NEURAL CONTROL OF THE BLADDER IN RELATION TO GYNAECOLOGY

P. W. NATHAN

There are two sorts of disturbance of the bladder induced by gynecologists or by gynecological disorders: the bladder can be made to empty too often or be made to empty too rarely. This is what one might expect; for the repertoire of bladder behaviour is limited. All a bladder can do is hold urine or not hold urine. If we introduce the factor of time into these activities, we then come back to the first statement, that the bladder does not pass urine when it should or that it often passes urine when it shouldn't.

Principal Structures used for Retaining and Expelling Urine

Somatic Muscles of Pelvis and Perineum

The floor of the pelvis consists of a sheet of muscle arising from the walls of the pelvis and inserted into the urethra, bladder, vagina, rectum, coccyx, and sacrum. This sheet of muscle is divided by the authors of most general anatomy textbooks into two, the levator ani and the coccygeus. Those more concerned with this region of the body name the parts of the sheet in accordance with the origin and insertion of each part, thus pubococcygeus, puborectalis, iliococcygeus.

This sheet of muscle supports the urethra, bladder, vagina and rectum. To do this, the muscle is kept in constant contraction. When micturition starts, the muscle ceases to contract, and the base of the bladder descends in the pelvis. The descent of the bladder is shown radiologically in Figure 1. When micturition is finished, the reverse occurs: the base of the bladder rises, returning to its original position. This is shown in Figure 2. The return of the bladder to the position in which it is kept for storing urine is due to contraction of the levator ani, and particularly of the two pubococcygeus muscles.

The nerve supply of the entire levator ani muscle and coccygeus muscles comes from the 3rd and 4th sacral roots. After the nerves leave the sacrum and coccyx they lie on the superior or intra-abdominal surface of the muscles before they penetrate them. These muscles are striated and are classified as somatic; their nerve-supply is similar in all respects to that of other somatic muscles.

The perineal striated muscles are the external sphincter of the urethra, the external sphincter of the anus, the bulbo- and ischio-cavernosus, and the two transverse perineal muscles. In the female the bulbo-cavernosi encircle the lower end of the vagina. Of this group of small muscles, those of particular importance for micturition and defaecation are the sphincters of the anus and urethra; they too are kept in constant contraction. When micturition or defaecation have to occur, these muscles are relaxed, and at the end of these actions, they resume their contraction.

The nerve supply to the perineal group of muscles is from the same segments of the sacral cord as that of the muscles of the pelvic floor; the nerve fibres reach the muscles via the pudendal nerve.

Visceral Muscles of the Bladder

The bladder is essentially a balloon made of muscle. The main muscle is the detrusor; the other muscle is small, flat, and triangular, the trigonal muscle. The

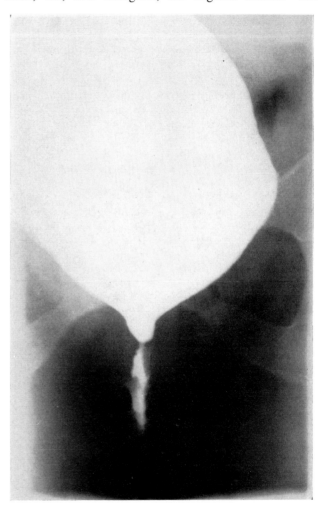

FIG. 1. Radiogram showing the onset of micturition. The base of the bladder has descended and in this view is well below the pubic arch. The neck of the bladder is open and funnel-shaped.

detrusor, the bladder neck, and the urethra form one smooth muscular structure in the female. Around the neck of the bladder, there is a great increase in elastic tissue, which is arranged circularly. For details of the anatomy of these muscles, the reader is referred to Uhlenhuth (1953), Bors (1957) and Woodburne (1967).

When the detrusor contracts, it actively pulls open the bladder neck. This results from the arrangement of the muscle fibres of the detrusor and the urethra, and it is not an example of reciprocal inhibition of antagonists. When the detrusor relaxes, the neck of the bladder is closed. The relaxed and even the dead bladder holds urine.

The nerve supply of the bladder is mainly parasympathetic, the transmitter being acetylcholine. The nerve fibres reach the bladder, and the vesical end of the ureter in the pelvic nerves. They originate mainly in the 3rd and 4th sacral roots, and to a lesser extent and in only some

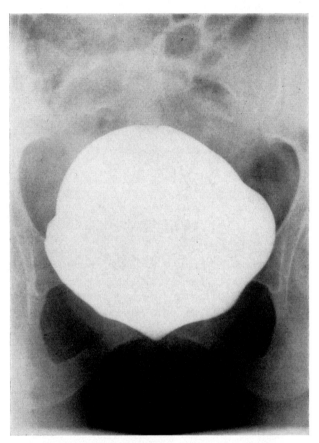

Fig. 2. Radiogram of the bladder storing urine. The neck of the bladder is closed and in this view it is immediately below the public arch. The patient is standing. We are most grateful to Mr. K. E. D. Shuttleworth for lending us these radiograms (Figs. 1 and 2) for reproduction.

subjects in the 2nd and 5th sacral roots. In addition to the parasympathetic nerve supply, there are sympathetic nerve fibres, which mainly run to the trigonal muscle. These fibres originate in the 11th and 12th thoracic and 1st and 2nd lumbar roots; they descend into the pelvis as the presacral nerve, and then join the pelvic nerves as the pelvic plexus, of which there is one on each side of the bladder.

It will be realized that apart from the sympathetic nerves, the nerve supply for all the visceral and somatic muscles concerned with micturition and defaecation comes from the same segments of the spinal cord. These segments are outside the pelvis, being enclosed by the 1st lumbar vertebrae. The nerves from these segments descend within the spinal canal until they reach their designated intervertebral foramina.

The role of the sympathetic nerve supply in the storage and expulsion of urine in man is not completely understood. In the male, by its action in contracting the trigonal sphincter, it prevents the products of the seminal vesicles from going into the bladder. Its action is essential during coitus to ensure the emission of semen out of the urethra. Following a bilateral sympathectomy affecting the sympathetic supply to the bladder, the male patient is rendered sterile. Whether there is any comparable or other action in the female is not yet known.

The role of the parasympathetic nerves to the bladder is to contract the whole musculature of the bladder, and thus to empty the organ. To do this in a fully efficient manner, it is necessary to have afferent nerves from the viscus to the segments of the sacral cord as well as efferent parasympathetic nerves from the same segments running to the bladder.

The Urethra

The entire urethra of the female is surrounded by muscle which acts as a sphincter. The proximal 3 cm. consists of visceral muscle fibres of the bladder. These muscle fibres descend longitudinally from the bladder neck to constitute the urethra. The distal 2 cm. of the urethra is supported and kept closed by the pubococcygeus and perineal muscles. The somatic and visceral muscles are intertwined.

The resistance of the urethra differs throughout its length, according to the researches of Lapides, Ajemian, Stewart, Breakley and Lichtwardt (1960). With the bladder containing urine and the patient in the lithotomy position they found that the pressure of the urethra averaged 28 cm. of water immediately below the bladder. Below the urogenital diaphragm, it averaged 21 cm. of water. The maximal pressure was found to be at the part of the urethra where the fibres of the pubococcygeus are inserted and which is surrounded by the urogenital diaphragm. Here the pressure averaged 51 cm. of water.

The length of the female urethra, according to Lapides, Ajemian, Stewart and Lichtwardt (1959) depends on the contraction of the striated muscles inserted into it. When they are contracted, the urethra is 4 cm. and when they are relaxed it is 3·8 cm. long. When the detrusor contracts, the urethra shortens still further.

The resistance offered by the urethra to the passage of urine is not only neurogenic; the turgor of the tissues and the proper position are also important. Both of these may deteriorate in old age.

Micturition

After the first two years or so of life, micturition occurs when the subject feels her bladder is full or when she considers that the time and place are suitable.

The ability to micturate even when the bladder contains only a very small amount of urine is not only a human ability. As every observer of dogs must have noticed, the male dog, using his urine to mark out his territory, may find the amount insufficient for his purpose; and so he often cocks a leg and induces the micturition reflex, only to find that he passes a few drops or none at all. Monkeys, like uninhibited boys, use micturition aggressively; travellers in Africa and South America confirm the accuracy of their aim.

Usually we do not micturate until we experience the sensation informing us that our bladders are full. This sensation originates from stretch and/or contraction of the detrusor muscle. In an investigation of the afferent nerves from the bladder of the cat, Iggo (1955) found that the same nerve fibres conduct impulses when the bladder is passively distended and when it actively contracts. In the human these afferent nerves run with the sacral parasympathetic efferent nerves to the 3rd and 4th sacral segments of the cord. From these segments nerve fibres soon cross the cord and ascend in the spino-thalamic tracts. In the same part of the spino-thalamic tract run the fibres subserving pain in the bladder, the vesical end of the ureter and the vagina, and pain and thermal sensibility in the urethra and anus (Nathan and Smith, 1951). It was shown later by the same workers (1953) that the pathway conducting impulses underlying the desire to defaecate occupies the same region of the spinothalamic tract.

The feeling that micturition is imminent is a different sensation from that underlying the desire to micturate; it has a larger urethral component and is more perineal than pelvic. This sensation, according to Nathan (1956), originates in the urethra and perineal muscles and in the two pubococcygeus muscles. The impulses subserving this sensation ascend the spinal cord in the posterior columns.

When we have the feeling that the bladder is full, we can either micturate or avoid micturition and continue to store urine in the bladder.

How micturition starts differs according to whether one merely decides that this is a suitable time and place to empty the bladder and the desire to micturate is not very strong or whether one has an urgent need to micturate. In the first case, the subject voluntarily relaxes the levator ani muscles; the detrusor contracts, the neck of the bladder is opened to form a funnel shape, so that the base of the bladder forms an almost straight line with the long axis of the urethra. In the second case, the micturition reflex is released and the detrusor contraction with opening up of the neck of the bladder occurs before the descent of the bladder in the pelvis due to the relaxation of the levatores ani. In both cases, the last act of the start of micturition is relaxation of the external sphincter of the urethra. The first act of ending micturition is contraction of this muscle; then the detrusor relaxes and the levator ani contracts. If micturition is avoided, detrusor contractions are stilled, and when further contractions do occur, they are not permitted to start off the micturition reflex.

The micturition reflex is a polysynaptic reflex of which the afferent limb is in the muscle fibres (and possibly the mucosa) of the bladder and of which the efferent limb is in the same bladder muscle fibres and the muscle fibres of the levator ani and perineal muscles. The reflex is excitatory to the smooth muscle of the bladder and inhibitory

to the somatic muscles of the pelvic floor and perineum. The effect of the reflex is to empty the bladder.

Conscious control of the bladder is organized mainly within a medial anterior region of the frontal lobes (Andrew and Nathan, 1964).

Increased Input to the Sacral Centre for Micturition

The threshold of the micturition reflex can be influenced by changes in the input to the sacral centres for micturition. This input comes from three directions: there is the input from supraspinal regions of the central nervous constantly coming in via the encephalo-spinal tracts; there is the input from the peripheral nerves coming from the bladder, the rectum and the somatic muscles concerned with micturition and defaecation; and there is an input arriving via interneuronal pathways from other sacral segments of the cord.

Many parts of the brain can change the threshold of the micturition reflex. They can make it fire off with only a small amount or else with a large amount of urine in the bladder. This is how psychological and emotional factors affect the frequency of micturition. If the spinal cord has been cut across and spasticity has developed, the parasympathetic motoneurons, like somatic motoneurons, have a lower threshold to excitation; and the micturition reflex may occur with as little as 50 ml. of urine in the bladder. If there is infection in the pelvis, such as cystitis or proctitis, then the threshold for the micturition reflex is lowered, and frequency and nocturia result.

It is known to all gynecologists and surgeons who operate upon the rectum and bladder that operations in this region of the body may cause retention of urine and of faeces. If there is a painful condition of the anus, such as a fissure, the patient is most unwilling to relax the external sphincter of the urethra for she cannot do so without relaxing the external sphincter of the anus. This muscle may be in spasm; and any movement of the muscle increases her pain. Any increase in the pain is a reflection of an increase in nerve impulses arriving at the sacral centres for defaecation and micturition.

The input to the sacral cord from the bladder is probably the most important factor controlling the output to the pelvic and perineal muscles. When the bladder is empty, the discharge of nerve impulses to the external sphincter of the urethra is minimal. As the bladder fills, this discharge increases, and when the bladder is full, the discharge becomes large and the muscle is held firmly contracted. This contraction can be further increased for brief periods by purposely contracting the perineal and pelvic muscles. One can easily observe in oneself that one cannot aid continence by a purposeful contraction of these muscles for very long; indeed it is difficult to keep these muscles contracted consciously for as long as a minute. In disorders of the central nervous system, the co-ordination of somatic and visceral muscles is disturbed. In addition to this, the somatic musculature involved in the storage and expulsion of urine is affected by the various disorders affecting other somatic musculature of the body. For example, it may become rigid in Parkinsonism and spastic with upper motor neuron lesions.

Division of Nerves between the Sacral Centre and Related Pelvic and Perineal Structures

As the storage and the elimination of urine and faeces are activities organized by the nervous system, it will be obvious that when the nerves between the sacral centre for these activities and the peripheral structures are divided, the activities cannot occur. When the structures are partially denervated, they will function only partially. As both the pelvic nerves and the sympathetic supply reach the bladder via the pelvic plexus, a lesion involving the pelvic plexus will almost certainly involve many sympathetic nerves as well.

Denervation of all muscles causes paralysis of flaccid type. This general principle applies here to the somatic muscles of the pelvic floor and perineum and to the visceral muscle of the detrusor. As has been mentioned above, a flaccid detrusor muscle is a bladder with the urethra closed. Following interference with the neural supply of the bladder at any level, changes in the bladder musculature commonly occur. Inco-ordination of muscular activity, stretching of the bladder, and infection probably all add a contribution. Hypertrophy of the bladder musculature may result. When it happens, the intravesical pressure rises and whenever a detrusor contraction occurs, there may be some expulsion of urine.

Division of Pelvic Nerves

When the pelvic nerves are cut through, then efferent and afferent nerve fibres supplying the musculature of the bladder have been interrupted: retention of urine ensues. Although there is an intramural plexus of autonomic ganglia and nerve fibres, this system cannot empty the bladder on its own. The micturition reflex no longer occurs; and none of the reflexes essential for the proper working of the bladder and for its total emptying can occur.

As the afferent nerve fibres from the bladder run in the pelvic nerves, the patient no longer experiences pain, strangury nor even the normal sensation giving her a desire to micturate. She is likely still to feel the sensation that micturition is imminent (unless the pudendal nerves are also divided) and she may experience a vague abdominal sensation associated with a full bladder. It needs careful questioning by the doctor and good observation by the patient to distinguish these various sensations. The two commonest conditions effectively dividing the afferent nerves from the bladder itself are tabes and diabetic neuropathy.

Division of Pudendal Nerves

As has been said above, the external sphincters of the urethra and of the anus and the two levatores ani muscles are kept in tonic contraction. Lapides, Ajemian, Stewart and Lichwardt (1959) found in women that voluntary and purposeful contraction of the levatores ani and perineal muscles "increased the intra-urethral resistance in the mid-urethra to 70 cm. of water." When a woman stands up, this pressure is reached without conscious contraction of these muscles. Sudden increases in intra-abdominal pressure caused, for instance, by coughing or sneezing, act as the stimulus to a reflex contraction of the external sphincter of the rectum and the urethra. This reflex can easily be examined by placing a finger in the rectum and getting the subject to cough. Coughing can cause a large increase in intravesical pressure. If this reflex is disrupted by division of the pudendal nerves, when the intravesical pressure rises above the intra-urethral pressure, stress incontinence results.

A cough may cause only a small rise in intravesical pressure; in this case, this is a reflection of the rise in intra-abdominal pressure. But at times coughing can induce a detrusor contraction. The difference between the two can be seen on cystometrography. If the column of fluid in the manometer is observed, when the detrusor contraction follows coughing, the rise in pressure continues to gather momentum after the coughing has stopped. A normal person under these circumstances has no leakage of urine. But if the control of the perineal muscles is insufficient, the rise in intravesical pressure causes a brief spurt of urine; for the intravesical pressure then exceeds the intra-urethral pressure. If the patient has deficient control of the detrusor muscle or of the sacral centre, then the detrusor contraction may go on to the complete micturition reflex and the bladder may expel a considerable amount of its contents.

The intravesical pressure rises when a woman changes position from lying to sitting or standing. This rise is about 12 to 40 cm. of water, being less than that induced by a good cough or sneeze, particularly if these cause a detrusor contraction. Warrell, Watson and Shelley (1963), who measured intravesical pressure by means of a radio-pill, found that walking increased intravesical pressure as it induced detrusor contractions; but the rise in pressure was only about 5 to 20 cm. of water, less than occurs with a detrusor contraction following a cough.

If one pudendal nerve is divided the effects on function are unimportant. If both nerves are divided, there are effects on continence and on starting and stopping micturition. If a bladder has either a functioning external sphincter of the urethra or a properly working detrusor muscle, it can still store urine. With both pudendal nerves divided, micturition can be started and stopped, though these acts take far longer than normally; and the ability to stop micturition in the middle of the act is no longer possible. With these nerves divided, the patient no longer feels urine passing and she no longer has the sensation that she has actively stopped micturating.

Division of All Nerves Between the Spinal Cord and Pelvic and Perineal Structures

Complete denervation of the bladder, the pelvic muscles, and the perineal muscles is most unlikely to occur as a consequence of a pelvic lesion. When it is found, the cause is probably neural; it is then a lesion of the sacral roots and/or the conus medullaris, which contains the sacral centres for the storage and the expulsion of urine.

When the pelvic floor is denervated, the muscles are relaxed. The perineum is seen to be bulging and to be in a descended position, and when the examiner feels the muscle per rectum he can observe that the patient is unable to contract it and move the rectum forwards. The descent of the pelvic floor and relaxation of the pubo-coccygeus muscles allows the base of the bladder to fall posteriorly towards the rectum. The bladder neck is relaxed so that it forms a straight line with the urethra, the position of readiness to start micturition and not the position for storage of urine.

When the bladder itself and the muscles of the pelvic floor and perineum are all denervated, there may be a feeble retention or there may be a continuous leaking of urine. On general principles, one might have expected to find a continuous leaking of urine, complete incontinence, the urethra not being closed by the perineal and pelvic muscles. But this is uncommon; a feeble retention of urine is commoner. This retention of urine with total denervation is unlike that which occurs with a transverse lesion of the spinal cord. It can be more easily overcome; urine can be expressed by pressure on the abdomen and it may pass whenever the patient moves or coughs. A catheter is very easily passed as the perineal muscles offer no resistance to its passage. If the detrusor does contract, it does so feebly as its contraction is not properly co-ordinated; only a small quantity of urine is passed, and the stream has no force.

Retention of Urine

Retention of urine occurs in the state of shock that follows acute division of the spinal cord. It nearly always occurs when there is any condition causing coma. It occurs when the afferent nerves and the efferent nerves to the detrusor are cut.

The eventual result of dividing the spinal cord from the brain is to cause all those motor effects we refer to as spasticity. The essential feature of this condition is a great increase in the activity of all motor neurons. With regard to the pelvic and perineal muscles and the detrusor musculature, this means that they react to insufficient stimuli and react exaggeratedly and for too long a time. This excessive activity overrides the principles of reciprocal innervation. The bladder may then start to empty and micturition be interrupted in midstream; or the detrusor may contract strongly, while the levator ani and external sphincter of the urethra remain tightly contracted.

If retention of urine comes on insidiously, the patient may not realize that she has it. She may just think that the urine is continuously leaking away. It is important to find out whether this is true or not. The urine does leak away almost continuously with retention of urine and overflow. With lesions of upper motor neuron type, it is more likely that the bladder is expelling its contents intermittently and incompletely at intervals of 5 to 35 minutes; but the patient usually thinks that urine is passing continuously. If urine is in fact continuously leaking away and the patient does not have retention with overflow, the likeliest cause is a fistula.

When there is evidence of some lesion in the central nervous system and the distended bladder is not recognized to be what it is, one of the classical errors in diagnosis is to consider that the distended bladder is a tumour arising from pelvic organs such as the uterus or the ovary, and that the neural lesion is a metastasis from this tumour.

The purpose of this chapter has not been to discuss the subject of disorders of micturition of neural origin (what is so often and so erroneously called "the neurogenic bladder"). It has been to relate the neurology of urology to gynecology.

REFERENCES

Andrew, J. and Nathan, P. W. (1964), *Brain*, **87**, 233.
Bors, E. (1957), *Urol. Surgery*, **7**, 177.
Iggo, A. (1955), *J. Physiol.*, **128**, 593.
Lapides, J., Ajemian, E. P., Stewart, B. H. and Lichtwardt, J. R. (1959), *Surg. Forum*, **10**, 896.
Lapides, J., Ajemian, E. P., Stewart, B. H., Breakley, B. A. and Lichtwardt, J. R. (1960), *J. Urol.*, **84**, 86.
Nathan, P. W. and Smith, M. C. (1951), *J. Neurol. Neurosurg. Psychiat.*, **14**, 262.
Nathan, P. W. and Smith, M. C. (1953), *Ibid.*, **16**, 245.
Nathan, P. W. (1956), *Brit. J. Urol.*, **28**, 126.
Uhlenhuth, E. (1953), *Problems in the Anatomy of the Pelvis*. Philadelphia: J. B. Lippincott.
Warrell, D. W., Watson, B. W. and Shelley, T. (1963), *J. Obst. Gyn. Brit. Commonwealth*, **70**, 959.
Woodburne, R. T. (1967), in *Neurogenic Bladder*, Chap. 1. Ed, S. Boyarsky. Baltimore: Williams and Wilkins.

4. PHARMACOLOGY OF THE UTERINE SYMPATHETIC NERVOUS SYSTEM

E. MARLEY and J. D. STEPHENSON

Introduction

The uterus is innervated through the autonomic nervous system, principally the sympathetic. The effects of autonomic nerves on uterine function were studied originally by nerve stimulation and isotonic recording of uterine contraction *in vivo*. Subsequently, isolated preparations of uterus or uterine horn bathed in an artificial salt medium were introduced; the effects of drugs on these isolated tissues were recorded isotonically or isometrically. The literature up to 1933 was reviewed by Gruber. More recently the effect of drugs on contractions evoked by transmural electrical stimulation of the isolated uterus or excitation of a hypogastric nerve have been examined. In the majority of studies, the system of recording permitted only measurement of changes in length and tone of longitudinal muscle, although there might be associated changes in tone of the circular and oblique muscles. Whereas in animals the entire uterus or a large part thereof is used for isolated preparations, from women only small sections of one of the muscle groups, usually the longitudinal are used.

The chemical transmitter at post-ganglionic sympathetic nerve terminals is noradrenaline, whereas that at the termination of parasympathetic nerves is acetylcholine. The molecules of transmitter are presumed to act on sites called receptors which are configuratively or electrostatically consonant with the shape or charge of the respective molecules. In the case of transmitter released on nerve stimulation this acts initially at the neuromuscular junctions but overflow occurs and the substance is then carried to other sites in the uterus and elsewhere in the body. The receptors involved can be characterized in a number of ways. One method is to compare the potency of the transmitter with that of a number of chemical congeners. By use of a series of closely allied congeners the most appropriate fit of a molecule at receptors is determined. Biological expediency has usually ensured that the most appropriately fitting molecule is the transmitter itself. This approach also allows interpretation of which part or parts of the molecule influence its activity, and it is thought that bonding of drug with receptors occurs first through the positively charged primary amino group in the case of noradrenaline and through the quaternary head in the case of acetylcholine. Another approach involves the use of selective antagonists. These antagonists are presumed to interact with receptors mediating the effects of the particular neurotransmitter so preventing its access to receptor sites.

The selective antagonists against the muscarinic action of acetylcholine at post-ganglionic receptor sites are atropine and hyoscine and against the nicotinic action of acetylcholine on ganglia are the ganglion-blocking agents. The position is also complicated for noradrenaline which acts on smooth muscle at two types of receptor

classified according to Ahlquist (1948) as α- and β-receptors for catecholamines. In general, excitatory effects such as contractions of a tissue are initiated through α-receptors whereas relaxor effects are mediated through β-receptors. Actions of catecholamines on α-receptors appear to be especially related to the interactions of the amino group and α-receptor, while the action on β-receptors is especially related to the interaction of the catechol group and β-receptor (Ariëns, 1961). Selective antagonists interacting at α-receptors are phentolamine and phenoxybenzamine; those at β-receptors are dichloroisoprenaline, pronethalol and propranolol (Fig. 1). These antagonists are selective in that they oppose only the particular transmitter and similarly-acting drugs. Whereas these selective antagonists are useful in indicating the transmitter released, the absolute criterion is collection of blood on nerve stimulation and identification of the transmitter. Ahlquist (1948) defined receptors not by using selective blocking agents but by testing the order of potency of four chemically allied amines (Fig. 1). An order of potency with noradrenaline the most potent and with descending order of noradrenaline > adrenaline > phenylephrine > isoprenaline indicated an action on α-receptors; an order of potency of isoprenaline > adrenaline > phenylephrine > noradrenaline indicated an action on β-receptors.

The literature concerning the effects of hypogastric nerve stimulation or catecholamines on uterine function abounds with conflicting statements, part of which is due to species difference in response. Four species are here considered; the coverage is intended to be illustrative rather than comprehensive. The effects of catecholamines and of nerve stimulation on uterine function are also influenced by oestrogen and progesterone and consequently by the different phases of the oestrous cycle and pregnancy. For example, in non-pregnant cats, adrenaline relaxes the uterus whereas during pregnancy, the uterus is contracted by it. Such antipodal effects were difficult to explain until recently and even led to the suggestion that a different transmitter was released during pregnancy. Introduction of selective antagonists at α- and β-receptors has clarified the phenomenon.

In this short review, contractor effects are synonymous with excitatory. A relaxor effect usually applies to relaxation of the uterus *in vivo* but also includes relaxation of spontaneous uterine contractions of isolated uteri; an inhibitory effect implies antagonism of acetylcholine-induced contractions of an isolated uterus.

UTERINE RESPONSE ACCORDING TO SPECIES

Rat

The inhibitory actions of adrenaline and noradrenaline on contractions elicited by acetylcholine of the rat's isolated uterus were first shown by de Jalon, Bayo and de Jalon'

1945. Various elaborations and improvements have been made subsequently for the isolated uterus to serve as an assay technique for adrenaline (Gaddum and Lembeck, 1949; Gaddum, Peart and Vogt, 1949). Antagonism of acetylcholine contractions are observed with other catecholamines, although their potencies differ, isoprenaline being

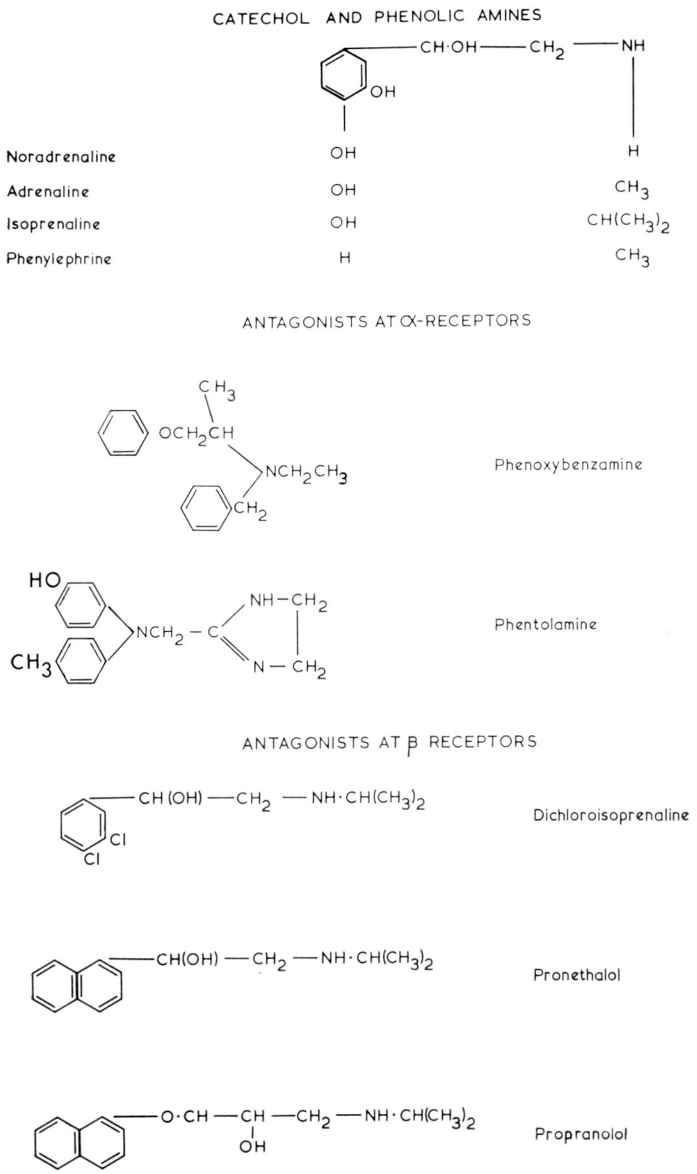

FIG. 1. Chemical structure of some catecholamines and their selective antagonists at α- and β-receptors.

more active than adrenaline. The order of potency in Ahlquist's (1948) experiments was isoprenaline > adrenaline > phenylephrine > noradrenaline. Since this order of potency was one ascribed to an action on β-receptors, Ahlquist considered rat uteri to possess mainly β-receptors. He later postulated (Ahlquist, 1962) that it was the inhibitory effects of catecholamines that were mediated in all uteri via β-receptors whereas α-receptors mediated the contractor effects. Sensitivity of rat's isolated uteri to adrenaline and isoprenaline is increased by Dibenamine or

phenoxybenzamine (Holzbauer and Vogt, 1955). On the basis of results with other tissues in which enhanced effects of catecholamines follow the use of an antagonist at α-receptors, a mixed action on α- and β-receptors was indicated. Rudzik and Miller (1962) also considered rat uteri to contain α- and β-receptors and suggested that both groups of receptors mediate uterine relaxation. However, Levy and Tozzi (1963) were unable to assure themselves that there were other than β-receptors. They found that the inhibitory effects of isoprenaline, adrenaline or phenylephrine were unaltered by an antagonist at α-receptors (phentolamine or phenoxybenzamine), but were abolished by an antagonist at β-receptors (dichloroisoprenaline). Moreover after pronethalol, another antagonist at β-receptors, adrenaline or phenylephrine did not evoke contractions as might have been anticipated if α-receptors were present. Tothill (1967) elegantly reinvestigated the matter in particular relation to the oestrus and progestational phases of the oestrous cycle and to pregnancy. The receptors mediating responses were studied both by selective antagonists and by the method of Butterworth (1963) in which repeated doses of isoprenaline are given until its inhibitory action is abolished. Under these circumstances the inhibitory effects of adrenaline, noradrenaline and phenylephrine were converted to contractor responses which were usually prevented by α-blockers but not by the β-blocker pronethalol. This could be accounted for by supposing that isoprenaline occupies β-receptors, thus allowing effects of adrenaline and allied amines upon α-receptors to emerge. These motor effects (after priming with isoprenaline) were obtained with uteri taken from pregnant rats or from those pretreated with diethylstilboestrol, but not with uteri from rats in natural oestrus or the progestational phase.

In work discussed hitherto, activity of whole uterine muscle or of a uterine horn was recorded. In experiments by Marshall (1959) electrical activity of single uterine fibres was recorded from isolated uterine horns of rats pretreated with oestradiol. In accord with its relaxor effect on the whole organ, adrenaline abolished action potential discharge and raised membrane potential.

Rabbit

Work on rabbit uteri antedates that on rats. Langley and Anderson (1895) observed contraction and pallor of a uterine horn on stimulating in vivo the corresponding hypogastric nerve. Pregnant and non-pregnant rabbit uteri also contracted to suprarenal extract, a mixture of adrenaline and noradrenaline (Langley, 1901), as did the isolated uterus with adrenaline (Kurdinowsky, 1904; Biagi, 1905). However, after ergot extract adrenaline, instead of contracting the uterus, inhibited rhythmic uterine contractions in vivo (Dale, 1906). Moreover, uterine relaxation α-receptors prevented myometrial contraction on hypogastric stimulation from which Cushny (1906) deduced that the nerve contained inhibitory and excitatory fibres; Mann (1950) considered the vasodilatation to be the result of anoxia after the intense vasoconstriction. Apart from differing effects on nerve stimulation, uterine tone may be paramount in determining the response to adrenaline for if tone was raised by immersing an isolated uterus in serum then adrenaline was relaxant (Falta and Fleming, 1911). Thus a contracted uterus might be more likely to relax to adrenaline and a relaxed uterus to contract, and indeed after increasing tone with pituitrin or histamine, adrenaline became relaxor (McSwiney and Brown, 1926). Ergotamine, whilst not altering uterine tone, converted the excitatory effect of adrenaline into a relaxant one, presumably by blockading α-receptors.

Evidence of sympathetic uterine innervation was provided by the increase of noradrenaline in uterine venous blood during stimulation of a hypogastric nerve (Mann, 1950); adrenaline was also increased but this probably came from the adrenal medullae. In further support of a sympathetic innervation, uterine contraction on hypogastric nerve stimulation was abolished by Dibenamine; Setekliev (1964) also demonstrated that antagonists at α-receptors prevented myometrial contraction on hypogastric nerve stimulation. Finally, bretylium which paralyzes sympathetic post-ganglionic nerves abolished the effects of hypogastric nerve stimulation on the rabbit's isolated nerve-uterus preparation. (Boura and Green, 1959).

Willems, Bernard, Delaunois and de Schaepdryver (1965) inferred the presence of α- and β-receptors in the progesterone dominated rabbit uterus in vivo. In this preparation adrenaline increased uterine activity, an effect on α-receptors since it was blocked by phenoxybenzamine after which adrenaline was relaxor. Miller and Marshall (1965) using an isolated nerve-uterus preparation from oestrogen pre-treated rabbits showed that hypogastric stimulation contracted the uterus whereas in uteri from oestrogen-plus-progesterone-treated animals, hypogastric stimulation inhibited spontaneous contractions, an effect on β-receptors since it was abolished by propranolol. Uterine catecholamine content was unaffected by oestrogen or oestrogen plus progesterone treatment. According to Shabanah, Toth and Maughan (1964) progesterone in moderate amounts rendered the excitatory (α) effect dominant whereas in large amounts the inhibitory (β) effect became dominant. This could account for the discrepancy between the results of Willems et al (1965) and Miller and Marshall (1965) and it would seem that during pregnancy the large amounts of circulating progesterone help to keep the uterus quiescent.

In 1954, Lewis studied a series of sympathomimetic amines on the isolated rabbit uterus but was unable to relate the degree of ionization (pKa value) of an amine with its pharmacological activity, possibly as a result of the amines having a mixed action on α- and β-receptors. With the availability now of β- receptor blocking agents, the effects of these amines might be again examined but in the presence of propranolol and a better relation between pKa and pharmacological activity established. With the exception of Lewis (1954) and Barger and Dale (1910), most work with sympathomimetic amines appears unfortunately to be restricted to the catecholamines.

In an excellent histochemical and pharmacological study of the rabbit fallopian tube, Brundin (1965) showed that hypogastric nerve stimulation and noradrenaline contract the isthmus, an effect localized to the circular muscle layer which has a rich adrenergic innervation. Results using pentamethonium (for ganglion-blocking action) and chronic hypogastric nerve section (to obtain post-ganglionic denervation) indicated that some preganglionic sympathetic fibres passed through the inferior mesenteric ganglia and synapsed in the hypogastric nerve and/or in the immediate vicinity of the fallopian tube.

Cat

Langley and Anderson (1895) described uterine pallor caused by stimulating "sympathetic nerves", adding that uterine contraction was much less constant and pronounced in cats than rabbits. Langley (1901) observed the same effect with suprarenal extract. The observation that stimulation of a hypogastric nerve in non-pregnant cats elicits relaxation of the uterus in situ whereas stimulation of the same nerve in pregnant cats elicits strong uterine contraction dates from the independent and almost simultaneous discovery of this phenomenon by Cushny and Dale (1906). The interpretation proved baffling until the recent introduction of drugs that blockade β-receptors. Indeed Dale assumed there was a mixture of motor and inhibitor elements in the sympathetic nerve supply of which one became functionally predominant according to whether the animal was or was not pregnant.

Vogt (1965) determined, after chromatographic separation, the amount of adrenaline or noradrenaline released into an ovarian vein on hypogastric nerve stimulation in anaesthetized, eviscerated and adrenalectomized cats. The amount determined represents "overflow", and is the difference between the amount released and that reabsorbed into nerve stores. The highest amount liberated per min. into the circulation on nerve stimulation was noradrenaline 5 μg and adrenaline 0·6 μg, the adrenaline probably having extra-uterine origin. Similar results were obtained in pregnant cats, so any changes taking place during pregnancy in response to hypogastric nerve stimulation appear not to involve changes in the transmitter.

Turning from experiments in vivo to those in vitro, Dale and Laidlaw (1912) noted relaxation by adrenaline of the isolated uterus of a virgin cat. One of the difficulties with this type of experiment in which response is altered by pregnancy is to obtain animals in the required physiological state. The appropriate condition can however be achieved by injection of oestrogen or progesterone. This was done by Robson and Schild (1938) who observed in vivo and in vitro that adrenaline relaxed the uterus of the spayed or oestrone-treated animals whereas it contracted the uterus of progesterone-treated or pregnant cats.

Graham and Gurd (1960) carried the work with isolated uteri a stage further. They confirmed that in the oestrous or oestrogen-injected cats, adrenaline stopped spontaneous rhythm and relaxed the uterus; with pregnant or pseudopregnant uteri (cat pretreated with oestrogen and then progesterone) addition of adrenaline caused spontaneous rhythm to develop or speed up and larger doses elicited contractions. Effects were obtained with smaller doses of adrenaline in the case of pregnant or pseudo-pregnant uteri than with uteri from oestrogen-injected cats or those in oestrus. In addition when a larger strip of a pregnant cat uterus was mounted in the same organ bath with a smaller strip of a non-pregnant uterus from a parous cat and left for 2–3 hr., the pregnant uterus contracted as before to adrenaline but so also did the non-pregnant uterus which had previously relaxed. The results implied that a substance was present in pregnant or progesterone-proliferated cat uteri which could be extracted by water and which diffused into a bath.

Dale (1906) who had postulated a dual mechanism subserving the motor and inhibitory effects of adrenaline on the cat's uterus based this partly on the different uterine response under differing physiological conditions and partly on his observation that the contractor effect of adrenaline on pregnant uteri *in situ* became relaxant after ergot. Ahlquist (1948) found an order of potency of isoprenaline > adrenaline > phenylephrine > noradrenaline on non-pregnant cats' uteri *in vivo* or *in vitro* suggesting activation of β-receptors. An order of potency isoprenaline > adrenaline > noradrenaline on isolated uteri was also found by Tsai and Fleming (1964) who further observed that the relaxant effect of adrenaline on the uteri of virgin cats was abolished by dichloroisoprenaline, an antagonist at β-receptors. In contrast the contractor effect of adrenaline or noradrenaline on pregnant cats' uteri was abolished by phenoxy-benzamine implying an action on α-receptors; indeed, a relaxant effect of adrenaline was then unmasked which was abolished by dichloroisoprenaline. Similar results were obtained with uteri of cats pretreated with oestrogen and progesterone.

Man

Adrenaline or noradrenaline contract strips of isolated uteri at any stage of the menstrual cycle, after the menopause, during pregnancy or at parturition (Garrett, 1955). Thus isolated uterine muscles of man and of rabbit react similarly to adrenaline. In patients close to term, *l*-noradrenaline infused intravenously increased uterine activity and tone (Cibils, Pose and Zuspan, 1962). Adrenaline given intravenously to pregnant subjects can have a dual effect (Kaiser, 1950); at low doses tone was reduced whereas at high doses it was increased. This work was extended by Garrett (1954) and Pose, Cibils and Zuspan, (1962). These last workers infused *l*-adrenaline at various rates for up to 3 hr. Spontaneous or Syntocinon induced uterine activity was significantly diminished, due mainly to a decrease in intensity of contraction though a reduction in contraction frequency was also noted. Strips of human isolated fallopian tube also contract to adrenaline, noradrenaline and isoprenaline (Hawkins, 1964; Rosenblum and Stein, 1966), and there are histochemical similarities in the adrenergic innervation of rabbit and human fallopian tubes (Brundin, 1965; Brundin and Wirsén, 1964).

β-receptors can be assumed to be present in the human uterus. In three patients close to term, isoprenaline infused intravenously abolished uterine contractions induced by Syntocinon or due to labour (Mahon *et al*, 1967). These effects and those on blood pressure and heart rate were blocked by propranolol indicating that they were due to β-receptor stimulation.

By using microelectrode techniques, Kumar, Wagatsuma and Barnes (1965) showed that adrenaline raised the resting membrane potential of myometrial cells from pregnant and non-pregnant human myometrial strips. Although the usual response of human isolated myometrial tissues is contractor, (presumably an α excitatory effect), these results suggest an action on β-receptors since elevation of the resting membrane potential is linked with relaxation (Bülbring, 1961). It is unfortunate that a simultaneous record of muscle tension was not taken. With rat uteri, relaxation and increase in resting membrane potential occur simultaneously with adrenaline (Marshall, 1959).

Therapeutic applications. Relaxation of uterine smooth muscle by amines activating β-receptors has been used in the treatment of threatened abortion. Isoxsuprine [2-(phenoxy-2-propylamino-1-(p-hydroxyphenyl)-1 propranol] is such an amine and a potent relaxant of smooth muscle (Lish, Dungan and Peters, 1960). In 1961, Hendricks, Cibils, Pose and Eskes demonstrated its effectiveness in reducing uterine activity during late pregnancy and in labour. In 9 subjects in premature labour, but with intact membranes, 6 pregnancies were significantly prolonged (11–126 days). The most important side effect was hypotension due to activation of β-receptors in vascular smooth muscle. The ($\pm$)isomer was the more potent uterine relaxant, and the ($-$)isomer the more potent on blood pressure (Ericksson and Wiquist, 1965).

Isoxsuprine may also act directly on the uterus, independently of β-receptor activation (Lish, Hillyard and Dungan, 1960). The uterine relaxant action of isoxsuprine on strips of pregnant human isolated uterus was not blocked by concentrations of the potent β-receptor blocking agent MJ 1999 [4-(2 isopropyl-amino-1-hydroxyethyl) methanesulphonamide] which prevented relaxation to isoprenaline (Stander, 1966). Cc.25(p-hydroxyphenyl-isopropylnoradrenaline) possesses similar properties to isoxsuprine on the uterine smooth muscle but is less active on vascular smooth muscle (Eskes, Stolte, Seelen, Moed and Vogelsang, 1965; Stolte, Eskes, Seelon, Moed and Vogelsang, 1965).

Summary

The effects of noradrenaline, adrenaline and isoprenaline on the uteri of four species are summarized in Table 1.

TABLE 1

THE EFFECTS OF NORADRENALINE (NAd), ADRENALINE (Ad) AND ISOPRENALINE (Isop) ON UTERI OF FOUR SPECIES

+ = contractor; − = relaxor.

Species		NAd	Ad	Isop
HUMAN	*in vivo*	+	−	−
	in vitro	+	+	−
RABBIT		+	+	−
CAT	non-pregnant	−	−	−
	pregnant	+	+	no effect
RAT		−	−	−

The uteri may be classed into two separate groups on the basis of their response to noradrenaline; those which are contracted (man, rabbit and pregnant cat) and those which are relaxed (rat and non-pregnant cat). Adrenaline B.P. prepared from natural sources was used in early experiments but contains 15–20 per cent noradrenaline; this makes early results difficult to interpret. Recognition that adrenaline possessed antipodal types of action on separate α and β receptors made interpretation simpler. Significant advances did not occur until selective α blocking agents (e.g. phenoxybenzamine), β blocking agents (e.g. propranolol) and the ovarian hormones, oestrogen and progesterone became available. The pharmacologist was then better equipped to study responses of the uterus to drugs under controlled hormonal conditions.

REFERENCES

Ahlquist, R. P. (1948), "A study of the Adrenotropic Receptors," *Amer. J. Physiol.*, **153**, 586–600.

Ahlquist, R. P. (1962), "The Adrentropic Receptor-detector," *Arch. int. pharmacodyn.*, **139**, 38–41.

Ariëns, E. J. (1961), "Sympathomimetic Drugs and their Receptors," in *Adrenergic Mechanisms* Ciba Foundation Symposium 1960 (Eds. J. R. Vane, G. E. W. Wolstenholme and M. O'Connor) pp. 253–263. Churchill, London.

Barger, G. and Dale, H. H. (1910), "Chemical Structure and Sympathomimetic Amines," *J. Physiol. (Lond.)*, **41**, 19–59.

Biagi (1905 quoted by Gruber, C. M. (1933) from "The Autonomic Innervation of the Genito-urinary System," *Physiol. Rev.*, **13**, 497–609.

Boura, A. L. A., and Green, A. F. (1959), "The Actions of Bretylium: Adrenergic Neurone Blocking and Other Effects," *Brit. J. Pharmac. Chemother.*, **14**, 536–548.

Brundin, J. (1965), "Distribution and Function of Adrenergic Nerves in the Rabbit Fallopian Tube," *Acta Physiol. Scand.*, **66**, Suppl., **259**, 1–57.

Brundin, J. and Wirsén, C. (1964), "Adrenergic Nerve Terminals in the Human Fallopian Tube by Fluorescence Microscopy," *Acta Physiol. Scand.*, **61**, 505–506.

Bülbring, E. (1961), "Biophysical Changes Produced by Adrenaline and Noradrenaline," in *Adrenergic Mechanisms* Ciba Foundation Symposium 1960 (Eds. J. R. Vane, G. E. W. Wolstenholme, and M. O'Connor) pp. 275–287. Churchill, London.

Butterworth, K. R. (1963), "The β-adrenergic Blocking and Pressor Actions of Isoprenaline in the Cat," *Brit. J. Pharmac. Chemother.*, **21**, 378–392.

Cibils, L. A., Pose, S. V., and Zuspan, F. P. (1962), "Effect of *l*-norepinephrine Infusion on Uterine Contractility and Cardiovascular System," *Am. J. Obstet. Gynec.*, **84**, 307–317.

Cushny, A. R. (1906), "On the Movements of the Uterus," *J. Physiol. (Lond.)*, **35**, 1–19.

Dale, H. H. (1906), "On Some Physiological Actions of Ergot," *J. Physiol. (Lond.)*, **34**, 163–206.

Dale, H. H. and Laidlaw, P. P. (1912), "The Significance of the Supra-renal Capsules in the Action of Certain Alkaloids," *J. Physiol. (Lond.)*, **45**, 1–26.

Eriksson, G. and Wiquist, N. (1965), "Action of Isoxsuprine and Its (+)isomer on the Pregnant Human Uterus; an Experimental Study, *Amer. J. Obstet. Gynec.*, **91**, 1076–1083.

Eskes, T., Stolte, L., Seelen, J., Moed, H. D. and Vogelsang, C. (1965), "Epinephrine Derivates and the Activity of the Human Uterus: II. The Influence of Pronethalol and Propanolol on the Uterine and Systemic Activity of *p*-hydroxyphenylisopropylarterenol (Cc. 25)," *Amer. J. Obstet. Gynec.* **92**, 871–881.

Falta and Flemming (1911) quoted by Gruber, C. M. (1933) from "The Autonomic Innervation of the Genito urinary System," *Physiol. Rev.*, **13**, 497–609.

Gaddum, J. H. and Lembeck, F. (1949), "The Assay of Substances from the Adrenal Medulla," *Brit. J. Pharmac. Chemother.*, **4**, 401–408.

Gaddum, J. H., Peart, W. S. and Vogt, M. (1949), "The Estimation of Adrenaline and Allied Substances in the Blood," *J. Physiol. (Lond.)*, **108**, 476–481.

Garrett, W. J. (1954), "The Effects of Adrenaline and Noradrenaline on the Intact Human Uterus in Late Pregnancy and Labour," *J. Obstet. and Gynaec. Brit. Emp.*, **61**, 586–589.

Garrett, W. J. (1955), "The Effects of Adrenaline, Noradrenaline and Dihydroergotamine on Excised Human Myometrium," *Brit. J. Pharmac. Chemother.*, **10**, 39–44.

Graham, J. D. P. and Gurd, M. R. (1960), "Effects of Adrenaline on the Isolated Uterus of the Cat," *J. Physiol. (Lond.)*, **152**, 243–249.

Gruber, C. M. (1933), "The Autonomic Innervation of the Genito-urinary System, "*Physiol. Rev.*, **13**, 497–609.

Hawkins, D. F. (1964), "Some Pharmacological Reactions of Isolated Rings of Human Fallopian Tube, *Arch. int. pharmacodyn.*, **152**, 474–478.

Hendricks, C. H., Cibils, L. A., Pose, S. V. and Eskes, T. K. (1961), "The Pharmacologic Control of Excessive Uterine Activity with Isoxsuprine," *Amer. J. Obstet. Gynec.*, **82**, 1064–1078.

Holzbauer, M. and Vogt, M. (1955), "Modification by drugs of the response of the Rat Uterus to Adrenaline, *Brit. J. Pharmac. Chemother.*, **10**, 186–190.

De Jalon, P. G., Bayo, J. B. and De Jalon, M. G. (1945), "Sensible y nuevo método de valoración de adrenaline en útero aislado de rata," *Farmacoter. actual*, **2**, 313–318.

Kaiser, I. H. (1950), "The Effect of Epinephrine and Norepinephrine on the Contractions of the Human Uterus in Labour," *Surg. Gynec. Obstet.*, **90**, 649–654.

Kumar, D., Wagatsuma, T. and Barnes, A. C. (1965), "*In vitro* hyperpolarizing Effect of Adrenaline on Human Myometrial Cell," *Amer. J. Obstet. Gynec.*, **91**, 575–576.

Kurdinowsky (1904) quoted by Gruber, C. M. (1933) from "The Autonomic Innervation of the Genito-urinary System," *Physiol. Rev.*, **13**, 497–609.

Langley, J. N. (1901), "Observations on the Physiological Action of Extracts of the Suprarenal Bodies," *J. Physiol. (Lond.)* **27**, 237–256.

Langley, J. N. and Anderson, H. K. (1895), "The Innervation of the Pelvic and Adjoining Viscera: Part IV, The Internal Generative Organs." *J. Physiol. (Lond.)*, **19**, 122–130.

Lewis, G. P. (1954), "The Importance of Ionization in the Activity of Sympathomimetic Amines," *Brit. J. Pharmac. Chemother.*, **9**, 488–493.

Levy, B. and Tozzi, S. (1963), "The Adrenergic Receptive Mechanism of the Rat Uterus," *J. Pharmacol. Exp. Therap.*, **142**, 178–184.

Lish, P. M., Dungan, K. W. and Peters, E. L. (1960), "A Survey of the Effects of Isoxsuprine on Nonvascular Smooth Muscle," *J. Pharmacol. Exp. Therap.*, **129**, 191–199.

Lish, P. M., Hillyard, I. W. and Dungan, K. W. (1960), "The Uterine Relaxant Properties of Isoxsuprine," *J. Pharmacol. Exp. Therap.*, **129**, 438–444.

McSwiney, B. A. and Brown, G. L. (1926), "Reversal of the Action of Adrenaline," *J. Physiol. (Lond.)*, **62**, 52–63.

Mann, M. R. (1950), "An Investigation as to the Constitution and Action of Sympathin," Ph.D. Thesis, Univ. London.

Marshall, J. M. (1959), "Effects of Estrogen and Progesterone on Single Uterine Muscle Fibers in the Rat," *Amer. J. Physiol.*, **197**, 935–942.

Mahon, W. A., Reid, D. W. and Day, R. A. (1967), "The *in vivo* Effects of Beta Adrenergic Stimulation and Blockade on the Human Uterus at Term," *J. Pharmacol. Exp. Therap.*, **156**, 178–185.

Miller, M. D. and Marshall, J. M. (1965), "Uterine Response to Nerve Stimulation; Relation to Hormonal Status and Catecholamines," *Amer. J. Physiol.*, **209**, 859–865.

Pose, S. V., Cibils, L. A. and Zuspan, F. P. (1962), "Effect of *l*-epinephrine Infusion on Uterine Contractility and Cardiovascular System," *Amer. J. Obstet. Gynec.*, **84**, 297–306.

Robson, J. M. and Schild, H. O. (1938), "Response of the Cat's Uterus to the Hormones of the Posterior Pituitary Lobe," *J. Physiol. (Lond.)*, **92**, 1–8.

Rosenblum, I. and Stein, A. A. (1966), "Autonomic Responses of the Circular Muscles of the Isolated Human Fallopian Tube," *Amer. Physiol.*, **210**, 1127–1129.

Rudzik, A. D. and Miller, J. W. (1962), "The Effect of Altering the Catecholamine Content of the Uterus on the Rate of Contraction and the Sensitivity of the Myometrium to Relaxin," *J. Pharmacol. Exp. Therap.*, **38**, 88–95.

Setekleiv, J. (1964), "Uterine Mobility of the Estrogenized Rabbit: 3. Response to Hypogastric and Splanchnic Nerve Stimulation," *Acta physiol. scand.*, **62**, 137–149.

Shabanah, E. H., Toth, A, and Maughan, G. B. (1964), "The Role of the Autonomic Nervous System in Uterine Contractility and Blood Flow: 1. The Interaction Between Neurohormones and Sex Steroids in the Intact and Isolated Uterus," *Amer. J. Obstet. Gynec.*, **89**, 841–859.

Stander, R. W. (1966), "Phenethanolamines and Inhibition of Human Myometrium," *Amer. J. Obstet. Gynec.* **94**, 749–765.

Stolte, L., Eskes, T., Seelen, J. Moed, H. D. and Vogelsang, C. (1965), "Epinephrine Derivates and the Activity of the Human Uterus: 1. The Inhibiting Effect of the ρ-hydroxyphenylisopropylarterenol (Cc./25) upon Uterine Activity in Human Pregnancy, *Amer. J. Obstet. Gynec.*, **92**, 865–870.

Tothill, A. (1967), "Investigation of Adrenaline Reversal in the Rat Uterus by the Induction of Resistance to Isoprenaline," *Brit. J. Pharmac. Chemother.*, **29**, 291–301.

Tsai, T. H., and Fleming, W. W. (1964), "The Adrenotropic Receptors of the Cat Uterus," *J. Pharmacol. Exp. Therap.*, **143**, 268–272.

Vogt, M. (1965), "Transmitter Released in the Cat Uterus by Stimulation of the Hypogastric Nerves," *J. Physiol. (Lond.)* **179**, 163–171.

Willems, J. L., Bernard, P. J., Delaunois, A. L., and Schaepdryver, A. F. De (1965), "Adrenergic Receptors in the Progesterone Dominated Rabbit Uterus," *Arch. int. Pharmacodyn.*, **157**, 243–250.

5. THE MECHANISM OF URINARY CONTINENCE AND OF INCONTINENCE

AXEL INGELMAN-SUNDBERG

CONDITIONS PRECEDENT FOR CONTINENCE

The general hydraulic laws are applicable to the urine in the bladder, in the urethra and in the ureters. This means, that the pressure of the enclosed fluid is transmitted equally to all parts, to which direct liquid communication exists, for instance between the urinary bladder and the posterior part of the urethra, which sometimes remains open even in continent women. The prerequisite condition for urine to remain inside the bladder is that the surrounding pressure must be higher than the pressure of the urine. This means that the pressure in some part of the urethra must always be higher than the pressure of urine inside the bladder; except on voiding.

CONDITIONS PRECEDENT FOR INCONTINENCE

When pressure, lower than that of the urine in the ureter, the bladder or the urethra, appears at any point, urine flows towards this point at the same time as levelling of pressure takes place. When there is a fistula to another organ, as for instance the vagina, the difference in pressure between the two organs and the size of the fistula determines the urinary flow through the fistula. Thus, for instance, a vesico-vaginal fistula with a diameter of a few millimeters is usually big enough to keep the bladder empty in an upright position. When there is an incontinence through the urethra, corresponding laws are valid, and the flow is regulated by the width of the urethra and the difference in pressure between the urethra and the urine in the bladder.

Physiology

Investigations by Enhörning (1960, 1964), later on confirmed by others (Beck and Hsu, 1964; Beck and Maugham, 1964) have shown, that simple hydraulic laws are valid for urinary continence. In continent women there is always a higher pressure in the middle part of the urethra, corresponding to the site of the deep transverse perineal muscle, than in the bladder. The difference between the pressure inside the bladder and the highest pressure found in the urethra is called *the closing pressure* of the urethra. As long as this pressure has positive values, the patient is continent; when the value is zero or negative, incontinence appears. The amount of urine leaking out depends on the difference in pressure, the width of the urcthra, and the period of time during which the negative difference in pressure exists, i.e. during a cough, for a very short period of time.

In experiments on female volunteers the musculature was paralyzed with succinylcholinchloride, and the intra-abdominal pressure regulated by means of a pressure chamber around the abdomen (Enhörning, 1961). An increase in the intra-abdominal pressure caused an increase in the intra-urethral pressure in the same way as when the patient coughed. The rise of pressure in the urethra during coughing and similar stress is therefore chiefly caused by the transmission of the increased abdominal pressure. The increase in pressure is, however, chiefly localized to the proximal half of the urethra, whereas the rise in pressure, caused by transmitted intra-abdominal pressure, is less in the distal half of the urethra. This means, that from a functional point of view, only the proximal half can be regarded as an intra-abdmoinal organ.

When, however, a woman with a normal urethra and normal musculature of the pelvic floor holds on, in order to retain urine, a considerable increase in pressure can be measured along the whole urethra, caused by the contraction of the muscles.

The pressure inside the bladder normally consists of the tonus of the bladder musculature and of the intra-abdominal pressure in the low part of the abdomen. This pressure varies with the position of the body, because of the weight of the intra-abdominal viscera and their mobility. In an upright position it is high, reaching values of

50–100 cm. H_2O. In the lithotomy position or the knee-elbow position, the pressure is often less than the surrounding air pressure. At a cough, or when bearing down in a standing position, on the other hand, values of almost 200 cm. H_2O are reached.

The pressure inside the urethra consists of the tone in the mucous membrane, and in the cavernous tissue, the tone of the musculature of the urethra, and of the musculature of the surrounding part of the pelvic floor, plus the transmitted part of the intra-abdominal pressure. In continent women the total pressure in the middle part of the urethra is always higher than the pressure inside the bladder which means, that the closing pressure is higher than zero.

Pathophysiology

The simplest and most common type of urinary incontinence is seen in women, following child-birth. In these women one finds a rotatory drop of the urethra and the anterior vaginal wall, when coughing at the same time as urinary leakage appears. Sometimes the leakage takes place merely at a cough in an upright position, as only in this position does the intra-vesical pressure reach values high enough for leakage. The rotatory drop of the urethra and the anterior vaginal wall, as well as of the bladder, is caused by a deficiency of the pelvic floor, created by the passage of the foetal head. If the vaginal wall is supported without compressing the urethra during the cough, no leakage occurs. Figuratively speaking, this is caused by the fact that the intra-abdominal pressure can now compress the urethra against the supporting finger. This phenomenon was already described in 1923 by Bonney, and ought therefore to be called Bonney's test. If the patient becomes continent, when the anterior vaginal wall is supported in the direction front—cranially, Bonney's test is positive. Under these circumstances the incontinence is chiefly caused by an incomplete transmission of the intra-abdominal pressure to the lumen of the urethra, because the urethra, figuratively speaking, slips away because of the increase in pressure. A positive Bonney's test is typical for a deficient pelvic floor, and is a very important sign, as it shows that the patient will be cured, when the support of the urethra and the bladder neck is restored.

Incomplete transmission of the intra-abdominal pressure to the lumen of the urethra may also be caused by the urethral wall being so scarified through inflammatory processes or previous operations, that the increase in pressure is absorbed by the wall itself, and can therefore not reach the lumen of the urethra. In such cases the urethra resembles a stiff soil tube, which cannot be compressed (Jeffcoate, 1961). The same effect may be caused by scar tissue around the urethra, which prevents the intra-abdominal rise in pressure from reaching the urethra. From a functional point of view in such cases the urethra is situated completely extra-abdominally.

In those cases, where scar tissue causes the incontinence, Bonney's test usually is negative, which means, that the patient is still incontinent when coughing, in spite of the fact that the vaginal wall is elevated. The therapy under these circumstances must be directed against the scar tissue, which must be removed. If this is impossible, closure of the urethra might be obtained by the urethra kinking operation (Ingelman-Sundberg, 1951).

The blood flow through the cavernous tissue, as well as turgor of the urethral mucous membrane, and contractile power of the musculature, are of great importance for the pressure inside the urethra. In young women this pressure varies parallel with the arterial pulse, but such variations in pressure cannot be demonstrated after the menopause (Enhörning, 1961). With increasing age the contractile power of the urethral musculature also decreases. In declining years therefore restoration of the circulation and vaginal estrogenic treatment, as well as the prescription of a small dose of androgenic hormone (Youssef, 1959) or an anabolic preparation to strengthen the musculature, are of great value for the cure.

In pre-climacteric women the cause of incontinence is therefore often a combination of an insufficiency of the pelvic floor, caused by delivery, and changes in the connective tissue, due to ageing as well as atrophy of the urethral mucous membrane. The pressure inside the urethra is then diminished, due to incomplete transmission of the intra-abdominal pressure, as well as a decrease of urethral tone.

If the urethral musculature is paralyzed, urinary incontinence can appear in spite of the fact that the transmission of the intra-abdominal pressure is normal. As a rule, however, the turgor of the tissue around the urethra is sufficient for fairly good continence. Due to the same circumstances it is possible to achieve sufficient continence through the use of a urethral transplant without musculature, if it is supported well enough for complete transmission of the intra-abdominal pressure to its lumen.

Incontinence of urine can be caused in a very special way, if adhesions exist between the urethral wall and the pubococcygeus muscles. When these muscles contract, a pull is transmitted through the adhesions to the urethral wall, and its lumen is opened (Ingelman-Sunberg, 1952; Hartl, 1953; Youssef, 1957). Bonney's test is usually negative.

However, urinary incontinence can appear in spite of a normal urethra and a normally functioning pelvic floor. The cause then is one of the following:

1. The tone of the bladder is too high.

2. A tumour, or for instance a pregnant uterus, compresses the bladder and thus increases the intra-vesical pressure.

3. Un-inhibited bladder contractions appear as in neural lesions, which elevate the pressure inside the bladder to values higher than the pressure in the urethra.

4. Maximum filling of the bladder is established, because of obstruction to the outflow, or because of paralysis of the bladder musculature, followed by an increase of pressure in the bladder, until the resistance of the urethra has been forced and an over-flow appears.

Under the conditions mentioned Bonney's test is negative, and therapy has to be directed against the primary cause.

Sometimes the patient cannot differentiate between urinary incontinence and urgency, as if she has an "irritable bladder," whereby the micturition reflex is released earlier than normally. Under these circumstances the cause may be an insufficient cerebral motor inhibition or urethritis; but food allergy or a hyper-sensitivity of some other kind may be the cause. At cystoscopy in these cases one often finds local oedema and redness in the trigone. It must be kept in mind, however, that a papilloma of the bladder, or an ovarian carcinoma, can give similar symptoms, before any infiltration of the bladder wall itself has taken place.

Urgency is often caused by cystitis, urethritis or urinary calculi. If these explanations can be excluded, the origin is usually neurogenic; often incomplete motor inhibition of the bladder occurs, as for instance in multiple sclerosis or in arteriosclerotic or diabetogenic changes in the spinal nerve tracts. Sometimes there is increased irritability in the bladder musculature. Under these circumstances ordinary walking (Warrel, Watson, Shelley, 1963), repeated coughing or jumping, may cause contraction of the bladder musculature, which may cause urinary leakage (Hodgkinson, Ayers, Drucker, 1963; Beck, Thomas, Maugham, 1966). Not seldom the cause is also psychogenic (Jeffcoate, Francis, 1966).

Also in polyuria, caused by polydipsia, diabetes, renal insufficiency or simply by nervous tension, it sometimes happens, that women interpret their pollakiuria as incontinence. This is often seen in elderly patients with a circulatory insufficiency, who excrete their oedema at night.

A decrease in the capacity of the urinary bladder, caused by shrinking after operations, radiation treatment or chronic inflammation, can give the same experience. If a patient has a greater amount of residual urine, the same effect can appear in spite of the fact that the volume of the bladder is normal. It is then caused by the decrease in effective bladder capacity.

Urinary leakage after micturition indicates that urine remains in the distal part of the urethra. In women the cause then almost always is a diverticulum. Diverticula are filled during micturition and later on emptied by an increase of pressure in the vagina, as for instance when the patient gets up or has coitus.

Under the different circumstances mentioned the therapy must be directed against the primary disease, and not against the incontinence which is a symptom.

NEUROGENIC URINARY INCONTINENCE AND SIMILAR CONDITIONS

In the aetiology of urinary incontinence there is often a combination of neurogenic and mechanical causes.

Neurogenic bladder disturbances are usually classified according to the site of the damage in relation to the spinal cord, and are divided into supra-nuclear and infra-nuclear lesions. The symptoms also vary according to what extent sensory or motor nerves are involved (see Section IX, Chap. 3).

Classification of Urinary Leakage

From the survey presented it is evident, that an involuntary flow of urine from the genital region may have many different causes. Valuable information can, however, be obtained on taking the case history. In the following scheme (Ingelman-Sundberg, 1953) the symptoms are graded and their appearance taken into consideration, giving the possibility for a rough primary classification of the cases for their future investigation and treatment.

A. Urinary Incontinence only at Stress: Stress Incontinence

Grade 1: Incontinent only when coughing or sneezing etc.

Grade 2: Incontinent also at sudden movements; when lifting, walking upstairs, etc.

Grade 3: Always incontinent in an upright position, continent when lying down.

B. Incontinence Independent of Stress

C. Continuous Incontinence

Group A contains most cases of urinary incontinence. In Group B we find the cases of psychogenic, neurogenic and inflammatory incontinence, and Group C includes the fistulae and those cases, where incontinence is caused by malformations.

REFERENCES

Beck, R. P. and Hsu, Nora (1964), "Relationship of Urethral Length and Anterior Wall Relaxation to Urinary Stress Incontinence," *Amer. J. Obstet. Gynec.*, **89**, 738.

Beck, R. P. and Maugham, G. B. (1964), "Simultaneous Intraurethral and Intra-vesical Pressure Studies in Normal Women and Those with Stress Incontinence," *Amer. J. Obstet. Gynec.*, **89**, 746.

Beck, R. P., Thomas, E. A. and Maugham, G. B. (1966), "The Detrusor Muscle and Urinary Incontinence," *Amer. J. Obstet. Gynec.*, **94**, 483.

Bonney, V. (1923), "On Diurnal Incontinence of Urine in Women," *J. Obst. Gyn. Brit. Emp.*, **30**, 358.

Enhörning, G. (1960), "Closing Mechanism of the Female Urethra," *Lancet*, 1414.

Enhörning, G. (1961), "Simultaneous Recording of Intravesical and Intraurethral Pressure," *Acta. Chir. Scandinav. Suppl.*, 276.

Enhörning, G. and Hurman, F., Jr. (1964), "Urethral Closure Studied with Cineroentgenography and Simultaneous Bladderurethra Pressure Recording," *Surg. Gynec. and Obst.*, **118**, 507.

Hartl, H. (1953), *Die funktionelle Harninkontinenz der Frau.* Stuttgart: Ferdinand Enke Verlag.

Hodgkinson, C. P., Ayers, M. A. and Drucker, B. H. (1963), "Dyssynergic Detrusor Dysfunction in the Apparently Normal Female," *Amer. J. Obstet. Gynec.*, **87**, 717.

Ingelman-Sundberg, A. (1952), "Urinary Incontinence in Women, Excluding Fistulas," *Acta Obstet. et Gynecol. Scandinav.*, **31**, 266.

Ingelman-Sundberg, A. (1953), "Urininkontinens hos kvinnan," *Nord. Med.*, **50**, 1149.

Jeffcoate, T. N. A. (1961), "Functional Disturbances of the Female Bladder and Urethra," *J. Roy. Coll. Surgeons, Edinburgh*, **7**, 28.

Warrell, D. W., Watson, B. W. and Shelley, T. (1963), "Intravesical Pressure Measurements in Women during Movement Using a Radio Pill and an Air-probe," *J. Obst. Gyn. Brit. Cmwth.*, **70**, 959.

Youssef, A. F. (1957), "Sphincter Incontinence of Urine in the Female: A New Approach to its Classification, Diagnosis and Treatment," *Acta Obst. Gynec. Scandinav.*, **36**, 759.

Youssef, A. F. (1959), "Drug Effect on the Female Bladder and its Sphincter Mechanism," *Obst. and Gynec.* **13** 61.

6. THE FEMALE URETHRA, OBSERVATIONS ON THE ANATOMY, PATHOLOGY AND TREATMENT OF ITS OCCLUSION MECHANISM

W. LANGREDER

The urethra is the canal through which urine is voided; it thus regulates the filling and emptying mechanism of the bladder through active closure and passive opening.

With the object of elucidating this system studies of anatomical sections have been made. The mechanism of urinary continence depends on the combination of the structures in the urethral wall and the peri-urethral tissues. The single symptom of urinary incontinence can be demonstrated as caused by manifold variations in structure as seen in longitudinal and transverse sections through the urethra and the surrounding tissue.

The various structures concerned in the mechanism of urinary continence are set out in Table 1.

TABLE 1

The mechanism of closure of the urethra consists of:

A. *Structures in the wall of the urethra*
1. The epithelium (with its folds and glands).
2. The submucosa (with venous sinuses, erectile tissue and elastic fascia).
3. The intrinsic muscle (with longitudinal and spiral muscle fibres but no distinct internal spincter).

B. *Surrounding structures which fix the urethra (the so-called para-urethrium)*
4. The muscle and fascia of the levator ani (or pelvic fascia).
5. The deep transverse perineal muscle (the so-called pelvic diaphragm, but without the formerly described picture of an external sphincter).
6. The bulbo-cavernosus muscle (the vaginal sphincter).
7. Fixation to the symphysis pubis (urethro-pubic fascia).
8. Fixation to the vulva (basal fixation).
9. Fixation to the vaginal wall (urethro-vaginal fascia).
10. Fixation to the paravaginal tissues (through the so-called urethro-vaginal sphincter).
11. Fixation to the parametrium (through the urethro-parametrial fascia).
12. Fixation to the cervix uteri (cervico-urethral fascia).
13. Fixation to the bladder, especially to the trigone (cranial fixation).

This summary makes clear the complex nature of the means by which the urethra is occluded. The importance of the para-urethral tissue becomes evident, consisting as it does of collagenous, elastic and smooth muscle tissue. In the pathogenesis of incontinence there may be a pure urethral or a pure para-urethral cause or it may arise from a combination of both.

The Sphincter Mechanism of the Urethra Itself

1. The epithelium itself has an important occlusive role. Its folds are prominent and in the inner cranial third it is lined with transitional epithelium, resembling that of the bladder. Sometimes a thick fold, or "uvula," is seen. In the middle third, the epithelial folds are not so thick. In some cases, a navicular fossa is found in the distal third.

These thick folds are mainly encountered in adult women and are smaller in children and the aged. During menstrual life cyclical changes take place in the urethral epithelium. During the follicular phase, there is desquamation; changes take place in the cells similar to those in the vagina at the same phase. In the progestational phase the epithelium becomes thicker with elongated cells and cell nest formation.

2. The subepithelial occlusion mechanism.

The subepithelial layer lies between the mucosa and the muscle of the urethral wall. In the proximal part of the urethra there is a complex venous plexus. There is believed to be a common haemodynamic mechanism in the urethra, cervix and anus.

The blood flow through the submucosa can be augmented by oestrogens and androgens. A deep and extensive coagulation of the bladder neck causes marked oedema of the submucosa, with later, marked scarring.

3. The occlusion mechanism of the urethral smooth muscle.

There is no doubt that the smooth muscle of the urethra itself is the most powerful agent in occlusion of the urethra. The arrangement of this muscle is described; the muscle fibres are arranged spirally, enclosing the whole urethra. At the cranial end, they are continuous with the muscle of the bladder. Outside the spiral layer, there is a layer of longitudinal muscle fibres also continuous with those of the bladder. Occlusion of the flow of urine is effected by contraction of these muscles and those of the bladder base. Atony of the muscles in this region or a prolapse of the bladder base, disturbs the mechanism of occlusion. In the menstrual cycle the muscle is more contractile during the follicular phase, with a decline in the secretory phase. Peri-urethral fixation is an important factor in facilitating the action of these muscles.

The powerful influence of the smooth muscle mechanism is recognized when operations are performed to raise the trigone and approximate the longitudinal muscle of the urethra. This operative procedure also affects the levator, the cervix and the bladder wall.

4. The occlusion mechanism of the levator ani muscle and its pelvic fascia.

A powerful and rapidly effective part of the whole occlusion mechanism is seen in the interlacing fibres of the various pelvic muscles. These muscle groups directly compress the urethra itself. In young women, the pubo-coccygeal component of the levator is directly related to the urethral muscle wall. The collagenous fibres of the urethral fascia blend directly with the fascia of the levator ani. Strengthening of the levator by remedial exercises may help cases of urinary incontinence. The "Perineo-meter" was invented to measure the compressive effect of the levator muscle. Operative elevation of the pelvic diaphragm may have a direct effect in curing urinary incontinence.

5. The occlusion mechanism of the deep transverse perineal muscle (or urogenital diaphragm).

Lateral to the urethra are found the transverse fibres of the deep perineal muscle. Horizontal sections through the urethra show these striated muscle fibres running transversely. Ventrally they are attached to the symphysis. In longitudinal sections it is also possible to show the interlacing fibres of the muscle. This "urogenital diaphragm" may be described as the "external sphincter of the urethra." Weakness of this muscle is rare as a cause of urinary incontinence unless the levator is also inefficient. Improvement of the tone of the transverse perineal muscle by exercises may help some cases of incontinence.

6. The occlusion mechanism of fixation by the bulbo-cavernosus muscle.

The bulbo-cavernosus, often called the vaginal sphincter, has the effect of compressing the distal urethra. It consists of striated muscle, running between the transverse perineal muscle and the levator ani. The corpora cavernosa of the clitoris and various para-urethral fixing tissues lie between the bulbo-cavernosus and the urethra itself. From the point of view of treatment, suturing or restoring the bulbo-cavernosus muscles has the effect of curing urinary incontinence. This is an essential part of the operation of colpo-perineorrhaphy or repair of episiotomy. Active interposition of the bulbo-cavernosus is also practised in the treatment of urinary incontinence.

7. The occlusion mechanism by fixation of the urethro-pubic structures to the symphysis.

The urethra is fixed most firmly to the back of the symphysis pubis, through the short strong, collagenous fibres of the urethro-pubic fascia. The arcuate ligament can normally bear a strain of one kilogramme. The bladder is also fixed by fascial attachments to the symphysis. In a case of prolapse the cranial urethra is detached from the symphysis, and incontinence of urine results. This is the basis of operations such as those of Marshall, Marchetti and others, designed to fix the urethra and bladder base to the symphysis by "retro-pubic suspension." Above the pelvic fascia and in front of and above the bladder neck, is the cave of Retzius which contains a fine mesh of elastic and muscle fibres, continuous with those of the pubo-vesical or pubo-cervical ligament.

8. The occlusion mechanism through fixation to the vulva.

The urethra is fixed to the vulva by interlacing fibres of fascial tissue, continuous with the erectile tissue of the corpora cavernosa and with the fascia of bulbo-cavernosus. Attempts have been made to treat incontinence of urine by advancing the urethra and attaching it to the clitoris.

9. The occlusion mechanism through attachment to the vagina.

There is a very close anatomical and functional relationship between the urethra and the vagina; the attachment is generally more firm in the caudal than in the cranial part of the urethra. In fact, the urethra appears to lie in the wall of the vagina in its upper one third. On examina-tion of the relationship between the urethra and the vagina, it is found that the lateral and dorsal fascia of the urethra blends with the anterior vaginal wall, and with the tissue lateral to the vagina. The tense attachment between the caudal part of the urethra and the vaginal wall is often described as the "urethro-vaginal sphincter." The muscle fibres found here act in antagonism to those of the deep transverse perineal muscle. The combination of these muscles has a powerful effect in closing the urethra. After childbirth, this urethro-vaginal attachment may become slack with the result that the transverse perineal muscle becomes much stronger in proportion. The tissue which binds the urethra to the vagina is described in many books as "fascia." In fact these tissues contain neither fascia nor striated muscle, but consist mainly of smooth muscle. There exists a difficulty in terminology, similar to that encountered in relation to the uterine ligaments. They are best described as "fixation fibres or the urogenital fixation layer."

During pregnancy the vagina increases not only in width, as is well known, but also in length. This process facilitates the passage of the child but leads to a looseness of the vaginal wall in the region of the urethra.

In the puerperium this active increase in size of the vagina is most in evidence. The labia are widely open, the vaginal introitus gapes and the vaginal wall is slack, giving the appearance of pseudo-urethrocoele and cysto-coele with marked looseness of the urethra and vagina. Epithelial proliferation occurs and this combined with a weakness of the fixing structures of the vagina, predisposes to incontinence of urine later in life.

10. The occlusion mechanism through fixation to the paravaginal tissues.

Above the attachment of the urethra to the anterior vaginal wall there is a large sheet of tissue running laterally and fixing the vagina to the lateral pelvic wall; this tissue consists mainly of smooth muscle. This muscle holds the urethra centrally above the anterior vaginal wall. Suture of this tissue is an important part of the cure of incontinence, especially when there is prolapse. It is then essential to restore the normal topography of the pelvic tissues.

11. The occlusion mechanism through fixation to the parametrium.

Through the anchoring of the cranial part of the urethra to the trigone of the bladder, there are tissues which attach it to the parametrium. These more laterally placed structures consist of relatively strong strands of fascia, connecting with the urethro-cervical fascia at the bladder neck. This ventral parametrium is often called the vesico-uterine ligament. This tissue has a powerful effect in elevating the base and neck of the bladder. Relaxation of this tissue may be associated with a small cystocele and ordinary incontinence. In more severe degrees of prolapse, as described by Donald and Fothergill, fixation of the lateral urethro-parametrial tissues is essential. Suture of the parametrial and paraurethral tissues has the effect of raising the uterus above the level of the levator ani and also of elevating the vaginal wall and urethra.

12. The occlusion effect of suture of the urethro-cervical and cervico-trigonal fixing tissues.

The arrangement of the fascia between the urethra and the cervix and between the cervix and the trigone of the bladder is described and illustrated. This is the tissue which is shortened and tightened in the Manchester operation by Donald and Fothergill. Normally there is a firm fascial layer between the bladder neck and the cervix. This fixation becomes loosened in pregnancy and may be torn by the foetal head descending forcibly against the pelvic wall. This will result in obliteration of the posterior urethral angle, as described by Jeffcoate and Roberts in cases of stress incontinence. When the angle is greater than 120 degrees, the occlusion mechanism of the bladder is disturbed and incontinence results.

The lateral X-ray, with the bladder outlined by radio-opaque material, is of value in showing the anatomical structure of the normal opening and closing mechanism of the bladder; posterior angulation of the urethra during micturition is all-important.

The histological grounds for this angulation are described. The intrinsic muscle of the urethra and bladder runs parallel with the urethro-cervical fixing layer. At rest, the intrinsic muscle and the fixing tissues work in opposition to each other. During micturition, the urethro-cervical fascia and the longitudinal and spiral muscles of the urethra are relaxed. These run parallel with the powerful levator ani, which holds the bladder base and neck in position in the true pelvis. If this is weakened, or if there is weakness of the smooth muscle of the fixing tissues, the normal topography of the urogenital apparatus is disturbed.

13. The occlusion mechanism through fixation to the bladder.

The attachment of the urethra to the bladder is closely connected with the vulva. At the cranial end of the urethra, the spiral and longitudinal muscles of the urethra are continuous with those of the bladder wall. The mean distance between the vulva and the bladder is a relatively good measure of the length of the urethra muscle. In prolapse, the length of the urethra is reduced and this in itself may be important in causing incontinence. During micturition, the urethra is shortened, and radiological studies show that the cranial part of the urethra is taken up into the bladder base.

This widening of the bladder neck resembles the taking up of the cervix and isthmus and the uterus during the first stage of labour. It necessitates a powerful fixation of the tissues in the paraurethium, and is made possible by the fibres which attach the urethra to the cave of Retzius and by the dorsal urethro-vaginal and urethro-cervical tissues. The upper part of the urethra thus controls the movements of the bladder in filling and emptying.

After childbirth and in first and second degree prolapse, this mechanism may become disturbed.

The operator, attempting to correct the condition must ensure proper fixation of the bladder within the true pelvis.

Good results may be obtained by a combination of abdominal and vaginal procedures.

Diagnostic Features

Urinary incontinence must not be considered as a single symptom, but as a complex picture demanding exact elucidation. The various structures responsible for closure of the urethra must be taken into account in the individual case. Incontinence may arise from a variety of factors, and these are important in deciding on the operation likely to prove must successful.

The mechanisms responsible for normal continence of urine are again outlined.

In the investigation of incontinence, clinical features such as the presence or absence of prolapse must be taken into account with the findings on radiographic examination, including cystography and urethrography. The bladder outline by radio-opaque material must be examined during straining and at rest. Accurate diagnosis of the functional and anatomical cause of incontinence enables the surgeon to choose among the various procedures described for its cure.

Summary of Treatment

In summing up the treatment, the object of restoring the normal shape, length and width of the urethra is stressed. Detailed knowledge of the anatomy of the urogenital apparatus is essential, and the supporting and fixing mechanism of the urethra is finally summed up and illustrated.

General Summary

1. The functional anatomy of the urethra and its various "fixing" tissues, the so-called "Paraurethrium" are described.

2. Various observations are made on the direct and indirect mechanisms of occlusion of the urinary flow.

3. The numerous possibilities of simple or combined disturbances of the occlusion mechanism that may be responsible for the single symptom of urinary incontinence are expounded in relation to their physiology and diagnosis.

4. The basis for the various conservative and operative methods of treatment is summed up from the point of view of the anatomy, functional aspects and pathogenesis of urinary incontinence.

Note: This article was adapted by the Editors with the permission of Professor Langreder from his article which appeared in *Zentralblatt für Gynäkologie*, 15 (1956).

1. HYPOTHALAMIC RELEASING FACTORS

MAY REED

Over the last 45 years evidence of control of the endocrine system—at least in part—by the higher centres of the brain, has slowly emerged. In 1920 Camus and Roussy found that atrophy of the genitalia had occurred in dogs where the hypothalamus had been damaged and Bailey and Bremer (1921) reported atrophy of the gonads and genitalia in dogs with lesions in the hypothalamus but whose pituitary glands were apparently unaffected. Hohlweg and Junkmann (1932) postulated a "sex centre" in the hypothalamus and suggested that the female sex cycle rhythm was dependent upon an anterior pituitary-hypothalamus relationship. Marshall and Verney (1936) showed that stimuli from the central nervous system could act upon the anterior pituitary and so effect ovulation in the rabbit and Harris (1937) postulated an hypothalamic control of the luteinizing hormone (LH) in this animal. Dempsey (1937) suggested that a periodic release of LH in the guinea-pig might be due to a rhythmic discharge from some part of the central nervous system. Later, in 1947, Green and Harris (on anatomical as well as physiological evidence) proposed a neurohumoral control mechanism

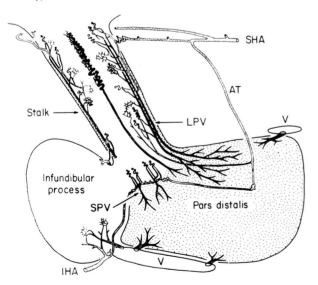

FIG. 1. Diagram of human pituitary gland, in the sagittal plane, showing the main features of its blood supply. Note in particular the long portal vessels (LPV) and the short portal vessels (SPV) which between them provide the sole blood supply to pars distalis. The artery of the trabecula (AT) runs through pars distalis without supplying the parenchymal cells. SHA, superior hypophysial artery; IHA, inferior hypophysial artery; V, venous sinus. *Neuroendocrinology*, **1**, 193–213 (1965–66). Observations on the portal circulation of the pituitary gland. J. H. Adams. P. M. Daniel and Marjorie M. L. Prichard.

of anterior pituitary function. In earlier work Popa and Fielding (1930, 1933) had described the hypothalamo-hypophysial portal vessels in the human and Wislocki and King (1936) had indicated that blood collected in a capillary network in the median eminence and was drained into vessels which pass down the pituitary stalk and thence into the sinusoids of the anterior lobe of the pituitary.

Experimental Evidence for Releasing Factors

Experimental evidence in support of the concept of a neurohumoral control of anterior pituitary function has been obtained from four main experimental procedures, viz. (i) Electrical stimulation of different areas of the brain, (ii) Stalk section, (iii) Lesions in various sites of the central nervous system and (iv) Transplantation of the anterior pituitary gland to some other part of the body. For reviews see Harris (1955), Benoit and Assenmacher (1955), Everett (1964), Adams, Daniel and Prichard (1966) and Reichlin (1966).

However, it must be borne in mind that some of the evidence is by no means conclusive. Whilst the results of experiments involving electrical stimulation and brain lesions indicate the involvement of a neuro-humoral mechanism, they could also indicate stimulation or interruption of a direct nervous pathway from the central nervous system to the anterior pituitary gland. Also the possibility of chemical effects of ions due to the passage of a current and the spread of current to adjacent areas should be taken into consideration. Stalk sectioning could affect formation and release of anterior pituitary hormones by damage to the blood supply of the gland as well as by interrupting the passage of releasing factors via the portal vessels. More positive evidence for a neuro-humoral control is provided by pituitary transplants to sites distant from the median eminence and the retransplantation studies.

Classical work by Smith (1926) and Smith and Engle (1927) indicated the important relationship between a functional anterior pituitary gland and a secreting ovary. Later workers (Westman and Jacobsohn, 1940; Harris and Jacobsohn, 1952; and Nikitovitch-Winer and Everett, 1958) have demonstrated that gonadotrophic activity is not maintained when the anterior pituitary is transplanted to a site remote from the sella turcica. Furthermore the gonadotrophic activity of the gland is dependent upon the integrity of the portal blood system enabling humoral stimuli from the hypothalamus to reach the gland cells.

Hypothalamic Releasing Factors

It is thought that releasing factors from the hypothalamic nerves pass into the capillary network of the median eminence and then into the portal vessels. As yet the mode of action of these factors is not clearly defined. They may effect the synthesis as well as the release of the trophic hormones. During the last few years interest has centred on the isolation and purification of the releasing factors. Activity has been found in extracts of stalk-median eminence tissue from a number of mammals including primates, bullocks, sheep, pigs, dogs, rabbits, rats and guinea-pigs. Extracts made from other parts of the brain have not proved to be active. Early work in the field includes that of corticotrophin releasing factor (CRF) activity by Guillemin and Rosenberg (1955) and Saffran and Schally (1955); luteinizing hormone releasing factor (LRF) by Campbell, Feuer and Harris in 1960 (see Harris, 1961) and McCann, Taleisnik and Friedman (1960), thyrotrophin releasing factor (TRF) by Schreiber, Rybák and Kmentová (1960) and Guillemin, Yamazaki, Jutisz and Sakiz (1962); follicular stimulating hormone releasing factor (FRF) by Igarashi and McCann (1964); somato-trophin releasing factor (SRF) by Pecile, Müller, Falconi and Martini (1965). Prolactin appears to have an inhibiting factor (PIF) as shown by Grosvenor, McCann and Nallar (1965). For reviews of hypothalamic releasing factors see Guillemin (1965) and Harris, Reed and Fawcett (1966).

Releasing factors are thought to be low molecular weight substances in minute concentration, and purification involves the processing of vast quantities of stalk-median eminence fragments in order to obtain sufficient material for identification. The chemical composition of the releasing factors is as yet not clear as none has been isolated pure. LRF and FRF appear to be separate entities (Schally and Bowers, 1964; Dhariwal, Nallar, Batt and McCann, 1965). Several workers have suggested that these factors are small basic peptides with a molecular weight of between 1,400 and 2,000 (Schally and Bowers, 1964; Dhariwal *et al.*, 1965 and Fawcett, Reed, Charlton and Harris, 1968). In a recent paper, however, Schally, Saito, Arimura, Sawano, Bowers, White and Cohen (1967) have expressed doubts about the peptide nature of LRF and FRF.

Physiological Evidence of Activity of Releasing Factors Concerned in Reproduction

In order to establish that a particular substance isolated from the median eminence and completely free from the relevant anterior pituitary hormone is a releasing factor, several criteria must be established. The factor must be shown to have a specific action in causing the release of the relevant trophic hormone from the gland into the peripheral circulation and under different physiological states of the animal the concentration of releasing factor in portal blood must be seen to vary with the degree of pituitary activation (e.g. an abrupt rise in LRF just prior to ovulation). As yet this has not been accomplished.

Crude and purified extracts from the hypothalamus have been tested for releasing factor activity by *in vivo* and *in vitro* methods. In the former an active factor, introduced into the test animal, acts upon the anterior pituitary tissue causing the release of the relevant trophic hormone into the circulation. Ideally the releasing factor should be applied directly to the anterior pituitary gland in the "normal" animal and the concentration of trophic hormone, released from the gland into the peripheral circulation, estimated chemically. To date suitable microchemical methods are not available and the anterior pituitary hormone liberated as a result of the action of the releasing factor can only be evaluated indirectly by its action upon the target organ in the test animal.

Fragments of anterior pituitary tissue can be incubated with the extract under test and after incubation both the incubation medium and the anterior pituitary tissue can be tested in the assay animal. In these *in vitro* methods the test substance is applied directly to the anterior pituitary tissue and, as in intrapituitary infusion (see later) a low concentration of the active substance should be effective in causing the release of the trophin. Results due to damage of the cell wall must be eliminated before estimating the changes in concentration of the anterior pituitary hormone in the incubation medium—since this could mask an action due to the releasing factor itself. However, once pure releasing factors are available it will be possible, by the use of suitable *in vitro* methods, to differentiate between the two mechanisms of action—that of effecting the release of the trophin from the pituitary tissue into the peripheral circulation, or that of effecting an increase in the formation of the trophin which would then lead to an increase in its release.

Luteinizing Hormone Releasing Factor
In vivo

Extracts believed to contain LRF have been introduced directly into the anterior pituitary tissue of oestrous rabbits, by infusion through a microcannula chronically implanted in the gland (see Campbell, Feuer and Harris, 1964 and Fawcett, Harris and Reed, 1965), and ovulation has been obtained. Similarly Nikitovitch-Winer (1962) evoked ovulation in the nembutal-blocked rat by infusing extracts of rat median eminence tissue. The advantages of this method are that small quantities produce an effect since the test substance is not diluted by the animal's blood, and the result of the test is based upon the physiological response of ovulation.

Other workers have used the ovarian ascorbic acid depletion test of Parlow (1958), a sensitive method of assessing the amount of LH released from the anterior pituitary after the intravenous introduction of an extract into the test animal (see McCann, Taleisnik and Friedman (1960) and McCann (1962)). These workers found that crude extracts of rat stalk-median eminence tissue, active in the intact animal, were inactive in hypophysectomized animals. Extracts of dorsal, lateral and posterior hypothalamus had little or no effect. Courrier, Guillemin, Jutisz, Sakiz and Aschheim (1961) showed that crude extracts of rat or sheep hypothalamus active in the Parlow test could also induce ovulation in the permanent oestrous rat but were inactive in the hypophysectomized rat. Active extracts of sheep hypothalamic tissue were effective in inducing ovulation in rats where hypothalamic lesions had inhibited the spontaneous cyclic release of LH (Schiavi, Justisz, Sakiz and Guillemin, 1963). In the ovariectomized adult rat, pretreated with oestrogens and progesterone to prevent the increase in circulating LH, which occurs after ovariectomy, Ramirez and McCann (1963) found a rise in LH activity in plasma within 10 mins. of an intravenous injection of rat stalk-median eminence tissue. Plasma of normal and ovariectomized rats, in which LH release had been blocked by lesions in the median eminence, showed a similar activity after injection of the extract.

In vitro

After two weeks' cultivation *in vitro* rat anterior pituitary tissue or single cells lose their gonadotrophic activity. The addition of crude extract of rat hypothalamic tissue to the culture medium at this time will cause an increase in gonadotrophins in both cells and culture medium, as assayed in the immature mouse uterine weight test. Hypothalamic tissue extracts themselves are not active in this test. Kobayashi (1965) showed that cells incubated with hypothalamic extracts had positive periodic acid-Schiff (PAS) staining whilst those incubated with cortical extracts had not—and there was an increase in the number of cytoplasmic granules in the cells. Autoradiographic studies with [3H] leucine added support to the concept that it is in the PAS positive cells that gonadotrophins are formed. The addition of hypothalamic extracts to the culture medium led to an increase in the uptake of [3H] leucine in the PAS positive cells but not in the acidophils or chromophobes—whilst in cells cultivated without the extract there was a significantly lower uptake in the PAS positive cells.

Follicular Stimulating Hormone Releasing Factor

Some evidence for a follicular stimulating hormone releasing factor (FRF) has been obtained from *in vivo* and *in vitro* experiments. In the former, plasma from donor rats injected with stalk-median eminence extracts had a significant effect in increasing ovarian and uterine weights in recipient immature mice (Igarashi, Nallar and McCann, 1964; Dhariwal, Nallar, Batt and McCann, 1965). The extracts themselves, or plasma from hypophysectomized rats injected with the extracts, were not effective. Hypothalamic extracts from ovariectomized female rats when added to the medium of adult female rat anterior pituitary cultures *in vitro* caused a significant release of FSH into the medium as assayed in the immature animal (Mittler and Meites, 1964).

Prolactin Inhibiting Factor

There is some evidence also of a prolactin inhibiting factor. The central nervous system appears to have a restraining action on the anterior pituitary secretion of prolactin. *In vivo* work in rats indicates that extracts of stalk median eminence tissue can prevent the usual reduction in the prolactin content of the anterior pituitary normally evoked by the action of suckling (Grosvenor, McCann and Nallar, 1965). Female rat anterior pituitary fragments incubated *in vitro* (Talwalker, Ratner and Meities, 1963) showed an increase in prolactin in the fragments and in the incubation medium—suggesting that the formation and release of the hormone was not depen-dent upon any influence from the hypothalamus. The addition of rat hypothalamic extracts to the incubation medium inhibited prolactin both in the medium and in the pituitary tissue. Extracts of cerebral cortex had no effect.

LRF as an Important Factor Concerned in the Mechanism of Ovulation

Since in the normal animal there is a delicate balance of circulating hormones, it is possible that CRF, TRF and SRF may play some minor role in reproduction, but as yet there is little evidence that this is so. A marked increase in the release of LRF probably occurs a few hours before ovulation, causing LH to be released from the anterior pituitary gland and rupture of the ripe ovarian follicle occurs—followed by the formation of a corpus luteum. The hypothesis of Moore and Price (1932) of a simple "feed-back" mechanism from gonads to anterior pituitary is no longer tenable. The concept of regulation of hormonal function by an increase or decrease in the concentrations of hormones circulating in the blood at certain times and at particular sites in the hypothalamus as well as in the anterior pituitary must be considered. Several workers have postulated two types of control of gonadotrophic function by neural elements in the hypothalamus: (i) a tonic control of basal formation and secretion of the hormones and (ii) a cyclic control of the release (principally of LH) just prior to ovulation (see Barraclough and Gorski, 1961, and Tejasen and Everett, 1967). Flerkó has suggested that neural elements in one area may respond to varying levels of sex hormones in the blood by a release regulating mechanism and a second "hypophyseotrophic area" (see Hálasz, Pupp and Ularik, 1962) may regulate the production and maintenance of a basal secretion of FSH and LH.

Studies in the guinea-pig indicate that there is probably a basal secretion of LH and FSH throughout most of the cycle but just before ovulation occurs an abrupt release of LRF may initiate a sudden rise in the concentration of LH circulating through the ovary. Of all the small laboratory mammals the guinea-pig most resembles the human in that it has a long cycle, ovulates spontaneously and has corpora lutea which actively secrete progesterone throughout most of the cycle—the level dropping a few days before the next ovulation is due. Ovulation can be induced in the guinea-pig by one single injection of LH (National Institutes of Health, Bethesda) before the animal shows anatomical oestrus (i.e. before the vagina begins to open) provided the ovaries contain ripe follicles. These are present at about 2-3 days before ovulation is due to occur. An injection of LH given in the middle of the anoestrous period has a destructive effect on the follicles and ovulation is not induced. Histological sections of the ovaries show degenerating follicles resembling those seen just after ovulation in the untreated animal (Plate I) (as also described in the monkey by Sturgis, 1961) and may be due to the action of LH on all the follicles which it cannot stimulate to rupture.

A single injection of LH at 5-6 days before ovulation is due does not cause rupture of the follicles but luteinization occurs and the ovum is entrapped—indicating that there is no increase in the level of LH even at this time late in the cycle in the untreated animal (Plate 2).

In the guinea-pig the basal secretion of FSH and LH throughout the cycle probably stimulates the growth and maturation of the follicles. A high level of progesterone

ovulation in the guinea-pig probably by preventing the release of LH but does not stop the follicles from maturing (Reed, 1966). Daily injections started just before oestrus fail to inhibit opening of the vagina but ovulation does not occur.

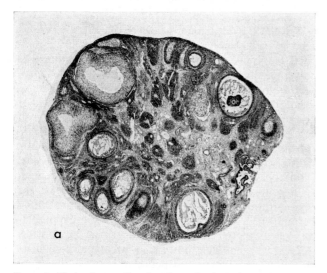

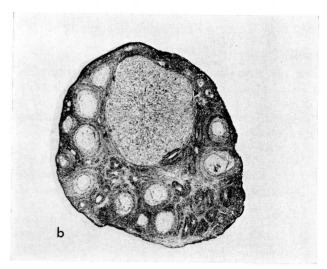

PLATE 1. Photomicrographs of sections of guinea-pig ovaries ×40. (a) Ovary of uninjected animal just after ovulation has occurred. Two ruptured follicles and some degenerating follicles. (b) Ovary of animal injected in the middle of the anoestrous period with LH (250 μg N.I.H.) and killed 48 hours later. All follicles are degenerating.

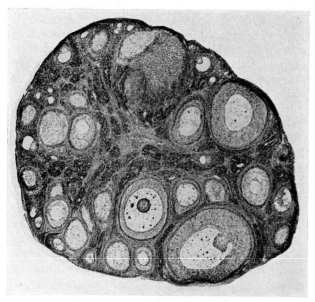

PLATE 2. Photomicrograph of section of guinea-pig ovary ×40. Ovary of animal injected at about 5 days before oestrus with LH (500 μg N.I.H.) and killed 48 hours later. Several luteinized follicles with extrapped ova.

secreted in the ovary does not prevent this maturation but there are indications that it is only when the circulating level of progesterone in the anterior pituitary and hypothalamus drops can ovulation occur—presumably by allowing the release of LH.

Studies with norethandrolone (Nilevar, Searle), a progestational steroid, add to the evidence that the release of LH is an abrupt mechanism. This steroid inhibits

The pituitaries of animals in which ovulation has been inhibited for some weeks contain gonadotrophins comparable in amount with those of untreated animals and homogenates of single anterior pituitaries from donor norethandrolone-inhibited pigs will induce ovulation when injected into recipient animals a day or two before oestrus (Plate 3). This suggests that the pituitaries of guinea-pigs, where ovulation has been inhibited, contain sufficient LH to induce ovulation but that norethandrolone has prevented its release.

Within a few days of stopping a course of daily injections of norethandrolone ovulation does occur—indicating that once the inhibition is removed the release of LH is made possible.

Inhibition of Ovulation

In the rabbit Hillard, Hayward, Croxatto and Sawyer (1966a) have shown that norethindrone injected subcutaneously 15–24 hrs. before mating prevents ovulation. The inhibition did not appear to be at the ovarian level since "subovulatory" amounts of LH injected intravenously activated ovarian progesterone output. Whilst intrapituitary or intraventricular infusions of median eminence extracts (1966b) induced ovulation in control animals they were ineffective in all animals pretreated with norethindrone—indicating an inhibition of LH release from sites in the anterior pituitary or median eminence.

Evidence from *in vitro* studies (Minaguchi and Meites, 1967) indicates that the antifertility action of Enavid in rats is mediated primarily through the hypothalamus although an action at the anterior pituitary level may also

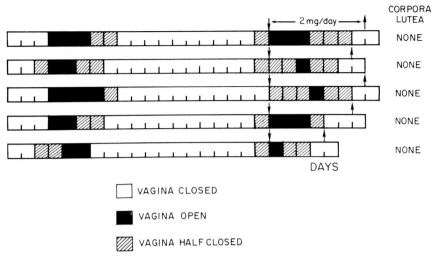

FIG. 2. Vaginal examinations of guinea-pigs. Each division represents one day. Norethandrolone (2 mg./day) injected just before oestrus and continued until the vagina closed. At autopsy there were no corpora lutea in the ovaries.

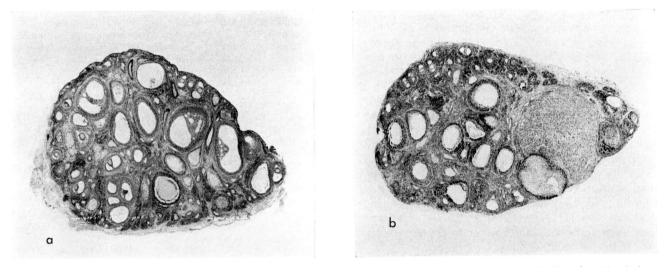

PLATE 3. Photomicrographs of guinea-pig ovaries × 40. (a) Ovary of animal where ovulation has been inhibited by daily injections of norethandrolone (2 mg./day/3 weeks, Nilevar, Searle). There are maturing follicles but no corpora lutea. (b) Ovary of recipient animal injected at about 3 days before oestrus with homogenate of anterior pituitary of guinea-pig where ovulation was inhibited (a). Freshly ruptured follicle is seen next to corpus luteum of present cycle.

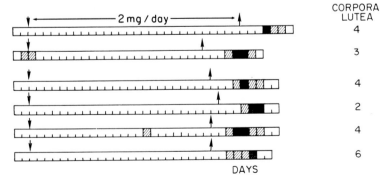

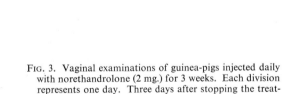

FIG. 3. Vaginal examinations of guinea-pigs injected daily with norethandrolone (2 mg.) for 3 weeks. Each division represents one day. Three days after stopping the treatment oestrus and ovulation occurred.

obtain. Hypothalamic extracts from adult female rats treated for twenty days with this steroid, when incubated with adult male rat pituitaries released significantly less LRF, FRF and PIF than extracts from control rats.

As yet little is known about the mechanisms whereby the various contraceptive drugs inhibit fertility (Diczfalusy, 1965, 1968). In women, preliminary studies with the long acting drug medroxyprogesterone acetate show that the mid-cycle peak of LH excretion, which normally occurs at about the time of ovulation, is abolished—indicating that this drug inhibits the release of LH (Mishell, 1967). The release of LH could be prevented at the hypothalamic level—where releasing factors might be "inactivated" or their formation restricted, or at the pituitary level where the release of LH from the gland could be inhibited. The formation of LH (if as it is believed releasing factors do affect the synthesis of trophins as well as their release) might also be prevented.

In contrast to rats where antigonadotrophic effects were observed (Holtkamp, Greslin, Root and Lerner, 1960) clomiphene citrate can cause ovulation in women. This may be because the clomiphene competes with natural oestrogens, which under certain circumstances can inhibit ovulation (Sturgis and Albright, 1940; Gual, Becerra, Rice-Wray and Goldzieher, 1967) and displaces it from binding sites in the pituitary and hypothalamus whence it is excreted in the urine—thus allowing the release of gonadotrophins (Kempers, Decker and Lee, 1967; Jones and de Moraes-Ruehsen, 1967). In the rat (Everett, 1947) there is evidence that oestrogen is concerned in the release of LH prior to ovulation. This could account for the opposite effects of clomiphene in women and rats—since in the work quoted above (Holtkamp et al., 1960) normal oestrous cycles were interrupted but the drug did not appear to have any effect upon the rat pituitary gonadotrophin content. This suggests that in the rat, clomiphene may have prevented the endogenous oestrogens from effecting the release of pituitary gonadotrophin.

Summary

Anatomical and experimental studies support the concept of a neurohumoral control of anterior pituitary function. Releasing factors are thought to pass from the hypothalamic nerves into the anterior pituitary gland via the portal blood vessels. Each factor is probably specific but as yet the mode of action is not clearly defined. In animals ovulation has been induced by purified extracts of LRF (Luteinizing Hormone Releasing Factor) and extracts of FRF (Follicle Stimulating Releasing Factor) have stimulated ovarian and uterine weight. Hormonal function is probably controlled by the varying concentrations of hormones circulating in the hypothalamus as well as in the anterior pituitary gland. Just before ovulation an abrupt release of LRF may initiate a sudden rise in the concentration of LH circulating through the ovary. In mammals with a sexual cycle there is evidence that LH can only be released when the level of progesterone in the hypothalamus as well as in the anterior pituitary drops to a low level. When final purification and synthesis of releasing factors is achieved in sufficient quantities for biological testing, the events leading to ovulation itself will be more clearly understood.

REFERENCES

Adams, J. H., Daniel, P. M. and Prichard, Marjorie M. L. (1965/1966), *Neuroendocrinology*, **1**, 193.

Bailey, P. and Bremer, F. (1921), *Arch. intern. Med.*, **28**, 773.

Barraclough, C. A. and Gorski, R. A. (1961), *Endocrinology*, **68**, 68.

Benoit, J. and Assenmacher, I. (1955), *J. Physiol. (Paris)*, **47**, 427.

Campbell, H. J., Feuer, G. and Harris, G. W. (1964), *J. Physiol. (Lond.)*, **170**, 474.

Camus, J. and Roussy, G. (1920), *Endocrinology*, **4**, 507.

Courrier, R., Guillemin, R., Jutisz, M., Sakiz, E. and Aschheim, P. (1961), *C.R. Acad. Sci. (Paris)*, **253**, 922.

Dempsey, E. W. (1937), *Amer. J. Physiol.*, **120**, 126.

Dhariwal, A. P. S., Nallar, R., Batt, M. and McCann, S. M. (1965), *Endocrinology*, **76**, 290.

Diczfalusy, E. (1965), *Brit. med. J.*, **2**, 1394.

Diczfalusy, E. (1968), *Amer. J. Obstet. Gynec.*, **100**, 136.

Everett, J. W. (1947), *Endocrinology*, **41**, 364.

Everett, J. W. (1964), *Physiol. Rev.*, **44**, 373.

Fawcett, C. P., Harris, G. W. and Reed, May (1965), *Proceedings of the 23rd International Congress of Physiological Sciences*, Tokyo, **4**, 300.

Fawcett, C. P., Reed, May, Charlton, H. M. and Harris, G. W. (1968), *Biochem. J.*, **106**, 229.

Flerkó, B. (1963), "Central Nervous System and the Secretion and Release of Luteinizing Hormone and Follicle Stimulating Hormone," in *Advances in Neuroendocrinology*, p. 211. Edited A. V. Nalbandov, University of Illinois Press.

Green, J. D. and Harris, G. W. (1947), *J. Endocr.*, **5**, 136.

Grosvenor, C. E., McCann, S. M. and Nallar, R. (1965), *Endocrinology*, **76**, 883.

Gual, C., Becerra, C., Rice-Wray, E. and Goldzieher, J. W. (1967), *Obstet. Gynec.*, **97**, 443.

Guillemin, R. (1964), *Recent Progress in Hormone Research*, **20**, 89.

Guillemin, R. and Rosenberg, B. (1955), *Endocrinology*, **57**, 599.

Guillemin, R., Yamazaki, E., Jutisz, M. and Sakiz, E. (1962), *C.R. Acad. Sci.*, (Paris), **255**, 1018.

Halász, B., Pupp, L. and Ularik, S. (1962), *J. Endocr.*, **25**, 147.

Harris, G. W. (1937), *Proc. roy. Soc. (Series B)*, **122**, 374.

Harris, G. W. (1955), *Neural Control of the Pituitary Gland*. Monographs of the Physiological Society, Edward Arnold (Publishers) Ltd.

Harris, G. W. (1961), "The Pituitary Stalk and Ovulation," in *Control of Ovulation*, p. 56. Edited C. A. Villee. Oxford: Pergamon Press.

Harris, G. W. and Jacobsohn, Dora (1952), *Proc. roy. Soc. (Series B)*, **139**, 263.

Harris, G. W., Reed, May and Fawcett, C. P. (1966), "Hypothalamic Releasing Factors," *Brit. med. Bull.*, **22**, 266.

Hilliard, J., Croxatto, H. B., Hayward, J. N. and Sawyer, C. H. (1966b), *Endocrinology*, **79**, 411.

Hilliard, J., Hayward, J. N., Croxatto, H. B. and Sawyer, C. H. (1966a), *Endocrinology*, **78**, 151.

Hohlweg, W. and Junkmann, K. (1932), *Klin. Wschr.*, **11**, 321.

Holtkamp, D. E., Greslin, J. G., Root, C. A. and Lerner, L. J. (1960), *Proc. Soc. exp. Biol.*, **105**, 197.

Igarashi, M. and McCann, S. M. (1964), *Endocrinology*, **74**, 446.

Igarashi, M., Nallar, R. and McCann, S. M. (1964), *Endocrinology*, **75**, 901.

Jones, Georgeanna, S. and de Moraes-Ruehsen, Maria, D. (1967), *Amer. J. Obstet. Gynec.*, **99**, 814.

Kempers, R. D., Decker, D. G. and Lee, R. A. (1967), *Obstet. Gynec.*, **30**, 699.

Kobayashi, T. (1965), *Proceedings of the 23rd International Congress of Physiological Sciences, Tokyo*, **4**, 306.

Marshall, F. H. A. and Verney, A. B. (1936), *J. Physiol. (Lond.)*, **86**, 327.

McCann, S. M. (1962), *Amer. J. Physiol.*, **202**, 395.

McCann, S. M., Taleisnik, S. and Friedman, H. M. (1960), *Proc. Soc. exp. Biol.*, **104**, 432.

Minaguchi, H. and Meites, J. (1967), *Endocrinology*, **81**, 826.

Mishell, D. R. Jr. (1967), *Amer. J. Obstet. Gynec.*, **99**, 86.

Mitler, J. C. and Meites, J. (1964), *Proc. Soc. exp. Biol.*, **117**, 309.

Moore, C. R. and Price, Dorothy (1932), *Amer. J. Anat.*, **50**, 13.

Nikitovich-Winer, Miroslava, B. (1962), *Endocrinology*, **70**, 350.

Nikitovich-Winer, Miroslava, B. and Everett, J. W. (1958), *Endocrinology*, **63**, 916.

Parlow, A. F. (1958), *Fed. Proc.*, **17**, 402.

Pecile, A., Müller, E., Falconi, G. and Martini, L. (1965), *Endocrinology*, **77**, 241.

Popa, G. and Fielding, Una (1930), *J. Anat.*, **65**, 88.

Popa, G. and Fielding, Una (1933), *J. Anat.*, **67**, 227.

Ramirez, V. D. and McCann, S. M. (1963), *Endocrinology*, **72**, 452.

Reed, May (1966), *J. Reprod. Fertil.*, **12**, 489.

Reichlin, S. (1966), *New Engl. J. Med.*, **275**, 600.

Saffran, M. and Schally, A. V. (1955), *Canad. J. Biochem.*, **33**, 408.

Schally, A. V. and Bowers, C. Y. (1964), *Endocrinology*, **75**, 608.

Schally, A. V., Saito, T., Arimura, A., Sawano, S., Bowers, C. Y., White, W. F. and Cohen, A. I. (1967), *Endocrinology*, **81**, 882.

Schiavi, R., Jutisz, M., Sakiz, E. and Guillemin, R. (1963), *Proc. Soc. exp. Biol.*, **114**, 426.

Schreiber, V., Rybák, M. and Kmentová, V. (1960), *Experientia*, **16**, 466.

Smith, P. E. (1926), *Anat. Rec.*, **32**, 221. (Abstract.)

Smith, P. E. and Engle, E. T. (1927), *Amer. J. Anat.*, **40**, 159.

Sturgis, S. H. (1961), "Factors Influencing Ovulation and Atresia of Ovarian Follicles," in *Control of Ovulation*, p. 213, edited C. A. Villee. Oxford: Pergamon Press.

Sturgis, S. H. and Albright, F. (1940), *Endocrinology*, **26**, 68.

Talwalker, P. K., Ratner, A. and Meites, J. (1963), *Amer. J. Physiol.*, **205**, 213.

Tejasen, T. and Everett, J. W. (1967), *Endocrinology*, **81**, 1387.

Westman, A. and Jacobsohn, D. (1940), *Acta path. microbiol. scand.*, **17**, 328.

Wislocki, G. B. and King, L. S. (1936), *Amer. J. Anat.*, **58**, 421.

2. HUMAN GONADOTROPHINS

A. C. CROOKE

INTRODUCTION

The milestones along the road to an understanding of hypothalamico adenohypophyseal gonadal relationships are incised with the names of Harvey Cushing, Herbert MacLean Evans, Philip Smith, Bernard Zondek, and more recently Geoffrey Harris, and their collaborators. In 1910 Crowe, Cushing and Homans first demonstrated atrophy of the reproductive organs after hypohysectomy in the dog and in 1921 Evans and Long reported excessive luteinization of the ovaries of normal rats by injection of crude anterior pituitary extracts.

In 1927 Smith showed that implantation of pituitary grafts into hypophysectomized rats repaired the gonadal atrophy and at about this time Zondek (1930) began to publish a series of papers on gonadotrophic substances culminating in the recognition of two separate factors, one obtained from the urine of menopausal women and the other from the urine of pregnant women. The former which they called prolan A stimulated the ovarian follicle and the latter which they called prolan B caused ovulation and luteinization. In 1931 Fevold, Hisaw and Leonard first showed with crude procedures that follicle stimulating hormone (FSH) and luteinizing hormone (LH) activities could be partially separated from one another in pituitary extracts and many others subsequently confirmed and extended this observation.

These terms FSH and LH have been criticized by many workers because they imply an activity in the ovary only whereas they are equally necessary for testicular function and many authorities prefer the term interstitial cell stimulating hormone (ICSH) for LH. The final chapter on the control of pituitary function by the hypothalamus has been subscribed to by many workers led by Harris. It remains for others to fill in the details.

The Hypothalamic Releasing Factors

The elaborate system of portal blood vessels which connect the hypothalamus with the anterior lobe of the pituitary gland through the infundibulum led to much speculation on the functional relationship between the hypothalamus and the anterior lobe. When the infundibulum is cut and the blood supply stopped there is only a brief interruption of the oestrus cycle in the rat. Harris (1950) showed that this is due to rapid repair but that if a plate is inserted between the cut ends of the infundibulum the cycle is halted for a prolonged period of time. Then it was found that extracts of hypothalamus, especially from the region of the median eminence contained substances which were capable of stimulating the pituitary to release gonadotrophins. These releasing factors (RF) have since been separated and are known as follicle stimulating hormone RF (FRF) and luteinizing hormone RF (LRF) respectively. They are apparently substances of relatively small molecular weights and are capable of releasing many times their weight of gonadotrophins (Schally, Saito, Arimura, Sawano, Bowers, White and Cohen, 1967). They are probably much less specific than the gonadotrophic hormones themselves and a number of other substances act as releasing factors at much higher dosages.

The factors which control the hypothalamus are not fully understood but there are many agents like light and warmth which, acting in different species, initiate the secretion of gonadotrophins. In women psychological stress is a potent inhibitor of sexual function. Abnormal loss of or gain in weight are others but the most important factors controlling the sexual cycle are the steroid hormones themselves. Thus an increase in the amount of circulating oestrogen will suppress the release of gonadotrophins while a reduction will stimulate it. This is the so called push-pull mechanism of control of the cycle. It is evidently a delicate mechanism and it is perhaps surprising that it is not more readily upset. A fuller knowledge about these activities awaits the development of more sensitive and specific assays for FSH and LH and of their releasing factors.

Human Gonadotrophins

The gonadotrophic hormones are relatively species specific and are often capable of inducing the formation of antibodies in other species. The interest of the clinician is therefore centred on human FSH and LH and on human chorionic gonadotrophin (HCG). FSH and LH are obtained from two sources: from human pituitary glands and from the urine of postmenopausal women (Human Menopausal Gonadotrophin—HMG). Large numbers of human pituitary glands obtained at autopsy are being collected in several centres. They are most easily preserved in 10 volumes of acetone which inhibits enzymic destruction of activity. The glands are then ground and the acetone dried powder can be stored indefinitely at 4°C. Several satisfactory methods of extraction have been described by different workers using preparations of very different potencies for clinical trials (see Butt, 1967). The Birmingham trials have depended on a preparation called CP1 which is of relatively high potency and reasonably constant from batch to batch. This material was chosen because of the need to make comparisons between different treatment schedules using similar preparations. Such pituitary preparations are not available commercially owing to the problems involved in the purchase of human glands. Commercial preparations are essentially dependent on the collection and extraction of great volumes of suitable urine.

Assay of Gonadotrophins

In the early clinical trials the dosages were expressed as mg. of crude preparations of unknown potency. At first workers generally relied upon the uterine weight assay in rodents but this is not specific and the results are strikingly influenced by the joint action of FSH and LH. The results therefore depended not only on the concentration of hormone present but also on the ratio FSH:LH. This unsatisfactory state of affairs was eventually overcome by the use of specific assays in which the extract was compared with a standard preparation. The majority of people now use the so-called augmentation assay of Steelman and Pohley (1953) in rats or of Brown (1955) in mice for FSH and the ovarian ascorbic acid depletion assay of Parlow (1958) for LH.

Several standards have been used in the past but most authorities now rely on the new international units (i.u.) of FSH and LH in a standard HMG. This is also described as the 2nd International Reference Preparation (IRP) of HMG—an unnecessary confusion once the i.u. have been accepted. HMG contains both FSH and LH and one ampoule of the new standard is defined as containing 40 i.u. FSH and 40 i.u. LH. The relative potencies of the different standards are given in Table 1 from Butt

TABLE 1
RELATIVE POTENCIES OF STANDARD PREPARATIONS OF GONADOTROPHINS

Designation	Assays for FSH (ovarian augmentation)		Assays for LH (OAAD method)	
	Equivalent amounts	i.u. per mg.	Equivalent amounts	i.u. per mg.
The International Standard 2nd IRP–HMG (Also working standard: Pergonal)	1 ampoule (40 i.u.)	(1) —	1 ampoule (40 i.u.)	(1) —
1st IRP–HMG Also HMG 24	280 mg.	0·14	80 mg.	0·5
NIH–FSH–S1 (2)	1·56 mg.	26	—	—
Armour 264–151X (3)	2·8–4·2 mg.	9·6–14·2	—	—
NIH–LH–S1	—	—	0·0264 mg.	1500
Armour 227–80	—	—	0·0264 mg.	1500

(1) The ampoule of the second IRP–HMG contains HMG and lactose (5 mg. of each).
(2) Some 5 mg. ampoules of this standard, packaged in 1959, have deteriorated and are no longer completely soluble in water.
(3) This standard has been variously estimated to be 37–55 per cent of NIH–FSH–S1.
(Butt (1967), *The Chemistry of the Gonadotrophins*, p. 16, American Lecture Series. Charles C. Thomas, Springfield, Ill.).

(1967) but owing to the joint action of FSH and LH in the uterine weight assay it is never right to express the results of this assay in i.u.

Extraction, Purification and Analysis of Gonadotrophins

Much has been written about different methods of extraction of gonadotrophins from urine. The method in most general use depends on adsorption on kaolin and purification by ion exchange chromatography on Permutit. Some separation of FSH and LH can then be effected by chromatography on CM cellulose and DEAE cellulose and gel filtration on Sephadex G100. Basically similar methods have been used for the extraction of pituitary gonadotrophins and several methods have been described which yield preparations of FSH and LH which are essentially free from each other and from other contaminants (see Butt, 1967). They are all glycoproteins. FSH stored in a medium of low ionic strength consists of a mixture of species of different molecular weights of about 17,000, 34,000 and 68,000 respectively based on their behaviour on various gel filtration media. These species are interconvertible by changing the ionic strength of the medium with no loss of biological activity, the monomer being predominant at high ionic strength and the dimer and tetramer at low ionic strength (Gray, 1967). The component analyses of both FSH and LH have been reported (see Butt, 1967). FSH contains about 21 per cent carbohydrate and structural studies are now in progress. These indicate that there are three different carbohydrate chains having N-acetyl neuraminic acid (NANA), fucose and galactose respectively at their termini. NANA is essential for biological activity but galactose can be removed completely without loss of activity (Butt, Jenkins and Somers, 1967). Amino-acid degradation by the method of Edman reveals no N-terminal amino-acid (Gray, 1968). It is probable that there is a single amino-acid chain since there is only one cysteine residue per molecular weight of 17,000.

The effects of various other chemical reactions on the biological activity have been investigated and it is evident that different groups in the molecule are concerned with biological and with immunological responses (see Butt, 1967).

Immunology of Gonadotrophins

There has been a great deal of work done on the immunology of gonadotrophins starting with the so called-anti-hormones of Zondek, of H. M. Evans and of Collip and their co-workers. These were thought to be specific substances which balanced the activities of the hormones affecting a mechanism of control. Later they were recognized as true antibodies but they often form antigen-antibody complexes which precipitate with some difficulty. The biggest problem, however, has been their tendency to cross react with other gonadotrophins of the same species. Thus antibodies to HCG cross react with LH and vice versa and antibodies to both cross react with HMG. Antibodies to very highly purified FSH also cross react with LH and HCG, although very occasionally it has been found that a guinea-pig or rabbit has formed specific antibodies to FSH (Midgley, 1967; Faiman and Ryan, 1967). These rare antisera are of great value.

The haemagglutination inhibition method has been used extensively for measuring urinary HCG but notoriously it gives much higher readings than are obtained by bioassay during the second and third trimesters of pregnancy evidently because of cross reactions with proteins closely related to HCG. The radioimmunoassay method using ^{131}I labelled HCG as antigen is now being used for the measurement of LH in urine and, in general, radioimmunoassay seems to offer the best hope for the future but the same problems of cross reactions apply to this as to the other immunological methods.

Cross reactions must indicate that identical immunoreceptor sites occur on each of these hormones. It is of great interest therefore that with the complement fixation method there is no cross reaction between antiserum to FSH and LH or HCG (Butt, 1967). This is believed to indicate a difference in spatial configuration of the proteins which disregards the similarity of immunoreceptor sites. It is in keeping with some of the known chemical characteristics of the hormones. Cysteine and proline are considerably higher in LH than in FSH indicating a high degree of cross linking with little or no α-helix formation in the configuration of the former compared with the latter. Unfortunately this technique is not sensitive enough for use in body fluids.

Gonadotrophins in Body Fluids

Nearly all the data on gonadotrophins in body fluids are derived from excretion in urine since only recently have sensitive enough methods become available for blood. Moreover most of the data on urinary excretion are based on the mouse uterine weight assay which is unsatisfactory because the response is sensitive to the joint action of FSH and LH. With this method it is difficult to demonstrate much change during the normal menstrual cycle. Using specific assays for FSH and LH, however, Stevens (1967) has shown striking changes. FSH is high at the beginning and then falls steadily towards the end of the cycle while LH is high at mid cycle, presumably in association with ovulation (Fig. 1). There is, however, great variation between patients and between cycles in the same patient. These changes serve to emphasize the fact that isolated estimations of either gonadotrophin taken at random, which are commonly requested by the clinician, can have little meaning. Indeed the widest fluctuations often occur in patients with irregular or infrequent menstruation and anovular cycles and they are sometimes observed in women with quite prolonged amenorrhoea shortly before spontaneous resumption of normal menstruation. An isolated high reading for FSH or LH within the menopausal range should not be taken as an indication that the patient will not respond to treatment with gonadotrophins but a series of sustained high readings is evidence of failure at the ovarian level. Patients showing such findings are unsuitable for treatment and it is not unusual to observe women change from the former to the latter in the course of a year or two while under observation. From an endocrinological point of view therefore the determination of gonadotrophins is the most important investigation for deciding on the suitability of a patient for treatment with gonadotrophins.

The estimation of HCG by the haemagglutination inhibition method has a great advantage in speed and cost over bioassays and this has led to its increasing use in spite of the much higher readings which it gives during the second and third trimesters. Excretion normally reaches a peak at about the tenth week of pregnancy and then falls to about a quarter of this value which it maintains throughout the rest of pregnancy (Fig. 2). A fall before the time of peak excretion or an abnormally rapid fall at the time when a fall is normally expected is commonly a warning of impending abortion. Since there is a great variation in peak values from patient to patient, however, serial estimations are imperative for prognosis. Estimations during the second and third trimesters of pregnancy appear to have little clinical value.

Clinical Effects of Gonadotrophins

Engle showed in 1938 that follicular growth and rupture could be caused in primates by gonadotrophins from pregnant mare's serum (PMS) followed by HCG, the former having mainly FSH activity and the latter luteinizing activity. Many attempts have since been made to utilize these substances to induce ovulation in the human but it is commonly considered that they are ineffective partly because gonadotrophins are thought to be species

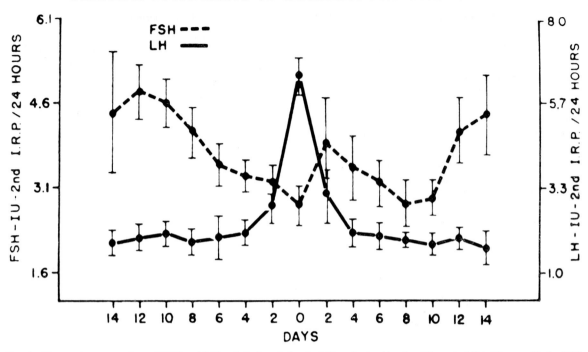

FIG. 1. Mean urinary excretion of FSH and LH activity in relation to LH peak at midcycle. (Mean ± S.E.) (Stevens, V. S., 1967, *In Recent Research on Gonadotrophins*, p. 227, Livingstone, Edinburgh and London).

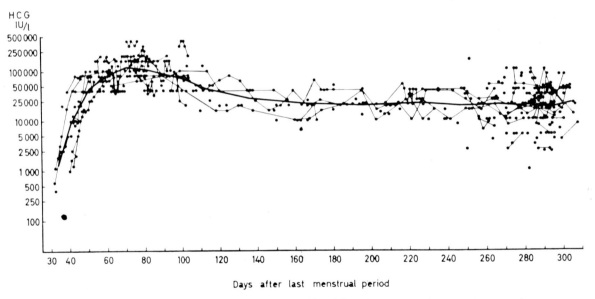

FIG. 2. Immunological HCG activity in 522 first morning urines collected from 240 women with normal pregnancies. The heavy line represents the mean values. (Wide, L., 1962, *Acta endocr.*, (Kbh.) Suppl. **70**, p. 81).

specific and partly because of their well authenticated activity as antigens. It is clear from perusal of the literature, however, that PMS followed by HCG does induce ovulation in the human and may indeed produce excessive responses which have on occasions proved fatal (Béclere, 1960; Matsumoto and Tohma, 1965). Experience with human FSH and HCG suggests that one reason why PMS has failed to become recognized as an effective agent for inducing ovulation in the human is that it has never been used systematically in planned experiments. Human gonadotrophins, however, have little tendency to induce

the formation of antibodies in the human and are obviously preferable.

There is now a considerable literature on the clinical response to human gonadotrophins (Crooke and Gemzell, 1968). The parameters used to assess the response and the dosage schedules have varied widely between different groups of workers. Gemzell, Diczfalusy and Tillinger (1958) who initiated this form of treatment relied on a collection of data including ovarian palpation or inspection by culdoscopy, vaginal cytology, endometrial biopsy and the estimation of oestrogens and pregnanediol in urine, the final evidence of ovulation of course being pregnancy. Several other groups led by Lunenfeld (Rabau, David, Serr, Mashiach, Lunenfeld and Gan, 1967) while using some of these parameters have relied mainly on the fern test. The Birmingham group have depended on the estimation of oestriol and pregnanediol in selected samples of urine (Crooke, Butt, Palmer, Morris, Edwards and Anson, 1963), while the Australian workers have used a new rapid but less specific method for measuring total oestrogens (Townsend, Brown, Johnstone, Adey, Evans and Taft, 1966; Shearman, 1966).

There has been a considerable controversy about the merits of these different parameters which is far from resolved. Those who rely mainly on vaginal cytology or the fern test consider that steroid analyses are too costly and too slow while those who rely on steroid analyses believe that the simpler methods are not sufficiently quantitative. The problem may be solved by a National Trial now being undertaken in Britain under the auspices of the Medical Research Council in which these different parameters are being compared.

In their original trials Gemzell, *et al.*, (1958) gave a constant daily dose of FSH for ten days. This was followed by 6,000 i.u. HCG daily for a further four days and they have varied little from this regime since. At an early stage they encountered patients who developed symptoms of severe overdosage and in consequence they restricted their dosage to a low range by comparison with that used by other workers. This appears to have reduced the incidence of severe symptoms but not of multiple pregnancies which continue to occur in about 50 per cent of the patients who conceive (Gemzell and Roos, 1966).

Lunenfeld, Rabau, Sulimovici and Eshkol (1963) developed a different system of treatment using a commercial preparation of HMG. They varied the daily dose and length of treatment according to their daily clinical findings. They commonly started with a single ampoule of HMG increasing to two and if necessary to three ampoules daily until they got evidence of a response. They then reduced the number of ampoules and added HCG for another day or two and finally gave HCG alone for the last day or two of treatment. This very flexible system resulted in a large number of pregnancies but there were excessive responses with severe symptoms in a considerable number of patients. Basically similar methods of treatment with minor modifications have been used by most other workers (Vande Wiele and Turksoy, 1965; Townsend, *et al.*, 1966; Shearman, 1966; Pasetto and Montanino, 1967; Bettendorf, Breckwoldt, Czygan and Groot, 1967; Taymor, Sturgis, Goldstein and Liberman, 1967).

Shearman (1968) (Personal communication) claims that using Brown's rapid method for determining the excretion of total oestrogens which gives a result on the same day has led to greatly increased control of dosage of FSH. He now gives only a single injection of HCG after FSH and if the excretion of oestrogens doubles from one day to the next he omits treatment with HCG altogether. He claims that this avoids severe symptoms of overdosage. An analysis of results obtained with this modification of treatment will be interesting.

It is apparent from the literature that at the same daily dose there is a possibility that a patient will respond excessively, normally or not at all. This is the justification for varying the dose from day to day or extending the length of treatment according to the daily clinical response. It leaves numerous questions unanswered, however, since there are many variables in treatment. The most important of these is the variation between patients but other factors are differences in dose and length of treatment with FSH, differences in preparations of FSH especially in the amount of LH with which they are contaminated, differences in dose, numbers of injections and timing of treatment with HCG and reproducibility of response from month to month. The Birmingham group have systematically examined these variables in a series of experiments of factorial design and gradually eliminated the less important ones (Crooke, *et al.*, 1963; Crooke, Butt, Palmer, Bertrand, Carrington, Edwards and Anson, 1964; Crooke, Butt and Bertrand, 1966(a), (b); Crooke, Butt, Bertrand and Morris, 1967(a), (b)). The parameters used were the estimation of oestriol (Brown, 1955; Palmer, 1964) and pregnanediol (Klopper, Michie

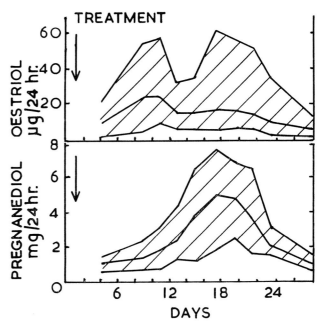

FIG. 3. Mean, maximum and minimum figures (shaded) for excretion of oestriol and pregnanediol by healthy women. The figures are adjusted for menstruation beginning on day 24. (Crooke, A. C. 1967). In *Modern Trends in Endocrinology*, 3, p. 115, Butterworths, London).

and Brown, 1955). The same methods have been used throughout in order that the results of one experiment can be compared with another. It appears that the more recent rapid methods have many advantages but they do not measure the same substances.

The excretion of oestriol and of pregnanediol by normal healthy women is shown in Fig. 3. This has been adjusted for menstruation starting on day 25 since this is the day on which menstruation occurred most commonly after starting treatment with FSH on day 1. Here the *mid cycle peak* in excretion of oestriol occurs on days 10 to 12.

This is followed by a fall and then often a secondary rise to a peak on about day 18. Pregnanediol rises when the oestriol falls and also reaches a peak on about day 18. Then both fall to control levels again before the end of the month. The initial rise of oestriol to the *mid cycle peak* is presumably caused by secretion of oestrogen by the leading follicle. The subsequent fall presumably results from rupture of this follicle and the simultaneous rise of pregnanediol is evidence of its conversion to a corpus luteum producing progesterone. The secondary rise in excretion of oestriol in association with the rise of pregnanediol is more puzzling. The suggestion that it is also derived from the corpus luteum is not convincing since it does not occur constantly and does not always reach a peak on the same day. It is more likely to be derived from secondary follicles which may not rupture.

Treatment with gonadotrophins may produce a similar normal steroid pattern or it may produce certain rather characteristic qualitative and quantitative variations from it. Figure 4A shows a qualitatively similar but quantitatively very exaggerated response in excretion of oestriol and pregnanediol in a patient treated with a succesion of decreasing doses of FSH followed by HCG. There is a *mid cycle peak* of oestriol at the same time as in the control in Fig. 3. It is followed by a fall which coincides with the rise of pregnanediol. Then there is a

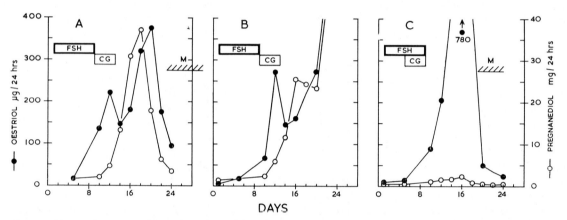

FIG. 4. Abnormal patterns of excretion of oestriol and pregnanediol after treatment with FSH and HCG. (a) Multiple ovulation; (b) multiple ovulation with pregnancy; (c) multiple follicular development without ovulation. M = menstruation. (Crooke, A. C., 1967. *In Modern Trends in Endocrinology*, 3, p. 116, Butterworths, London, and *Proc. R. Soc. Med.*, 1964, 57, p. 113).

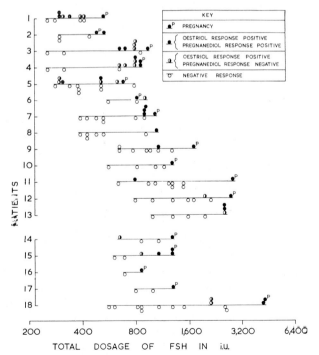

FIG. 5. Positive and negative responses to different dosages of FSH in thirteen patients with secondary amenorrhoea (numbers 1 to 13) and five patients with anovular cycles (numbers 14 to 18). (Crooke *et al*, 1966, *Acta endocr.*, (Kbh.) Suppl., p. 7).

secondary rise of oestriol to a peak at about day 18 when the peak in pregnanediol also occurs and finally both steroids fall to control levels. The patient subsequently menstruated. Figure 4B shows an almost identical response in the same patient given the same total amount of FSH but in equal daily doses and followed by the same dose of HCG as before. Her steroid pattern is remarkably similar except that both oestriol and pregnanediol show a continuous rise to the end of the month. She failed to menstruate and was pregnant and she subsequently gave birth to twins. Pregnancy can thus be diagnosed before the end of the first month. These two patterns form an interesting contrast with the one seen in Fig. 4C from another patient. This shows a qualitatively and quantitatively abnormal response. There is a greatly exaggerated rise in excretion of oestriol to a peak on about day 18 without a break at mid cycle and with no corresponding rise in pregnanediol. This pattern can occur with unsuitable treatment and is characteristic of the development of multiple follicles without ovulation. It has been confirmed by laparotomy.

These qualitatively abnormal patterns must always be taken into consideration although the variables in treatment were investigated initially by their quantitative effects only. In the early experiments allowance had to be made for differences between patients while less complex variables were examined first. One of these was differences between preparations of FSH. It appeared that too highly purified FSH or too much contamination with LH was undesirable but there seemed to be considerable latitude in between, and preparations of pituitary FSH and of HMG with only moderate differences in the ratio of FSH to LH gave essentially similar results.

Variation in the number of injections of FSH proved to be of considerable importance not only in saving expensive material but, more important, in the light thrown on the physiology of ovarian stimulation. It has been found that a given dose is twice as effective in a single injection as it is when divided into eight equal daily injections.

Variation between patients presents a difficult problem. Figure 5 shows the responses of 18 patients to different doses of FSH with positive responses marked above each line and negative responses below. The positive responses are subdivided into those with an increase in oestriol excretion only representing the development of follicles without ovulation, those with an increase in oestriol and pregnanediol representing ovulation, and those in which a response was followed by pregnancy. The first 13 patients had prolonged secondary amenorrhoea and the remaining five had anovular cycles (Crooke, et al., 1966(a)).

It is obvious from a glance at the figure that there is a wide difference in sensitivity to FSH between patients in both groups. Subsequent experience has confirmed this and shown that the range is even greater, several patients having never responded until a dose of 8,000 i.u. was reached while several others have become pregnant following a dose of only 500 i.u.—a sixteenfold range. It is also obvious that in general negative responses recurred at the lower doses, positive responses at the higher ones and pregnancy after the highest dose.

Many instances have been reported of patients developing severe symptoms with an excessive reponse to FSH and many authorities seemed to regard them as frequently unavoidable. In order to minimize such risks it is necessary to establish a dose-response relationship but methods normally employed for bioassays are unsuitable because of the great variation in sensitivity between patients. In order to overcome this difficulty the ED 50 was estimated for each patient by a standard technique—the ED 50 being that dose which, if repeated many times, would be expected to give a positive response 50 per cent and a negative response 50 per cent of the times it was given. Each dose given to each patient was then expressed as a percentage of that patient's ED 50. Since the ED 50's of the two groups of patients were not significantly different from one another all ED 50's were superimposed and all doses given to all patients plotted on the same graph. This is shown in Fig. 6 where the ED 50 is expressed as 100 and all positive responses are recorded above the upper line and all negative ones below the lower line. With these data it is possible to calculate a dose-probability of response relationship and this is shown as a curved line on the graph. It is clear that for any patient a dose of twice her ED 50 is likely to produce a positive response in more than nine in ten treatments.

In Fig. 7 the probabilities of different types of response are shown. Line A is the same as that in Fig. 6 and represents the probability of all responses. Line B represents the probability of responses with ovulation, line C with pregnancy and line D with symptoms of an excessive response. Each line was drawn by making the area under it proportional to the number of patients in the corresponding category. In this instance there were only three patients

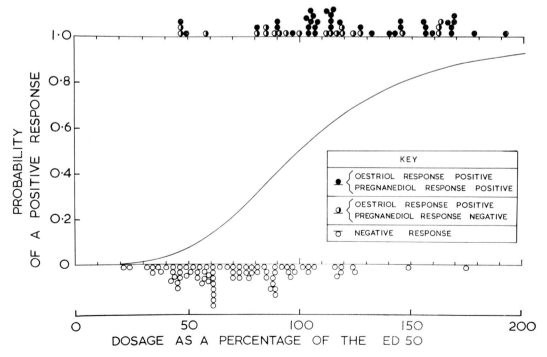

FIG. 6. Positive and negative responses of the eighteen patients at dosages expressed as percentages of each patient's ED 50, and the resulting dose-response line. (*Ibidem*, p. 11).

with symptoms of excessive response in 140 treatments so that it was considered that this estimate could only be very approximate. It has been supported by subsequent experience, however, since there have now been six cases in over 600 treatments or about one per cent. If line D in Fig. 7 is a fair estimate of the probability of an excessive response occurring at different doses then it is apparent

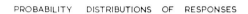

PROBABILITY   DISTRIBUTIONS   OF   RESPONSES

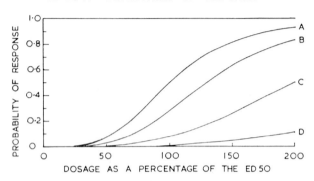

FIG. 7. Probability distributions of responses. A, probability of a positive response; B, of ovulation; C, of pregnancy and D, of hyperstimulation syndrome. The areas under curves between 0 and 200 are proportional to the number of responses of each type. (Crooke, A. C. (1967), In *Recent Research on Gonadotrophins*, p. 281, Livingstone, Edinburgh and London).

that at a dose of 200 per cent or twice a patient's ED 50 the probability is about ten per cent. This dose, therefore, is getting dangerously high.

The method of treatment used in Birmingham to reduce the risk of an excessive response is simple and economical. It consists of giving three equal injections of FSH on days, 1, 4 and 8 followed by 4,000 i.u. HCG on day 10. The practice of giving the whole dose of FSH in a single injection on day 1 followed by HCG on day 10 was abandoned since the peak of excretion of oestrogen was considerably earlier and the pregnancy rate was reduced to a half of the previous rate (Crooke and Bertrand, 1968). Treatment is begun with a dose of 500 i.u. FSH and this dose is increased by a factor of about 30 per cent each month until a positive response is obtained. The dosage schedule is given in Table 2. In the middle is the treatment schedule used with three equal doses of FSH given on days 1, 4 and 8. The equivalent total dosage in three injections is 1·5 times greater than the total dosage given as a single injection, for reasons given on page 501. On the right is the corresponding schedule for commercial preparations of HMG, in ampoules of 75 i.u. each and given on the same days. This treatment with FSH is followed by 4,000 i.u. HCG given on day 10.

Dr. John Marshall (personal communication) working at the National Institutes of Health, Bethesda, and using different patients, different parameters and different preparations of FSH, namely commercial preparations of HMG, has obtained a dose response relationship

TABLE 2

DOSAGE SCHEDULE FOR TREATMENT WITH FSH

Single injections Total dosage as FSH i.u.	Triple injections			
	as FSH i.u.		as FHS i.u.	
	Split	Total	Split	Total
350	3 × 175	525	3, 2, 2	7
500	3 × 250	750	4, 3, 3	10
650	3 × 325	975	5, 4, 4	13
850	3 × 425	1275	6, 6, 5	17
1100	3 × 550	1650	8, 7, 7	22
1400	3 × 700	2100	10, 9, 9	28

which is almost identical with that of the Birmingham workers. He relies on purely clinical findings for assessing the response but uses the same system of treatment described above. Full details however have not yet appeared in print.

A positive response is one in which the excretion of oestriol at mid cycle rises 15 μg. per 24 hours above the control level on day 1 regardless of changes in excretion of pregnanediol. Ovulation is judged to have occurred

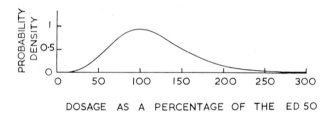

FIG. 8. The estimated distributions about the ED 50 of effective test dosages, with dosage increments of 50 per cent. (Crooke *et al.* 1966. *Acta endocr.* (Kbh.) Suppl. 111, p. 14).

when the excretion of pregnanediol on day 18 is 1 mg. more than twice the control level of pregnanediol on day 1. These criteria are based on data from months in which pregnancies occurred. It will be observed that with this notation the control 24 hour sample of urine is collected from zero to day 1 and treatment is given on day 1 when this collection is completed. HCG is given nine days later, that is on day 10 and the mid cycle peak in excretion of oestriol is typically found in one of three 48 hour samples of urine completed on days 8, 10 and 12. Further 24 hour samples of urine are collected on day 18 for pregnanediol and on day 29, which is day 1 of the next cycle if conception has not occurred.

The first dose of FSH at which a patient gives a positive response will not necessarily be identical with that patient's ED 50. It is possible, however, to calculate the probability of the first positive response occurring at various doses of FSH in terms of the ED 50. This is shown in Fig. 8 for doses increasing by a factor of 50 per cent each month. From this it can be seen that there is a probability of about six per cent that a patient will not have a positive response until she has been given a dose of twice her ED 50. But in Fig. 7 it was shown that the probability of a patient developing symptoms of an excessive response at a dose of twice her ED 50 was about ten per cent. Taking these data together it seems that this dosage schedule does not involve an unreasonable risk. If pregnancy fails to occur after the first positive response subsequent dosages must be judged by the magnitude of that response. An increase is only justified if the next response at the same dose level is negative. It now remains to be seen whether a simpler method of assessing a positive response can be relied upon.

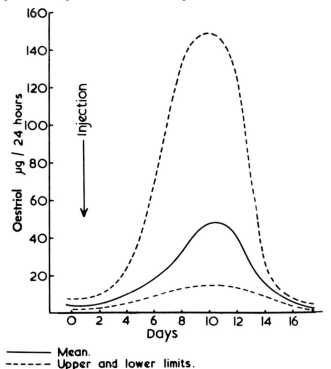

—— Mean.
------ Upper and lower limits.

FIG. 9. The average excretion of oestriol following injection of effective dose of FSH and 12,000 i.u. HCG in eighteen patients with secondary amenorrhoea. (Butt, W. R., 1967. *The Chemistry of the Gonadotrophins*, p. 5, American Lecture Series. C. C. Thomas, Springfield, Ill.)

This form of treatment is in striking contrast to that used by most other workers and described earlier in this chapter. Their method of giving daily injections of FSH and adjusting the dose according to the daily clinical response would seem to be the rational approach but it overlooks the fact that the excretion of oestriol continues to increase for up to ten days after an effective dose has been given. This is shown in Fig. 9 where the daily excretion of oestriol by a group of 18 patients with secondary amenorrhoea is plotted after a single effective dose of FSH given with HCG (Butt, 1967). The explanation is not clear but the FSH itself is excreted rapidly and cleared from the urine in about three days. This is shown in Fig. 10 (Morell, Crooke and Butt, 1968) which bears a resemblance to the excretion of FSH in the normal menstrual cycle shown in Fig. 1. It suggests that a follicle once stimulated to grow beyond a certain point continues to grow spontaneously. It may explain why FSH is more

effective when given as a single injection than when it is divided into eight or ten equal daily injections. It also sheds doubt on the validity of altering the daily dose of FSH in accordance with the daily clinical response and suggests that increasing the dose at intervals of less than a week or ten days would be dangerous.

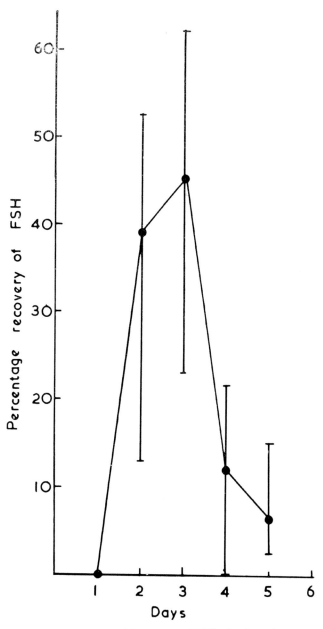

FIG. 10. Percentage daily recovery of FSH in 5 patients given FSH on day 1. ● represents mean daily recovery I represents range of daily recovery. (Morell *et al*, 1968 *J. Endocr.*) **41**. 571.

The results of treatment of the whole group of patients in Birmingham are awaiting analysis but, of the smaller group illustrated in Fig. 5, 16 out of 18 became pregnant. One of the two who failed to conceive gave up because of dysmenorrhoea after the first effective course of treatment and the other because she adopted a baby. This high pregnancy rate with FSH has fallen since the introduction of clomiphene (Greenblatt, Barfield, Jungck and Ray, 1961). All patients are now given an extensive trial with this drug before starting treatment with gonadotrophins. Those who are eventually given gonadotrophins seem to be more difficult to treat and tend to require higher doses of FSH. Nevertheless a considerable number who fail to respond to clomiphene eventually respond to gonadotrophins.

A group of 36 patients in Birmingham have had both kinds of treatment at different times and the results are shown in Table 3 (Tsapoulis and Crooke, 1968). Six of the 36 patients were given FSH first and the other 30

severe symptoms compared with one in the six which have occurred in Birmingham.

Symptoms associated with an excessive response to treatment with gonadotrophins have been called the *"hyperstimulation syndrome"* by Gemzell, Diczfalusy and Tillinger (1960), Pasetto and Montanino (1964), Buxton and Herrmann (1964) and Mozes, Bogokowski, Antebi, Lunenfeld, Rabau, Serr, David and Salomy (1965). About two weeks after beginning treatment patients complain of lower abdominal pain, vomiting and often diarrhoea with swelling of the abdomen and on physical examination the ovaries are greatly enlarged and cystic.

TABLE 3

RESPONSE OF PATIENTS TO CLOMIPHENE AND TO FSH/HCG

	No. of patients	No. responding		No. of cycles		Average minimum effective dose	
		Clomid	FSH	Clomid	FSH	Clomid	FSH
Primary amenorrhoea	4	0	0	12	30	—	—
Premature menopause	3	0	0	10	14	—	—
Secondary amenorrhoea	15	2	14	54	106	100	2750 i.u. (860–8000)
Anovular menstruation	8	6	8	29	50	150	940 i.u. (500–2200)
Stein–Leventhal syndrome Secondary amenorrhoea	2	1	2	10	18	200	4225 i.u. (3750–4750)
Stein–Leventhal syndrome Anovular menstruation	4	3	4	23	17	120	930 (500–1700)

(Tsapoulis and Crooke, 1968, *Lancet* ii, 1321).

received clomiphene first. Some of the latter had responded well to clomiphene as judged by the biphasic character of their basal temperature records, but they had failed to conceive. Most, however, were given FSH because they had failed to respond at all to clomiphene. There was no instance of a patient who failed to respond to FSH responding satisfactorily to clomiphene.

The table shows that patients with anovular cycles including those with Stein–Leventhal syndrome responded almost as well to Clomiphene as to FSH. Women with secondary amenorrhoea of more than six months duration including those with Stein–Leventhal syndrome responded poorly to clomiphene but well to FSH although the average minimum effective dosage of FSH was nearly three times as high in the latter as it was in the former.

The incidence of miscarriage and placental failure is high in the Birmingham series as it is in other reported series. The incidence of twins or more appears to be about half as high as in most of the other reported series and the incidence of symptoms of an excessive response is considerably lower than in the only other series in which sufficient data are available for comparison. Lunenfeld (1967) reported 14 cases in the course of 230 months of treatment or six per cent compared with less than one per cent in Birmingham. Moreover seven of his 14 patients had

This is *hyperstimulation syndrome* of moderate severity and the symptoms usually subside within a week or two. In the severe form these symptoms are associated with ascites and sometimes pleural effusions and, in extreme cases, with haemoconcentration, increased coagulability and thrombosis which may lead to gangrene and death (Mozes, *et al.*, 1965). There is no evidence of cardiac or renal failure and the water retention is evidently a direct result of endocrine disturbance but the exact mechanism is not understood. The best line of treatment is, therefore, uncertain. It seems to be generally agreed that if there is evidence of an excessively rapid rise in excretion of oestrogen after FSH then HCG should be withheld and care taken to avoid rupturing the greatly enlarged and tense follicles during examination. Severe symptoms are said then not to develop. Symptoms of moderate severity subside spontaneously with rest in bed in two or three weeks. If pregnancy ensues, however, the ovarian enlargement may persist throughout most of the first trimester and ovarian rupture has been reported (Pasetto and Montanino, 9641. Acsites and pleural effusions also subside spontaneously and rapidly but may require aspiration if they are causing distress. The main concern is the development of haemoconcentration and the risk of thrombosis. This is probably best treated in a potentially pregnant woman by a prolonged infusion of heparin, if necessary for many days, until danger is past.

Simmonds' Disease

There have been several reports of patients with Simmonds' disease treated with FSH and HCG who ovulated and became pregnant but the type of response may be related to the severity of the pituitary failure. It sometimes happens that the excretion of oestrogen will rise to a high figure without evidence of ovulation. Fig. 4C shows an example of the response of a patient with Simmonds' disease to gonadotrophins. This patient was given the same doses of FSH and HCG on many occasions but in different months they were supplemented with a variety of other pituitary trophic hormones none of which enabled ovulation to occur in the doses in which they were tried (Crooke, Butt, Palmer, Morris and Morgan, 1964). Five of the six patients with Simmonds' disease who have been treated with gonadotrophins in Birmingham responded in a similar way.

Stein–Leventhal Syndrome

Many authorities have stated that it is unsafe to treat patients who have Stein–Leventhal Syndrome with gonadotrophins because they are exceptionally sensitive. Indeed the first patient to develop hyperstimulation syndrome in Birmingham had Stein–Leventhal syndrome and her response is shown below (see Fig. 13). Many others, however, have proved to be remarkably insensitive.

The effect of treatment on the steroids in the fluid from the cysts in polycystic ovaries is striking. Short (1964) has shown that typically there is a high concentration of androstenedione, little progesterone and no oestrogens in the ovarian cyst fluid in Stein–Leventhal syndrome. Treatment restores the steroid pattern to normal as shown in Fig. 11 (Crooke, 1967). In this patient oestriol rose to 290 μg. per 24 hours and laparotomy was performed 18 hours after giving her HCG. No corpus luteum was found but nine follicular cysts were aspirated and the steroid content of each measured separately. The results are given on the right of the figure and show a very high concentration of progesterone, high oestrogens and little androstenedione. The similarity of the steroid patterns in the different cysts is remarkable.

The result of treating another patient is shown in Fig. 12. Here laparotomy was performed six days after giving HCG and a corpus luteum was present. The cystic follicles were small and insufficient fluid could be obtained for separate determinations. Fluid was therefore pooled from the follicles in the left and right ovaries separately. The steroid contents of the two samples are shown on the right of the figure and again there is a striking similarity between the two samples. At this time interval after treatment, however, the tiny follicles were luteinized

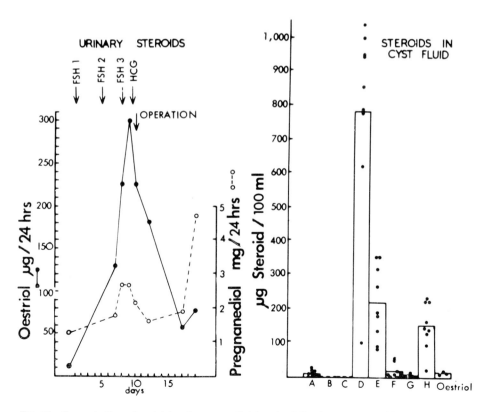

Fig. 11. Concentration of oestriol and pregnanediol in urine following treatment with FSH and HCG and concentrations of steroids in cyst fluid removed at operation 18 hr. after giving HCG. Key to cyst fluid steroids in this and following figures: A = Pregnenolone, B = 17α-hydroxypregnenolone, C = Dehydroepiandrosterone, D = Progesterone, E = 17α-hydroxyprogesterone, F = Androstenedione, G = Oestrone, H = Oestradiol-17β. (Crooke, A. C. 1967, Proc. 5th World Congress on Fertility and Sterility, ICS No. 133, p. 57. Excerpta Medica Foundation, Amsterdam).

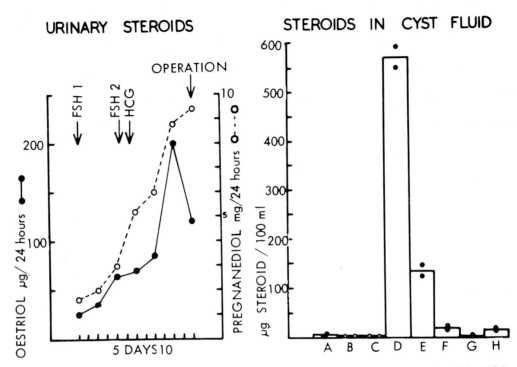

Fig. 12. Concentration of steroids in urine, and in cyst fluid removed at operation, 6 days after giving HCG. (*Ibidem*, p. 58).

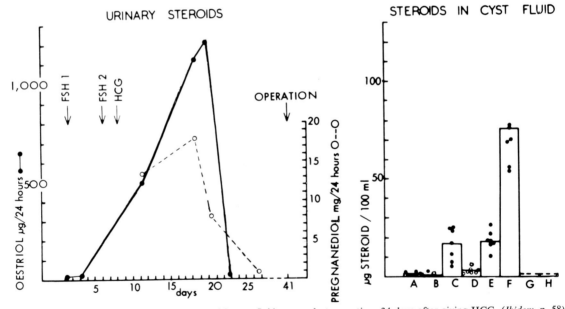

Fig. 13. Concentration of steroids in urine, and in cyst fluid removed at operation, 34 days after giving HCG. (*Ibidem*, p. 58).

and they contained a high concentration of progesterone but little oestrogen or androstenedione. This pattern differs from that of the previous patient and reflects the different time interval after treatment when samples were taken. Many other patients treated similarly have shown essentially the same pictures differing only with the time of sampling.

A very different pattern is seen in Fig. 13. This shows the steroid excretion of a patient who developed hyperstimulation syndrome. Her oestriol reached 1,200 µg.

and her pregnanediol 18 mg. per 24 hours and she had massive enlargement of her ovaries. She had no treatment other than rest in bed until laparotomy was performed 41 days after starting treatment and 35 days after having HCG. Her urinary steroids had returned to control levels 23 days after starting treatment but her ovaries were still considerably enlarged (12·5 × 10 and 7·5 × 5 cm.). They contained numerous large follicular cysts seven of which were aspirated. The steroid patterns of the samples of fluid from these follicles were strikingly similar and typical of that found in Stein–Leventhal syndrome. There was high androstenedione, little progesterone and no oestrogen.

These findings are interpreted as evidence that a follicle stimulated to the point of producing measurable amounts of oestrogen can only continue to secrete oestrogen for about three weeks. After this synthesis breaks down and androstenedione accumulates in the ageing follicles. If, however, the follicle ruptures after about ten days growth the resulting corpus luteum only secretes progesterone for the next ten or twelve days unless pregnancy ensues. The length of the secretory cycle of the follicle which fails to rupture is therefore about the same as that of the follicle and corpus luteum together in the normal cycle. If this is confirmed it must be assumed that when prolonged treatment with FSH causes prolonged secretion of oestrogens it acts by stimulating successive crops of follicles. This is undesirable because of the increased risk of multiple pregnancies and of hyperstimulation syndrome.

Since normal ovulation can be readily induced in the polycystic ovary by treatment with FSH and HCG and since the steroid pattern rapidly reverts when ovulation fails to occur it seems that Stein–Leventhal syndrome is not a disease entity but rather a condition of altered physiology. This condition is essentially a time related breakdown of the synthesis of oestrogens at *androstenedione* in a *polycystic ovary* associated with deficient or disordered gonadotrophin stimulation.

CONCLUSION

Knowledge of the gonadotrophic hormones has made great progress since the identity of separate follicle stimulating and luteinizing activities were first described about 40 years ago. The control of gonadotrophic secretion by hypothalamic releasing factors has been established and details of this mechanism are being worked out. The chemical constitution of human FSH and LH and of HCG is under intensive study which is beginning to yield results. The immunological properties of the hormones have been investigated and methods of immunoassay in body fluids have been developed.

Alongside these academic studies extensive clinical trials of the human gonadotrophic hormones have been undertaken. These have revealed great differences in sensitivity to FSH between patients but after adjustment has been made for this variable a dose-response relationship has been established. This has enabled a more detailed study to be made of the causation of multiple births and of hyperstimulation syndrome. A satisfactory sensitivity test has been described in which progressively increasing doses are given at monthly intervals until a satisfactory response has occurred. The test doses of FSH are invariably followed by HCG so that the first effective test dose can lead to ovulation and be followed by pregnancy.

Gonadotrophin therapy has been used to elucidate the chemical pathology of the polycystic ovary. It has demonstrated that the condition is reversible and it appears to be due either to defective gonadotrophin secretion or to diminished ovarian sensitivity to the hormones.

REFERENCES

Béclère, C. (1960), "Acute Complications of Massive Ovarian Luteinization. Posology of the gonadotrophins in gynaecology." *Presse med.*, **68**, 31.

Bettendorf, G., Breckwoldt, M., Czygan, P. J. and Groot, K. (1967), "Dangers of Ovarian Overstimulation with Human Gonadotrophins," *Gynaecologia*, **163**, (3), 134.

Brown, J. B. (1955), "Chemical Method for the Determination of Oestriol, Oestrone and Oestradiol in Human Urine," *J. biol. Chem.*, **60**, 185.

Brown, P. S. (1955), "The Assay of Gonadotrophin from Urine of Non-pregnant Human Subjects," *J. Endocr.*, **13**, 59.

Butt, W. R. (1967), "The Chemistry of the Gonadotrophins," *American Lecture Series No.* 678. Springfield, Ill.: C. C. Thomas.

Butt, W. R., Jenkins, J. F. and Somers, P. J. (1967), "Some Observations on the Chemical Properties of Human Pituitary Follicle-stimulating Hormone," *J. Endocr.*, **38**, xi.

Buxton, C. L. and Herrmann, W. (1964), "Induction of Ovulation in the Human with Human Gonadotropins," *Amer. J. Obstet. Gynec.*, **81**, 584.

Crooke, A. C. (1967), "Proceedings of the 5th World Congress on Fertility and Sterility, ICS No. 133," *Excerpta Medica Foundation Amsterdam.*

Crooke, A. C. and Bertrand, P. V. (1968), "Comparison of the Effects of Pergonal and Human Pituitary Follicle-stimulating Hormone", in "Developments in the Pharmacology and Clinical Uses of Human Gonadotrophins." A meeting organized by G. D. Searle and Co. Ltd., on 15th March 1968, at the Royal Society of Medicine.

Crooke, A. C., Butt, W. R. and Bertrand, P. V. (1966a), "Clinical Trial of Human Gonadotrophins. 3. Variation in Sensitivity between patients and standardization of treatment," *Acta endocr. (Kbh.)*, **53**, Supplement 111.

Crooke, A. C., Butt, W. R. and Bertrand, P. V. (1966b), "Treatment of Idiopathic Secondary Amenorrhoea with Single Injections of Follicle-stimulating Hormone and Human Chorionic Gonadotrophin," *Lancet*, ii, 514.

Crooke, A. C., Butt, W. R., Bertrand, P. V. and Morris, R. (1967a), "Current Trends in the Treatment of Amenorrhoea with Human Gonadotrophin," *Proc. roy. Soc. Med.*, **60**, 656.

Crooke, A. C., Butt, W. R., Bertrand, P. V. and Morris, R. (1967b), "Treatment of Infertility and Secondary Amenorrhoea with Follicle-stimulating Hormone and Human Chorionic Gonadotrophin," *Lancet*, ii, 636.

Crooke, A. C., Butt, W. R., Palmer, R. F., Bertrand, P. V., Carrington, S. P., Edwards, R. L. and Anson, C. J. (1964), "Clinical Trial of Human Gonadotrophins. 2. Effect of pituitary and urinary follicle-stimulating hormone and human chorionic gonadotrophin on patients with idiopathic secondary amenorrhoea," *J. Obstet. Gynaec. Brit. Commonwealth*, **71**, 571.

Crooke, A. C., Butt, W. R., Palmer, R. F., Morris, R., Edwards, R. L. and Anson, C. J. (1963), "Clinical Trial of Human Gonadotrophins. 1. Effect of pituitary and urinary follicle-stimulating hormone and human chorionic gonadotrophin on patients with idiopathic secondary amenorrhoea," *J. Obstet. Gynaec. Brit. Commonwealth*, **70**, 604.

Crooke, A. C., Butt, W. R., Palmer, R. F., Morris, R. and Morgan, D. B. (1964), "The Effect of Human Gonadotrophins on a Patient with Simmonds' Disease," *Acta endocr. (Kbh.)*, **46**, 292.

Crooke, A. C. and Gemzell, C. A. (1968), "Induction of Ovulation in Humans with Human Gonadotrophins," *Bibliography of Reproduction*, **11**, 1.

Crowe, S. J., Cushing, H. and Homans, J. (1910), "Experimental Hypophysectomy," *Johns Hopk. Hosp. Bull.*, **21**, 127.

Engle, E. T. (1938), "Gonadotrophin stoffe in blut, harn und in anderen körperflussigkeiten," *Arch. Gynäk.*, **166**, 131.

Evans, H. M. and Long, J. A. (1921), "The Effect of Anterior Lobe Administered Intraperitoneally upon Growth, Maturity and Oestrus Cycles of the Rat," *Anat. Rec.*, **21**, 62.

Faiman, C. and Ryan, R. J. (1967), "Serum Follicle-stimulating Hormone and Luteinizing Hormone Concentrations during the Menstrual Cycle as Determined by Radioimmunoassays," *J. clin. Endocrin.*, **27**, 1711.

Fevold, M. L., Hisaw, F. L. and Leonard, S. L. (1931), "The Gonad Stimulating and the Luteinizing Hormones of the Anterior Pituitary," *Amer. J. Physiol.*, **97**, 159.

Gemzell, C. A., Diczfalusy, E. and Tillinger, K. G. (1958), "Clinical Effect of Human Pituitary Follicle-stimulating Hormone (FSH)," *J. clin. Endocrin.*, **18**, 1333.

Gemzell, C. A., Diczfalusy, E. and Tillinger, K. G. (1960), "Human Pituitary Follicle-stimulating Hormone. 1. Clinical effects of a partially purified preparation." *Ciba Foundation Colloquia on Endocrinology*, **13**, 191. London: Churchill.

Gemzell, C. A. and Roos, P. (1966), "Pregnancies following Treatment with Human Gonadotrophins," *Amer. J. Obstet. Gynec.*, **94**, 490.

Gray, C. J. (1968), unpublished.

Gray, C. J. (1967), "Molecular Weight of Human Follicle-stimulating Hormone," *Nature*, **216**, 1112.

Greenblatt, R. B., Barfield, W. E., Jungck, E. C. and Ray, A. W. (1961), "Induction of Ovulation with MRL 41," *J. Amer. med. Ass.*, **178**, 101.

Harris, G. W. (1950), "Oestrous Rhythm. Pseudopregnancy and the pituitary stalk in the rat." *J. Physiol.*, **111**, 347.

Klopper, A. I., Michie, E. A. and Brown, J. B. (1955), "A Method for the Determination of Urinary Pregnanediol," *J. Endocr.*, **12**, 209.

Lunenfeld, B., Rabau, E., Sulimovici, S. and Eshkol, A. (1963), "Treatment of Amenorrhoea by Gonadotrophic Substances from Women's Urine," *Harefuah*, **64**, 289, Hebrew.

Lunenfeld, B. (1967), In *Recent Research on Gonadotrophic Hormones*, p. 257. Edinburgh: Livingstone.

Marshall, J. R. (1968), Personal communication, in "Developments in the Pharmacology and Clinical Uses of Human Gonadotrophins." A meeting organized by G. D. Searle & Co. Ltd., on 15th March 1968 at the Royal Society of Medicine.

Mastsumoto, S. and Tohma, K. (1965), "Case who became Pregnant with Symptom of Acute Abdomen as the Result of Ovulation Induced with PMS and HCG," *J. Endocr.*, (*Japan*), **12**, 159.

Midgley, A. R. (1967), "Radioimmunoassay for Human Follicle-stimulating Hormone," *J. clin. Endocr.*, **27**, 295, Preliminary communication.

Morell, M., Crooke, A. C. and Butt, W. R. (1968), *J. Endocr.*, **41**, 571.

Mozes, M., Bogokowski, H., Antebi, E., Lunenfeld, B., Rabau, E., Serr, D. M., David, A. and Salomy, M. (1965), "Thromboembolic Phenomena after Ovarian Stimulation with Human Gonadotrophins," *Lancet*, **ii**, 1213.

Palmer, R. F. (1964), "A Short Method for the Estimation of Oestriol in Urine," *J. Obstet. Gynaec. Brit. Commonwealth*, **71**, 744.

Parlow, A. F. (1958), "Rapid Bioassay Method for LH and Factors Stimulating LH Secretion," *Fed. Proc.*, **17**, 402.

Pasetto, N. and Montanino, G. (1964), "Human Urinary Gonadotrophins (HMG and HCG) in the Therapy of Amenorrhoeas," *Minerva ginec.*, **16**, 337.

Pasetto, N. and Montanino, G. (1967), "Pregnancy after Combined HMG-HCG Treatment in Amenorrhoeic Patients," *Fertil. and Steril.*, **18**, 685.

Rabau, E., David, A., Serr, D. M., Mashiach, S., Lunenfeld, B. and Gan, R. (1967), "Human Menopausal Gonadotropins for Anovulation and Sterility," *Amer. J. Obstet. Gynec.*, **98**, 92.

Schally, A. V., Saito, T., Arimura, A., Sawano, S., Bowers, C. Y., White, W. F. and Cohen, A. I. (1967), "Purification and *in vitro* and *in vivo* Studies with Porcine Hypothalamic Follicle-stimulating Hormone-releasing Factor," *Endocrinology*, **81**, 882.

Shearman, R. P. (1966), "Induction of Ovulation," *A review. Australasian Annals of Medicine*, **15**, 266.

Short, R. V. (1964), "Steroid Concentrations in the Fluid from Normal and Polycystic (Stein–Leventhal) Ovaries." Proceedings of the Second International Congress of Endocrinology, London, Part II, p. 940, *Excerpta Medica Congress. series No. 83*.

Smith, P. E. (1927), "The Disabilities caused by Hypophysectomy and their Repair," *J. Amer. med. Ass.*, **88**, 158.

Steelman, S. L. and Pohley, F. M. (1953), "Assay of the Follicle-stimulating Hormone Based on the Augmentation with Human Chorionic Gonadotropin," *Endocrinology*, **53**, 604.

Stevens, V. S. (1967), *In Recent Research on Gonadotrophic Hormones*, p. 227. Edinburgh: Livingstone.

Taymor, M. L., Sturgis, S. H., Goldstein, D. P., Liebermann, B. (1967), "Induction of Ovulation with Human Postmenopausal Gonadotropin. 3. Effect of varying dosage schedules on oestrogen and pregnanediol excretion levels," *Fertil. and Steril.*, **18**, 181.

Townsend, S. L., Brown, J. B., Johnstone, J. W., Adey, F. D., Evans, J. H. and Taft, H. P. (1966), "Induction of Ovulation," *J. Obstet. Gynaec. Brit. Commonwealth*, **73**, 529.

Tsapoulis, A. D. and Crooke, A. C. (1968), "A Comparison of Clomiphene and of Human Gonadotrophins in the Treatment of Anovulation," *Lancet*, **ii**, 1321.

Vande Wiele, R. L. and Turksoy, R. N. (1965), "Use of Human Menopausal and Chorionic Gonadotropins in Patients with Infertility due to Ovulatory Failure," *Amer. J. Obstet. Gynec.*, **93**, 632.

Zondek, B. (1930), "Über die hormone des hypophysen vorderlappers." *Klin. Wschr.*, **9**, 679.

3. IMMUNOLOGICAL DETERMINATION OF HUMAN GONADOTROPHINS

LEIF WIDE

Introduction

In the field of reproductive endocrinology many discoveries have been made by the use of classic experimental methods in endocrinology such as the surgical removal of tissues or glands, by replacement therapy, by transplantation of glands and by the administration of crude extracts and more purified hormone preparations. It soon became apparent that these methods were unable to give a satisfactory understanding of the role played by hormones in reproductive physiology. There was a need for methods of measuring the concentration of the hormones involved in blood and urine in order to obtain estimates of hormonal secretion.

As far as gonadotrophins are concerned, the molecular structures of these hormones are still unknown in detail, and these hormones therefore are still defined only by their biological effects when injected into animals. Although a number of more or less ingenious biological methods were developed for the assay of gonadotrophins in body fluids they could not fulfill the requirements of elucidating the complete role of these hormones in reproductive physiology. Bioassays were insufficiently sensitive to permit estimation of low concentrations of gonadotrophins in blood. Gonadotrophins in urine could only be assayed after the preparation of atoxic extracts from larger amounts of urine. Furthermore, the specificity of several of these methods in common use is very low, and the results therefore are of questionable value.

It should however, be emphasized that so long as we define these hormones by their biological effect, biological methods will be a prerequisite for evaluation of the specificity of every new chemical or immunochemical gonadotrophin assay method. It has not yet been possible to assay these hormones with classical chemical methods. For about ten years now immunological methods have been applied to the assay of a great number of protein hormones (Arquilla and Stavitsky, 1956; Read and Stone, 1958; Yalow and Berson, 1960).

Historical Review

The idea of using immunological techniques for the detection of a protein hormone is old, and encouraging attempts to detect gonadotrophins in the urine of pregnant women by immunological means were already made in 1934 by Erlich and in 1950 by Schuyler, Anderson, Serlow and Erickson. The improvement in immunological techniques, the purification of protein hormones and the recognition of their species specificity have been contributing factors to the later rapid development of immunoassay methods for most of the human protein and polypeptide hormones.

Since 1960, immunological pregnancy tests and immunological methods for the quantitative assay of human chorionic gonadotrophin—HCG (Brody and Carlström, 1960; McKean, 1960; Swierczynska and Samochowiec, 1960; Wide and Gemzell, 1960) and luteinizing hormone—LH (Wide, Roos and Gemzell, 1961; Wide and Gemzell, 1962) have been widely used. A detailed review of the results from immunoassay of gonadotrophins reported before 1966 was recently published (Wide, 1967). Since then various radio-immunological techniques have been developed for assaying LH (Bagshawe, Wilde and Orr, 1966; Franchimont, 1966a, b; Midgley, 1966; Odell, Ross and Rayford, 1966; Wide and Porath, 1966) and follicle-stimulating hormone—FSH (Franchimont, 1966a, b; Faiman and Ryan, 1967a; Midgley, 1967; Rosselin and Dolais, 1967) in blood and urine from non-pregnant individuals.

In the past two years about a hundred publications have appeared where immunological techniques have been used for the assay of gonadotrophins, and the results are in many cases conflicting. A number of different characteristics of gonadotrophins have now been revealed, which suggest explanations for the unexpected difficulties in developing highly specific immunoassay methods for these hormones. This chapter will mainly discuss the possibilities and limitations in obtaining reliable and practical immunological methods for the assay of the various gonadotrophins.

Immunological Techniques

The human gonadotrophins, HCG, LH and FSH are species specific glycoproteins with a molecular weight of between 25,000 and 45,000. Antibodies directed against these hormones can be produced in various animals by the injection of the hormones. A number of different immunological techniques are then available for the detection and assay of the gonadotrophins. Some of these techniques are used mainly for qualitative analyses as the different gel diffusion methods.

For quantitative estimations the choice of technique will depend on the concentration of the hormones in the body fluids. Haemagglutination inhibition methods or complement fixation tests are suitable and widely used in assaying HCG in urine or blood during pregnancy. However, the concentration of LH or FSH in blood and urine is about a thousand times lower than HCG, and for these radio-immunoassay procedures are preferable as they provide much higher sensitivities. A detailed review of the various immunological techniques for the assay of protein hormones has been published by Berson and Yalow (1964). Many of the immunological methods, and especially the radio-immunological variants, combine adequate sensitivity with acceptable precision and high specificity.

Biological Specificity

Immunological specificity has in general very little to do with the biologically specific action of the hormone. One of the difficulties with the gonadotrophins is that definitions for FSH, LH or HCG are somewhat vague.

As mentioned above the molecular structures of these hormones are still unknown, and they are defined from certain biological effects that they present. These effects are assayed in animals, and for each gonadotrophin there are several assay methods which are claimed to be specific for that particular hormonal effect (Loraine and Bell, 1967). When several "specific" methods for a certain gonadotrophic effect have been compared quite different results have been obtained (Parlow and Reichert, 1963; Rosenberg, Solod and Albert, 1964; Hamashige, Astor, Arquilla and Van Thiel, 1967).

The divergencies between the different methods appear to present a complex problem. It has, for instance, been shown that from an HCG preparation at least six different homogenous components could be isolated with biological potencies ranging from 4000 to 19000 IU/mg (Van Hell, Goverde, Schuurs, De Jager, Matthijsen and Homan, 1966). The biological potencies of these different compounds increased proportionally to their content of sialic acid, when the assays were based upon gonadal stimulation in rats. However, the effect on spermiation in frogs seemed to be independent of the sialic acid (Hamashige et al., 1967).

Thus, it can be postulated that the hormonal effect defined as HCG may be derived from a number of components with different specific activities. Two "specific" biological methods having two different indices of response may not be sensitive to the same active sites on a population of "HCG" molecules. These problems become even more complicated considering that various kinds of gonadotrophin inhibitors (Soffer and Fogel, 1963; Pavel and Petrescu, 1966; Sairam, Madhwa Raj and Moudgal, 1966) and/or substances augmenting the biological effect may be present (e.g. Parlow, 1963; Wide and Hobson, 1967).

Furthermore, it is necessary to extract the hormones to assay gonadotrophins in human body fluids. Different extraction methods may concentrate different groups of molecules of varying gonadotrophic specific activity (Van Hell et al., 1966; Hamashige et al., 1967). The potency then estimated represents a summation dependent on the content and ratios of the various components with gonadotrophic activity. Thus it can be concluded that when we define a certain gonadotrophin, biological methods are used which determine certain characteristic configurations of some parts of the molecules. Furthermore, different bioassays may differ in sensitivity to smaller changes in these configurations. It should also be emphasized that the effect of the human gonadotrophins as measured in animals may considerably differ from their effect in the human being.

Immunological Specificity

Immunologically, molecules the size of gonadotrophins cannot be regarded as single antigens but as molecules with several antigenic sites. Most antisera contain several populations of antibodies which are directed against different antigenic sites on the molecules. These antigenic sites may be specific for the hormone in question. However as far as the gonadotrophins are concerned one of the great problems has been the fact that at least four different hormones, all glycoproteins: FSH, LH, HCG and TSH seem to have at least one antigenic site in common (Odell, Wilber and Paul, 1965; Robyn, Hubinont and Diczfalusy, 1966; Faiman and Ryan, 1967a; Midgley, 1967; Odell, Reichert and Bates, 1968; Rosen, Schlaff and Roth, 1968). This means that when immunizing with one of these hormones one may easily obtain antibodies which react not only with this hormone but also with one, two or three other hormones.

In the case of HCG and LH it seems to be a complete cross-reaction (Moudgal and Li, 1961; Wide et al., 1961) and quantitative immunoassays which can distinguish between these two hormones do not seem yet to have been reported. It is possible however, to separate the two hormones by gelfiltration and a subsequent immunoassay of the different fractions can give an estimate of the content of the two hormones in a mixture (Midgley, Fong and Jaffe, 1967).

It seems as if animals injected with FSH more commonly produce antibodies cross-reacting with LH and HCG than antibodies that are directed against sites specific for FSH. In our experience of 17 animals (12 rabbits and 5 guinea-pigs) ten have given rise to antibodies which cross-react while only two animals gave a high titer of FSH specific antibodies (one rabbit and one guinea-pig). One of these latter antisera (guinea-pig) contained negligible amounts of cross-reacting antibodies and gave identical results before and after absorption with HCG or LH. The other antiserum containing both cross-reacting and specific antibodies could be used only after absorption with HCG or LH. Difficulties in obtaining specific antibodies against FSH have been reported from several laboratories.

It seems wise to use randomly bred instead of inbred animals as the chances of obtaining a high titer of specific antibodies is then greater, and the antiserum from one animal can in general be used for several hundred thousand reactions. The problems of cross-reactivity may be solved through the selection of antisera, and if necessary by absorption with other hormones. The fact that these gonadotrophins have several antigenic sites and that some of them are in common with those of other hormones or non-hormonal substances have been important factors contributing to the discrepancies in results obtained by different laboratories.

Even with the use of the same antiserum there are some reports that different immunological methods may give different results. It was recently reported that an antiserum to FSH which showed a cross-reaction with LH in the radioimmunoassay, failed to do so in the complement fixation technique (Butt and Lynch, 1968).

The use of highly purified antigens is one of the prerequisites for obtaining specific radio-immunological assays. It is interesting that highly purified FSH preparations from human pituitaries and human post-menopausal urine differ considerably both in regard to aminoacid composition and in regard to specific biological activity. Pituitary FSH has been purified to a specific activity of about 14000 IU/mg and urinary FSH to 780 IU/mg (Roos, 1967). It has nevertheless been possible to use antisera to pituitary FSH for immunoassay of both urinary and pituitary FSH.

While immunization with the pituitary FSH preparations has given rise to specific antibodies to FSH we have not in our laboratory up till now been able to obtain specific antibodies to urinary FSH preparations (500–600 IU/mg). Successful immunizations with crude urinary FSH preparations have however, been reported from other laboratories (Mori, 1967; Tamada, Soper and Taymor, 1967). The great difference in molecular structure between urinary and pituitary FSH is not in agreement with the concept that urinary FSH represents a main fragment of pituitary FSH. It has therefore, been suggested that formation of urinary FSH from pituitary has involved both subtraction and addition of glycopeptides and/or peptides (Roos, 1967).

It has been shown that immunological differences exist between urinary and pituitary FSH (Roos, 1967; Taymor, Tamada, Soper and Blatt, 1967). The two hormones however, seem to have at least one antigenic site in common. Comparable investigations on aminoacid composition of urinary and pituitary LH has not yet been reported. There is no doubt that LH in human pituitaries, serum and urine have antigenic sites in common although certain differences seem to exist in some antigenic sites between urinary and pituitary LH (Mori, 1968).

Immunological versus Biological Gonadotrophic Activity

As the gonadotrophins are defined by their biological effect it has been postulated that immunological assays for gonadotrophins are only acceptable if they give values numerically similar to bioassay. From the facts presented above on specificity problems it can be concluded that an absolute agreement between the results of bioassay and immunoassay is rather unlikely to occur. It has been shown that when an HCG preparation is heated it retains its immunological activity while losing its hormonal activity (Wide, 1962).

Furthermore, it was shown that results from parallel immunological and biological estimations did not agree when HCG in the urine of pregnant women was assayed (Wide, 1962). Immunologically active substances with no or very little biological activity were present in the urine (Hobson and Wide, 1964). It is thus most probable that biologically and immunologically active sites on a gonadotrophin molecule may exist independently. In an HCG preparation where six different components with different biological activities were isolated they were all immunochemically homogeneous (Van Hell et al., 1966). The immunological reactivity seemed to be independent of the sialic acid content (Van Hell et al., 1966; Hamashige et al., 1967). It is not clear whether these components with lower biological activity originate from the chorion or if some of them are degradation products.

It has been shown that immunological methods sometimes measure biologically inactive material derived from the gonadotrophin, and it is conceivable that immunoassay in this situation may give a better estimate of hormonal secretion than bioassay. It has also been shown that the ratio between immunologically and biologically HCG active components produced by hydatidiform moles or invasive trophoblast varies (Wide and Hobson, 1967; Hobson and Wide, 1968). The ratio biological/immunological activity seemed to be related to the degree of malignancy of the trophoblast, a high ratio is associated with a good prognosis and a low ratio with a poor one.

As the cross-reactivity between the four glycoprotein hormones FSH, LH, HCG and TSH is a serious complication for obtaining specific reactions, control analyses on the capacity of antisera to neutralize the different biological activities are of great value (Robyn, Diczfalusy and Finney, 1968).

Immunological methods should thus not be rejected, just because they do not, in all body fluids, measure the same activities as bioassays. Similarly, they cannot replace bioassays for estimation of hormonal effects. Both types of methods have their advantages, and the problem is to characterize the specificity of each particular system used.

Physiological Studies and Clinical Application

Immunological methods have many advantages as compared with biological when applied to clinical studies, due to the combination of high sensitivity, precision and practicability. Immunological techniques for detection of HCG are now widely used as pregnancy tests. Quantitative immunoassays of HCG have shown to be of great diagnostic value in cases of ectopic pregnancy, threatened abortion, hydatidiform mole, and invasive trophoblast (reviewed by Wide, 1967).

Immunoassays for LH and FSH in blood and urine have hitherto mainly been used to clarify the physiological concentrations in normal men, women and children (e.g. Midgley and Jaffe, 1966; Franchimont, 1966b; Faiman and Ryan, 1967b; Odell, Ross and Rayford, 1967; Saxena, Demura, Gandy and Peterson, 1968). Due to differences in specificity of the immunological systems used it seems necessary for every laboratory to establish its "normal" ranges for the gonadotrophin concentrations as measured by each particular system; at least until standardized antigens and antisera are available.

Concerning LH, there is a good agreement between the data obtained by bioassay methods (McArthur, Worcester and Ingersoll, 1958) and immunological methods both in urine (Wide, 1966) and in plasma (Midgley and Jaffe, 1966). In all studies there is a marked mid-cycle peak, which appears more sharply in plasma than in urine. Concerning FSH, the results obtained by bioassays (Rosenberg and Keller, 1965; Steven and Vorys, 1967) and immunoassays (Franchimont, 1966b; Faiman and Ryan, 1967b; Saxena et al., 1968) do not agree so well as for LH. The divergencies here are probably both due to differences in specificity in the techniques, and to individual variation. The most extensive investigation hitherto reported on FSH excretion in urine as estimated by bioassay is the one by Steven and Vorys (1967) which shows a broad menstrual peak, followed by another less pronounced postovulatory maximum.

It is conceivable that gonadotrophin assay methods will

be of great clinical value when the physiological inter-relationships between hypophyseal and gonadal function is more fully clarified. The endocrine regulation of the menstrual cycle is still a matter of controversy. The effect of various steroids, including those used in contraceptive drugs, on the secretion of gonadotrophins is at present being intensively studied (reviewed by Diczfalusy, 1968).

of both bioassay and immunoassay methods. An interesting difference in the metabolic clearance rates for LH (24 ml./min.) and for HCG (4 ml./min.) was found.

As the normal variation in the secretion of the gonadotrophins during the menstrual cycle has still not been fully investigated, very few data on immunoassay of gonadotrophins in gynaecological disorders have as yet

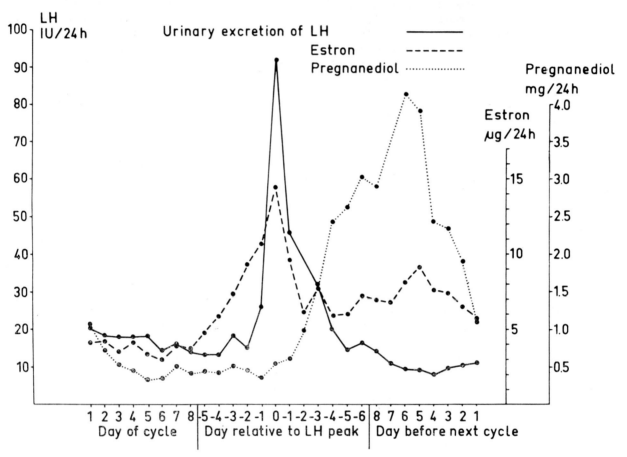

FIG. 1. The relationship between the mean excretion of LH, oestrone and pregnanediol in urine of six women with normal menstrual cycles.

The relationship between the plasma levels of luteinizing hormone and progesterone during the normal menstrual cycle was studied by Neill, Johansson, Datta and Knobil (1967). The rise in the plasma progesterone levels did not start until after the midcycle surge of LH became fully evident. The relationship between the mean excretion of LH, oestrone and pregnanediol in urine of six women with normal menstrual cycles is shown in Figure 1). The oestrone excretion started about 5 days before the LH peak. The first oestrone peak and the LH peak coincided in all six cycles.

With the limitations in specificity in mind, the immuno-assays are excellent tools for measuring secretion rates, metabolism and renal elimination of the gonadotrophins. The metabolic clearance and the production rates of luteinizing hormone were studied by Kohler, Ross and Odell (1968) by radio-immunoassays, and the metabolic clearance and renal clearance rates for HCG by Wide, Johannisson, Tillinger and Diczfalusy (1968) with the use

been published. Immunoassay of LH has been suggested to be of value in infertility cases both for the diagnosis of certain gynaecological endocrinopathies, especially associated with failure of ovulation (Mishell, 1966) and for the detection of the day of ovulation (Bermes, Heffernan and Isaacs, 1965; Wide, 1966). It is conceivable that immunological methods for the determination of gonadotrophins will be of great value in the future, not only for the diagnosis of pregnancy, of HCG producing tumours and of various disorders during pregnancy, but also for the diagnosis of gynaecological disorders with abnormal hypophyseal gonadotrophin secretion.

REFERENCES

Arquilla, E. R. and Stavitsky, A. B. (1956), "The Production and Identification of Antibodies to Insulin and Their Use in Assaying Insulin," *J. clin. Invest.*, **35**, 458.
Bagshawe, K., Wilde, C. and Orr, A. (1966), "Radio-immunoassay of HCG and LH," *Lancet*, **290**, 1118.

Bermes, E. W., Heffernan, B. T. and Isaacs, J. H. (1965), "Immunochemical Detection of Ovulation," *Obstet. Gynec.*, **25**, 792.

Berson, S. A. and Yalow, R. S. (1964), "Immunoassay of Protein Hormones," in Pincus, G., Thimann, K. V. and Artwood, E. B. (eds.), *The Hormones*, Vol. IV, p. 557. New York and London: Academic Press, Inc.

Brody, S. and Carlström, G. (1960), "Estimation of Human Chorionic Gonadotrophin in Biological Fluids by Complement Fixation," *Lancet*, **2**, 99.

Butt, W. R. and Lynch, S. S. (1968), "Some Observations on the Radio-immunoassay of Follicle Stimulating Hormone," in Margoulies, M. (ed.), *Protein and Polypeptide Hormones*, p. 134. Amsterdam, New York, London, Paris, Milan, Tokyo, Buenos Aires: Excerpta Medica Foundation.

Diczfalusy, E. (1968), "Mode of Action of Contraceptive Drugs," *Amer. J. Obstet. Gynec.*, **100**, 136.

Ehrlich, H. (1934), "Immunisierungsversuche mit gonadotropen hormonen," *Wien. klin. Wschr.*, **47**, 1323.

Faiman, C. and Ryan, R. (1967a), "Radio-immunoassay for Human Follicle Stimulating Hormone," *J. clin. Endocr.*, **27**, 444.

Faiman, C. and Ryan, R. J. (1967b), "Serum Follicle-stimulating Hormone and Luteinizing Hormone Concentrations during the Menstrual Cycle as Determined by Radio-immunoassays," *J. clin. Endocr.*, **27**, 1711.

Franchimont, P. (1966a), "Dosage radio-immunologique des gonadotrophines folliculo-stimulante et lutéinisante," *Journal of Labelled Compounds*, **2**, 303.

Franchimont, P. (1966b), "Le dosage des hormones hypophysaires somatotropes et gonadotropes et son application en clinique." Brussels: Editions Arscia S. A.

Hamashige, S., Astor, M. A., Arquilla, E. R. and Van Thiel, D. H. (1967), "Human Chorionic Gonadotropin: A Hormone Complex," *J. clin. Endocr.*, **27**, 1690.

Hobson, B. M. and Wide, L. (1964), "The Immunological and Biological Activity of Human Chorionic Gonadotrophin in Urine," *Acta Endocr.*, **46**, 632.

Hobson, B. M. and Wide, L. (1968), "Human Chorionic Gonadotrophin Excretion in Men and Women with Invasive Trophoblast Assayed by an Immunological and a Biological Method," *Acta Endocr.*, **58**, 473.

Kohler, P. O., Ross, G. T. and Odell, W. D. (1968), "Metabolic Clearance and Production Rates of Human Luteinizing Hormone in Pre- and Postmenopausal Women," *J. clin. Invest.*, **47**, 38.

Loraine, J. A. and Bell, E. T. (1966), *Hormone Assays and their Clinical Application*. Edinburgh and London: E. and S. Livingstone Ltd.

McArthur, J. W., Worcester, J. and Ingersoll, F. M. (1958), "The Urinary Excretion of Interstitial-cell and Follicle-stimulating Hormone Activity during the Normal Menstrual Cycle," *J. clin. Endocr.*, **18**, 1186.

McKean, C. M. (1960), 'Preparation and Use of Antisera to Human Chorionic Gonadotrophin," *Amer. J. Obstet. Gynec.*, **80**, 596.

Midgley, R. A. (1966), "Radio-immunoassay: a Method for Human Chorionic Gonadotrophin and Human Luteinizing Hormone," *Endocrinology*, **79**, 10.

Midgley, R. A. (1967), "Radio-immunoassay for Human Follicle Stimulating Hormone," *J. clin. Endocr.*, **27**, 295.

Midgley, R. A. and Jaffe, R. B. (1966), "Human Luteinizing Hormone in Serum during the Menstrual Cycle: Determination by Radio-immunoassay," *J. clin. Endocr.*, **26**, 1375.

Midgley, R. A., Fong, I. F. and Jaffe, R. B. (1967), "Gel Filtration Radio-immunoassay to Distinguish Human Chorionic Gonadotrophin from Luteinizing Hormone," *Nature*, **213**, 733.

Mishell, D. R. (1966), "Daily Urinary Assay of Luteinizing Hormone by an Immunologic Method," *Amer. J. Obstet. Gynec.*, **95**, 747.

Mori, K. F. (1967), "Immunologic Studies with Follicle-stimulating Hormone from Human Postmenopausal Gonadotrophin," *Endocrinology*, **81**, 1241.

Mori, K. F. (1968), "Immunologic Reaction between Human Luteinizing Hormones and Antiserum to Urinary Luteinizing Hormone," *Endocrinology*, **82**, 945.

Moudgal, N. R. and Li, C. H. (1961), "An Immunological Study of a Human Pituitary Interstitial Cell-stimulating Hormone," *Nature*, **191**, 192.

Neill, J. D., Johansson, E. D. B., Datta, J. K. and Knobil, E. (1967), "Relationship between the Plasma Levels of Luteinizing Hormone and Progesterone during the Normal Menstrual Cycle," *J. clin. Endocr.*, **27**, 1167.

Odell, W. D., Wilber, J. F. and Paul, W. E. (1965), "Radio-immunoassay of Thyrotrophin in Human Serum," *J. clin. Endocr.*, **25**, 1179.

Odell, W., Ross, G. and Rayford, P. (1966), "Radio-immunoassay for HLH," *Metabolism*, **15**, 287.

Odell, W. D., Ross, G. T. and Rayford, P. L. (1967), "Radio-immunoassay for Luteinizing Hormone in Human Plasma or Serum: Physiological Studies," *J. clin. Invest.*, **46**, 248.

Odell, W. D., Reichert, L. E. and Bates, R. W. (1968), "Pitfalls in the Radio-immunoassay of Carbohydrate Containing Polypeptide Hormones," in Margoulies, M. (ed.), *Protein and Polypeptide Hormones*, p. 124. Amsterdam, New York, London, Paris, Milan, Tokyo, Buenos Aires: Excerpta Medica Foundation.

Parlow, A. F. (1963), "Influence of Serum on the Prostate Assay of Luteinizing Hormone (LH, ICSH)," *Endocrinology*, **73**, 456.

Parlow, A. F. and Reichert, L. E. (1963), "Influence of Follicle-stimulating Hormone on the Prostate Assay of Luteinizing Hormone (LH, ICSH)," *Endocrinology*, **73**, 377.

Pavel, S. and Petrescu, S. (1966), "Inhibition of Gonadotrophin by a Highly Purified Pineal Peptide and by Synthetic Arginin Vasotocin," *Nature*, **212**, 1054.

Read, C. H. and Stone, D. B. (1958), "An Immunologic Assay for Minute Amounts of Human Pituitary Growth Hormone," *Amer. J. Dis. Child.*, **96**, 538.

Robyn, C., Hubinont, P. O. and Diczfalusy, E. (1966), "Immunological Cross Reaction between Human Chorionic Gonadotrophin and Human Pituitary Gonadotrophins," *Acta endocr.*, **53**, 420.

Robyn, C., Diczfalusy, E. and Finney, D. J. (1968), "Bioassay of Antigonadotrophic Sera," *Acta endocr.*, **58**, 593.

Roos, P. (1967), *Human Follicle-stimulating Hormone*, pp. 1–93. Uppsala: Almqvist and Wiksells A. B.

Rosen, S. W., Schlaff, S. and Roth, J. (1968), "Anti-human Follicle Stimulating Hormone: Complete Cross Reactivity with Three Other Human Glycoprotein Trophic Hormones, Luteinizing Hormone, Human Chorionic Gonadotrophin and Thyrotropin," in Margoulies, M. (ed.), *Protein and Polypeptide Hormones*, p. 396. Amsterdam, New York, London, Paris, Milan, Tokyo, Buenos Aires: Excerpta Medica Foundation.

Rosemberg, E., Solod, E. A. and Albert A. (1964), "Luteinizing Hormone Activity of Human Pituitary Gonadotrophin as Determined by the Ventral Prostate Weight and the Ovarian Ascorbic Acid Depletion Methods of Assay," *J. clin. Endocr.*, **24**, 714.

Rosemberg, E. and Keller, P. (1965), "Studies on the Urinary Excretion of FSH and LH during the Menstrual Cycle," *J. clin. Endocr.*, **25**, 1262.

Rosemberg, E., Keller, P., Lewis, W. B., Albert, A., Carl, G. and Bennett, D. (1965), "Influence of Follicle-stimulating Hormone on the Estimation of Luteinizing Hormone in the Ventral Prostate and Ovarian Ascorbic Acid Depletion Assays," *Endocrinology*, **76**, 1150.

Rosselin, G. and Dolais, J. (1967), "Dosage de l'hormone folliculo-stimulante humaine par méthode radio-immunologique," *La Presse Medicale*, **75**, 2027.

Sairam, M. R., Madhwa Raj, H. G. and Moudgal, N. R. (1966), "Presence of a Gonadotrophin Inhibitor in the Urine of the Bonnet Monkey, Macaca Radiata," *Endocrinology*, **78**, 923.

Saxena, B. B., Demura, H., Gandy, H. M. and Peterson, R. E. (1968), "Radio-immunoassay of Human Follicle-stimulating and Luteinizing Hormones in Plasma," *J. clin. Endocr.*, **28**, 519.

Schuyler, L. H., Anderson, K., Serlow, S. and Erickson, C. A. (1950). "A Serologic Study of Chorionic Gonadotrophin," *Proc. Soc. exp, Biol.*, **75**, 552.

Soffer, L. J. and Fogel, M. (1963), "Effect of Urinary Gonadotrophin-inhibiting Substance upon the Action of Human Chorionic Gonadotrophin (APL) and on Human Postmenopausal Urinary Gonadotrophin (Pergonal)," *J. clin. Endocr.*, **23**, 870.

Stevens, V. C. and Vorys, N. (1967), "The Regulation of Pituitary Function by Sex Steroids," *Obstet. gynec. Surv.*, **22**, 781.

Swierczynska, Z. and Samochowiec (1960), "Serologic Detection of Chorionic Gonadotropin in Urine. Its Value in the Diagnosis of Pregnancy," *Pol. Tyg. lek.*, **15**, 1217.

Tamada, T., Soper, M. and Taymor, M. L. (1967), "Immunologic Studies with Urinary Follicle Stimulating Hormone," *J. clin. Endocr.*, **27**, 379.

Taymor, M. L., Tamada, T., Soper, M. and Blatt, W. F. (1967), "Immunologic Relationships between Urinary and Pituitary Follicle-stimulating Hormone," *J. clin. Endocr.*, **27**, 709.

Van Hell, H., Goverde, B. C., Schuurs, A. H. W. M., De Jager, E., Matthijsen, R. and Homan, J. D. H. (1966), "Purification, Characterization and Immunochemical Properties of Human Chorionic Gonadotropin," *Nature*, **212**, 261.

Wide, L. (1962), "An Immunological Method for the Assay of Human Chorionic Gonadotrophin," pp. 1–111, *Acta Endocr.*, Supplement **70**.

Wide, L. (1966), "Immunoassay of Human LH for the Detection of Ovulation," in Greenblatt, R. (ed.), *Ovulation*, p. 283. Philadelphia: J. B. Lippincott Co.

Wide, L. (1967), "Immunoassay of Human Gonadotrophins. Specificity Problems and Clinical Application," in Marcus, S. and Marcus, L. (eds.), *Advances in Obstetrics and Gynecology*, Vol. I, p. 56. Baltimore: Williams and Wilkins Co.

Wide, L. and Gemzell, C. A. (1960), "An Immunological Pregnancy Test," *Acta Endocr.*, **35**, 261.

Wide, L. and Gemzell, C. A. (1962), "Immunological Determination of Pituitary Luteinizing Hormone in the Urine of Fertile and Post-menopausal Women and Adult Men," *Acta Endocr.*, **39**, 539.

Wide, L. and Porath, J. (1966), "Radio-immunoassay of Proteins with the Use of Sephadex-coupled Antibodies," *Biochim. biophys. Acta*, **130**, 257.

Wide, L. and Hobson, B. M. (1967), "Immunological and Biological Activity of Human Chorionic Gonadotrophin in Urine and Serum of Pregnant Women and Women with a Hydatidiform Mole," *Acta Endocr.*, **54**, 105.

Wide, L., Roos, P. and Gemzell, C. A. (1961), "Immunological Determination of Human Pituitary Luteinizing Hormone (LH)," *Acta Endocr.*, **37**, 445.

Wide, L., Johannisson, E., Tillinger, K.-G. and Diczfalusy, E. (1968), "Metabolic Clearance of Human Chorionic Gonadotrophin Administered to Non-pregnant Women," *Acta Endocr.*, (in the press).

Yalow, R. S. and Berson, S. A. (1960), "Immunoassay of Endogenous Plasma Insulin in Man," *J. clin. Invest.*, **39**, 1157.

4. THE NEUROHYPOPHYSIS AND LABOUR

G. W. THEOBALD

For the purpose of preparing the blood the soul has established in the cerebrum an illustrious chymical laboratory, which it has arranged into members and organs and by the ministry of these it destils and elaborates a lymph animated by the animal spirit, whereby it imbues the blood with its own inmost essence, nature and life.

Swedenborg, 1741

It is little more than 10 years ago that it became established that neurosecretions, elaborated both in the paraventricular and in the supraoptic nuclei, are transported along nerve axons and stored in the neurohypophysis until, as the result of specific chemical or nervous stimuli, they are released into the blood stream. It is thought that vasopressin and oxytocin may be carried in separate particles although most adequate stimuli bring about release of both, albeit in varying ratios (Barer, Heller and Lederis, 1963; Stutinsky, 1966), (Fig. 1). Their separate release in man has been recorded (Theobald, 1959).

The hypophysis cerebri measures approximately $10 \times 10 \times 5$ mm., weighs about 0·6 g., and enlarges during pregnancy. It consists of two parts, the adenohypophysis which derives from the somatic ectoderm of the bucco-pharyngeal pouch and pushes upwards towards the third ventricle, and the neurohypophysis developing in the opposite direction from the floor of the diencephalon towards the base of the skull. The neurohypophysis stores both vasopressin (antidiuretin or ADH) and oxytocin in a manner not yet fully understood.

The adenohypophysis elaborates several different hormones and is discussed on page 460 *et seq.* The fact, however, that lactation is dependent on the adenohypophysis and milk ejection on the neurohypophysis illustrates interrelation as well as propinquity. It is moreover thought that some of the hormones secreted in the adenohypophysis have different actions depending on the target organ on

which they act, and this concept of specificity of target organ reaction is vitally important to the understanding of pregnancy and labour.

Posterior Pituitary Extract

Dr. G. Oliver, a wealthy medical practitioner, called on Prof. Schäfer in the autumn of 1893 and persuaded him to try the effect of suprarenal extract on the blood pressure in a cat. The startling vasopressor effect of both suprarenal and posterior pituitary extracts was later reported by Oliver and Schäfer (1895a, b) and this was the virtual beginning of the physiology of the ductless glands.

The diuretic activity of posterior pituitary extract was reported in 1901 (Magnus and Schäfer, 1901; Schäfer and Herring, 1906), its oxytocic activity in 1906 (Dale, 1906), its galactobolic effect in 1910 (Ott and Scott, 1910) and its antidiuretic activity in 1913 (von den Velden, 1913; Konschegg and Schuster, 1915). It is noteworthy that posterior pituitary extract was thought to be diuretic for 12 years simply because all tests were made on anaesthetized animals, and it was not until it was injected into man and other conscious animals that its potent antidiuretic activity was recognized. Indeed, the first clinical application of this extract was in the form of *diuretic* tablets given by mouth. Its earliest use in obstetrics was in the treatment of "shock, uterine atony, and intestinal paresis" (Blair Bell, 1909). Hofbauer (1911) injected the extract both intramuscularly and intravenously and in 1927,

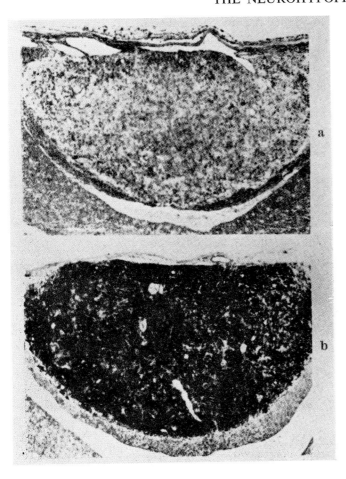

FIG. 1(A). Shows cross-sections of the neurohypophysis of the rat. The one above (a) is from a thirsting rat and shows depletion of neurosecretory substance, while that below (b) is from a control animal which had received as much water as it wanted. Gomori's chrome-haematoxylin. After Eichner, 1953. In, *British Obstetric Practice*, Ed. A. Claye, Heinemann, London, 3rd ed., 1963.

and du Vigneaud *et al.*, (1953); its synthesis was achieved a year later (du Vigneaud *et al.*, 1954), followed shortly afterwards by its synthesis on a commercial scale (Boissonas *et al.*, 1955). This latter achievement ensured not only an adequate commercial supply of pure oxytocin for both clinical and research purposes but paved the way to the preparation of a large number of analogues which have contributed greatly to our understanding of the relation between chemical structure and pharmacological function.

Both these hormones are octapeptide amides and their nine amino-acid residues are numbered in the generally accepted sequence.

Vasopressin is therefore phenylalanyl[3]-arginyl[8]-oxytocin (phe[3]-arg[8]-oxytocin). Conversely, oxytocin is ileu[3]-leu[8]-vasopressin. Lysine vasopressin (phe[3]-lys[8]-oxytocin) occurs naturally in the neurohypophyses of the pig, hippopotamus and the peccary, and so far as is known in no other animal. Because of ease of extraction commercial vasopressin is now exclusively extracted from pigs' posterior pituitary glands and "beef" vasopressin, similar to that occurring in man, is virtually unobtainable, because synthetic argenine vasopressin is unstable. The "standdard" vasopressin powder is therefore only standard for pigs and hippopotami.

It may here be observed that interference with the amino-acids in positions 4, 5, 6 and 7 destroys the activity of both oxytocin and vasopressin whereas alterations in positions 1, 2, 3 and 8 result in varying compounds which have activities intermediate between those of oxytocin and vasopressin (Berde, Cerletti and Konzett, 1961; van Dyke, 1961; Berde, 1965).

The results obtained from these analogues are compatible with the drug-receptor interaction hypothesis which in its simplest form suggests that the response to a drug is proportional to the number of receptors activated by it. Vasopressin, for example, is more than 10 times more potent than oxytocin on water diuresis in man and in the dog, whereas oxytocin has more than ten times the effect of vasopressin on uterine activity in man at term. Further, oxytocin lowers avian blood pressure far more effectively than does vasopressin, which in fact may cause it to rise after it has been lowered by oxytocin. It has, moreover, just been reported that both 1 Penicillamine-oxytocin and 1-deaminopenicillamine-oxytocin inhibit the oxytocic response to oxytocin in the rat as well *in vivo* as *in vitro*, without affecting spontaneous uterine activity or uterine response to either angiotensin or bradykinin. The following activities characteristic of oxytocin; rabbit milk-ejectory, avian depressor, rat vasopressor and rat anti-

together with Hoerner, tried the buccal route but discarded it in favour of its intranasal application (see Knaus, 1926).

Oxytocin and Vasopressin (A D H)

The virtually complete separation of oxytocin from vasopressin was effected in 1928 by Kamm *et al.*; its structure was determined independently by Tuppy (1953)

OXYTOCIN

1	2	3	4	5	6	7	8	9
Cy S	Tyr	Ileu	Glu (NH2)	Asp (NH2)	Cy S	Pro	Leu	Gly (NH2)

VASOPRESSIN

Cy S	Tyr	PHE	Glu (NH2)	Asp (NH2)	Cy S	Pro	ARG	Gly (NH2)

diuretic were not caused by these analogues (Chan, Fear and du Vigneaud, 1967).

These points are illustrated in Fig. 2 showing the key (oxytocin, vasopressin) and the levers or detainers in the lock which represent tissue receptors. Removal of the central steps of the key renders it useless. If the detainers or tissue receptors are absent or otherwise occupied, as

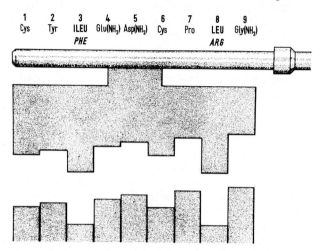

FIG. 2. Oxytocin shown as a key. Changing of steps 3 and 8 turns it into vasopressin. Alteration of steps 4 to 7 destroys its efficacy. Substituting penicillamine for cystine in position 1 so changes the key that it inhibits oxytocin activity. Other changes in positions 1, 2, 3 and 8 result in compounds having activities intermediate between oxytocin and vasopressin. The levers or detainers of the lock illustrated beneath the key represent the tissue receptors.

for example by 1 Penicillamine-oxytocin, the key is relatively useless. Rapid destruction or inactivation of any substance in the blood likewise prevents it from operating.

Oxytocinase or Vasopressinase

Fekete (1930) reported that the serum of pregnant women inactivated oxytocin. It was later established that the substance concerned was oxytocinase, an aminopeptidase which acts equally effectively on both oxytocin and vasopressin. It only occurs in the blood of pregnant women and of pregnant anthropoid apes. In women it can be detected shortly after the 16th day of pregnancy and thereafter increases some 60 fold to reach its maximum at term (Tuppy, 1961; Semm, 1961). Plasma obtained from 18 women at term was found to inactivate 50 per cent of added Syntocinon in 4.54 ± 1.13 (SD) min. (Mendez-Bauer et al., 1961). More recently Glendening et al., (1965) have shown that starch gel electrophoresis of sera from normal pregnant women has consistently resulted in the separation of three components which can be demonstrated by incubation with L-leucyl-beta-naphthylamide. Leucine amino-peptidase (LAP) occurs in both pregnant and non-pregnant women but the two cystine aminopeptidases (CAP_1 and CAP_2) are characteristic of human pregnancy and are capable of destroying both oxytocin and vasopressin.

The maximum myometrial sensitivity to oxytocin occurs when the amount of oxytocinase in the blood is

at its highest, and water diuresis in a pregnant woman at term is as well inhibited by the intravenous infusion of 0.5 m-u. ADH/min. as in the non-pregnant state or in the male. Further, nonspecific oxytocin-inactivating enzymes have been found in the sera of non-pregnant animals (including men and women) and have been demonstrated in extracts of erythrocytes, ovaries, pancreas, liver and uterus. The half-life of oxytocin in the male varies between 4.4 and 6.1 min. (mean, 4.8 min.) and that of lysine vasopressin from 4 to 6 min. (Lee, 1968). These times differ little from those reported for pregnant women at term.

It is therefore difficult to envisage the function, if any, of oxytocinase, and it may be that it is designed to prevent the accumulation of these octapeptide amides in the placental tissues, and more particularly of vasopressin (Mathur and Walker, 1968).

Vasopressin

Following the discovery of the antidiuretic activity of posterior pituitary extract it was noted that the urine secreted in a heart-lung-kidney preparation was very similar to plasma ultrafiltrate and that it could be concentrated either by adding posterior pituitary extract to the circulating blood or by including the head in the circuit (Verney and Starling, 1922; Starling and Verney, 1925; Verney, 1926). Later Verney and his associates (Klisiecki, Pickford, Rothschild and Verney, 1933) showed that there was a time lag of 15 minutes between peak water load of the tissues and the peak of the water diuresis curve; that the ingestion and absorption of water results in decrease in blood osmolarity, inhibition of ADH release and a consequent diuresis which does not begin until after the hormone already in the blood stream has either been removed or inactivated. A year later Simon and Kardos demonstrated that the neurohypophyses of rabbits, guinea-pigs and cats kept for four days on a dry diet became largely depleted of their hormone contents (see Fig. 1). Subsequently the late results of lesions placed in the hypothalamus on water diuresis were tabulated. This type of experiment was followed by observing the direct effects caused by stimulation of certain points in the supraoptic area on both water diuresis and uterine activity. The elegance of the technique of remote control of such stimulation in conscious rabbits contrasts somewhat sharply with the rather haphazard manner in which the results were assessed (Harris, 1947, 1948).

In 1926 Molitor and Pick affirmed that the injection of posterior-pituitary extract into dogs under chloralose narcosis had no effect on water diuresis, and that its intrathecal injection had a more profound effect on water diuresis than when it was injected intravenously. At about the same time Anselmino, Hoffmann and Kennedy (1932) maintained that eclampsia could be attributed to hyperactivity of the neurohypophysis. The curious thing is that nobody had attempted any quantitative estimate of the minimal amount of antidiuretic hormone which when injected intravenously would achieve its physiological effect. Theobald (1934a, b) working with dogs found: that water diuresis in the dog, man and pregnant woman at term was inhibited by a single intravenous injection of from 0·5 to 10 m-u. posterior pituitary extract, Fig. 3; that chloralose narcosis did not affect the efficacy of this extract to inhibit diuresis in the dog; that an amount of this extract which when injected intrathecally has no effect may nevertheless be effective in inhibiting water diuresis when given intravenously; that posterior pituitary extract added to blood may be adsorbed to red blood corpuscles and to plasma proteins; and that water diuresis may be completely inhibited both by afferent nerve stimuli

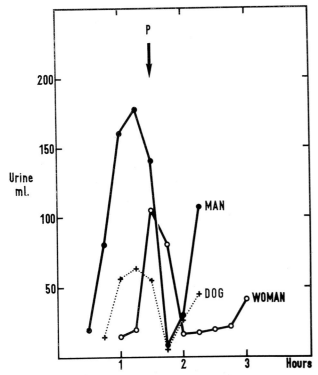

FIG. 3. Graph showing the effects of a single intravenous injection of posterior pituitary extract on water diuresis in a dog, a male medical student and a pregnant woman at term. The dog had been previously hydrated and given 250 ml. water through a stomach tube, the student had drunk 1,000 ml. and the pregnant woman 500 ml. water. The urine was collected and measured at 15 min. intervals. A catheter was used for this purpose in the dog and in the woman. At point P an intravenous injection of posterior pituitary extract was made, 5 m-u. into the dog and 10 m-u. into both the student and the pregnant woman. This provoked an immediate fall in the amount of urine secreted in all three subjects. Composite graph made from two appearing in Theobald, (1934), *Clinical Science*, **1**, 225.

and by emotional disturbances. Subsequently Theobald and Verney (1935) showed that afferent nerve impulses inhibited water diuresis after complete denervation of the kidney.

Theobald (1955) later showed that water diuresis in man could be inhibited by the intravenous infusion of 0·25 m-u. Pitressin/min. and conversely that the intravenous infusion of 50,000 m-u. Pitressin over a period of two hours failed to inhibit water diuresis completely or to maintain an elevated blood pressure. It is unlikely that such a prolonged fall in blood pressure following its initial elevation could be attributed to coronary con-

striction. It also seemed improbable that nature would use the same hormone to inhibit water diuresis and in vastly greater concentration to cause a fleeting rise of blood pressure. The term "vasopressin" so far as it applies to man, dog or bird is therefore as unfortunate and misleading as that of "toxaemia" of pregnancy.

By exteriorizing the carotid artery Verney and his associates showed that water diuresis was inhibited by the intracarotid infusion of hypertonic solutions of sodium and sucrose, but not of urea. They concluded that the osmoreceptors lie somewhere in the peripheral supply of the carotid arteries, probably in the vicinity of the supraoptic nucleus and that they are permeable to urea and semipermeable to glucose (Verney, 1947). It was calculated that an increase of osmotic pressure in blood plasma of 2 per cent equalled a rise in concentration of $Na+$ of 3 milli-equiv/litre and caused a release of 1 μ-u. ADH/sec.

The following facts can be tabulated: Water diuresis is unaccompanied by any change in blood flow through the kidney, and the flow through a denervated kidney runs parallel with that through the innervated kidney.

Human kidneys can reabsorb, without the aid of ADH, some 80 per cent of the 200 litres which are daily filtered through the glomeruli. ADH probably exerts its fine regulating effect mainly on the distal convoluted tubules. It enhances the power of the tubular cells to absorb water against an osmotic gradient, possibly by stimulating local release of hyaluronidase which affects the intracellular cement substance.

There is a definite diurnal rhythm in the secretion of urine as there is in the concentration of steroids in the blood, all part of the activity of the somewhat mysterious biological clock.

Further studies concerning the effect of emotional stress on water diuresis were made by O'Connor and Verney (1942, 1945) and it seems probable that ADH release is more frequently effected by nervous impulses than by changes in blood osmolarity.

A reversible state of diabetes insipidus was provoked in dogs by the injection of di-isopropyl-flurophosphate (DFP) directly into their supraoptic nuclei. DFP inhibits the formation of cholinesterase and it may therefore be concluded that cholinergic afferent fibres play some part in the control of the supraoptic nuclei (Duke, Pickford and Watt, 1950).

It is thus clear that ADH plays an important part in the fine regulation of the amount of water released by the kidneys, but the control of the total amount of water in the body is a very complicated matter which is discussed more fully on page 440. It may however be observed that the excretion in urine of sodium, potassium and water are closely interrelated. Water drunk in quantity "overflows" from the circulation into the tissue spaces until the kidneys are ready to excrete it and the return of the excess water from the tissue spaces into the circulation is usually rapid. Women who routinely take a diuretic twice weekly because of some degree of oedema sometimes find that they may not be able to remove rings from their fingers until several hours after the diuresis is finished so that there is often a delay in readjustment between the fluid compartments of the body. Aldosterone release, controlled by angiotensin, causes sodium retention. The complicated feed back mechanisms involved can be illustrated by two facts. The first is that both oxytocin and ADH release can be prevented by the previous administration of adrenalin. Secondly; the addition of aldosterone to the cat heart-lung-kidney preparation results in the net loss of sodium but its normal action can be restored by adding oxytocin to the circulating blood (Davy and Lockett, 1960).

The Therapeutic Uses of ADH

ADH serves two useful purposes, the one therapeutic and the other diagnostic. Severe diabetes insipidus is associated with the excretion of over six and up to 20 litres of urine daily (up to one tenth of the total glomerular ultrafiltrate). The usual method of controlling this condition is by the intramuscular injection of Pitressin tannate in oil. More recently synthetic lysine-vasopressin nasal spray has been used with considerable success, particularly in the milder cases and also as an adjuvant by patients who either prefer or are forced to give themselves Pitressin injections (Fraser and Scott, 1963; Sjöberg and Luft, 1963; Martin and Mathew, 1964).

It is also used as a test of pituitary-adrenal function. Corticotrophin releasing factors in man are polypeptides formed in the hypothalamus and labelled α and β. It so happens that ADH resembles the β factor and can cause release of corticotrophin. An extensive literature has accumulated concerning the use of ADH for this purpose and was well summarized in a leading article in the British Medical Journal (1966, **2**, 425).

Standardization of Oxytocin

In 1925 a Committee of the League of Nations adopted the U.S.P. Standard Reference Powder as the international standard for posterior pituitary extracts, 0·5 mg. of this powder being equivalent to one international unit. This powder was made from the whole posterior lobes of cattle, collected immediately after death and ground in acetone to remove water and fat. Syntocinon is standardized by the rat uterus method and stabilized by buffering to an acid pH of between 3·0 and 4·0. Small quantities of chlorbutol and ethanol are added as preservatives. One milligram of Syntocinon has an oxytocic activity of about 450 IU and is therefore more than 200 times more potent than the Reference Powder.

The Genesis of the Oxytocin Drip

The intravenous injection of minimal amounts of posterior pituitary extract into hydrated dogs caused such strictly reproducible effects on water diuresis that it was possible by looking at the graphs to pick out those relating to each dog. Seeing that the extract was standardized for its oxytocic activity it was postulated, that if oxytocin were concerned either with instituting or controlling labour, it would be effective in a concentration in the blood strictly comparable with that of ADH which inhibited water diuresis. This concept is implicit in the title "A

centre, or centres, in the hypothalamus controlling menstruation, ovulation, pregnancy and parturition" (Theobald, 1936), and involves the assumption that the human myometrium must become exquisitely sensitive to oxytocin before labour can start.

This concept has been challenged from two different quarters. Caldeyro-Barcia (1961) has advanced the diametrically opposite view that "increased secretion of oxytocin by the neurohypophysis is one of the important factors causing the augmentation in the intensity and frequency of the uterine contractions during pre-labour . . ." and that the work so done dilates the cervix and institutes the onset of true labour. He also believes that the amount of oxytocin released increases as labour advances. The other challenge is that "oxytocin release" triggered by uterine or cervical distension, "plays a role in the expulsion of the foetus" but not in initiating the onset of labour (Fitzpatrick and Walmsley, 1965; Folley and Knaggs, 1964, 1965).

Changes in Myometrial Sensitivity to Oxytocin in Man during the last four weeks of pregnancy

Previous studies have assumed that the average of uterine activity obtained from different women at varying stages of pregnancy can be extrapolated to present a composite picture showing gradually increasing spontaneous uterine activity from the 34th week until term. In the following study spontaneous uterine activity and the effect on it caused by the intravenous infusion of 1 m-u. Syntocinon/min. followed by 2 m-u./min. (each for 30 minutes) were recorded in the same woman at roughly weekly intervals, from the 32nd week of pregnancy until the spontaneous onset of labour. This study was limited to primigravidae (Farr, Robards and Theobald, 1968). Steady increase in spontaneous uterine activity did not occur in a single subject, but increasing response to oxytocin was evident. Effective response to it only became evident shortly before the onset of labour and the intravenous infusion of 0·5 m-u. Syntocinon/min. sufficed on some occasions to put a woman into labour. Oxytocin contractions often persisted for an hour or longer after the infusion was stopped. There appeared to be a random variation in the diurnal pattern of uterine activity and sensitivity tests were useless if marked uterine activity was occurring. All uterine activity is spontaneous and is only affected by oxytocin for brief intervals in a woman's life, immediately before and after, and during labour. It is beyond dispute that increasing sensitivity of the myometrium to oxytocin has been demonstrated in some women but cannot always be recorded and for two reasons. The first is that it may occur suddenly and be missed, and the second is that it may be completely masked by spontaneous uterine activity (Figs. 4-8) (Theobald, Robards, Suter, 1969).

It has previously been reported: that the sensitivity of the myometrium to oxytocin may remain low in those patients who fail to go into labour subsequent to amniotomy and may not increase adequately until four or five days later; that labour may be restarted in patients with secondary uterine inertia by means of an intravenous infusion of 0·5 m-u. Syntocinon/min.; and that on the 4th day of the puerperium both uterine contractions and milk ejection can be caused by the intravenous infusion of 0·2 m-u. Oxytocin/min. (Theobald, Kelsey and Muirhead, 1956; Theobald, 1959). Strips of myometrium from the non-pregnant human uterus do not contract in an oxytocin bath, but those taken from pregnant women become increasingly susceptible to oxytocin as pregnancy advances (Fuchs and Fuchs, 1963). Smyth's sensitivity test is not precise enough for research studies (Smyth, 1965; Turnbull and Anderson, 1968).

Action of Oxytocin on Structures other than the Uterus

The amount of glucose in the blood rises during normal spontaneous labour in women, but this expected rise is prevented by an intravenous oxytocin infusion (Fairweather, 1965). Oxytocin modifies urinary secretion and

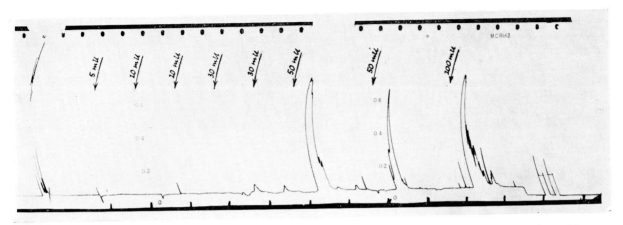

FIG. 4. Sensitivity test by the Bradford method on a woman at term. A glucose water drip was started and traces of uterine activity were made with Smyth's guard-ring tokograph. Time markers register 5 minute intervals. At similar intervals increasing amounts of Syntocinon were injected rapidly into the rubber tubing close to the needle in the vein, while the tube from the drip bottle was temporarily clamped. It was concluded that in this particular woman, during the period of the test, the myometrium was sensitive to between 50 and 100 m-u. Syntocinon. In one patient at term the rapid injection of 2,000 m-u. Syntocinon failed to cause a single uterine contraction. The trace would of course be different if the Syntocinon were given in a continuing intravenous infusion. From Theobald, (1968). Obstetrical and Gynaecological Survey, 23, 109. The traces in the following four figures were also made with Smyth's tokograph.

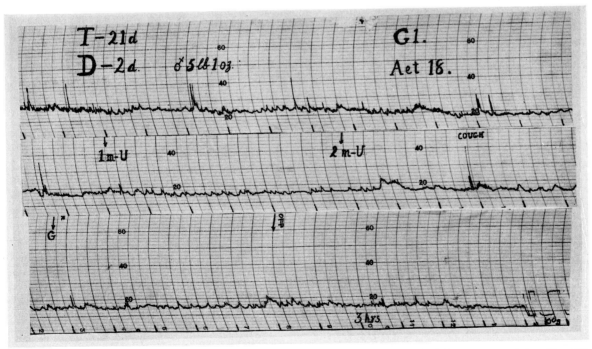

FIG. 5. This trace continues from above downwards and lasts about 3½ hours. It was obtained from a young primigravida, aged 18, some three weeks before labour was due. No significant uterine activity was recorded neither was there any response to the intravenous infusion of 2 m-u. Syntocinon/min. Seeing that she was unexpectedly delivered two days later it must be supposed that a sudden increase in spontaneous activity, and probably in myometrial sensitivity to oxytocin, must have occurred. T denotes term; D, day of delivery, G, glucose infusion, and the arrows show where the Syntocinon infusions were started. The upstroke of the pen when the patient was asked to cough proves that the tokograph was working satisfactorily.

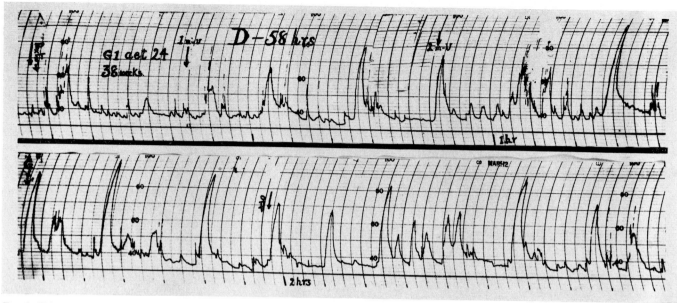

FIG. 6. This trace was obtained from a young primigravida at 38 weeks. There was little spontaneous activity of the uterus either before the glucose drip was started or while it was running. The intravenous infusion of 1 m-u. Syntocinon/min. caused a marked increase in uterine activity and it is a pity that 2 m-u./min. were given. She was due for another sensitivity test three days later, but it was remarked in the notes that she was likely to go into premature labour before then, and she did. This trace provides a marked contrast with that in Fig. 5.

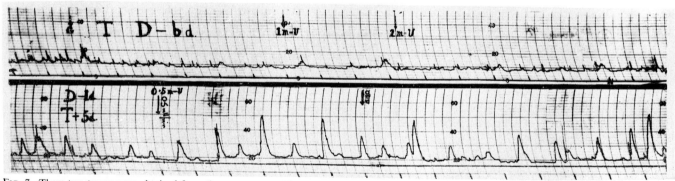

FIG. 7. These two traces were obtained from the same woman, the upper one 6 days and the lower one the day before delivery occurred. There is no sign of any significant activity during the 1½ hours of the first trace, neither did the intravenous infusion of 2 m-u. Syntocinon/min. have any effect on it. The lower trace shows slightly increased spontaneous activity during the glucose-water infusion, and a very definite increase in activity subsequent to the intravenous infusion of 0·5 m-u. Syntocinon/min.

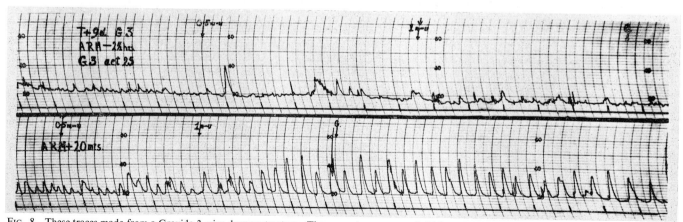

FIG. 8. These traces made from a Gravida 3, nine days postmature. The upper trace was made 2½ hours before amniotomy and shows neither significant spontaneous activity nor response to the intravenous infusion of 1 m-u. Syntocinon/min. The lower trace was made 20 min. after she had returned from having amniotomy done. It shows a slight increase in spontaneous activity, some response to the intravenous infusion of 0·5 m-u. and marked response to the infusion of 1 m-u. Syntocinon/min.

renal clearance in dogs and increases renal plasma flow (RPF) without affecting either glomerular filtration rate (GFR) or the systemic blood pressure (Dicker and Heller, 1943; Berde, 1959; Pickford, 1961). It has an anti-diuretic effect in rats (van Dyke et al., 1955), and in man (Theobald, 1956, 1959) and its effect on water diuresis in the woman varies during the different phases of the menstrual cycle and causes responses at the end of pregnancy which differ from those obtained during the puerperium (Howarth et al., 1963).

When injected intravenously it usually causes vascular dilatation in man, dog and cat, but this action is reversed by the previous administration of oestrogen (Haigh et al., 1963; Deis and Pickford, 1964). Posterior pituitary extract decreases the rate of oedema formation in man (Sacks, 1924) and this action is probably due to the oxytocin fraction (Ferguson, 1962). Both GFR and RPF as well as tubular maxima were said to be reduced in dogs after neurohypophysectomy and the normal renal haemodynamics could be restored by oxytocin but not by vasopressin (Demunbrum et al., 1954). All the above effects, with the possible exception of the first, require pharmacological amounts of oxytocin. There appears to be no experimental evidence to support the view that oxytocin facilitates the ascent of spermatozoa in the uterus.

Milk Ejection

See Section VII by Folley and Cowie.

Pressure in the Human Mammary Gland during Pregnancy, Labour and Parturition

Members of the Montevideo school (Caldeyro-Barcia, 1965) have introduced a polyethylene catheter into a mammary duct and by means of a pressure transducer have recorded intramammary pressures during pregnancy, labour and the puerperium. They stressed three points. The first was that the rhythm of mammary contractions was not identical with that of the uterus. Independence of rhythm of contractions affecting round ligaments and uterus was noted by Hendricks and Moawad, (1965). The second was that the average intramammary pressure rose from 1 mm. Hg. during pregnancy to 20 mm. Hg. between the 5th and 8th days of the puerperium. The third was that the threshold amount of oxytocin which produced a detectable response in intramammary pressure decreased from 100 m-u. during early pregnancy to 1 m-u. during mid-pregnancy and thereafter showed no further change.

It seemed reasonable to conclude that emptying the mammary glands might be a feed back mechanism to promote lactogenesis, for it is well known that in the total lactational performance of an animal these events are closely linked. This hypothesis was tested in man by Haeger and Jacobsohn (1953) with favourable results and it is noteworthy that striking increases in milk yield occurred following one injection and that thereafter lactation usually proceeded normally. Favourable results have been reported by a number of authors including Newton and Egli (1958); Berde (1959), Huntingford (1961), and Kretzschmar and Stoddard (1962). In a fairly extensive

double blind experiment at Bradford it was concluded that the oxytocin nasal spray was clinically ineffective and some even maintain that it does harm. The oxytocin nasal spray indubitably causes milk ejection in normal lactating women and it is claimed by some that if it is used prophylactically it will prevent engorgement and ease the onset of lactation. This may well be true but for many reasons is difficult to prove, because psychological factors are involved. It can be asserted that poor lactation is not often primarily due to unsatisfactory milk ejection and that the intranasal oxytocin spray is at present little used for this purpose in this country and is not used at all in many important centres in the U.S.A. and in Europe.

This may be a convenient point to refer to the use of oxytocin in pharmacological amounts in the prevention and treatment of postpartum haemorrhage. Ergometrine may kill an unsuspected twin and is said from time to time to cause a serious rise in blood pressure. In some Units oxytocin is preferred before the expulsion of the placenta has taken place and in recent years Syntometrine (0·5 mg. ergometrine maleate plus 5 U Syntocinon) has been increasingly used (Fliegner and Hibbard, 1966).

The Action of Oxytocin on the Uterus

The isolated guinea-pig uterus preparation for evaluating posterior pituitary extracts was the first standardized bio-assay procedure (Dale and Laidlaw, 1912). Oxytocin causes the isolated uterus of most laboratory animals to contract, provided the hormonal state of the animal was appropriate when the organ was removed and the ionic composition of the fluid in the organ bath is physiological. The pregnant rabbit uterus does not respond to oxytocin until the very end of pregnancy (Knaus, 1925–6) and this fact has been used as a method for quantitative comparison of oxytocin and related polypeptides (Berde and Cerletti, 1958).

No method of bio-assay gives a reliable guide as to the effect of any of the analogues of oxytocin on the human uterus in vivo (Saameli, 1964). Further, oxytocin has no demonstrable effect on the human myocardium or ureter (Caldeyro-Barcia, 1964) or on the non-pregnant human uterus, whether in vivo or in vitro. It actually exerts an inhibiting effect on intestinal motility in the anaesthetized dog, on the guinea-pig's tracheal chain and on the isolated ileum, both of the guinea-pig and of the rabbit (Levy, 1963).

Mode of Action of Oxytocin

It is crystal clear that oxytocin does not stimulate all plain muscle and the remarkable thing is that whereas the human myometrium is made sensitive to oxytocin by pregnancy, the rabit uterus is rendered insensitive to it by pregnancy, except at its very end. It is therefore the specific response of the plain muscle target organ to it that determines whether or not oxytocin will cause it to contract and this specific response is hormonally determined.

Oxytocin acts by lowering membrane potential and increasing the frequency of the trains of impulses and of the discharges composing each train. It can still cause contractions of strips of plain muscle after the membrane has been completely depolarized by immersion in potassium-Ringer's solution, and can presumably activate the contractile elements of plain muscle apart from the mediation of membrane depolarization (Evans, Schild and Thesleff, (1958).

The Amount of Oxytocin in the Blood

Oxytocin is either eliminated or inactivated in the body in an exponential manner, and many problems would be solved if a reliable method of measuring the amount of this hormone in the blood could be devised. Much painstaking research has been devoted to this problem. The extraction of oxytocin from blood plasma is effected by its application to a dextran gel column (Sephadex G-25, medium grade) and by this method the mean recovery rate was 85 per cent (Folley and Knaggs, 1965). The oxytocin content of the extract thus obtained is

TABLE 1

CLARIFICATION OF NOMENCLATURE

One gram Syntocinon	One gram Standard Powder
1,000 mg.	1,000 mg.
450,000 I.U. (International units)	2,000 I.U.
450,000,000 m-u.	2,000,000 m-u.
450,000,000,000 μ-u.	2,000,000,000 μ-u.
450,000,000,000,000 nano-u.	2,000,000,000,000 nano-u.

The intravenous infusion of 0·5 m-u. Syntocinon/min. would add 100 nano-u./min./ml. blood.

measured by one of four methods: its milk ejection activity on the lactating mammary gland of (a) a guinea-pig and (b) a rat, and its mammatonic effect on strips of either rat or mouse uterus. Retrograde cannulation of the rat's saphenous artery is possible if it is first relaxed with papaverine, and it is important to identify the lactiferous sinus at the base of the nipple and to make sure that the tip of the catheter enters it. The mammatonic method

is much simpler and apparently equally sensitive (Fabian et al., 1968). Whatever method of bioassay has been used it has so far been impossible to detect less than 10 μ-u./ml. plasma, and it is unlikely that these methods can be much further refined.*

It is relatively simple to collect internal jugular vein (into which blood from the neurohypophysis drains) blood from the cow, mare, ewe or goat. It is claimed that considerable quantities of oxytocin are present in such blood from these animals immediately before and during the ejection of their foetuses (see Table 2) but little or none at the onset of parturition. This has led Folley and Knaggs (1964, 1965) to conclude that oxytocin may play no part in the initiation of parturition but only in the ejection of the foetus. It is noteworthy that these and other veterinarians have no experience of the effect of the intravenous infusion of small amounts of oxytocin on the uterine activity of these domestic animals at the onset of parturition.

It is not possible to withdraw blood from the internal jugular vein in man but Coch et al., (1965) found up to 900 μ-u. oxytocin in each ml. blood plasma removed from the external jugular vein of a woman in the second stage of labour; and 300 μ-u. oxytocin on the second day and 100 μ-u. oxytocin/ml. in the *peripheral* blood plasma on the 8th day of the puerperium. Warren and Hawker (1967) claimed to have found up to 2,650 μ-u. oxytocin/ml. in peripheral blood taken from a normal menstruating woman at a time when other observers could find none. Taking the figures of Coch et al., there can be at least 600 m-u. oxytocin circulating in the blood of a woman on the second day of the puerperium at a time when the intravenous infusion of 0·5 m-u. Syntocinon/min. causes increased uterine activity.

Saameli (1963) estimated that the concentration of exogenous oxytocin in the blood which sufficed to cause

---

* Since this chapter was written a radioimmunoassay for oxytocin has been developed (Chard, Forsling and Kitau, 1969).

TABLE 2   MEASUREMENTS OF OXYTOCIN IN BLOOD IN MAN

Authors	Blood from	Amount of oxytocin in one ml. blood in micro-units
Bisset (1961)	Central blood from a man after intravenous injection of nicotine.	4,100
Coch et al. (1965)	Blood *plasma* from external jugular vein.	
	During or just before expulsion of baby.	900
	Peripheral blood *plasma*: 2nd day puerperium.	300
Warren and Hawker (1967)	Peripheral blood: during menstruation.	2,650
	IN ANIMALS *Internal jugular vein blood: during expulsion of foetus*	
Fitzpatrick (1961)	Ewe	3,000
Folley and Knaggs (1964)	Goat	90–300
Fitzpatrick and Walmsley (1965)	Cow	350–1,000
	Mare	12–800

uterine activity during the last three weeks of pregnancy was of the order of 3 μ-u./ml. blood, and Theobald concluded that it might be as little as 70 nano-u./ml. blood at the onset of true labour. In any case the intravenous infusion of 0·5 m-u. Syntocinon/min. often suffices to cause effective uterine contractions at term and may even put a woman into labour. It is quite unreasonable to expect a tocographically detected variation in uterine activity to be caused by a mere fraction of the previously existing level of endogenous oxytocin. It is still more unreasonable to believe that 600 or more m-u. oxytocin circulate in the blood of a woman on the second day of the puerperium. Published results concerning the bioassay of oxytocin in blood vary widely and are in any event unrealistic when applied to man, but some obstetricians have been deluded by them.

Myometrial Changes occurring apart from Pregnancy

The proper study of the uterus must begin and end with the non-pregnant state. All uterine activity is spontaneous, begins at or before puberty, lasts well into the menopause and is but modified by the milieu in which it operates. Unlike other plain muscle the length of the myometrial fibre alters but little during contraction, except during labour, and unlike all other structures the effects caused by stimulation of the nerves which supply it vary with its hormonal state. Changes in the myometrium and cervix which precede the onset of labour in man include: (1) alteration in electrolyte and water content, both within and without the cells (Hawkins and Nixon, 1958, 1961; Cibils and Schweid, 1964), (2) increase in intramyometrial actomyosin and of high energy phosphates (Csapo, 1961; Kumar, Russell and Barnes, 1962), (3) marked increase in extensibility and in length-tension relation in myometrial strips (Schofield, 1966; Schofield and Wood, 1964), (4) alterations in electrical conductivity in the myometrium (Csapo, 1961; Jung, 1961, 1962), (5) changes in the physical structure of the cervix (Cullen and Harkness, 1958, 1959), and (6) increase in the sensitivity of the myometrium to oxytocin (Theobald, 1936, 1959; Theobald, Kelsey and Muirhead, 1956; Caldeyro-Barcia and Theobald, 1968). All these changes, with the exception of the last, can be provoked in spayed animals by giving hormones but never to the same degree as seen at the end of pregnancy.

Similar changes, but never to the same degree, can be studied in the non-pregnant human uterus during the menstrual cycle. At the fourth day of the cycle the contractions are frequent (about three a minute), of low amplitude and were called A waves by Moir (1934). These gradually merge into what he described as B waves, which are of high amplitude and low frequency, and are in fact indistinguishable from those seen in pregnant women before the onset of labour. Hendricks has described a technique which has made it possible to make such studies in depth (Hendricks, 1964, 1965; Bengtsson and Theobald, 1965, 1966; Cibils, 1967). Seeing that effective uterine contractions can occur in the non-pregnant state apart altogether from oxytocin, it is unrealistic to assume that oxytocin is essential *merely* to cause efficient uterine activity.

The Initiation of Labour

"The genetic interaction in the Holstein-Friesian may prolong pregnancy to 90 days past term with a foetus living *in utero;* among Guernseys, such a combination may result in a pregnancy of 510 days, the normal gestation being 280 days. In all instances reported, the foetus is alive. At no time during pregnancy, at term, and at no time during the post-term period, is there any attempt at labor" (Holm, 1965). "The fetus as a factor in the initiation of labor", and also "The role of immune phenomena in labor" are discussed in "Initiation of Labor", pp. 159–92. It must, however be born in mind that after removal or destruction of the foetus in the monkey, rat or mouse, "physiological" pregnancy persists, and in the monkey for as long as three calendar months (van Wagenen and Newton, 1943). In man labour may not start until several weeks after the death of the foetus, nearer indeed to the expected date of delivery than to that on which the foetus died. The main problem is why the uterus not only tolerates but accelerates growth at an unnecessary rate to accommodate the embryo, and the factors concerned cannot include as yet unformed foetal structures. It is reasonable to suppose that the cessation of these selfsame factors will result in the onset of labour. The genetic interactions described by Holm must therefore be regarded as abnormal.

THE OXYTOCIN DRIP

The amount of oxytocin in the first drip given to induce labour was *calculated* and is still recommended (Theobald, Graham, Campbell, Gange and Driscoll, 1948). A year later Hellman (1949) mentioned the intravenous infusion of posterior pituitary extract in the treatment of uterine dystocia but it was not until 1950 that he and his colleagues recognized the full significance of this discovery (Hellman, Harris and Reynolds, 1950). Page (1943) in a short communication on "pitocin tannate in oil", in the treatment of uterine inertia, stated that he had found that the intravenous infusion of from 10 to 20 units of Pitocin in one litre of normal saline gave more physiological responses than did Pitocin tannate. He gave no indication that this infusion was continued for any length of time in the one subject or was repeated in another. Since 1950 an extensive world literature has accumulated on this subject.

Broadly speaking the oxytocin infusion has been more frequently used in "private" patients in North America where the obstetrician stays with the patient until she is delivered, and in "hospital" patients in the British Isles where 80 per cent of all confinements are conducted by midwives. In this country the Bradford method is largely followed and consists of amniotomy followed the next day by an intravenous oxytocin drip if the patient is not by then in labour. Quicker delivery is achieved by starting the drip immediately after amniotomy, but this involves greater expenditure of money and increased work for house surgeons, and is reserved for patients who need speedy delivery. The main variations, and they are but variations, consist in the amount of oxytocin given, the system by which the increase in dosage is regulated, and whether the actual dosage which causes efficient uterine activity is maintained or reduced. It is not clear whether the writers who advocate large amounts of oxytocin actually believe that oxytocin induced contractions play any part in the expulsion of the foetus, but they are careful to exclude patients with cephalo-pelvic disproportion and other stigmata. Evidence has already been given to suggest that a woman does not go into labour until her myometrium becomes exquisitely sensitive to oxytocin, and if this be true it is highly dangerous to give oxytocin in pharmacological amounts without adequate monitoring.

Barnes (1965) increases the amount of oxytocin infused intravenously until satisfactory uterine contractions occur, and states that there is no "God-given dosage". "We often can't tell when we are overdosing unless we have an intraamniotic catheter present and a pressure tracing available". In such hands and with such monitoring pharmacological amounts of oxytocin *may* be given safely by means of some electrically driven mechanical pump, even though they are quite unnecessary. It is significant that Caldeyro-Barcia (1964) rarely finds it necessary to give more than 8 m-u. Syntocinon/min. and that Hendricks (1963) affirms that for 80 per cent of his time he does not exceed 5 m-u./min. and in only 3 per cent of the time does he exceed 10 m-u./min. Neither of these writers leaves the woman until she is delivered, and both invariably monitor their patients with electronic equipment.

It is therefore disturbing that Turnbull and Anderson (1968) advocate giving up to 137 m-u. Syntocinon/min. with but "constant supervision" afforded by medical *or* nursing staff who assess "uterine contractility by simple palpation". One ruptured uterus occurred in 1965 and at least three babies in the first three months of 1964 died "in part at least to the effects of the increased dose of oxytocin used".

Transbuccal Oxytocin

Buccal oxytocin was reintroduced into obstetrics, after an interval of some 30 years, by Dillon, Douglas, du Vigneaud and Barber (1960). The original tablet contained 200 units and a day's course of 22 tablets took about five hours to complete. During this time the subject was advised to refrain from eating or drinking and to restrict conversation. Many patients were given 8,800 or more units of oxytocin, enough to induce labour in about 4,000 women if given intravenously. This course has been modified in different centres, but the dosage is always high.

It is difficult to assess results as in many of the reported series amniotomy was also done. It is however clear that the rate of the transbuccal absorption of oxytocin is both unpredictable and incalculable. It is idle to pretend that the removal of the tablet can prevent the continuing activity of the amount already absorbed.

The advantage claimed for the method is that it avoids operative interference but an unknown, and probably high, percentage of these women will have to submit to operative interference after having endured the tablet for two days. On the other hand only 20 per cent of women who have their membranes ruptured need an oxytocin infusion, and only 7 per cent will need it for more than one day. A pharmacological intravenous oxytocin infusion can kill, but the danger can be greatly minimized by careful monitoring, whereas no such care can overcome the risks of buccal oxytocin. The gravamen of the charge against buccal oxytocin is that a very potent and dangerous substance is administered by a route which defies absorption analysis.

INDUCTION OF LABOUR: RESULTS

Many careful tocographic studies have been made showing the effects of oxytocin on the uterus immediately before and during labour, but until the report of Turnbull and Anderson (1968) no series, other than those published from Bradford (Theobald, Kelsey and Muirhead, 1956; Theobald, 1963) have shown in detail what happened to a given section of a hospital population in whom labour was induced. The last significant paper on induction of labour by amniotomy without using oxytocin was published by Tennent and Black (1954) and this will stand for all time as the most important record of results which flow from low amniotomy and also as a tribute to impeccable obstetrics. It is therefore proposed to report the main features of the Bradford results and with those published by Turnbull and Anderson, and compare them with those published by Tennent and Black and thus to evaluate the overall significance of oxytocin.

Bradford is a large industrial city with a fairly rapidly changing population which has included high numbers of "displaced" persons and presently accommodates a considerable immigrant population, notably from Pakistan. Half the women were initially booked for domiciliary confinement. By the end of 1960 labour had been induced in over 5,000 women without a single rupture of the uterus and without caesarean section having to be done because of foetal distress caused by uterine hypercontractility due to oxytocin. The induction studies were prospective and when amniotomy was done the woman was provided with a green card filled in with all relevant information which was completed after delivery was complete, and filed separately after she was discharged so that information about the baby could be included. The membranes were ruptured in the operating theatre, not in the labour ward, with elaborate antiseptic precautions, usually between 1200 and 1800 hrs. An oxytocin drip was started the next morning if the woman was not by then in labour and she was then furnished with a white card which was also filed separately as soon after the patient was discharged as possible.

No contraindication to induction of labour was recognized and amongst the 3,131 patients induced the head was "high" in 266 and was in many of them associated with cephalo-pelvic disproportion. Labour was induced in many women who had previously been delivered by caesarean section and 38 per cent of all sections done in the "oxytocin group" were done in Gravidae 2 and 3.

At least one Gravida 20 had an oxytocin drip. If the cervix was long (2 inches), hard and would not admit the tip of a finger (such cases occurred very rarely) induction was delayed unless the indication for it was urgent. In such cases a Drew Smyth catheter was used to rupture the membranes. It may be added in parenthesis that patients with hypertension and proteinuria (pregnancy

The amniotomy-delivery times in women who did not require oxytocin are shown in Table 4 and the results reported are strictly comparable with those reported by Turnbull and Anderson save for the fact that they did a number of caesarean sections in this group. The methods of delivery in women induced because of postmaturity are shown in Table 5. The figures for 1957–8 and 1959–60

TABLE 3

INDUCTION OF LABOUR IN WOMEN 215 OR MORE DAYS PREGNANT. METHODS OF DELIVERY, 1957–60 (INCLUSIVE)

	Total Numbers	Number of cases of			
		Oxytocin Drip	Spontaneous Delivery	Caesarean Section	Forceps Extraction
Primigravidae	1,187	273 (23)	928 (78)	48 (4)	211 (18)
Gravidae 2 and 3	1,260	210 (17)	1,183 (94)	36 (3)	41 (3)
Gravidae 4 and 4 plus	684	180 (26)	658 (96)	13 (2)	13 (2)
Totals	3,131	663 (21)	2,769 (89)	97 (3·1)	265 (8·5)

Percentage figures in brackets.

(This Table, together with Tables 4 and 5, is reproduced from *British Obstetric and Gynaecological Practice*, Claye and Bourne, Heinemann Medical Books Ltd., 1963.)

"toxaemia") often proved to be the most difficult subjects in whom to start labour, and this fact was noted by Tennent and Black (1954) and also by Turnbull and Anderson (1968). This clinical fact in no way supports the claim that "toxaemia" is associated with hypercontractility of the uterus, (Cobo, 1964).

The overall results are clearly shown in Table 3: 79 per cent of all women went into labour as the result of amniotomy alone; the caesarean section rate was 3·1 per cent; the forceps rate was 8·5 per cent and only 7 per cent of all women induced required a drip for more than 8 hours. During the years 1959–60 there were 1,674 inductions and only 10 perinatal deaths in babies weighing 5 lb. (2·3 kg.) or over, and of these 10, only 5 were born to women who had oxytocin. It may be observed that if amniotomy were done at 1200 hrs., the drip would be stopped at 2100 hrs. on the following day, 33 hours after amniotomy, and would be stopped the next day 57 hours after the membranes were ruptured. If amniotomy were done at 1800 hrs. the corresponding figures would be 27 and 51 hours. Amniotomy-delivery times were not recorded for the women who had oxytocin but it can be stated that just over 2 per cent of all inductions received a drip more than 51 hours after amniotomy. If these women, who delivered spontaneously, had been delivered by caesarean section, the section rate for the series would have been increased from 3·1 per cent to just over 5 per cent and would have included most of the women with cephalo-pelvic disproportion.

are shown separately just to illustrate the consistency of the results.

It can be calculated from Table 3 that 40 per cent of the total number induced were Gravidae 2 and 3, whereas it is

TABLE 4

HOURS BETWEEN AMNIOTOMY AND DELIVERY IN PATIENTS WHO DID NOT REQUIRE AN OXYTOCIN DRIP

1957

Total Numbers	6 hours and less	7–10	11–12	13–18	19–24	25–26	36+
523	95 (18)	157 (30)	68 (13)	97 (19)	58 (11)	42 (8)	6 (1·0)

61 per cent

1960

645	159 (25)	197 (31)	70 (11)	132 (20)	47 (7)	24 (4)	16 (2·5)

67 per cent

Percentage figures in brackets.

TABLE 5

INDUCTION OF LABOUR: METHODS OF DELIVERY IN POSTMATURE WOMEN

| | 1957 *and* 1958 | | | | | 1959 *and* 1960 | | | | |
| | Total Nos. | *Number of cases of* | | | | Total Nos. | *Number of cases of* | | | |
		Oxytocin Drip	*Spontaneous Delivery*	*Caesarean Section*	*Forceps Extraction*		*Oxytocin Drip*	*Spontaneous Delivery*	*Caesarean Section*	*Forceps Delivery*
Primigravidae	294	55 (19)	246 (84)	13 (4·5)	35 (12)	328	67 (20)	264 (80)	10 (3)	54 (16)
Gravidae 2 and 3	261	34 (13)	254 (97)	2 (0·8)	5 (2)	289	42 (15)	269 (93)	9 (3)	11 (4)
Gravidae 4 and 4+	125	30 (24)	122 (98)	1 (0·8)	2 (1·5)	197	48 (25)	192 (97)	1 (0·5)	4 (2)
Totals	680	119 (17·5)	622 (92)	16 (2·3)	42 (6)	814	157 (19)	725 (89)	20 (2·4)	69 (8·5)

Percentage figures in brackets.

shown in Table 6 that only 14 per cent of the total number of Gravidae 2 and 3 delivered in the city required labour to be induced. It may be added that Gravidae 4 and 4 plus usually had rapid labours and provided the highest number of those which occurred within 6 hours of amniotomy. They also provided the highest moiety of those in whom labour was most difficult to start. The essential difference between the results published by Tennent and Black (1954) and those published from Bradford are shown in Figures 9 and 10. It will be seen from Fig. 9 that the number of women in labour within 24 hours of amniotomy was very similar in all three series. The significant feature is what happened to the women who did not go into labour during that period; 25 per cent in Lanark

and 21 per cent in Bradford. It is shown in Fig. 10 that nearly 70 per cent of the Lanark and 90 per cent of the Bradford women who were not in labour within 24 hours, had started labour within 72 hours of amniotomy. In other words 10 per cent of the total Lanark inductions took more than 72 hours in which to start labour compared with just over 2 per cent in Bradford. These figures

TABLE 6

BRADFORD 1957–60

PERCENTAGES OF PARITIES SHOWN IN TABLE 3
COMPARED WITH THOSE OF TOTAL DELIVERIES IN CITY

| | Total Number | *Percentages of parities* | | |
		Primigravidae	*Gravidae 2 and 3*	*Gravidae 4 and 4 plus*
Deliveries in city (1961)	5177	29	45	26
Numbers induced (1957–60)	3131	38	40	22
Percentages of total deliveries in whom labour was induced		21	14	15
Percentages of total deliveries given an oxytocin drip		5	2·4	4

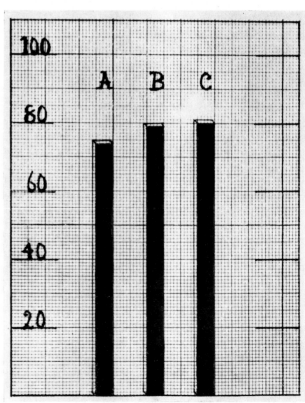

FIG. 9. Histogram indicating percentages of women who went into labour within 24 hours of amniotomy: A, Lanark, B, Bradford, and C, Aberdeen.

show two things clearly: that the main contribution of exogenous oxytocin is to shorten the time interval between amniotomy and the onset of labour and in consequence to lower perinatal mortality, and that those who advocate pharmacological oxytocin infusions do not stand on very sure ground.

Aberdeen is a sheltered non-industrial city with a stable and relatively homogeneous population, and a high hospital delivery rate. During 1964 labour was induced in 1,284 women after all those with suspected cephalo-

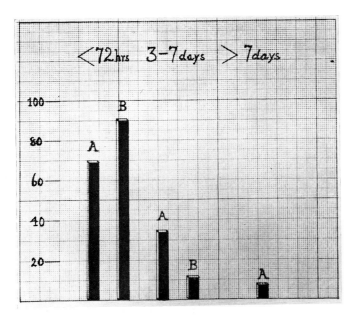

Fig. 10. Histogram showing what happened to the 25 per cent of women at Lanark and the 21 per cent at Bradford who did not go into labour within 24 hours of amniotomy. Column A (Lanark) shows that 70 per cent of these women went into labour between 24 and 72 hours after amniotomy. The corresponding figure for Bradford was 90 per cent.

pelvic disproportion had been excluded. The caesarean section rate was 4·4 per cent, the vaginal operative rate 18·7 per cent and the perinatal mortality rate was 17·3, which probably included babies weighing less than 5 lb. (2·34 kg.). Turnbull and Anderson (1968) claim that "the efficacy of induction of labour can best be judged by the time interval between rupture of the membranes and delivery of the baby". An alternative view is that efficient induction means safe delivery of a healthy infant with the lowest operative interference rate.

Just over 2 per cent of the Bradford women were given oxytocin after more than 57 hours had elapsed from amniotomy. It is difficult to believe that the overall time interval between amniotomy and delivery varied greatly between the Bradford and Aberdeen patients. The thing that did vary was the amount of oxytocin given; for whereas in Bradford in 1960 only 3·4 per cent of all the women who had an oxytocin drip received more than 5 m-u. Syntocinon/min., Turnbull and Anderson (1968) gave up to 137 m-u. Syntocinon/min. In a comparatively small series they

had one ruptured uterus and the loss of three babies attributable in part or in whole to oxytocin. It seems reasonable to postulate that if extreme pharmacological amounts of oxytocin are advocated they should be given through an electrically driven mechanical pump and be monitored by electronic devices and not by palpation by the nursing staff. The oxytocin drip should be reserved for "physiological" amounts of oxytocin.

CONCLUSIONS

There is no proof that oxytocin is necessary for normal delivery, neither is there convincing evidence that it can occur without it, either in laboratory animals or in man. In the small number of women who have become pregnant, or delivered subsequent to hypophysectomy, effective labour has occurred, but these women were probably not devoid of oxytocin and in any case an adequate amount for the purpose could have been supplied by the foetus.

The uterus shows spontaneous activity throughout the reproductive life of the woman, but the pattern of its unceasing activity changes during each menstrual cycle. The contractions during menstruation vary little from those that occur at the beginning of labour, but owe nothing to oxytocin. Indeed it has been clearly shown that oxytocin has relatively little effect on plain muscle and may even cause it to relax.

It is true that uterine strips from most laboratory animals contract when placed in an oxytocin bath, but for the purpose of this discussion attention will be focussed on two significant facts. The first is that whereas oxytocin causes the non-pregnant rabbit uterus to contract it has no effect on the pregnant rabbit uterus whether tested *in vitro* or *in vivo*, until a few hours before the onset of labour. Conversely, oxytocin has no effect on the non-pregnant human uterus, whether *in vitro* or *in vivo*, but the myometrium becomes sensitized to it both *in vitro* and *in vivo* by (or during) pregnancy. Whereas spontaneous uterine activity occurs unceasingly by day and by night throughout the reproductive life of the woman and is modified by hormonal influences, endogenous oxytocin affects its contractility pattern for but a few hours in a woman's life, immediately before and after, and during labour.

It can therefore be stated categorically that oxytocin acts on the pregnant uterus, not because of its inherent ability to do so, but because of the specific sensitivity of the target organ to it. Pregnancy, in some at present unknown way, decreases the sensitivity of the rabbit uterus and increases that of the human uterus to oxytocin. It has been shown that up to 75 per cent of the changes in the various parameters characteristic of pregnancy (such as alterations in electrolyte and water content both within and without the myometrial cell, increase in intramyometrial actomyosin, marked increase in extensibility in myometrial strips, alteration in electrical conductivity of the myometrium, and changes in the physical structure of the cervix) can be provoked in spayed animals by giving oestrogen, progesterone and relaxin, but it is not known what causes the remaining 25 per cent of changes, or what alters the sensitivity of the myometrium to oxytocin. It seems clear that the physico-chemical changes associated with pregnancy cause the changes both in the cervix and in the myometrium and that together with unknown factors they cause increased spontaneous activity and increased myometrial sensitivity to oxytocin. It is probable that changes in the cervix precede and are not caused by uterine contractions.

It is generally conceded that the sensitivity of the human myometrium to oxytocin increases as pregnancy advances to the 34th week, and evidence has been provided above that at least in some women this sensitivity becomes exquisite just before the onset of true labour. In addition to this evidence it may be noted that 80 per cent of all women in whom labour is induced go into labour within 24 hours of amniotomy and in all such cases respond to the infusion of 5 m-u. Syntocinon/min.; that the myometrium has been shown to be relatively insensitive to oxytocin in those women who fail to go into labour after amniotomy and that this sensitivity increases before the onset of labour; and that all women will ultimately go into labour whether or not their membranes are ruptured. It must also be asked why both the myometrium and the mammary myoepithelial cells become sensitive to oxytocin during pregnancy. The fact that a few women have a myometrium insensitive to oxytocin at the time the obstetrician wants to induce labour must not be allowed to cloud the overwhelming evidence that oxytocin has been provided as a fine regulator of coordination of uterine activity just as ADH is a fine regulator of renal water metabolism.

It therefore seems unreasonable to attempt to cause accouchement forcé by flogging the uterus with oxytocin. The danger of the pharmacological intravenous infusion of oxytocin is that the dose of the hormone may be increased at the very moment that the sensitivity of the myometrium to it is increasing. There is little evidence either that oxytocin contractions can expel a foetus or that increasing sensitivity of the myometrium to endogenous oxytocin occurs much faster while strong oxytocin contractions are occurring. On the other hand there is clear evidence that 90 per cent of all women 37 or more weeks pregnant will go into labour within 72 hours of amniotomy, without receiving any exogenous oxytocin. If oxytocin is involved in causing and regulating parturition, the above fact can only mean that the myometrium ultimately becomes sensitive to that amount of oxytocin which is released by the neurohypophysis, and there is no evidence that this amount is augmented above the normal non-pregnant level.

REFERENCES

Anselmino, K. J., Hoffmann, F. and Kennedy, W. P. (1932), "Relation of Hyperfunction of Posterior Lobe of Hypophysis to Eclampsia and Nephropathy of Pregnancy," *Edinb. med. J.*, **39**, 376.

Barer, R., Heller, H. and Lederis, K. (1963), "The Isolation, Identification and Properties of the Hormonal Granules of the Neurohypophysis," *Proc. roy. Soc. (B)*, **158**, 388.

Barnes, A. C. (1965), "Clinical Circumstances at the Time of Labour," p. 214, in *Initiation of Labor*, eds. J. M. Marshall and W. M. Burnett, U.S. Public Health Service Publication, No. 1390, Washington, D.C.

Bell, W. Blair (1909), "Therapeutic Value of the Infundibular Extract in Shock, Uterine Atony and Intestinal Paresis," *Brit. med. J.*, **2**, 1609.

Bengtsson, L. Ph. and Theobald, G. W. (1966), "The Effects of Oestrogen and Gestagen on the Non-pregnant Human Uterus," *J. Obstet. Gynaec. Brit. Cwlth.*, **73**, 273.

Berde, B. (1959), *Recent Progress in Oxytocin Research*. Springfield: Charles C. Thomas.

Berde, B. (1965), "Some Observations on the Circulatory Effects of Oxytocin, Vasopressin, and Similar Polypeptides," pp. 11–34, in *Advances in Oxytocin Research*, ed. J. M. Pinkerton. Oxford: Pergamon Press.

Berde, B. and Cerletti, A. (1958), "Quantitative Comparison of Substances Related to Oxytocin: a New Test," *Acta endocr.*, **27**, 314.

Berde, B., Cerletti, A. and Konzett, H. (1961), "The Biologica, Activity of a Series of Peptides Related to Oxytocin," pp. 247–2641 in *Oxytocin*, eds. R. Caldeyro-Barcia and H. Heller. Oxford: Pergamon Press.

Bisset, G. W. (1961), "The Assay of Oxytocin and Vasopressin in the Blood and the Mechanism of Inactivation of these Hormones by Sodium Thioglycollate," pp. 380–398, in *Oxytocin*, eds. R. Caldeyro-Barcia and H. Heller. Oxford: Pergamon Press.

Boissonas, R. A., Guttman, St., Jacquenod, P. -A. and Waller, J. -P. (1955), "Une nouvelle synthèse de l'oxytocine," *Helv. chim. acta*, **38**, 1491.

British Medical Journal (1966), "Test of Pituitary-Adrenal Function," Leading Article, **2**, 425.

Caldeyro-Barcia, R. (1964), personal communication.

Caldeyro-Barcia, R. (1961), "Actions of Pregnant Uterus," pp. 73–84, in *Physiology of Prematurity*, ed. M. Kowlessar. New York: John Macy Jr. Foundation.

Caldeyro-Barcia, R. (1965), in *Initiation of Labor*, eds. J. M. Marshall and W. M. Burnett. U.S. Public Health Service Publication, No. 1390, Washington, D.C., pp. 29–34, 63.

Caldeyro-Barcia, R. and Alvarez, H. (1954), "Effect of Presacral Nerve Stimulation on Contractility of Non-pregnant Human Uterus," *J. appl. Physiol.*, **6**, 556.

Caldeyro-Barcia, R. and Theobald, G. W. (1968), "Sensitivity of the Pregnant Human Myometrium to Oxytocin," *Amer. J. Obstet. Gynec.*, **102**, 1181.

Chan, W. Y., Fear, R. and du Vigneaud, V. (1967), "Some Pharmacologic Studies on 1-L-Penicillamine-oxytocin and 1-Deamino-penicillamine-oxytocin: Two Potent Oxytocin Inhibitors," *Endocrinology*, **81**, 1267.

Chard, T. (1969), Personal communication.

Chard, T., Forsling, M. L. and Kitau, M. J. (1969), "Development of a Radio-immunoassay for Oxytocin," *J. Endocrin.*, **43**, lxi–lxii.

Cibils, L. A. (1967), "Contractility of the Non-pregnant Human Uterus," *Views and Reviews*, **30**, 441.

Cibils, L. A. and Schweid, D. E., "Electrolyte Content and Distribution in Human Myometrium." (1) 1964. "Postmenopausal Age Group," *Amer. J. Obstet. Gynec.*, **88**, 715. (2) 1966. "Childbearing Age Group," *Amer. J. Obstet. Gynec.*, **94**, 619.

Cobo, E. (1964), "Uterine Hypercontractility in Toxemia of Pregnancy," *Amer. J. Obstet. Gynec.*, **90**, 505.

Coch, J. A., Brovetto, J., Cabot, H. M., Fielitz, C. A. and Caldeyro-Barcia, R. (1965), "Oxytocin-equivalent Activity in the Plasma of Women in Labor and During the Puerperium," *Amer. J. Obstet. Gynec.*, **91**, 10.

Cross, B. A. and van Dyke, H. B. (1953), "The Effects of Highly Purified Posterior Pituitary Principles on the Lactating Mammary Gland of the Rabbit," *J. Endocr.*, **9**, 232.

Csapo, A. (1961), "Defence Mechanism of Pregnancy," pp. 3–27, in *Progesterone and the Defence Mechanism of Pregnancy*. Eds. G. E. W. Wolstenholme and M. P. Cameron. London: Churchill.

Cullen, B. M. and Harkness, R. D. (1958), "Effect of Oestradiol, Progesterone and Relaxin on the Physical Properties of the Uterine Cervix," *J. Physiol.*, 46P.

Cullen, B. M. and Harkness, R. D. (1959), "The Effect of Hormones on the Physical Properties and Collagen Content of the Rat's Uterine Cervix," *J. Physiol.*, **152**, 419.

Dale, H. H. (1906), "On Some Physiological Actions of Ergot," *J. Physiol.*, **34**, 163.

Dale, H. H. and Laidlaw, P. P. (1912), "A Method of Standardizing Pituitary (Infundibular) Extracts," *J. Pharmacol. exper. Ther.*, **4**, 75.

Davy, M. J. and Lockett, M. F. (1960), "Actions and Interactions of Aldosterone Monoacetate and Neurohypophysial Hormones on the Isolated Cat Kidney," *J. Physiol.*, **152**, 206.

Deis, R. P. and Pickford, M. (1964), "The Effect of Autonomic Blocking Agents on Uterine Contractions of the Rat and Guinea-pig," *J. Physiol.*, **173**, 215.

Demunbrum, T. W., Keller, A. D., Levkoff, H. H. and Purser, R. M. Jr. (1954), "Pitocin Restoration of Renal Hemodynamics to Pre-neurohypophysectomy Levels," *Amer. J. Physiol.*, **179**, 429.

Denamur, R. (1965), "The Hypothalamic-Neurohypophysial System and the Milk Ejection Reflex," Rev. Article No. 129. *Dairy Sci. Abstr.*, **27**, (5), pp. 193–224; (b) pp. 263–280.

Dicker, H. B. and Heller, H. (1946), "The Renal Action of Posterior Pituitary Extract and its Fractions as Analysed by Clearance Experiments in Rats," *J. Physiol.*, **104**, 353.

Dillon, T. F., Douglas, R. G., du Vigneaud, V. and Barber, M. L. (1960). *J. Obstet. Gynae.*, **15**, 587.

Duke, H. N., Pickford, M. and Watt, J. A. (1950), "The Immedaite and Delayed Effects of Diisopropylfluorophosphate Injected into the Supraoptic Nuclei of Dogs," *J. Physiol.*, **111**, 81.

van Dyke, H. B., Adamsons, K. (Jr.) and Engel, S. L. (1955), "Aspects of the Biochemistry and Physiology of the Neurohypophysial Hormones," *Recent Progr. Hormone Res.*, *N.Y.*, **11**, 1.

van Dyke, H. B. (1961), "Some Features of the Pharmacology of Oxytocin, pp. 48–66, in *Oxytocin*, eds. R. Caldeyro-Barcia and H. Heller. Oxford: Pergamon Press.

Embrey, M. P. and Moir, J. C. (1967), "A Comparison of the Oxytocic Effects of Synthetic Vasopressin and Oxytocin," *J. Obstet. Gynaec. Brit. Cwlth.*, **74**, 648.

Evans, D. H. L., Schild, H. O. and Thesleff, S. (1958), "Effects of Drugs on Depolarized Plain Muscle," *J. Physiol.*, **143**, 474.

Fabian, M., Forsling, M. L., Jones, J. J. and Lee, J. (1968), "Oxytocin Assay with the Rat Mammary Gland *in vivo* and *in vitro*," *J. Physiol. Proc.*, 12–13th Jan.

Fairweather, D. V. I. (1965), "Changes in Serum Non-esterified Fatty Acid Levels in Spontaneous and Oxytocin Induced Labour," *J. Obstet. Gynaec. Brit. Cwlth.*, **72**, 408.

Farr, C. J., Robards, M. F. and Theobald, G. W. (1968), "Changes in the Myometrial Sensitivity to Oxytocin in Man during the Last Six Weeks of Pregnancy," *J. Physiol.*, **196**, 58–59.

Fekete, K. (1930), "Beiträge zur Physiologie der Gravidität," *Endokrinologie*, **7**, 364.

Ferguson, J. K. W. (1962), personal communication.

Fitzpatrick, R. J. (1961), "The Estimation of Small Amounts of Oxytocin in Blood," pp. 358–377, in *Oxytocin*, eds. R. Caldeyro-Barcia and H. Heller. Oxford: Pergamon Press.

Fitzpatrick, R. J. and Walmsley, C. F. (1965), "Release of Oxytocin during Parturition, 51–72, in *Advances in Oxytocin Research*, ed. J. H. M. Pinkerton. Oxford: Pergamon Press.

Fliegner, J. R. and Hibbard, B. M. (1966), "Active Management of the Third Stage of Labour," *Brit. med. J.*, **2**, 622.

Folley, S. J. (1956), *The Physiology and Biochemistry of Lactation*, Edinburgh: Oliver and Boyd.

Folley, S. J. and Knaggs, G. S. (1964), "Observations on Oxytocin Release in Ruminants," *J. Reprod. Fertil.*, **8**, 265.

Folley, S. J. and Knaggs, G. S. (1965), "Levels of Oxytocin in the Jugular Vein Blood of Goats during Parturition," *J. Endocr.*, **33**, 301.

Fraser, R. and Scott, D. J. (1963), *Lancet*, **1**, 1159.

Fuchs, A.-R. and Fuchs, F. (1963), "Spontaneous Motility and Oxytocin Response of the Pregnant and Non-pregnant Human Muscle in Vitro," *J. Obstet. Gynaec. Brit. Cwlth.*, **70**, 658.

Glendening, M. B., Titus, M. A., Schroeder, S. A., Mohun, G. and Page, E. W. (1965), "The Destruction of Oxytocin and Vasopressin by the Aminopeptidases in Sera from Pregnant Women," *Amer. J. Obstet. Gynec.*, **92**, 814.

Haeger, K. and Jacobsohn, D. (1953), "A Contribution to the Study of Milk Ejection in Women," *Acta physiol. scand.*, **30**, Suppl. 3, 152.

Haigh, A. L., Kitchin, A. H. and Pickford, M. (1963), "The Effect of Oxytocin on Hand Blood Flow in Man following the Administration of an Oestrogen and Isoprenaline," *J. Physiol.*, **169**, 161.

Harris, G. W. (1947), "The Innervation and Actions of the Neurohypophysis; an Investigation using the Method of Remote-control Stimulation," *Philos. Trans. B.*, **232**, 385.

Harris, G. W. (1948), "The Excretion of an Antidiuretic Substance by the Kidney, after Electrical Stimulation of the Neurohypophysis in the Unanaesthetized Rabbit," *J. Physiol.*, **107**, 430.

Hawkins, D. F. and Nixon, W. C. W. (1961), "The Influence of Oestrogen and Progesterone on the Electrolytes of the Human Uterus," *J. Obstet. Gynaec. Brit. Cwlth.*, **68**, 62.

Hellman, L. M. (1949), "Factors Influencing Successful Posterior Pituitary Treatment of Functional Uterine Dystocia with Particular Consideration of its Intravenous Administration," *Amer. J. Obstet. Gynec.*, **57**, 364.

Hellman, L. M., Harris, J. S. and Reynolds, S. R. M. (1950), "Intravenous Pituitary Extract in Labor with Patterns of Uterine Contractility," *Amer. J. Obstet. Gynec.*, **59**, 41.

Hendricks, C. H. (1963), personal communication.

Hendricks, C. H. (1965), "Activity Patterns in the Non-pregnant Human Uterus," pp. 349–362, in *Muscle*, eds. W. M. Paul, E. E. Daniel, C. M. Kay and G. Monkton. Oxford: Pergamon Press.

Hendricks, C. H. (1964), "A New Technique for the Study of Motility in the Non-pregnant Human Uterus," *J. Obstet. Gynaec. Brit. Cwlth.*, **96**, 824.

Hendricks, C. H. and Moawad, A. H. (1965), "Round Ligament Motility *in vivo* Studies in Man," *J. Obstet. Gynaec. Brit. Cwlth.*, **72**, 618.

Hofbauer, J. (1911), "Hypophysenextrakt als Wehemittel," *Zbl. Gynäk.*, **35**, 137.

Hofbauer, J. and Hoerner, J. K. (1927), "The Nasal Application of Pituitary Extract for the Induction of Labor," *Amer. J. Obsett. Gynec.*, **14**, 137.

Holm, L. W. (1965), "The Fetus as a Factor in the Initiation of Labor," pp. 159–178, in *Initiation of Labor*, eds. J. M. Marshall and W. M. Burnett, U.S. Public Health Service Publication, No. 1390, Washington.

Howarth, A. T., Lundborg, R. A. and Theobald, G. W. (1963), "The Antidiuretic Effect of Oxytocin in Man," *J. Physiol.*, **168**, 16.

Huntingford, P. J. (1961), "Intranasal Use of Synthetic Oxytocin in Management of Breast Feeding," *Brit. med. J.*, **1**, 709.

Initiation of Labor (1965), eds. J. M. Marshall and W. M. Burnett, U.S. Public Health Service Publication, No. 1390, Washington, D.C.

IVth International Symposium on Neurosecretion (1966), ed. F. Stutinsky. Berlin: Springer.

Jung, H. (1961), "The Effect of Oxytocin on the Mechanism of Uterine Excitation," 87–99, in *Oxytocin*, eds. R. Caldeyro-Barcia and H. Heller. Oxford: Pergamon Press.

Jung, H. (1965), "Effects of Progesterone on Uterine Activity," 75–93, in *Induction of Labor*, eds. J. M. Marshall and W. M. Burnett, U.S. Public Health Service Publication, No. 1390, Washington, D.C.

Kamm, O., Aldrich, T. B., Grote, I. W., Rowe, L. W. and Bugbee, E. P. (1928), "The Active Principles of the Posterior Lobe of the Pituitary Gland: (1) The Demonstration of the Presence of Two Active Principles. (2) The Separation of the Two Principles and Their Concentration in the Form of Potent Solid Preparations," *J. Amer. chem. Soc.*, **50**, 573.

Klisiecki, A., Pickford, M., Rothschild, P. and Verney, E. B. (1933), "The Absorption and Excretion of Water by the Mammal; Part 1: The Relation between Absorption of Water and its Excretion by the Innervated and Denervated Kidney. Part 2: Factors Influencing the Response of the Kidney to Water Ingestion," *Proc. Roy. Soc. B.*, **112**, 496 and 521.

Knaus, H. (1925–26), "On the Active Principles of the Pituitary Extract," *J. Pharm. exp. Ther.*, **26**, 337.

Knaus, H. (1926), "The Action of Pituitary Extract Administered by the Alimentary Canal," *Brit. med. J.*, **1**, 234.

Konschegg, A. and Schuster, E. (1915), "Ueber die Beieinflussing der diurese durch Hypophysenextrakte," *Dtsch. med. Wschr.*, **41**, 1091.

Kretzschmar, W. A. and Stoddard, F. J. (1962), "Milk Stimulation with Oxytocin," *Amer. J. Obstet. Gynec.*, **84**, 265.

Kumar, D., Russell, J. J.and Barnes, A. C. (1962), "Studies in Human Myometrium during Pregnancy," *Amer. J. Obstet. Gynec.*, **84**, 586.

Lee, J. (1968), personal communication.

Levy, B. (1963), "The Intestinal Inhibitory Response to Oxytocin, Vasopressin and Bradykinin," *J. Pharmacol. exp. Ther.*, **140**, 356.

Magnus, R. and Schäfer, E. A. (1901), "The Action of Pituitary Extracts upon the Kidney," *J. Physiol.*, **27**, 9.

Martin, F. I. R. and Mathew, T. H. (1964), "The Treatment of Diabetes Insipidus with Synthetic Lysine-vasopressin by Inhalation," *Med. J. Aust.*, **2**, 984.

Mathur, V. S. and Walker, J. M. (1968), "Oxytocinase in Plasma and Placenta in Normal and Prolonged Labour," *Brit. med. J.*, **3**, 96–97.

Méndez-Bauer, C. J., Carballo, M. A., Cabot, H. M., Negreiros de Paiva, C. E. and González-Panizza, V. H. (1961), "Studies on Plasma Oxytocinase, pp. 325–335, in *Oxytocin*, eds. R. Caldeyro-Barcia and H. Heller. Oxford: Pergamon Press.

Miller, M. D. and Marshall, J. M. (1965), "Uterine Response to Nerve Stimulation, Relation to Hormonal Status and Catecholamines," *Amer. J. Physiol.*, **209**, 859.

Moir, J. C. (1933–34), "Recording Contractions of Human Pregnant and Non-pregnant Uterus," *Trans. Edinb. obstet. Soc.*, in *Edinb. med. J.*, p. 93.

Molitor, H. and Pick, E. (1926), "Ueber zentrale Regulation des Wasserwechsels. III. Ueber den zentralen Angriffspunkt der Diuresehemmung durch Hypophysenextrakte," *Arch. exper. Path. Pharmakol.*, **112**, 113.

Newton, M. and Egli, G. E. (1958), "The Effect of Intranasal Administration of Oxytocin on the Let-down of Milk in Lactating Women," *Amer. J. Obstet. Gynec.*, **76**, 103.

O'Connor, W. J. and Verney, E. B. (1942), "The Effect of Removal of the Posterior Lobe of the Pituitary on the Inhibition of Water Diuresis by Emotional Stress," *Quart. J. exp. Physiol.*, **31**, 393.

O'Connor, W. J. and Verney, E. B. (1945), "The Effect of Increased Activity of the Sympathetic System on the Inhibition of Water Diuresis by Emotional Stress," *Quart. J. exp. Physiol.*, **33**, 77.

Oliver, G. and Schäfer, E. A. (1895a), "The Physiological Effects of Extracts of the Suprarenal Capsules," *J. Physiol.*, **18**, 230.

Oliver, G. and Schäfer, E. A. (1895b), "On the Physiological Action of Extracts of Pituitary Body and Certain Other Glandular Organs," *J. Physiol.*, **18**, 277.

Ott, I. and Scott, J. C. (1910), "The Action of Infundibulin upon the Mammary Secretion," *Proc. Soc. exp. Biol. Med.*, **8**, 48.

Page, E. W. (1943), "Response of Human Pregnant Uterus to Pitocin Tannate in Oil," *Proc. Soc. exp. Biol. N.Y.*, **52**, 195.

Petersen, W. E. (1944), "Lactation," *Physiol. Rev.*, **24**, 340.

Pickford, M. (1961), "Some Extra-uterine Actions of Oxytocin," pp. 68–79, in *Oxytocin*, eds. R. Caldeyro-Barcia and H. Heller. Oxford: Pergamon Press.

Saameli, K. (1963), "An Indirect Method for the Estimation of Oxytocin Blood Concentration and Half-life in Pregnant Women near Term," *Amer. J. Obstet. Gynec.*, **85**, 186.

Saameli, K. (1964), "Quantitative Comparison between Oxytocin and Four Related Neurohypophysial Peptides on the Human Uterus *in situ*," *Brit. J. Pharmacol.*, **23**, 176.

Sacks, B. (1924), "Observations upon the Vascular Reactions in Man in Response to Infundin, with Special Reference to the Behaviour of the Capillaries and Venules," *Heart*, **11**, 353.

Schäfer, E. A. and Herring, P. T. (1906), "The Action of Pituitary Extracts upon the Kidney," *Proc. roy. Soc. B.*, **77**, 571.

Schofield, B. M. (1966), "The Increased Extensibility of Pregnant Myometrium," *J. Physiol.*, **182**, 690.

Schofield, B. M. and Wood, C. (1964), "Length-tension Relation in Rabbit and Human Myometrium," *J. Physiol.*, **175**, 125.

Semm, K. (1961), "The Significance of Oxytocinase in Pregnancy and Labour," pp. 336–340, in *Oxytocin*, eds. R. Caldeyro-Barcia and H. Heller. Oxford: Pergamon Press.

Simon, A. and Kardoz, Z. (1934), "Ueber den Gehalt der Hypophysenhinterlappen normaler und durstender Tiere an Blutdruck- und Uterus-wirksamen Stoffen," *Arch. exp. Path. Pharmakol.*, **176**, 238.

Sjöberg, H. and Luft, R. (1963), *Lancet*, **1**, 1160.

Smyth, C. N. (1965), "The Oxytocin Sensitivity Test," pp. 115–123, in *Advances in Oxytocin Research*, ed. J. H. M. Pinkerton. Oxford: Pergamon Press.

Starling, E. H. and Verney, E. B. (1925), "The Secretion of Urine as Studied on the Isolated Kidney," *Proc. roy. Soc. B.*, **97**, 321.

Stutinsky, F. (1966), Editor, *IVth International Symposium on Neurosecretion, q.v.*

Tennent, R. A. and Black, M. D. (1954), "Surgical Induction of Labour in Modern Obstetric Practice," *Brit. med. J.*, **2**, 833.

Theobald, G. W. (1934), *Clin. Sci.*, **1**, 225.

Theobald, G. W. (1934b), *J. Physiol.*, **81**, 243.

Theobald, G. W. (1936), "A Centre, or Centres, in the Hypothalamus Controlling Menstruation, Ovulation, Pregnancy and Parturition," *Brit. med. J.*, **1**, 1038.

Theobald, G. W. (1955), *The Pregnancy Toxaemias: or the Encymonic Atelositeses*, London: Kimpton, p. 80.

Theobald, G. W. (1959), "The Separate Release of Oxytocin and Antidiuretic Hormone," *J. Physiol.*, **149**, 443.

Theobald, G. W. (1963), "Induction of Labour and of Premature Labour," pp. 1055–1088, in *British Obstetric Practice*, ed. A. Claye. London: Heinemann.

Theobald, G. W. (1968), "The Nervous Control of Uterine Activity," **2**, 15, in *Physiology of Labor*, ed. E. J. Quilligan. *Clin. Obstet. Gynec.*, **2**, 15.

Theobald, G. W., Graham, A., Campbell, J., Gange, P. D. and Driscoll, W. J. (1948), "The Use of Post-pituitary Extract in Physiological Amounts in Obstetrics: A Preliminary Report," *Brit. med. J.*, **2**, 123.

Theobald, G. W. Kelsey, H. A. and Muirhead, J. M. B. (1956), "The Pitocin Drip," *J. Obstet. Gynaec. Brit. Emp.*, **63**, 641.

Theobald, G. W. and Lundborg, R. A. (1962), "Changes in Myometrial Sensitivity to Oxytocin Provoked in Different Ways," *J. Obstet. Gynaec. Brit. Cwlth.*, **69**, 417.

Theobald, G. W., Robards, M. P., and Suter, P. E. N. (1969). *J. Obst. Gynae. Brit. Cwlth.*, **76**, 385.

Theobald, G. W. and Verney, E. B. (1935), "The Inhibition of Water Diuresis by Afferent Nerve Stimuli after Complete Denervation of the Kidney," *J. Physiol.*, **83**, 341.

Tuppy, H. (1953), "The Amino-acid Sequence in Oxytocin," *Biochim. biophys. Acta*, **11**, 449.

Tuppy, H. (1961), "Biochemical Studies of Oxytocinase," pp. 315–324, in *Oxytocin*, eds. R. Caldeyro-Barcia and H. Heller. Oxford: Pergamon Press.

Turnbull, A. C. and Anderson, A. B. M., *"Induction of Labour"*: Part 1 (1967), "Amniotomy," *J. Obstet. Gynaec. Brit. Cwlth.*, **74**, 849. Part 2 (1968), "Intravenous Oxytocin Infusion," *J. Obstet. Gynaec. Brit. Cwlth.*, **75**, 24. Part 3 (1968), "Results with Amniotomy and Oxytocin Titration," *J. Obstet. Gynaec. Brit. Cwlth.*, **75**, 32.

Velden, R. von den (1913), "Die Nierenwirkung von Hypophysenextrakten beim Menschen," *Berl. klin. Wschr.*, **50**, 2083.

Verney, E. B. (1926), "The Secretion of Pituitrin in Mammals, as shown by Perfusion of the Isolated Kidney of the Dog," *Proc. roy. Soc. B.*, **135**, 25.

Verney, E. B. (1947), "The Antidiuretic Hormone and the Factors which Determine its Release," *Proc. roy. Soc. B.*, **135**, 25.

Verney, E. B. and Starling, E. H. (1922), "On Secretion by the Isolated Kidney," *J. Physiol.*, **56**, 353.

du Vigneaud, V., Ressler, C. and Trippett, S. (1953), "The Sequence of Amino-acids in Oxytocin, with a Proposal for the Structure of Oxytocin," *J. biol. Chem.*, **205**, 949.

du Vigneaud, V., Ressler, C., Swan, J. M., Roberts, C. W., Katsoyannis, P. G. and Gordon, S. (1954), "The Synthesis of an Octapeptide Amide with the Hormonal Activity of Oxytocin," *J. Amer. chem. Soc.*, **75**, 4879.

van Wagenen, G. and Newton, W. H. (1943), "Pregnancy in the Monkey after Removal of the Fetus," *Surg. Gynec. Obstet.*, **77**, 539.

Warren, N. L. and Hawker, R. W. (1967), "Blood Oxytocin in Dysmenorrhoea," *Aust. N.Z. J. Obstet. Gynaec.*, **7**, 78.

5. THE THYROID

A. STUART MASON

Even in ancient times a relationship between the thyroid and pregnancy had been established by observation. The physiological enlargement of the thyroid in early pregnancy was used as a crude test for pregnancy, the change in neck measurement being made obvious by tying a cord or reed round the woman's neck: a bas-relief of 5000 B.C. shows the Queen of Assyria with a reed round her neck. To-day, the development of sophisticated methods of studying the thyroid has led to an impressive corpus of knowledge that gives a scientific basis for the detailed study of the effects of the female sexual cycle upon the thyroid. However, only relatively crude techniques are available for the investigation of the sexual cycle so that the influence of the thyroid on this aspect of physiology is more a matter of clinical observation than of scientific explanation. Indeed, there are many valid clinical facts in this relationship between the thyroid and the sexual cycle that have not yet been described in a proper scientific manner. Consequently this chapter will deal mainly with scientific observations on thyroid function, but it will also draw attention to certain clinical states that require further investigation.

THYROID FUNCTION

Good modern reviews of thyroid function abound: the interested reader will profit from consulting the books edited by Pitt–Rivers and Trotter (1964), or written by Wayne, Koutras and Alexander (1964). Briefly speaking, the thyroid depends on a daily intake of about 150 μg of iodine in the diet. On entering the blood stream, after rapid and complete absorption from the gut, iodine in the form of iodide, will be trapped by the thyroid or eliminated from the body by the kidney. The disappearance rate of plasma iodide is the sum of the thyroid and renal clearance rates, which are roughly equal. It is important to realize that the renal clearance of iodine is not part of the body's mechanisms for the conservation of iodine; it is proportional to the glomerular filtration rate (Hlad and Bricker (1954).)

The thyroid is, in a sense, always competing against the kidney for the available iodide. This is of no physiological concern when the dietary supplies of iodide are more than adequate. However, increases in the renal loss of iodine can be significant if the dietary iodide is low, for this may lead to thyroid iodine deficiency and the formation of goitre under the influence of an increased pituitary output of thyroid stimulating hormone (TSH) which increases the thyroid's capacity to trap iodine and also increases thyroid size. Minimal amounts of iodide are also lost in sweat. The salivary glands have a considerable capacity for iodide trapping, but this iodide re-enters the circulation after absorption from the gut so that there is no net loss of

iodide from the body. During lactation iodide is trapped by the mammary glands, their clearance rate being about half that of the normal thyroid rate. This constitutes a significant change in the iodine balance of the body and may contribute to a state of thyroid iodide deficiency. About 20 per cent of a mother's daily iodine intake may be lost in her milk (Wayne, et al., 1964).

The organification of iodine within the thyroid to form mono- and di-iodothyrosine and the subsequent combination of these compounds to form tri-iodothyronine and thyroxine (tetra-iodothyronine) are not events of direct interest to the gynaecologist.

The release of thyroid hormones from their intrathyroidal association with thyroglobulin is accompanied by proteolysis of this globulin moeity. Both thyroxine and tri-iodothyronine are released into the blood stream; their transport in plasma is of the greatest importance to those who wish to correlate ovarian and thyroid function. Circulating thyroxine is bound to a specific thyroxine binding globulin (TBG), which moves between the alpha 1 and alpha 2 globulin fractions and has an isoelectric point close to pH 4·0. Some thyroxine is also bound to prealbumen, which appears to have a genuine role in the transport of thyroid hormone and is not a technical artifact; a little is also bound to albumen. Less than 0·1 per cent of thyroxine circulates in an unbound form. The availability of free thyroxine, which is the form required for actual hormonal action at cellular level, will depend on the rate of dissociation of thyroxine from its protein binding in the plasma and the amount of TBG. In contrast, tri-iodothyronine is mainly present in a free form, and TBG has a far greater affinity for thyroxine than for tri-iodothyronine. Osorio (1967) has given an excellent account of the carriage of thyroid hormones in plasma. The difference in the binding properties of the two thyroid hormones explains the differences in their potency, speed of action and rate of disappearance from the blood stream. Tri-iodothyronine is about five times more potent than thyroxine. Although its concentration in blood is very low compared to that of thyroxine, its contribution in terms of biological activity is probably considerable; in rats the plasma concentration of tri-iodothyronine is one-twentieth of that of thyroxine, but the metabolic activities of the two hormones are approximately equal. (Pitt–Rivers and Rall, 1961).

For the gynaecologist the amount of circulating TBG is of paramount importance because it is greatly influenced by ovarian hormones. There is a marked rise of TBG in pregnancy which results in an increase in the total concentration of circulating thyroxine with a normal amount of the free hormone. The same phenomenon can be induced by oestrogen therapy (Dowling, Freinkel and Ingbar, 1956a and b).

Tests of Thyroid Function

It scarcely needs emphasizing that there is no such thing as a test of thyroid function which can give an overall diagnostic result. There are very valuable tests, each of which measures some aspect of iodine metabolism. Each test requires understanding in a physiological context, and the interpretation of results depends on this and a knowledge of factors that may alter the result.

Radio-iodine Uptake

The accumulation of radio-iodine as iodide by the thyroid is a measure of thyroidal avidity for iodine. It gives an indication of the iodide "trap". The rate at which radio-iodine is concentrated in the thyroid is measured best soon after the dose is given because later measurements record the balance between uptake by and discharge from the thyroid and do not measure the actual initial accumulation of iodide as trapped by the gland. For example, the thyrotoxic gland has a marked avidity for iodine which is trapped very quickly and in high concentration by the thyroid. This can be demonstrated in the first three hours after giving the isotopic iodine. After this time a rising amount of isotopic iodine will be leaving the gland as thyroxine so that the radioactivity within the thyroid no longer measures the trapping capacity of the gland. The iodide trap will be increased if the dietary iodide is too low (endemic iodine deficient goitre), or in states of congenital dyshormonogenesis in which there are defects in the efficient organification of iodine and in thyrotoxicosis when large amounts of iodine are necessary for the increased secretion of thyroxine. It is important to remember that the foetal thyroid will concentrate iodine at about the twelfth week of embryogenesis, before the synthetic mechanisms for the making of thyroxine are developed. Consequently the administration of radio-iodine to the pregnant woman is to be avoided as a test of thyroid function.

Protein Bound Iodine (PBI)

This is the common standby for the estimation of circulating thyroid hormone. The techniques required are not easy, and the results will be of no value unless the laboratory concerned is really experienced and performing enough estimations to give constant quality control. Iodinated compounds, as used for contrast radiography and for therapy (e.g. enterovioform, and other organic iodide medicaments used for various symptoms including diarrhoea) will give falsely high values for protein bound iodine; heavy metals, as in mercurial diuretics, will give erroneously low results by inhibiting the chemical reactions on which the measurement depends. Determination of the plasma iodine extractable with butanol is a more direct measure of thyroid hormonal iodine as iodinated compounds other than thyroxine and tri-iodothyronine are not extracted; however, the method is tedious and difficult.

As the total concentration of thyroid hormones is measured in the PBI there is no indication of the amount of free thyroxine. If the amount of TBG is increased the PBI will be elevated; thus, in pregnancy the PBI rises by about 2 μg. per cent, and the rise may be up to 4 μg. per cent.

Tri-iodothyronine Uptake Tests in vivo

When radio-active tri-iodothyronine (T_3) is incubated with a patient's blood, it is partitioned between red cells and plasma in such a way that the uptake of red cells is high in thyrotoxicosis and low in myxoedema (Hamolsky, Stein and Freedberg, 1957). The red cell uptake has been shown to be inversely related to the number of free binding sites available in TBG (Osorio, Jackson, Gartside and Goolden, 1961). Hence the increased amount of thyroxine in thyrotoxicosis will have taken up most of the TBG capacity for binding and the T_3 will cling to the red cells; the reverse occurs in myxoedema when the small amount of thyroxine does not fill the available binding sites. It would be anticipated that an increase in the amount of TBG in the presence of a normal amount of thyroxine would be indicated by a low uptake of T_3 by red cells as there would be more binding sites available. This is exactly what is found in pregnancy. More practical methods are now in use for this type of measurement. Anion exchange resin can be used in lieu of red cells so that the plasma is incubated with resin and tri-iodothyronine (Mitchell, Harden and O'Rourke, 1961).

By measuring the PBI and the T_3 resin uptake a formula can be applied which will give an index of circulating free thyroxine. This correlates well with actual measurement of free thyroxine, a most difficult experimental technique. In pregnancy it can be shown that the level of free thyroxine is normal, the PBI being raised and the T_3 uptake being lowered. To quote from Clark (1964), who discussed modern techniques of measurement, "free thyroxine concentration in plasma is currently considered to be the major determinant of thyroid status. It depends upon the total thyroxine concentration in plasma, and on the free or unsaturated capacity of the plasma proteins for thyroxine.

Free thyroxine concentration can be measured in absolute terms from the product of total thyroxine concentration in plasma (or PBI) and the percentage of free ^{131}I thyroxine derived from equilibration dialysis, gel filtration, etc. Alternatively, it can be measured in relative terms from the PBI and the tri-iodothyronine uptake by red cells or resin which allows for the degree of protein binding".

EFFECTS OF OVARIAN FUNCTION ON THE THYROID

Pregnancy is the obvious situation in which to study the effects of high concentrations of oestrogens and progestogens on the thyroid. Similar but less marked changes in thyroid status are caused by oestrogen/progestogen mixtures used in therapy or for contraception. The onset of the sexual cycle at puberty is a further example of ovarian influence on the thyroid.

The renal clearance of iodine is increased in pregnancy, leading to a net loss of iodide in the urine (Cassano, Baschieri and Andreani, 1957). This alteration in the economy of the iodine cycle is met by an increase in thyroidal clearance of iodide (Halnan and Pochin, 1958). These changes are not of importance if the dietary iodide is more than adequate, but a state of iodine deficiency will be induced if the intake is at the lower limit of normal and a further strain is put on the thyroid if existing iodine deficiency is made worse by the renal loss of iodide in pregnancy.

The degree to which the thyroid can trap sufficient iodine for adequate hormone synthesis will depend on the stimulus of TSH which increases the iodide trap and also increases thyroid size. Thus goitre due to iodine deficiency becomes common in pregnancy in areas of endemic goitre, or thyroid enlargement becomes noticeable in those whose iodine intake has been at the borderline of normality and in those whose thyroid's capacity for increasing its trapping power can only be exercised by an increase in thyroid cells. The whole sequence of renal loss of iodide and increasing iodide trapping by the thyroid has been shown to operate in the genesis of pregnancy goitre by Aboul–Khair, Crooks, Turnbull and Hytten (1964). Adequate supplies of dietary iodine will prevent the formation of goitre, but if the thyroid has enlarged the administration of thyroxine, by diminishing the secretion of TSH will bring down the size of the thyroid. It must be remembered that lactation, with the loss of iodine in the milk, will put the thyroid under strain after the end of pregnancy and is an event that may be associated with the initiation or exaggeration of a goitre.

One clinical aspect of the effect of pregnancy on the thyroid is the difficulty of finding valid tests of thyroid function for the detection of thyroid disorder. Fortunately, most cases of thyrotoxicosis or myxoedema that are associated with pregnancy are diagnosed on straightforward clinical grounds, but there are bound to be cases in which laboratory aids are very desirable. Radio iodine should not be administered to any pregnant woman because of the danger of the foetal thyroid receiving damaging radiation. The PBI, raised in normal pregnancy, has to be very high (above 20 μg. per cent) before it can be held to be diagnostic of thyrotoxicosis, and in these cases the diagnosis would be clinically obvious. However, a PBI measured before and after the administration of tri-iodothyronine (usually 120 μg. daily for four or five days) is of diagnostic use because the level of PBI will remain unchanged if the patient is thyrotoxic, but will fall if thyroid function is normal (Misra and Hamburger, 1965). On the other hand, the T_3 resin uptake is very low in normal pregnancy and will not come up to the levels seen in the non-pregnant myxoedemic. These difficulties can be resolved most satisfactorily by using the PBI together with the T_3 resin uptake and from these results calculating the free thyroxine factor. This remains normal in cyesis and its elevation during pregnancy indicates thyrotoxicosis and subnormal values are consistent with the diagnosis of myxoedema (Goolden, Gartside and Sanderson, 1967).

The changes in thyroid function during the menstrual cycle are so small as to defy significant quantitation, but they are likely to be influenced by the rising concentrations of oestrogen and progesterone in the luteal phase; indeed, some patients notice the swelling of their thyroid at that time. Oestrogen therapy certainly increases the amount of circulating TBG so that the PBI rises and the T_3 resin uptake falls and this is more apparent under the influence of the oestrogen/progestogen mixtures used for contraception (Williams, Denardo and Zelinik, 1966). (Goolden, et al., 1967). However, the 24-hour uptake of radio iodine is not altered by such medication (Irizarry, Parriagua, Pincus, Janer and Frias, 1966). This is not a very accurate test of thyroid iodide trap, but will be of significance in the diagnosis of thyroid dysfunction in patients taking any combination or single type of ovarian like hormones. It is important for the clinician to remember that good history taking must always include an enquiry about the "pill".

THYROID DISORDERS

Thyrotoxicosis may arise in pregnancy, but there is no good evidence to suggest that there is any causal relationship of pregnancy to hyperthyroidism. Indeed, the course of thyrotoxicosis is ameliorated by pregnancy as the increased amounts of TBG bind some of the excess thyroxine and thereby diminish the amount of hormone that is free to damage the patient.

One interesting facet of physiology is the fact that pituitary TSH does not pass the placental barrier, but the Long Acting Thyroid Stimulator (LATS), the probable cause of thyrotoxicosis, does pass to enter the foetal circulation and cause neonatal thyrotoxicosis, (McKenzie, 1964). This is a self-limiting disease which lasts as long as there is a significant titre of LATS in the baby's circulation; the half life of LATS being about two weeks in this situation. It should also be remembered by the clinician that antithyroid drugs, such as methyl thiouracil or carbimazole, used in the treatment of maternal thyrotoxicosis will pass the placental barrier and may induce enlargement of the foetal thyroid if present in large doses.

Fortunately, the doses required for therapy in pregnancy are not sufficient to cause a foetal goitre and this event is only seen when the mother has been treated with more enthusiasm than skill. During the puerperium the level of TBG falls so that the thyrotoxic process may appear to be more active. At this stage it must be remembered that anti-thyroid drugs are secreted in the mother's milk so that lactation should be inhibited to prevent the baby from developing a drug induced hypothyroidism.

Menstrual irregularities are a common feature in thyrotoxic women before the menopause. The type of irregularity is variable, but amenorrhoea or oligomenorrhoea are seen more frequently than polymenorrhoea or menorrhagia. The disturbance of physiology underlying these changes is not known.

Myxoedema is usually associated with menorrhagia, but the menstrual cycle may be unchanged or irregular. Few patients with untreated myxoedema become pregnant. If they do, there is a tendency to post-partum haemorrhage, a clinical observation of some antiquity that remains unexplained. The treated myxoedemic is not infertile, but will require an increase in the dose of thyroxine in order to keep up the blood level of free thyroxine in the face of an increase in TBG. There is evidence from work on rats that hypothyroidism tends to decrease the gonadotrophic activity of the pituitary (Contopoulos, Simpson and Koneff, 1958). The overall lowering of metabolic rate might affect the pituitary response to the hypothalamic gonadotrophin releasing factors which in turn would give an irregular non-cyclical stimulus to the ovaries. On the other hand, there may well be an impaired ovarian response to gonadotrophin. The sophistication of methods available for testing out these ideas in a valid experimental programme in women will allow a solution to a teasing physiological problem indicated by clinical observation. There is evidence that alterations in the level of circulating thyroid hormone will affect the metabolism of human oestrogens (Brown and Strong, 1965). To make matters more complicated, there are reported cases of precocious puberty associated with juvenile hypothyroidism (Jenkins, 1965). It has been suggested that such cases have an "over-lap" on the pituitary feed-back so that the increased TSH of hypothyroidism leads to an increase in gonadotrophic activity. This is a concept that should be matched against the fact that very few cases of hypothyroidism go through puberty at an abnormal age and if they do, a late onset of puberty is the more likely abnormality. It may well be, as suggested by Donovan and van der Werfften Bosch (1965) that the hypothyroidism and sexual precocity are due to a common cause.

As more advanced methods of investigation become available they can be employed to advantage in determining the physiological abnormalities that give rise to the clinically observed abnormalities of the sexual cycle seen with disorders of thyroid function.

REFERENCES

Aboul-Khair, S. A., Crooks, J., Turnbull, A. C. and Hytten, F. E. (1964), *Clin. Sci.*, **27**, 195.

Brown, J. B. and Strong, J. A. (1965), "The Effect of Nutritional Status and Thyroid Function on the Metabolism of Oestradiol," *J. Endocr.*, **32**, 107.

Cassano, C., Baschieri, L. and Andreani, D. (1957), "Rilievi sui gozzi du eccessiva perdita urinaria di iodo Rass," *Fisiopat. clin. Ter.*, **29**, 253.

Clark, F. (1967), "The Estimation of Thyroid Hormone Binding by Plasma Proteins and of unbound levels of Thyroxine in Plasma.

Dowling, J. T., Freinkel, N. and Ingbar, S. H. (1956), (a) "Thyroxine binding by Sera of Pregnant Women," *J. Clin. Endocr.*, **16**, 280. (b) "Effects of diethylstilboestrol on the Binding of Thyroxine in Serum," *J. clin. Endocr.*, **16**, 1491.

Goolden, A. W. G., Gartside, J. M. and Sanderson, C. (1967), "Thyroid Status in Pregnancy and in Women taking Oral Contraceptives," *Lancet*, **I**, 12.

Halnan, K. E. and Pochin, E. E. (1958), "The use of [132]I for Thyroid Function Tests," *Brit. J. Radiol.*, **31**, 581.

Hamolsky, M. W., Stein, M. and Freedberg, A. S. (1957), "The Thyroid Hormone-plasma Protein Complex in man. II. A New Method for the Study of 'uptake' of labelled Hormonal Components by Human Erythrocytes," *J. clin. Endocr.*, **19**, 103.

Hlad, C. J. and Bricker, N. S. (1954), "Renal Function and [131]I Clearance in Hyperthyroidism and Myxoedema," *J. clin. Endocr.*, **14**, 1537.

Irizarry, S., Parriagua, M., Pincus, G., Janer, J. L. and Frias, Z. (1966), "Effect of Cyclic Administration of Certain Progestogen Oestrogen combinations on the 24-hour Radio-iodine Thyroid Uptake, *J. clin. Endocr.*, **26**, 6.

Jenkins, M. E. (1965), "Precocious Menstruation in Hypothyroidism," *Am. J. Dis. Child.*, **109**, 252.

McKenzie, J. M. (1964), "Neonatal Graves' Disease," *J. clin. Endocr.*, **24**, 660.

Misra, S. and Hamburger, J. I. (1965), "Liothyronine Suppression of Protein Bound Iodine." A test for Hyperthyroidism in pregnancy, *Obstet. and Gynec.*, **26**, 165.

Mitchell, M. L., O'Rourke, M. E., and Harden, A. B. (1961), "Resin Uptake of Radiothyroxine from Serum in Thyroid Disease and Pregnancy."

Osorio, C. (1976), "Carriage of Circulating Thyroid Hormones and the Estimation of Total Plasma Hormones Levels," *Suppl. J. Clin. Path.*, **20**, 335.

Osorio, C., Jackson, D. J., Gartside, J. M. and Goolden, A. W. G. (1961), "The Uptake of [131]I Triiodothyronine by Red Cells in Relation to the Binding of Thyroid Hormones by Plasma Proteins," *Clin. Sci.*, **21**, 355.

Pitt-Rivers, R. and Rall, J. E. (1961), "Radioiodine Equilibrium Studies of Thyroid and Blood," *Endocrinol.*, **68**, 309.

Pitt-Rivers, R. and Trotter, W. R. (editors) (1964), *The Thyroid Gland*, 2 vols. London: Butterworths.

Wayne, E. J., Koutras, D. A. and Alexander, W. D. (1964), *Clinical Aspects of Iodine Metabolism*. Oxford: Blackwells.

6. THE ADRENAL

JOHN BIGGS and ARNOLD KLOPPER

Steroid hormones are becoming ever more important in the practice of gynaecology and of obstetrics. The adrenocortical steroids are of particular interest in virilism and the involvement of the adrenal cortex in oestrogen production during pregnancy. These topics will be discussed after a review of the hormones and methods for their estimation. The adrenal medulla, which is a modified part of the sympathetic nervous system is not of present concern.

The chemical names used in this chapter are the trivial ones.* The conventions of steroid nomenclature are detailed in "The Chemistry of the Steroids" by Klyne (1965). This book can be recommended for readers who seek to understand the terms used in papers with a biochemical bias.

Adrenocortical Hormones

The adrenal cortex produces steroid hormones which may be considered in four groups: glucocorticoids, androgens, mineralocorticoids and oestrogens.

The adrenal glucocorticoids consist of cortisol (formerly called "hydrocortisone") and a smaller amount of corticosterone. These hormones are mainly concerned with water and electrolyte balance, exerting much of their effect through the glomerulus. They also help in maintaining normal blood pressure and are concerned in suppression of inflammatory reactions. The raised cortisol levels obtaining in pregnancy are thought to be the cause of the improvement in rheumatoid arthritis and bronchial asthma which has been observed in pregnancy. Control of carbohydrate metabolism seems to be one of the lesser functions of this group of hormones but the term "glucocorticoids" is widely used and will be applied in this chapter.

* The trivial names used and their chemical equivalents are as follows:
aldosterone, 11β, 21-Dihydroxy-3, 20-dioxopregn-4-en-18-al
androstenedione, Androst-4-ene-3, 17-dione
corticosterone, 11β, 21-Dihydroxypregn-4-ene-3, 20-dione
cortisol, 11β, 17α, 21-Trihydroxypregn-4-ene-3, 20-dione
dehydroepiandrosterone, *DHA*, 3β-Hydroxyandrost-5-en-17-one
dehydroepiandrosterone sulphate, *DHAS*, 3β-Hydroxyandrost-5-en-17-one sulphate
11 *deoxycortisol*, 17α, 21-Dihydroxypregn-4-ene-3, 20-dione
dexamethasone, 9α-Fluoro-16α-methyl-11β, 17α, 21-trihydroxypregn-1, 4-diene-3, 20-dione
epitestosterone, 17α-Hydroxyandrost-4-en-3-one
11β-*hydroxyandrostenedione*, 11β-Hydroxyandrost-4-ene-3, 17-dione
16-*hydroxydehydroepiandrosterone*, 16-*hydroxy DHA*, 3β, 16α-Dihydroxyandrost-5-en-17-one
17α-*hydroxyprogesterone*, 17α-Hydroxypregn-4-ene-3, 20-dione
pregnanediol, 5β-Pregnane-3α, 20α-diol
pregnanetriol, 5β-Pregnane-3α, 17α, 20α-triol
oestriol, Oestra-1, 3, 5(10)-triene-3, 16α, 17β-triol
oestrone, 3-Hydroxyoestra-1, 3, 5(10)-trien-17-one
testosterone, 17β-Hydroxyandrost-4-en-3 one
tetrahydro-11-*deoxycortisol*, 3α, 17α, 21-Trihydroxy-5β-pregnan-20-one

The second group consists of androgenic hormones. There has been dispute over which androgens are actually produced in the adrenal cortex. Recent work showing *in vitro* and *in vivo* interconversion of androgens brings new possibilities (Blaquier, Forchielli and Dorfman, 1967; Horton and Tait, 1966). Testosterone, dehydroepiandrosterone (DHA), dehydroepiandrosterone sulphate (DHAS), androstenedione and 11β-hydroxyandrostenedione have been found in higher concentration in blood from the adrenal vein than in peripheral blood (Prunty, 1966) and are believed to be produced in the adrenal cortex. Unlike the glucocorticoids which have 21 carbon atoms, the adrenal androgens all have only 19 carbon atoms and are sometimes referred to as C19 steroids.

With the possible exception of 11-hydroxylated or 11-oxygenated compounds all of the androgenic hormones are produced in the ovary as well as in the adrenal. In the former these androgens are intermediates in the biogenesis of other steroids rather than secretory products in their own right.

The androgens and their metabolites vary considerably in their androgenic potency and the information in humans on this subject is incomplete. Most of what is known has come from animal experiments and the results may not be wholly applicable to man. Goldzeiher (1964) has written:

"chick combs are one thing and androgenic effects in the human . . . are another."

The consensus of opinion is that testosterone is the most potent androgen in humans. This subject has been reviewed by Prunty (1966).

Studies of androgen production have often been based on concentrations of metabolites in urine or blood. Among the problems that arise are the origin of most of the androgens from more than one gland and the fact that several different hormones may give the same metabolite. In addition, the greater part of the steroids are promptly conjugated, that is combined with glucuronic acid or sulphuric acid so that they are present in the blood stream as glucuronides or sulphates. The conjugation process occurs mostly in the liver and many steroids are excreted in the bile, becoming involved in an entero-hepatic circulation. Faecal excretion of pregnanediol has been demonstrated and probably occurs with all of the steroid hormones.

The third, mineralocorticoid, group is centred upon aldosterone. This hormone is produced by the outer zona glomerulosa in the cortex and unlike the other hormones is not stimulated by corticotrophin from the anterior pituitary gland. Despite this, aldosterone is produced along the same pathways as the other adrenocortical hormones, being the result of changes at the 18-position of corticosterone. Aldosterone is present in higher concentration in late pregnancy (Martin and Mills, 1956). It will not be discussed further.

Oestrogens are produced in small amounts by the adrenal cortex. Urinary oestrone assays in post-menopausal women with ovarian ablation gave levels of the order of 0·9 μg. per 24 hours in 47 women (Nissen-Meyer and Sanner, 1963). Adrenal tumours may give higher levels (Brown, Bulbrook and Greenwood, 1957). Brown, Falconer and Strong (1959) showed that when adrenocorticotrophin (ACTH) was given to patients whose ovaries had been removed there was an increase of 3 to 9 times in oestrogen output. The response was lost after adrenalectomy.

In considering the adrenal hormones, it should be pointed out that the adrenal, ovary, placenta and the testis have much the same potentials for steroid biogenesis. They differ in the relative amounts of steroid which they direct down different metabolic pathways, and this direction is determined by the enzyme concentrations present.

Measurement of Adrenocortical Function

Important developments in understanding of the adrenal cortex have accompanied the introduction of new methods of steroid assay. The appearance of more sophisticated

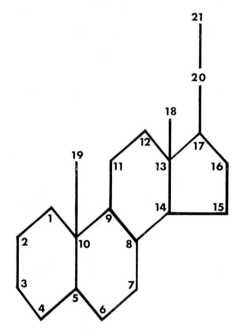

FIG. 1. The steroid nucleus as conventionally drawn, showing numbering of the carbon atoms. The true shape of the nucleus is a partially folded flat plane. The methyl groups (CH₃) at positions 18 and 19 lie above this plane. Substituents on the same side of the plane as these methyl groups are designated β and drawn with a solid line; those on the opposite side are designated α and indicated by an interrupted line.

methods has brought an increasing awareness of the shortcomings of older methods and adrenocortical function can now be better defined.

Earlier assessments were based on urinary methods. Collection of urine over 24 hours gives a summation of adrenocortical function over that time. There are many problems of urine collection, however, and in acute clinical conditions such as adrenal insufficiency it may be impossible to wait 24 hours for an answer.

Blood assays have the advantage of certainty and simplicity in collection. The very fact that blood can be so quickly obtained also means that the results of assay are applicable only to the moment when the blood was withdrawn. The findings may give an inadequate picture of continuing adrenal function and this is borne out by the considerable diurnal variation that is found in plasma corticosteroid levels. Collection of blood samples at a specific time in the day overcomes part of the problem.

Urinary 17-oxosteroids (formerly 17-ketosteroids). The measurement of 17-oxosteroids was the first commonly used biochemical test of adrenal function and it remains in wide use today. The 17-oxosteroids are a variety of closely related compounds, for the most part physiologically inactive metabolites of adrenal or gonadal hormones. They are C19 steroids characterized by an oxygen atom attached to the 17-carbon atom. (See Fig. 1).

The measurement of these compounds as a group came into use in the 1930's when the Zimmermann colour reaction was evolved. Although not specific for the C=O group at C-17 it has proved very useful in the assessment of adrenocortical function. Included in the 17-oxosteroids are DHA, DHAS and androstenedione, together with their metabolites. Cortisol, corticosterone and testosterone are among the active hormones whose breakdown products give rise to urinary 17-oxosteroids.

Recent criticism of the test has come from Goldzeiher (1964). He believes that increasing "simplification" of the test as performed in many routine laboratories has resulted in serious loss of specificity. Up to 90 per cent of the colour reaction by which the 17-oxosteroids are measured may be due to non-specific chromogens.

Despite reservations, the test remains of value in giving a general assessment of adrenocortical function where more specific tests are not yet available. It is also of value in dynamic tests of adrenal function, in determining the response to stimulation, as with ACTH or to suppression, as with dexamethasone. The normal values have been reviewed by Lorraine and Bell (1966). There is a change with age but these workers give 3–20 mg. per 24 hours as the normal range for women between 20 and 40 years of age.

The compounds measured, however poorly, by the 17-oxosteroid estimation are derived in part from extra-adrenal sources. In seeking a better assessment of adrenocortical function, methods have been sought which measure compounds of purely adrenal origin. Early attempts centred on measuring cortisol and its metabolites. These compounds have 21 carbon atoms and have a hydroxyl (OH) group at C-17 in addition to the side chain. The term "17-hydroxycorticosteroids" was applied to these substances and many methods were devised for measuring them.

Different methods of assay for these compounds have measured different segments of the wide range of steroid metabolites associated with cortisol and different results have been obtained. Some laboratories have adopted one method and some another. The practice in the U.S.A., for example, differs from that in Britain. The important thing is that the clinician should be aware of the method used in his centre and know its limitations as well as its normal values.

17-oxogenic steroids (formerly 17-ketogenic steroids). Norymberski, Stubbs and West (1953) described a method in which sodium bismuthate was used to remove the side chain at C-17 and thus convert cortisol and allied compounds into 17-oxosteroids. The 17-oxosteroids could then be measured by the well established Zimmermann reaction. The naturally occurring 17-oxosteroids had first to be determined and then subtracted from the results obtained after bismuthate oxidation. The double measurement of oxosteroids magnifies the errors inherent in this assay. Normal values for 17-oxogenic steroids in urine of adult females are 6–16 mg. per 24 hours.

Total 17-hydroxycorticosteroids. Appleby, Gibson, Norymberski and Stubbs (1955) introduced a preliminary reduction step, using sodium borohydride, into the hydroxycorticosteroid assay. This effectively altered the originally present 17-oxosteroids so that they no longer took part in the colour reaction and did not have to be separately determined and subtracted. The end result is again measured by the Zimmermann reaction. The term "total" 17-hydroxycorticosteroids was coined to distinguish this determination. Normal values for females between 20 and 40 years of age are 4–15 mg. per 24 hours.

17-Hydroxycorticosteroids—Porter Silber Chromogens. Porter and Silber (1960) described a colour reaction for the dihydroxy-acetone side chain at C-17 which is common to cortisol and most of its metabolites. The reaction involves phenylhydrazine and sulphuric acid and gives a red colour. Estimations by this method are often referred to as "17-hydroxycorticosteroids" but because of the relatively poor specificity of the colour reaction "Porter-Silber Chromogens" has been advocated as a more appropriate term. Modifications to earlier methods have brought improvements in reproducibility. The normal range for adult females is 4–10 mg. per 24 hours.

In reviewing all of these methods, Cope (1964) found that they gave similar results and had similar shortcomings. Estimations by these methods appear to be meaningful only when the levels are at least twice normal—as in florid Cushing's syndrome. Low, normal or slightly elevated levels are of much less significance as there is a wide scatter in normal subjects. In addition, there are many reports in the literature of incongruous results in clinical adrenal disorders.

Earlier methods for estimating plasma corticosteroids were often adaptations of the urinary methods described above. The concentrations of steroids in plasma are lower than in urine and problems of specificity arise. Methods involving paper, column or gas-liquid chromatography allowed separation of individual steroids but these are too demanding of time, training and resources for routine clinical use.

11-hydroxycorticosteroids. One of the features common to cortisol and corticosterone is the presence of a hydroxyl (OH) group at C-11. Hydroxylation at this position occurs only in the adrenal cortex, and estimation of 11-hydroxy-lated corticosteroid compounds provides a valuable index of adrenocortical function. A method for determining these compounds in plasma has proved of much value (Mattingly, 1963). The simplicity and specificity of the method have led to its wide use in clinical problems.

Secretion Rate Studies

A recent development in assessing adrenocortical function is the steroid secretion rate test. This can be applied to any steroid which has a unique and measurable urinary metabolite. The metabolite must originate from the steroid alone and not be contributed to from any other source.

The patient is given a physiologically insignificant injection of the isotopically labelled steroid. The total urinary metabolite and its radioactivity in a 24 or 48 hour urine collection are measured. The ratio of total metabolite excreted to hormone secreted by the adrenal in the period of study is equal to the ratio of radioactive metabolite excreted to radioactive steroid injected. Three of the four values are known and the secretion rate of the steroid can thus be calculated. Secretion rates for cortisol and aldosterone have been most widely studied (Cope, 1966a, b). Secretion rates of androgens are complicated by the fact that none of the androgens has a specific metabolite unique to it. The subject has been discussed in detail by Lieberman and Gurpide (1966).

Adrenal Factors in Virilism and Hirsutism

Virilism is the development of masculine characteristics in the female. The changes of virilism include clitoral hypertrophy, breast atrophy, loss of female body contour and a deepening of the voice. The most common symptom, whose significance is often difficult to assess, is hirsutism or the growth of excess and unwanted body hair. A few patients will be seen with several of these features. A diagnosis of virilism may be made and a source of excess androgens sought. Many patients will present with hirsutism alone when the chance of finding a correctable cause are much less. Virilism and hirsutism will be considered separately, though it must be realized that these may be phases of the same pathological process whereby more and more male characteristics are imposed on a female organism.

Virilism and Congenital Adrenal Hyperplasia

Congenital adrenal hyperplasia is due to an inborn defect of steroid hormone biogenesis. The expanding study of this condition has shed new light on several phases of steroid metabolism (Bongiovanni, Eberlein, Goldman and New, 1967). The most common feature of the disorder is virilism, presenting at birth in the female or from about 2 years of age in the male. In the newborn female there are likely to be clitoral enlargement and fusion of the labio-scrotal folds. The urethra may traverse the enlarged clitoris in severe cases and chromosome analysis may be needed to decide the true sex of the infant. Many patients have an associated salt-losing tendency. Addisonian crisis may occur and result in early death.

Surviving patients, if untreated, will develop pubic and axillary hair from about 2 years onwards. Rapid muscular and skeletal growth will occur but premature closure of the epiphyses will result in short adult stature. Severe hypertension is a feature of some forms of the disease. The disorder may be suspected because of the features of intersex at birth, rapidly developing water and electrolyte imbalance, or a suggestive family history.

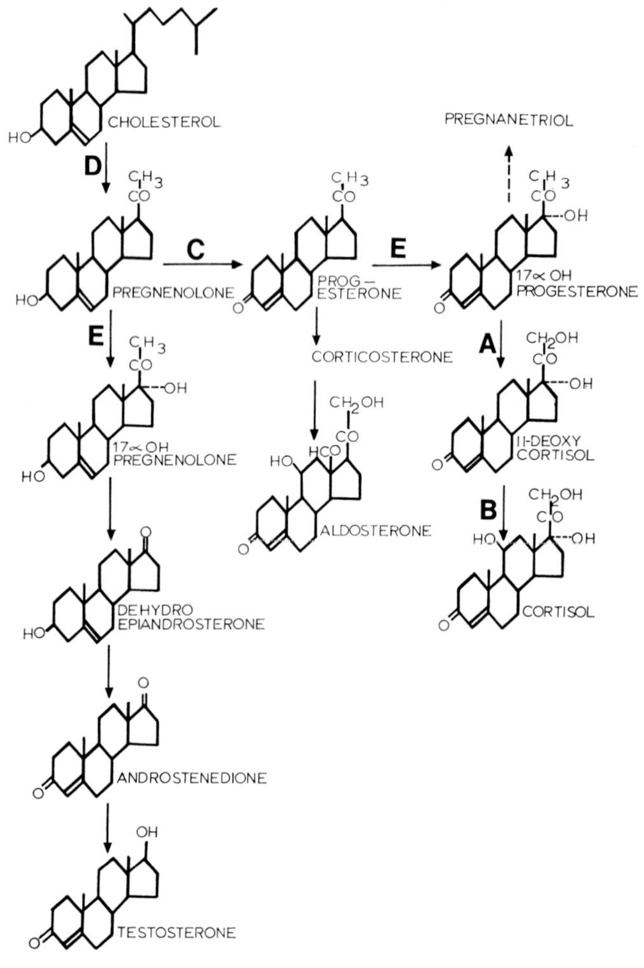

Fig. 2. Metabolic pathways in cortisol production. A, B, C, D and E refer to the enzyme systems necessary for these reactions. A is 21-hydroxylase and deficiency of this enzyme is responsible for the most common type of congenital adrenal hyperplasia (C.A.H.). B is 11β-hydroxylase, deficiency of which causes the less common hypertensive form of C.A.H. C refers to 3β-hydroxysteroid dehydrogenase. D is cholesterol desmolase and E is 17α hydroxylase.

Diagnosis will require assays of urinary pregnanetriol, 17-hydroxycorticosteroids and 17-oxosteroids.

The basic defect in congenital adrenal hyperplasia is deficiency of an enzyme necessary for the production of cortisol. In an attempt to overcome the resulting low circulating levels of cortisol, the pituitary secretes a continuously high level of ACTH. This stimulates adrenocortical activity and the increased androgens which result are responsible for virilism. As cortisol production is blocked its precursors either accumulate or are directed down little used pathways. An example of the latter response is the considerable rise that occurs in pregnanetriol excretion in the common form of the disease. Urine assays will show low levels of 17-hydroxycorticosteroids. There will be raised levels of 17-oxosteroids.

At least five enzyme defects have been described and each has characteristic clinical features. The salt-losing tendency occurs with varying frequency in four forms of the disorder. The sites of enzyme defect are shown in Figure 2.

The most common form of the condition results from deficiency of the enzyme 21-hydroxylase (A in Figure 2). The conversion of 17α-hydroxyprogesterone to 11-deoxycortisol is blocked and some of the accumulating precursor is metabolised to pregnanetriol. Cox (1962) has shown a wide range in levels of pregnanetriol excretion in patients with congenital adrenal hyperplasia and has reviewed other urinary metabolites which are found in this condition.

Figures quoted by Bongiovanni et al. (1967) show that 90–95 per cent of patients with congenital adrenal hyperplasia have a deficiency of 21-hydroxylase. Virilism is a constant feature of these patients and salt-losing problems occur in about a third of them.

A second form of congenital adrenal hyperplasia is due to 11β-hydroxylase deficiency (B in Figure 2). Virilization is seen, but hypertension is also commonly present. Salt-losing is rarely seen. Since 21-hydroxylation is not impeded there is very little elevation in pregnanetriol. As before, there will be low cortisol output and raised urinary 17-oxosteroids.

In a third form of the disorder there is a deficiency of 3β-hydroxysteroid dehydrogenase (C in Figure 2). This defect blocks cortisol production but also interferes with testosterone production, so that the new-born male infant may have incompletely developed male genitalia. The female infant may show moderate virilization, probably as a result of other, weaker androgens than testosterone. The salt-losing tendency is common and there is a high mortality.

Two other forms of congenital adrenal hyperplasia have been suggested. A deficiency of cholesterol desmolase (D in Figure 2) may be responsible for a rapidly fatal condition in which there is low adrenocortical output of all hormones, and in which the adrenal cells are found to be filled with cholesterol. A deficiency of 17α-hydroxylase may also occur (E in Figure 2). There is very low production of androgens as well as cortisol.

In the majority of cases the effects of the disorder can be overcome by adequate cortisol replacement therapy. Excess ACTH secretion is then suppressed and adrenal androgen production is reduced to normal levels. Operative reconstruction of female genitalia may be necessary.

Cases of virilism in older children and young adults have been described in which the biochemical features are identical to those in congenital adrenal hyperplasia. Brooks, Mattingly, Mills and Prunty (1960) described three such cases. Lipsett and Riter (1961) described another and both groups suggested that these patients had partial defects of steroid metabolism which only became clinically evident with growth or the changes of puberty.

Virilism—Adrenocortical Carcinoma

The rapid development of virilism in postpubertal females should bring to mind the likelihood of adreno-cortical carcinoma. In this rare condition, in which Cushingoid features may also be seen, the 17-oxosteroid excretion is considerably raised, often to more than 100 mg. per 24 hours. Attempts to suppress these high levels by corticosteroid administration are unlikely to succeed. If levels do fall they are unlikely to come down to normal. Radiology after perirenal air insufflation may help in the diagnosis. Estimation of the metabolites of 11-deoxycortisol, especially tetrahydro-11-deoxycortisol have been suggested as being valuable in diagnosis. Lipsett, Hertz and Ross (1963) have recently reviewed this condition.

Virilism: Adrenocortical Hyperplasia

Having dealt with some defined causes of excessive adrenal activity we are left with a large group of patients where virilism is due to adrenocortical overactivity of uncertain aetiology. Upon occasion signs of adreno-cortical overactivity other than virilism may also be present as in Cushing's syndrome. On the other hand, the only evidence of hyperactivity may be an increased sensitivity to ACTH stimulation.

The severity of virilism in overt Cushing's syndrome varies considerably. This may be due to variability in the selective overproduction of glucocorticoids. Mills (1968) has reviewed the evidence for a pituitary factor which acts synergistically with ACTH in stimulating androgen production in the adrenal. Such a factor might be present to different degrees in patients with Cushing's syndrome, giving rise to different grades of virilism. The varying severity may also be due to altered peripheral response to secreted androgens. Such a varying response is supported by some workers (Goldzeiher, 1964; Greenblatt and Mahesh, 1964) and rejected by others (Prunty, 1967).

Adult adrenal hyperplasia in which androgen over-production is the dominant abnormality—with resulting virilism—has been discussed by Goldzeiher (1964). He describes patients with this condition as having a gradual onset of virilization as compared with the acute onset in patients with adrenal neoplasms. The excretion of 17-oxosteroids is high—up to 100 mg. per 24 hours—but adrenal suppression is usually achieved with relatively small doses of corticosteroids. This, too, provides a distinction from adrenal carcinoma in which suppression of excess oxosteroid excretion by corticoid administration is difficult if not impossible.

Hirsutism

The most common presenting complaint in the whole field of virilism is an increase in hair growth where the patient, guided by present-day advertising and social mores, believes there should be none. The hair may just be on the upper lip and this may bring the sensitive, introspective girl to seek advice. Often there is hair growth on the chin and neck and this is more difficult for a girl to disguise or overlook. Too often these girls present to the doctor with extensive inflammation and scarring of the face and neck as a result of the prior ministrations of the commercial electrolysist.

Hairiness may cause distress when it is limited to the legs and arms although widely known patent measures are usually effective if this is the only problem. Occasionally, a girl complains of hair around the areolae of the breasts or between the breasts or an excessive growth on the abdomen. These symptoms often mask the patient's real concern, that they may be early evidence that she is losing her femininity or that worse may be in store.

So many patients are distressed by unwanted hair that the first task of the physician is to assess whether the increase in hair is pathological or within the bounds of normal. The patient's complexion and her racial and family background are of great importance in this respect (Hamilton, 1964). Several methods have been described for obtaining a more quantitative estimate of hair growth. The man who regularly shaves with a safety razor and without lather will find a remarkably constant amount of hair on his razor after each 24 hour period. This principle has been applied by Hamilton (1964) who measured the hair from the right axilla of normal and hirsute patients and by Casey, Burger, Kent, Kellie, Moxham, Nabarro and Nabarro (1966) who weighed the hair after shaving measured areas of the thigh, forearm or face in normal and hirsute women. Such quantitative measures as these deserve wider use in the initial assessment of hirsute patients and in studying the reponse to treatment.

Aetiology of Hirsutism

The term "simple hirsutism" has been applied to patients who have no other evidence of virilism. The adjective "idiopathic" has also been applied. In the usual sense—"occurring without known cause"—the word is apt. It might be better to say that many possible causes for simple hirsutism are known but that in most patients the cause is not able to be determined. Once again, racial and other hereditary factors play a large part in simple hirsutism and the dividing line between these physiological causes of hairiness and the pathological causes is very difficult to determine.

An increase in circulating androgens is often associated with hirsutism. The androgens may be of ovarian or adrenal origin and in many cases it is difficult to tell the source. Various tests have been devised for successively suppressing one source while stimulating the other. The interactions of the suppressing and stimulating hormones may annul any results obtained (Goldzeiher, 1967). Increases in 11-hydroxylated compounds are believed to show increased adreno-cortical activity, since 11-hydroxyla-tion appears to occur only in the adrenal. In hirsutism, however, even the pattern of these metabolites may not be constant (Mahesh, Greenblatt, Aydar, Roy, Puebla and Ellegood, 1964).

The polycystic ovary syndrome provides an example of hirsutism associated with an ovarian source of excess androgen. The urinary excretion of 17-oxosteroids is generally around the upper limits of the normal range and urinary and plasma testosterone are usually raised in this condition. Hirsutism was present in 69 per cent of over a thousand proven cases reviewed by Goldzeiher and Green (1962). There are recent review articles on this subject by Shearman and Cox (1966) and Goldzeiher (1967).

In simple hirsutism without ovarian abnormality there is only limited evidence for adrenal involvement. As has been emphasized already the 17-oxosteroid assay has many drawbacks. In particular it measures androgenic substances of varying potency from both ovary and adrenal. Nevertheless, Mills, Brooks and Prunty (1962) showed that in hirsute women who had received ACTH there was a greater increase in 17-oxosteroids than in 17-oxogenic steroids—when compared with normal women. This observation that the adrenals of women with idiopathic hirsutism were in some way different—that the androgen producing mechanism was particularly sensitive to ACTH stimulation—had previously been made by Goldzeiher and Laitin (1960).

Testosterone has been shown to be the most potent androgen in humans. Since it does not have a carbonyl group $(C=O)$ attached to the 17-position it is not itself one of the 17-oxosteroid group. Such is its relative potency, however, that a small increase in concentration would have a greater androgenic effect than larger increases in 17-oxosteroid concentration. The development of methods for estimation of testosterone gave new possibilities in the study of hirsutism (Finkelstein, Forchielli and Dorfman, 1961; Finkelstein, 1964).

Some workers found raised testosterone levels in hirsute women (Dorfman, Forchielli and Gut, 1963; Gandy, Moody and Peterson, 1965) while others found no increase (Conti, Sorcini, Sciarra, Concolino and Lotti, 1964). The value of testosterone assays in the assessment of hirsutism is still open to question. On the one hand the assay may provide a useful clue to the agent responsible for the excess hair growth and thus help to distinguish the condition from those due to racial, genetic or non-hormonal factors. On the other hand a raised testosterone level tells one nothing about the source of the hormone or the pathological process leading to its production.

Epitestosterone, an isomer of testosterone which differs only in having the 17-hydroxyl group in a different spatial position relative to the rest of the molecule, may also be present in increased concentration in hirsute patients. The significance of this compound has recently been considered by de Nicola, Dorfman and Forchielli (1966) and has been reviewed by Klopper and Jeffery (1968).

Management of Hirsute Patients

The importance of the initial assessment of the patient who complains of excess hair has already been stressed. After a careful history, taking into account the relevant facts about hirsutes in the family, and a general examination directed particularly toward the features of Cushing's syndrome, a vaginal examination is mandatory. Many of these patients will be virgins and it may be best to defer the examination until it can be done with the patient anaesthetized. Recording of the findings and particularly of the hair distribution is aided by the use of a special chart with blank body diagrams that can be shaded in. The availability of that most precious commodity, time, for assessing such patients as this is of great importance. They are particularly unsuited for assessment in the rushed conditions of an ordinary gynaecological clinic, and there is much to be said for the creation of a special venue where these women can be dealt with.

Urine collections should be made over two consecutive 24 hour periods. This is best done in hospital under supervision but adequate instructions, given verbally and reinforced by a printed sheet, may allow the collection to be done at home. Provision of light plastic bottles, inconspicuous bags and a large plastic funnel make for greater co-operation from the patient. The urine specimens should be analyzed for 17-oxosteroids and if these are elevated a suppression test should be carried out. Of many suggested tests, one that has been widely used is to give 2 mg. of dexamethasone every 6 hours for 4 days. Urine collections before, during and after dexamethasone are assayed for 17-oxosteroids. In simple hirsutism the basal levels of 17-oxosteroid will usually be in the normal range (3–20 mg. per 24 hours). The value of the suggested tests is in distinguishing patients with gross adrenal pathology as a cause of their virilism.

As mentioned above, it may be necessary to admit the patient to hospital for examination under an anaesthetic. Although bimanual examination is open to quantitative error, it gives a valuable qualitative indication of ovarian size. Air insufflation studies or gynaecography have been advocated as a means of determining ovarian size and thus indicating a possible ovarian contribution to hirsutism. But the most likely ovarian cause is the polycystic ovary and in this disorder there may be no overall enlargement. The wider use of laparoscopy should be considered. By this means the ovary can be seen and photographed. A marked probe or a pair of callipers which opened when inserted into the peritoneal cavity would allow accurate ovarian measurement.

In many hirsute patients no clear evidence of adrenal or ovarian involvement can be obtained and one is obliged to resort to the diagnosis of "idiopathic hirsutism." The treatment of these patients is unsatisfactory. The dermatologist is able to offer something by way of cosmetic improvement. Depilatory preparations, judicious shaving and electrolysis all have a place in treatment. Greenblatt and Mahesh (1964) have suggested the daily bathing of areas of unwanted hair with 50 per cent hydrogen peroxide solution as a means of bleaching the hairs to make them less noticeable. Hair growth may be retarded a little by this means.

Adrenal suppression, sometimes combined with ovarian suppression has been used in the treatment of simple hirsutism. Greenblatt and Mahesh (1964) described the use of prolonged courses of oestrogens in adolescent girls with hirsutism. Promising results were also obtained with ovarian suppression by Casey et al. (1966). Whether of adrenal or ovarian origin, hirsutes can seldom be reversed and the best that the endocrinologist can offer is suppressive treatment which will prevent any advance in hair growth. This is a very unsatisfactory state of affairs. Although hirsutes may not be a disease threatening life in the same way as an infection or a neoplasm, it is a physiological malfunction bringing a great deal of distress in its train and eminently worthy of thoughtful medical consideration.

Adrenocortical Influence on Oestrogens in Pregnancy

The estimation of urinary oestriol has come to be widely accepted as a valuable test of foeto-placental function (Klopper, 1968). There have been suggestions that alterations in adrenal activity or the giving of adrenocortical steroids in pregnancy might affect urinary oestrogen excretion and thus devalue the test. The evidence for these suggestions requires examination.

Outside of pregnancy normal females have been shown to excrete increased amounts of urinary oestrogen after both ACTH and dexamethasone (Barlow, 1964). The changes were only seen during the follicular phase of the menstrual cycle and it was postulated that most of the increased oestrogen was of ovarian origin, but resulted from increased adrenal production of DHA.

In pregnancy two effects must be considered. The first is the purely methodological one, of chemical interference with the oestrogen assay by cortisol and its synthetic analogues. Brown, Bulbrook and Greenwood (1957) showed that cortisone interfered in the chemical assay of urinary oestrogens and described an improved method to overcome this difficulty. Adlercreutz (1968) has shown that ACTH administration will also interfere with the Kober reaction in oestriol estimation.

More important than these methodological problems is a real reduction in urinary oestrogen output which occurs after glucocorticoid administration (Simmer, Dignam, Easterling, Frankland and Naftolin, 1966; MacLeod, Brown, Beischer and Smith, 1967; Warren and Cheatum, 1967). The main precursors for oestrogens in pregnancy are DHA-sulphate and 16-hydroxy-DHA-sulphate. These compounds are converted to oestrogens by the placenta, the maternal sources being predominant in early pregnancy and the foetal sources in the latter half of pregnancy (Bolte, 1967). It is reasonable to believe that adrenal suppression by glucocorticoids reduces the production of oestrogen precursors, and thus of oestrogen. This sequence of events has been demonstrated by Lauritzen (1967).

Just as adrenal suppression gives decreased precursors and oestrogens so adrenal stimulation might be expected to give increased secretion of precursors and thus of oestrogens. Lauritzen (1967) found such increases as did Dassler (1966). Adlercreutz (1968) while investigating conditions for hydrolysis of oestrogens, gave ACTH to 7 subjects with normal pregnancies. He found slight falls in oestriol execretion which he attributed to problems in the method of assay. Jeffery (1968, personal communication) is unable to show any increase in urinary oestriols in normal pregnancy after ACTH administration.

The effect of ACTH stimulation on urinary oestriol excretion is thus in doubt. Whether stimulation and suppression affect the foetal adrenal in the same way as the maternal adrenal is not known.

The most important clinical result of these studies is that oestriol estimations cannot be accepted as guides to satisfactory foetoplacental function when the mother is receiving ACTH, cortisol or its synthetic analogues.

Effects of Corticosteroids on the Foetus

Congenital defects have been suggested as a side effect of long-term glucocorticoid therapy in the mother. The possibility first arose from animal experiments in which cleft palate was more frequently observed after administration of cortisone. Bongiovanni and McPadden (1960) reviewed the evidence for similar effects in humans. They found that vigorous steroid therapy in early pregnancy carried an increased risk of foetal abnormality, but concluded that the problem was not a significant one. Warrell and Taylor (1968) in a retrospective study showed an increase in perinatal mortality in babies born to mothers on long term prednisolone therapy. The use of corticosteroids in such conditions as asthma and skin disorders appears to be increasing. There is an important place for further studies—preferably prospective ones—of the effects of corticosteroids in pregnancy.

REFERENCES

Adlercreutz, H. (1968), "Studies on the Hydrolysis of Gel-filtered Urinary Oestrogens," *Acta endocr., Copenhagen*, **57**, 49.

Appleby, J. I., Gibson, G., Norymberski, J. K. and Stubbs, R. D. (1955), "Indirect Analysis of Corticosteroids, 1. The Determination of 17-hydroxycorticosteroids." *Biochem. J.*, **60**, 453.

Barlow, J. J. (1964), "Adrenocortical Influence on Estrogen Metabolism in Normal Females," *J. clin. Endocrin.*, **24**, 586.

Blaquier, J., Forchielli, E. and Dorfman, R. I. (1967), "In Vitro Metabolism of Androgens in Whole Human Blood." *Acta Endocr., Copenhagen*, **55**, 697.

Bolte, E. (1967), "Precursors of Placental Estrogens," *Clinical Obstetrics and Gynecology*, **10**, 60.

Bongiovanni, A. M. and McPadden, A. J. (1960), "Steroids during Pregnancy and Possible Fetal Consequences," *Fertil. and Steril.*, **11**, 181.

Bongiovanni, A. M., Eberlein, W. R., Goldman, A. S. and New, M. (1967), "Disorders of Adrenal Steroid Biogenesis," *Recent Progress in Hormone Research*, **23**, 375.

Brooks, R. V., Mattingly, D., Mills, I. H. and Prunty, F. T. G. (1960), 'Post-pubertal Adrenal Virilism with Biochemical Disturbance of the Congenital Type of Adrenal Hyperplasia." *Brit. med. J.*, **1**, 1294.

Brown, J. B., Bulbrook, R. D. and Greenwood, F. C. (1967), "An Additional Purification Step for a Method for Estimating Oestriol, Oestrone and Oestradiol-17β in Human Urine." *J. Endocr.*, **16**, 49.

Brown, J. B., Falconer, C. W. A. and Strong, J. A. (1959), "Urinary Oestrogens of Adrenal Origin in Woman with Breast Cancer." *J. Endocr.*, **19**, 52.

Casey, J. H., Burger, H. G., Kent, J. R., Kellie, A. E., Moxham, A., Nabarro, J. and Nabarro, J. D. N. (1966), "Treatment of Hirsutism by Adrenal and Ovarian Suppression." *J. clin. Endocr.*, **26**, 1370.

Conti, C., Sorcini, G., Sciarra, F., Concolino, G. and Lotti, P. (1964), "Plasma Testosterone Levels in Normal Subjects and in Hirsute Women during Adrenal and Gonadal Function Tests." *Research on Steroids*, **1**, 77. Edited by Cassano, C. Rome. Il Pensiero Scientifico.

Cope, C. L. (1964), *Adrenal Steroids and Disease*, p. 192, London. Pitman Medical Publishing Co.

Cope, C. L. (1966a), "The Adrenal Cortex in Internal Medicine—Part 1," *Brit. med. J.*, **2**, 847.

Cope, C. L. (1966b), "The Adrenal Cortex in Internal Medicine—Part 2," *Brit. med. J.*, **2**, 914.

Cox, R. I. (1962), "Steroid Metabolites in Congenital Adrenal Hyperplasia," In *The Human Adrenal Cortex*, p. 383. Currie, A. R., Symington, T. and Grant, J. K. (Editors) Edinburgh: Livingstone.

Dassler, C. G. (1966), "Der Einfluss Von Corticotrophin Auf Die Östrogenausscheidung in Der Schwangerschaft Und Bei Intrauterinem Fruchttod," *Acta Endocr., Copenhagen*, **53**, 401.

de Nicola, A. F., Dorfman, R. I. and Forchielli, E. (1966), "Urinary Excretion of Epitestosterone and Testosterone in Normal Individuals and Virilized Females, *Steroids*, **7**, 351.

Dorfman, R. I., Forchielli, E. and Gut, M. (1963), "Androgen Biosynthesis and Related Studies," *Recent Progress in Hormone Research*, **19**, 251.

Finkelstein, M., Forchielli, E. and Dorfman, R. I. (1961), "Estimation of Testosterone in Human Plasma," *J. Clin. Endocrin.*, **21**, 98.

Finkelstein, M. (1964), "Pregnanetriolone, Estrogens and Testosterone Assays," *Research on Steroids*, **1**, 67. Edited by Cassano, C. Rome: Il Pensiero Scientifico.

Gandy, H. M., Moody, C. B. and Peterson, R. E. (1965), "Androgen Levels in Ovarian and Adrenal Venous Plasma," *Excerpta Medica International Congress Series No. 112*, p. 223.

Goldzieher, J. W. and Laitin, H. (1960), "Evaluation of the Pituitary—Adrenal Axis in Simple Hirsutism," *J. clin. Endocrin.*, **20**, 967.

Goldzieher, J. W. and Green, J. A. (1962), "The Polycystic Ovary 1. Clinical and Histological Features," *J. clin. Endocrin.*, **22**, 325.

Goldzieher, J. W. (1964), "Adrenal Cortical Dysfunction," *Clinical Obstetrics and Gynecology*, **7**, 1136.

Goldzieher, J. W. (1967), "Polycystic Ovarian Disease," In *Advances in Obstetrics and Gynecology*, p. 354, Edited by Marcus, S. L. and Marcus, C. C. Baltimore: Williams and Wilkins.

Greenblatt, R. B. and Mahesh, V. B. (1964), "Clinical Evaluation and Treatment of the Hirsute Female," *Clinical Obstetrics and Gynecology*, **7**, 1109.

Hamilton, J. B. (1964), "Racial and Genetic Predisposition (to Hirsutism)" *Clinical Obstetrics and Gynaecology*, **7**, 1075.

Horton, R. and Tait, J. F. (1966), "Androstenedione Production and Interconversion Rates Measured in Peripheral Blood and Studies on the Possible Site of its Conversion to Testosterone," *J. clin. Invest.*, **45**, 301.

Klopper, A. (1968), "The Assessment of Feto-placental Function by Estriol Assay," *Obstet. gynec. Surv.* **23**, 813.

Klopper, A. and Jeffery, J. d'A. (1968), "Ovarian Steroidogenesis: Normal and Abnormal," In *Modern Trends in Gynaecology*, **4**, Edited by Keller, R. J. London: Butterworths. In press.

Klyne, W. (1965), "The Chemistry of the Steroids," London: Methuen.

Lauritzen, C. (1967), "A Clinical Test for Placental Functional Activity using DHEA-sulphate and ACTH Injections in the Pregnant Woman," *Acta Endocr. Supplementum*, **119**, 188.

Lieberman, S. and Gurpide, E. (1966), "Isotopic Dilution Methods for the Estimation of Rates of Secretion of the Steroid Hormones," In *Steroid Dynamics*, p. 531, Edited by Pincus, G., Nakao, T. and Tait, J. F. New York: Academic Press.

Lipsett, M. B. and Riter, B. D. (1961), "Urinary Steroids in Postnatal Adrenal Hyperplasia with Virilism," *Acta endocr., Copenhagen*, **38**, 481.

Lipsett, M. B., Hertz, R. and Ross, G. T. (1963), "Clinical and Patho-physiologic Aspects of Adrenocortical Carcinoma," *Amer. J. Med.*, **35**, 374.

Loraine, J. A. and Bell, E. T. (1966), "Hormone Assays and Their Clinical Application," Second Edition, p. 430, Edinburgh: Livingstone.

Macleod, S. C., Brown, J. B., Beischer, N. A. and Smith, M. A. (1967), "The Value of Urinary Oestriol Measurements During Pregnancy," *Aust. and N.Z. J. Obstet. Gynaec.*, **7**, 25.

Mahesh, V. B., Greenblatt, R. B., Aydar, C. K., Roy, S., Puebla, R. A. and Ellegood, J. O. (1964), "Urinary Steroid Excretion Patterns in Hirsuitism, 1. Use of Adrenal and Ovarian Suppression Tests in the Study of Hirsuitism," *J. clin. Endocrin.*, **24**, 1283.

Martin, J. D. and Mills, I. H. (1956), "Aldosterone Excretion in Normal and Toxæmic Pregnancies," *Brit. med. J.*, **2**, 571.

Mattingly, D. (1963), "Plasma Steroid Levels as a Measure of Adrenocortical Activity," *Proc. R. Soc. Med.*, **56**, 717.

Mills, I. H., Brooks, R. V. and Prunty, F. T. G. (1962), "The Relationship between the Production of Cortisol and of Androgen by the Human Adrenal," In *The Human Adrenal Cortex*, p. 204. Editors, Currie, A. R., Symington, T. and Grant, J. K. Edinburgh: Livingstone.

Mills, I. H. (1968), "The Control of the Adrenal Precursors of 17-oxosteroids," In *The Investigation of Hypothalamic-Pituitary-Adrenal Function*, p. 83. Edited by James, V. H. T. and Landon, J. Memoirs of the Society for Endocrinology, **17**, Cambridge University Press.

Nissen-Meyer, R. and Sanner, T. (1963), "The Excretion of Oestrone, Pregnanediol and Pregnanetriol in Breast Cancer Patients," *Acta Endocr., Copenhagen*, **44**, 334.

Norymberski, J. K., Stubbs, R. D. and West, H. F. (1953), "Assessment of Adrenocortical Activity by Assay of 17-ketogenic Steroids in Urine," *Lancet*, **1**, 1276.

Porter, C. C. and Silber, R. H. (1950), "A Quantitative Color Reaction for Cortisone and Related 17,21-Dihydroxy-20-Ketosteroids," *J. biol. Chem.*, **185**, 201.

Prunty, F. T. G. (1966), "Androgen metabolism in Man—Some Current Concepts," *Brit. med. J.*, **2**, 605.

Prunty, F. T. G. (1967), "Hirsutism, Virilism and Apparent Virilism and their Gonadal Relationship," *J. Endocr.*, **38**, 85.

Shearman, R. P. and Cox, R. I. (1966), "The Enigmatic Polycystic Ovary," *Obstet. Gynec. Surv.*, **21**, 1.

Simmer, H. H., Dignam, W. J., Easterling, W. E., Frankland, M. V. and Naftolin, F. (1966), "Neutral C-19 Steroids and Steroid Sulphates in Human Pregnancy, 3," *Steroids*, **8**, 179.

Warrell, D. W. and Taylor, R. (1968), "Outcome for the Foetus of Mothers receiving Prednisolone during Pregnancy," *Lancet*, **1**, 117.

Warren, J. C. and Cheatum, S. G. (1967), "Maternal Urinary Estrogen Excretion: Effect of Adrenal Suppression," *J. clin. Endocrin.*, **27**, 433.

7. THE PANCREAS

C. W. H. HAVARD

Anatomy

The pancreas lies immediately behind the peritoneum on the posterior abdominal wall. The head is moulded into the concavity of the duodenum. The head of the pancreas is supplied by the superior and inferior pancreatico-duodenal arteries, and the body and tail by the splenic artery. The veins drain into the portal, superior mesenteric, and splenic veins. The pancreatic duct extends from the tail to the head increasing in size as it receives numerous tributaries on the way. It joins the common bile duct at the ampulla of Vater and opens onto the surface of the duodenum, (Fig. 1). The acces-

or pancreatic juice is the product of secretory units or acini, the cells of which resemble those of salivary glands.

Pancreatin is the watery secretion of the pancreas and it is slightly alkaline due to the presence of sodium bicarbonate. The alkalinity enables the acidity of gastric contents to be neutralized. With increased rates of secretion the juice becomes more alkaline. The organic matter of the juice consists of mucin and the digestive enzymes or their inactive precursors. The enzymes are proteolytic, lipolytic and amylolytic. The daily output of juice is 500 to 1500 ml. in man. The protein content of 0·1–3 per cent is chiefly enzymes, and may amount to several

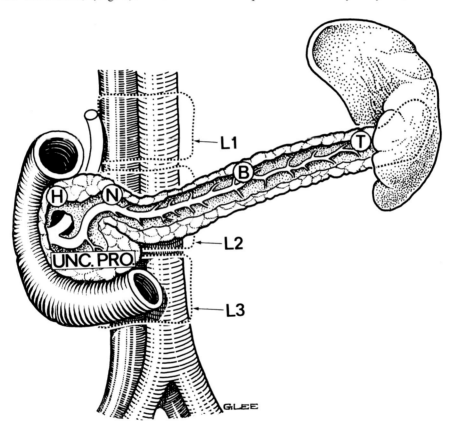

Fig. 1. The anatomy of the pancreas.

sory pancreatic duct, which drains the lower part of the head, opens into the duodenum 2 cm. proximal to the main duct, although frequently the two ducts communicate.

Physiology

The pancreas is a compound racemose gland and produces both external and internal secretions. The internal secretions or hormones are insulin and glucagon. They are both concerned with carbohydrate metabolism and are dealt with elsewhere (p. 343). The external secretion

grammes a day. The concentration of various pancreatic enzymes runs in parallel. Thus if trypsin is increased other enzymes are also increased—though not necessarily to the same degree. Trypsin exists as its precursor trypsinogen, which must be activated by intestinal enzymes called kinases. The pancreas also contains trypsin inhibitors to prevent minute amounts of trypsin activating more trypsinogen. Trypsin is slowly destroyed and there is little tryptic activity in the lower part of the intestine of adults. Trypsin is a powerful protein-splitting enzyme, converting them into polypeptides. Lipase hydrolyses fats to fatty acids and monoglycerides, but acts best when the fat is in a suitable physical state, as that produced by the action of bile salts. Amylase hydrolyses starch to maltose. A certain amount of pancreatic amylase is absorbed into the blood and secreted into the urine. The urine thus has starch splitting or diastatic properties. Blood also contains tryptic activity but it is greatly reduced by the presence of inhibitors.

Control of Pancreatic Secretion

Although there is a small continuous flow of pancreatic juice, three mechanisms control pancreatic secretion.

1. Secretin. This is a humoral agent liberated by the duodenal mucosa when the acid gastric contents enter the duodenum. Secretin promotes the secretion of water and salts (bicarbonate). It is extremely potent, for one mg. of secretin will produce 12 litres of pancreatic juice. Patients with achlorhydria have adequate pancreatic secretion.

2. Pancreozymin. This is another humoral agent liberated from the mucosa of the upper intestine. It promotes the secretion of the pancreatic enzymes and has little if any affect on the volume of juice. Pancreozymin is secreted into the blood in response to the presence of fat and other foods in the duodenum and upper jejunum. It also causes contraction of the gall bladder and increases both pepsin secretion by the stomach and motor activity of the gut.

3. Vagus Nerve. Stimulation of the vagus nerve causes the production of a secretion rich in enzymes, similar to that following pancreozymin. It is, however, inhibited by atropine. The act of eating is the stimulus and there is no need for food to enter the stomach for the vagal effect on the pancreas. The parasympathetic nerves also enhance the hormonal stimuli of the pancreas.

The juice secreted in response to fat is particularly rich in enzymes, that to protein a little less rich and that in response to carbohydrate is the juice least in volume and enzyme content.

INVESTIGATION OF PANCREATIC FUNCTION

The investigation of pancreatic disease is notoriously difficult. The glucose tolerance test is a poor guide to the presence of chronic pancreatitis and the serum concentrations of amylase are only useful in cases of active acute pancreatitis. The electrophoretic separation of amylase into its pancreatic and salivary components has recently been achieved and this will probably enhance the value of serum concentrations in pancreatic disease. It is possible that the ratio of salivary to pancreatic amylase may provide a screening test for pancreatic disease.

The investigation of pancreatic function includes:

1. Tests of the Secretory Activity of the Pancreas.
2. Tests of Intestinal Malabsorption.
3. Specialized Tests for specific pancreatic disorders, e.g., sweat tests for mucoviscidosis.
4. Radiology.
5. Radioactive Scanning. The choice of test will depend on the pancreatic disorder being considered.

1. Tests Involving Studies of Secretory Activity

The two enzymes amylase and lipase may be measured in (1) Serum (2) Urine, (3) Duodenal juice. The first two methods are used in the diagnosis of pancreatitis and the third to determine pancreatic insufficiency.

Serum and Urine Enzymes

Amylase activity is measured by the ability of the serum or urine to break down starch. This used to be assessed in terms of disappearance of the iodine-starch blue colour as hydrolysis of starch progresses, but it is now better determined by the appearance of sugar. The amount of sugar appearing after a given time being the measure of amylase activity. The normal serum level is 50–180 Somogyi units and it may be raised severalfold in acute pancreatitis. It must be remembered that the pancreas is not the only source of amylase. Indeed the serum level is little affected by pancreatectomy. Amylase originates also from the salivary glands, the liver and the Fallopian tubes. The liver is probably the most important source of blood amylase under normal circumstances.

The serum level may be raised after rupture of a tubal pregnancy. In normal pregnancy there is a steady rise in the later months. The serum level is, however, the net result of the amount of enzyme entering the blood from tissue sources and the amount being excreted by the kidneys. Thus in chronic renal failure or in any shocked patient when glomerular filtration is reduced, high serum levels may occur. Intestinal obstruction below the entrance of the pancreatic duct will also raise the serum concentration. High levels are common in abdominal catastrophies such as perforation of a peptic ulcer, empyema of the gall bladder and gangrene of the small intestine. Drugs such as morphine may also be responsible, presumably by inducing spasm of the sphincter of Oddi. Mumps parotitis without pancreatitis may raise the serum amylase. A normal concentration does not exclude a diagnosis of pancreatitis absolutely. Levels of more than 900 units are highly suggestive.

Lipase is more specific to the pancreas and is, therefore, a more reliable measure of pancreatic function. There are, however, technical difficulties surrounding its estimation and these detract from its value. The time required for the determination is much longer. Raised serum concentrations of lipase also occur in intestinal obstruction, peritonitis and renal failure.

Enzymes in Duodenal Juice

Duodenal juice is not the same as pancreatic juice for it contains trypsin, not trypsinogen and it is contaminated by gastric juice, bile and the secretion of Brunner's glands. When attempting aspiration of the duodenal juice a double lumen tube (such as Dreiling or Lagerlof tube) should be used to separate gastric from duodenal contents, by a special technique.

The samples should be kept at freezing point as lipase is sensitive to temperature. The volume of juice and the concentration of bicarbonate, amylase, lipase and tryspin should be examined and the presence of blood sought.

This test has the disadvantage of requiring accurate intubation of the stomach and duodenum and the careful collection of all specimens.

Recently a new test of secretory activity has been introduced. It utilizes a synthetic substrate to estimate the tryptic activity in duodenal aspirates after a standard test meal. Total collections of secretions are not required, nor are any injections necessary.

2. Tests of Intestinal Malabsorption

As the pancreas has a large reserve capacity steatorrhoea does not occur until pancreatic function is severely impaired. In chronic pancreatitis the symptom triad of steatorrhoea, pancreatic calcification and diabetes mellitus is a late manifestation. Even then malnutrition is an unusual feature of pancreatic disease. This is because the defect of absorption is largely confined to fat and the patients have a good appetite so that their intake of food remains adequate. Although 80 per cent of the dietary fat may appear in the faeces nutritional defects are uncommon.

An average daily diet contains 100 g. fat. Faecal excretion does not normally exceed 7 g. daily. Even on a fat free diet 3 g. daily will be excreted from endogenous sources such as desquamated mucosal cells. The best test of intestinal malabsorption is the quantitative chemical determination of faecal fat excreted over a period of three days. If a diagnosis of steatorrhoea is established the next problem is to decide whether it is due to a disorder of digestion or whether it is due to a defect in intestinal absorption. The D-Xylose excretion is often helpful.

Disorders of intestinal digestion are not all the result of pancreatic disease. They may be due to lack of bile as a result of obstructive jaundice or due to impaired mixing of ferments with food as a result of previous gastrectomy or gastro-jejunostomy.

3. Specialized Tests for Specific Pancreatic Disorders. Sweat Test for Mucoviscidosis

The most useful and specific test for mucoviscidosis is the demonstration of an excessive concentration of sodium and chloride in the sweat. Mucoviscidosis affects all the exocrine glands of the body including the sweat glands.

4. Radiology

There is unfortunately no excretory pancreaticogram comparable to the intravenous pyelogram. The pancreas thus remains one of the few organs defying radiological demonstration. The diagnosis of pancreatic tumours remains notoriously difficult. A plain X-ray of the abdomen may reveal pancreatic calcification suggesting chronic pancreatitis (Fig. 2). It occurs in 20 to 25 per cent of cases. Barium studies are of no help in the diagnosis of pancreatic disorders. Arteriography is a valuable method of diagnosing tumours of brain and kidney because of the vascular displacement and pooling of the contrast medium that is characteristic of tumours in these organs. These signs rarely occur in tumours of the pancreas. Islet cell tumours however hold on to the contrast medium in about one third of the patients, so that they may become demon-

strable in the late parenchymatous phase. Those radiologists adept at this procedure have been able to demonstrate vessel narrowing or a tumour circulation in a large proportion of patients with carcinoma of the pancreas.

5. Scanning

The aminoacid, methionine, is rapidly taken up by the pancreas as a substrate for the synthesis of pancreatic enzymes. The substitution of 75–Selenium for the sulphur in methionine does not alter its physiological properties. Photoscanning 30 minutes after giving $3 \mu C$ per kg. of 75–Selenium will visualize the pancreas. The liver also takes up the isotope and therefore, the liver must first be scanned with radioactive colloidal gold, so that the areas where the liver overlaps the pancreas can be identified. Cold areas in the pancreatic scan indicate nonfunctioning tissue and are likely to indicate areas of neoplasia or cysts.

DISORDERS OF THE PANCREAS
Acute Pancreatitis

There is evidence that pregnancy predisposes to acute pancreatitis. It occurs more commonly in pregnancy and in the puerperium than would be expected by chance alone, and when attacks occur during pregnancy 70 per cent of the patients relapse during the puerperium. The majority of these patients are primigravida in the third decade of life, which contrasts with a mean age of over 50 for non-pregnant patients with acute pancreatitis. It is often important to exclude pancreatitis in hyperemesis gravidarum. An awareness of the possibility of pancreatitis is the most essential prerequisite to a diagnosis. Acute pancreatitis presents with upper abdominal pain, often severe, radiating through to the back. It is associated with nausea, vomiting and collapse. It is thus an important differential diagnosis for the obstetrician as nausea, vomiting and epigastric discomfort are common complaints during pregnancy. When the onset of these symptoms is sudden and associated with abdominal tenderness, acute pancreatitis must be considered.

Aetiology

Non-bacterial inflammation of the pancreas can occur in association with a number of endocrine, metabolic, mechanical and vascular disorders, and there does not appear to be any connecting link between them. Infection itself is rarely of importance except as an unusual complication of mumps. Activation of the pancreatic ferment trypsinogen with subsequent digestion of the pancreas is an important factor in the aetiology of pancreatitis. This leads to extensive acinar necrosis, cellular infiltration with interstitial oedema and haemorrhage into pancreatic tissue. The changes may be general throughout the pancreas or limited to a part of the gland. Any injury to the acinar cells of the pancreas may cause the release of trypsinogen and other enzymes which are responsible for these tissue changes. Activation of the potent circulatory enzymes bradykinin and kallikrein contributes to the severe shock characteristic of acute pancreatitis. If the patient survives,

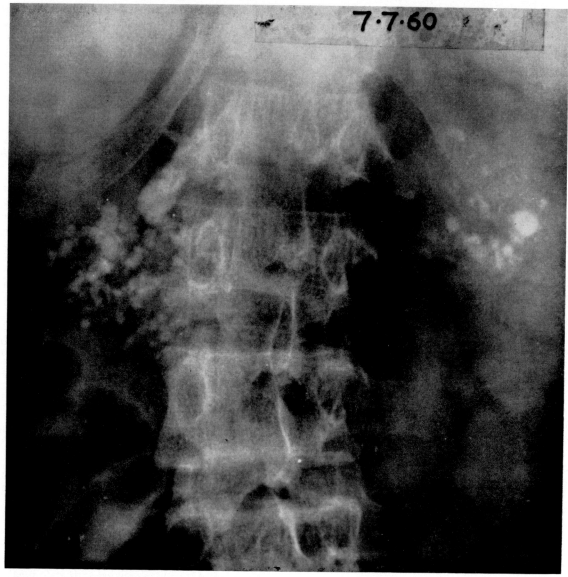

Fig. 2. Plain X-ray of abdomen of a woman aged 54 years with pancreatic calcification due to hyperparathyroidism.

secondary infection of necrotic tissue with suppuration and abscess formation may occur.

Although the precise mechanism is not understood a number of disorders are known to predispose to non-bacterial inflammation of the pancreas:

1. Disease of the Biliary Tract. In one third to one half of patients with acute pancreatitis in Britain the disorder is associated with disease of the gall bladder, particularly gall stones and cholecystitis. It is uncertain how gall bladder disease causes pancreatitis but in the experimental animal, regurgitation of bile down the pancreatic duct precipitates pancreatitis.

2. Alcohol. In Britain 10 to 20 per cent of cases of acute pancreatitis are secondary to alcoholism. In America the proportion is much higher. Alcohol causes an increase in pancreatic secretion and spasm of the sphincter of Oddi, a combination of events which predisposes towards auto-digestion.

3. Miscellaneous. Pancreatitis may occur secondary to a variety of metabolic, endocrine, traumatic and vascular disorders such as:

(a) Trauma (including post-operative pancreatitis)
(b) Pregnancy
(c) Hyperparathyroidism
(d) Hyperlipidaemia
(e) Hypothermia
(f) Disseminated Lupus Erythematosus (D.L.E.)
(g) Ascariasis
(h) Drugs such as chlorothiazide and tetracycline.

Traumatic and post-operative pancreatitis and that associated with D.L.E., may be explained on a vascular basis, arterial thrombosis resulting in local ischaemia to an area of the gland. The way in which metabolic abnormalities predispose to pancreatitis is unknown. In hyperparathyroidism it has been suggested that the raised tissue concentration of calcium activates trypsinogen. In pancreatitis associated with chlorothiazide administration the relationship is probably causal, as pancreatitis can be induced in a large proportion of mice treated with comparable doses.

Clinical and Biochemical Features

The symptoms of pancreatitis have been described. The patient is usually febrile and the pulse is rapid. There is abdominal tenderness and guarding and rebound tenderness is frequent. In severe cases the pulse is thready, the patient shocked and the abdomen distended. Chest signs are common and a pleural effusion, especially on the left side, may occur in 40 per cent of cases.

Leucocytosis is frequent and hypocalcaemia often develops on the second day due to the combination of calcium with fatty acids formed by digestion in and around the pancreas. A serum calcium concentration of less than 7 mg. per 100 ml. is of grave prognosis. The serum may be milky due to hyperlipidaemia and the concentration of amylase is raised, (p. 544). The concentration of amylase in the peritoneal fluid is even higher than that in the serum and it rises early in the disease. It is also high in associated pleural effusions. The enzyme concentration in peritoneal fluid is 8,000 to 19,000 units compared with 200 to 5,000 units in cases of peptic ulcer perforation. The blood sugar may be raised due to destruction of pancreatic islet cells with consequent loss of insulin production. An X-ray of the abdomen will not show pathognomonic evidence of pancreatitis but it may show pancreatic calcification or it may reveal evidence of peptic ulcer perforation such as air under the diaphragm.

The important differential diagnoses include perforation of a peptic ulcer, acute cholecystitis, mesenteric artery thrombosis, pericarditis, myocardial infarction and dissection of the aorta. In pancreatitis the serum amylase is usually over 500 Somogyi units and when over 1,000 units it is usually diagnostic. There remain a proportion of patients with acute pancreatitis in whom the serum amylase is not raised, and in many patients with peptic ulcer perforation and intestinal obstruction the serum amylase is raised though rarely over 800 units.

Management

The principles of management consist of:

1. The alleviation of pain, and the prevention and treatment of shock. Pethidine is the analgesic of choice.
2. The suppression of pancreatic secretion, by restriction of oral feeding and by suction of gastric juice.
3. The maintenance of electrolyte balance.

Trasylol is an inhibitor of trypsin and kallikrein that has been isolated from bovine parotid gland. It also inhibits chymotrypsin and fibrinolysis. Once necrosis of the pancreas is well established this anti-enzyme may not be effective but it has been shown to offer protection when given early. It may be given intravenously in a dose of 150,000 to 300,000 units daily.

Electrolyte imbalance is likely to occur in acute pancreatitis. In particular hypokalaemia, hypocalcaemia and a metabolic acidosis are real dangers. A close watch on the serum electrolytes is required as losses of potassium especially may be considerable. Observation of the blood sugar is also indicated as diabetic ketosis may be a complication of pancreatic islet cell destruction.

A broad spectrum antibiotic is advisable to control secondary bacterial infection.

Relapsing and Chronic Pancreatitis

A careful study of patients who survived an acute attack of pancreatitis suggests that a further attack occurs in 55 per cent over the subsequent three years. The relapsing and chronic forms of pancreatitis are of less interest to the obstetrician as they are more common in men and this may reflect the importance of alcohol as an aetiological agent. The disease is characterized by recurrent attacks of subacute pancreatitis lasting about 24 hours. Progressive destruction of the gland occurs and it becomes hard and fibrotic. The best test of pancreatic failure is the estimation of duodenal enzymes. As the pancreas has an immense reserve, the symptom triad of steatorrhoea, diabetes mellitus and pancreatic calcification does not occur until late in the disease. Repeated attacks of acute pancreatitis do not however always lead to chronic pancreatitis, and chronic pancreatitis may occur without previous acute attacks.

Mucoviscidosis

Mucoviscidosis is a genetically determined inborn error of metabolism, in which a widespread disorder of mucus secreting glands occurs. These glands include the pancreas, and mucous glands of the intestine, bronchial mucosa and biliary tract. The mucus produced by these glands is abnormally viscid and blocks the acini and ducts of the glands. The disorder is inherited as an autosomal recessive characteristic and its relevance to the obstetrician is that 10 per cent of cases present in the neonatal period as meconium ileus. Intestinal obstruction occurs in the newborn child from viscid meconium. Destruction and fibrosis of the pancreas occurs later and bronchial obstruction from viscid mucous leads to recurrent respiratory infections, bronchiectasis and recurrent pneumonia. From these causes young infants may present with a failure to thrive. Obstruction of the biliary ducts predisposes to infection and biliary cirrhosis. Less commonly the disease may present with pancreatic steatorrhoea coinciding with the introduction of mixed feeding. The commonest presentation is undoubtedly recurrent respiratory disease in childhood. The diagnosis is made by a sweat test (p. 545) and the evidence of impaired duodenal concentration of pancreatic enzymes.

Tumours of the Pancreas

In discussing the physiology of the pancreas it was pointed out that the pancreas produces both internal secretions or hormones (insulin and glucagon) as well as its external secretion pancreatic juice. The cells of these two components of pancreatic function are distinct in both structure and function so that the tumours of these cells will be considered separately.

Carcinoma of Pancreas. Tumours of the acinar cells of the pancreas are rare. The common cancer of the pancreas is an adenocarcinoma of the duct cells. Laparotomy is often necessary to confirm the diagnosis and a cholecysto-jejunostomy to relieve the jaundice. Curative operations are rarely possible.

The diagnosis of a carcinoma in the body or tail of the pancreas is much more difficult than one in the head of the pancreas because jaundice is not a feature. The symptom of back pain aggravated by lying down should arouse suspicion and this is often associated with a variety of non-specific symptoms such as anorexia, loss of weight and lethargy. Multiple phlebothromboses are sometimes a feature though they are not specific for pancreatic neoplasms. There are no pathognomic tests but photo-scanning of the pancreas following administration of radioactive seleno-methionine promises to be helpful (p. 545). Secondary metastases may appear in the ovaries.

Hormone Secreting Tumours of the Pancreas

The islet cells of the pancreas secrete insulin and glucagon. Tumours of islet cells can be found in one to two per cent of routine autopsies but hypersecretion occurs only in a small minority. When it does insulin is nearly always the hormone secreted, only a few instances of glucagon-secreting tumours having been recorded. Adenoma formation of islet cells, which are not beta cells may also occur and these cells secrete gastrin. The excess gastrin causes gastric acid hypersecretion and peptic ulceration, a syndrome bearing the name of Zollinger and Ellison who first described it. Occasionally islet cell tumours are part of a more general adenoma formation in endocrine glands—a syndrome described as Multiple Endocrine Adenopathy. Multiple endocrine adenopathy is a familial disorder characterized by the occurrence of multiple tumours or hyperplasia involving endocrine glands. The parathyroid, pancreatic islets and anterior pituitary are the glands most often involved. Less frequently the adrenal and thyroid glands may be affected. The adenomas may be hormonally active in any one or more of the glands affected. In more than 50 per cent of the reported cases peptic ulceration has been present. The disorder is inherited as a dominant characteristic.

Organic Hyperinsulinism (Insulinoma). Organic hyperinsulinism is due to excessive insulin production by islet-cell tumours of beta cells. These tumours may be multiple and usually occur in the body or tail of the pancreas. In one third of cases they are histologically malignant but they are rarely invasive and long term survival is common. Both sexes are equally affected and the disease usually presents in middle age. The clinical features are provoked by attacks of hypoglycaemia, which are particularly prone to occur during periods of fasting. They are therefore most common in the early morning, and late afternoon.

Hypoglycaemia produces central nervous symptoms directly related to the low blood glucose. In addition it causes symptoms of sympathetic nervous system hyperactivity as the output of adrenaline from the adrenal medulla is increased to promote glycogenolysis and to restore the blood sugar to normal. Faintness, confusion, dysarthria, blurred vision, convulsions and coma are manifestations of the low blood glucose. Sweating, trembling, anxiety, weakness, hunger pains and tachycardia are due to excessive sympathetic nervous activity. The most frequently encountered symptoms are weakness, confusion, sweating and hunger pains, and characteristically they appear with fasting and are aggravated by exercise.

The condition is often mistaken for psychiatric illness, encephalitis, subdural haematoma and cerebral arterial disease. Emotional disturbances are common during pregnancy, the puerperium and at the menopause and it is particularly easy for the gynaecologist to ascribe such symptoms to the time of life. When, however, the symptoms are intermittent and sometimes even when they are not, hypoglycaemia deserves serious consideration.

The diagnosis of hypoglycaemia can be confirmed during an attack by the demonstration of a blood glucose below 30 mg. per 100 ml. (blood sugar below 50 mg. per 100 ml.) and by the relief of symptoms following an injection of intravenous glucose. If attacks of hypoglycaemia are infrequent provocative tests may be required. The most useful test is a prolonged fast during which only water and black coffee are allowed by mouth. Physical activity should be maintained and the blood glucose determined at intervals of three hours. Seventy five per cent of patients with organic hyperinsulinism develop symptoms within 24 hours and 98 per cent within 48 hours. A blood glucose should then be taken and intravenous glucose given. Another provocative test is the Tolbutamide Test. Tolbutamide causes release of insulin from insulinomas as well as from normal islet cells. If one gramme is given intravenously there is an excessive fall in blood glucose within 30 minutes.

The management of organic hyperinsulinism is surgical. The tumours, which are often multiple, should be removed. If no tumour is found the body and tail of the pancreas should be removed. When surgery is not possible or fails, glucagon may be used to control hypoglycaemia but it has to be given by intramuscular injection. Diazoxide is an oral diabetogenic agent, chemically related to the thiazide diuretics, and it has proved useful in the control of attacks of hypoglycaemia.

Zollinger-Ellison Syndrome. A syndrome of gastric hypersecretion and peptic ulceration was described in 1955. It is due to an islet cell tumour which does not produce insulin, but gastrin. If peptic ulcers recur after adequate surgery the disorder should be seriously considered. It is important to confirm the clinical suspicion by demonstrating gross gastric hypersecretion, especially a high resting secretion.

It has been mentioned that patients with islet cell tumours commonly have tumours of other endocrine glands and this is particularly true of patients with the Zollinger–Ellison syndrome, in whom associated endocrine adenomas are found in 20 per cent. As the syndrome is so commonly part of a multiple endocrine adenopathy, skull X-rays, determination of the serum concentration of calcium and phosphate and the urinary excretion of oxogenic steroids should be done to seek evidence of adenomas of pituitary, parathyroid and adrenal glands.

8. THE INVESTIGATION OF GONADAL ENDOCRINE FUNCTION

MAX-F. JAYLE

The ovaries are endocrine glands of a complex order due to their cyclical function, the variety of independent endocrine compartments involved and the multitude of pathological changes to which they themselves are subject. In spite of improved methods of quantitative analysis that are now available for testing urinary steroids, the results can lead to false information. The level of oestrogens for instance depends on the stage in the menstrual cycle at which the urine is tested, and as for the pregnanediol rate which is a firm indication of the presence of a corpus luteum, it is not in any way superior to the temperature curve, to vaginal smears or to endometrial biopsy. As for the level of plasma steroid hormones, this subject still belongs to medical research and not to practical application.

At present we have available substances that specifically stimulate or inhibit the adrenal cortex and the ovaries and these now allow us to carry out tests that open up new fields for investigating what we will call the dynamic testing of the endocrine functions of the gonads of both sexes. We will in turn describe the test that depends on stimulation with chorionic gonadotropin (HCG), the sequential use of human menopausal gonadotropin (HMG) and human pituitary gonadotropin (HPG), and tests resulting from the suppression of ovarian secretions. As an introduction we will briefly review the latest publications concerning the ovarian secretion of different hormones.

According to Savard and his colleagues (1965, 1967) we can visualize the ovary as made up of three endocrine compartments. The use of radioactive acetate has shown that while each is capable of producing several steroids they are nevertheless moderately specialized. Thus oestrogens are mainly elaborated by thecal tissue, gestagens by the corpus luteum and androgens by the stroma which does not produce germ cells. The hormones thus produced are oestradiol, oestrone, progesterone, 20-dihydro-progesterone, 17-hydroxy-progesterone, androstenedione (the main ovarian androgen) and small quantities of dehydro-epiandrosterone. Although most of the testosterone found in women in the plasma is formed by the peripheral breakdown of androstenedione as reported by Horton and Tait (1966), and Bardin and Lipset (1967) we do know that small quantities of testosterone do come from the ovary as Gandy, Moody and Peterson showed (1965) by finding trace levels in the ovarian vein. The rate of production for oestrogens varies between 30 and 350 μg./24 hours as shown by Goering, Matsuda and Herrmann (1965) whose work confirms the figures that had been produced by Brown (1955). As for the C-19 group of steroids, the ovaries secrete 2·3 mg. of dehydroepiandrosterone in 24 hours according to MacDonald, VandeWiele and Lieberman (1963) and the rates of secretion of androstenedione and testosterone are respectively 3·30 ± 1·86

mg./24 h. and 0·230 ± 0·073 mg./24 h. (Bardin and Lipsett, 1967).

The metabolism of ovarian steroids mainly occurs in the liver. Oestrone (E_1) and oestradiol (E) are in a reversible equilibrium and therefore have the same clinical significance. Oestriol (E_3) is the product into which they are partially changed, the remaining portion being destroyed by the liver. The three main oestrogens are for the most part excreted in the urine, mainly in the form of glucuronides, the proportion being E_3 approximately equal to $E_1 + E_2$. Progesterone and 20-dihydro-progesterone are excreted as pregnanediol glucuronide (PG), the 17 α-hydroxy-progesterone being transformed to pregnanetriol (PGT). Finally all the androgens derived from the ovary are converted to androsterone (A) and etiocholanolone (E).

Action of Human Chorionic Gonadotropin

Human chorionic gonadotropin (HCG) has all the properties of the pituitary luteinizing hormone (LH, or interstitial-cell stimulating hormone, ICSH). It can moreover transform the normal cyclic corpus luteum into a pseudo-pregnant corpus luteum. These properties can be used pharmacologically either to bring about a pseudo-pregnant state or to stimulate production of androgens by testes or polycystic ovaries.

HCG-Dexamethasone Test

In the last fifteen years we have standardized a dynamic test of the human corpus luteum (Jayle, 1967) in order to determine its function under maximal stimulation. This compares with the test that Thorn and others worked out with ACTH to investigate metabolic and androgenic function of the adrenocortical glands.

The human corpus luteum is of mixed structure—partly being composed of luteinised granulosa cells and partly of thecal tissue. In our early studies we found that it was necessary to wait 5 to 6 days before the normal cyclical corpus luteum could become transformed into that of the pseudo-pregnancy state. It required 15,000 IU of HCG given in three intramuscular injections in normal women and 30,000 IU in obese women to achieve maximum stimulation. Figure 1 demonstrates the conditions for standardizing this test. To appraise the adrenocortical activity, the 17-oxo-steroids and corticosteroids (Porter and Silber chromogens) are estimated in a 24 hour sample of urine collected before the start of the test. If the concentration of 17-oxo-steroids is more than 20 mg., we have to carry out chromatographic separation. The test must start on the third day of the luteal temperature plateau. 1 mg. of dexamethasone is given every 8 hours, i.e. 3 mg. daily during the six days of the test, to suppress the production of corticosteroids from the adrenal. The HCG is administered on the first, third and fifth days. On the sixth day of the test a second 24 hour specimen of urine is collected. The creatinine level is calculated on both samples, which allows us to have a control because in normal women the variation should not be more than ±10 per cent. When the Porter and Silber

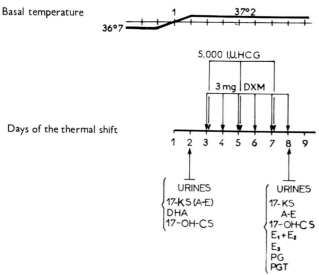

Fig. 1. The conditions under which the HCb-Dexamethasone Test is performed.

chromogens have fallen below 1 mg., we confirm that the suppression of adrenal steroid excretion has been achieved. We use the second sample of urine to evaluate by rapid chromatographic methods $E_1 + E_2$ and E_3 (Scholler, Heron and Jayle, 1962), PG and PGT (Jayle, Scholler and

Del Pozo, 1962) as well as the residual fraction A + E (Drosdowsky, Scholler and Jayle, 1962).

All those assays can be realized rapidly enough to allow a clinical application of the test. Relative variation, when the assays are carried out in duplicates, is less than 10 per cent. The reproducibility is good as shown when the tests are performed twice or three times in the same patient, even with an interval of a few months between them. Differences between normal and pathological results are very significant for each category of the evaluated steroids.

To date, after having carried out nearly 20,000 tests, we have never had any case of intraperitoneal trauma and only very rarely have minor complications ensued. So the result of this test can be summarized as:

1. On the sixth day of the test, each patient's normal limits of steroid excretion can be determined providing that the test was started at the beginning of the luteal phase. In other words, this test reveals whether the corpus luteum is normal.

2. Any deviation from the normal range above or below the standard levels indicates that the ovaries are either insufficiently active or over-active as far as their oestrogen, luteal or androgenic functions are concerned.

3. Abnormalities of endocrine function in the ovaries can be associated or independent from one another. For instance, one can discover a total ovarian insufficiency by finding very low levels of pregnanediol and oestrogens beside separate insufficiencies affecting solely oestrogenic or progestational activity.

Table 1 summarizes the different types of normal or pathological response to the HCG-dexamethasone test. In 107 normal women, we found, at the sixth day of the test, levels of pregnanediol and of oestrogens similar to those found in early pregnancy, 4 weeks after the last menstruation. The rate of the fraction A + E corresponds

TABLE 1

DIFFERENT CATEGORIES OF RESPONSES TO THE HCG–DEXAMETHASONE TEST

	A–E fraction mg./24 hr.	PGT mg./24 hr.	PG mg./24 hr.	$E_1 + E_2$ μg./24 hr.	E_3 μg./24 hr.
Normal response	1·6 (1–2·2)	1·5 (1–2)	6·5 (5–9)	33 (25–40)	48 (30–60)
Castration, panhypopituitarism mental anorexia	0·3 (0–0·7)	0	0·2 (0–0·6)	3 (0–5)	7 (5–10)
Oestrogenic insufficiency associated with luteal insufficiency	1·5 (0·7–2)	0·9 (0·5–1·8)	3·1 (1–4·5)	18 (10–25)	25 (15–35)
Oestrogenic insufficiency	1·4 (1–2)	1·1 (1–1·8)	6·4 (5–8·3)	17 (10–20)	25 (20–30)
Luteal insufficiency	1·7 (1·2–2)	1·2 (1–2)	3·3 (2–4·5)	31 (25–40)	41 (35–50)
Anovulatory cycles	1·5 (0·7–2)	0·2 (0·1–1)	0–0·5	5–40	10–50
Hyperandrogenism	3·0 (2·5–5·5)	1·6 (0·6–2·7)	5·7 (2–14·5)	34 (10–75)	50 (20–100)
Hyperoestrogenism	2·0 (1·6–2·4)	2·0 (1·5–2·4)	5·4 (0·5–9)	45 (30–60)	80 (40–100)
Hyperluteinism	1·7 (1–2)	1·5 (1·2–2)	12 (9·5–16)	32 (25–40)	43 (30–60)
Total hyperplasia	3·0 (2·6–3·4)	2·2 (1·8–2·7)	12·0 (9·5–14·0)	43 (35–60)	90 (55–110)

to that found after adrenocortical inhibition by dexamethasone. HCG administration doubles the excretion of PG, PGT, E_1, E_2 and E_3, although it does not modify that of the fraction A + E.

What is true for different forms of ovarian diminished activity is equally true for the different forms of over-activity. When hyperplasia affects the whole organ it modifies the three endocrine functions. The HCG-dexamethasone test results in a highly increased response in contrast to the "hormonal vacuum" found in total ovarian insufficiency. In this case, the levels of PG and PGT as well as of $E_1 + E_2 + E_3$ are higher than the upper limits of the normal range. This usually occurs in women with enlarged ovaries. We might imagine that this total ovarian hyperactivity is caused by an over-production of FSH and LH by the pituitary. Indeed, as we will see later on, it can be reproduced by the sequential administration of these two stimulants. The most important criteria of ovarian endocrine deficiency and over-activity are related to the level of oestrogens and pregnanetriol on the sixth day of the dynamic test.

We find in women who have been castrated, or who have had their menopause long ago, or are in a state of hypopituitarism, or are suffering from anorexia nervosa, absence or hypoplasia of the ovaries demonstrated by minimal quantities of oestrogens and undetectable quantities of pregnanediol. The residual level of the fraction A + E is less than 0·5 mg. and far lower than in normal women ($p < 0.01$). The exact opposite is found when there is endocrine over-activity in the ovaries: the sum of the three oestrogens is found to be between 100 and 200 μg. and that of pregnanetriol between 2·5 and 5 mg. Let us in passing say that there are rare forms of over-activity of the ovaries where the level of pregnanediol is alone raised (lutein cyst) and others where urinary hyperexcretion of oestrogens occurs by itself.

Taking these results all together we have to reappraise several classic ideas. In this way we find that there is no increase of urinary oestrogens in the pre-menstrual syndrome and that over-production of oestrogens is rare in menorrhagia.

Similarly it is usual to equate the "Swiss cheese" cystic hyperplasia of the endometrium in menometrorrhagia with over-production of oestrogens. It is true that this form of hyperoestrogenism exists, but it is very rare. Weak but persistent secretion of oestrogens without luteal phase interruption results in the end in a hyperplasia of the endometrium in which the determining factor is the absence of the corpus luteum.

We have to reconsider as well the pathology of repeated abortions and sterility of endocrine origin. A statistical survey has enabled us to establish that deficient secretion of progesterone by the corpus luteum is just one secondary cause of these troubles. On the other hand, diminished oestrogen secretion as proved by the HCG-dexamethasone test and demonstrated by levels of $E_1 + E_2 + E_3 < 55$ μg. is the most important cause of repeated abortions and sterility of endocrine origin. We have found in over 95 per cent of women with too low oestrogenic activity as proved by this test that the level of pregnanediol is normal

(isolated oestrogenic insufficiency) or insufficient (total luteal insufficiency).

Comparison between Ovarian Hyperandrogenism and the Androgenic Activity of the Testis

Ovarian hyperandrogenic activity is often confused with the Stein–Leventhal syndrome which, apart from its anatomico-pathologic features, is associated with amenorrhoea or anovular oligomenorrhoea together with sterility and often with hirsutism. Simple blocking with dexamethasone results in very small quantities of oestrogens (5 to 15 μg.) and a residual level of the A + E fraction between 2 and 4 mg., which means that it is significantly increased above the upper limits of the normal range, (Jayle and others, 1962 and Mahesh, 1966). Stimulation with HCG causes an increase in the oestrogen level to between 30 and 40 μg. and sometimes even above this. The residual fraction of A + E is twice as high as is found after simple blocking with dexamethasone—it rises to between 3 and 7 mg. The pregnanetriol level is about 1 mg. and there are only small traces of pregnanediol.

The increase of the A + E fraction under HCG stimulation high above the levels of the controls can be considered to be characteristic of gonadal hyperandrogenism. Normal women do not show any rise in the residual level of that fraction under the effects of HCG (Jayle and Mauvais–Jarvis, 1965).

Although there are similarities between the Stein–Leventhal syndrome and testicular function, when we look at them from a point of response to HCG-dexamethasone they differ from one another in the nature of the androgens. Leydig cells of the male gonads produce testosterone, and according to most authors the level of secretion is between 5 and 7 mg. On the other hand, the secretion of the male hormone in ovarian hyperandrogenism is low, although it is slightly higher than that of normal ovaries. According to Bardin and Lipsett (1967) polycystic ovaries show a range of testosterone secretion from 0.23 ± 0.073 mg. to 1.180 ± 0.210 mg. and these results agree with MacDonald and others (1963). Corticotropin has no influence on the secretion rate in either sex. As we see from Table 2 modified from MacDonald (1965) dexamethasone

TABLE 2

	TESTOSTERONE mg./24 hr.	ANDROSTENEDIONE mg./24 hr.
Base	4·1	3
ACTH	4·7	8
DXM	5·6	0
DXM + HCG	8·5	14
Norethindrone Ac.	0·4	—

TESTOSTERONE AND ANDROSTENEDIONE SECRETION RATES IN A NORMAL MAN—MacDonald *et al.* (1965).

does not influence the rate of secretion of testosterone in the male. It doubles under the effect of HCG whereas suppression by oestrogens or norethindrone brings it down to very low values. In the Stein–Leventhal syndrome the precursors of urinary androsterone and etiocholanolone are steroids of the C-19 group which have very weak androgenic activity, such as androstenedione and dehydro-epiandrosterone (Bardin and Lipsett, 1967) and (MacDonald, 1963). It is therefore necessary to see that there is a difference between hirsutism and virilism. In the Stein–Leventhal syndrome virilism scarcely exists or is very rare, but it definitely does exist in women who have certain kinds of ovarian tumours, (Kase and Conrad, 1964, Savard and others, 1961).

In women the level of plasma testosterone is five to ten times lower than in men where the range is 0·5 to 1·5 μg. per 100 ml. In ovarian hyperandrogenism, the plasma levels are slightly raised in women but do not reach levels anywhere near those of men. In neither sex does ACTH or dexamethasone have any significant effect on the level of male hormone in the blood. The administration of HCG doubles or triples the levels found in men but has no affect in normal women and only slightly raises the level of testosterone in women with polycystic ovaries (Table 3).

above the level of 30 μg. in 24 hours provides the most valuable pointer to the activity of Leydig cells. Where we are dealing with cases of primary testicular insufficiency and in castrated subjects (Jayle and others, 1959 and 1962) there are only small traces of oestrogens both before and after the test. In elderly patients as during puberty there is an increase of the fraction A + E, with no significant change in the oestrogen level. We have found that same effect in some pathologic conditions of the testis. The estimation of urinary testosterone can give extra information before and after HCG (Vermeulen, 1966). The estimation is more difficult and cannot be used in daily clinical routine. As far as the level of plasma testosterone goes, this also still seems to be restricted to the field of research.

So far we have pointed out the similarities and the differences between gonadal hyperandrogenism and Stein-Leventhal syndrome, and androgenic activity in testicular Leydig tissue. In fact, the Stein-Leventhal syndrome is just an outstanding form of ovarian hyperandrogenism while its anatomical, pathological, and clinical definition

TABLE 3

Subjects	Base μg./100 ml.	HCG Δ	ACTH Δ	CS Δ	References
Normal men	0·86 (0·45–1·30)	+1·12	+0·13	−0·18	Kirschner et al. (1965)
Normal women	0·042 ± 0·012	0	0	0	Lloyd et al. (1966)
PCO* with hirsutism	0·135 ± 0·128	+0·103	0	−0·056	,, ,,
Idiopathic hirsutism	0·085 ± 0·064	+0·074	+0·017	−0·038	,, ,,

* PCO: Polycystic ovary.

PLASMA TESTOSTERONE LEVELS IN NORMAL SUBJECTS AND WOMEN WITH HIRSUTISM; VARIATIONS (Δ) AFTER HCG. ACTH OR CORTICOSTEROIDS (CS).

The level of urinary testosterone which is less than 10 μg. in 24 hours in women is found to be between 50 and 150 μg. in men. Furthermore, in men it rises very much under the influence of HCG. Many authors consider that an estimate of the plasma testosterone is the best indication of androgenic activity of the testis. This seems to be debatable when we consider that Crepy, Dray and Sebaoun (1967) have shown that plasma testosterone levels are closely linked to the production of testosterone binding protein (TBP) the concentration of which seems to be controlled by thyroid hormones.

We believe from our observations that we can test the hormone capacity of Leydig cells with the help of the HCG stimulation text. We have now simplified the standard test previously reported (Jayle, Scholler, Sfikakis and Héron, 1962). We find it adequate to administer to the male 5,000 IU of HCG on three consecutive days and to estimate before the start of the test the levels of creatinine, of the fraction A + E and E_1, E_2 and E_3 in 24 hours specimens, repeating these estimations after the third injection of HCG. The levels of the fraction A + E as well as those of oestrogens are increased after HCG administration. Strange as it may seem, a rise in oestrogens

differs from author to author. Some of these state that it is congenital, supporting this theory with descriptions of the presence of biochemical lesions and even of anomalies of karyotype (Jayle 1967, Jayle, 1965, and Prunty, 1967). So far we cannot prove or disprove the congenital nature of this disease. We do however think that there can be an acquired form in which the syndrome evolves through successive stages:

1. The cycle is regular and ovulation occurs. We carry out the HCG-dexamethasone test in the luteal phase of the cycle, we find a normal excretion of E_1, E_2 and E_3 and PG, and we also find that the residual level of fraction A + E is increased significantly on an average between 2·5 and 5 mg. per 24 hours. Often this hyperandrogenism goes with an increase in oestrogen excretion.

2. In the second stage degeneration of the ovaries starts. The level of PG becomes progressively smaller and oligomenorrhoea is noted.

3. Where as in stage 2 the oligomenorrhoea was ovular, now it is anovular. The levels of PG, PGT and E_1, E_2 and E_3 are very low on the sixth day of the test

and the only feature that remains is the rise in the residual level of fraction A + E.

4. In the fourth stage we have amenorrhoea and the ovary on laparoscopy looks typical of the Stein–Leventhal syndrome.

Most people think that over-production of ovarian androgens is one cause of sterility. A statistical study on ovular cycles together with hyperandrogenism (Jayle and Engler, 1967), failed to confirm this. We think that sterility is due to the fibrous shell that imprisons the follicles and so stops their evolution. According to Kase it is the androgens, whether they are of ovarian or adrenal origin, that cause the fibrosis of the outer layers of the ovary, (Kase, 1964).

Sequential Stimulation with HMG and HCG

In the normal menstrual cycle the ovaries are stimulated by the two pituitary gonadotropins FSH and LH. The former has a mixed action of morphological origin, bringing the egg to the surface and causing it to mature, whereas the latter is responsible for ovulation, the formation of the corpus luteum and plays a dominate role in the biogenesis of the steroid hormones. Sequential stimulation of the ovaries brings into play successively a gonadotropin with follicle stimulating activity and a gonadotropin with a luteo-stimulating activity. For the first we can use pregnant mare's serum (PMSG), human pituitary gonadotropin (HPG) or human menopausal urine gonadotropin (HMG). The pregnant mare serum may cause an antibody formation; HPG is not commercially available, so we prefer to use HMG. This stimulant is associated with HCG which has a similar action to LH.

Whereas the test that we have described earlier is innocuous, sequential stimulation carries risks for patients. In several cases the ovaries have formed multiple cysts with acute peritoneal catastrophes and thrombo-emboli have occurred whereas often, twins, triplets and even quintuplets have been delivered after this form of therapy. We cannot therefore use it as a day to day routine method of investigation of function, but must reserve it for treatment of certain forms of sterility and then under the most stringent gynaecological and biological controls. We can lessen the risks of the sequential therapy greatly by biochemical analyses. We have in fact pointed out that catastrophes are specially likely to happen when the preliminary test with HCG-dexamethasone has shown either hyperandrogenism of ovarian origins or hyperoestrogenism or a rise in the level of urinary PGT. Moreover, and on the other hand, when the levels of PGT, of E_1, E_2 and E_3 and of the A + E fraction are very low in the last day of the test we have described, the likelihood of a catastrophe is very small. We can lessen them still more if we carry out rapid fluorimetric estimations of the levels of oestrogens in the urine collected on the fourth or fifth day between 8 p.m. and 8 a.m. (Scholler and others, 1966).

This control too allows us to decide the exact moment to administer the HCG. We would advise that it should be given when the level of oestrogens expressed as oestrone equivalent is between 50 and 100 μg. in 24 hours.

A scheme of therapy can be recommended entailing the daily administration of 150 units IRP_2 of HMG* for 10 consecutive days and 5,000 IU of HCG on each of the three following days. Where we are treating a case of amenorrhoea with ovarian hyperandrogenism, the daily does of HMG must never exceed 75 units IRP_2 of HMG. When we are treating a case of hypothalamic amenorrhoea with low levels of urinary steroids as found after the HCG-dexamethasone test, we start with 150 units IRP_2 HMG a day. We can increase the dose to 225 units between the tenth and the fifteenth day if the level of oestrogens has not risen above the base line. No HCG should be given until the oestrogen level has risen to between 50 and 100 μg. in 24 hours. The dose of HCG should not exceed 1,500 to 3,000 units when the oestrogen level is above 150 μg. on the last day of treatment with HMG. Working with Mauvais–Jarvis, Decourt and others (1967) we have found a relationship between the level of plasma LH and the response to sequential stimulation as determined by the suppression of adrenal activity with dexamethasone, (Table 4). In Table 4 we have together with these authors classified patients into two categories according to the level of plasma LH as expressed by OAAD† according to the method of Parlow. Most of the patients in the first group had polycystic ovaries whereas those in the second group had hypothalamic amenorrhoea. From these observations we can make the following statements:

1. At the end of a course of treatment with HMG together with administration of dexamethasone we find substantial quantities of PGT, a slight but significant rise in the oestrogen level and a rise in the residual level of the fraction A + E in the group with polycystic ovaries. On the other hand there are only traces of PG.

2. After stimulation with HCG we find a marked rise in the level of E_1, E_2, E_3 and PGT and PG.

3. There is a relationship between the levels of oestrogens at the end of the treatment with HMG and those that we find after HCG treatment.

When there is a polycystic reaction of the ovaries together with an acute peritoneal reaction, the excretion of oestrogens becomes very high indeed, rising to and even exceeding 5,000 μg. with a level of PGT between 15 and 25 mg. These results confirm the research of Gemzell and Diczfalusy who were the originators of the treatment of sterility by stimulation with HPG–HCG. (Gemzell and others, 1958). They found an enormous increase in 17-oxo-steroids, 17-ketogenic steroids and oestrogens in patients with polycystic ovaries. Brooks and others (1966) who estimated the steroid production in the case of Stein-Leventhal syndrome after administration of HPG, found 12 mg. of oestrogens, 25 mg. of steroids in the C-19 form and 2·8 mg. of testosterone. This proves that polycystic ovaries can produce the same quantities of oestrogens as those produced by the placenta during a pregnancy as well as producing androgens and 17-hydroxy-progesterone.

---

* 75 units IRP_2 of HMG is equivalent to 500 units of IRP standard.
† Ovarian Ascorbic Acid Depletion.

TABLE 4

RESPONSES TO THE HMG–HCG SEQUENTIAL TEST ASSOCIATED WITH DEXAMETHASONE (DXM), IN RELATION WITH THE PLASMA LH LEVEL, EXPRESSED AS OAAD. Mauvais-Jarvis *et al.* (1967).

	LH OAAD* %	$E_1 + E_2$ μg./24 hr.	E_3 μg./24 hr.	PG mg./24 hr.	PGT mg./24 hr.	A + E mg./24 hr.
POLYCYSTIC OVARIES						
Base	35·5 (25–54)	6·9 (5–10)	6·9 (tr–10)	tr**	0·4 (tr–0·9)	—
DXM + HMG 1500 U ↓	—	196 (30–600)	205 (40–700)	tr	2·1 (1·5–5·5)	3·5 (3–4·2)
DXM + HCG 15,000 UI	—	1510 (100 – 6500)	417 (75–1300)	10·2 (4–19)	10·5 (3–19·5)	5·1 (3·5–11)
HYPOTHALAMIC AMENORRHOEA						
Base	12·1 (0–22)	2·5 (tr–5)	3·0 (tr–5)	tr	0·3 (tr–0·7)	—
DXM + HMG 1500 U ↓	—	21 (10–50)	37·5 (15–100)	tr	1·1 (0·1–11)	0·6 (0·2–0·8)
DXM + HCG 15,000 UI	—	45 (20–90)	52·5 (20–125)	5 (2–8·5)	2·8 (2–5)	0·4 (0·2–0·6)

* OAAD: Ovarian Ascorbic Acid Depletion.
** tr: trace level.

$E_1 + E_2$ = Oestrone + Oestradiol E_3 = Oestriol
PG = Pregnanediol   A + E = Androsterone + Etiocholanolone
PGT = Pregnanetriol

Test of Inhibition of Gonadal Activity

There are now on the market a large variety of drugs with contraceptive properties which are able to inhibit the secretory activity of the different endocrine functions of the gonads of both sexes. If we administer them together with dexamethasone these drugs reduce the steroids in the urine to very low levels. The diagnostic value of the association of oestrogen and gestagens is far less important than their therapeutic value. Indeed, in polycystic changes of the ovaries as demonstrated by global hyperplasia of the three endocrine compartments in the HCG-dexamethasone test, the treatment can be found to be very useful. Not only will it bring the size of the ovaries back to normal, but also return their endocrine activity to normal, so long as the treatment is started soon enough.

Summary

The different aspects of the dynamic investigation of the gonads of both sexes in both normal and abnormal conditions has been reviewed. Far the most valuable information concerning the functional activity of the gonads is obtained by stimulating the gonads with HGG and inhibiting the adrenal activity with dexamethasone.

This test brings about a biochemical symptomatology which has caused us to reconsider many of the generally accepted ideas on gonadal function and to produce a new classification of the gonadal pathology of the ovaries.

REFERENCES

Bardin, C. W. and Lipsett, M. B. (1967), "Testosterone and Androstenedione Blood Production Rates in Normal Women and Women with Idiopathic Hirsutism or Polycystic Ovaries," *J. clin. Invest.*, **46**, 891.

Brooks, R. V., Jeffcoate, S. L., London, D. R., Prunty, F. T. G. and Smith, P. M. (1966), "Studies of Ovarian Androgen Secretion," in "Androgens in normal and pathological conditions," *Excerpta medica Found. intern. Congr. Ser. No.* **101**, 108.

Brown, J. B. (1955), "A Chemical Method for the Determination of Oestriol, Oestrone and Oestradiol in Human Urine," *Biochem. J.*, **60**, 185.

Crepy, O., Dray, F. and Sebaoun, J. (1967), "Rôle des hormones thyroïdiennes dans les interactions entre la testostérone et les protéines sériques," *C. R. Acad. Sci., Paris*, Série D, **264**, 2651.

Drosdowsky, M., Scholler, R. and Jayle, M. F. (1962), "Séparation chromatographique et dosage des trois fractions des 17-cétostéroïdes," in *Analyse des stéroïdes hormonaux, tome 2: méthodes de dosage*, Masson publ., Paris, **2**, 64.

Gandy, H. M., Moody, C. B. and Peterson, R. E., "Androgens Levels in Ovarian and Adrenal Venous Plasma," in Proc. 6th

Pan-American Congr. Endocr., Mexico 1965, *Excerpta medica Found., intern. Congr., Ser. No.* **112**, 223.

Gemzell, C. A., Diczfalusy, E. and Tillinger, G. (1958), "Clinical Effect of Human Pituitary Follicle-Stimulating Hormone (F.S.H.)," *J. clin. Endocr. Metab.*, **18**, 1333.

Goering, R. S., Matsuda, S. and Herrmann, W. (1965), "Oestrogen Secretion Rates in Normal Women," *Amer. J. Obstet. Gynec.*, **92**, 441.

Horton, R. and Tait, J. F. (1966), "Androstenedione Production and Interconversion Rates Measured in Peripheral Blood and Studies on the Possible Site of its Conversion to Testosterone," *J. clin. Invest.*, **45**, 301.

Jayle, M. F. (1967), "Dynamic Investigation of Ovarian Endocrine Functions," in *"Endocrine Functions of the Ovary, Part 2,"* M. F. Jayle, ed., Pergamon Press publ., **2**, 377.

Jayle, M. F., Decourt, J. and Doumic, J. (1959), "Action des gonadotropines chorioniques sur l'excrétion des stéroïdes urinaires chez 3 hommes castrés," *Ann. Endocr.*, **20**, 617.

Jayle, M. F. and Engler, R. (1967), "Biochemical Diagnosis of Ovarian Hyperandrogenism," in *Endocrine Functions of the Ovary, Part 2*, M. F. Jayle, ed., Pergamon Press publ., **2**, 501.

Jayle, M. F. and Mauvais-Jarvis, P. (1965), "Anomalies de la biogénèse et du métabolisme des hormones stéroïdes au cours des affections congénitales ovariennes," in *Les troubles congénitaux de l'hormonogénèse, Rapport de la 8e réunion des endocrinologues de langue française*, Masson publ., Paris, 65.

Jayle, M. F., Scholler, R. and Del Pozo, D. (1962), "Dosage chromatographique rapide du prégnandiol et du prégnanetriol par la méthode de Jayle, Judas et Crépy," in *Analyse des stéroïdes hormonaux, tome 2: méthodes de dosage*, Masson publ., Paris, **2**, 295.

Jayle, M. F., Scholler, R., Mauvais-Jarvis, P. and Szper, M. (1962), "Investigation of Ovarian Function by Means of Chorionic Gonadotropins in Combination with Dexamethasone: Application to the Diagnosis of Ovarian Virilism," *Clin. chim. Acta*, 7, 322.

Jayle, M. F., Scholler, R., Sfikakis, A. and Heron, M. (1962), "Excrétion des phénolsteroïdes et des *17*-cétostéroïdes après administration de gonadotropines chorioniques à des hommes," *Clin. chim. Acta.*, 7, 212.

Kase, N. (1964), "Steroid Synthesis in Abnormal Ovaries: III. Polycystic Ovaries," *Amer. J. Obstet. Gynec.*, **90**, 1268.

Kase, N. and Conrad, S. H. (1964), "Steroid Synthesis in Abnormal Ovaries: I. Arrhenoblastoma," *Amer. J. Obstet. Gynec.*, **90**, 1251.

Kirschner, M. A., Lipsett, M. B. and Collins, D. R. (1965), "Plasma Ketosteroids and Testosterone in Man: a Study of the Pituitary-testicular Axis," *J. clin. Invest.*, **44**, 657.

Lloyd, C. W., Lobotsky, J., Segre, E. J., Kobayashi, T., Taymor, M. L. and Batt, R. E. (1966), "Plasma Testosterone and Urinary 17-KS in Women with Hirsutism and Polycystic Ovaries," *J. clin. Endocr. Metab.*, **26**, 314.

MacDonald, P. C., Chapdelaine, A., Gonzalez, O., Gurpide, E., VandeWiele, R. L. and Lieberman, S. (1965), "Studies on the Secretion and Interconversion of the Androgens: IV. Quantitative Results in a Normal Man whose Gonadal and Adrenal Function were Altered Experimentally," *J. clin. Endocr. Metab.*, **25**, 1569.

MacDonald, P. C., VandeWiele, R. L. and Lieberman, S. (1963), "Precursors of the Urinary 11-desoxy-17-ketosteroids of Ovarian Origin," *Amer. J. Obstet. Gynec.*, **86**, 1.

Mahesh, V. B. (1966), "Response of the Ovary to Suppressing and Stimulating Agents," in *Ovulation—Stimulation, Suppression, Detection*. R. B. Greenblatt, ed., Lippincott & Co. publ., Philadelphia (Toronto) 166.

Mauvais-Jarvis, P., Louchart, J., Jayle, M. F. and Decourt, J., Etude du mode réactionnel de l'ovaire à la stimulation par les gonadotropines humaines (HMG et HCG). *Presse médicale—* (1967), **75**, 1971.

Prunty, F. T. G. (1967), "Hirsutism, Virilism and Apparent Virilism and Their Gonadal Relationship: Part II, *J. Endocr.*, **38**, 203.

Savard, K. (1967), "Role of Gonadotropins in the Biogenesis of Steroids in the Ovary," in *"Endocrine Functions of the Ovary, Part 2,"* M. F. Jayle, ed., Pergamon Press publ., **2**, 189.

Savard, K., Gut, M., Dorfman, R. I., Gabrilove, J. L. and Soffer, L. J. (1961), "Formation of Androgens by Human Arrhenoblastoma Tissue *in vitro*," *J. clin. Endocr. Metab.*, **21**, 165.

Savard, K., Marsh, J. M. and Rice, B. F. (1965), "Gonadotropins and Ovarian Steroidogenesis," *Recent Progr. Hormone Res.*, **21**, 285.

Scholler, R., Heron, M. and Jayle, M. F. (1962), "Analyse Chromatographique rapide de la fraction oestrone + oestradiol et de l'oestriol," in *Analyse des stéroïdes hormonaux, tome 2: méthodes de dosage*, Masson publ., Paris, **2**, 397.

Scholler, R., Leymarie, P., Heron, M. and Jayle, M. F. (1966), "A Study of Estrogen Fluorescence using Ittrich's Procedure," *Acta Endocr.*, **52**, suppl. 107.

Scholler, R., Metay, S., Herbin, S. and Jayle, M. F. (1966), "Hydrolyse enzymatique rapide des oestrogènes conjugués urinaires: I. Oestrogènes totaux (1) (concentration supérieure a 5000 μg/1000 ml)," *Eur. J. Steroids*, **1**, 1373.

Vermeulen, A. (1966), "Urinary Excretion of Testosterone," in *"Androgens in Normal and Pathological Conditions," Excerpta medica Found. intern. Congr. Ser. No.* **101**, 71.

9. THE ENDOCRINE FUNCTIONS OF THE PLACENTA

E. C. AMOROSO and D. G. PORTER

Introduction

The subject of this chapter has been analysed and reviewed on many occasions (Newton, 1938, 1939, 1949; Courrier, 1945; Amoroso, 1955a, 1960a; Mayer and Klein, 1955; Diczfalusy and Troen, 1961; Deanesly, 1966). In this account an attempt will be made to review briefly the measurable changes of secretion, metabolism, and excretion of hormones during pregnancy and to ascertain to what extent these changes should be considered as consequences of the products of conception, or are of significance for the proper development of the offspring.

Although references to books and journals outline the foundation on which the text is laid, they are no more than a series of clues to the vast literature that exists. Hence a review or paper with a good bibliography is frequently cited in place of the original contribution, a practice open to criticism but not, it is hoped, indulged in to excess.

The State of Pregnancy

The view has gained ground that pregnancy is characterized by an endocrine readjustment on the part of the mother in which the placenta holds a key position. Today, a certain amount of direct evidence is also available that the endocrine functions of the pregnant female, the placenta and the foetus interact complexly to control the course of embryonic development (Amoroso, 1956; Block, Benirscke, Rosenberg, 1956). The maternal hormones are essential for the progestational transformation of the endometrium and for the initiation of pregnancy, but with advancing gestation their relative importance diminishes as ovarian and hypophysial functions are gradually taken over by the placenta.

This concept of attributing responsibility to the placenta, rather than to altered functions of pre-existing glands has a long history in so far as biologists and clinicians have long been aware of the variable necessity of the ovaries in pregnancy, from species to species (see Amoroso, 1955a, 1960a; Amoroso and Finn, 1962; Deanesly, 1966). It has also become obvious that under certain conditions the placenta secretes substances which affect processes normally associated with the secretions of the hypophysis, the adrenal cortex and other endocrinologically active tissues.

Generally speaking, the idea of pregnancy assumes the continued presence of a developing embryo. Perhaps this has been so because death of the human foetus usually is followed by spontaneous emptying of the uterus, although this need not be a precipitate event. On the other hand, experiments with rabbits (Weymeersch, 1912; Hammond, 1917; Klein, 1933), rats (Klein, 1935; Selye, Collip and Thompson, 1935), mice (Newton, 1935; Brooksby and Newton, 1938), hamsters (Klein, 1938b) and monkeys (Dorfman and van Wagenen, 1941; van Wagenen and

Newton, 1940, 1943; van Wagenen and Jenkins, 1943) bring out the fact that pregnancy, in terms of the altered maternal physiology, can be independent of the presence of the foetus for the greater part of its length. Also during the later part of gestation in these species, the relative importance of the placenta as an organ of internal secretion is emphasized and a second phenomenon, the onset of labour, is shown to be unquestionably independent of the immediate presence of the foetus (see, however, Liggins, Kennedy and Holm, 1967).

It is thus evident that the developing organism grows prenatally in a complicated hormonal environment and that the satisfactory and economical relationship between mother and foetus, which must be the basis of pregnancy, is brought about by a change in the physiological organization of the mother, whereby the wants of the foetus are largely anticipated. From the time of implantation to the end of pregnancy, hormones from the placenta may be available to the foetus and at certain periods the placenta is permeable to hormones. These hormones vary quantitatively and qualitatively during pregnancy, and may reach the foetus, at least in some species, in effective amounts. But while many of these hormones are undoubtedly derived from the placenta or from the mother, there is evidence which points to function of the foetal endocrine glands and indicates the establishment of their hormonal inter-relationships before birth.

At birth the new-born mammal is dependent upon its mother's milk, which has been shown in several species to contain oestrogenic and gonadotrophic hormones for a period of time. This adds a source of exogenous hormones, and suckling young have been found to be affected by such maternal hormones. In post-natal development the various endocrine glands reach (or have already reached at birth) their functional state; the complicated inter-relationship of gonads, hypophysis, thyroids and adrenals are established; and hormones from the gonads assume the major role in the development of the contrasting somatic characteristics in adult individuals.

Endocrine Activity of the Foetal Placenta

Evidence from Experiments on Laboratory Animals

While it was the discontinuance of pregnancy following removal of the corpora lutea which offered the first experimental evidence that these bodies are necessary for implantation and maintenance of embryos in the uterus (Magnus, 1901; Fraenkel and Cohen, 1901), indications that the pregnant uterus might itself produce hormones, came from the study of species such as the human female (Halban, 1905; Asdell and others, 1928), the guinea pig (Loeb and Hesselberg, 1917; Loeb and others 1923), the horse (Hart and Cole, 1934; Amoroso and Finn, 1962) and the cat (Courrier and Gros, 1935; Gros, 1936) which tolerate bilateral removal of the ovaries after a certain stage without aborting. That it is the placenta, however, rather than the uterus itself, the decidua or the foetus that is concerned in the maintenance of luteal function became clear when the effects of foetal dissociation in laboratory animals were compared with those following removal of the whole pregnant uterus. Thus, it has been shown that total hysterectomy in the gravid female, or removal of the pregnant horn in unilateral pregnancy (rabbits, Hammond, 1917; Knaus, 1930; but see also, Klein, 1933; rats, Klein, 1938a; hamsters, Klein, 1938b; cats, Amoroso, unpublished data), results in the rapid involution of the corpora lutea, the reappearance of oestrus and an immediate return of the endometrium of the sterile horn to the resting condition. When, however, a similar operation is performed on ferrets (Deanesly, 1967) or on the badger (Canivenc, Bonnin-Laffargue and Relexans, 1962) the functional survival of the corpora lutea remains unimpaired, suggesting that in these mustelids the luteal bodies are independent of any placental luteotrophin. On the other hand, removal of, or killing the foetuses in a series of rabbits (Weymeersch, 1912), mice (Newton, 1935; Brooksby and Newton, 1938), monkeys (van Wagenen and Newton, 1940, 1943; Dorfman and van Wagenen, 1941; van Wagenen and Jenkins, 1943), rats (Selye *et al.*, 1935; Huggett and Pritchard, 1945) and cats (Amoroso, unpublished data) leaving the placentae *in situ*, did not alter the course of pregnancy. In these experiments the corpora lutea survived; body weight was maintained; the placentae were retained and continued to grow; mammary development was complete and parturition (expulsion of the placentae) occurred at the normal time. In short, mice, rats, monkeys and cats remain physiologically pregnant despite the absence of the foetuses. It would be a mistake, however, to imagine that the foetus is altogether a passenger, since Liggins, Kennedy and Holm (1966) have shown that following hypophysectomy of the foetus, parturition is suppressed in the sheep. Even in the mouse, in which placental pregnancy so closely resembles the normal, pubic separation does not occur (Newton and Lits, 1938), the act of parturition may be sluggish and lactation occasionally fails to occur.

From the foregoing results it would thus appear that by transforming the cyclic corpus luteum into the corpus luteum of pregnancy, the uterus exerts a sustaining influence on the luteal bodies during pregnancy which it is prevented from exercising during the previous phases of the cycle. They indicate, moreover, that neither the myometrium itself nor the decidua nor the metrial glands are directly implicated in luteal stimulation. They do not, however, exclude the effects of uterine distension in pregnancy, nor the possibility that the physical presence of the placenta itself may release the neural signals necessary for the continued maintenance of the corpora lutea. In other words, it is possible that a reflex mechanism (Nalbandov, Moore and Norton, 1955; Inskeep *et al.*, 1962), not unlike that associated with the post-coital discharge of ovulating hormones, might be involved (Deanesly, Fee and Parkes, 1930). The conclusive experiment has yet to be made, but Mayer and Klein (1955) find that uterine distension has no endocrine effect on the duration of pregnancy in rodents.

These experiments, together with various scattered observations by other investigators on the effects of retained placentae, are sufficient to prove that the foetal placenta is the active element in the maintenance of the hormone balance of pregnancy in most species.

Relationship Between the Pituitary Gland and the Placenta

According to current theory the pituitary gland is directly implicated in the induction of uterine function adequate for the initiation, and the maintenance of pregnancy through the stimulation of ovarian secretions. Hence, ablation of the pituitary during pregnancy might be expected to yield information regarding the function of this gland in the gravid female. Intolerant of the operation at any time are the goat, bitch, cat and ferret, whereas, in others which include the human female, monkeys, mice, rats and the guinea pig, pregnancy is interrupted only if ablation is performed during early pregnancy (*see*, Amoroso, 1955a, and also Amoroso and Porter, 1966). In the monkey (Smith, 1954) and mouse (Selye, Collip and Thompson, 1935; Newton and Beck, 1939; Gardner and Allen, 1942), delivery of young occurs at the normal time, body weight is maintained, and mammary development is complete, but absence of pituitary function becomes apparent after parturition, when lactation fails to occur (Smith, 1946; Newton and Richardson, 1940).

The position of the rabbit is equivocal. White (1933) reported that hypophysectomy up to day 26 in the pregnant rabbit caused abortion, but that pregnancy continued to term when the ablation was performed later. Similarly, Robson (1937) reported that rabbits hypophysectomized on the 23rd day carried litters to term. However, upon this evidence, and that of Firor (1933) whose ablations were confined to day 3 it has been concluded (Amoroso and Porter, 1966; Keys and Nalbandov, 1967) that the adenohypophysis is essential throughout pregnancy in this species. The possibility exists though that the pituitary may be dispensable for the last third of pregnancy in the rabbit. If so, this would be consistent with the increasing evidence of a luteotrophic role for the rabbit placenta (*vide infra*).

In hypophysectomized mice in which the products of conception are reduced to placentae, full mammary development is sometimes impaired, but body weight is maintained, luteal function is sustained (Deanesly and Newton, 1941) and the resorption of the interpubic ligament proceeds normally (Newton and Beck, 1939). In monkeys, Smith (1954) was unable to establish, with certainty, the earliest time in gestation when the gland could be removed without causing abortion but the postpartum behaviour of the gravid females was abnormal only in so far as they did not consume the after-birth, as is the case with normal mothers (Hartman, 1932). In other respects the mothers displayed normal maternal behaviour towards the infants, suggesting that hypophysial secretions do not appear to be involved in the protective behaviour towards the young. In the human female placental endocrine secretions were maintained after hypophysectomy in a patient with cancer of the breast and pregnancy went to term (Little *et al.*, 1958; Kaplan, 1961).

These considerations make it clear that in animals like the goat, bitch, cat, ferret, hypophysectomy of the gravid female removes the normal stimulus to corpus luteum maintenance and progesterone secretion, whereas, in species like the rat and mouse, the continuation of pregnancy after hypophysectomy must depend on the functional activity of the corpora lutea and this by stimulation from sources other than the pituitary, since these are among the animals in which ovariectomy terminates pregnancy (*see* below). The main feature of the relationship would thus appear to be the luteotrophic activity of the placenta. But, since the ovaries can be removed from women, monkeys, guinea pigs, sheep and mares, without terminating pregnancy, any function of the placenta as an ovarian stimulant is not essential in these species.

Although the evidence here summarized falls short of actual proof, it points strongly to the existence of a reciprocal functional relationship between the pituitary and the placenta, the main feature of which is the luteotrophic activity of the placenta. The important discovery of Philipp (1930) in the human female and of Evans and Simpson (1929) and others in rodents that the anterior pituitary seems to discontinue gonadotrophin production further emphasizes the wide functional significance of the foeto-maternal connection.

The Placenta as a Source of Gonadotrophic Hormones

The question which must now concern us is whether the placenta itself secretes the substances which lends it similar properties to that of pituitary tissue. It may be stated at once that there is a good deal of information pointing more and more to the placenta as the focus, but as Newton (1938, p. 419) put it "the unifying conception which would make everything fall into place is elusive".

Hirose (1919) was one of the first to suggest that the human placenta was responsible for maintaining the corpus luteum of pregnancy by the secretions of the trophoblastic covering of the villi. With human placental extract he stimulated the formation of corpora lutea in rabbits, and a few years later, Murata and Adachi (1927), using a similar extract, produced sexual maturity in the young rabbit. They showed, moreover, that a pulmonary choriocarcinoma contained a similarly active substance. In 1927 also, Aschheim and Zondek demonstrated in the blood and urine of pregnant women large amounts of a gonadotrophin which was also present in placental tissue but which they believed was produced by the maternal pituitary. Shortly thereafter Klein (1929) and Philipp (1929) proposed that this gonadotrophin was produced by the placenta.

Later Astwood and Greep (1938) prepared luteotrophic extracts from rat placenta, and these findings were confirmed by Astwood (1941) and by Lyons and his collaborators (Averill *et al.*, 1950; Ray *et al.*, 1955). In addition to confirming the presence of a placental gonadotrophin

concerned with the maintenance of pregnancy in the hypophysectomized rat, by means of placental implants, Averill *et al.* (1950) and Ray *et al.* (1955) were able to elicit mammotrophic, lactogenic and crop-stimulating activities with injections of extracts of 12-day rat placenta. They showed, moreover, that when compared with pituitary mammotrophin (prolactin), the rat placenta is potent in regard to its luteotrophic, mammotrophic and lactogenic properties, but weak in its crop-stimulating activity. Matthies (1965) confirmed the earlier findings of a placental luteotrophin in the rat and further showed that it was probably a protein of a molecular weight in excess of 30,000. Similarly, the discovery of a potent luteotrophic hormone in the mouse placenta (Cerruti and Lyons, 1960) would explain the findings of Pencharz and Long (1931), that pregnancy can be maintained and mammary development can proceed in animals hypophysectomized in mid-pregnancy. It must, of course, be emphasized that mere presence is not evidence of secretion.

The ability of the trophoblast to maintain luteal function in the mouse has been demonstrated by Zeilmaker (1968) using transplants of ova to non-uterine sites. Similar evidence of an early luteotrophic effect of the conceptus in the sheep had been furnished by Moor and Rowson (1966), through experiments in which conceptuses had been removed at various times after mating.

The study of heterotransplants of the human placenta into the anterior chamber of the eye of the mouse (Voss, 1927) or the rabbit (Kido, 1937; Gurchot *et al.*, 1947; Stewart, 1951) have likewise yielded information regarding the secretion of placental gonadotrophins as indicated by evidence of oestrogenic stimulation of the uterus. So, too, have the results of Mayer and Canivenc (1950) which indicate that a homograft of rat placenta placed under the kidney capsule in an unmated female was capable of eliciting luteotrophic, mammotrophic and lactogenic effects. This evidence is, however, inconclusive since the secretions of the animal's own pituitary might be responsible for the observed effects, and only a repetition of the experiments with suitable precautions in hypophysectomized animals could finally settle this point (*see*, however, Averill *et al.*, 1950).

There is some indirect evidence of a luteotrophic function of the rabbit placenta. Placental dislocation is known to cause prompt abortion (Csapo and Lloyd-Jacob, 1961) and administration of oestrogen, which has been shown to be luteotrophic in the rabbit (Westman and Jacobsohn, 1937; Robson, 1937, 1939; Heckel and Allen, 1939; Hammond and Robson, 1951; Keyes and Nalbandov, 1967) will prevent such abortion (Porter, Becker and Csapo, 1968). That it is the placenta, and not the foetus, which is responsible for maintaining luteal function is revealed by the fact that removal of the foetuses alone, or severance of the umbilical cords does not interrupt pregnancy (Weymeersch, 1912; Klein, 1933). The crucial question whether the luteotrophic factor is placental oestrogen, or a substance which stimulates ovarian secretion of oestrogen has yet to be decided.

The best direct evidence of the production of gonadotrophins by the human placenta is provided by Stewart,

Sano and Montgomery (1948). Their results show that human placental cells of approximately three months of age, grown in continuous tissue culture *in vitro*, secrete gonadotrophic hormone as assayed qualitatively in rabbits and infantile mice. A direct correlation was noted between the growth of the Langhan's cells and the production of the hormone suggesting an origin from these cells, but this has now been disproved (Midgley and Pierce, 1962).

Placental Gonadotrophins

During the course of pregnancy, gonadotrophins similar to, but distinct from those elaborated by the pituitary have been demonstrated in the body fluids and in the placenta of various animals. The best known of these are the luteotrophic hormones of the rat and mouse (LTH), to which we have already alluded; human chorionic gonadotrophin, or urine of pregnancy (HCG); rhesus chorionic gonadotrophin (MCG); chorionic growth hormone-prolactin (CGP) and pregnant mare's serum or equine gonadotrophin (PMSG).

These substances, as obtained from the three groups of mammals represented, namely, rodents, ungulates and primates, all possess the biological properties of the gonadotrophic principles of the pituitary and appear to represent evolutionary steps in the adoption of pituitary function by the placenta (Hisaw and Astwood, 1942; Hisaw, 1944; Amoroso, 1955a, b, c, 1968). In rodents, the emphasis is on furtherance of luteal function adequate for the maintenance of normal gestation, whereas in the mare the emphasis is on the follicle-stimulating component, and in women they resemble the luteinizing hormone in most of their effects. Their function in these species, as well as their apparent absence in others, present an unsolved puzzle.

In this connection, it is perhaps as well to recall, that Lyons, Simpson and Evans (1953) have demonstrated qualitative difference in the urinary gonadotrophins as obtained from pregnant women. Tested by the response of the hypophysectomized immature female rat's ovaries, the urine from the earliest period of human pregnancy, 12 days after ovulation, caused only interstitial tissue repair, but by the 33rd day of gestation, urinary concentrates in large amounts caused stimulation of follicular growth in addition to repair of hypertrophy of the interstitial cells.

Human Chorionic Gonadotrophins (HCG).
Human chorionic gonadotrophin, which was also present in placental tissue, was first discovered by Aschheim and Zondek (1927) more than 40 years ago in the urine and blood of pregnant women.

They assumed that it was produced by the maternal hypophysis, but subsequently it was shown that it is made by cells covering the chorionic villi. The fact that this hormone is found in the urine of pregnant women is the basis of most pregnancy tests.

Despite an abundant literature on the subject, the relative importance of cytotrophoblast and syncytiotrophoblast in the production of human chorionic gonadotrophin remains controversial. Reviewing the evidence up to 1960, Diczfalusy and Troen (1961), concluded that the cytotrophoblast is probably the major, if not exclusive source of the gonadotrophic hormone in the blood and urine of pregnant women and monkeys. Support for this view has been provided by Pattillo and Gey (1968), who, in tissue culture studies established a cell line of human trophoblastic cells capable of synthesizing HCG similar to that produced by the normal human placenta and by its malignant counterpart, choriocarcinoma.

Attempts to confirm this theory histochemically have confused rather than clarified the problem, stainable mucoprotein having been reported in cytotrophoblast (Pearse, 1948), in syncytiotrophoblast (Pali and Lajos, 1952), and in both cell types (Zilliacus, 1953). On the other hand, by employing the fluorescent antibody technique, Midgley and Pierce (1962) have localized HCG in syncytiotrophoblastic tissues with an antiserum which had previously been shown to react specifically with biologically active HCG (Midgley *et al.*, 1961). Midgley and his associates (Pierce *et al.*, 1959) discount an origin from cytotrophoblast and suggest that part, at least, of the well-developed endoplasmic reticulum of the syncytiotrophoblast may be implicated in the synthesis of the hormone.

This trophic hormone of pregnancy is described as appearing in the urine a few days prior to the expected menstrual period (Smith, Albert and Randall, 1951), within a few days of implantation (Lyons, Simpson and Evans, 1953), or in the third week of the cycle (Browne and Venning, 1936; Tenney and Parker, 1937). By present assay methods, pregnancy gonadotrophin is now detectable at 7 days after fertilization (Hammond *et al.*, 1967). After this time the amount of the hormone in the urine begins to increase. Following a somewhat slow start, the concentration rises abruptly to a maximum (Fig. 1), which is usually described as occurring between 50 and 70 days after the last menstrual period (Browne and Venning, 1936; Evans, Kohl and Wonder, 1937; Boycott and Rowlands, 1937; Smith, Albert and Randall, 1951; Venning, 1955). Venning (1955) gives 50,000–150,000 I.U./24 hours as the maximum excretion in pregnancy, whereas other workers (e.g. Lyons, Simpson and Evans, 1953) obtained values of 400,000 I.U./24 hours or more at the peak. By the 120th day, that is, prior to the time at which overall placental function reaches its peak, which it does at approximately 36–38 weeks (Hellman *et al.*, 1948), the chorionic gonadotrophin levels have usually decreased to 3,000–10,000 I.U./24 hours. Thereafter the level of excretion remains constant till the expulsion of the placenta when it disappears from the urine. Finally, Diczfalusy (1953) has shown that the curve of HCG in placental tissue (cf. Figs. 1, 2, 3) throughout gestation closely resembles that of HCG in pregnancy serum (Jones, Delfs and Stran, 1944; Albert and Berkson, 1951) or urine (Loraine, 1950; Albert and Berkson, 1951; Venning, 1955) indicating that the level of HCG in these body fluids probably reflects the release of the hormone by the placenta.

If it be true that the placenta produces the hormone, any increase in the quantity or activity of this tissue would augment the levels of the hormone in the urine or serum. Extremely high levels have been reported in multiple pregnancies and in the toxaemias of pregnancy as well as in cases of hydatidiform moles and in choriocarcinomas (Hinglais and Hinglais, 1949; Hamburger, 1944; Haskins

mole pregnancies the urinary excretion of HCG falls within the normal range.

Moderate increases in the level of serum HCG are likewise observed in a proportion of diabetic pregnancies (Smith and Smith, 1941a, b; White, 1952; Loraine and

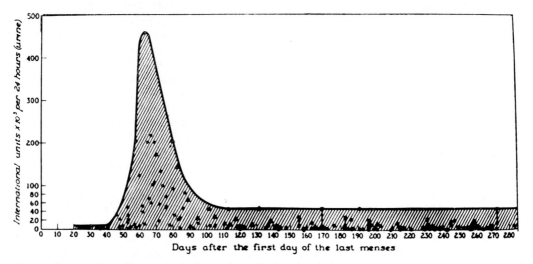

FIG. 1. Concentration of human chorionic gonadotrophin in urine during normal pregnancy. From Albert and Berkson (1951).

and Sherman, 1951; Hobson, 1955; Diczfalusy, 1958). Hobson (1955) as well as Diczfalusy, Nillson and Westman (1958) have also shown that moles exhibit a higher concentration of HCG per unit weight than normal placentae from a corresponding stage of pregnancy, but they emphasize, nevertheless, that in a considerable number of

Matthew, 1954), and as in patients with eclampsia and severe pre-eclamptic toxaemia (Smith and Smith, 1935; Loraine and Matthew, 1953) placental concentrations of HCG tend to be increased (Loraine and Matthew, 1953) and renal clearances to be decreased (Loraine, 1950). Loraine (1949) noted an appreciable, but transient, fall in

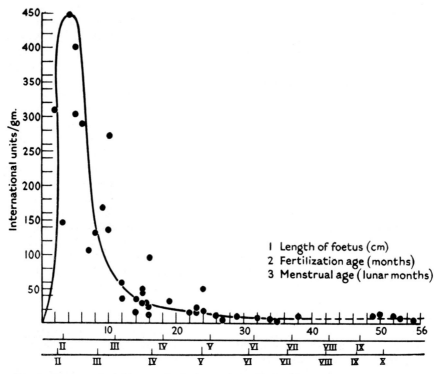

FIG. 2. Concentration of human chorionic gonadotrophin in placental tissue during normal pregnancy. International units per gram of wet tissue. From Diczfalusy et al. (1958).

urinary HCG excretion during the course of oestrogen therapy.

According to White (1952), a deficiency of oestrogen and corpus luteum hormone in pregnant diabetic women, which appears after about the twenty-first week of pregnancy is the cause of an abnormal increase in the concentration of chorionic gonadotrophin in the blood which is frequently accompanied by signs of toxaemia of pregnancy. The excess of this hormone as well as the environmental changes induced by the toxaemia are considered by White to be the cause of the over-development and incapacity for

and Gray, 1968) chorionic gonadotrophin (HCG) is demonstrable in the urine throughout most of pregnancy. The presence of MCG in the urine of pregnant hypophysectomized rhesus monkeys excludes the pituitary as a source of the hormone.

Chorionic Growth Hormone–Prolactin (CGP). A human polypeptide hormone that is chemically and immunologically similar to human pituitary growth hormone and that has prolactin and growth hormone-like activity has been demonstrated in the blood of pregnant women. It was first isolated by Josimovich and his collaborators

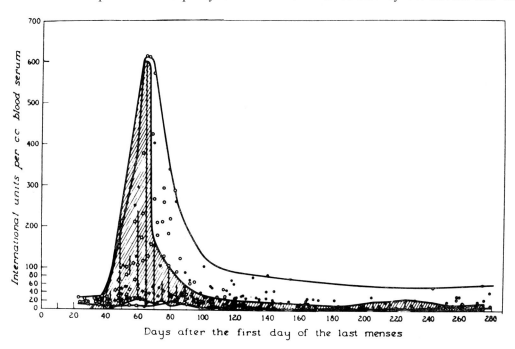

FIG. 3. Concentration of human chorionic gonadotrophin in blood serum during normal pregnancy. From Albert and Berkson (1951).

survival of the foetus in pregnancies complicated by diabetes mellitus. Such conditions are similar to those found in animal experiments, where the administration of human chorionic gonadotrophin results in the typical features of diabetes mellitus, namely, over-development, death and maceration of the animal foetuses (Snyder, 1934, 1936, 1938).

Rhesus Chorionic Gonadotrophin (MCG). The presence of a chorionic gonadotrophin in the urine and blood of the pregnant rhesus monkey and in the urine of the gravid chimpanzee has been demonstrated several times (monkey, Hamlett, 1937; van Wagenen and Simpson, 1954; Tullner and Hertz, 1966a; chimpanzee, Zuckermann, 1935; Schultze and Snyder, 1935). Rhesus chorionic gonadotrophin (MCG) is first detectable in the serum on the 15th post-mating day and in the urine between the 18th and 25th day of pregnancy (Tullner and Hertz, 1966a). In both the monkey and chimpanzee the elimination of chorionic gonadotrophin ceases before the end of pregnancy and is limited to a brief period at its beginning. In contrast, in the human (*op cit*) and in the gorilla (Tullner

(Josimovich and MacLaren, 1962; Josimovich and Astwood, 1964) who emphasized its luteotrophic and lactogenic activity in the rabbit, rat and pigeon. It has now been extensively studied by Kaplan and Grumbach (1965a). *See also* Grumbach and Kaplan, 1964; Grumbach *et al.*, 1968) and it has been suggested that this placental polypeptide (at least in part), rather than pituitary growth hormone functions as an important metabolic hormone of late pregnancy. The demonstration by Samaan, Yen, Friesen and Pearson (1965) of chorionic growth hormone prolactin in the sera of patients with hydatidiform moles, as well as in male individuals with choriocarcinoma of the testis, further strengthens a placental origin for this hormone. Radioimmunoassay and other assay procedures for the quantitative measurement of the hormone (Fig. 4) have been reported recently (Beek *et al.*, 1965; Samaan *et al.*, 1965; Kaplan and Grumbach, 1965b).

A comparable simian placental hormone to the chorionic growth hormone prolactin (CGP) found in the blood of pregnant women has likewise been identified in the monkey placenta (Kaplan and Grumbach, 1964). This polypeptide hormone bears an even closer immuno-chemical relationship to the human placental hormone than either has to its respective pituitary growth hormone and may, like its human counterpart act as a metabolic hormone of late pregnancy.

Pregnant Mare's Serum Gonadotrophin (PMSG). Nearly forty years ago Cole and Hart (1930a, b) demonstrated that the blood of pregnant mares contained large amounts of a gonadotrophin which appeared only infrequently or in traces in the urine (Cole, Howell and Hart, 1931). This hormone, which is also found in the lymph in high concentration (Amoroso, 1960) appears in the blood stream of the mare in large quantities only over a relatively variation in maximum hormone concentration, both within and between the two groups.

Available evidence seems to indicate that the major portion of the PMSG is slowly metabolized in the body rather than excreted in the urine and milk, but the exact site remains unknown (Cole, Bigelow, Finkel and Rupp, 1967). A half-life of six days has been reported for exogenous PMSG in the gelding (Catchpole, Cole and Pearson, 1938) and of about 24 hours in the rabbit and rat (Parlow and Ward, 1961). Similarly, in the mare hysterectomized during pregnancy, the half-life of endogenous PMSG was found to be about the same as reported previously for the gelding (Cole *et al.*, 1967) suggesting that the gonads may

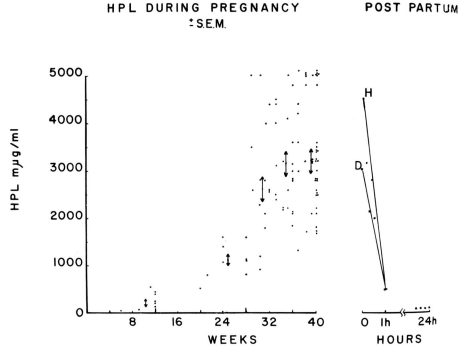

Fig. 4. Serum chorionic growth hormone-prolactin (CGP) levels during the various periods of gestation and post-partum. The dots represent individual values and the arrows indicate the standard error of the mean at various periods of gestation. From Samaan, Yen, Friesen and Pearson (1966).

limited span of gestation (Cole and Saunders, 1935). Its appearance in the blood and in the lymph corresponds to the time of implantation of the blastocyst (Amoroso, 1952).

Equine or pregnant mare's serum gonadotrophin (PMSG) first appears in the blood and lymph at about the 40th day of pregnancy, reaches a peak at about 90 days, remains high for another month and then gradually disappears. The levels are extremely variable and bear no relation to the age or parity of the animal, the diet or the concentration of gonadal hormones in the blood (Cole, 1938; Day and Rowlands, 1947; Rowlands, 1949). Its presence in the blood provides an effective means of pregnancy diagnosis (Glud *et al.*, 1933). Figures 5 and 6, reproduced from Allen (1969) show the concentrations of PMSG in two groups of mares of different breed and different size, an interesting feature of which is the marked not be directly concerned with the disappearance of the hormone (see also Fitko, 1965). The long half-life of PMSG has been attributed to its high molecular weight of about 68,000, a suggestion which is consistent with the fact that a single injection of the hormone is as effective as multiple injections (Cole, Guilbert and Goss, 1932; Connell, 1965).

Pregnant mare's serum gonadotrophin appears to be derived from cup-like structures in the fertile endometrium (Cole and Goss, 1943; Amoroso, 1952, 1955a, 1959; Clegg, Boda and Cole, 1954) rather than from the chorion. The cups occupy an area of the endometrium in the neighbourhood of the insertion of the yolk-sac, suggesting that the stimulus for cup-formation comes from the chorio-vitelline placenta and not, as Clegg *et al.* (1954) and Deanesly (1966) maintain from the allanto-chorion. The cups contain a viscous gel derived from the disintegrating

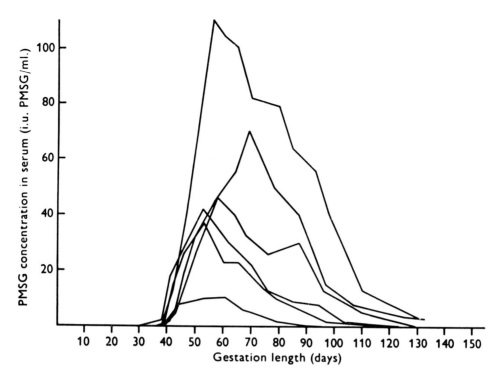

**Pregnant mare serum gonadotrophin (PMSG) concentration
in the serum of six Welsh Mountain pony mares.**

Fig. 5

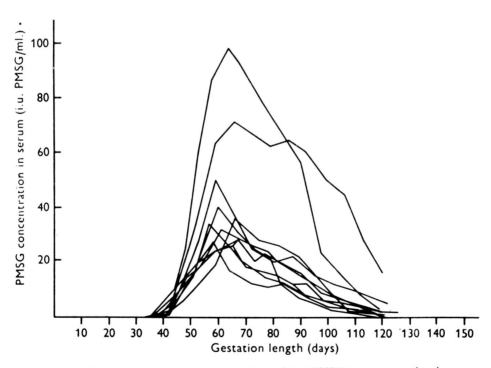

**Pregnant mare serum gonadotrophin (PMSG) concentration in
the serum of ten thoroughbred mares.**

Fig. 6

tissues of the endometrium. Amoroso (1952, 1955a, 1959) and Clegg, Boda and Cole (1954), review earlier work and illustrate the growth and regression of the cups, a feature of which is the profusion of lymphatic tissue and lymphatic vessels in the basal parts of these transient structures (Amoroso, 1955a).

The concentration of gonad stimulating hormone in the serum of the pregnant mare is, in general, inversely proportional to the size of the mare (Cole, 1938; Day and Rowlands, 1940, 1947; Rowlands, 1949) and is uniformly higher in twin-pregnant mares having two sets of endometrial cups. A sudden fall in serum potency occurs after abortion (Aylward and Ottaway, 1945; Rowlands, 1949). Moreover, the maintenance of a high blood level in an instance of foetal resorption suggests that the conceptus may be necessary for the preservation of the functional activity of the endometrial cups (Rowlands, 1949).

The view that the cups constitute the site of formation of PMSG is supported by the following observations: (1) The appearance of the hormone in the blood coincides with the development of the cups and its disappearance with their regression; (2) when two sets of cups are present, as in twin pregnancies, the concentration of PMSG in the serum is higher than in that of mares carrying only one foal (Rowlands, 1949); (3) in the early stages of their development, the cups contain the hormone in a concentration higher than that of the blood or lymph; and (4) the uterine mucosa contains gonadotrophin only in the cup area. Finally, cytological and histochemical studies (Amoroso, 1955a) strongly suggest that it is the cup cells themselves, rather than the glandular epithelium in the neighbourhood of the cups, that are principally concerned in the production of the hormone (see, however, Cole and Goss, 1943; also Clegg, Boda and Cole, 1954).

Although the function of PMSG in the pregnant mare remains unknown it may be significant that the time of its onset coincides with the fixation of the blastocyst and the appearance of numerous accessory corpora lutea, and its disappearance, roughly, with the time when the ovaries contain neither corpora lutea nor large follicles and when ovariectomy no longer interrupts pregnancy (Amoroso, Hancock and Rowlands, 1948; Amoroso and Finn, 1962). Gonadotrophic hormone is present in the blood serum of non-pregnant mares at all stages of the oestrous cycle, the greatest concentration being reached during the metoestrum (Cole and Goss, 1939). The amounts are, however, small compared with those of pregnancy.

Gonadotrophic Hormones in other Mammals. Pregnancy gonadotrophins with similar properties to that of pregnant mare's serum gonadotrophin (PMSG) have also been detected in the serum of the donkey (for references, *see below*), zebra (Zondek, 1935) and fallow deer (Unterberger, 1932), and in the urine of the pregnant giraffe (Wilkinson and de Fremery, 1940). There is, furthermore, suggestive evidence for the occurrence of a gonadotrophin in the body fluids of the nilgai (*Boselaphus tragocamelus*) and the rhinoceros, but whether or not the biological activity of the postulated gonadotrophin corresponds to that produced by the pregnant mare remains unknown.

Between the 40th and the 200th day of pregnancy, the blood of the donkey, like that of the mare, contains demonstrable gonadotrophic activity (Samodelkin, 1940; Zondek and Sulman, 1945; Calisti and Oliva, 1955; Oliva, 1957; Oliva and Chicchini, 1961), but after the 150th day of gestation the levels are so reduced as to be unreliable for pregnancy diagnosis.

A series of experiments on hybrid donkey and horse pregnancies by Bielanski, Ewy and Pigoniowa (1955) in Poland and by Clegg, Cole, Howard and Pigon (1962) in California brings out the point that the genotype of the foetus may influence hormone production. The Californian workers showed that when a mare is sired by a jack donkey and is carrying a mule foetus, gonadotrophin is secreted, but at a reduced rate, whereas the Polish investigators failed to detect any activity in the endometrial cup tissues of mares similarly mated. The disagreement in results have not yet been unequivocally answered, but may be due partly to differences in the assay procedures employed by the Americans and the Europeans. (Cf. Allen, 1969.)

The presence of a gonad-stimulating substance has been reported in the urine of a pregnant giraffe (Wilkinson and de Fremery, 1940), though it would appear that its elimination in the urine ceases before the end of pregnancy (Amoroso and Kellas, unpublished data). It is difficult to assess the comparative significance of these findings, because of the limited observations. However, as judged by the extensive follicular development and lutcinization in the foetal ovaries, a relationship between hormone production and foetal gonadal activity in this species is suspected (Amoroso, 1955a, 1959; Kellas *et al.*, 1958).

Increased Production of Oestrogens during Pregnancy

One of the outstanding features of pregnancy in many mammals (e.g. women, cows, mares) is the steady increase in the production and excretion of oestrogens, the values at term far exceeding that in the non-pregnant female (Aschheim and Zondek, 1927; Hart and Cole, 1934; Cohen and Marrian, 1935; Smith and Smith, 1935a, b; Bradshaw and Jessop, 1953 and others).

In the human female, oestrogen is excreted in the urine after the first week of pregnancy in increasing quantities up to the time of parturition, after which it disappears abruptly. In non-pregnant women, urinary oestriol approximates the sum of oestrone and oestradiol, its metabolic precursors (Brown, 1955) but during pregnancy the increase of oestriol far exceeds the sum of oestrone and oestradiol (Heusghem, 1956; Brown, 1957; Fishman and Brown, 1962). The increased urinary excretion of oestrogens seems to parallel the increase in weight of the placenta (Fig. 7) as well as the increase in size of the foetus and its adrenals (Frandsen, 1963). Worthy of note also is the fact that as pregnancy advances urinary oestriol excretion increases at a rate greater than that of oestrone and oestradiol, 17-β (Hengshem, 1957). Diczfalusy and Troen (1961) estimate that at the end of human pregnancy, oestrone plus oestradiol excretion is of the magnitude of 1·0–3·5 mg. whilst oestriol seems to range between about 15–50 mg. In terms of rat units, the final maximum rate of excretion may approach 100,000–200,000 R.U., compared with a maximum excretion of about 250 R.U. during the cycle, representing a 1000-fold increase (Hengshem, 1956; Brown, 1957).

This excretion cannot be due to a lowering of the kidney threshold, for after the eighth week oestrogen is demonstrable in the blood (Figs. 8 and 9) in quantities greater than those obtaining at any other time (Nachtigall, *et al.*, 1966). It must, therefore, be due to lack of usage or to increased production as removal of the ovaries from pregnant women does not stop the excretion (Diczfalusy and Toren, 1961) and placental extracts have oestrogenic properties (Fellner, 1913). It is possible that the placenta secretes the bulk of the oestrogen. On the other hand, the rate of excretion may not be abnormal, but instead of being used it may be

sensus of opinion (which may yet be wrong), is that the greatly increased amounts of the hormones excreted by the mother are synthesized by the placenta—probably by the syncytiotrophoblast—from precursors originating in the foetus and/or the mother, suggesting that the placenta may be dependent, in some way, upon the foetus for maximum production. Most of the available evidence is consistent with this idea and frequently points to it very directly. The subject is fully discussed by Newton (1938, 1939) and by Diczfalusy and Troen (1961).

The most suggestive facts are as follows:

(a) Oestrogens continue to be excreted after double oophorectomy or removal of the corpus luteum from pregnant women (Halbanp, 1905; Ask-Umark, 1926;

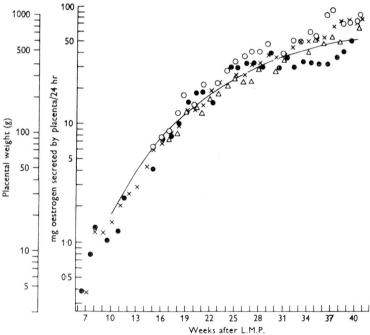

FIG. 7. Scatter-diagram of values for placental secretion of oestrone plus oestradiol plus oestriol throughout four normal pregnancies (calculated from the urine figures; Brown, 1956). Superimposed on the diagram is a line fitting the mean weights of placentae found at various times during pregnancy.

converted into a physiologically inactive and non-metabolizable form (Cohen and Marrian, 1936).

Although Cohen, Marrian and Watson (1935) reported that the ratio of "free" oestrogen excreted in the urine, to conjugated (i.e. glucuronidates) increases dramatically at term, this was subsequently found to be erroneous and had been caused by the artefactual hydrolysis of the conjugated oestrogen during urine collection (Clayton and Marrian, 1950). Thus all oestrogens excreted by the human female during pregnancy are conjugated and such conjugated oestrogens have little physiological potency. In blood, oestrone and oestriol are also largely bound although oestradiol appears to be free (Smith and Arai, 1963).

The Placenta as a Source of Oestrogens

The source of oestrogens, oestrone, oestradiol and oestriol during pregnancy is controversial but the con-

Asdell, 1928; Tulsky and Koff, 1957; Diczfalusy and Troen, 1961; Amoroso and Finn, 1962; Deanesly, 1966. Also Dorfman and van Wagenen (1941) and others found the removal of ovaries and foetus ineffective in altering the excretion rate in pregnant monkeys, but expulsion of the placenta caused a drop to non-pregnant levels.

(b) The excretion of oestrogen is definitely associated with chorionic tissue even when this is present in the absence of a foetus, as in retained placenta, hydatidiform mole or choriocarcinoma (MacDonald and Siiteri, 1964; van Lewsden and Villee, 1966).

(c) Oestrogen excretion is not appreciably altered by the occurrence of Addison's disease during pregnancy (Samuels, Evans and McKelvey, 1943; Knowlton, Mudge and Jailer, 1949) indicating that the maternal adrenal cortex is not an important source of the oestrogens excreted during pregnancy.

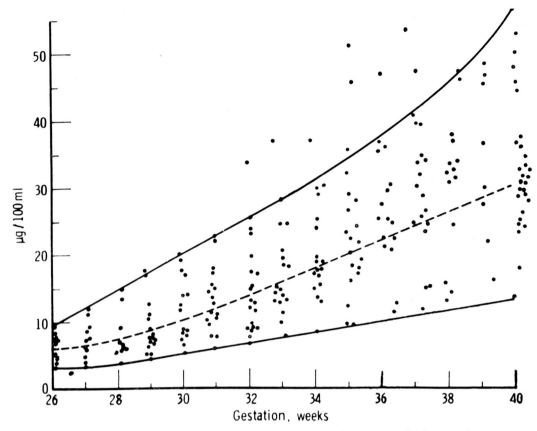

Fig. 8. Mean (broken line) and approximate upper and lower limits of plasma oestriol in normal pregnancy. From Nachtigall, Bassett, Hogsander, Slagle and Levitz (1966).

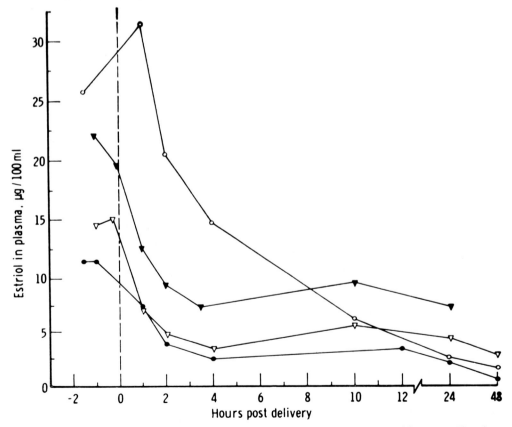

Fig. 9. Comparison of post-partum and prenatal plasma oestriol levels in normal gravid women. There is a rapid fall off in the early post partum period to values one half those obtained just prior to delivery. After Nachtigall, Bassett, Hogsander, Slagle and Levitz (1966).

(d) The best indirect evidence in favour of oestrogen production by the placenta is provided by Stewart (1951), who demonstrated oestrogenic stimulation of the uterus in ovariectomized rabbits with intra-ocular implants of full-term human placenta; HCG *per se* did not produce such an effect. Moreover, the histological examination of the implants established the occurrence of syncytium, which, from histochemical evidence Wislocki and Bennett (1943), Dempsey and Wislocki (1944), Wislocki and Dempsey (1948) and Wislocki and Padykula (1963) believe to be in some way associated with the synthesis of the steroid hormones.

(e) While neither the maternal ovary nor the maternal adrenal is essential for oestriol production, urinary oestriol levels are regarded as useful indices of foetal viability (Smith and Smith, 1948; Greene and Touchstone, 1963). In many instances of intrauterine foetal death (Lenters, 1958), urinary oestrogen excretion drops rapidly to levels which are of the same order as those reported in the urine of women bearing a live anencephalic foetus with defective adrenals (Frandsen and Stakemann, 1962; Coyle, 1962; Michie, 1965). This would seem to implicate the foetus and suggests adrenal involvement. On the other hand, the fact that the maternal urinary oestrogen levels found in anencephaly are much higher than the levels measured in nonpregnant women bespeaks placental participation (*see* Siiteri and MacDonald, 1966).

It has been suggested, however, that it is the interruption of the foetal circulation to the placenta, rather than the absence of the foetus which is the important factor in the production of oestrogens, since *in vivo* perfusion of the placenta from the foetal side with maternal blood after removal of the foetus promptly restores the preoperative levels of oestrin in the urine (Cassmer, 1959).

While agreeing with the importance of the foetal circulation for the maintenance of normal placental function, MacDonald and Siiteri (1964) point out, nevertheless, that Cassmer's results may also indicate that when the placenta is adequately perfused, a substance produced in the maternal organism and circulated via the maternal vessels may, under normal circumstances serve as an oestrogen precursor in the placenta. This thesis, they regard as particularly attractive during the early stages of gestation when the foetal contribution is negligible. Of immediate relevance in this connection also, is the genesis of the large amounts of urinary oestrogens excreted by women with hydatidiform moles, in which there is no circulation in the chorionic villi and the foetus is absent. In these circumstances it has been shown that the oestrogens produced by the molar tissue do not arise by *de novo* synthesis, but that moles, like the term placenta, can utilize dehydroisoandrosterone as a precursor of oestrone and oestriol, but lack the enzymes to convert C_{21} to C_{19} steroids (MacDonald and Siiteri, 1964; van Leusden and Villee, 1966).

Oestrogen Synthesis and Metabolism in the Placenta

The *in vivo* conversion of oestrone and oestradiol to oestriol is now well established and is considered the major source of oestriol production (Dorfman, 1957).

The predominant pathway of oestriol biosynthesis during pregnancy appears to be aromatization by the placenta of a precursor such as 3β-hydroxy-5-androsten-17-one (dehydroxyisoandrosterone) via the reactions shown in Fig. 10 (Magendantz and Ryan, 1964). It is highly probable that the bulk of placental oestradiol is derived from this adrenal steroid which is present in the two circulations and which, in all probability, is formed both in the maternal and foetal adrenals from placental pregnenolone; these two sources of precursor DS contribute about equally to urinary oestrone and oestradiol. The oestrone and oestradiol thus formed can enter the maternal circulation where they are in part metabolized to oestriol. The major portions of the oestrone and oestradiol reaching the foetus are conjugated with sulphuric acid and/or glucuronic acid and it is as conjugates that they are transported back to the placenta prior to their excretion in the urine. The finding of a significantly higher mean concentration of oestrone and oestradiol $17-\beta$ in umbilical venous than in umbilical arterial plasma, is evidence of the secretion of these hormones into the foetal circulation by the placenta and their subsequent metabolism by the foetus (Manner *et al.*, 1963).

Conjugates are poorly transferred to the mother. However, the placenta and foetal membranes are endowed with active sulphatases which hydrolyse sulphates to the free form, thus facilitating transfer to the mother (Levitz, 1966) where they contribute to the urinary oestradiol and oestriol. Figure 11 taken from Solomon (1966) attempts to summarize some of these steps. Conjugation is probably the major metabolic mode of inactivation, and doubtless is a safety factor in shielding the human foetus from the rising level of steroids as pregnancy advances. The ability of the foetus to metabolize conjugates directly without prior hydrolysis is another possible mechanism of inactivation. Because of these metabolic relations oestriol levels are a reliable index of foetal placental function in patients suspected of bearing a dead foetus.

Notwithstanding the foregoing account, the possibility exists that oestriol can also be produced by the foetoplacental unit from a non-oestrogenic precursor without involving the classic biosynthetic conversion from oestrone and oestradiol (Ryan, 1958, 1959; Siiteri and MacDonald, 1963; Bolte *et al.*, 1964; Hobkirk and Nilsen, 1966). It has been suggested that placental aromatization of 16-oxygenated C_{19} neutral steroids could be responsible for the formation of the excess oestriol which dilutes the urinary oestriol formed by peripheral metabolism of oestrone and oestradiol in maternal tissues. It has been claimed that oestrone is made by the foetus and not by the mother (Gurpide *et al.*, 1966; *see also* Mikhail, Wiquist and Diczfalusy, 1963).

The factors controlling oestrogen production are not surely known, but it would appear that urinary excretion of oestrogens can be maintained within normal limits during pregnancy in the absence of the pituitary (Little *et al.*, 1958; Kaplan, 1961). It is also known that the premature ageing of the placental syncytium in cases of toxaemia of pregnancy (Wislocki and Bennett, 1943) is accompanied by a marked drop in oestrogen production

(Smith and Smith, 1948; Hinglais and Hinglais, 1953). The daily production of placental oestrogen is not surely known, but may be of the order of 50–100 mg. (Diczfalusy, 1960).

Oestrogenic activity has been reported in both red cells and plasma (Albrieux, 1941) and it has been suggested that both may contain enzymes for oestrone-oestradiol interconversion and other steroid metabolic conversions. In this connection the possible role of the profusion of eosinophils in the endometrial cups of the mare, as an additional pathway for the removal of oestrogens is worthy of further study.

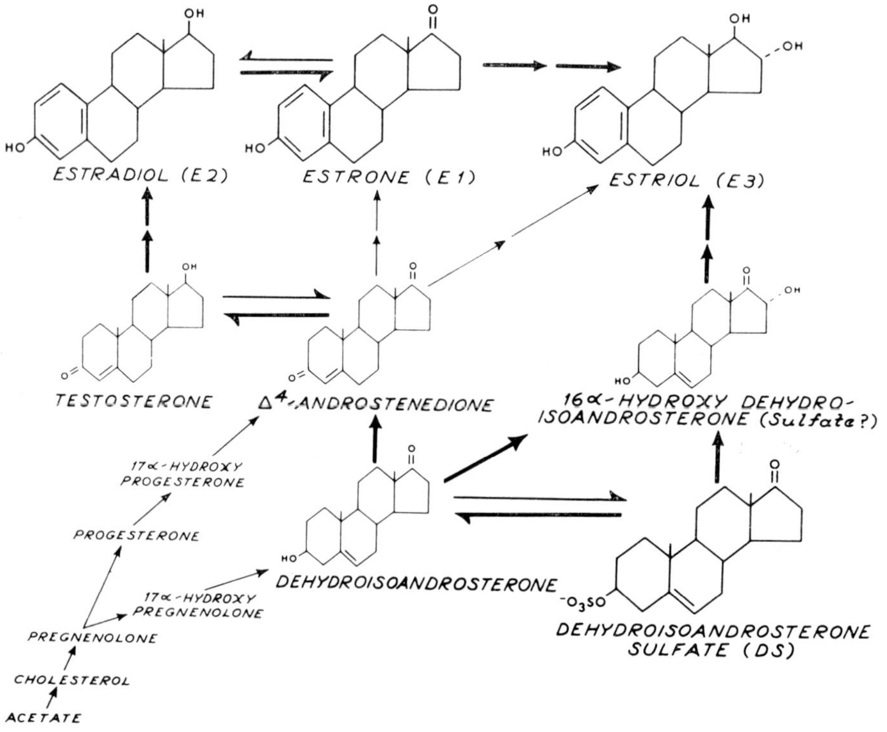

during pregnancy (Corner, 1947) and evidence that the synthesis of uterine actomyosin is regulated by oestrogen was furnished by Csapo (1950). Courrier (1945; 1950) had suggested earlier that progesterone and oestrogen might act synergistically to promote uterine growth, and this has been supported recently (DeMattos, Kempson, Erdos and Csapo, 1967).

In view of the apparent stimulatory effect of oestrogens upon uterine muscular activity (Parkes, 1930; Robson, 1935, etc.) the concept arose that oestrogen might act as an antagonist to progesterone and that uterine activity might be determined at any given time by the prevailing

Fig. 10. The possible biochemical pathways and some of the important intermediates leading to the three classic oestrogens, oestrone, oestriol, and oestradiol. From Siiteri and MacDonald, (1966) after Magendantz and Ryan (1964).

The probable role of human chorionic gonadotrophin in oestrogen production is discussed by Diczfalusy and Troen (1961).

Role of Oestrogens in Pregnancy

Although it is becoming increasingly evident that oestrogens exert a profound effect on a variety of biochemical processes in the reproductive tract (e.g. carbohydrate and lipid metabolism, Aizawa and Mueller, 1961; Leonard, 1958; Hall, 1965; Eckstein and Villee, 1966; Williams and Provine, 1966; Barker and Warren, 1966; protein and nucleic acid synthesis, Hamilton, 1963, 1964; Wilson, 1963; Jervill et al., 1958) and elsewhere (e.g. erythropoiesis, Mirand and Gordon, 1966), the physiological significance of the large amounts of oestrogens produced by the placenta is by no means clear. It has been suggested that oestrogens are involved in the rapid growth of the uterus

ratio of the two hormones (Robson, 1935; Reynolds, 1935, etc.). However, evidence that oestrogen can overcome progesterone dominance has not been forthcoming (Klopper and Dennis, 1962) and studies have revealed that there is no decline in progesterone titres in the blood (Llauro, Runnebaum and Zander, 1968) nor rise in oestrogen levels in urine (Smith and Smith, 1941a) immediately prior to the onset of labour. Nevertheless, recent work in the human female (Turnbull, Anderson and Wilson, 1967; Turnbull and Anderson, 1968) has indicated a negative correlation between the level of oestriol excretion at 34 weeks of pregnancy and gestation length. Puck and Hubner (1956) claimed that oestrogens increase the sensitivity of the myometrium to oxytocin preparatory to parturition. It has been suggested moreover, that oestrogenic substances are involved in the continued secretion of progesterone by acting directly on the ovary

(Robson, 1937, 1939; Hammond and Robson, 1951; Hammond, 1956) or, by way of the pituitary gland (Klein and Mayer, 1942, 1950) and may thus influence mammary development through prolactin secretion (Lyons, 1951).

Since placental oestrogen may enter the foetal organism directly (e.g. guinea-pig, Levitz et al., 1960; human, Manner et al., 1965), the question arises whether it has any important function in the regulation of foetal development. Foetal gonadal development has been studied in the horse (Cole, Hart, Lyons and Catchpole, 1933; Amoroso and Rowlands, 1951) where pregnancy lasts for about eleven months and oestrogens and gonadotrophins are abundant. The evidence points to the existence of an association between the concentration of urinary oestrogens and the quantitative development and regression of the foetal gonads.

Growth begins during the phase of maximum concentration of oestrogens in the urine of the mother at about the fourth month when gonadotrophins are no longer present in quantity in the circulation. The foetal gonads, at their maximum, weigh twice as much as those of the mother (Amoroso and Rowlands, 1951) and the gonadal enlargement has been shown to be due to a tremendous development of the interstitial tissue with little evidence of germinal activity (Amoroso and Rowlands, 1951; Amoroso and Finn, 1962); regression sets in at about the eighth month when the interstitial tissue disintegrates. In the newborn female the accessory organs also show characteristic signs of oestrogen stimulation and the mammary glands may secrete at birth (Courrier, 1945).

Similar quantitative changes have been described in the gonads of the Grey and Common Seal at birth (Amoroso and Matthews, 1951; Amoroso et al., 1951, 1965), but as yet no correlation between urinary oestrogens and gonadal development have been reported. In the females the ovaries at birth are far larger than those of the mother and the histological changes in the reproductive tract suggest the action of progesterone, possibly derived from the maternal ovaries, acting on an oestrogen stimulated genital tract (Amoroso and Matthews, 1951; Amoroso et al., 1951, 1965). In the new-born male grey seal, the testes are also enlarged and the prostate appears active and shows evidence of androgenic stimulation, but by the end of the first month of post-natal life it has regressed and is no longer so (Amoroso et al., 1951, 1965; Parkes, 1954).

Relationship between the Corpus Luteum and the Placenta

That progesterone plays an essential role in conditioning uterine reactions during pseudopregnancy and during gestation is a fact well known to biologists and clinicians alike. It is generally believed, moreover, that very early in pregnancy the corpus luteum is the source of progesterone and that the placenta, in some species, fairly soon takes place over the major role in the production of this gestagen: For example, removal of the corpus luteum from pregnant women (Kulseng-Hanssen, 1951; Glasser, 1952; Tulsky and Koff, 1957), or bilateral oophorectomy (Halban, 1905; Blair Bell, 1920; Ask-Upmark, 1926;

Pratt, 1927; Asdell, 1928; Benazzi, 1933; Guldberg, 1936; Calatroni et al., 1945; Venning, 1957; Diczfalusy and Borell, 1961) does not interrupt pregnancy, not even when performed as early as the first or second month (see also, Buchanan, Enders and Talmage, 1956). However, although the corpus luteum does not appear to be essential for the maintenance of gestation after the first or second month, it should not be assumed that it is without function. On the contrary, several investigators suggest that it functions throughout pregnancy. At mid-pregnancy, for example, the corpus luteum has been shown to synthesize cholesterol from acetate at a high rate (Davis and Plotz, 1957) and progesterone has been demonstrated in corpora lutea of pregnancy to the very end of gestation (Zander et al., 1958).

As with the human female, the results of experiments performed in rhesus monkeys demonstrate that these animals can maintain pregnancy, deliver normal young and provide adequate lactation even though ovariectomized as early as the twenty-first day after mating (Tullner and Hertz, 1966b) in a pregnancy which normally varies in length from 146–182 days (Hartman, 1932; van Wagenen and Newton, 1943).

The mechanism responsible for the interruption of pregnancy after bilateral removal of the ovaries, on the one hand, and the maintenance of it on the other, is not surely known. However, the common inference is that since in many of the mammals so far investigated the corpus luteum is necessary throughout gestation, those few species, such as the guinea pig (Daels, 1908; Herrick, 1928; Deanesly, 1960a), mare (Hart and Cole, 1934; Amoroso and Finn, 1962), monkey (Hartman, 1941; Hartman and Corner, 1947; Tullner and Hertz, 1966b) and the human female, which can dispense with it, must have some alternative source of oestrogen as well as progesterone. It is generally assumed that the extra-ovarian source is the placenta and not the foetal adrenal ovary or testis (Diczfalusy and Troen, 1961). Furthermore, the demonstration that the placenta not only contains but secretes the two hormones (e.g. human, Zander and von Münstermann, 1954; Lurie et al., 1966; monkey, Short and Eckstein, 1961; ewe, Short and Moore, 1959; guinea-pig, Deanesly, 1960b) and that the life span of this organ coincides with the excretion of their derivatives (Susuki, 1947; Venning, 1957) supports this.

The Placenta as a Source of Progesterone

That progesterone is the most abundant neutral steroid elaborated during pregnancy is now very generally recognized (Solomon, 1966). It is also generally agreed that in animals, progesterone is formed directly from pregnenolone (Heftmann and Mosettig, 1960; Pion, Jabbe, Eriksson, Wiquist and Diczfalusy, 1965) and that the biosynthetic sequence leading to progesterone is the same in plants as in animals (Bennett and Heftmann, 1965). It has been suggested, moreover. that maternal cholesterol is a major source of the progesterone (and also pregnenolone) elaborated by the human placenta (van de Wiele and Jailer, 1959; Solomon, 1966), that the in vivo human placenta at term can utilize pregnenolone sulphate as an efficient and significant precursor for progesterone production (Pion, Conrad and Wolff, 1966), and that women carrying twin pregnancies secrete more progesterone than those carrying singles (Short and Elton, 1959).

From a quantitative point of view, the most important urinary metabolite of progesterone is pregnanediol. This reduction product which was first obtained from human pregnancy urine by Marrian (1929) is inactive as a gestagen, and occurs in conjugation with glucuronic acid (Venning and Browne, 1936; Venning, 1957). With the exception of the pregnant mare (Suzuki, 1947) it has not yet been found in the urine of any species except man. Progesterone metabolism may therefore not follow an identical course in all mammalian species (Fig. 11).

early pregnancy by the corpus luteum, whereas, an additional source is provided by the placenta after the second month. Similarly, Amoroso (1956 unpublished observations) found the removal of ovaries ineffective in altering the excretion rate of pregnanediol in pregnant mares (cf. Amoroso and Finn, 1962), whereas expulsion of the placenta caused a precipitate drop to nonpregnant levels (Suzuki, 1947).

Very low concentrations of plasma progesterone have been found during late pregnancy in the cow (Gorski, Erb, Dickson and Butler, 1958) and none was detected in the placenta (Short, 1957; Gorski, Dominguez, Samuel and Erb, 1958). Furthermore, although the bovine corpus luteum at term (Wickersham and Tanabe, 1967) is capable

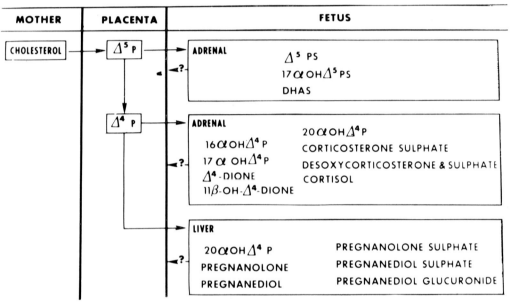

FIG. 11.   Biosynthesis of neutral steroids in the foeto-placental unit at midpregnancy.   From Solomon (1966).

The excretion of pregnanediol appears to be influenced by a number of factors, both known and unknown (Smith, Smith and Schiller, 1941; Guterman and Tulsky, 1949; Klopper and Billewicz, 1963). In addition to the endogenous factors which affect pregnanediol metabolism in undetermined ways (e.g. contribution of pregnanolone, Arcos et al., 1964; and other steroids; variations in hepatic metabolism of progesterone etc.), other factors such as variations in diuresis appear to affect the concentrations of the metabolite. These considerations, therefore, render pregnanediol estimations a useful yardstick of progesterone secretion but a poor inchtape.

Like oestriol, pregnanediol excretion begins to rise in concentration in pregnancy urine at about the eighth week and from less than 10 mg. per litre may attain 80 mg. per litre during the last month of pregnancy, but falls precipitously after parturition (Browne, Henry and Venning, 1937; Venning, 1955, 1957 and others). Likewise, Jones and Weil (1938) having obtained the pregnanediol complex from the urine of a pregnant woman following ovariectomy on the fifty-eight day after the last menstrual flow, concluded that progesterone is produced during

of synthesizing progesterone in vitro, removal of the corpora lutea after the 200th day did not induce abortion (McDonald, McNutt and Nichols, 1953), and progesterone levels did not fall until some nine days after ovariectomy (Erb, Gomes, Randel, Estergreen and Frost, 1967; Gupta and Pole, 1968). Indeed, Plotka, Estergreen and Frost (1967) found a positive correlation between the stage of pregnancy and the peripheral blood progesterone levels, but a negative correlation between the stage of pregnancy and ovarian vein titres. The possibility exists therefore of either the presence of an unidentified progestogen (Gorski, Erb, Dickson and Bulter, 1958) or, since progesterone has been identified in the gland, that the adrenals are the main source.

In this connection it may be worth while recalling the observations of Haterius (1936) and those of Selye et al. (1935) and of Newton (1938, 1939) and many others, that even in those species, like the rabbit, mouse and rat in which the ovaries are essential throughout gestation, pregnancy may be maintained after bilateral oophorectomy if most of the foetuses are removed and the placentae retained, thus assuring a high placental-foetal ratio. Worthy of note also is the suggestion that neither in *Mustelus canis*, a viviparous elasmobranch fish (Hisaw, 1959), nor in the viviparous garter and water snakes (Bragdon *et al.*, 1954) are the ovaries essential for the maintenance of pregnancy. The latter investigators also record the occurrence of progesterone-like agents in the circulating plasma of the reptiles. Progesterone has, likewise, been discovered in the African plant *Holarrhena floribunda* (Le Boeuf *et al.*, 1964), as well as in *Xysmalobium undulatum* (Tschesche and Snatzke, 1960) and *Trachycalymna fimbriatum* (von Euw and Reichstein, 1964) but, its physiological role, if any, in plants remains unknown.

One of the most striking actions of placental progesterone is the profound effect it exerts on myometrial function, blocking propagation (Csapo, 1962; Csapo and Takeda, 1965) of electrical and mechanical activity, reducing sensitivity to oxytocin (Knaus, 1926; 1934), and increasing extensibility (Schofield, 1966a) of the uterine muscle. These effects upon the musculature may be more important than those upon the endometrium as pregnancy advances, (Reynolds, 1949; Courrier, 1952). In recent years there has been considerable controversy (*see*, Bengtsson, 1967; Csapo and Wood, 1968; Kao, 1967 for reviews) over the significance of progesterone in myo-

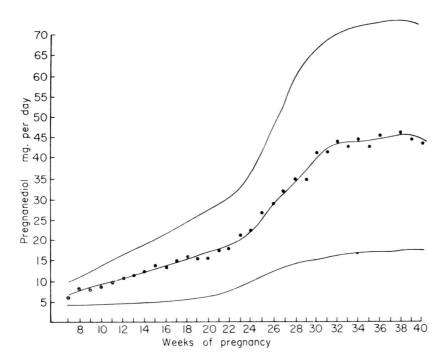

FIG. 12. Urinary excretion of pregnanediol in normal pregnancy. The upper and lower lines show the limit of 95 per cent probability. From Shearman (1950).

Insofar as progesterone has been found to be necessary in many viviparous animals for the maintenance of pregnancy, its occurrence presents less of a problem than that of either oestrogen or HCG. A fairly recent critical evaluation of the evidence has been made by Deanesly (1966), and it is clear that many of the effects produced by the luteal hormone under physiological conditions involve the simultaneous action of the oestrogenic hormone as well (Courrier, 1950).

Functions of Progesterone

It is now known that in addition to its role in the nutrition and transportation of ova and in the full differentiation of the reproductive tract and mammary glands, progesterone is also necessary to maintain the life of the foetus and placenta *in utero*. It is also believed to exert a profound influence on the activity of the anterior pituitary and is an important precursor of corticoids, and androgens, and indirectly also of oestrogens.

metrial regulation in animals in which the placenta is the main source of progesterone. The theory of Csapo (1956) that placental progesterone exerts a local as well as a systemic effect meets many of the objections to a systemically operative block mechanism, and is supported by a growing body of evidence (e.g. Kuriyama and Csapo, 1961; Schofield, 1966b; Porter, 1968). However, in an attempt to simulate a local effect of placental progesterone in the guinea-pig, by intra-uterine implants of the steroid Porter (1969a and b) was unable to prolong pregnancy. Furthermore, in the non-pregnant guinea-pig, neither systemic nor intra-uterine progesterone was capable of suppressing spontaneous uterine activity.

In certain rodents, notably the guinea-pig, Deanesly (1960a, 1963) has shown that while an ovarian or an exogenous progestagen is not required for ovo-implantation, lack of it affects embryonic growth with the subsequent death of many embryos. It appears, moreover, that the arrest of development, and death, is not at any time a direct result of uterine compression but is more probably due to nutritional deficiencies associated with the absence of luteal secretions. Finally, it seems probable that water retention by progesterone is a factor operating in pregnant rodents and is fundamentally responsible for the extra-uterine weight gain in mice. Thus Dewar (1957) has shown that the weight gain of pregnant mice could be maintained after hysterectomy (as a means of removing the placentae) with or without removal of the ovaries, by administering progesterone in *physiological* amounts. Oestrogens alone failed to have this effect and did not augment the action of progesterone.

The Biosynthesis and Metabolism of Progesterone during Pregnancy

Naturally, the elaboration of large amounts of progesterone (approximately 0·25–0·28 gm. per day) during human pregnancy (Pearlman, 1957; Zander, 1959) raises the question of its fate in the body. All of the evidence available at present supports the concept that progesterone, synthesized from cholesterol in the human placenta through the intermediate pregnenolone (Solomon *et al.*, 1965), is converted into a large number of metabolites, sizeable quantities of which continuously reach the foetus. The tissues of the latter constitute an important site for the metabolism of placental progesterone as early as the third month of pregnancy (Zander, 1959, 1961, 1965). It has been estimated that approximately 70 µg. of the hormone passes from the placenta to the foetus in a 24-hour period (Zander, 1959) where it may be utilized by the foetal adrenal and liver as a major precursor for the synthesis of 17-hydroxyprogesterone, androstene-dione, hydrocortisone, and other steroids (Troen, 1961; Zander, 1959, 1961; Villee and Villee, 1965; Bird *et al.*, 1966; Wilson *et al.*, 1966). There is evidence that the metabolic changes of progesterone in the liver are more of a reductive and those in tissues other than the liver more of an oxidative nature. Furthermore, both endogenous and exogenous progesterone have been shown to pass into the adipose tissue of the human female, the concentration of the hormone in fat during gestation being higher than in the peripheral blood (Kaufman and Zander, 1956). Studies on the turnover time of progesterone in the human female indicate a half-life of about four minutes (Short, 1961).

The nature of the steroids present in umbilical cord blood and the arterio-venous differences are indicative of the types of steroids produced by the placenta. The increasing levels of progesterone in the peripheral venous blood of the mother during pregnancy and the higher concentration of progesterone in umbilical venous blood than in umbilical arterial blood, suggests placental production and transport from that tissue to the foetus. It implies, moreover, a net transfer of progesterone from mother to foetus and the metabolism of that progesterone (Zander, 1959, 1961). Harbert *et al.* (1964), estimate that the human foetus can metabolize approximately 30 µg. of progesterone/100 ml. of plasma reaching it. By contrast, there is, at the time of delivery a higher concentration of such steroids as dehydroisoandrosterone, 16α-hydroxydehydroisoandrosterone, 17α-hydroxyprogesterone, Δ⁴-pregnene-20α-ol-3-one, Δ⁴-pregnene-20β-ol-3-one, etc. in the umbilical artery than in the vein, indicating that the foetus produces sizeable amounts of these substances which are then transported towards the placenta (Runnebaum and Zander, 1962).

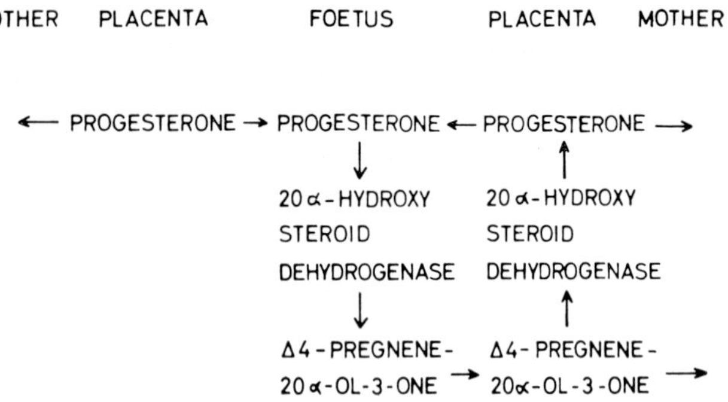

MOTHER   PLACENTA   FOETUS   PLACENTA   MOTHER

←— PROGESTERONE → PROGESTERONE ←— PROGESTERONE —→

$$\downarrow \qquad\qquad \uparrow$$

20α-HYDROXY   20α-HYDROXY
STEROID   STEROID
DEHYDROGENASE   DEHYDROGENASE

$$\downarrow \qquad\qquad \uparrow$$

Δ4-PREGNENE-   Δ4-PREGNENE-
20α-OL-3-ONE → 20α-OL-3-ONE —→

FIG. 13. The placental-foetal circulation of progesterone. From Zander (1965).

In the steroid metabolism of the foeto-placental unit, not only the metabolic fate of the placental steroids in the foetus is involved, but also the metabolic conversion of the foetal metabolites in the placenta, and even in the uterus. In this connection the conversion of progesterone to 17-hydroxyprogesterone (Little and Shaw, 1961) is of particular interest because of the central role this compound may play in steroid synthesis. It has been suggested (Davis and Plotz, 1957; Solomon, 1960) that 17-hydroxyprogesterone may be an intermediate in the synthesis of androgens, oestrogen and corticosteroids.

More evidence of the metabolic conversion of foetal metabolites of placental steroids is provided by the results of *in vivo* and *in vitro* experiments of Zander (1965) in which he showed that Δ⁴-pregnene-20α-ol-3-one, one of the major foetal metabolites of placental progesterone returning to the placenta in the umbilical arteries, can be reoxidized to progesterone in the placenta and thus be available to return to the foetus (Fig. 13).

Pregnanetriol in Pregnancy

The excretion of pregnanetriol in pregnancy has been investigated many times in recent years since this steroid was first shown to be the primary urinary metabolite of 17-hydroxyprogesterone (Jailer *et al.*, 1955). This latter substance constitutes, as we have already observed, an important intermediary in the biosynthesis of both adrenal and gonadal steroids.

Although no accurate data are available indicating the conversion rate of 17α-hydroxyprogesterone to pregnanetriol, one may assume that within certain limits, increased urinary pregnanetriol excretion reflects increased renal activity and perhaps also increased conversion of progesterone to androgens and oestrogens. An increase in the excretion of urinary pregnanetriol, during the last trimester of pregnancy, has been reported by several investigators in both the intact and adrenalectomized human female (Herman and Silverman, 1957; Ronan *et al.*, 1960; Fotherby *et al.*, 1965; Harkness and Love,

1966). It has been suggested (Harkness and Love, 1966) that in the absence of the adrenal the foeto-placental unit is probably the source of the increased amounts of this compound in the urine and presumably it is also the origin of some of the increase observed in normal pregnancy. The occurrence of the rise in the last trimester would, likewise, tend to support the view that the foetal component of the placenta may be the more important source (*see* Diczfalusy, 1965).

Relationship between the Adrenal Gland and the Placenta

It has long been known that during late pregnancy in the rat (Andersen and Sperry, 1937) and in women (Venning, 1946; Jones *et al.*, 1953; Davis and Plotz, 1956; Plotz and Davis, 1956), secretory activity of the adrenal cortex of the mother appears to be high and also that adrenalectomy during pregnancy in rats results in foetal adrenal hyperplasia (Firor and Grollman, 1933; Ingle and Fisher, 1938; Houssay, 1945; Davis and Plotz, 1954; Jost *et al.*, 1955, 1960). Pregnancy is also known to prolong the survival time of adrenalectomized animals (*see* Amoroso and Finn, 1962) and to relieve temporarily the symptoms of Addison's disease in the human female (Davis and Plotz, 1954; Angervall, 1962).

Jost and his associates (Jost *et al.*, 1955; Jost, 1961) have suggested that the enlarged adrenals of the foetus following adrenalectomy of the mother or in women with Addison's disease, can secrete sufficient amounts of cortical hormones to maintain the life of the gravid female. While this suggestion may not be completely disregarded, the alternative hypothesis, that the beneficial effect on the symptoms of adrenal cortical insufficiency imposed on the mother by bilateral adrenalectomy is due to the secretion of progesterone or of corticosteroids by the placenta, must be considered.

Experiments with rats have shown that pseudopregnancy (Collings, 1941) as well as the administration of progesterone (Bourne, 1939; Emery and Greco, 1940) can maintain adrenalectomized animals in good health, while intensive stimulation and luteinization of the ovaries by different gonadotrophins increased the survival period (Emery and Schwabe, 1936; D'Amour and D'Amour, 1939). Moreover, since it is known that the rat placenta at an early stage of development contains a substance that stimulates the corpus luteum to secrete progesterone, it is possible that the sustaining effect of pregnancy in adrenalectomized rats is accomplished chiefly through the luteotrophic action of the placenta on the corpus luteum (Emery and Schwabe, 1936).

Corticosteroid Production in Human Pregnancy

Among changes in maternal environment that result from pregnancy in the human female is the spectacular rise in corticosteroids (Gold, 1957; Nelson *et al.*, 1960; Telegdy *et al.*, 1963; Plager *et al.*, 1964). In the rat, this change in plasma corticosteroid levels, which affects not only bound but also the unbound corticosteroids, is the result not only of increased binding, which decreases

clearance, but also of stimulation of corticosteroid secretion evoked by oestrogens (Kitay, 1963; Telegdy *et al.*, 1964). In addition, there may be secretion of corticosteroids by the placenta (Little and Rossi, 1957). Thus, the quantity of corticosteroids extractable from rat placentae increased following adrenalectomy of the mother and remained unchanged when, in addition, the foetuses were removed (Ratsimamanga *et al.*, 1964). A fuller discussion of this aspect of the subject is to be found in the review by Parkes and Deanesly (1966).

17-Hydroxycorticosteroids

While there is a good deal of evidence suggesting increase in the urinary excretion of adrenocortical C_{21} steroids in human pregnancy (Venning, 1946, 1957; Jailer, 1951) the excretion of androgenic or 17-ketosteroids is equivocal. It would appear, nevertheless, that plasma levels of free 17-hydroxycorticosteroids (17-OHCS) rise

PLASMA 17-HYDROXYCORTICOSTEROID LEVELS IN NON-PREGNANT AND PREGNANT WOMEN IN THE THIRD TRIMESTER

	Micrograms 17-OHCS/ml. of Plasma	
	Non-pregnant Women	Pregnant Women
Gemzell (1953, 1954)	6.6 ± 0.95	25.0
Robinson *et al.* (1955)	12.0 ± 1.1	33.0 ± 1.4
Bayliss *et al.* (1955)	9.5	24.0 ± 1.6
Migeon *et al.* (1957b)	15.5 ± 6.3	23.3 ± 9.2
Assali *et al.* (1955)	$7.0 - 15.0$	$34.6 (25.6 - 47.5)$

progressively during pregnancy, reach a maximum some time in the third trimester and gradually return to the normal range after parturition (Table 1, *see also* Martin and Mills, 1958; Little *et al.*, 1958a; Kawahara, 1958; Doe *et al.*, 1960); labour is also known to cause an acute elevation (Migeon *et al.*, 1956; Nichols *et al.*, 1958). In contrast, the urinary 17-OHCS are usually normal, but may increase slightly during late pregnancy, due primarily to increase in the unconjugated fraction (Migeon *et al.*, 1957a, b; Martin and Mills, 1958). However, in a pregnancy, complicated by Cushing's syndrome, Kreines, Perin and Salzer (1964), reported absence of diurnal variation of the elevated plasma 17-OHCS and increased urinary excretion of 17-OHCS. But despite this, it is well to remember that the 17-ketosteroids may be falsely elevated, due to the fact that there may be an increased excretion of 20-ketosteroids, which also react with the Zimmermann reagents (Martin and Mills, 1958).

Although the foetal adrenal gland can synthesize such steroids (Block *et al.*, 1956), the finding of normal values of 17-OHCS in cord blood of anencephalic foetuses precludes the possibility that these hormones are secreted by the foetal zone (Migeon *et al.*, 1957a, b). However, since $4C^1$, cortisol as well as the non-isotopic steroid, can cross the placental barrier (Migeon *et al.*, 1957a, b), the cord levels of plasma 17-OHCS may merely be a reflexion of those of the mother, suggesting that the foetal glands, near term produce little or no corticosteroids.

Bayliss, Browne, Round and Steinbeck (1955) also dismiss the foetus as well as the placenta as being responsible for the elevated levels of 17-OHCS. They state that the main site of production is the maternal adrenals because the glands are hypertrophied (Aschner, 1912) and during the puerperium the steroid level falls gradually and not precipitately, as would be the case if the foetus and placenta were directly involved (see also Robinson et al., 1955). Migeon, Bertrand and Wall (1957) and Cohen et al. (1958), on the other hand, present evidence which indicates that the rise in plasma levels of cortisol during pregnancy is due neither to secretions from the placenta or the foetus, nor to increased production by the maternal adrenals but to a diminished ability of pregnant women to transform cortisol to certain of its metabolites and to an alteration in the distribution of cortisol in pregnancy.

Another possible explanation for the elevation of the 17-OHCS in pregnancy has been advanced by Staunwhite and Sandberg (1959). Since it is known that the preponderant part of plasma cortisol is bound to a special protein transcortin (Bush, 1957; Sandberg et al., 1957) it has been postulated that transcortin-bound cortisol is biologically inactive and not available for metabolism. Moreover, since the levels of transcortin have been shown to be elevated in pregnancy, especially in the last trimester, this finding may explain the elevated 17-OHCS in pregnancy and the lack of any real signs of hypercorticism.

Adrenocortical and other Androgens in Pregnancy

The plasma levels of 17-ketosteroids (17-KS) in normal pregnancy usually decrease, but urinary excretion of 17-KS may increase, especially during the last trimester (Venning, 1955; Martin and Mills, 1958). These investigators point out, however, that the 17-KS may be falsely elevated due to the fact that there may be an increased excretion of pregnanolone and other 20-ketosteroids derived from progesterone which also react with the Zimmermann reagents. Thus, except for the progressive increase in total 17-ketosteroids in pregnant Addisonian women (Samuels et al., 1943; Jailer and Knowlton, 1950; Klotz, 1955; but see Baulieu et al., 1956, 1957), and the presence of androgens in extracts of placental tissue (Salhanick et al., 1952, 1956; Berliner et al., 1956; Troen, 1959 and others), which is denied by Dorfman (1948), there is little evidence to suggest that the human placenta contributes significantly to androgen production.

As with the human female, studies on monkeys indicate that the excretion of androgens, like that of oestrogens increases during the course of pregnancy and more especially towards full term (Dorfman and van Wagenen, 1941); this excretion is unaffected by ovariectomy. But whereas this excretion of androgens persists at a high level, after ovariectomy, early in gestation, and for a month after parturition, the oestrogens decrease at once to normal values after parturition or expulsion of the placenta. It may thus be concluded that in women andmonkeys, at least, that the placenta is not a major source of androgen production and that the androgens excreted in pregnancy are of adrenal origin, being the result of hypophysial stimulation of the adrenal cortex, perhaps through the circulating oestrogens.

Allusion has already been made to changes in the prostate of newborn male seals (Amoroso and Matthews, 1951; Amoroso et al., 1951, 1965; Parkes, 1954) suggesting androgenic stimulation of these accessory structures. Deanesly (1966) states that androgens also circulate during at least the first pregnancy in the mouse and she believes the increase in androgen output may be attributed as in other species, to the action of ACTH on the adrenal cortex. In the pregnant guinea-pig, on the other hand, Brooks, Clayton and Hammant (1960) have shown that the excretion of androgens is increased even after ovariectomy or adrenalectomy, indicating that some, at any rate of the 17-ketosteroids are of placental derivation.

Aldosterone Production in Human Pregnancy

There are many reports of high urinary values of aldosterone during the course of normal human pregnancy (see Assali and Hamermesz, 1954; Venning and Dyrenfurth, 1956; Jones et al., 1959; van de Wiele et al., 1960; Wanatabe et al., 1965) and after hypophysectomy during the twelfth week of gestation (Kaplan, 1961) but the source of the hormone remains uncertain. The foregoing results are in keeping with a placental origin, but in the light of results demonstrating very low urinary excretion of aldosterone by pregnant women with Addison's disease (Baulieu et al., 1958; Christy and Jailer, 1959; Moses et al., 1959) or after bilateral adrenalectomy (Laidlaw, Cohen, Gormall, 1958; Angervall, 1962) it is tempting to suggest that the hormone in normal pregnancy is adrenal rather than placental. However, when the foetus dies in utero, there is a concomitant drop in aldosterone secretion as compared with the characteristically elevated rates observed in normal pregnancy implying foetal participation. But since neither the foetal adrenal, nor other foetal tissues converts progesterone reaching it to aldosterone (Solomon et al., 1965) foetal participation can only be indirect. Because oestrogens (Layne et al., 1962) and progesterone (Laidlaw et al., 1962) are known to stimulate the synthesis of aldosterone by the maternal adrenal however, their decrease after intra-uterine foetal death may be an important factor in the lowered aldosterone production observed. On the other hand, the hypersecretion has been considered compensatory to the natriuretic effect of the elevated levels of progesterone elaborated during gestation (Martin and Mills, 1956). Other studies have failed to demonstrate placental production of aldosterone in vitro (Sybulski, 1959).

That some adrenocortical-like material is formed in the placenta is suggested by the gradual increase in the excretion of 17-ketosteroids, which attains normal levels during the last trimester in Addisonian women (Samuels et al., 1943; Knowlton et al., 1949; Jailer and Knowlton, 1950) and also by the fact that a hormone with cortical-like activity can be extracted from the placenta (Johnson and Haines 1952; De Courcy et al., 1952).

Pituitary, Adrenal and Placental Interrelationships

While there are no obvious indications of adrenal-cortical insufficiency in pregnant rodents hypophysectomized during the second half of gestation (Amoroso and Porter, 1966), the pregnant uterus and its contents do not completely compensate for hypophysial function. In gravid mice and rats, for example, the adrenal glands regress as rapidly as they do following hypophysectomy in non-pregnant animals (Gardner and Allen, 1942; Greer, 1949; Contopoulos and Simpson, 1959). In monkeys, on the other hand, the adrenal cortex of animals hypophysectomized during pregnancy do not undergo the involution that invariably occurs in non-pregnant females. Adrenal weight is well maintained but declines rapidly after parturition (Smith, 1954) suggesting an alternative source of ACTH other than the maternal hypophysis.

The extent to which the foetal pituitary, the placenta or both are implicated in these changes in the monkey remains uncertain. The late maturation of the hypophysial-adrenal axis in the foetus as well as the impermeability of the placental membrane to ACTH make it improbable, however, that the foetus supplies ACTH to the mother (see Smith, 1954; also Amoroso, 1960a, b). On the other hand, strong support for placental production of ACTH-like material has come both from assay studies of extracts from the placenta (Jailer and Knowlton, 1950; Opsahl and Long, 1951; Cohen and Kleinberg, 1952; Assali and Hamermesz, 1954) and from the observations by Smith (1954) of the maintenance of adrenal weight and structure in his hypophysectomized monkeys during gestation. Similarly, Tuchmann-Duplessis et al. (1952) found that a human placental extract would increase the weight of the adrenals in 14-day hypophysectomised rats, but mere occurrence cannot in this case be lightly accepted as proof of secretion (Strobel, 1961).

The presence of an adrenal-weight factor, distinct from ACTH, in the blood from pregnant women was first demonstrated by Jailer, Longson and Christy (1957). This was later confirmed by Lanman and Dinerstein (1959) who presented evidence that the factor responsible for the effect was chorionic gonadotrophin, which they showed to be effective in maintaining adrenal weight in hypophysectomized male rats. In these experiments it has been suggested that HCG does not act directly upon the adrenal glands, but stimulates androgen production by the testes, which in turn, partially protects the adrenal cortex after hypophysectomy (Zizine, Simpson and Evans, 1950). That the placenta itself may, nevertheless, contribute to androgen production is suggested by the experiments of Brooks, Clayton and Hammant (1960) cited above.

The Placenta in Relation to Mammary Development and Pelvic Relaxation

Because of the pre-eminent role of the anterior pituitary in the successful control of luteal function and mammary development it may be presumed that species in which pregnancy is not interrupted by hypophysectomy would yield information concerning the trophic effect of the placenta upon the progress of mammary growth during normal pregnancy.

Numerous observations on several species of pregnant females including the cat, rat, mouse, guinea-pig, monkey and woman (for a list of references, see Amoroso and Finn, 1962), show that the pituitary is not essential for full differentiation of the mammary gland, and that involution of the gland occurs only when the placenta is removed at the same time. However, lack of pituitary function promptly makes itself felt after parturition when lactation fails to occur, or at the most makes a transient appearance (Allan and Wiles, 1932; McPhail, 1935; Newton and Richardson, 1940). It would thus appear that, in rats and mice at least, the placenta plays a significant role in mammary development which is largely independent of both ovaries and pituitary (Lyons, 1951; Ray et al., 1955).

In the human female (Kaplan, 1961) and in the rhesus monkey (Agate, 1952; Smith 1954) on the other hand pregnancy can be successfully maintained and lactation can occur in the total absence of the pituitary. In both secretion of milk occurred a few days after delivery; it was minimal in amount and of short duration (Kaplan, 1961; Agate, 1952). This is not surprising since the reproductive process of women and monkeys are so similar, extending to the production of chorionic gonadotrophin (Noble and Plunkett, 1955). The question as to why lactation is not normally initiated during pregnancy has been ably discussed by Deanesly (1966).

Relaxin a Hormone of Pregnancy

It is now more or less taken for granted that in addition to the gonadal hormones, there is present in the ovaries (especially the corpora lutea) and placentae of many mammals, relatively large amounts of a polypeptide hormone relaxin. The hormone has been prepared in a relatively pure state (Abramowitz et al., 1944) and found to be associated with the pseudoglobulin fraction of serum and to have a peptide structure, though the N content of 11 per cent was somewhat low. The claim of relaxin to individuality rests on its speed of action—its chemical difference from the other two hormones, oestrogen and progesterone—its lack of oestrogenic or progestational effect; and its ability to bring about pubic separation by active bone resorption and ligament formation.

Until fairly recently relaxin was considered to be concerned primarily with relaxation of the pelvic ligaments during late pregnancy. It is now believed that it may have additional roles during pregnancy and parturition. For example, it has been shown to be capable of inhibiting spontaneous uterine motility in vivo in prepubertal and adult mice and in vitro (Felton et al., 1953; Miller et al., 1957; Bloom et al., 1958; Kroc et al., 1958) and of inducing spontaneous delivery of living young in pregnant mice spayed and maintained on progesterone (Smithberg and Runner, 1956; Hall, 1956, 1957). Relaxin is reported to inhibit uterine activity without impairing its sensitivity to oxytocin (Sawyer, Frieden and Martin, 1953). In addition, although it is itself devoid of oestrogenic or progestational activity, relaxin has a synergistic action with oestrogen and progesterone on the growth of the virgin rat and mouse mammary gland (Hamolsky and Sparrow, 1945; Hall, 1956, 1957; Wada and Turner, 1959a, b) and with progesterone in the maintenance of pregnancy in the spayed mouse.

The ovary, uterus and placenta have been suggested as possible sites for the production of relaxin. In the sow (Hisaw and Zarrow, 1950), mouse (Newton and Beck, 1939; Hall and Newton, 1947) and the Fin and Blue whale (Steinetz et al., 1959) the ovaries appear to be the principal source, whereas in the guinea-pig, the placenta plays a more significant role (Herrick, 1928; Zarrow, 1948). In the rabbit, under suitable conditions, the ovaries, uterus, vagina, placenta and even the mammary glands may all secrete relaxin (Zarrow and Rosenberg, 1953). Relaxin activity was also found in the testes of birds and in homogenates of ovaries from a gravid shark, but none was found in assays of ripe ovaries of a bony fish (Steinitz et al., 1959).

Newton and his collaborators were chiefly responsible for the view that the production of relaxin in the mouse is apparently different from that observed in guinea-pigs and rabbits. When the ovaries are present in pregnant mice, pubic separation is normal, but in their absence it does not occur (Newton and Lits, 1938). On the other hand, hypophysectomy during pregnancy does not influence pubic separation, provided the placentae are not lost, hence a placental-ovarian relationship must be presumed (Newton and Beck, 1939). In pregnant guinea pigs, neither of these operations interferes with normal pubic relaxation so that the relaxative hormone appears to be of placental origin. However, that the placenta is not the only source in the guinea-pig is suggested by the occurrence of pubic separation at oestrus, when the animal is non-pregnant. Hall and Newton (1947) suggest that in the mouse the placenta acts by stimulating the production of relaxin in the ovary, probably by means of a luteotrophic principle (Cerruti and Lyons, 1960). Smithberg and Runner (1956, 1957) assert, on the other hand, that oestrogen, produced by the mouse placenta can account for the trophic influence. The mode of action of relaxin is not clear and any presumed function in whales can certainly not be concerned with pubic relaxation. For a full account of the biology of relaxin the reader should consult the reviews of Hisaw and Zarrow (1950), and of Hall (1960).

Production of Other Non-steroid Hormones by the Placenta

Except for their presence in placental extracts, there is, as yet, insufficient evidence to indicate whether such non-steroid substances as thyroxine, serotonin, oxytocin, vasopressin and the melanocyte stimulating hormone (MSH) are produced by the human placenta or merely stored there (Diczfalusy and Troen, 1961). There is, furthermore, no acceptable evidence that Thyroid-stimulating Hormone (TSH) activity is increased during normal pregnancy (Greer, 1949; Yamazaki, Nogouchi and Slingerland, 1961; and others), though Koch, van Kessel,

Stolte, and van Leusden (1966) state that in molar pregnancies PBI values where much higher than in normal gravid women.

Comment

The foregoing account together with various other scattered observations on the effects of retained placentae raise important issues, even though, as Newton (1939) pointed out more than a quarter of a century ago, and as Diczfalusy (1960) has forcibly argued recently "we still have only a limited knowledge of the factors influencing production, transport, maintenance of the proper concentration at the target organs and disappearance of the hormones", serves to prove that the foetus and the state of pregnancy are not inseparable and that besides its role as a vital link between mother and infant, the placenta provides a certain degree of biological autonomy to the reproductive process during gestation. Indeed, as De Snoo put it as long ago as 1919, "In my opinion the fact is most striking that the uterine decidua is expelled a few hours after the removal of an extra-uterine ovum, without regard of whether the foetus is alive or dead. These observations strongly suggested to me that the placenta exerts an *inhibiting* influence on uterine contractions. I decided to test this hypothesis. I reasoned that if the placenta does exert such an influence, labour should begin sooner and proceed more speedily in women with total abruptio than in patients with subtotal abruptio. for the latter retain normal placental function to a considerable extent.

"My observations showed that in patients with complete abruptio, labour started earlier and was also completed quicker than in patients with incomplete abruptio. It may be argued that in patients with total abruptio, bleeding is generally more severe and the retroplacental haematoma is larger, resulting in a greater degree of stretching (and consequent stimulation) of the uterus. However, the significance of this fact is limited by the frequent observation that in patients with incomplete abruptio, labour was often delayed for weeks in spite of such excessive haematomas of one kilogramme or more.

"In my opinion the striking difference in the rapidity of the clinical events after complete and incomplete abruptio is best explained by supposing, that the ovum exerts an *inhibiting* effect upon the uterus which is suddenly *eliminated* in cases of total abruptio, while the effect persists to some degree in patients with subtotal abruptio. Even if other maternal inhibitions exist, the inhibition by the ovum is the most important one. The experience with foetal death *in utero* and specifically that of missed abortion shows, that this inhibiting influence does not originate from a living foetus. Consequently, the inhibiting influence must be of placental origin, more precisely an effect of the foetal placenta, the chorionic villi."

In an important paper, published twenty-five years ago, Hisaw (1944) provides an hypothesis for the relationship between placenta and ovaries in primates. In this paper and elsewhere (Hisaw and Astwood, 1942) he postulates for the monkey and human female a chain of hormone combinations leading up to the complete dominance of the placenta. The exact nature of the pregnancy-maintaining mechanism remains to be determined nevertheless, but it is evidently dependent on some, or all of the hormones secreted by the placenta.

REFERENCES

Abramowitz, A. V., Money, W. L., Zarrow, M. X., Talmage, R. C., Kleinholz, L. H. and Hisaw, F. L. (1944), "Preparation, Biological Assay and Properties of Relaxin," *Endocrinology*, **34**, 103.

Agate, F. J. Jr. (1952), "The Growth and Secretory Activity of the Mammary Glands of the Pregnant Rhesus Monkey (*Macaca mulatta*) following Hypophysectomy," *Amer. J. Anat.*, **90**, 257.

Aizawa, Y. and Mueller, G. C. (1961), "The Effect *in vivo* and *in vitro* of Oestrogens on Lipid Synthesis in the Rat Uterus," *J. biol. Chem.*, **236**, 381.

Albert, A. and Berkson, J. (1951), "A Clinical Bio-assay for Chorionic Gonadotropin," *J. clin. Endocr. Metab.*, **11**, 805.

Albrieux, A. S. (1941), "The Distribution of Estrogens in the Blood of Pregnant and Non-pregnant Women," *J. clin. Endocr. Metab.*, **1**, 893.

Allan, H. and Wiles, P. (1932), "The Role of the Pituitary Gland in Pregnancy and Parturition. I. Hypophysectomy," *J. Physiol.*, **75**, 23.

Allen, W. R. (1969), "The Immunological Measurement of Pregnant Mare Serum Gonadotrophin," *J. Endocr.*, **43**, 593.

Amoroso, E. C. (1952), "Placentation." In: *Marshall's Physiology of Reproduction*. (A. S. Parkes, Ed.). Vol. II, Chap. 15, p. 127. London: Longmans.

Amoroso, E. C. (1955a), "Endocrinology of Pregnancy," *Brit. med. Bull.*, **11**, 117.

Amoroso, E. C. (1955b), "The Comparative Anatomy and Histology of the Placenta." In: *Gestation* (L. B. Flexner, Ed.), Vol. I, p. 119. New York: Josiah Macy, Jr. Foundation.

Amoroso, E. C. (1955c), "De la signification du placenta dans l'evolution de la gestation chez les animaux vivipares," *Ann. Endocr. Paris*, **16**, 435.

Amoroso, E. C. (1956), "The Endocrine Environment of the Foetus," *Proc. 3rd Congr. Anim. Reprod., Cambridge*, I, 25.

Amoroso, E. C. (1959), "The Biology of the Placenta." In: *Gestation* (C. A. Villee, Ed.), Vol. V, p. 13. New York: Josiah Macy, Jr. Foundation.

Amoroso, E. C. (1960a), "Comparative Aspects of the Hormonal Functions." In: *The Placenta and Fetal Membranes* (C. A. Villee, Ed.), p. 3. Baltimore: Williams and Wilkins.

Amoroso, E. C. (1960b), "Viviparity in Fishes." In: *Hormones in Fishes* (I. Chester-Jones, Ed.), *Symp. zool. Soc., Lond.*, No. 1, p. 153.

Amoroso, E. C. (1968), "The Evolution of Viviparity." In: *Life before Birth, Symp. No. 10, Proc. roy. Soc. Med.*, **61**, 1188.

Amoroso, E. C., Bourne, G. H., Harrison, R. T., Matthews, L. H., Rowlands, I. W. and Sloper, J. C. (1965), "Reproductive and Endocrine Organs of Foetal, Newborn and Adult Seals," *J. Zool.*, **147**, 430.

Amoroso, E. C. and Finn, C. A. (1962), "Ovarian Activity during Pregnancy, Ovum Transport and Implantation." In: *The Ovary* (S. Zuckerman, Ed.), Vol. I, p. 431. London: Academic Press.

Amoroso, E. C., Hancock, J. L. and Rowlands, I. W. (1948), "Ovarian Activity in the Pregnant Mare," *Nature, Lond.*, **161**, 355.

Amoroso, E. C., Harrison, R. J., Matthews, L. H. and Rowlands, I. W. (1951), "Reproductive Organs of Near Term and Newborn Seals," *Nature, Lond.*, **168**, 771.

Amoroso, E. C. and Matthews, L. H. (1951), "The Growth of the Grey Seal *Halichoerus grypus* (Fabricius) from Birth to Weaning," *J. Anat., Lond.*, **85**, 427.

Amoroso, E. C. and Porter, D. G. (1966), "Anterior Pituitary Function in Pregnancy." In: *The Pituitary Gland* (G. W. Harris and B. T. Donovan, Eds.), Vol. I, Chap. 12, p. 364.

Amoroso, E. C. and Rowlands, I. W. (1951), "Hormonal Effects in the Pregnant Mare and Foetal Foal," *J. Endocrine*, **7**, 1.

Andersen, D. H. and Sperry, W. M. (1937), "A Study of Cholesterol in the Adrenal Gland in Different Phases of Reproduction in the Female Rat," *J. Physiol.*, **90**, 296.

Angervall, L. (1962), "Adrenalectomy in Pregnant Rats: Effects on Offspring," *Acta endocr., Copenh.*, **41**, 546.

Arcos, M., Gurpide, E., Van de Wiele, R. L. and Lieberman, S. (1964), "Precursors of Urinary Pregnanediol and their Influence in the Determination of the Secretory Rate of Progesterone," *J. clin. Endocr. Metab.*, **24**, 237.

Artunkal, T. and Colonge, R. A. (1949), "Action de L'ovariectomie sur la Gestation du Cobaye," *C.R. Soc. Biol., Paris*, **143**, 1590.

Aschheim, S. and Zondek, B. (1927), "Ei und Hormon. Hypophysenvorder-lappenhormon und Ovarialhormon im Harn von Schwangeren," *Klin. Wschr.*, **6**, 1321.

Aschner, I. (1912), "Uber die Funktion der Hypophyse," *Pflüg. Arch. ges. Physiol.*, **146**, 1.

Asdell, S. A. (1928), "The Growth and Function of the Corpus Luteum," *Physiol. Rev.*, **8**, 813.

Ask-upmark, M. E. (1926), "Le Corps Jaune est-il Nécessaire pour L'accomplissement Physiologique de la Gravité Humaine?" *Acta obstet. gynec. scand.*, **5**, 211.

Assali, N. S., Garst, J. B. and Voskian, J. (1955), "Blood Levels of 17-hydroxycorticosteroids in Normal and Toxemic Pregnancies," *J. Lab. Clin. Med.*, **46**, 385.

Assali, N. S. and Hamermesz, J. (1954), "Adrenocorticotropic Substances from Human Placenta," *Endocrinology*, **55**, 561.

Astwood, E. B. (1941), "The Regulation of Corpus Luteum Function by Hypophysial Luteotrophin," *Endocrinology*, **28**, 309.

Astwood, E. B. and Greep, R. O. (1938), "A Corpus Luteum Stimulating Substance in the Rat Placenta," *Proc. Soc. exp. Biol., N.Y.*, **38**, 715.

Averill, S. C., Ray, E. W. and Lyons, W. R. (1950), "Maintenance of Pregnancy in Hypophysectomized Rats with Placental Implants," *Proc. Soc. Exp. Biol., N.Y.*, **75**, 3.

Aylward, F. and Ottoway, C. W. (1945), "The Collection and Examination of Plasma from Pregnant Mares for Gonadotrophic Hormone," *J. comp. Path. Therap.*, **55**, 159.

Baker, K. L. and Warren, J. C. (1966), "Estrogen Control of Carbohydrate Metabolism in the Rat Uterus: Pathways of Glucose Metabolism," *Endocrinology*, **78**, 1205.

Baulieu, E. E., Bricaire, H. and Jayle, M. F. (1956), "Lack of Secretion of 17-hydroxycorticosteroids in a Pregnant Woman with Addison's Disease," *J. clin. Endocr. Metab.*, **16**, 690.

Baulieu, E. E., Vigan, M. de, Bricaire, H. and Jayle, M. F. (1957), "Lack of Plasma Cortisol and Urinary Aldosterone in a Pregnant Woman with Addison's Disease," *J. clin. Endocr. Metab.*, **17**, 1479.

Bayliss, R. I. S., Browne, J. C. M., Round, B. P. and Steinbeck, A. W. (1955), "Plasma 17-hydroxycorticosteroids in Pregnancy," *Lancet*, **1**, 62.

Beck, P., Parker, M. L. and Daughaday, W. H. (1965), "Radioimmunologic Measurement of Human Placental Lactogen in Plasma by a Double Antibody Method during Normal and Diabetic Pregnancies," *J. clin. Endcor. Metab.*, **25**, 1457.

Benazzi, M. (1933), "Sulla Funzione Ovarica in Gravidanza," *Arch. Sci. Biol.*, **18**, 409.

Bengtsson, L. Ph. (1967), "Progesterone and the Myometrium in Human Pregnancy." Chap. 7. In: *Advances in Obstetrics and Gynecology* (S. L. Marcus, and C. C. Marcus, Eds.). Baltimore: Williams and Wilkins.

Bennett, R. D. and Heftmann, E. (1965), "Progesterone: Biosynthesis from Pregnenolone in *Holarrhena floribunda*," *Science*, **149**, 652.

Berliner, D. L., Jones, J. E. and Salhanick, H. A. (1956), "The Isolation of Adrenal-like Steroids from the Human Placenta," *J. biol. Chem.*, **223**, 1043.

Bielanski, W., Ewy, Z. and Pigoniowa, H. (1955), "Differences in Endocrine Secretion of Mares Pregnant with Stallion or Jack," *Bull. Acad. Polonaise Sci. Ch.*, **111**, 37.

Bird, C. E., Wiqvist, N., Diczfalusy, E. and Solomon, S. (1966), "Metabolism of Progesterone by the Perfused Previable Human Fetus," *J. clin. Endocr. Metab.*, **26**, 1144.

Blair-Bell, W. (1920), *The Sex Complex*. London.

Block, E., Benirschke, K. and Rosemberg, E. (1956), "C$_{14}$ Steroids, 17-α-hydroxycorticosterone and a Sodium Releasing Factor in Human Foetal Adrenal Glands," *Endocrinology*, **58**, 626.

Bloom, G., Paul, K. G. and Wiqvist, N. (1958), "A Uterine-relaxing Factor of the Pregnant Rat," *Acta endocr., Copenh.*, **28**, 112.

Bolte, E., Mancuso, S., Eriksson, G., Wiqvist, N. and Diczfalusy, E. (1964), "Studies on the Aromatization of Neutral Steroids in Pregnant Women. 3. Over-all Aromatization of Dehydro-dehydroepiandrosterone Sulfate Circulating in the Foetal and Maternal Compartments," *Acta Endocr. Copenh.*, **45**, 576.

Bourne, G. (1939), "The Effect of Progesterone on the Survival of Adrenalectomized Rats," *J. Physiol.*, **95**, 12P.

Boycott, M. and Rowlands, I. W. (1938), "The Biological Nature and Quantitative Variation of Pregnant Mare's Serum," *Brit. Med. J.*, **1**, 1097.

Bradshaw, T. E. T. and Jessop, W. J. E. (1953), "The Urinary Excretion of Oestrogens and Pregnanediol at the End of Pregnancy, during Labour and during the Early Puerperium," *J. Endocr.*, **9**, 427.

Bragdon, D. E., Lazo-Wasem, E. A., Zarrow, M. X. and Hisaw, F. L. (1954), "Progesterone-like Activity in the Plasma of Ovoviviparous Snakes," *Proc. Soc. exp. Biol., N.Y.*, **86**, 477.

Brooks, R. V., Clayton, B. E. and Hammant, J. E. (1960), "Some Observations on the Excretion of 17-ketosteroids and 17-ketogenic Steroids by Guinea-pigs," *J. Endocr.*, **20**, 24.

Brooksby, J. B. and Newton, W. H. (1938), "The Effect of the Placenta on the Body Weight of the Mouse," *J. Physiol.*, **92**, 136.

Brown, J. B. (1955), "Urinary Excretion of Oestrogens during the Menstrual Cycle," *Lancet*, **1**, 320.

Brown, J. B. (1957), "The Relationship between Urinary Oestrogens and Oestrogens Produced in the Body," *J. Endocr.*, **16**, 202.

Browne, J. S. L., Henry, J. S. and Venning, E. H. (1937), "The Corpus Luteum in Pregnancy," *J. clin. Invest.*, **16**, 678.

Browne, J. S. L. and Venning, E. M. (1936), "Excretion of Gonadotrophic Substances in the Urine during Pregnancy," *Lancet*, **231**, 1507.

Buchanan, G. D., Enders, A. C. and Talmage, T. V. (1956), "Implantation in Armadillos Ovariectomized during the Period of Delayed Implantation," *J. Endocr.*, **14**, 121.

Bush, I. E. (1957), "The Physiochemical State of Cortisol in Blood." In: *Hormones in Blood* (G. E. W. Wolstenholme and C. E. P. Miller, Eds.). Ciba Foundation Colloquia on Endocrinology, Vol. 11, p. 263. London: Churchill.

Calatroni, C. J., Ruiz, V. and Paola, G. (1945), "La Castración en el Embarazo," *Obst. y Ginec., Latino-Am.*, **3**, 145.

Calisti, V. and Oliva, O. (1955), "Ricerca Istochimica sulla Localizazio ne delle Gonadotropina nella Placenta Degli Equini," *Clin. Vet.*, **78**, 65.

Canivenc, R., Bonnin-Laffargue, M. and Relexans, M. C. (1962), "L'uterus gravide a-t-il une fonction luteotrope chez le Blaireau europeen *Meles meles*?" *C.r.Seanc. Soc. Biol.*, **156**, 1372.

Cassmer, O. (1959), "Hormone Production of the Isolated Human Placenta. Studies of the Role of the Foetus in the Endocrine Functions of the Placenta," *Acta endocr., Copenh.*, **32**, Supp. 45, 5.

Catchpole, H. R., Cole, H. H. and Pearson, F. B. (1938), "Studies on the Rate of Disappearance and Fate of Mare Gonadotropic Hormone following Intravenous Injection." *Amer. J. Physiol.*, **112**, 21.

Cerruti, R. A. and Lyons, W. R. (1960), "Mammogenic Activities of the Mid-gestational Mouse Placenta," *Endocrinology*, **67**, 884.

Christy, N. P. and Jailer, J. W. (1959), "Failure to Demonstrate Hydrocortisone and Aldosterone during Pregnancy in Addison's Disease," *J. Clin. Endocr. Metab.*, **19**, 263.

Clayton, B. E. and Marrian, G. F. (1950), "Urinary Oestrogen Excretion during Labour," *J. Endocr.*, **6**, 332.

Clegg, M. T., Boda, J. M. and Cole, H. H. (1954), "The Endometrial Cups and Allanto-chorionic Pouches in the Mare with Emphasis on the Source of Equine Gonadotropin," *Endocrinology*, **54**, 448.

Clegg, M. T., Cole, H. H., Howard, C. B. and Pigon, H. (1962), "The Influence of Fetal Genotype on Equine Gonadotrophin Secretion," *J. Endocr.*, **25**, 245.

Cohen, H. and Kleinberg, W. (1952), "Placental Content of A.C.T.H.," *Lancet*, **2**, 201.

Cohen, M., Stiefel, M., Reddy, W. J. and Laidlaw, J. C. (1958), "The Secretion and Disposition of Cortisol during Pregnancy," *J. clin. Endocr. Metab.*, **18**, 1076.

Cohen, S. L. and Marrian, G. F. (1935), "The Hydrolysis of the Combined Forms of Oestrone and Oestriol Present in Human Pregnancy Urine," *Biochem. J.*, **29**, 1577.

Cohen, S. L. and Marrian, G. F. (1936), "The Isolation and Identification of a Combined Form of Oestriol in Human Pregnancy Urine," *Biochem. J.*, **30**, 57.

Cohen, S. L., Marrian, G. F. and Watson, M. (1935), "Excretion of Oestrin during Pregnancy," *Lancet*, (i), 674.

Cole, H. H. (1938), "High Gonadotropic Hormone Concentration in Pregnant Ponies," *Soc. exp. Biol. Med., N.Y.*, **38**, 193.

Cole, H. H., Bigelow, M., Finkel, J. and Rupp, C. R. (1967), "Biological Half-life of Endogenous PMS following Hysterectomy and Studies on Losses in Urine and Milk," *Endocrinology*, **81**, 927.

Cole, H. H. and Goss, H. (1939), "Gonadotropic Hormone in the Non-pregnant Mare," *Am. J. Physiol.*, **127**, 702.

Cole, H. H. and Goss, H. (1943), "The Source of Equine Gonadotropin." In: *Essays in Biology*, p. 107. University of California Press.

Cole, H. H., Guilbert, H. R. and Goss, H. (1932), "Further Considerations of the Properties of the Gonad-stimulating Principle of Mare Serum," *Amer. J. Physiol.*, **102**, 227.

Cole, H. H. and Hart, G. H. (1930a), "Sex Hormones in the Blood Serum of Mares: The Sera of Mares from the 222nd day of Pregnancy to the First Heat Period Post-partum," *Amer. J. Physiol.*, **94**, 597.

Cole, H. H. and Hart, G. H. (1930b), "The Potency of Blood Serum of Mares in Progressive Stages of Pregnancy in effecting the Sexual Maturity of the Immature Rat," *Amer. J. Physiol.*, **93**, 57.

Cole, H. H., Hart, G. H., Lyons, W. R. and Catchpole, H. R. (1933), "The Development and Hormonal Content of Fetal Horse Gonads," *Anat. Rec.*, **56**, 275.

Cole, H. H., Howell, C. E. and Hart, G. H. (1931), "The Changes occurring in the Ovary of the Mare during Pregnancy," *Anat. Rec.*, **49**, 199.

Cole, H. H. and Saunders, F. J. (1935), "The Concentration of Gonad Stimulating Hormone in Blood Serum and of Oestrin in the Urine throughout Pregnancy in the Mare," *Endocrinology*, **19**, 199.

Collings, W. D. (1941), "The Effect of Experimentally Induced Pseudo-pregnancy upon the Survival of Adrenalectomized Rats," *Endocrinology*, **28**, 75.

Connell, G. M. (1965), "Pregnant Mare Serum Gonadotrophin Potency: Effect of Single and Multiple Injections," *Nature, Lond.*, **207**, 412.

Contopoulos, A. N. and Simpson, M. E. (1959), "Growth Promoting Activity of Pregnant Rat Plasma after Hypophysectomy and after Thyroidectomy," *Endocrinology*, **64**, 1023.

Corner, G. W. (1947), *The Hormones in Human Reproduction*, p. 204 Princeton, New Jersey: Princeton University Press.

Courrier, R. (1945), *Endocrinologie de la Gestation*. Paris: Masson.

Courrier, R. (1950), "Interactions between Estrogens and Progesterone," *Vitamins and Hormones*, **8**, 179.

Courrier, R. (1952), "Sur Quelques Anomalies de la Gestation Obtenues par Méchanisme Hormonal," *Arch. Anat., Strasbourg*, **34**, 145.

Courrier, R. and Gros, G. (1935), "Contribution à L'endocrinologie de la Grossesse Chez la Chatte," *C.R. Soc. Biol., Paris*, **120**, 5.

Coyle, M. G. (1962), "The Urinary Excretion of Oestrogen in Four Cases of Anencephaly and One Case of Foetal Death from Cirrhosis of the Liver," *J. Endocr.*, **25**, VIII.

Csapo, A. I. (1950), "Actomyosin Formation by Oestrogen Action," *Am. J. Physiol.*, **162**, 406.

Csapo, A. (1956a), "Progesterone 'block'," *Amer. J. Anat.*, **98**, 273.

Csapo, A. (1956b), "The Mechanism of Effect of Ovarian Steroids," *Recent Progr. Hormone Res.*, **12**, 405.

Csapo, A. (1962), "Smoth Muscle as a Contractile Unit," *Physiol. Rev.*, **42**, 7–33.

Csapo, A. (1965), "The Placenta and the Initiation of Labour," *Ned. T. Verlosk.*, **65**, 229.

Csapo, A. and Lloyd-Jacob, M. (1961), "Delayed and Prolonged Labor, Placental Retention and Haemorrhage in Rabbits," *Am. J. Obstet. and Gynec.*, **82**, 1349.

Csapo, A. and Takeda, H. (1965), "Effect of Progesterone on the Electric Activity and Intra-uterine Pressure of Pregnant and Parturient Rabbits," *Am. J. Obstet. Gynec.*, **91**, 221.

Csapo, A. and Wood, C. (1968), "The Endocrine Control of the Initiation of Labor in the Human." In: *Recent Advances in Endocrinology*. (V. H. T. Jones, Ed.). London: J. and A. Churchill.

Daels, F. (1908), "On the Relations between the Ovaries and the Uterus," *Surg. Gynec. Obstet.*, **6**, 153.

D'Amour, M. C. and D'Amour, F. E. (1939), "Effect of Luteinization on the Survival of Adrenalectomized Rats," *Proc. Soc. exp. Biol., N.Y.*, **40**, 417.

Davis, M. E. and Plotz, E. J. (1954), "Effects of Cortisone Acetate on Intact and Adrenalectomized Rats during Pregnancy," *Endocrinology*, **54**, 384.

Davis, M. E. and Plotz, E. J. (1956), "The Excretion of Neutral Steroids in the Urine of Normal non-pregnant Women," *Acta endocr., Copenh.*, **21**, 245.

Davis, M. E. and Plotz, J. (1957), "The Metabolism of Progesterone in Pregnancy," *Recent Progr. Hormone Research*, **13**, 347.

Day, F. T. and Rowlands, I. W. (1940), "The Time and Rate of Appearance of Gonadotrophin in the serum of Pregnant Mares," *J. Endocr.*, **2**, 255.

Day, F. T. and Rowlands, I. W. (1947), "Serum Gonadotrophin in Welsh and Shetland Ponies," *J. Endocr.*, **5**, 1.

Deanesly, R. (1960a), "Implantation and Early Pregnancy in Ovariectomized Guinea-pigs," *J. Reprod. Fertil.*, **1**, 242.

Deanesly, R. (1960b), "Endocrine Activity of the Early Placenta of the Guinea-pig," *J. Endocr.*, **21**, 235.

Deanesly, R. (1963), "Early Embryonic Growth and Progestagen Function in Ovariectomized Guinea-pigs," *J. Reprod. Fert.*, **6**, 143.

Deanesly, R. (1966), "The Endocrinology of Pregnancy and Foetal Life." In: *Marshall's Physiology of Reproduction* (A. S. Parkes, Ed.). Vol. 3, Chap. 32, p. 891. London: Longmans Green.

Deanesly, R. (1967), "Experimental Observations on the Ferret Corpus Luteum of Pregnancy," *J. Reprod. Fert.*, **13**, 183.

Deanesly, R., Fee, A. R. and Parkes, A. S. (1930), "Studies on Ovulation. II. The Effect of Hypophysectomy on the Formation of the Corpus Luteum," *J. Physiol.*, **70**, 38.

Deanesly, R. and Newton, W. H. (1941), "The Influence of the Placenta on the Corpus Luteum of Pregnancy in the Mouse," *J. Endocr.*, **2**, 317.

De Courcy, C., Gray, C. and Lunnon, J. B. (1952), "Adrenal Cortical Hormones in Human Placenta," *Nature, Lond.*, **170**, 494.

De Mahos, C. E. R., Kempson, R. L., Erdos, T. and Csapo, A. I. (1967), "Stretch Induced Myometrial Hypertrophy," *Fertil. and Steril.*, **18**, 545–556.

Dempsey, E. W. and Wislocki, G. B. (1944), "Observations on some Histochemical Reactions in the Human Placenta, with Special Reference to the Significance of the Lipoids, Glycogen and Iron," *Endocrinology*, **35**, 409.

Desclin, L. (1932), "A Propos des Interactions entre L'utérus et le Corps Jaune au Cours de la Grossesse Chez le Cobaye," *C.R. Soc. Biol., Paris*, **109**, 972.

De Snoo (1919). Quoted by Csapo, A. (1965) from Kloosterman's (1963), translation of De Snoo's text.

Dewar, A. D. (1957), "The Endocrine Control of the Extra-uterine Weight Gain of Pregnancy in the Mouse," *J. Endocr.*, **15**, 216.

Diczfalusy, E. (1953), "Chorionic Gonadotrophin and Oestrogens in the Human Placenta," *Acta endocr. Copenh.*, **12**, Suppl. 12, p. 1.

Diczfalusy, E. (1958), "Chorionic Gonadotrophin in Hydatidiform Moles," *Acta endocr., Copenh.*, **28**, 137.

Diczfalusy, E. (1960), "Endocrine Function of the Human Placenta," *1st Int. Congr. Endocrinology, Copenhagen, Symposium* lecture, 129.

Diczfalusy, E. (1965), "*In vivo* Biogenesis and Metabolism of Oestrogens in the Foeto-placental Unit," *Proc. 2nd Int. Congr. Endocrinology, London*, **2**· 732.

Diczfalusy, E. and Borell, U. (1961), "Influence of Oophorectomy on Steroid Excretion in Early Pregnancy," *J. clin. Endocr. Metab.*, **21**, 1119.

Diczfalusy, E. and Lindqvist, P. (1956), "Isolation and Estimation of 'Free' Oestrogens in Human Placentae," *Acta endocrin., Copenh.*, **22**, 203.

Diczfalusy, E., Nilsson, L. and Westman, A. (1958), "Chorionic Gonadotrophin in Hydatidiform Moles," *Acta endocr. Copenh.*, **28**, 137.

Diczfalusy, E. and Troen, P. (1961), "Endocrine Functions of the Human Placenta," *Vitamins and Hormones*, **19**, 229.

Doe, R. P., Zinneman, H. H., Flink, E. B. and Ulstrom, R. A. (1960), "Significance of the Concentration of Non-protein-bound Plasma Cortisol, in Normal Subjects, Cushing's Syndrome, Pregnancy and during Estrogen Therapy," *J. clin. Endocr. Metab.*, **20**, 1484.

Dorfman, R. I. (1948), "Biochemistry of Androgens." In: *The Hormones* (G. Pincus and Thimann, Eds.), Vol. 1, p. 469. New York.

Dorfman, R. I. (1957), "Biochemistry of the Steroid Hormones," *Ann. Rev. Biochem.*, **26**, 523.

Dorfman, R. I. and van Wagenen, G. (1941), "The Sex Hormone Excretion of Adult Female and Pregnant Monkeys," *Surg. Gynec. Obstet.*, **73**, 545.

Eckstein, B. and Villee, C. A. (1966), "Effect of Estradiol on Enzymes of Carbohydrate Metabolism of Rat Uterus," *Endocrinology*, **78**, 409.

Emery, F. E. and Greco, P. A. (1940), "The Comparative Activity of Desoxycorticosterone Acetate and Progesterone in Adrenalectomized Rats," *Endocrinology*, **27**, 473.

Emery, F. E. and Schwabe, E. L. (1936), "The Rôle of the Corpora Lutea in Prolonging the Life of Adrenalectomized Rats," *Endocrinology*, **20**, 550.

Endröczi, E., Telegdy, G. and Martin, J. (1958), "Analysis of Δ⁴-3-ketosteroids in Human Placenta by Paper Chromatography," *Acta physiol. Acad. Sc. Hung.*, **14**, 311.

Engel, L. L. and Cameron, C. B. (1960), "Estrogen in Plasma." In: *Hormones in Human Plasma* (H. N. Antoniades, Ed.), p. 399. London: Churchill.

Erb, R. E., Gomes, W. R., Randel, R. D., Estergreen, V. L. and Frost, O. L. (1967), "Effect of Ovariectomy on Concentration of Progesterone in Blood Plasma and Urinary Oestrogen Excretion Rate in the Pregnant Bovine," *J. Dairy. Sci.*, **51**, 420.

Euw, J. von and Reichstein, I. (1964), quoted by Bennett and Heftmann (1965).

Evans, H. M., Kohls, C. L. and Wonder, D. H. (1937), "Gonadotrophic Hormone in the Blood and Urine of Early Pregnancy," *J. Amer. med. Ass.*, **108**, 287.

Evans, H. M. and Simpson, M. E. (1929), "The Effect of Pregnancy on the Anterior Hypophysis of the Rat and Cow as Judged by the Capacity of Implants to Produce Precocious Maturity," *Amer. J. Physiol.*, **89**, 379.

Fellner, O. O. (1913), "Experimentelle Untersuchungen über die Wirkung von Gewebsextrakten aus der Plazenta und den weiblichen Sexualorganen auf das Genitale," *Arch. Gynaek.*, **5**, 234.

Felton, L. C., Frieden, F. H. and Bryant, H. H. (1953), "The Effect of Ovarian Extracts upon Activity of the Guinea-pig Uterus *in situ*," *J. Pharmacol.*, **107**, 160.

Firor, W. M. (1933), "Hypophysectomy in Pregnant Rabbits," *Amer. J. Physiol.*, **104**, 204.

Firor, W. M. and Grollman, A. (1933), "Studies on the Adrenals: I. Adrenalectomy in Mammals with Particular Reference to the White Rat (*Mus norvegicus*)," *Amer. J. Physiol.*, **103**, 686.

Fitko, R. (1965), Quoted by Cole, H. H. (1969). In: *Reproduction in Domestic Mammals* (H. H. Cole and P. T. Cupps, Eds.). Academic Press.

Forbes, T. R. and Wagenen, G. van (1959), "Progestin in the amniotic Fluid of Monkeys," *Endocrinology*, **65**, 528.

Fotherby, K., James, F., Kamyab, S., Klopper, A. I. and Wilson, G. R. (1965), "Excretion of 6-oxygenated Metabolites of Progesterone and 5β-pregnane, 3α, 17α, 20α-triol during Pregnancy," *J. Endocr.*, **33**, 133.

Frandsen, V. A. (1963), *The Excretion of Oestriol in Normal Human Pregnancy*. Copenhagen: Munksgaard.

Frandsen, V. A. and Stakemann, G. (1962), "The Site of Production of Oestrogenic Hormones in Human Pregnancy," *Acta Endocr., Copenh.*, **38**, 383.

Fränkel, L. and Cohn, F. (1901), "Experimentelle Untersuchungen über den Einfluss des Corpus Luteum und die Insertion des Eies," *Anat. Anz.*, **20**, 294.

Gardner, W. V. and Allen, E. (1942), "Effects of Hypophysectomy at Mid-pregnancy in the Mouse," *Anat. Rec.*, **83**, 75.

Gemzell, C. A. (1952), "Increase in the Formation and Secretion of ACTH in Rats following Administration of Oestradiolbenzoate," *Acta endocr., Copenh.*, **11**, 221.

Gemzell, C. A. (1953), "Blood Levels of 17-hydroxycorticosteroids in Normal Pregnancy," *J. clin. Endocr. Metab.*, **13**, 898.

Gemzell, C. A. (1954), "Variations in Plasma Levels of 17-hydroxy-corticosteroids in Mother and Infant following Parturition," *Acta endocr., Copenh.*, **17**, 100.

Glasser, J. W. H. (1952), "Early Removal of the Corpus Luteum of Pregnancy," *Bull. Margaret Hague Maternity Hosp.*, **5**, 112.

Glud, P., Pedersen-Bjergaard, K. and Portman, K. (1933), "Uber Graviditätsreaktion bei der Stute," *Endokrinolgie*, **13**, 21.

Gold, J. J. (1957), "Blood Corticoids: Their Measurement and Significance. A Review," *J. clin. Endocr. Metab.*, **17**, 296.

Gorski, J., Domingues, O. V., Samuels, L. T. and Erb, R. E. (1958), "Progestins of the Bovine Ovary," *Endocrinology*, **62**, 234.

Gorski, J., Erb, R. E., Dickson, W. M. and Butler, H. C. (1958), "Sources of Progestins in the Pregnant Cow," *J. Dairy Sci.*, **41**, 1380–1386.

Greene, J. W. Jr. and Touchstone, J. C. (1963), "Urinary Estriol as an Index of Placental Function," *Amer. J. Obst. Gynec.*, **85**, 1.

Greer, M. A. (1949), "Trophic Hormones of the Placenta: Failure to Demonstrate Thyrotrophin or Adreno-corticotrophin Production in the Hypophysectomized Pregnant Rat," *Endocrinology*, **45**, 178.

Gros, G. (1936), "Contribution à L'endocrinologie Sexuelle. Le Cycle Génitale de la Chatte," *Thèse*, Université d'Alger, **140**, 21.

Grumbach, M. M. and Kaplan, S. L. (1964), "On the Placental Origin and Purification of Chorionic 'Growth Hormone-prolactin' and its Immunoassay in Pregnancy," *Trans. N.Y. Acad. Sci.*, **27**, 167.

Grumbach, M. M., Kaplan, S. L., Sciarra, J. J. and Burr, I. M. (1968), "Chorionic growth Hormone-prolactin (CGP): Secretion, Disposition, Biologic Activity in Man, and Postulated Function as the 'Growth-hormone' of the Second Half of Pregnancy," *Ann. N.Y. Acad. Sci.*, **148**, 501.

Guldberg, E. (1936), "Die Produktionsstätten der Sexualhormone im normalen graviden weiblechen Organismus im Lichte der Hormonanalyse des ovariopriven graviden Zustandes," *Acta obst. gynec., Scand.*, **15**, 345.

Gupta, S. K. and Pope, G. S. (1968), "Variation in the Level of Progesterone in the Systemic Plama of the Cow," *J. Endocr.*, **40**, xii.

Gurchot, C., Krebs, E. T. Jr. and Krebs, E. T. (1947), "Growth of Human Trophoblast in the Eye of the Rabbit. Its Relationship to the Origin of Cancer," *Surg. Gynec. Obstet.*, **84**, 301.

Gurpide, E., Schwers, J., Welch, M. T., van de Wiele, R. L. and Lieberman, S. (1966), "Fetal and Maternal Metabolism of Estradiol during Pregnancy," *J. clin. Endocr. Metab.*, **26**, 1355.

Guterman, H. S. and Tulsky, A. S. (1949), "Observations on the use of Progesterone in Threatened Abortion," *Amer. J. Obstet. and Gynec.*, **58**, 495.

Halban, J. (1905), "Die innere Sekretion von Ovarium und Plazenta und ihre Bedeutung für die Funktion der Milchdrüse," *Arch. Gynäk. Jahrg.*, **75**, 353.

Hall, K. (1956), "An Evaluation of the Roles of Oestrogen, Progesterone, and Relaxin in producing Relaxation of the Symphysis Pubis of the Ovariectomized Mouse, using the Technique of Metachromatic Staining with Toluidine Blue," *J. Endocr.*, **13**, 384.

Hall, K. (1957), "The Effect of Relaxin Extracts, Progesterone, and Oestriol on Maintenance of Pregnancy, Parturition and Rearing of Young after Ovariectomy in Mice," *J. Endocrin.*, **15**, 108.

Hall, K. (1960), "Relaxin," *J. Reprod. Fertil.*, **1**, 368.

Hall, K. (1965), "Histochemical Investigation of the Effects of Oestrogen, Progesterone and Relaxin on Glycogen, Amylophosphorylase, Transglycosylase and Uridine Diphosphate Glucose-glucogen Transferase in Uteri of Mice," *J. Endocr.*, **32**, 245.

Hall, K. and Newton, W. H. (1946), "The Action of Relaxin in the Mouse," *Lancet*, **1**, 54.

Hall, K. and Newton, W. H. (1947), "The Effect of Oestrone and Relaxin on the X-ray Appearance of the Pelvis of the Mouse," *J. Physiol.*, **106**, 18.

Hamburger, C. (1944), "Contribution to the Hormonal Diagnosis of Hydatidiform Mole and Chorionepithelioma Based on 76 Cases with Hormonal Analyses," *Acta obstet. gynec., Scand.*, **24**, 45.

Hamilton, T. H. (1963), "Isotopic Studies on Estrogen-induced Accelerations of Ribonucleic Acid and Protein Synthesis," *Proc. Nat. Acad. Sci., U.S.A.*, **49**, 373.

Hamilton, T. H. (1964), "Sequences of RNA and Protein Synthesis during Early Estrogen Action," *Proc. Nat. Acad. Sci., U.S.A.*, **51**, 83.

Hamlett, G. W. D. (1937), "Positive Friedman tests in the Pregnant Rhesus Monkey, *Macaca mulatta*," *Amer. J. Physiol.*, **118**, 664.

Hammond, C. B., Marshall, J. R., Ross, G. I. and Odell, W. D. U. (1967), "Plasma Human Chorionic Gonadotropin (HCG) and Urinary Total Gonadotropin Levels in very Early Pregnancy," *Obstet. Gynecol.*, **29**, 430.

Hammond, J. (1917), "On the Causes Responsible for the Developmental Progress of the Mammary Glands in the Rabbit during the Latter Part of Pregnancy," *Proc. Roy. Soc.*, B, **89**, 534.

Hammond, J. Jr. (1956), "The Rabbit Corpus Luteum: Oestrogen Prolongation and the Accompanying Changes in the Genitalia," *Acta endocr., Copenh.*, **21**, 307.

Hammond, J. Jr. and Robson, J. M. (1951), "Local Maintenance of the Rabbit Corpus Luteum with Oestrogen," *Endocrinology*, **49**, 384.

Hamolsky, M. and Sparrow, R. C. (1945), "Influence of Relaxin in Mammary Development in Sexually Immature Female Rats," *Proc. Soc. exp. Biol., N.Y.*, **60**, 8.

Harbert, G. M. Jr., McGaughey, H. S. Jr., Scoggin, W. A. and Thorton, W. M. Jr. (1964), "Concentration of Progesterone in Newborn and Maternal Circulation at Delivery," *Obstet. Gynec.*, **23**, 413.

Harkness, R. A. and Love, D. N. (1966), "Studies on the Estimation of Urinary Pregnanetriol during Pregnancy and Childhood," *Acta endocr., Copenh.*, **51**, 526.

Hart, G. H. and Cole, H. H. (1934), "The Source of Oestrin in the Pregnant Mare," *Amer. J. Physiol.*, **109**, 320.

Hartman, C. G. (1932), "Studies in the Reproduction of the Monkey (*Macacus (Pithecus) rhesus*) with Special Reference to Menstruation," *Contr. Embryol. Carneg. Instn.*, **23**, 1.

Hartman, C. G. (1941), "Non-effect of Ovariectomy on the 25th day of Pregnancy in the Rhesus Monkey," *Proc. Soc. exp. Biol., N.Y.*, **48**, 221.

Hartman, C. G. and Corner, G. W. (1947), "Removal of the Corpus Luteum and of the Ovaries of the Rhesus Monkey during Pregnancy: Observations and Cautions," *Anat. Rec.*, **98**, 539.

Haskins, A. L. and Sherman, A. I. (1952), "The Quantitative Assay of Serum Chorionic Gonadotropin in Pregnancy, using the Modified Male Frog Technique," *J. clin. Endocr. Metab.*, **12**, 385.

Haterius, H. O. (1936), "Reduction of Litter Size and Maintenance of Pregnancy in the Oophorectomized Rat: Evidence Concerning the Endocrine Role of the Placenta," *Amer. J. Physiol.*, **114**, 399.

Heap, R. B. and Deanesly, R. (1966), "Progesterone in Systemic Blood of Intact and Ovariectomized Pregnant Guinea-pigs," *J. Endocr.*, **34**, 417.

Heckel, G. and Allen, W. M. (1939), "Maintenance of the Corpus Luteum and Inhibition of Parturition in the Rabbit by Injection of Oestrogenic Hormone," *Endocrinology*, **24**, 137.

Heftmann, E. and Mosettig, E. (1960), *Biochemistry of the Steroids*. New York: Reinhold.

Hellman, L. M., Flexner, L. B., Wilde, W. S., Vosburgh, G. J. and Proctor, N. K. (1948), "The Permeability of the Human Placenta to Water and the Supply of Water to the Human Foetus as Determined with Deuterium Oxide," *Amer. J. Obst. and Gynec.*, **56**, 861.

Herrick, E. H. (1928), "Duration of Pregnancy in Guinea-pigs after removal and also after Transplantation of Ovaries," *Anat. Rec.*, **39**, 193.

Herrmann, W. and Silverman, L. (1957), "Excretion of Pregnane-3α, 17α, 20α-triol in Pregnancy," *J. clinl Endocr. Metab.*, **17**, 1482.

Heusghem, C. (1956), *Contributions à l'Étude Analytique et Biochimique des Oestrogènes Naturels*. Liège: Thone.

Heusghem, C. (1957), *Contributions à l'Étude Analytique et Biochimique des Oestrogènes Naturels*. Paris: Masson.

Hinglais, H. and Hinglais, M. (1949), "Étude hormonale de la môle hydatiforme. Prolan, oestrogènes, pregnanediol dans les cas de môle active en évolution," *C.R. Soc. Biol.*, **143**, 61.

Hinglais, H. and Hinglais, M. (1953), "Action prénatrice des oestrogènes sur le trophoblastome. Nouvelles données pour le traitement médical éventuel du chorio-épithéliome post-molaire à son extrême début," *C.R. Soc. Biol., Paris*, **147**, 555.

Hirose, T. (1919), "Experimentelle histologische Studie zur Genese Corpus Luteum," *Mitt. a. d. med. Fak. Univ., Tokyo*, **23**, 63.

Hisaw, F. L. (1944), "The Placental Gonadotropin and Luteal Function in Monkeys (*Macacus mulatta*)," *Yale J. Biol. Med.*, **17**, 119.

Hisaw, F. L. (1959), "Endocrine Adaptations of the Mammalian Estrous Cycle and Gestation." In: *Comparative Endocrinology* (A. Gornman, Ed.), p. 533. New York: Academic Press.

Hisaw, F. L. and Astwood, E. B. (1942), "The Physiology of Reproduction," *Ann. Rev. Physiol.*, **4**, 542.

Hisaw, F. L. and Zarrow, M. X. (1950), "The Physiology of Relaxin," *Vitamins and Hormones*, **8**, 151.

Hobkirk, R. and Nilsen, M. (1966), "Specific Activities of Seven Urinary Metabolites of Estradiol 17β-6,7-³H in Pregnant Women," *J. clin. Endocr. Metab.*, **26**, 625.

Hobson, B. M. (1955), "The Excretion of Chorionic Gonadotrophin in Normal Pregnancy and in Women with Hydatidiform Mole," *J. Obstet. Gynaec., Brit. Emp.*, **62**, 354.

Houssay, B. A. (1945), "Acción de la insuficiencia suprarenal durante la preñez sobre la madre y el hijo," *Rev. Soc. argent. Biol.*, **21**, 316.

Huggett, A. St. G. and Pritchard, J. J. (1945), "Placental Growth after Foetal Death in the Rat," *J. Physiol.*, **104**, 4 P.

Ingle, D. J. and Fisher, G. T. (1938), "Effects of Adrenalectomy during Gestation on the Size of the Adrenal Glands of New-born Rats," *Proc. Soc. exp. Biol., N.Y.*, **39**, 149.

Inskeep, E. K., Oloufa, M. M., Howland, B. E., Pope, A. L. and Cassida, L. F. (1962), "Effect of Experimental Uterine Distension on Oestrual Cycle Lengths in Ewes," *J. Anim. Sci.*, **21**, 331.

Jailer, J. W. (1951), In *Proceedings of the Second Clinical ACTH Conference* (J. E. Mote, Ed.), Vol. 1, p. 77. Philadelphia.

Jailer, J. W., Gold, J. J., van de Wiele, R. and Lieberman, S. (1955), "17α-Hydroxyprogesterone and Desoxyhydrocortisone: Their Metabolism and possible Role in Congenital Adrenal Hyperplasia," *J. clin. Invest.*, **34**, 1639.

Jailer, J. W. and Knowlton, A. I. (1950), "Simulated Adrenocortical Activity during Pregnancy in an Adisonian Patient," *J. clin. Invest.*, **29**, 1430.

Jailer, J. W., Longson, D. and Christy, N. P. (1957), "Cushing's Syndrome. II. Adrenal Weight-stimulating Activity in the Plasma of Patients with Cushing's Syndrome," *J. Clin. Invest.*, **36**, 1608.

Jervill, K. F., Diñiz, C. R. and Mueller, G. C. (1958), "Early Effects of Estradiol on Nucleic Acid Metabolism in the Rat Uterus," *J. biol. Chem.*, **231**, 945.

Johnson, R. H. and Haines, W. J. (1952), "Extraction of Adrenal Cortex Hormone Activity from Placental Tissue," *Science*, **116**, 456.

Jones, G. E. S., Delfs, É. and Stran, H. M. (1944), "Chorionic Gonadotropin and Pregnanediol Values in Normal Pregnancy," *Bull Johns Hopkins Hosp.*, **75**, 359.

Jones, H. L. and Weil, P. G. (1938), "The Corpus Luteum Hormone in Early Pregnancy. Report on a Case in which there was Early Removal of the Corpus Luteum," *J.A.M.A.*, **111**, 519.

Jones, J. M., Lloyd, C. W. and Wyatt, T. C. (1953), "A Study of the Interrelationship of Maternal and Fetal Adrenal Glands of Rats," *Endocrinology*, **53**, 152.

Jones, K. M., Lloyd-Jones, R., Riondel, A., Tait, J. F., Tait, S. A. S., Bulbrook, R. D. and Greenwood, F. C. (1959), "Aldosterone Secretion and Metabolism in Normal Men and Women and in Pregnancy," *Acta Endocr., Copenh.*, **30**, 321.

Josimovich, J. B. and Atwood, B. L. (1964), "Human Placenta Lactogen (HPL), a Trophoblastic Hormone Synergizing with a Chorionic Gonadotropin and Potentiating the Anabolic Effects of Pituitary Growth Hormone," *Amer. J. Obstet. Gynec.*, **88**, 867.

Josimovich, J. B. and MacLaren, J. A. (1962), "Presence in the Human Placenta and Term Serum of a Highly Lactogenic Substance Immunologically Related to Pituitary Growth Hormone," *Endocrinology*, **71**, 209.

Jost, A. (1961), "The Role of Fetal Hormones in Development," *The Harvey Lectures*, **55**, 201.

Jost, A., Jacquot, R. and Cohen, A. (1955), "Sur les interrelations entre les hormones corticosurrénaliennes maternelles et la surrénale du foetus de rat," *C.R. Soc. Biol., Paris*, **149**, 1319.

Kao, C. Y. (1967), "Ionic Basis of Electrical Activity in Uterine Smooth Muscle." Ch. II in *Cellular Biology of the Uterus*, (R. M. Wynn, Ed.). Amsterdam: North-Holland.

Kaplan, N. M. (1961), "Successful Pregnancy following Hypophysectomy during the Twelfth Week of Gestation," *J. clin. Endocr. Metab.*, **21**, 1139.

Kaplan, S. L. and Grumbach, M. M. (1964), "Studies of a Human and Simian Placental Hormone with Growth Hormone-like and Prolactin-like Activities," *J. clin. Endocr. Metab.*, **24**, 80.

Kaplan, S. L. and Grumbach, M. M. (1965a), "Serum Chorionic 'Growth Hormone Prolactin' and Serum Pituitary Growth Hormone in Mother and Fetus at Term," *J. clin. Endocr. Metab.*, **25**, 1370.

Kaplan, S. L. and Grumbach, M. M. (1965b), "Immunoassay for Human Chorionic Growth-Hormone-Prolactin in Serum and Urine," *Science*, **147**, 751.

Kaufman, C. and Zander, J. (1956), "Progesteron in menschlichen Blut und Gewebe. II. Progesteron in Fettgewebe," *Klin. Wschr.*, **34**, 7.

Kawahara, H. (1958), "Plasma Levels of 17-hydroxycorticosteroids in Umbilical Cord Blood; with Special Reference to Variations of the Level between A. umbilicalis and V. umbilicalis," *J. clin. Endocr. Metab.*, **18**, 325.

Kellas, L. M., Van Lennep, E. W. and Amoroso, E. C. (1958), "Ovaries of some Foetal and Prepubertal Giraffes (*Giraffa camelopardalis, Linnaeus*)," *Nature, Lond.*, **181**, 487.

Keyes, P. L. and Nalbandov, A. V. (1967), "Maintenance and Function of Corpora Lutea in Rabbits depend on Estrogen," *Endocrinology*, **80**, 938–946.

Kido, I. (1937), "Die Menschliche Plazenta als Produktionsstätte des sogenannten Hypophysenvorderlappenhormons," *Zbl. Gynäk.*, **61**, 1551.

Kitay, J. I. (1963), "Effects of Estradiol on Pituitary-adrenal Function in Male and Female Rats," *Endocrinology*, **72**, 947.

Klein, M. (1929), "La substance du placenta qui est active sur l'ovaire, est-elle une hormone pre-hypophysaire?" *C. r. Soc. Biol., Paris*, **102**, 1070.

Klein, M. (1933), "Sur l'ablation des embryons chez la lapine gravide et sur les facteurs qui déterminent le maintien du corps jaune pendant la deuxième partie de la grossesse," *C.R. Soc. Biol.*, **113**, 441.

Klein, M. (1935), "Recherches sur le rôle du placenta dans l'arrêt des manifestations du cycle ovarien au cours de la grossesse," *Arch. anat. micr.*, **31**, 397.

Klein, M. (1938a), "Sur les facteurs qui maintiennent l'activité functionelle du corps jaune gravidique," *Hormones sexuelles, Coll. Singer Polignac*, p. 86, Paris.

Klein, M. (1938b), "Relation between the Uterus and the Ovaries in the Pregnant Hamster," *Proc. Roy. Soc.*, B, **125**, 148.

Klein, M. and Mayer, G. (1942), "Effèts d'injections d'oestrogènes sur l'ovaire gestatif de la rate. Maintien de l'état gestatif de l'ovaire après ablation de l'utérus gravide par des injections d'oestrogènes chez la rate," *Arch. Phys. biol.*, **16**, 125.

Klein, M. and Mayer, G. (1950), "Sur les oestrogènes et sur la prolactine comme facteurs de maintien des crops jaunes ovariens," *J. Physiol. Path. gén.*, **42**, 620.

Kloosterman, G. J. (1963), "The Placenta, the Duration of Pregnancy and Perinatal Mortality. Margaret Orford Lecturer for 1963," *Trans. College Phys. and Surg. Gynec. S. Africa*, **1**, 181.

Klopper, A. and Billewicz, W. (1963), "Urinary Excretion of Oestriol and Pregnanediol during Normal Pregnancy," *J. Obstet. and Gynec. Brit. Cwlth.*, **70**, 1024.

Klopper, A. and Dennis, K. (1962), "Effect of Oestrogens on Myometrial Contractions," *Brit. Med. J.*, **ii**, 1157.

Klotz, H. P. (1955), "Forte Hypersécrétoin d'androgènes avec Virilisme pilaire au cours d'une grossesse," *Ann. Endocr., Paris*, **16**, 342.

Klyne, A. and Wright, A. A. (1959), "Steroids and other Lipids of Pregnant Cow's Urine," *J. Endocr.*, **18**, 32.

Knaus, H. (1926), "Action of Pituitary Extract upon the Pregnant Uterus of the Rabbit," *J. Physiol.*, **61**, 383.

Knaus, H. (1930), "Zur Physiologie des Corpus luteum," *Arch. Gynaek.*, **141**, 374.

Knaus, H. (1934), *Periodic Fertility and Sterility in Women.* Vienna: Mandrich.

Knowlton, A. L., Mudge, G. H. and Jailer, J. W. (1949), "Pregnancy in Addison's Disease," *J. clin. Endocr. Metab.*, **9**, 514.

Koch, H., Kessel, H. van., Stolte, L. and Leusden, H. van (1966), "Thyroid Function in Molar Pregnancy," *J. clin. Endocr. Metab.*, **26**, 1128.

Kreines, K., Perin, E. and Salzer, R. (1964), "Pregnancy in Cushing's Syndrome," *J. clin. Endocr. Metab.*, **24**, 75.

Krieger, D. T., Gabrilove, J. L. and Soffer, L. J. (1960), "Adrenal Function in a Pregnant Bilaterally Adrenalectomized Woman," *J. Clin. Endocr.*, **20**, 1493.

Kroc, R. L., Steinetz, B. G. and Beach, V. L. (1958), "The Effects of Oestrogens, Progestagens and Relaxin in Pregnant and Non-pregnant Laboratory Rodents," *Ann. N.Y. Acad. Sci.*, **75**, 942.

Kulseng-Hanssen, K. (1951), "Maintenance of Early Pregnancy Despite Extirpation of the Corpora Lutea," *Acta obst. et gynec. Scand.*, **30**, 420.

Kuriyama, A. and Csapo, A. I. (1961), "Placenta and Myometrial Block," *Am. J. Obstet. and Gynec.*, **82**, 592–599.

Laidlaw, J. C., Cohen, M. and Gornall, A. G. (1958), "Studies on the Origin of Aldosterone during Human Pregnancy," *J. clin. Endocr. Metab.*, **18**, 222.

Laidlaw, J. C., Ruse, J. and Gornall, A. G. (1962), "The Influence of Estrogen and Progesterone on Aldosterone Excretion," *J. clin. Endocr. Metab.*, **22**, 161.

Lanman, A. J. and Dinerstein, J. (1959), "The Adrenotropic Action of Human Pregnancy Plasma," *Endocrinology*, **64**, 494.

Layne, D. S., Meyer, C. J., Vaishwaner, P. S. and Pincus, G. (1962), "The Secretion and Metabolism of Cortisol and Aldosterone in Normal and in Steroid Treated Women," *J. clin. Endocr. Metab.*, **22**, 107.

Le Boeuf, M., Cave, A. and Goutarel, R. (1964), quoted by Bennett and Heftmann (1965).

Lenters, G. J. W. N. (1958), *Oestrioluitscheiding in de urine en de anatomische Toestand van de Placenta.* Groningen: Thesis, Wolters.

Leonard, S. L. (1958), "Hormonal Effects on Phosphorylase Activity in the Rat Uterus," *Endocrinology*, **63**, 853.

Leusden, H. A. van and Villee, C. A. (1966), "Formation of Estogens by Hydatidiform Moles *in vitro*," *J. clin. Endocr. Metab.*, **26**, 842.

Levitz, M. (1966), "Conjugation and Transfer of Fetal-placental Steroid Hormones," *J. clin. Endocr. Metab.*, **26**, 773.

Levitz, M., Condon, G. P., Money, W. L. and Dancis, J. (1960), "The Relative Transfer of Estrogens and their Sulfates across the Guinea-pig Placenta: Sulfurylation of Estrogens by the Placenta," *J. biol. Chem.*, **23.**, 973.

Liggins, G. C., Kennedy, P. C. and Holm, L. W. (1967), "Failure of Initiation of Partuirition after Electrocoagulation of the Pituitary of the Foetal Lamb," *Am. J. Obstet. and Gynec.*, **98**, 1080–1086.

Little, B. and Rossi, E. (1957), "Production of Porter-Silber Reactive Material by Human Placenta Incubated *in vitro*," *Endocrinology*, **61**, 109.

Little, B., Smith, D. W., Kessiman, A. G., Selenkow, H. A., Van't Hoff, W., Eglin, J. M. and Moore, F. D. (1958a), "Hypophysectomy during Pregnancy in a Patient with Cancer of the Breast," *J. clin. Endocr. Metab.*, **18**, 425.

Little, B., Vance, V. K. and Rossi, E. (1958b), "Plasma 17-hydroxy-corticosteroid Levels in Patients with Abnormal Glucose Tolerance during Pregnancy," *J. clin. Endocr. Metab.*, **18**, 49.

Little, R. and Shaw, A. (1961), "The Conversion of Progesterone to 17α-hydroxyprogesterone by Human Placenta *in vitro*," *Acta endocr., Copenh.*, **36**, 455.

Llauro, J. L., Runnebaum, B. R. and Zander, J. (1968), "Progesterone in Human Blood, befoer, during and after Labour," *Am. J. Obstet. and Gynec.*, **101**, 867–873.

Loeb, L. (1923), "Mechanism of the Sexual Cycle with Special Reference to the Corpus Luteum," *Amer. J. Anat.*, **32**, 305.

Loeb, L. and Hesselberg, C. (1917), "The Cyclic Changes in the Mammary Gland under Normal and Pathologic Conditions," *J. exp. Med.*, **25**, 295.

Loraine, J. A. (1949), "The Excretion of Chorionic Gonadotrophin by Pregnant Diabetics," *Brit. med. J.*, **2**, 1496.

Loraine, J. A. (1950a), "The Renal Clearance of Chorionic Gonado-trophin in Normal and Pathological Pregnancies," *Quart. J. exp. Physiol.*, **36**, 11.

Loraine, J. A. (1950b), "The Estimation of Chorionic Gonado-trophin in the Urine of Pregnant Women," *J. Endocr.*, **6**, 319.

Loraine, J. A. and Matthew, G. D. (1953), "The Placental Concentration of Chorionic Gonadotrophin in Normal and Abnormal Pregnancy," *J. Obstet. Gynaec. Brit. Empire*, **60**, 640.

Loraine, J. A. and Matthew, G. D. (1954), "Essais hormonaux dans la grossesse diabétique," *Le Diabète*, **2**, 43.

Lurie, A. O., Reid, D. and Villee, C. (1966), "The Role of the Fetus and Placenta in Maintenance of Plasma Progesterone," *Amer. J. Obstet. Gynec.*, **96**, 670.

Lyons, W. R. (1951), "Lobule-alveolar Mammary Growth in the Rat." *Colloq. int. Cent. nat. Rech. sci., Méchanisme physiologique de la séecrétion lactée*, p. 29, Strassbourg, 1950.

Lyons, R. A., Simpson, M. E. and Evans, H. M. (1953), "Qualitative changes in Urinary Gonadotropins in Human Pregnancy during the Period of Rapid Increase in Hormone Titer," *Endocrinology*, **53**, 674.

McDonald, E. E., McNutt, S. H. and Nichols, R. E. (1953), "On the Essentiality of the Bovine Corpus Luteum of Pregnancy," *Am. J. Vet. Res.*, **14**, 539–541.

MacDonald, P. C. and Siiteri, P. K. (1964), "Study of Oestrogen Production in Women with Hydatidiform Mole," *J. clin. Endocr. Metab.*, **24**, 685.

Macedo-Costa, L. and Csapo, A. I. (1959), "Asymmetrical Delivery in Rabbits," *Nature, Lond.*, **184**, 144.

McPhail, M. K. (1935), "Hypophysectomy in the Cat," *Proc. Roy. Soc., B.*, **117**, 45.

Magendantz, H. G. and Ryan, K. J. (1964), "Isolation of an Estriol Precursor, 16-hydroxydehydroepiandrosterone, from Human Umbilical Sera," *J. clin. Endorc. Metab.*, **24**, 1155.

Magnus, V. (1901), "Ovariets betydning for svangerskabet med saerligt hensyn til corpora lutea," *Norsk. Mag. Laegevidensk.*, **62**, 1128.

Manner, T. D., Saffan, B. D., Wiggins, R. A., Thompson, J. D. and Preedy, J. R. K. (1963), "Interrelationship of Estrogen Concentrations in the Maternal Circulation, Fetal Circulation and Maternal Urine in Late Pregnancy," *J. clin. Endocr. Metab.*, **23**, 445.

Marrian, G. F. (1938), "The Chemistry of the Oestrogenic Hormones," *Ergeb. Vitam- u.Hormonforsch.*, **1**, 419.

Martin, J. D. and Mills, I. H. (1956), "Aldosterone Excretion in Normal and Toxaemic Pregnancies," *Brit. med. J.*, **2**, 571.

Martin, J. D. and Mills, I. H. (1958).

Mathies, D. L. (1967), "Studies of the Luteotropic and Mammo-tropic Factor found in Trophoblast and Maternal Peripheral Blood of the Rat at Mid-pregnancy," *Anat. Rec.*, **157**, 55.

Mayer, G. and Canivenc, R. (1950), "Autogreffes du placenta chez la ratte," *C.R. Soc. Biol., Paris*, **144**, 410.

Mayer, G. and Klein, M. (1955), "Les hormones du placenta." In: *L'Équilibre Hormonal de la Gestation; les Androgènes dans l'Organisme Féminin; la cortisone dans l'Équilibre Hormonal. Rapports de la 111e réunion des endocrinologistes de langue français. Paris.*

Michie, E. A. (1966), "Oestrogen Levels in Urine and Amniotic Fluid in Pregnancy with Live Anancephalic Foetus and the Effect of Intra-amniotic Injection of Sodium Dehydroepiandrosterone Sulphate on these Levels," *Acta Endocr. Copenh.*, **51**, 535.

Midgley, A. R., Jr. and Pierce, G. B., Jr. (1962), "Immunohisto-chemical Localization of Human Chorionic Gonadotropin," *J. exp. Med.*, **11.**, 289.

Midgley, A. R., Jr., Pierce, G. B., Jr. and Weigle, W. O. (1961), "Immunobiological Identification of Human Chorionic Gonadotropin," *Proc. Soc. exp. Biol. Med.*, **108**, 85.

Migeon, C. J., Bertrand, J. and Wall, P. E. (1967a), "Physiological Disposition of 4-C^{14} Cortisol during Late Pregnancy," *J. clin. Invest.*, **36**, 1350.

Migeon, C. J., Bertrand, J., Wall, P. E., Stempfel, R. S. and Prystowsky, H. (1957b), "Metabolism and Placental Transmission of Cortisol during Pregnancy near Term," *Ciba. Colloq. Endocrinol.*, **11**, 338.

Migeon, C. J., Prystowsky, H., Grumbach, M. M. and Byron, M. C. (1956), "Placental Passage of 17-hydrocorticosteroids; Comparison of the Levels in Maternal and Fetal Plasma and Effect of ACTH and Hydrocortisone Administration," *J. clin. Invest.*, **35**, 488.

Mikhail, G., Wiqvist, N. and Diczfalusy, E. (1963), "Oestriol Metabolism in the Human Foeto-placental Unit," *Acta endocr., Copenh.*, **43**, 213.

Miller, J. W., Kisley, A. and Murray, W. J. (1951), "The Effects of Relaxin-containing Ovarian Extracts on Various Types of Smooth Muscle," *J. Pharmacol.*, **120**, 426.

Mirand, E. A. and Gordon, A. S. (1966), "Mechanism of Estrogen Action in Erythropoiesis," *Endocrinology*, **78**, 325.

Moor, R. M. and Rowson, L. E. A. (1966), "The Corpus Luteum of the Sheep: Effect of Removal of Embryos on Luteal Function," *J. Endocrin.*, **34**, 497.

Moses, A. M., Lobotsky, J. and Lloyd, C. W. (1959), "The Occurrence of Pre-eclampsia in a Bilaterally Adrenalectomized Woman," *J. clin. Endocr. Metab.*, **19**, 987.

Murata, M. and Adachi, K. (1927), "Uber die künstliche Erzeugung des Corpus Luteum durch Injection der Plazentarsubstanz aus frühen Schwangerschaftsmonaten," *Z. Geburtsh. Gynäk.*, **92**, 45.

Nachtigall, L., Bassett, M., Hogsander, U., Slagle, S. and Levitz, M. (1966), "A Rapid Method for the Assay of Plasma Estriol in Pregnancy," *J. clin. Endocr. Metab.*, **26**, 941.

Nalbandov, A. V., Moore, W. W. and Norton, H. W. (1955), "Further Studies on the Neurogenic Control of the Oestrous Cycle by Uterine Distension," *Endocrinology*, **56**, 225.

Nelson, D. H., Eik-Nes, E. and Sanberg, A. A. (1960), "Corticosteroids in Blood." In: *Hormones in Human Plasma* (H. N. Antoniades, Ed.), Chap. XI, p. 333. London: Churchill.

Nelson, W. O. (1934), "Studies on the Physiology of Lactation. III. The Reciprocal Hypophysial-ovarian Relationship as a Factor in the Control of Lactation," *Endocrinology*, **18**, 33.

Newton, W. H. (1935), "Pseudo-parturition in the Mouse and the Relation of the Placenta to the Post-partum Oestrus," *J. Physiol.*, **84**, 196.

Newton, W. H. (1938), "Hormones and the Placenta," *Physiol. Rev.*, **18**, 419.

Newton, W. H. (1939), "Some Problems of Endocrine Function in Pregnancy." In: Allen's *Sex and Internal Secretion*, 2nd Edition, Chap. X, p. 720. London: Baillière, Tindall and Cox.

Newton, W. H. (1949), *Recent Advances in Physiology*. London: Churchill.

Newton, W. H. and Beck, N. (1939), "Placental Activity in the Mouse in the Absence of the Pituitary Gland," *J. Endocr.*, **1**, 65.

Newton, W. H. and Lits, F. J. (1938), "Criteria of Placental Endocrine Activity in the Mouse," *Anat. Rec.*, **72**, 333.

Newton, W. H. and Richardson, K. C. (1940), "The Secretion of Milk in Hypophysectomized Pregnant Mice," *J. Endocr.*, **2**, 322.

Nichols, J., Lescure, O. L. and Migeon, C. J. (1958), "Levels of 17-hydrocorticosteroids and 17-ketosteroids in Maternal and Cord Plasma in Term Anancephaly," *J. clin. Endocr. Metab.*, **19**, 444.

Noble, R. L. and Plunkett, E. R. (1955), "Biology of the Gonadotrophins," *Brit. Med. Bull.*, **11**, 98.

Oliva, O. (1957), "Sul contenuto in ormone gonadotropo della placenta di Asina," *Boll. Soc. Eustachiana*, **50**, 31.

Oliva, O. and Chicchini, U. (1961), "Comportamento electroforetico di un estratto gonadotropo da placenta di Asina," *Atti. Soc. Ital. Sci. Vet.*, **15**, 305.

Pali, K. and Lajos, L. (1952), "Histochemische Untersuchungen der innersekretorischen Tätigkeit der Hypophyse und der Plazenta," *Gynaecologia*, **133**, 37.

Parkes, A. S. (1930), "On the Synergism between Oestrin and Oxytocin," *J. Physiol.*, **612**, 463–472.

Parkes, A. S. (1954), "The Mammalian Foetus: Physiological Aspects of Development. Endocrine Environment of the Foetus," *Cold Spr. Harb. Symp. quant. Biol.*, **19**, 1.

Parkes, A. S. and Deanesly, R. (1966), "Relation between the Gonads and the Adrenal Glands." In: *Marshall's Physiology of Reproduction* (A. S. Parkes, Ed.), Vol. 3, Chap. 33. London: Longmans.

Parlow, A. F. and Ward, D. N. (1961). In: *Human Pituitary Gonadotropins*. (A. Albert, Ed.), 204. Springfield, Illinois: Thomas.

Pattillo, R. A. and Gey, G. O. (1968), "The Establishment of a Cell Line of Human Hormone-synthesizing Trophoblastic Cells *in vitro*," *Cancer Res.*, **28**, 1231.

Pearlman, W. H. (1957), "Circulating Steroid Hormone Levels in Relation to Steroid Hormone Production," *Ciba Foundation Colloquia on Endocrinology*, **11**, 233.

Pearlman, W. H. (1960), "Progesterone." In: *Hormones in Human Plasma*. Hl Antoniades (Ed.), p. 415. London.

Pearse, A. G. E. (1948), "Cytochemistry of the Gonadotrophic Hormones," *Nature, Lond.*, **162**, 651.

Pencharz, R. I. and Long, J. A. (1931), "The Effect of Hypophysectomy on Gestation of the Rat," *Science*, **74**, 206.

Pencharz, R. I. and Lyons, W. R. (1934), "Hypophysectomy in the Pregnant Guinea-pig," *Proc. Soc. exp. Biol.*, *N.Y.*, **31**, 1131.

Philipp, E. (1929), "Sexualhormone, Plazenta und Neugeboren experimentelle Studie," *Zbl. Gynäk.*, **53**, 2386.

Philipp, E. (1930), "Hypophysenvorderlappen und Plazenta," *Zbl. Gynäk.*, **54**, 450.

Philipp, E. (1945), In: *Biologie und Pathologie des Weibes*. (L. Seitz and A. J. Amreich), Fds. 2nd ed., p. 375.

Philipp, E. (1956). In: *Probleme der foetalen Endokrinologie*. (Ed. H. Nowakowski), p. 132. Heidelberg: Julius Springer.

Pierce, G. B., Dixon, F. J., Jr. and Verney, E. (1959), "Endocrine Function of a Heterotransplantable Human Embryonal Carcinoma," *Arcg. Path.*, **67**, 204.

Pion, R., Conrad, S. H. and Wolf, B. J. (1966), "Pregnenolone Sulphate—An Efficient Precursor for the Placental Production of Progesterone," *J. clin. Endocr.*, **26**, 225.

Pion, R. J., Jaffe, R., Eriksson, G., Wiqvist, N. and Diczfalusy, E. (1965), "Studies on the Metabolism of C-21 Steroids in the Human Foeto-Placental Unit," *Acta endocr., Copenh.*, **48**, 234.

Plager, J. E., Schmidt, K. G. and Staubitz, W. J. (1964). *J. clin. Invest.*, **43**, 1066.

Plotka, E. D., Estergreen, V. and Frost, O. L. (1967), "Relationships between Progesterone Levels in Peripheral and Ovarian Venous Blood Plasma, Corpora Lutea, and Ovaries during Pregnancy," *J. Dairy. Sci.*, **50**, 1001.

Plotz, E. J. and Davis, M. E. (1956), "The Excretion of Neutral Steroids in the Urine of Pregnant Women, following the Administration of Large Doses of Progesterone," *Acta endocr., Copenh.*, **21**, 259.

Porter, D. G. (1968), "The Local Effect of Intra-uterine Progesterone Treatment on Myometrial Activity in Rabbits," *J. Reprod. Fert.*, **1**, 437.

Porter, D. G. (1969a), "Studies in the Regulation of Uterine Activity," *Postgrad. med. J.*, **45**, 70.

Porter, D. G. (1969b). In press.

Porter, D. G., Becker, R. and Csapo, A. I. (1968), "On the Mechanism of Action of Intra-amniotic Hypertonic Saline Treatment in Rabbits," *J. Reprod. and Fert.*, **17**, 433–442.

Pratt, J. P. (1927), "Corpus Luteum in its Relation to Menstruation and Pregnancy," *Endocrinology*, **11**, 195.

Puck, A. and Hübner, K. A. (1956), "Die Wirkungen des Oestriols auf Uterus und Vagina des Kaninchens und Meerschweinchens und auf die Symphyse des Meerschweinchens," *Acta endocr., Copenh.*, **22**, 291.

Ratsimamanga, A. R., Rabinowicz, M. and Jacquard, S. (1964), "Synthèse possible des corticosteroides par la placenta chez le rat," *C.R. Soc. Biol., Paris*, **158**, 1798.

Ray, E. W., Averill, S. C., Lyons, W. R. and Johnson, R. E. (1955), "Rat Placental Hormonal Activities corresponding to those of Pituitary Mammotropin," *Endocrinology*, **56**, 359.

Reynolds, S. R. M. (1935), "A Predisposing Factor for the Normal Onset of Labor: the Probable Role of Oestrin," *Amer. J. Obstet. and Gynec.*, **29**, 630–638.

Reynolds, S. R. M. (1949), *Physiology of the Uterus.* New York.

Robinson, H. J., Bernhard, W. G., Grubin, H., Wanner, H., Sewekow, G. W. and Silber, R. H. (1955), "17,21-Dihydroxy-20-ketosteroids in Plasma during and after Pregnancy," *J. clin. Endocr. Metab.*, **15**, 317.

Robson, J. M. (1937), "Maintenance by Oestrin of the Luteal Function in Hypophysectomized Rabbits," *J. Physiol.*, **90**, 435.

Robson, J. M. (1935), "Effect of Oestrin on Uterine Reactivity and its Relation to Experimental Abortion and Parturition," *J. Physiol.*, **84**, 121.

Robson, J. M. (1938), "Mechanism of Oestrus Inhibition in the Mouse during Pregnancy," *Quart. J. exp. Physiol.*, **28**, 195.

Robson, J. M. (1939), "Maintenance of Pregnancy in the Hypophysectomized Rabbit by the Administration of Oestrin," *J. Physiol.*, **95**, 83.

Robson, J. M. (1947), *Recent Advances in Sex and Reproductive Physiology.* London: Churchill.

Ronan, F. F., Parsons, L., Namiot, R. and Wotiz, H. H. (1960), "Studies in Steroid Metabolism. IX. The Excretion of Pregnane-3α, 17α, 20α-triol during Pregnancy," *J. clin. Endocr. Metab.*, **20**, 355.

Rowlands, I. W. (1949), "Serum Gonadotrophin and Ovarian Activity in the Pregnant Mare," *J. Endocr.*, **6**, 184.

Rowlands, I. W. (1963), "Levels of Gonadotropins in Tissues and Fluids with Emphasis on Domestic Animals. Ch. 3. In: *Gonadotropins.* Cole, H. H. (Ed.). San Francisco and London: Freeman and Co.

Runnebaum, B. and Zander, J. (1962), "Progesteron; Δ⁴-Pregnen-20α-ol-3on, Δ⁴-Pregnen-20β-ol-3on, 17α-Hydroxyprogesteron im Plasma der Nabelvene, und der Nabelarterien," *Klin. Wschr.*, **40**, 453.

Ryan, K. J. (1958), "Conversion of Δ⁵-Androstene-3β, 16α, 17β-triol to Estriol by Human Placenta," *Endocrinology*, **63**, 392.

Ryan, K. J. (1959), "Metabolism of C-16-oxygenated Steroids by Human Placenta: the Formation of Estriol," *J. biol. Chem.*, **234**, 2006.

Salhanick, H. A., Neal, L. M. and Mahoney, J. P. (1956), "Blood Content of Human Placenta," *J. clin. Endocr. Metab.*, **16**, 1120.

Salhanick, H. A., Noall, M. W., Zarrow, M. X. and Samuels, L. T. (1952), "The Isolation of Progesterone from Human Placentae," *Science*, **115**, 708.

Samaan, N., Yen, S. C. C., Friesen, H. and Pearson, O. H. (1966), "Serum Placental Lactogen Levels during Pregnancy and in Trophoblastic Disease," *J. clin. Endocr. Metab.*, **26**, 1303.

Samodelkin, P. A. (1940), "Hormonal Methods of Pregnancy Diagnosis in the Asses," *Aminal Breeding Abstracts*, **8**, 225.

Samuels, L. T., Evans, G. T. and McKelvey, J. L. (1943), "Ovarian and Placental Function in Addison's Disease," *Endocrinology*, **32**, 422.

Sandberg, A. A., Slaunwhite, W. R., Jr. and Antoniades, H. N. (1957), "The Binding of Steroids and Steroid Conjugates to Human Plasma Proteins," *Recent. Progr. Hormone Research*, **13**, 209.

Savard, K. (1961), "The Estrogens of the Pregnant Mare," *Endocrinology*, **68**, 411.

Sawyer, W. H., Frieden, E. H. and Martin, A. S. (1953), "*In vitro* Inhibition of Spontaneous Contractions of the Rat Uterus by Relaxin-containing Extracts of Sow Ovaries," *Amer. J. Physiol.*, **172**, 547–552.

Schofield, B. M. (1961), "The Acute Effect of Progestational Compounds on Intact Rabbit Myometrium," *J. Physiol., Lond.*, **157**, 117.

Schofield, B. M. (1963), "The 'Local' Effect of the Placenta on Myometrial Activity in the Rabbit," *J. Physiol., Lond.*, **166**, 191.

Schofield, B. M. (1966a), "The Increased Extensibility of Pregnant Myometrium," *J. Physiol.*, **182**, 690–694.

Schofield, B. M. (1966b), "The Local Influence of the Placenta on Myometrial Activity," *Mem. Soc. Endocr.*, **14**, 221.

Schultze, A. H. and Snyder, F. F. (1935), "Observations on Reproduction in the Chimpanzee," *Bull. Johns Hopkins Hosp.*, **57**, 193.

Seegar, G. E. and Delfs, E. (1940), "Preganediol Excretion following Bilateral Oophorectomy in Early Pregnancy," *J.A.M.A.*, **115**, 1267.

Selye, H. and Collip, J. B. (1936), "Fundamental Factors in the Interpretation of Stimuli Influencing Endocrine Glands," *Endocrinology*, **20**, 667.

Selye, H., Collip, J. B. and Thompson, D. L. (1935), "Endocrine Inter-relations during Pregnancy," *Endocrinology*, **19**, 151.

Short, R. B. (1957), "Progesterone and Related Steroids in the Blood of Domestic Animals," *Colloq. on Endocr. Ciba Foundation*, **11**, 362.

Short, R. V. (1961), "Progesterone." In: *Hormones in Blood* (Gray, C. H. and Bacharach, A. L., Eds.). New York.

Short, R. V. and Eckstein, P. (1961), "Oestrogen and Progesterone Levels in Pregnant Rhesus Monkeys," *J. Endocr.*, **22**, 15.

Short, R. V. and Eton, B. (1959), "Progesterone in Blood. III. Progesterone in the Peripheral Blood of Pregnant Women," *J. Endocr.*, **18**, 418.

Short, R. V. and Moore, N. W. (1959), "Progesterone in Blood. Progesterone and 20α-hydroxy-pregn-4-en-3-one in the Placenta and Blood of Ewes," *J. Endocr.*, **19**, 288.

Siiteri, P. K. and MacDonald, P. D. (1966), "Placental Estrogen Biosynthesis during Human Pregnancy," *J. clin. Endocr. Metab.*, **26**, 751.

Smith, G. V. S. and Smith, O. W. (1934), "Excessive Gonad-stimulating Hormone and Subnormal Amounts of Oestrin in the Toxaemias of late Pregnancy," *Amer. J. Physiol.*, **107**, 128.

Smith, G. V. S. and Smith O. W. (1935a), "The Quantitative Determination of Urinary Oestrin," *Amer. J. Physiol.*, **112**, 340.

Smith, G. van and Smith, O. W. (1935b), "Evidence for the Placental Origin of the Excessive Prolan of Late Pregnancy Toxaemia and Eclampsia," *Surg. Obstet. Gynec.*, **61**, 175.

Smith, G. van and Smith, O. W. (1941a), "Estrogen and Progestin Metabolism in Pregnancy: Endocrine Imbalance of Pre-eclampsia and Eclampsia. Summary of Findings to February, 1941," *J. clin. Endocr. Metab.*, **1**, 470.

Smith, G. van and Smith, O. W. (1941b), "Estrogen and Progestin Metabolism in Pregnancy: The Effect of Hormone Administration in Pre-eclampsia," *J. clin. Endocr. Metab.*, **1**, 472.

Smith, G. V. S. and Smith O. W. (1948), "Internal Secretions and Toxemia of Late Pregnancy," *Physiol. Rev.*, **28**, 1.

Smith, O. W. and Arai, K. (1963), "Blood Estrogens in Late Pregnancy: An Evaluation of Methods with Improved Recovery," *J. clin. Endocr. Metab.*, **23**, 1141.

Smith, O. W. and Smith, G. van S. (1958), "Oestrogens in the Urine of Women with Special Reference to Hydrolytic Procedures. Part III. Biologically Active Material in Pregnancy not Accounted for by Oestradiol, Oestrone and Oestriol," *Acta endocr., Copenh.*, **28**, 479.

Smith, O. W., Smith, G. S. and Schiller, S. (1941), "Estrogen and Progestin Metabolism in Pregnancy: Spontaneous and Induced Labor," *J. clin. Endocr. Metab.*, **1**, 461.

Smith, P. E. (1946), "Non-essentiality of Hypophysis in the Maintenance of Pregnancy in Rhesus Monkeys," *Anat. Rec.*, **94**, 497.

Smith, P. E. (1954), "Continuation of Pregnancy in Rhesus Monkeys (*Macaca mulatta*) following Hypophysectomy," *Endocrinology*, **55**, 655.

Smith, R. A., Albert, A. and Randall, L. M. (1951), "Chorionic Gonadotropin in the Blood and Urine during Early Pregnancy," *Amer. J. Obstet. Gynec.*, **61**, 514.

Smithberg, M. and Runner, M. N. (1956), "The Induction and Maintenance of Pregnancy in Prepubertal Mice," *J. exp. Zool.*, **133**, 441.

Smithberg, M. and Runner, M. N. (1951), "Pregnancy Induced in Genetically Sterile Mice," *J. Hered.*, **48**, 97.

Snyder, F. F. (1934), "The Prolongation of Pregnancy and Complications of Parturition in the Rabbit following Induction of Ovulation near Term," *Johns Hopk. Hosp. Bull.*, **54**, 1.

Snyder, F. F. (1936), "Further Observations in Experimental Superfetation," *Anat. Rec.*, **64**, 46, Abs.

Snyder, F. F. (1938), "Factors Concerned in the Duration of Pregnancy," *Physiol. Rev.*, **18**, 578.

Solomon, S. (1960), *The Placenta and Fetal Membranes* (C. A. Villee, Ed.). Baltimore: Williams and Wilkins.

Solomon, S. (1966), "Formation and Metabolism of Neutral Steroids in the Human Placenta and Fetus," *J. clin. Endocr. Metab.*, **26**, 762.

Solomon, S., Bird, C. E., Wilson, B., Wiqvist, N. and Diczfalusy, E. (1965), "Progesterone Metabolism in the Fetal-placental Unit," *Proc. 2nd Int. Congr. Endocr., London*, **2**, 721.

Staunwhite, W. R., Jr. and Sandberg, A. A. (1959), "Transcortin, a Corticosteroid Binding Protein in Plasma," *J. clin. Invest.*, **38**, 384.

Steinetz, H. G., Beach, V. L. and Kroc, R. L. (1959), "The Physiology of Relaxin in Laboratory Animals." In: *Recent Progress in Endocrinology of Reproduction*, C. W. Lloyd (Ed.), p. 390. London.

Stewart, H. L., Jr. (1951), "Hormone Secretion by Human Placenta Grown in the Eyes of Rabbits," *Amer. J. Obstet. Gynec.*, **61**, 990.

Stewart, H. L., Sano, M. E. and Montgomery, T. L. (1948), "Hormone Secretion by Human Placenta Grown in Tissue Culture," *J. clin. Endocr. Metab.*, **8**, 175.

Strobel, E. (1961), "I. ACTH Activity of Rat Placenta and Foetus. II. Influence of Hypophysectomy on the ACTH Activity of Rat Placenta and Foetus," *Endocrinology*, **41**, 45.

Suzuki, Y. (1947), "Studies on the Physiology of the Corpus Luteum Hormone. 2. The Fate of the Corpus Luteum Hormone during Pregnancy in Mares," *Jap. J. vet. Sci.*, **9**, 149.

Sybulski, S. (1956), *The Production and Metabolism of Corticoids in Pregnancy*. Ph.D. Thesis, McGill University, Montreal, Canada.

Telegdy, G., Endröczi, E. and Lissak, K. (1963), "Ovarian Progesterone Secretion during the Oestrous Cycle, Pregnancy and Lactation in Dogs," *Acta endocr., Copenh.*, **44**, 461.

Tenney, B., Jr. and Parker, F., Jr. (1937), "Some Observations of the Gonadotrophic Hormones of Pregnancy," *Endocrinology*, **21**, 687.

Troen, P. (1959), "Perfusion Studies of the Human Placenta. In: *Recent Progress in the Endocrinology of Reproduction* (C. W. Lloyd, Ed.), p. 299. London: Academic Press.

Troen, P. (1961), "Perfusion Studies of the Human Placenta. III. Production of Free and Conjugated Porter-Silber Chromogens,' *J. clin. Endocr. Metab.*, **21**, 1551.

Tschesche, R. and Snetzke, G. (1960), quoted by Bennett and Heftmann (1965).

Tuchmann-Duplessis, H., Mayer, M., Quelet, J. and Sary, A. (1952), "Sur la présence d'une substance corticostimulante du placenta humain," *C.R. Acad. Sci., Paris*, **235**, 209.

Tullner, W. W. and Hertz, R. (1966a), "Chorionic Gonadotropin Levels in the Rhesus Monkey during Early Pregnancy," *Endocrinology*, **78**, 204.

Tullner, W. W. and Hertz, R. (1966b), "Normal Gestation and Chorionic Gonadotropin Levels in the Monkey after Ovariectomy in Early Pregnancy," *Endocrinology*, **78**, 1076.

Tullner, W. W. and Gray, C. W. (1968), "Chorionic Gonadotropin Excretion during Pregnancy in a Gorilla," *Proc. Soc. Exp. Biol. Med.*, **128**, 954.

Tulsky, A. S. and Koff, A. K. (1957), "Some Observations on the Role of the Corpus Luteum in Early Pregnancy," *Fertil. and Steril.*, **8**, 118.

Turnbull, A. C. and Anderson, A. B. M. (1968), "Uterine Contractility and Oxytocin Sensitivity during Human Pregnancy in Relation to the Onset of Labour," *J. Obstet. Gynaec. Brit. Cwlth.*, **75**, 278–288.

Turnbull, A. C., Anderson, A. and Wilson, G. R. (1967), "Maternal Urinary Oestrogen Excretion as Evidence of a Foetal Role in Determining Gestation at Labour," *Lancet*, **ii**, 627–629.

Unterberger, F. (1952), "Vergleichende Biologische Untersuchungen über das Hypophysenvorderlappenhormon der *Cerviden*," *Zbl. Gynäkol.*, **56**, 2112.

Vande Wiele, R. L., Gurpide, E., Kelly, W. G., Laragh, J. H. and Lieberman, S. (1960), "The Secretory Rate of Progesterone and Aldosterone in Normal and Abnormal Late Pregnancy," *Acta endocr. Copenh. Suppl.*, **51**, 159.

Van de Wiele, R. L. and Jailer, J. W. (1959), "Placental Steroids," *Ann. N.Y. Acad. Sci.*, **75**, 889.

Venning, E. H. (1946), "Adrenal Function in Pregnancy," *Endocrinology*, **39**, 203.

Venning, E. M. (1955), "Clinical Value of Hormone Estimations," *Brit. med. Bull.*, **11**, 140.

Venning, E. H. (1957), "The Secretion of Various Hormones and the Activity of the Adrenal Cortex in Pregnancy." In: *Gestation* (C. A. Villee, Ed.), *Proc. 3rd Conf. Josiah Macy, Jr. Foundation*. New York.

Venning, E. H. and Browne, J. S. L. (1936), "Isolation of a Water Soluble Pregnanediol Complex from Human Pregnancy Urine," *Proc. Soc. exp. Biol., N.Y.*, **34**, 292.

Venning, E. H. and Dyrenfurth, I. (1956), "Aldosterone Excretion in Pregnancy," *J. clin. Endocr. Metab.*, **16**, 426.

Villee, D. B. and Villee, C. A. (1965), "Synthesis of Corticosteroids in the Fetal-placental Unit," *Proc. 2nd Int. Congr. Endocrin.*, **2**, 709.

Voss, H. E. (1927), "Uber die Funktion endocriner Heterotransplantate als Kennzeichen ihrer Einheilung. In: *Biologia Generalis*, Vol. 111, p. 571.

Wada, H. and Turner, C. W. (1959a), "Effect of Relaxin on Mammary Gland Growth in Female Mice," *Proc. Soc. exp. Biol., N.Y.*, **101**, 707.

Wada, H. and Turner, C. W. (1959b), "Effect of Relaxin on Mammary Gland Growth in the Female Rat," *Proc. Soc. exp. Biol., N.Y.*, **102**, **568**.

Wagenen, G. van and Jenkins, R. H. (1943), "Pyelo-ureteral Dilatation in Successive Pregnancies," *J. Urol.*, **49**, 228.

Wagenen, G. van and Newton, W. H. (1940), "Maintenance of the Habits of Pregnancy and Timely Onset of Labor after Removal of the Fetus," *Amer. J. Physiol.*, **129**, 485.

Wagenen, G. van and Newton, W. H. (1943), "Pregnancy in the Monkey after Removal of the Fetus," *Surg. Gynec. Obstet.*, **77**, 539.

Wagenen, G. van and Simpson, M. E. (1954), "Gonadotrophic Hormone Excretion in the Pregnant Monkey (*Macaca mulatta*)," *Proc. Soc. exp. Biol., N.Y.*, **90**, 346.

Watanabe, M., Meeker, C. I., Gray, M. J., Sims, E. A. H. and Solomon, S. (1965), "Aldosterone Secretion Rates in Abnormal Pregnancy," *J. clin. Endocr. Metab.*, **25**, 1665.

Westman, A. and Jacobsohn, D. (1937), "Über Oestrin-Wirkungen auf die Corpus-luteum-Funktion," *Acta Obstet. Gynec. Scand.*, **17**, 1, 133.

Weymeersch, A. (1912), "Persistance de la placentation après excision des embryons chez la lapine," *Ann. Soc. Sci. méd. nat., Bruxelles*, **76**, 104.

White, P. (1952), "Pregnancy Complicating Diabetes." In: *Treatment of Diabetes Mellitus* (E. P. Joslin, H. F. Foot, P. White and A. Marble, Eds.), 9th Ed., Chap. 27. Philadelphia: Lea and Febiger.

White, W. E. (1933), "The Effect on Ovulation and Pregnancy of Blocking the Pituitary Circulation in the Rabbit." *Amer. J. Physiol.*, **102**, 505.

Wickersham, E. W. and Tanabe, T. Y. (1967), "Functional Status of Bovine Corpora Lutea of Pregnancy," *J. Dairy Sci.*, **50**, 1001.

Wilkinson, J. F. and De Fremery, P. (1940), "Gonadotrophic Hormones in the Urine of the Giraffe," *Nature, Lond.*, **146**, 491.

Williams, H. E. and Provine, H. T. (1966), "Effects of Estradiol on Glycogen Synthetase in the Rat Uterus," *Endocrinology*, **78**, 786.

Wilson, R., Bird, C. E., Wiqvist, N., Solomon, S. and Diczfalusy, E. (1966), "Metabolism of Progesterone by the Perfused Adrenalectomized Human Fetus," *J. clin. Endocr. Metab.*, **26**, 1155.

Wilson, J. D. (1963), "The Nature of the RNA Response to Estradiol Administration by the Uterus of the Rat," *Proc. Nat. Acad. Sci., U.S.A.*, **50**, 93.

Wislocki, G. B. and Bennett, H. S. (1943), "The Histology and Cytology of the Human and Monkey Placentae, with Special Reference to the Trophoblast," *Amer. J. Anat.*, **73**, 335.

Wislocki, G. B. and Dempsey, E. W. (1946), "Histochemical Age Changes in Normal and Pathological Villi (*Hydatidiform Mole, Eclampsia*)," *Endocrinology*, **38**, 90.

Wislocki, G. B. and Dempsey, E. W. (1948), "The Chemical Histology of Human Placenta and Decidua with Reference to Mucoproteins, Glycogen, Lipids and Acid Phosphatase," *Amer. J. Anat.*, **83**, 1.

Wislocki, G. B. and Padykula, H. A. (1961), "Histochemistry and Electron Microscopy of the Placenta." In: *Sex and Internal Secretions* (W. C. Young, Ed.), 3rd Ed., Vol. 2, p. 883.

Ymazaki, E., Noguchi, A. and Slingerland, D. W. (1961), "Thyrotropin in the Serum of Mother and Fetus," *J. clin. Endocr. Metab.*, **21**, 1013.

Zander, J. (1959), "Gestagens in Human Pregnancy." In: *Recent Progress in the Endocrinology of Reproduction* (Lloyd, G. W. Ed.), p. 255. New York: Academic Press.

Zander, J. (1961), "Relationship between Progesterone Production in the Human Placenta and the Foetus." In: *Ciba Foundation Study Group*, No. 9, G. E. W. Wolstenholme and M. P. Cameron (Eds.), p. 32. London: Churchill.

Zander, J. (1965), "Progesterone and its Metabolites in the Human Placentao-foetal Unit," *Proc. 2nd Int. Congr. Endocr.*, **2**, 715.

Zander, J., Forbes, T. R., von Münstermann, A. M. and Neher, R. (1958), "Δ⁴-3-ketopregnene-20α-ol, and Δ⁴-3-ketopregnene-20β-ol, two naturally occurring Metabolites of Progesterone. Isolation, Identification, Biologic Activity and Concentration in Human Tissues," *J. clin. Endocr. Metab.*, **18**, 337.

Zander, J. and von Münstermann, A. (1954), "Weitere Untersuchungen über Progesteron im menschlichen Blut und Geweben," *Klin. Wschr.*, **32**, 894.

Zarrow, M. X. (1948), "The Role of the Steroid Hormones in the Relaxation of the symphysis Pubis of the Guinea-pig," *Endocrinology*, **42**, 129.

Zarrow, M. X. and Rosenberg, B. (1953), "Sources of Relaxin in the Rabbit," *Endocrinology*, **53**, 593.

Zeilmaker, G. H. (1968), "Luteotrophic Activity of the Ectopic Mouse Trophoblast," *J. Endocr.*, **41**, 455.

Zilliacus, H. (1953), "Polysaccharide Structures in Normal Chorionic Villi, Hydatiform Mole and Chorioepithelioma, with Special Reference to the Chorionic Gonadotrophic Hormone," *Gynaecologia*, **135**, 161.

Zizine, L. A., Simpson, M. E. and Evans, H. M. (1950), "Direct Action of Male Sex Hormone on the Adrenal Cortex," *Endocrinology*, **47**, 97.

Zondek, B. (1935), *Die Hormone des Ovariums und des Hypophysenvorderlappens*, 2nd Ed. Vienna: Springer-Verlag.

Zondek, B. and Sulman, F. (1945), "A Twenty-four Hour Pregnancy Test for Equines," *Nature, Lond.*, **155**, 302.

Zuckerman, S. (1935), "The Aschheim-Zondek Diagnosis of Pregnancy in the Chimpanzee," *Amer. Physiol.*, **110**, 597.

10. ADOLESCENCE

H. BOUTOURLINE YOUNG

Adolescence may be defined as the period from the earliest signs of sexual maturation until the attainment of physical, mental and emotional maturity. This chapter will be confined to the events of physical maturation and to common departures from physical health during the adolescent period.

Girls come to puberty about two years ahead of boys, but there is a wide standard deviation so that there is some overlap and an early maturing boy may be more precocious than a late maturing girl of the same chronological age. Both girls and boys have been reaching puberty progressively earlier over the past century and in a number of recent studies the mean age of menarche in girls was to be found under thirteen years (Simons and Greulich, 1943; Nicolson and Hanley, 1953; Kinsey, Pomery, Martin and Gebhard, 1953; Thoma, 1960; Boutourline Young, Zoli and Gallagher, 1963; Zukowski, Kmietowicz-Zukowska and Gruska, 1964).

In boys the growth in height is somewhat more intense and longer, accounting in part for the adult sex differences. The remaining difference is mainly accounted for by the extra two years of growth which boys have enjoyed before the self limiting adolescent spurt begins. However, at all ages, adolescence included, the growth of girls seems less affected by stress such as illness or poor nutrition.

PHYSICAL MATURATION IN GIRLS

The Breast

The first evidence of sexual maturation in girls is usually the appearance of a breast bud. There is elevation of the papilla, enlargement of the areola and evident swelling of breast tissue. Reynolds and Wines (1948) have described breast development stages and their classification has been widely accepted. The following stages are described:

Stage

1. Pre-adolescent, confined to elevation of papilla;

2. Breast bud, elevation of breast and papilla and increased areola;

3. Progressive enlargement of and protuberence of breast and areola;

4. Protuberence of areola and papilla above breast, occurring in something more than one half of all subjects;

5. Maturation: further increase in breast tissue, projection of papilla only, recession of areola.

Garn (1952) has criticized this classification and maintains that the observations should be confined to the areola and nipple, ignoring the more variable mammary and fatty tissues. He describes four stages of development as follows:

(a) Infantile: everted nipple with small flat, lightly pigmented areola;

(b) 1st stage maturation: nipple absorbed into areola which has become larger, swollen and more pigmented;

(c) 2nd stage maturation: nipple still absorbed into areola which is still larger, more pigmented and elevated with a ring of peripheral pigmentation;

(d) 3rd stage maturation: regression of swelling of areola and emergence of nipple.

Plate 1 taken from Tanner, Ed. Lytt Gardiner (Endocrine and Genetic Diseases of Childhood, in press) shows the most recent breast standards and it is urged that these be accepted as they combine the best features of the previous classifications.

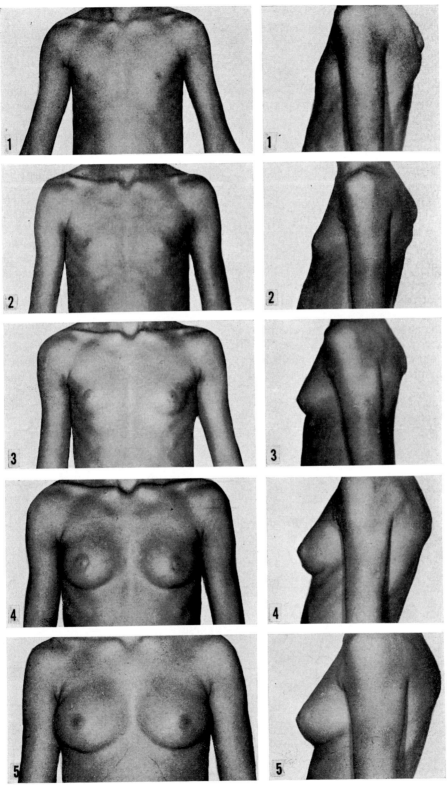

PLATE 1. Breast development in girls. Stages 1 to 5 according to the classification of Reynolds and Wines (modified by Tanner).

Pubic Hair

The first appearance of pigmented crinkly pubic hair is usually several months after Reynolds and Wines breast stage 2, but it *may* sometimes precede it. Pubic hair stages may be defined as follows:

Child	1.	In a child, any hair on pubes is no different from that on the abdominal wall;
Immediate prepuberal	2.	Growth on pubes of long, downy, non- or only slightly pigmented hair;
	3.	Appearance of coarse, pigmented, crinkly pubic hair in small quantity;
Puberal stages	4.	Coarse, pigmented, crinkly hair in moderate quantity;
	5.	Coarse, pigmented, crinkly pubic hair in considerable quantity with the female pattern of straight or concave upper level;
Adult	6.	Completion to adult form including hair on the inner side of the thigh.

Stage 2 may appear at any age from 8 to 14 and the process of development to stage 5 takes up to three years.

Figure 1 illustrates the appearance of the pubic hair in early, mid and late puberty corresponding to stages 3, 4 and 5 above. Plate 2 shows development of pubic hair in boys and girls from prepuberty to the last stage of puberty.

The sequence of some of the events at adolescence is presented in Figure 2 (Tanner, 1962).

Axillary Hair

Pigmented, crinkly hair appears in the axilla, usually one to two years after its first appearance on the pubes, but occasionally one may find an exception where it may take precedence. With the appearance of a moderate amount of axillary hair, axillary sweating with typical odour may first appear.

It should be remembered that the amount of hair pigmentation may vary in different parts of the world; in Northern Europe, for example, pigmentation in some individuals may be barely discernible.

Classification of Sexual Maturity

It is generally recognized that it is useful to evaluate the degree of sexual maturity during adolescence and for this a classification is necessary. A suggested classification is presented in Table 1 (Boutourline Young *et al.*, 1963).

Physicians should make detailed notes on sexual maturity which in turn permits a classification from 1 to 6 as shown in Table 1.

Linear Growth and Sexual Maturity

If height increments during puberty are plotted against chronological age we lose much of our perception of what is happening because of the large individual age differences at maturation. Instead when height increments are plotted against phases of puberty, relationships are clearly seen.

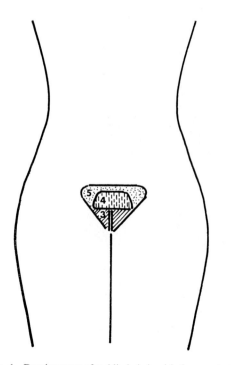

FIG. 1. Development of pubic hair in girls from early to late puberty.

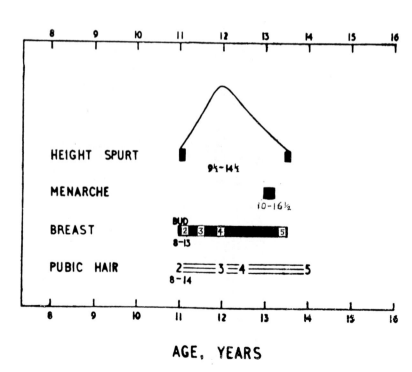

AGE, YEARS

FIG. 2. Relationships of height spurt, menarche, breast and pubic hair development in girls taken from *Growth at Adolescence*, J. M. Tanner, Second Edition Oxford Blackwell 1962.

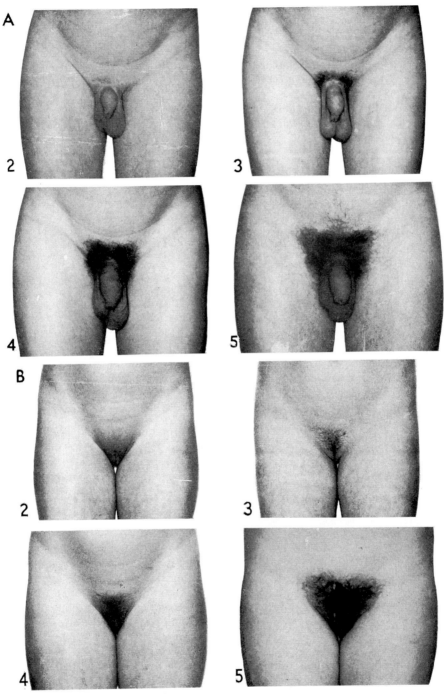

PLATE 2. Pubic hair development in boys and girls from prepuberal (stage 2) to final stage puberty (stage 5).

Figure 3 presents height increments (cm./year) (Boutourline Young *et al.*, 1963) against phases of puberty as classified in Table 1. It is seen that menarche occurs well on the down grade of height velocity and that the mean maximum height velocity is 7 cm./year. Girls grow fastest at stage 3 in the classification of sexual maturity (first stage puberty) when there is only a *small* amount of coarse early pigmented pubic hair.

Broadening of the hips and increase of subcutaneous tissue in that area becomes especially noticeable about the time of menarche.

It is believed that full reproductive efficiency does not occur for a year or two after menarche and that the cycles, until that time, are frequently anovulatory.

Body Build and Physical Maturation

Our own observations (Boutourline Young *et al.*, 1963) agree with those of others (Tanner, 1962; McNeill and Livson, 1963) that plumpness or endomorphy appears to be associated with earlier maturation. There is also some evidence (Tanner, 1962, pp. 95–104) that lean spare subjects, scoring high on linearity, tend to arrive later at

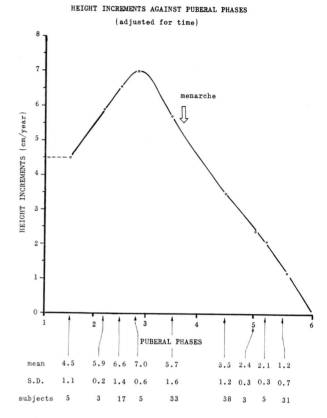

FIG. 3. Height increments in girls during the phases of puberty.

	mean	S.D.	subjects
	4.5	1.1	5
	5.9	0.2	3
	6.6	1.4	17
	7.0	0.6	5
	5.7	1.6	33
	3.5	1.2	38
	2.4	0.3	3
	2.1	0.3	5
	1.2	0.7	31

TABLE 1

CLASSIFICATION OF SEXUAL MATURITY

Classification	Characteristics
1. No change from a child	No growth of puberal hair, no growth spurt;
2. Prepuberal phase	Downy pubic hair; usually first evidence of growth spurt; elevation breast papilla; perhaps early budding;
3. First stage puberty	Pubic hair, pigmented, coarse and curly in small quantity; budding of breasts, areola enlargement; marked growth spurt; enlargement of labia;
4. Second stage puberty	Pubic hair as described above in moderate quantity; filling out of breasts, sometimes projection of areola and papilla to form a secondary mound; axillary hair as described above in small quantity; menarche usual in this phase; growth spurt marked, but already falling away; further growth labia;
5. Third stage puberty	Pubic hair further increased and approaching or reaching adult quantity and distribution; moderate quantity axillary hair; breasts approaching or reaching adult type configuration with recession of areola to level of the breast; labia approaching or reaching adult type; annual growth less than before puberty; menstruation usually well established;
6. Adult	Further growth axillary and perhaps pubic hair to adult type and distribution; breasts adult; labia adult; growth in height usually less than 1·5 cm. in previous 12 months.

puberty although in our limited series we could not confirm this. McNeill and Livson (1963) have demonstrated endomorphy as the major prediction of early maturation. Our own early maturers tended to be fatter throughout development and less linear as adults.

Changes in Body Composition

After the age of 8 the measured skin folds of girls increase until maturity. This is in contrast to boys where there is a decrease in the width of skin folds on the limbs during adolescence. The situation is illustrated in Figure 4 (Boutourline Young, 1965), where skin folds in groups of males and females are plotted against both chronological age and phase of maturity. The second part of this figure shows the divergence between the sexes after early puberty in bone and muscle. After this point the relatively small sex differences in strength and co-ordination become much more marked.

It is now possible to predict fairly accurately at the age of 8 the adult height of a person and such predictions are of potential value where height is attached to an occupation involving long training (e.g. ballerinas). Bayley's prediction tables (Bayley and Pinneau, 1952) involve consideration of actual height, actual age and skeletal age. If practicable methods were available for slowing down height, the methods would be of considerable value in dealing with the problem of very tall girls.

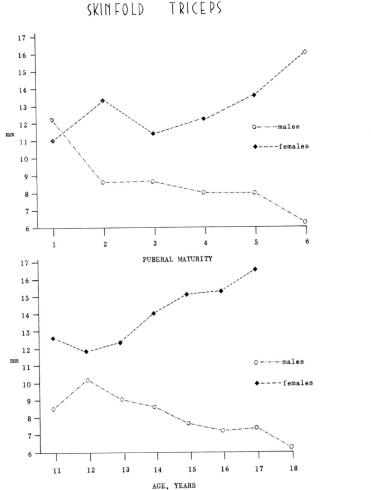

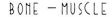

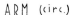

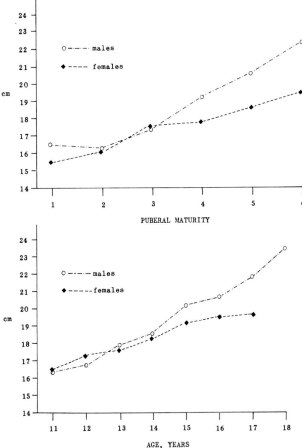

FIG. 4(a). Skinfold thickness (triceps) in males and females during puberty.

FIG. 4(b). Bone and muscle (arm) circumference in males and females during puberty.

Attempts to Suppress Excessive Growth in Girls

Oestrogens have been used for this purpose but Bayley, Gordan, Bayer, Goldberg and Storment (1962) appear to have demonstrated that there is no significant difference between mature height after treatment and that previously predicted. Oestrogen treatment accelerated the rate of skeletal maturation and since there was no change in predicted height the hormone must also have increased the rate of linear growth proportionately.

The Secular Change in Puberal Maturity

Girls have been reaching menarche more than three months earlier with each decade during the past 100 years in Western Europe. There is some evidence that the fall is less in the more privileged social classes. Whitehead (1847), cited by Tanner, (1962), observed social class differences of more than one year, whereas in our own work no significant social class differences were seen. Under stable economic circumstances there is a high correlation between time of arrival at menarche of mothers and daughters. Observation of the mean age of menarche of subjects and their mothers in relation to social mobility has shown a relationship between upward social mobility and a relative lowering of menarchal age in the daughters (Boutourline Young et al., 1963). The reporting by mothers is not very reliable being retrospective and possibly subject to systematic distortion in different social groups. but our results, together with those of others demonstrating significant social class differences in time of arrival at menarche (Wofinden and Smallwood, 1958; Bojlén, Rasch and Weis-Bentzon, 1954) do support better nutrition and improved hygiene as factors in the progressive lowering in the age of menarche (nutrition hygiene hypothesis).

There is some evidence that in the more privileged social classes menarche is more likely to occur early in the course of the development of secondary sexual characteristics. This is shown in Table 2 (Boutourline Young et al., 1963).

TABLE 2

MEAN AGES AT THE STAGES OF PUBERTY AND MEAN PUBERAL STAGE AT MENARCHE

Social Class	2		3		4		5		6		Mean point of puberal stage on arrival at menarche	
		No.		No.		No.		No.		No.		No.
1 and 2	11·48 (0·68)	8	12·15 (0·70)	23	12·77 (0·74)	27	13·65 (0·90)	20	14·76 (1·05)	9	3·71 (0·41)	32
3	11·72 (0·41)	13	12·43 (0·55)	22	12·74 (0·84)	31	13·65 (0·95)	27	15·10 (0·83)	17	3·85 (0·42)	35
4 and 5	11·67 (0·55)	4	12·48 (0·62)	6	12·53 (0·77)	11	13·49 (0·84)	13	14·62 (0·88)	10	3·92 (0·52)	13
TOTAL	11·33	25	12·31	51	12·72	69	13·61	60	14·88	36	3·81	80

Figures in parenthesis are standard deviations

The accuracy of recorded age at menarche has been discussed by Livson and McNeill (1962) who conclude that there may be expected an error of six months after an interval of 15–20 years. Evidence from a limited longitudinal study of Florentine girls supports this (Boutourline Young et al., 1963). Livson suggests that accuracy may be increased by improved questioning techniques.

Menarche comes later to girls in families where there are many children (Scott, 1961; Valsik, 1965; Stukowsky, Valsik and Bulai-Stirbu, 1967). This may be purely an economic effect although the reasons are not yet entirely clear.

Climate and Race and Menarche

A review of the evidence suggests that climate has little effect upon growth or maturation (Mills, 1942; Eveleth, 1966). Ellis (1950) reports menarche in economically privileged Nigerian girls as 14·3. With regard to race, there is some evidence (Ito, 1942) that there may be differences not accounted for by economic circumstances, but it is difficult to separate out the respective influences of race and body shape, already referred to as associated with time of arrival at menarche.

Seasonal Variation

Both girls and boys grow more in height in the spring and more in weight in the autumn, but there are wide individual differences, some children and adolescents fluctuating very little with season and others not corresponding to the general pattern. Valsik (1965) reports two peaks of increased incidence of menarche; one in July–September and the other, less marked, at mid winter. He also reports a retarding effect of altitude upon menarche, but it is not clear if socio-economic factors have been controlled.

Menstrual Symptoms, Socio-Cultural Factors and age of arrival at Menarche

It has been hypothesized that socio-cultural factors may so affect attitudes as to lead to markedly differing preva-

lence of dysmenorrhoea in different environments. Our own unpublished observations have failed to support this, but instead show an increased prevalence of dysmenorrhoea in the precocious girls. At least in the two cultures of Italy and the United States, the late developers appear to accept menarche as a gift, while those who arrive early demonstrate a tendency to attach symptoms to the function. If this work is confirmed, it may be helpful in indicating to school health educators where one of their investments should be.

Age at Menarche and Age at Marriage

Buck and Stavraky (1967) report a significant relationship in women less than 30 years old. This work needs to be confirmed in a sample not selected because of child bearing.

Physiological Changes

Shock (1943, 1946) has shown that physiological changes, such as in systolic blood pressure, oxygen consumption and heart rate, are in relation to menarche and not chronological age. Soon after menarche the blood pressure reaches adult female levels; there is a fall over 3 years of basal metabolic rate to adult values and a steady decline in resting heart rate. In contrast to boys, there is no rise in the number of red blood corpuscles or in haemoglobin level. Shock has also demonstrated that from age 13, there is a sex difference in alveolar CO_2 tension, boys being higher than girls. There does not yet appear to be sufficient information as to when the menstrual cycle fluctation in pCO_2 commences, a heralder of much greater changes which occur during pregnancy (Boutourline Young, H. and Boutourline Young, E., 1956), during which alveolar pCO_2 may progressively fall from 38 mm. to nearly 30 mm. Hg.

Another difference in sex patterns is in respect of gastric acidity (Vanzant, Alvarez, Eusterman, Dunn and Berkson, 1932). At puberty there is a much larger increase in boys in free HCl secreted in response to a test meal. The difference persists until after 40.

The mouth temperature of girls departs abruptly from

the male trend at the time of puberty (Iliff and Lee, 1952). Presumably the fluctuations in temperature with the menstrual cycle commence with ovulation.

Skeletal Age

This important biological indicator is used widely in clinical investigations of growth disturbance and in epidemiological studies. Different standards have been created for boys and girls because girls are consistently more mature (Greulich and Pyle, 1950; Tanner and Whitehouse, 1959; Tanner, Whitehouse and Healey, 1962).

Growth Disorders in Adolescent Girls

Patterns of growth and development depend a great deal on heredity and a first step in the assessment of apparent linear growth deficiency is a careful family history with time of arrival at puberty of parents and siblings and including a prediction of the adolescents' height from the mid parental height (Garn, unpublished work). It is important to bear in mind that such prediction tables are based upon the assumption of adequate environmental circumstances during growth for both generations. At the extremes of environmental pressure, mature body height may be reduced by as much as 10 per cent (Bloom, 1964). Further investigation of apparent growth failure will include observation of growth increments and a medical examination which will give special attention to presence of congenital defects, chronic infection or the long term results of previous infection and nutritional disorders. An X-ray of the hand and wrist and possibly other centres for skeletal age is part of this examination. Endocrine disorders such as hypothyroidism need to be excluded.

Exclusion of the above factors in the presence of marked retardation is an indication for referral to one of the special growth clinics, such as that conducted by Prof. J. M. Tanner at the Institute of Child Health of London University. Here it is possible to undertake further specialized investigations such as determination of 17-KS and FSH, blood glucose response to insulin, and chromosome studies. In a very small proportion of cases, patients may be identified as suitable for growth hormone treatment.

In Western societies, the majority of cases of growth failure will have been identified during childhood.

Growth of hair on the face and body may be a reason for seeking the advice of a gynaecologist. Tanner (1962) states that hair on the face has a relatively high threshold to adrenal androgens and is more influenced by testosterone. Women in the child bearing period with increased facial hair have a greater production of 17-ketosteroids and a more masculine body build.

Common Disorders in Adolescents

Acne provokes much concern amongst adolescents. The prevalence rises from zero in the prepuberal period to a peak of 30 per cent in American boys in the final phase of puberty (Masland, 1956). Due basically to oestrogen-androgen imbalance, it is more common in males than females. It usually continues for a year or two. The treatment of this has been discussed by Gallagher (1960) who also deals with other disorders such as defects of posture and the common orthopaedic disorders. Flat feet are frequently seen, but few of them are painful; these must be treated. Gallagher has found that self inspection in the nude by means of a long mirror will encourage an adolescent to ask for measures which may improve her posture. Improved posture and exercises for the pectoral muscles may also improve the figure, a desire of many adolescent girls. It is also important to distinguish functional from structural scoliosis to bring important early treatment to the latter. Epiphysitis, spondylolisthesis, epiphysiolysis of the femoral capital epiphysis and osteochondritis are also discussed by Gallagher.

Fatigue is another common complaint to be dealt with by a thorough physical examination with special attention to possible anaemia, after effects of acute disease, such as mononucleosis or hepatitis, and habits such as going to bed late. With medical and hygienic causes excluded, many cases will be found to have psychological origins.

Obesity is also a common problem in girls. Height and weight tables should be interpreted with care as some mesomorphic girls may have excess weight due to muscle and bone. Fat may be satisfactorily measured by skin calipers (Tanner and Whitehouse, 1955). Obesity occurs when intake of calories systematically exceeds body requirements. Appetite is regulated by a number of factors and it is important to remember that excess eating may not only be a bad habit but also may protect against many stresses. Many fat girls exercise little and motion picture studies of obese subjects at camps have confirmed habitual economy of movement in many of them. Before initiating treatment with diet and exercise, it is important to exclude metabolic defects and we should remember that fatness occurs in some families and here there may be limits to what may be achieved by diet and exercise.

There is a striking incidence of myopia at adolescence (Slataper, 1950) and also an increase in the severity of existing myopia (Gardiner, 1954). Regular vision testing is therefore particularly indicated at this time.

Adolescents are entitled to a confidential examination. Parents should be interviewed separately, preferably at a different time of day. In the examination, the adolescent should be given every chance to talk in an informal atmosphere and the results of the examination should be discussed with her so that a treatment partnership is built up.

I am grateful to The Grant Foundation of New York for the opportunity to study over a ten year period the events of adolescence. I would also like to express my gratitude to Dr. James L. Whittenberger for his support in this work and for his criticisms of this chapter.

I thank Prof. J. M. Tanner for permission to reproduce Plates 1 and 2 taken from *Endocrine and Genetic Diseases of Childhood*, Ed. Lytt Gardiner, W. B. Saunders, Philadelphia, in press, and Prof. Tanner and Blackwell Scientific Publications for permission to use Figure 2.

BIBLIOGRAPHY

Bayley, N. and Pinneau, S. R. (1952), "Tables for Predicting Adult Height from Skeletal Age: revised for use with the Greulich-Pyle Hand Standards," *J. Pediat.*, **40**, 423–41 (erratum corrected in *J. Pediat.*, **41**, 371).

Bayley, N., Gordon, G. S., Bayer, L. M., Goldberg, M. B. and Storment, A. (1962), "Attempt to Suppress Excessive Growth in Girls by Estrogen Treatment: Statistical Evaluation," *J. Clin. Endocr.*, **22**, 1127–1129.

Bloom, B. S. (1964), *Stability and Change in Human Characteristics.* New York: Wiley.

Bojlén, K. W., Rasch, G. and Weis-Bentzon, M. (1954), "The Age Incidence of the Menarche in Copenhagen," *Acta obstet. gynec. scand.*, **33**, 405–433.

Boutourline Young, H. and Boutourline Young, E. (1956), "Alveolar Carbon Dioxide Levels in Pregnant, Parturient and Lactating Subjects," *J. obstet. gynaec. Brit. Emp.*, **63**, 509–528.

Boutourline Young, H., Zoli, A. and Gallagher, J. R. (1963), "Events of Puberty in a Group of 111 Florentine Girls," *Amer. J. Dis. Child.*, **106**, 568–577.

Boutourline Young, H. (1965), *Body Composition, Culture and Sex. Human Body Composition*, pp. 139–159. Oxford: Pergamon Press.

Buck, C. and Stavraky, K. (1967), "The Relation Between Age at Menarche and Age at Marriage Among Childbearing Women," *Hum. Biol.*, **39**, 93–102.

Ellis, R. W. B. (1950), "Age of Puberty in the Tropics," *Brit. med. J.*, **1**, 85–89.

Eveleth, P. B. (1966), "Eruption of Permanent Teeth and Menarche of American Children Living in the Tropics," *Hum. Biol.*, **38**, 60–70.

Gallagher, J. R. (1960), *Medical Care of the Adolescent.* New York: Appleton Century Crofts.

Gardiner, L. (Editor) (in press) *Endocrine and Genetic Diseases of Childhood.* W. B. Saunders, Philadelphia.

Gardiner, P. A. (1954), "The Relation of Myopia to Growth," *Lancet*, **1**, 476–478.

Garn, S. M. (1952), "Changes in Areolar Size During the Steroid Growth Phase, *Child Develop.*, **23**, 55–60.

Garn, S. M. and Rohmann, C. G. (1966), "Interaction of Nutrition and Genetics in the Timing of Growth and Development," *Pediat. Clin. N. Amer.*, **13**, 353–379.

Greulich, W. W. and Pyle, S. I. (1950), *Radiographic Atlas of Skeletal Development of the Hand and Wrist.* 190 pp. Stanford, California: Stanford University Press.

Iliff, A. and Lee, V. A. (1952), "Pulse Rate, Respiratory Rate, and Body Temperature of Children Between Two months and Eighteen Years of Age," *Child Develop.*, **23**, 237–245.

Ito, P. K. (1942), "Comparative Biometrical Study of Physique of Japanese Women Born and Reared Under Different Environments," *Hum. Biol.*, **14**, 279–351.

Kinsey, A. C., Pomeroy, S. E., Martin, C. E. and Gebhard, P. H. (1953), *Sexual Behavior in the Human Female.* Philadelphia: Saunders.

Livson, N. and McNeill, D. (1962), "The Accuracy of Recalled Age of Menarche," *Hum. Biol.*, **34**, 218–221.

Masland, R. P., Heald, F. P., Hill, W. R. and Gallagher, J. R. (1956), "Some Comments on Acne Vulgaris in Adolescents," *J. Pediat.*, **49**, 680–684.

McNeill, D. and Livson, N. (1963), "Maturation Rate and Body Build in Women," *Child Develop.*, **34**, 25–32.

Mills, C. A. (1942), "Climatic Effects on Growth and Development with Particular Reference to the Effects of Tropical Residence," *Amer. Anthrop.*, **44**, 1–14.

Nicolson, A. B. and Hanley, C. (1953), "Indices of Physiological Maturity: Derivation and Inter-relationships," *Child Develop.*, **24**, 3–38.

Reynolds, E. L. and Wines, J. V. (1948), "Individual Differences in Physical Changes Associated with Adolescence in Girls," *Amer. J. Dis. Child.*, **75**, 329–350.

Scott, J. A. (1961), *Report on the Heights and Weights (and Other Measurements) of School Pupils in the County of London in 1959.* London: County Council.

Simmons, K. and Greulich, W. W. (1943), "Menarchal Age and the Height, Weight and Skeletal Age of Girls 7 to 17 Years," *Amer. J. Ped.*, **22**, 518–548.

Shock, N. W. (1943), "The Effect of Menarche on Basal Physiological Function in Girls," *Amer. J. Physiol.*, **139**, 288–292.

Shock, N. W. (1946), "Some Physiological Aspects of Adolescence," *Texas Rep. Biol. Med.*, **4**, 368–386.

Slataper, F. J. (1950), "Age Norms of Refraction and Vision," *Arch. Ophthal. (N.Y.) N.S.*, **43**, 466–481.

Stukowsky, R., Valsik, J. A. and Bulai-Stirbu, M. (1967), "Family Size and Menarchal Age in Constanza, Romania," *Hum. Biol.*, **39**, 277–283.

Tanner, J. M. (1962), *Growth at Adolescence*, 2nd ed., pp. 95–104. Oxford, England: Blackwell Scientific Publications.

Tanner, J. M. and Whitehouse, R. H. (1955), "The Harpenden Skin Fold Caliper," *Amer. J. phys. Anthrop. N.S.*, **13**, 743–746.

Tanner, J. M. and Whitehouse, R. H. (1959), *Standards for Skeletal Maturity*, Part 1. Paris: International Children's Centre.

Tanner, J. M., Whitehouse, R. H. and Healey, M. J. R. (1962), *A New System for Estimating Skeletal Maturity from the Hand and Wrist with Standards Derived from a Study of 2600 Healthy British Children*, Part 2, The Scoring System. Paris: International Children's Centre.

Tanner, J. M. and O'Keefe, B. (1962), "Age at Menarche in Nigerian Schoolgirls, with a Note on their Heights and Weights from Age 12 to 19," *Hum. Biol.*, **34**, 187–196.

Thoma, A. (1960), "Age at Menarche, Acceleration and Heritability," *Acta Biologica Acad. Sci. Hungaria*, **11**, 241–254.

Valsik, J. A. (1965), "The Seasonable Rhythm of Menarche: a Review," *Hum. Biol.*, **37**, 75–90.

Vanzant, F. R., Alvarez, W. C., Eusterman, G. B., Dunn, H. L. and Berkson, J. (1932), "The Normal Range of Gastric Acidity from Youth to Old Age," *Arch. int. Med.*, **49**, 345–359.

Whitehead, J. (1847), *On the Causes and Treatment of Abortion and Sterility.* London: Churchill. Manchester: Simms & Dinham.

Wofinden, R. C. and Smallwood, A. L. (1958), *School Health Service, Annual Report of the Principal School Medical Officer to City and County of Bristol Education Committee.* Bristol.

Zukowski, W., Kmietowicz-Zukowska, A. and Gruska, S. (1964), "The Age at Menarche in Polish Girls," *Hum. Biol.*, **36**, 233–234.

SECTION XI

BACTERIOLOGY

1. MICROBIOLOGY

ROSALINDE HURLEY

Normal Bacterial Flora of the Human Body
(Wilson and Miles, 1964)

The distribution of various types of bacteria in the human body has received little systematic study, save with respect to the incidence of a few important pathogens. Thus, at present, it is not possible to give a complete account, and the paragraphs that follow must be regarded as approximate descriptions of the true basal ecological state, and, moreover, pertaining chiefly to investigations carried out principally in temperate climates and amongst western communities.

Mouth and Saliva

Amongst the common bacteria isolated are (1) micrococci: some are anaerobic, some are pigment producing (2) *Staphylococcus albus* and *Staphylococcus aureus* (3) streptococci: of these, α haemolytic streptococci (*Str. viridans*) are constantly present, but *Str. pyogenes* (β haemolytic streptococcus Lancefield Group A) is exceedingly rare, if, indeed, it occurs in normal persons at all. Other β haemolytic streptococci (for example, of groups B, C, G, F or ungroupable) occur in 5–10 per cent of throat swabs. (4) lactobacilli, and aerobic spore bearers (*Bacillus*) (5) coliform bacilli, *Proteus* and other intestinal organisms (6) spirochaetes and fusiform bacilli (7) actinomycetes (8) pleuropneumonia-like organisms, and tiny, Gram-negative anaerobic cocci, *Veillonella* (9) yeasts, especially *Candida albicans* (10) *Corynebacterium spp.* (diphtheroids) (11) *Neisseria spp.* (12) *Nocardia* and *Leptotrichia*. In routine clinical bacteriological practice, in Southern England, the most commonly reported bacteria are *Str. viridans*, diphtheroids, *Neisseria* and staphylococci.

The infant's mouth becomes colonized within a few days of birth, and the main source of the colonizing organisms is the maternal vagina. Most of the normal mouth flora is sensitive to penicillin, and after treatment with this antibiotic, yeasts and coliform bacilli predominate.

The Intestine

At birth, the intestine may contain a few bacteria, and it is rapidly colonized. The flora of the breast fed infant consists largely of anaerobic lactobacilli, (about 99 per cent), but coliforms are also present. After weaning, the flora resembles that of the adult.

The empty stomach is usually sterile. Bacteria are ingested with food, but most are rapidly killed by the digestive juices. The jejunum and the upper ileum are practically sterile. The flora of the lower ileum is scanty but similar to that of the large intestine : obligatory

anaerobic, non-sporing species predominate, and bacteria, mostly dead, are said to make up $\frac{1}{4}$ to $\frac{1}{3}$ by weight of the faeces. *Clostridia*, coliforms, enterococci, staphylococci, fungi (especially *Candida spp.*) and *Proteus* also occur. *Staph. aureus*, *Pseudomonas aeruginosa*, *Klebsiella spp.* and anthracoids as well as β haemolytic streptococci (Lancefield Group D) are encountered. *Escherichia coli* is predominant amongst the coliforms. The organisms reported as occurring in routine specimens of faeces in Southern England are mainly lactose and non-lactose fermenting coliforms, staphylococci and enterococci and *Proteus* and *Pseudomonas*. This distribution reflects the cultural methods in routine use, which do not include anaerobic techniques.

Respiratory Tract

The bacterial flora of the nasal passages is less copious than that of the nasopharynx, and consists chiefly of *Staph. aureus*, *Staph. albus* and diphtheroids. *Str. viridans*, non-haemolytic streptococci, and Gram-negative cocci, often of *Neisseria pharyngis* type, are the basal flora of the naso- and oro-pharynx. The accessory nasal sinuses are normally sterile, and the trachea and bronchi contain few bacteria. There is little difference between bronchial swabs from healthy persons and from those with respiratory disease, and the frequency of *Str. viridans*, micrococci, Gram-negative cocci and *Haemophilus spp.* is substantial in both. *Str. pneumoniae* and yeasts are also cultivated from the respiratory tract, and *N. meningitidis* is carried in some populations.

Potentially pathogenic staphylococci are part of the normal flora of the nose, and carrier rates of up to 70 per cent have been recorded for healthy nurses, (Williams, *et al.*, 1966).

The upper respiratory tract of the infant is colonized soon after birth, particularly after close contact with the mother at the first feed, (about 12 hours).

The Vulva, Vestibulum and Vagina

The vulva and vestibulum of the newborn are sterile, organisms appearing in 7–8 hours. The commonest aerobic organisms are staphylococci, diphtheroids, enterococci, coliform bacilli and yeasts. Many anaerobes also occur, but pathogenic bacteria are uncommon. The vulval flora is distinct from the vaginal flora, save immediately after parturition and for the first few days of the puerperium.

The vagina of the newborn is sterile, and organisms appear in 12–14 hours. Staphylococci, enterococci and diphtheroids appear at first, but are replaced in 2–3 days by an almost pure culture of Döderlein's bacilli. At this time the vaginal secretion is acid, and glycogen is demonstrable in the vaginal epithelium. The occurrence of glycogen appears to be due to the presence of oestrin derived from the maternal circulation. Soon this is excreted in the urine, and the vaginal secretion becomes alkaline. Thereafter, until puberty, the secretion remains alkaline, and staphylococci, streptococci other than *Str. pyogenes*, coliforms and diphtheroid bacilli predominate. At puberty, glycogen is again deposited in the vaginal wall, the secretion becomes acid, and Döderlein's bacilli are re-established as the predominant organisms. The flora is mixed, and streptococci, diphtheroids and fungi are present. The streptococci of the vagina are varied and *Str. faecalis* (Lancefield Group D) is common; Lancefield Groups C, B, F, and G occur but are less frequent. *Str. viridans* is occasionally found, but it is doubtful whether anaerobic streptococci ever occur in the normal vagina. *Mycoplasma* (pleuro-pneumonia-like organisms) can be demonstrated occasionally. In addition to these organisms, numbers of Gram-negative rods, not all being members of the *Enterobacteriaceae*, are encountered, and some Gram-negative cocco-bacilli bearing a superficial resemblance to *Haemophilus spp.* are found.

The Urethra

The female urethra is either sterile or contains a few non-pathogenic cocci, and coryneform bacteria. The saprophytic acid fast bacillus *Mycobacterium smegmatis* may be present, and, if contaminating the urine, may be mistaken for *Mycobacterium tuberculosis*.

The Skin

The flora of the skin may be classified into the "resident" flora, those species that multiply freely, particularly in the sebaceous glands, and the "transient" flora. Staphylococci, including *Staph. albus* and *Staph. aureus*, and micrococci, are found, and Gram-negative bacilli (*Mima, Moraxella*, anitratus group of organisms) and diphtheroids, are also encountered. Coliforms, fungi, enterococci and *Proteus spp.* are seldom isolated. Anaerobic organisms outnumber the aerobic and are chiefly lactobacilli. In the newborn, *Staph. albus* and diphtheroids predominate.

Str. pyogenes (Lancefield Group A) can be transiently carried on the skin, as can other pathogenic bacteria, but healthy skin seems to have some natural self-disinfecting mechanism, so that implanted organisms are rapidly eliminated.

Human Milk

Large numbers of bacteria occur in human milk, but if this is collected under strictly aseptic conditions, the plate count should not exceed 2,500 organisms/ml. Micrococci, diphtheroids, occasional coliforms, staphylococci, non-haemolytic streptococci and anaerobic lactobacilli are isolated, and the milk of healthy nursing mothers delivered in hospital often contains appreciable numbers of *Staph. aureus*.

Abnormal Flora

Exogenous Microbes. In many bacterial diseases, for example, the epidemics associated with exogenous microbes, the demonstration of a particular microbe is an indication of morbidity, or, at the very least, of carriage, subsequent to infection, and likely to be harmful to others. The salmonellae and shigellae are never part of a normal flora, although some species may be carried for weeks or months after the original infection has subsided. *Pasteurella pestis* is never isolated from a normal flora, although very similar organisms may be found as secondary invaders of the respiratory tract, and *Pasteurella pseudotuberculosis* is sometimes isolated from the diseased appendix. *Neisseria gonorrhoeae* and *Treponema pallidum* are strict parasites. The isolation of *Mycobacterium tuberculosis* is pathognomonic of tuberculosis, although some other mycobacteria (the anonymous mycobacteria) may occur as commensals, principally in the respiratory tract. *Str. pyogenes* (Lancefield Group A) is not an inhabitant of the healthy vagina, or throat. When exogenous, or strictly parasitic, organisms are isolated, the interpretation of findings is easy and direct.

Endogenous Microbes isolated from sites normally sterile or sites remote from their normal habitat

In other diseases, commensal bacteria are isolated from sites that are remote from their customary habitat. This is an abnormal situation. If chance contamination can be excluded, it is usually associated with morbidity. Thus, the isolation of bacteria from sites normally sterile, such as the bloodstream, urinary tract, or body fluids is extremely strong presumptive evidence of infection. Occasionally, organisms generally regarded as "non-pathogenic", such as coagulase negative staphylococci, are isolated from the cerebrospinal fluid, the urine or the bloodstream. Careful consideration must be given to the clinical state of the patient before such organisms are discounted as laboratory contaminants. Again, while it is normal to isolate *Cl. welchii* from the stools or from a small percentage of vaginal swabs due to contamination from the perineum, it is abnormal to isolate it from wounds; however, even in this situation, its mere presence will not warrant a diagnosis of gas gangrene, in the absence of clinical signs of infection. The presence of the microbe may prognosticate gangrene.

Endogenous Microbes isolated from their normal habitat, but associated with Sepsis

Some commensals of man belong to the category of microbes that pathologists call "opportunistic" organisms. Only occasionally do they exert a hostile effect on their hosts, usually when general or local resistance is lowered as a consequence of debilitating disease, trauma, haemorrhage or other conditions, or in consequence of a particular physiological state such as the state of being newly born, or pregnant. When such microbes cause disease localized to body areas where they are usually, or often, demonstrable as commensals, the assignment to them of a pathogenic role cannot be inferred simply from the cultural findings. Thus staphylococci are normal denizens of the skin, conjunctiva, the naso-pharynx, the vagina and the alimentary tract. Their demonstration in these sites is to be expected. None the less, the newborn is especially prone to skin or conjunctival sepsis caused by staphylococci. *Candida albicans* is a normal inhabitant of the vagina, and its isolation from this site will not warrant a diagnosis of vaginitis in the absence of symptoms. During pregnancy, the incidence of candida vaginitis rises. Thus pregnancy provides the yeast with an opportunity for causing a morbid process, but we do not know the mechanism underlying the increased susceptibility of the host. Clearly, the proof that an organism, normally commensal in a given site, is responsible for disease in that particular site, cannot rest solely on demonstration of the microbe, but must be interpreted in conjunction with the clinical findings, and where appropriate, the results of other laboratory tests. The reaction of the host to the microbe must be shown to be abnormal, since the presence of the microbe is not.

GENERAL CONSIDERATIONS

Infections in Gynaecological Practice

Infections of the Reproductive Tract. Only one common infection is peculiar to the female reproductive organs: this is vaginitis caused by the protozoan, *Trichomonas vaginalis*, and occurs in the non-pregnant as well as in the pregnant.

Infections of the reproductive tract are rare in infancy and childhood, although epidemic vulvo-vaginitis caused by gonococci, streptococci and staphylococci can occur in institutions, and sporadic cases, often associated with *Str. pyogenes*, also occur. Acute infections of the vagina in adult women are usually caused by *Trichomonas* or *Candida spp.* These infections may prove resistant to treatment, and become chronic. Even with adequate treatment, relapse is frequent, and since both infections can be harboured by the sexual partner, reinfection is often venereal.

Bacteria rarely cause vaginitis in the mature female. Attempts have been made to equate "non-specific vaginitis" with particular microbes, the most recent and successful of these being the alleged association between vaginitis, and an organism named "Haemophilus vaginalis". However, taxonomists do not admit the existence of such an organism as a distinct species (Cowan and Steel, 1965) and critical appraisals of organisms labelled with this name have shown a diversity of bacteria, some being *Haemophilus spp.*, and others not. Small Gram-negative rods abound in the vagina, and belong to many genera. However, the distinctive epithelial cells described by Gardner and Dukes (1955) are certainly seen in cases of vaginitis not associated with *Trichomonas* and *Candida*, and the aetiology may well be infective, as they suggest. An infective role has been suggested for pleuro-pneumonia like organisms (*Mycoplasma*) (see Marmion, 1967). Bacterial vaginitis can occur in elderly women, and is caused by streptococci, and pyogenic organisms such as *Escherichia coli*, and staphylococci. Senile endometritis and pyometra also occur.

The gonococcus causes acute or chronic disease of the reproductive organs, and syphilis and tuberculosis both effect the reproductive tract.

Wound Infections are important causes of morbidity in surgical practice. Their prevention cannot be discussed here, and the reader is referred to the book by Williams *et al.* (1966).

Infections Complicating Pregnancy and the Puerperium

Any of the acute or chronic specific infectious diseases may be contracted during the course of pregnancy or the puerperium, and conception may occur in women already subject to infection. The co-existence of pregnancy may aggravate the risk to maternal life of the more serious of these diseases, and some constitute a hazard to the foetus, and the newborn. Foetal death may result from contagion, for some viruses, bacteria and protozoa are able to cross the placental barrier; or it may be caused by placental insufficiency, hyperpyrexia, or maternal exhaustion and toxaemia. The newborn may contract a transmissible disease from close contact with an infected mother shortly after birth, or, as a result of maternal infection, it may be born in a sickly and marasmic condition, and soon succumb to intercurrent infection. In the early part of the puerperium, parturient women are peculiarly susceptible to serious infections of the genital tract, and child bed fever has always been one of the most important causes of maternal death.

The incidence of infection is greatest in malnourished and unhygienic communities and in areas where serious epidemic and endemic microbial diseases are rife. Many of these diseases are preventable. Rigorous campaigns to improve the general standards of hygiene, and the introduction of measures specifically designed to control communicable disease are accompanied by a lessening of the maternal, foetal and perinatal mortality and morbidity rates. The importance of the public health services to maternal and foetal life and health cannot be exaggerated, and a good service provides the soundest scientific basis for the development of high standards of obstetric care and practice.

Pregnancy and the Puerperium

Fortuitous Infections: Acute. Casual or chance infections occurring during pregnancy range from mild illnesses to the major microbial diseases.

In the Far East and in other parts of Asia, in Africa and South America, pregnant women may be exposed to diseases such as smallpox, cholera, plague, dysenteries, and the enteric fevers. Pandemic viral diseases (influenza) also occur, and may be world wide. The untreated mortality rates of these diseases are high. Abortion or premature birth may occur in the course of the illness, and the baby, if born viable, may be sickly and weak. In parts of Africa, Asia and the Americas, severe, systemic fungal infections such as coccidioidomycosis, histoplasmosis and North and South American blastomycosis occur, and, rarely, may be transmitted to the foetus. Parasitic infestations with the organisms of hookworm, tapeworm, bilharzia and other diseases are common in many parts of the world, and it is important to bear in mind that as a world producer of death and morbidity, malaria is second to none.

Although serious microbial disease is well controlled in the United Kingdom, mothers of young children, particularly of those at school, are exposed to the specific infectious diseases of childhood, and, in addition to the common upper respiratory tract infections, may contract mumps, chickenpox, measles, rubella, scarlet fever, acute bacterial tonsillitis, whooping cough, dysentery or viral diarrhoeas. As young adults, the mothers may contract toxoplasmosis, or poliomyelitis. Some of these diseases have important consequences in obstetric practice but all pose a problem if the mother's antenatal condition necessitates admission to an obstetric unit.

The occurrence of highly infectious diseases in antenatal patients who require in-patient obstetric care is sometimes neglected by hospital planners, who are occasionally heard to deny the need for isolation facilities in maternity hospitals. This viewpoint is defensible only if the obstetric unit is part of a larger hospital, and an isolation unit is available nearby. Unaffected pregnant and parturient women and the newborn must be protected from exposure to the organisms of rubella, scarlet fever and the dysenteries, for infection may prove fatal to foetus, mother, or newborn. At the same time, proper obstetric care should not be denied to those already infected. If the need arises, they should be admitted to an obstetric unit, but they must be nursed in isolation, and the greatest care taken with the disposal of putatively or actually contaminated fomites and excreta. If the patients are to be taken to the operating theatre or delivery room, scrupulous arrangements must be made to avoid dissemination of the infection. The staff of the isolation wards must be thoroughly conversant with the principles underlying the control of communicable disease, and the patients should be nursed in separate rooms. Adequate and separate bathing and toilet facilities should be provided. The patients should not be admitted to the general wards of the obstetric unit until they are adjudged free of specific infection. Often this necessitates prolonged bacteriological tests, but these should not be avoided as the safety of other patients may depend upon them. The same general considerations apply to all patients in a maternity unit known or suspected to be suffering from a contagious disease, whether contracted within or outside the hospital.

The venereal diseases may be contracted at any time during pregnancy or the puerperium, and those that could have fatal or crippling effects on the foetus are sought during the antenatal period. Routine serological tests for syphilis are performed during pregnancy, usually at the first visit.

The other venereal diseases, gonorrhoea, chancroid, granuloma inguinale and lymphogranuloma venereum are sought during pregnancy at the routine antenatal clinical examinations, by the eliciting of the medical and social history, by physical examination and by appropriate laboratory tests. The occurrence of an acute fortuitous infection in the puerperium may be diagnosed during the lying in period or noted at the routine post-natal visit (6–8 weeks after delivery). Exacerbation of caries, and dental sepsis, occurs during pregnancy, and women with valvular disease of the heart are at risk of subacute bacterial endocarditis if dental surgery is necessitated.

Pregnancy

Fortuitous Infections: Chronic. Pregnancy may occur in the course of a chronic infection, or chronic infection may first be diagnosed during pregnancy. Its detection is one of the purposes of the general medical examination made at the first antenatal visit. Radiographic examination of the chest to diagnose or exclude pulmonary tuberculosis is standard practice in the United Kingdom, as are serological tests for syphilis. Other chronic infections are less commonly encountered, but actinomycosis, leprosy, gonorrhoea and other venereal diseases, brucellosis and chronic systemic fungal and parasitic diseases do occur. If the infection is open and communicable women with these diseases should be segregated from other patients and from their newborn children. Vectors of the diseases should be controlled.

Infections Associated with Pregnancy

These are all acute infections, although recrudescence of chronic infections may occur. None is peculiar to pregnancy, but their incidence is increased in the pregnant as compared with the non-pregnant women. Infections of the urinary tract are common complications of pregnancy, and increasing emphasis is being placed on their early diagnosis and treatment. Any part of the renal tract may be involved, and with modern bacteriological techniques infection by significant numbers of organisms can be detected before the onset of symptoms. These infections may be acute and primary, or a recrudescence of chronic infection. They range from urethritis to acute pyelonephritis, and the more common causes in pregnancy are members of the *Enterobacteriaceae*, and related genera of Gram-negative rods, as well as the pathogenic cocci. The relationship of urinary tract sepsis to abortion and stillbirth is not established.

The incidence of vulvo-vaginitis is increased in pregnancy, and the increase is occasioned largely by infections with members of the genus *Candida*, the fungi of thrush. The other important cause of vaginitis in pregnancy is the protozoan parasite *Trichomonas vaginalis*.

The Puerperium

Infections Associated with the Puerperium. These are acute infections and the most notorious is infection of the genital tract, which formerly accounted for the majority of deaths from infection in pregnancy and the puerperium, and is still the most important cause of death from infection in obstetric practice in the United Kingdom. Inflammation and suppuration of the lactating breast may occur in the puerperium, and urinary tract infections are fairly frequent. Women who have been subjected to surgery may develop bronchopneumonia, or wound infections. All are common causes of elevation of the temperature in the lying in period.

Infections in Intra-uterine and Neonatal Life (Schaffer, 1966;
Janeway, 1966)

The newborn is peculiarly prone to certain infections, and is less able to localize them than the adult. Conversely, the newborn is immune to some other infections and immunity continues for several months after birth. The immunological status of the newborn is the resultant of two systems: the first is active, and depends on his own capacity to develop immunity; the second is passive, and is derived from the transfer of maternal antibody during gestation. Immunity in the neonatal period, to diseases like mumps and measles is the consequence of transferred immunity from the mother. The infant is temporarily immune from certain diseases if the mother has suffered from them or is herself immune. Common diseases in which immunity is transferred from mother to foetus are measles, scarlet fever, diphtheria and poliomyelitis, chicken pox, smallpox and mumps; antitoxins to diphtheria, scarlet fever, and tetanus are often present in the same concentration as in maternal blood. Virus antibodies may confer on the child an immunity that lasts for from six to twelve months, although antibodies to bacterial antigens do not persist so long. The foetus begins to take up antibody by the fourth to the sixth month of gestation, and the quantity rises during the last months. Transmission of antibody from mother to foetus is an active, and a selective process; thus, some antibodies in cord blood may be equal to or higher than those in maternal blood, for example, tetanus or diphtheria antitoxin, while others, such as streptococcal agglutinins, may be considerably lower, or even absent.

At birth, the newborn is not fully competent to respond to all antigens in an adult fashion, although he can respond to some. This lack of full immunological competence is reflected in the physiological dysglobulinaemia of normal neonates. The foetus manufactures its own albumin and its own α and β globulin, but almost its entire store of γ globulin is maternally derived, and the total level in the newborn is about the same level as that of its mother, or even slightly higher. This falls rapidly during the first month of life and remains at a low level for about three months. After this, it rises slowly, reaching adult levels by about the age of two.

Most of the γ globulin of the newborn is maternally derived IgG (7S) globulin, and the infant starts elaborating this fraction of immune antibody at about four weeks, when plasma cells appear in the bone marrow, spleen and lymph nodes. A small proportion of neonatal γ globulin is IgM (19S), and is entirely of foetal origin, since maternal IgM does not cross the placental barrier. IgM continues to be elaborated after birth, and reaches adult levels by nine months. The third fraction, IgA (7S–12S) is not transferred *via* the placenta, or elaborated by the foetus, and thus is absent from cord blood. IgA begin to be elaborated at about three weeks of age, but adult levels are not reached until adolescence. The dysglobulinaemia of the newborn consists of lack of IgA, and paucity of IgM. In addition most of its store of IgG is derived from its mother.

The response of adults to antigenic stimulation consists of production of IgM, followed quickly by production of IgG. The pattern of response in the newborn is different; IgM is elaborated as a first response, but this response persists for several weeks before IgG is elaborated.

The reasons for the poor response of the newborn to certain infections are not clearly understood, but there is some evidence that in addition to the physiological dysglobulinaemia mentioned above, the cellular response to infection varies in the newborn, and the phagocytes are less active. The distribution of leucocytes in the blood of newborns also differs from that of the adult: the total white cell count varies from 5,000–25,000 per cmm., and of these from 30–70 per cent are polymorphonuclear leucocytes. In general the newborn responds to pyogenic infections by a rise in numbers of polymorphonuclear leucocytes. The percentage of mononuclear cells is high (5–17 per cent) in the first two weeks of neonatal life, but falls thereafter, while the eosinophilic leucocytes, initially low in numbers, rise to 5–6 per cent in the next 3–4 days, falling to adult levels after this.

Infections such as rubella, cytomegalic inclusion disease, toxoplasmosis and listeriosis may be disseminated and fatal in the newborn while rarely so in the adult; and certain bacteria, such as *Flavobacterium meningosepticum*, cause meningitis in the newborn but are never isolated as pathogens in adults. There is, therefore, in the newborn a proclivity towards severe infections with organisms that in the adult are usually of low virulence or even, perhaps, non-pathogenic, (e.g. some staphylococci); and there is furthermore a tendency for microbial diseases to disseminate, with fatal consequence.

The commonest source of infection in the newborn, and the only frequent source in the foetus, is the mother. Protozoa, viruses, bacteria and fungi can all pass the placental barrier, and cause congenital infections, or death *in utero*. Organisms notorious for transmission *via* this route include the pneumococcus, *Salmonella typhi*, malarial parasites, *Treponema pallidum*, the viruses of rubella and cytomegalic inclusion disease and *Toxoplasma gondii*. The foetus can be infected directly during operative procedures, such as intra-uterine blood transfusions, and is prone to infection *via* the amniotic fluid when the membranes have been ruptured longer than 24 hours. Infections transmitted postnatally, such as gonorrhoea or candidosis usually derive from the mother, but rarely the nurse or other human contact provides the source. Strict attention to regimes of personal and ward hygiene, and scrupulous care in the preparation of bottle feeds in nurseries, lowers the incidence of certain infections of the newborn (See Winner and Hurley, 1964, pp. 96–100). It is plain that the importance of nurses and nursery personnel as vectors of disease can be greatly diminished through the imposition of rigorous standards of hygiene. There is general agreement that prematurity, prolonged labour, prolonged rupture of the membranes, vigorous manipulative or operative delivery, and maternal infection all predispose to infection of the newborn. These are regarded by many physicians as indications for prophylaxis in the newborn period with non-toxic, broad-spectrum antibiotics.

The most frequent cause of neonatal sepsis in the United Kingdom is *Staphylococcus aureus*, but *Str. pyogenes* may occasionally cause septicaemia and meningitis and peritonitis. Meningitis and septicaemia may also be caused by *Escherichia coli*, and by other Gram-negative bacteria, including *Pseudomonas aeruginosa*, and poorly classified organisms in the *Achromobacter*, *Mima*, *Moraxella* groups, or *Alkaligenes* group. These infections often occur in premature babies, and may be associated with artificially raised humidity. The aetiology of severe forms of epidemic diarrhoea of the newborn is still disputed. Occasionally salmonellae are isolated, orpathogenic (typable) *Escherichia coli*, and, probably, other cases have a viral aetiology. Other forms may be non-infective (see Wilson and Miles, 1964, p. 1894–1909).

Because of the susceptibility of the newborn to infection rigorous aseptic and antiseptic techniques are used in hospital nurseries. The index of cross infection in hospitals in the United Kingdom is usually taken to be the coagulase positive staphylococcus, although infection with coagulase negative staphylococci almost certainly occurs in newborns. Williams *et al.*, (1966) give a full account of procedures used to control hospital infection, and Gordon (1965) discusses the control of communicable disease in general.

TYPES OF INFECTIONS AND SPECIFIC INFECTIONS

Since some broad classes of infection, for example, wound and puerperal infection, ophthalmia neonatorum, or urinary tract infections may be caused by diverse microbes, a general account of these precedes that of specific infections. The only specific infections discussed will be those occurring commonly in the United Kingdom, and apparently rare infections that are currently receiving intensive study.

Urinary Tract Infections

Urinary tract infections are common in women, and are particularly likely to occur during pregnancy, labour and the puerperium. Infections of all grades of severity are encountered and any part of the urinary tract may be involved. Thus the infections range from mild urethritis, through cystitis, and pyelitis to pyelonephritis.

At the beginning of the antibiotic era, the incidence of frank pyelitis of pregnancy was 1·2 per cent, and the maternal mortality 3·58 per cent (McLane, 1939). Foetal loss, from premature termination of the pregnancy, was 15·8 per cent, and in some series it was up to 30 per cent. The complete clinical picture of frank pyelitis is seen far less commonly nowadays, almost certainly owing to the prompt administration of antibiotics to women with signs or symptoms of infection of the urinary tract. Characteristically, the onset is about the 5th or 6th month of pregnancy, or in the 1st week of the puerperium; and the symptoms include fever, rigors, headache, pain in the renal angle, dysuria and frequency. Examination of the urine usually shows a strongly acid urine, loaded with organisms and pus cells, and, sometimes, with frank blood. Pro-

teinuria also occurs. Under 10 cases a year, in 3,500 deliveries, are now seen at Queen Charlotte's Maternity Hospital. Subacute, or low grade, infections are far more common than pyelitis, and between 2–4 per cent of all women under in-patient care at Queen Charlotte's Maternity Hospital are treated at some time during pregnancy, or the puerperium, for urinary tract infection.

The route of infection is probably an ascending one, and the risk of introducing infection by catheterization has long been recognized. Much hospital-acquired infection, following catheterization or operations on the bladder, is associated with organisms that are being disseminated in the wards (Wilson and Miles, 1964, p. 1801). Another route of infection is the lymphatic system; the right kidney has a direct connection, *via* the lymphatics, with the ascending colon to which it is directly related (Martius, 1941). Infection may be bloodborne, and blood cultures are frequently positive in pyelitis. Experimentally, organisms such as *Staph. aureus*, *Ps. aeruginosa*, and faecal streptococci, if injected into laboratory animals by the intravenous route, cause localized disease of the kidneys. Intravenous injection of *Esch. coli* will not produce renal lesions unless the ureter is ligated, or the kidney has been previously damaged.

Mechanical factors, particularly those factors that obstruct urinary flow, are important in promoting bacterial infection of the urinary tract, and the immediate predisposing cause of urinary tract infections in pregnancy is stasis. Progesterone causes dilation of the ureters, and oestrogens cause muscular hypertrophy, at a time when changing anatomical relationships in the pelvis and abdomen lead especially to compression of the right ureter.

Most of the infections that occur sporadically in the population are caused by *Esch. coli*, and this organism is the one most frequently isolated in obstetric and gynaecological practice. Organisms less frequently encountered include *Proteus spp.*, *Str. faecalis*, *Klebsiella spp.*, staphylococci and *Ps. aeruginosa*. Pyelitis may be recurrent and may be followed by chronic pyelonephritis, or the latter may develop without apparent acute episodes. Pyelitis of pregnancy is often a clinical manifestation of an inapparent infection, aggravated by the stasis of pregnancy. Such inapparent infections were, in the past, described as the asymptomatic bacteriuria of pregnancy. They occur throughout the population, but the incidence is highest in pregnant women.

Kass (1955) demonstrated that quantitative culture of urine specimens that were freshly voided was a reliable means of detecting urinary infection, and he accepted 100,000 organisms/ml. as presumptive evidence of urinary tract infection. If this number of organisms is detected in two successive specimens, a correct diagnosis of infection would be made in 96 per cent of cases. In about half of the infections detected in this way, there is no excess of leucocytes in the urine. Nearly all acute and active chronic infections can be detected by quantitative bacteriological methods, although some patients with long standing chronic pyelonephritis do not excrete organisms in the urine. An increase in the rate of excretion of white cells after the intravenous injection of predniso-lone may help in such cases. The biology of pyelonephritis is discussed by Quinn and Kass (1960).

The bacteriological diagnosis of urinary tract sepsis thus depends on quantitative examination of freshly voided urine. The urine sample is a mid stream specimen, which should be collected under aseptic, but not anti-septic, conditions and examined as soon as possible. If examination is to be delayed, the sample may be refri-gerated for short periods. In view of the risk of infection, catheter specimens of urine are no longer used for diagnos-tic work. The methods used to enumerate bacteria vary from laboratory to laboratory, but pour plate techniques, and surface inoculation of plates with measured quantities of urine are amongst the most frequently used. In addi-tion the urine is cultured aerobically on blood agar and on MacConkey's medium and the organisms are identified. If the growth is significant, antibiotic sensitivity tests are performed. The pH of the urine is then determined, urinary protein is measured, and the deposit is examined for the presence of casts, red cells and pus cells. Red cells and white cells are better enumerated in a counting chamber than assessed per high power field. An excess leucocyte count of more than 20 cells per ml. is likely to indicate sepsis, and the presence of microscopic blood is inferred from the differential red/white cell count.

Puerperal Sepsis and Wound Infections

Puerperal sepsis includes a series of febrile disorders of the lying-in period that share the common aetiology of being wound infections of the genital tract. It may occur after delivery or abortion, and is occasioned by several genera of pathogenic bacteria, of which the most notorious and dangerous are *Streptococcus* and *Clostridia*. Some of the infecting microbes may have been present in the genital tract before or during labour (endogenous infec-tion) but in the great majority of fatal cases, the organisms are introduced from without (exogenous infection); and such infections are preventable.

The contagiousness of child-bed or milk fever was postulated before the promulgation of the theory of "vegetable parasitism" by bacteria; and was, indeed, in part demonstrated. Charles White of Manchester (1793) and Robert Gordon, of Aberdeen (1785) believed puerperal fever to be infectious, and the pioneer epidemio-logical studies of Oliver Wendell Holmes in the United States and of Semmelweis in Vienna about 1840–1843 showed that puerperal sepsis could be carried from the dead house. Their work was contemporaneous with that of Agostino Bassi, who first showed the microbial aetiology of a contagious disease of an animal; and it preceded by some 30 years the work of Koch and Lister on bacterial infections (Major, 1954). The use of antiseptic solutions and attention to general hygiene, particularly that of the hands, diminished the ravages of puerperal sepsis, long before the aetiological agents were discovered in the era of scientific bacteriology.

In the time of Semmelweis, epidemics of puerperal sepsis frequently occurred in maternity hospitals, and were accompanied by a mortality of 60–75 per cent. In the late

twenties and early thirties of this century, mortality rates of up to 30 per cent in streptococcal puerperal sepsis are recorded (Colebrook, 1935). The mortality in the last 10 years in the United Kingdom has been about 10 cases a year (Registrar General's Reports).

Since the establishment of rigid techniques of asepsis and antisepsis in maternity units over the last century, and since the introduction of chemotherapeutic agents and the antibacterial antibiotics in the 1930's and after-wards, the aetiological pattern of puerperal sepsis has altered. Formerly, exogenous organisms accounted for the great majority of fatal cases, and were mainly Group A β haemolytic streptococci, originating from the atten-dants, the patient's own body outside the genital tract, and from visitors; they spread to the parturient patient by droplet infection, infected dust, infected hands, and fomites, such as bedding, bed pans, instruments, dressings and utensils. Nowadays, aerobic non-haemolytic strepto-cocci, anaerobic streptococci, members of the *Entero-bacteriaceae* (*Esch. coli*, *Proteus*, etc.) occasionally staphylo-cocci, *Cl. welchii*, *Str. faecalis*, or β haemolytic streptococci of other groups are more often encountered. All these are commensal organisms of the bowel, perineum, or lower vagina. Staphylococci, too, cause puerperal sepsis, and these may have an intrinsic or extrinsic origin.

Puerperal sepsis is a wound infection, and the factors predisposing to infection include premature rupture of the membranes, repeated examinations of the vagina and instrumentation, lacerations of the birth canal, episiotomy, manual rotation, forceps delivery, and sometimes Caesarean section. Factors tending to lower general resistance, such as anaemia, haemorrhage and maternal exhaustion are also operative. The retention of blood clot, or of fragments of membrane or placenta encourages infection by the provision of a suitable nidus for the multiplying bacteria.

The diagnosis of puerperal sepsis is made on clinical grounds, and the identity of the infecting microbes is established by the laboratory. Direct Gram-stained smears of exudate from the vagina, or from within the uterus, are examined, and the specimen is cultured. Media in routine use in laboratories in the United Kingdom include blood agar incubated aerobically and anaerobically and MacConkey's medium. The *in vitro* sensitivity to antibiotics of the organisms is determined by simple plate techniques, where necessary. In the case of organisms other than *Clostridia*, the nature and sensitivity of the pathogen is usually established in less than 48 hours.

The patient is treated with appropriate antibiotics (a safe, broad spectrum antibiotic should be chosen if the specific aetiology is completely unsuspected), by surgical measures when indicated, and by supportive therapy, including bedrest, isolation, fluids and oral and nasal hygiene.

Other Wound Infections. The organism most frequently found in septic wounds in gynaecological and obstetric practice is *Straphylococcus aureus*, followed by coliform and *Proteus* bacilli, and streptococci including *Str. pyogenes*, *Str. faecalis*, and anaerobic cocci. Infection with *Pseudomonas aeruginosa* ("pyocyanea") may also occur. Opinions differ on the relative importance of the operating theatre and the ward as the place of infection, and probably this differs from hospital to hospital. Certainly, the hands of the surgeon, the body of a member of the operating team, fomites surrounding the patient, such as blankets, air sucked into the theatre from other parts of the hospital, and the patient's own skin may be the source of the infection (See Wilson and Miles, 1964, p. 1805). Inexpert and clumsy surgery is undoubtedly a contributory factor.

Diagnosis

The diagnosis is established from the appearance of the wound, and the laboratory findings. Erythema and suppuration are the cardinal signs.

Treatment

The importance of surgical intervention promoting drainage in acute suppurative infections must be emphasized. Antibiotic therapy depends on the nature of the infection, and the sensitivity of the infecting microbe. The measures taken to control wound infections are many and diverse (Williams *et al.*, 1966).

Pneumonia in the New Born

Pneumonia is one of the important causes of perinatal death, but figures on its incidence are much complicated by the absence of universally acceptable criteria. Accepting neonatal pneumonia as the presence of "excess" of leucocytes in the alveolar or intestitial tissue, with no major lesions elsewhere, the 1958 Perinatal survey of the National Birthday Trust Fund (Butler and Bonham, 1963), established that one in 750 babies die of pneumonia in the first week of life; this comprised 10 per cent of all deaths in that period. An unequivocal relationship between morbid anatomical appearances and the presence of an infecting microbe is all too rarely demonstrated. It is difficult to obtain infective material from babies with clinical infections, and at necropsy, bacteriological or viral investigations are seldom made. If specimens are cultured, whether *ante* or *post mortem*, the interpretation of the findings poses difficulties, for there is uncertainty as to the normal bacteriological flora of the respiratory tract in the newborn. Some 58 per cent of specimens from the upper respiratory tract immediately after birth yield positive cultures (Glynn *et al.*, 1967), including staphylococci, streptococci, Gram-negative bacilli, candidas and other organisms.

Thus, although it is customary to regard deaths with morbid anatomical demonstration of pneumonia as deaths from infection, the microbiologist is seldom afforded an opportunity to investigate the assumed infective aetiology.

Not surprisingly, the organisms associated with pneumonia in the newborn include all the potentially pathogenic bacteria that can be isolated from the pharynx. Blood cultures are rarely positive.

Pneumonia may be acquired by the foetus in intrauterine life as the result of transplacental transfer of a pathogen, or it may follow prolonged rupture of the membranes, and be the result of an ascending intrauterine infection. Thus intra-uterine pneumococcal pneumonia may develop if the mother suffers a pneumococcal septicaemia. If the membranes are ruptured, and the patient is in labour, contamination of the liquor occurs with some frequency after 24 hours. Since the foetus swallows liquor, and will gasp if subject to asphyxia, the pathogens gain access through the foetal alimentary, or upper respiratory tract. Pneumonia may also be acquired during labour or postnatally, sometimes as a consequence of the aspiration of maternal faecal matter, food, or gastric contents.

Authorities are divided on the usefulness of prophylactic antibiotic therapy for babies born after prolonged membrane rupture time, or complicated delivery. Most controlled studies show no difference with respect to mortality or morbidity between the group receiving prophylaxis and the untreated group (Schaffer, 1966). However, the incidence of clinically recognizable pneumonia is certainly lessened by prompt treatment with a broad spectrum antibiotic of all babies that have respiratory difficulty in the first few days of life.

The parasite *Pneumocystis carinii* causes an interstitial plasma cell pneumonia of infants. Premature infants between 2 and 6 weeks are chiefly affected, and the case fatality rate is thought to be about 20 per cent (Wilson and Miles, 1964). The parasite forms cysts, or vacuoles in the alveolar exudate, and can be demonstrated by Giemsa's stain.

Meningitis

Schaffer (1966) quotes the incidence of neonatal meningitis in published series as ranging between 1–4 per cent of neonatal deaths, and 3 per 10,000 live births. The frequency, and, probably, also the distribution of bacteria, varies from community to community.

In most published series, the predominant organisms early in the neonatal period are Gram-negative rods (60–80 per cent) including common organisms like *Esch. coli* and rare bacteria like *Flavobacterium meningosepticum*. Gram-negative rods are also frequently isolated from septicaemias of the newborn, and positive blood cultures coexist with, or precede, meningitis in 60–70 per cent of cases. Infection with Gram-positive cocci is said to occur less frequently in the first two weeks of life, although these organisms predominate as causes of meningitis in the 3rd and 4th weeks of life. Amongst the Gram-negative rods species of *Klebsiella*, *Pseudomonas*, *Proteus* and *Salmonella* may cause meningitis, and amongst the Gram-positive cocci, streptococci, pneumococci and staphylococci. Meningitis caused by *Listeria monocytogenes* also occurs. *Haemophilus influenzae* and *Neisseria meningitidis* are rare causes in the United Kingdom. Meningitis and septicaemia caused by Gram-negative rods are rare in our experience at Queen Charlotte's Maternity Hospital, and of 5 recent cases encountered in the early neonatal period, from 4,000 deliveries, two were associated with staphylococci, two with streptococci (one Lancefield Group D, the other Lancefield Group B) and the fifth with a species of *Alkaligenes*. It is our practice to culture the bloodstream of all infants who fail to thrive, and bacteriological examinations are made routinely at necropsy. Premature birth, prolonged membrane rupture, difficult labour and operative delivery are causes predisposing to meningitis of the early neonatal period.

Meningitis may be acquired *in utero* as a consequence of maternal infection and transplacental transfer of the pathogen, or as a result of operative intervention such as intrauterine blood transfusion. If bacteria gain access to the liquor, they may enter the foetus as a result of swallowing, or of gasping if the foetus is asphyxiated. The infection may be acquired postnatally following respiratory tract infection, cord or skin or other infection.

The diagnosis is made from the clinical state, and from examination of the cerebro-spinal fluid, which shows an elevated cell count and protein content, and reduced sugar. Organisms are seen in the stained smear, and are grown on culture.

Meningo-encephalitis may be caused by *Toxoplasma gondii* and by the viruses of rubella and cytomegalic inclusion disease as well as by those of herpes simplex, zoster, poliomyelitis, mumps and chicken pox. Coxsackie viruses also affect the central nervous system.

Ophthalmia Neonatorum

Conjunctivitis (incidence 5–7 per cent) is the commonest of the superficial infections of the newborn at Queen Charlotte's Maternity Hospital and it is diagnosed when a purulent discharge, no matter how slight, is seen. *Staphylococcus aureus* was formerly the organism most commonly isolated, but coagulase negative staphylococci are now frequently encountered, and regarded as pathogens. Pneumococci, and α haemolytic and non-haemolytic streptococci and *Haemophilus spp.* are also isolated from mild cases, as are, occasionally, coliform bacilli. Some cultures are sterile, and, rarely, on staining with Giemsa, the cytoplasm of the epithelial cells shows the characteristic blue staining granules of inclusion blenorrhoea.

Ophthalmia caused by *Neisseria gonorrhoeae* is a serious condition. It occurs characteristically on the 2nd–3rd day of life, but the onset is occasionally delayed until the second week of life. Its incidence at Queen Charlotte's Maternity Hospital is about 1 in 5,000 deliveries, but the frequency of the disease varies from country to country, and within socio-economic groups. The source of the infection is the mother, and infection is usually acquired during passage through the birth canal. Formerly, chemical prophylaxis with silver nitrate drops was used to prevent it, but this was followed by cases of chemical conjunctivitis, and where the risk of gonococcal ophthalmia is slight, it is no longer used. In certain parts of the United States the instillation of penicillin or silver nitrate drops into the eyes of the newborn is required by law; and there is no doubt that where adequate surveillance of the newborn cannot be guaranteed, as, for example, following early discharge from hospital, there is a good case for insistence on chemical prophylaxis.

All forms of conjunctivitis respond rapidly to local antibiotic therapy, and systemic antibiotics should be used for gonococcal ophthalmia.

Umbilical Sepsis

Serous, sanguineous, or frankly purulent drainage from the umbilical stump occurs, and in some cases, umbilical phlebitis and septic arteritis initiate a fatal sepsis of the newborn. The cord of the newborn may represent a hazard to the mother if it becomes colonized with β haemolytic streptococci.

The organisms usually isolated are staphylococci, coliform organisms and *Proteus spp.* Tetanus neonatorum usually originates in an infected cord stump.

Neonatal Myocarditis

Group B coxsackie viruses are the chief cause of myocarditis in the newborn, and 54 cases were collected up to 1961 (Schaffer, 1966). Twenty-eight were infected during nursery outbreaks, and the mother was the original source of the infection in many cases. The majority of cases seem to have been acquired postnatally, but some patients seem to have acquired the infection *in utero.* Staphylococci, toxoplasma and rubella also cause myocarditis.

Trichomoniasis

The protozoan parasite *Trichomonas vaginalis*, a pear-shaped organism 9–13 μ long, is accepted as an aetiological agent of vaginitis. An extremely similar organism, *Trichomonas hominis*, inhabits the gastro-intestinal tract. The protozoan is freely mobile as a result of its undulating membrane, and the body has a tail-like axostyle at one end, and a cluster of 3–5 flagella at the opposite pole. The nucleus occupies about one sixth of the cell. Nowadays it is less frequent as a cause of vaginitis than species of *Candida*. Eastman and Hellman (1966) state that the organism is found in about 20–30 per cent of all women during antenatal examination; but that the infection is symptomatic in a much smaller percentage of patients.

There is evidence that the organism can be transmitted by venereal contact, whatever its primary source may be. This probably accounts in part for one of the most typical features of the disease, its tendency to recur. Relapses are frequent when the patient is fatigued and worried.

The infection is diagnosed when trichomonads are demonstrated in the vaginal discharge, and the patient has symptoms. The discharge is greenish yellow, frothy and irritant, with a musty odour.

The organism is recognized by its characteristic jerky movements in "wet" preparations. The vaginal secretion should be examined microspically with low magnification, and then with the 1/6 in. lens. Films stained with Leishman or Giemsa, or Papanicolaou's technique may also be used to demonstrate the parasite.

Candidosis (Winner and Hurley, 1964, 1966)

The fungi that cause candidosis belong to the genus *Candida* (M.R.C. Memo, 1967). This generic name replaces the incorrect *Monilia* long used in medical literature.

The most important pathogen of the genus is *Candida albicans*, but other species, notably *C. tropicalis, C. stellatoidea, C. pseudotropicalis, C. krusei, C. parapsilosis* and *C. guilliermondii* are associated with muco-cutaneous and deep seated candidosis in man. These fungi are dimorphic, and exist in the yeast phase, that is, as unicellular organisms (1·5–5 μ diam.) that reproduce by budding, and also in the mycelial, or filamentous phase. They are easy to cultivate, growing readily on Sabouraud's medium (glucose-peptone agar) at 22°C.–37°C. *C. albicans* is distinguished from other species by the readiness with which it produces chlamydospores. These are thick-walled refractile spherical structures (7–17 μ), growing on media such as corn-meal agar. *C. albicans* rapidly produces "germ tubes" or short filaments, in the presence of serum, and this propensity is also used in identifying the fungus. The other species are identified principally by their fermentative and assimilative biochemical reactions.

These fungi, and others of the genus *Candida*, are widely spread in nature, and are commensals of the gastro-intestinal tract, and the vagina. Numerous surveys attest to the predominant incidence of *C. albicans*, which can be found in up to 36 per cent of the vaginas of pregnant women, and up to 16 per cent of the non-pregnant. Yeast-like fungi, predominantly *C. albicans*, have been found in the mouths of up to 54 per cent of children aged 2–6 weeks. The organisms are rarely harboured on the skin (less than 1 per cent). In spite of their occurrence as commensals, infection by these organisms can still, on occasion, be exogenous: in the vagina, as the result of unclean instrumentation, and in the mouths of babes, as a result of contaminated teats or bottles. Conjugal infection can also occur. Thus, although usually endemic, vaginal candidosis and thrush can occur in epidemic form.

Vaginal Candidosis

Pregnancy and diabetes predispose to thrush vaginitis, as does administration of some broad spectrum anti-biotics in some women. Parous women are more often infected than multiparous. The incidence of vaginal yeasts rises in pregnancy, but there is general agreement that the number is greatly diminished after parturition, possibly as a consequence of the cleansing effect of the lochia. The overall incidence of vaginal thrush at Queen Charlotte's Hospital in pregnant women is about 10 per cent. The ratio of candida to trichomonal vaginitis is about 7:1 in non-pregnant patients, and 15:1 in the pregnant. The incidence is highest in the 3rd trimester, and during pregnancy there is no seasonal incidence. In the non-pregnant, the incidence is higher in the summer months, and exacerbations occur in the pre-menstrual period. Candida vulvo-vaginitis rarely occurs in little girls, but occurs fairly frequently after the menopause. The discharge is thin, and often highly acid in the acute stages, and vulvitis is a concomitant feature.

Oral Thrush

The incidence of oral thrush in maternity units varies between 0·5 and 19 per cent. Infection of the baby's mouth is thought to occur principally from the mother's vagina, and thrush is some 35 times more common in children born of women harbouring vaginal candidas. Infection can be conveyed by imperfectly sterilized teats and bottles after use in a common nursery, and the hands of nurses and mothers, as well as the breasts of nursing mothers, may convey the infection. Air-borne infection is not regarded as a likely route of infection, although candidas have been isolated from nursery fomites. The most recent surveys have failed to show a significant difference between bottle and breast fed babies, or in those with or without preceding antibiotic therapy. Low birth weight, prolonged labour, birth trauma and prematurity have also been discounted as relevant to the aetiology of thrush. There is no doubt that a low incidence of thrush is associated with scrupulous attention to the cleanliness and sterility of feeds.

Candidosis of the Skin

The premature infant is unduly susceptible to skin candidosis, the sources of infection being similar to those of oral thrush, with the added risk of imperfectly sterilized napkins. Skin thrush in the newborn is thought to be more common than was formerly supposed, and the results of a survey in one London obstetric hospital showed that at least 3 per cent of babies had been affected by the age of six months. *C. albicans* is an important cause of napkin rash, which may occur in epidemic form, and generalized cutaneous candidosis may occur in the newborn, though rarely. Candida onychia may also occur. Bloodstream infection with *Candida* species occurs in the newborn; it is rare, and uniformly fatal unless promptly diagnosed and treated. It always occurs in sickly and debilitated children.

Diagnosis

Because of the widespread occurrence of *Candida* species as commensals, the diagnosis of candidosis must be made on clinical grounds, and cultural evidence is confirmatory. Serological tests are without value save in the rare disseminated or gastro-intestinal forms, when the precipitin test is helpful.

Treatment

Polyene antifungal antibiotics for example, nystatin and amphotericin B, are effective in vaginal thrush. Nystatin is used both prophylactically and therapeutically in thrush of the newborn. The cure rate with nystatin in vaginal candidosis is of the order of 90 per cent, although more than one course may have to be given. Since the drug kills fungi by contact, care should be taken that the patient is tamponaded and the pessaries inserted well into the vaginal vault.

Syphilis (see Wilson and Miles, 1964, p. 2175 *et seq*.)

Syphilis is not primarily a disease of the genital tract, but the chancre of the primary stage usually occurs as a button-like induration of the skin of the clitoris or labia, and is associated with hard discrete inguinal glands that do not suppurate. Pregnancy masks the early stages of syphilis, and the chancre may appear as little more than an abrasion, which if situated on the cervix may be overlooked. Condylomata, that is, moist warty elevations around the anus and vulva, occur in the secondary stage.

Syphilis is important in obstetrics because the spirochaete can and does cross the placental barrier. If the infection arises before conception, abortion or premature labour may result; if coincident with conception, intra-uterine death with premature delivery of a macerated foetus is likely; and if infection occurs late in pregnancy, the child will be born with syphilis and may die in neonatal life.

The aetiological agent of syphilis is the strict parasite, *Treponema pallidum*, a spirochaete which is characterized by a number of regular, primary spirals, each about 1 μ long. Secondary spirals appear as the organism moves, but its differentiation from other spirochaetes by dark ground microscopy may be very difficult, particularly if the exudate being examined comes from a primary chancre of the lip, or of the female genital tract, where saprophytic spirochaetes occur. The difficulties of growing *Treponema pallidum in vitro* are so great that the organism is usually preserved by *in vivo* methods.

Serological tests have thus become of paramount importance in the diagnosis of syphilis, and are included in the routine tests made on pregnant women because of the danger of untreated syphilis to the foetus. The serological reactions of syphilis have been subjected to intensive study, and modifications of the standard Wasserman Reaction and Kahn tests have produced different results in the hands of different workers. The proportion of positive reactions varies widely in different stages and types of the disease, and rather higher proportions of negative results are found in primary and tertiary syphilis than in secondary syphilis or general paresis of the insane. The interpretation of serological tests of syphilis requires close co-operation between clinician and pathologist. In general, reactions occurring in both yaws and pinta are regarded as true positive reactions, indicating treponemal infection. False positive reactions may occur, either as the result of faulty technique, or in association with pathological or physiological states, such as leprosy, malaria, sleeping sickness, tuberculosis, glandular fever and pregnancy; the latter are referred to as "biological false positive" reactions.

The antigen used in the standard Wasserman Reaction and Kahn tests is of the same general type, and is an extract of heart muscle. Variability in the performance of complement fixation and flocculation tests was greatly diminished by the introduction of "cardiolipin" antigen, which is highly purified and for which an international reference preparation is available. In most laboratories cardiolipin antigen has replaced the crude tissue extracts formerly used. The Wasserman Reaction utilizes the principle of complement fixation, while the Kahn test is a precipitation reaction. Of recent years, a number of tests have been introduced that make use of treponemal antigens. The chief methods of testing comprise complement fixation, agglutination, immobilization of living treponemes, immune adherence and fluorescence microscopy.

In practice, screening of the blood of antenatal patients for antibodies suggestive of syphilis is performed by using more than one test: thus complement fixations with cardiolipin (heart extract antigen), and with an antigen of *Treponema pallidum* (often the Reiter Protein antigen) is combined with one or more precipitation tests such as the Kahn Test or the V.D.R.L. test. Sera giving positive reactions are usually re-examined, and may be referred for the Treponema Immobilization Test (T.P.I.) or other tests to specialist laboratories after discussion by the pathologist and clinician concerned. The T.P.I. test is accepted generally as the ultimate standard of reference, but the result is usually negative in the primary, and often in the secondary stage; and in patients not treated till late in the disease, as well as in congenital syphilis, the test remains positive. It is, however, useful in differentiating "biological false positive" tests in pregnancy.

Serological tests for syphilis are said to be positive in 0·35 per cent of pregnant women (Wilson Clyne, 1962).

Gonorrhoea

This is an acute, specific infectious disease, usually transmitted during sexual intercourse, and characterized, in adults, primarily by invasion of the genito-urinary tract, though secondary disturbances may complicate its course. In women the disease begins with an acute urethritis, infection of Skene's ducts, and spread to the cervix. After a few days, it becomes subacute, and the infection may spread to Bartholin's glands, the bladder, the Fallopian tubes, and the pelvic peritoneum. Unless treated promptly, the infection becomes chronic, resulting in Bartholin cyst or abscess, chronic cervicitis, chronic salpingo-oöphoritis, and occasionally, through bloodstream dissemination, in arthritis, tenosynovitis or ophthalmia. Rarely, the disease is disseminated and fatal from the beginning. Venereal warts affecting the thighs and labia are probably of viral aetiology, although often associated with gonorrhoea.

In neonates, gonococcal ophthalmia, which is rare in adults, is the most common manifestation of infection; and vulvo-vaginitis occurs in infants, spreading by contact with imperfectly sterilized fomites such as napkins, and assuming epidemic proportions in institutions. The gonococcus is not, however, the only cause of epidemic vulvo-vaginitis, which can be caused by streptococci or staphylococci.

Neisseria gonorrhoeae is a strict parasite, growing well on aerobic media containing serum, but poorly on ordinary media, and under anaerobic conditions. Growth is good in 5–10 per cent of carbon dioxide. The cocci are usually arranged in pairs, and are Gram-negative. Special media are often used for its isolation and the organism is differentiated from other *Neisseria* and other bacteria by its fermentation and other biochemical reactions.

The diagnosis depends, in the main, on demonstration of the parasite, and in acute infections, with typical signs and symptoms, direct examination of the Gram-stained smear shows the characteristic kidney or bean-shaped Gram-negative intracellular diplococci. However, these may be concealed by a heavy flora of commensal organisms and the resemblance of some of these to *N. gonorrhoeae* may give rise to difficulty. Experience is needed in identifying *N. gonorrhoeae* in stained films. Wherever possible cultures must be made. In chronic cases, the gonococcus is less easy to demonstrate and to cultivate, and specimens sent to the laboratory must be taken from the sites most likely to be the seat of chronic infection, such as Bartholin's glands, and the cervical glands. Fluid withdrawn from joint lesions, and pus from chronically inflamed Fallopian tubes are frequently sterile. The gonococcus is extremely susceptible to drying, and care must be taken with swabs sent to distant laboratories. These are usually placed in Stuart's Transport Medium, and the swabs themselves may require preliminary treatment (Wilson and Miles, 1964, p. 1758). In the face of all these difficulties failure to grow the gonococcus can not be looked upon as definite evidence against the diagnosis, and other methods of diagnosis must be used.

The gonococcal complement fixation test is difficult to perform and to interpret, and is usually referred to special laboratories. The reaction does not become positive for at least two weeks after infection, and is often negative in simple cases of gonococcal urethritis, though generally positive in complicated cases. In some patients the test may remain positive for years after clinical cure. A single negative reaction does not exclude the diagnosis, and the test should be repeated. The test is most likely to be positive in just those cases where the organism is least likely to be seen or cultivated, and is especially useful in chronic pelvic disease.

Penicillin, streptomycin and tetracycline are used in treatment, and the dosage must be adequate to avoid masking concomitant syphilitic infection.

Tuberculosis

Genital Tract

Tuberculosis of the genital tract commonly orginates in the lungs, whence the infection spreads *via* the bloodstream. Its incidence varies in published series between 1·1 to 5·6 per thousand admissions, and, as would be expected, the distribution is regional. A much higher incidence of genital tuberculosis occurs in patients complaining of sterility, an incidence of from 2·1 per cent (Scandinavia) to 14·8 per cent (Spain) (see Wilson Clyne, 1963).

Tuberculosis of the vulva is rare, but cervical tuberculosis occurs more frequently. Tuberculous endometritis is associated with sterility, but the Fallopian tubes are the primary site in the vast majority of cases of pelvic tuberculosis, being affected in over 90 per cent of cases.

The diagnosis is established from bacteriological and histological examinations of curettings, occasionally of menstrual discharge, and of biopsy specimens. Hysterosalpingography is sometimes helpful, and involvement of the lungs and kidneys should be excluded by Chest X ray, intravenous pyelogram, and bacteriological examination of sputum (if any) and urine.

Of the Newborn

Neonatal tuberculosis is usually acquired through contact with a tuberculous mother, although cases of true congenital tuberculosis, resulting from transplacental transmission, are on record. When infection is acquired at birth, probably from inhalation of infected amniotic fluid or vaginal secretions, or from contact with open respiratory tuberculosis, signs of morbidity do not appear until 6–8 weeks.

The tuberculin test is unreliable in the newborn, sometimes remaining negative for many months in the presence of the disease. The diagnosis is established by demonstration of *Mycobacterium tuberculosis* in gastric or bronchial washings, the cerebro-spinal fluid, or, rarely, in the bloodstream. Mothers with open tuberculosis should be segregated from their infants, who should be protected by vaccination with B.C.G. as early as possible.

Tuberculosis in Pregnancy

The average number of new cases of pulmonary tuberculosis discovered during pregnancy per year in England and Wales is about 700. In 1955, the number of fatal cases was four; it is now about one a year, and is thus a commoner cause of maternal death than tetanus (2 cases in the last 10 years), though less common than postdelivery puerperal sepsis (about 10 cases a year) (Figures from the Registrar General). Most of these diagnoses have been made as a result of chest X ray in the antenatal period, supported by bacteriological findings.

Laboratory Findings

Neutropaenia, and anaemia may both occur in association with tuberculosis. The causative organism is *Mycobacterium tuberculosis*, a slender acid fast rod. The rods are non-motile, and Gram-positive. They are aerobic, and extremely slow growing, and are cultured on special media, Dorset's egg medium, Lowenstein–Jensen medium and others being commonly used. On these media, growth of human *Myco. tuberculosis* takes about two weeks.

The organisms are pathogenic to laboratory animals. The guinea pig is highly susceptible to both human and bovine bacilli, and injection of suspected organisms, or injection or implantation of suitably treated specimens results in dissemination of the disease in a few weeks. Animals that do not die spontaneously, are killed at six weeks, necropsied, and, if lesions are present, smears are stained by the Ziehl–Neelson or other techniques.

Streptococcal Infections

The streptococci are Gram-positive, usually non-motile, chaining cocci that have always proved difficult to classify. The medical bacteriologist groups the organisms in the following manner:

α haemolytic streptococci, (usually *Str. viridans*)
β haemolytic streptococci, (including *Str. pyogenes*)
pneumococci, (*Str. pneumoniae*)
anaerobic streptococci

further identifying them, for epidemiological purposes, by serological methods. All these organisms are of importance in obstetrics and gynaecology, and many are commensals.

Str. viridans, the chief cause of subacute bacterial endocarditis, is pathogenic only if the heart valves are already the seat of a morbid process. During pregnancy, the teeth often show accelerated caries, necessitating dental surgery and sometimes extraction. Manipulations on the teeth are regularly accompanied by the entry of *Str. viridans* into the blood stream, an occurrence of no consequence in healthy people, but dangerous indeed to those with congenital or rheumatic valvular disease of the heart. The occurrence of subacute bacterial endocarditis is no rarity in obstetric practice in the United Kingdom. Despite antibiotic therapy, this disease still has a high morbidity, and a mortality rate of 10–20 per cent. Dental surgery for patients with valvular lesions must, therefore, be undertaken under cover of antibiotics, but antibiotic therapy should not be started long before the operation, because of the danger of selectively encouraging resistant strains. Penicillin is usually given so that the maximum concentration following the first dose is reached at the time of operation. The exact timing depends on the preparation used.

Invariably isolated from the stools of normal people, and, through anal contamination, an inhabitant of the perineum and the lower vagina, *Streptococcus faecalis*, though a commensal, may be pathogenic outside the alimentary tract. It causes urinary tract infections, wound infections, middle ear disease, and puerperal and skin infections. It differs from other streptococci in its greater resistance to heat and chemical germicides, and to antibacterial antibiotics, and unlike other α haemolytic streptococci and the β haemolytic streptococci is often resistant to penicillin.

Str. pneumoniae, a commensal of the nasopharynx in a variable proportion of adults and children (up to 40 per cent), is a cause of pneumonia which may complicate recovery from operation. Despite all antibiotics, pneumonia is still one of the most important causes of death in the United Kingdom, and lobar as well as bronchopneumonia may occur post-operatively, although the latter is more common.

Serious though these infections by named species of streptococci are, they pale to insignificance beside the epidemics that may be caused by *Str. pyogenes*. This decimator of populations has always been the most important pathogen in obstetric and surgical practice, and the elucidation of its epidemiological behaviour has been the peculiar province of obstetricians, and of scientific workers in Institutes of Obstetrics. It causes scarlet fever, scarlatina, erysipelas, surgical wound infections and peritonitis, middle ear disease and puerperal sepsis. It is also an occasional cause of vaginitis, especially in childhood.

The mortality rate of epidemics of puerperal sepsis in the time of Semmelweis (1818–1865) has already received comment, but there is no doubt that taking all the evidence as a whole, *Str. pyogenes* has been undergoing a steady decline in virulence over the last century. Much of the decline in the death rate from streptococcal puerperal sepsis can be attributed directly to the measures taken to control the infection. Semmelweis equated puerperal sepsis with hospital delivery, noting that mothers who had their children *en route* to, or outside, the hospital rarely succumbed to the disease. He noted that the pathological changes at autopsy of one of the professors who had died following injury received in the post-mortem room were similar to those seen in the victims of child bed fever, and became convinced that the disease was caused by transmission *via* the unclean hands of the examining physician. In 1847 he introduced the regulation that all who examined pregnant women, or cared for them during labour, should wash their hands in an antiseptic solution, probably calcium chloride. This was the first application of antisepsis in clinical practice. The mortality rate fell from 12·24 per cent in May to 2·38 per cent in June, and to 1·2 per cent in July (Major, 1954).

The work of Rebecca Lancefield in the 1930's on serological grouping of streptococci gave a new tool to epidemiologists, and promoted studies on the carriage of β haemolytic streptococci. It enabled workers at Queen Charlotte's Maternity Hospital to demonstrate that the source of the infection was not endogenous as had formerly been supposed, but exogenous (Colebrook, 1935). Surveys of the incidence of symptomless carriage of haemolytic streptococci showed that 5–10 per cent persons carried *Str. pyogenes* in the throat. The isolation of infected cases, with rigid exclusion of carriers, the liberal use of disinfectant hand creams and masks, and aseptic and antiseptic techniques used by those in attendance on women in labour and after delivery still further reduced the incidence of fatal puerperal sepsis, and the mortality was greatly reduced following the use of chemotherapeutics and antibiotics.

It is no longer customary, or necessary, to swab the throats of the personnel of large maternity units routinely to detect carriage of Group A β haemolytic streptococci. This does not mean that no control is exercised over the population of a maternity unit and a considerable degree of surveillance must be exercised if routine swabbing is not employed. All entrants, patients and staff alike, should be questioned for history of contact with, or symptoms of, streptococcal disease, and those with sore throats must be excluded from the lying-in wards. Should streptococcal sepsis occur, contacts must be throat swabbed to exclude "carriers" who may be incubating the disease.

Anaerobic streptococci also cause wound infections, and puerperal sepsis.

Diagnosis

Streptococci are easy to cultivate, and grow well on media containing blood, forming pinpoint, colourless colonies. They may be aerobic or anaerobic. Most strains are haemolytic, the narrow zones of α haemolysis appearing greenish, and opaque, and the broad zones of β haemolysis being transparent; some streptococci are non-haemolytic and some strains produce filterable haemolysins. The organisms form chains in culture, and these are longest in liquid media. Thirteen different serologically active polysaccharide antigens were described by Lancefield (Groups A–O) using precipitation techniques. It is customary to group only β haemolytic streptococci by the Lancefield technique. *Str. pyogenes* (Lancefield Group A) is most virulent, but Groups B, C and G may all cause mild puerperal sepsis, and these can be isolated from the genital tract as commensals. *Str. faecalis*, which ferments lactose, and can be α haemolytic, β haemolytic or non-haemolytic, contains the Lancefield D antigen. Groups F and K have occasionally been reported as pathogens.

Type specific proteins were studied by Griffiths, using predominantly Lancefield Group A strains. The number of types presently recognized is about 50, and they are studied by agglutination reactions. With the decline of streptococcal epidemics, these types are now little used in clinical obstetric practice.

Str. pyogenes combines the capacity for tissue invasion with the production of filterable exotoxins. Infections of the genital tract may spread, and pelvic cellulitis, salpingitis, peritonitis and septicaemia may occur as complications. The importance of control of *Str. pyogenes* infection is emphasized by the extreme rapidity of its fatal course, which is sometimes less than 6 hours from the onset of the first symptom. Both *Str. pyogenes* and *Str. viridans* are invariably sensitive to penicillin.

Clostridial Infections

Clostridia is a genus of Gram-positive, anaerobic or microaerophilic rods, producing endospores. They often vigorously decompose protein, and ferment carbohydrates The species most pathogenic in man produce exotoxins.

Their principal habitat is the soil, but some are common inhabitants of the intestinal tract of man and animals. *Cl. welchii* is uniformly present in human faeces, and *Cl. tetani* in about 10–40 per cent of faecal specimens from domestic animals. *Cl. sporogenes* and *Cl. histolyticum* also occur in faeces. They appear frequently in dust, milk and sewage. Organisms occurring so frequently in the intestinal tract are isolated from the vagina and perineum also, so that the rare presence of *Clostridia* in clinical specimens does not connote disease, but must be interpreted in conjunction with clinical findings. The fact that they are rarely reported as occurring in rectal swabs, or stools, in routine clinical practice is simply a reflection of the exclusive use of aerobic methods of culture in examining specimens from the gastro-intestinal tract. The *Clostridia* are endogenous microbes and the diseases they cause, though infectious, are not contagious, and consequently there is no need to isolate, or to barrier nurse, patients with gas gangrene or tetanus.

The *Clostridia* of importance in obstetric and gynaecological practice are pathogens of wounds, causing surgical and puerperal sepsis.

Cl. tetani is the cause of tetanus. Gas gangrene may be caused by a number of different anaerobic bacteria, usually clostridia, but sometimes by anaerobic streptococci; of these the three most important anaerobes are *Cl. welchii* (perfringens), *Cl. oedematiens* and *Cl. septicum*; of less importance are *Cl. bifermentans*, *Cl. fallax*, *Cl. histolyticum* and *Cl. sporogenes*. Pathogenic clostridia are often only simple contaminants of wounded tissues, sometimes associated only with cellulitis, and only infre-

quently with true gas gangrene, clostridial myositis. They tend to occur in association with each other, although sometimes they are present singly in wounds. *Cl. welchii* is usually responsible for the rare cases of post-operative, post-delivery and post-abortion gas gangrene.

Unlike streptococci, the clostridia have poorly developed powers of invasion and they multiply only in tissues previously damaged where anaerobic conditions prevail. When multiplication is established absorption of their toxins, the most poisonous substances known to us, may be lethal. Although the microbes are commensals of man, clostridial infection begins with the introduction of the bacteria, or their spores, directly into the wound, either by contact with soil, or *via* a contaminated instrument. Thus, in obstetric practice it is more common after instrumented (usually illegal) abortion, and in those parts of the world where delivery takes place in the open. Surgical tetanus and gas gangrene are rare and are invariably associated with contamination of instruments or dressings due to imperfect sterilization. The spores of bacteria are resistant to chemical and physical germicides and safe theatre practice must include methods of sterilizing that destroy the spores of *Clostridia*. Maternal deaths from tetanus in England and Wales in the last 10 years have been 2 (Registrar General's Figures). Tetanus neonatorum is usually associated with umbilical sepsis, signs appearing between the 6th and 14th day of birth.

Diagnosis: The diagnosis of clostridial disease must be made on clinical grounds. The chief reasons for this are (i) clostridia may be present as commensals, or contaminants only, (ii) if disease is established, treatment must be given at once and laboratory methods are too slow to do other than confirm the clinical diagnosis. Mixtures of clostridia can be extremely difficult to separate into pure cultures, which is a prerequisite practice for biochemical studies of organisms, but in routine bacteriological practice the identification of *Cl. tetani* and *Cl. welchii* can usually be made in 48 hours. The organisms can be seen in direct Gram-stained smears from the affected part and, if abundant, morphologically typical forms of *Cl. welchii* (capsulated stout, straight rods with truncated or rounded ends) can sometimes be recognized. If the smear has been made from the uterine cavity, and the patient has symptoms, a presumptive diagnosis of clostridial infection can be made. Blood culture may be positive, particularly if the infecting organism is *Cl. welchii* or *Cl. septicum*. *Cl. welchii* forms typical round, greyish white colonies 2–5 mm. in diameter, surrounded by a zone of β haemolysis, on blood agar anaerobically. Colonies of *Cl. tetani* are more effuse, with less marked, if any, haemolysis. The α toxin of *Cl. welchii* is a lecithinase. This fact is utilized in identifying the organisms on a Nagler plate. The culture medium incorporates lecithin and half the inoculated plate is treated with anti-*Cl. welchii* serum which neutralizes the effect of any lecithinase produced by the inoculated organism on that half of the plate. Organisms suspected of being *Cl. tetani* are injected into a pair of animals, one being protected with anti-tetanus serum. The unprotected animal will die of tetanus in 3–5 days if the suspect microbe is *Cl. tetani*.

Treatment

Radical surgery, or saucerisation of the wound, is indicated in established uncontrolled gas gangrene. The antibiotic of choice is penicillin by the intramuscular route; and therapeutic dosage of mixed antitoxins is 30–40,000 units each of *Cl. oedematiens* and *Cl. welchii* and 15–20,000 units of *Cl. septicum*, given intravenously if possible, otherwise intramuscularly, and repeated 4–6 hourly according to the response of the patient.

In tetanus infections also, everything must be done to avoid the persistence of necrotic tissue, and to control bacterial proliferation within the wound, and to this end radical surgery may be necessary, although wide excision of the umbilicus in neonatal tetanus does not materially improve the chances of recovery. Large doses of antitoxin (100,000–200,000 units) should be given very slowly by the intravenous route, with due precautions against allergic reactions in subjects likely to be hypersensitive to horse proteins. A dose of 10,000 units intramuscularly on two successive days should be adequate for a newborn. General measures such as paralysis by curarization, and positive pressure respiration (Ellis, 1963) greatly reduce the mortality rate, and adequate sedation must be given to control the spastic paralyses. Antibiotics such as penicillin, or the tetracyclines, may be given as an adjunct to antitoxin.

It is too early to assess the value of treatment of clostridial infections with hyperbaric oxygen, but some degree of success is claimed.

Staphylococcal Infections

The staphylococci are non-motile Gram-positive cocci. In Gram stains made from colonies on solid media they are arranged in characteristic grape-like clusters. They grow easily on common laboratory media forming colonies coloured white, beige or golden. The production of the enzyme coagulase is typical of pathogenic staphylococci, which belong chiefly to the golden group, *Staphylococcus aureus*. Non-producers of coagulase are usually *Staphylococcus albus*.

The staphylococci are important pathogens, not least because of their inhabitation of the nose, skin and intestine of normal persons. Up to 80 per cent of nursing personnel have been found to harbour potentially pathogenic staphylococci. Their danger as potential pathogens is enhanced by their propensity to become resistant to antibacterial antibiotics.

The similarity of staphylococci can be gauged crudely from their antibiotic sensitivity and resistance patterns, and coagulase positive organisms can be differentiated from each other by comparing the patterns of their susceptibility to a given series of phages (viruses). Phage typing of staphylococci is used to study the course and sources of epidemics of staphylococcal sepsis. In general, the phage type does not necessarily indicate the virulence of a particular isolate, but the 52, 52A, 80, 81, complex of strains is most frequently associated with outbreaks of severe sepsis in hospitals.

Since staphylococci are ubiquitous and carried on normal persons the measures taken to control staphylococcal cross infection are complex. All are designed to interrupt the cycle of cross infection, by the classical method of the interposition of multiple disrupting agents and physical barriers into the cycle. Thus, the use of antibiotics, and physical and chemical germicides, frequent cleansing of potentially contaminated fomites, and segregation of cases of frank sepsis are all used. Masks, gowns, and sterile gloves are used as barriers. Staphylococci are readily destroyed by heat, and by many germicides (see Williams *et al.*, 1966).

Staphylococcal Infections of the Newborn

Pemphigus neonatorum is a vesicular skin infection caused by *Staph. aureus*, and is characterized by flat blebs containing fluid that is clear at first but becomes turbid in a few days. Ritter's disease, an acute exfoliative dermatitis of infants, is an extreme form of pemphigus. Septic spots, not always vesicular, are one of the common manifestations of staphylococcal sepsis, and the more severe ones are like boils, often with an underlying cellulitis. The pustular type of lesion may be accompanied by serious lesions elsewhere, including deep abscesses, osteomyelitis and pneumonia. Paronychia also occurs, and *Staph. aureus* is one of the causes of neonatal conjunctivitis. All these infections may occur either sporadically, or in epidemic form, and minor sepsis is common in maternity units, affecting from 10–25 per cent of infants.

Staphylococcal Infections in Obstetrics and Gynaecology

Breast abscess in nursing mothers is almost always caused by *Staph. aureus*, and the development of acute mastitis is influenced by local predisposing factors, such as engorgement.

Post-operative wound sepsis is a serious problem, and the organism most frequently isolated is *Staph. aureus*. In the Public Health Laboratory Service Survey (Report 1960) *Staph. aureus* was isolated alone from 45 per cent of infected wounds, and, with other pathogens, mostly coliforms, in a further 15 per cent.

Toxoplasmosis (Harrison, 1966; Beattie, 1967)

Infection with the protozoan parasite *Toxoplasma gondii* is common and widespread in man, as shown by serological surveys. The organism is an obligatory, intracellular parasite, elongated or sickle-shaped, and approximately $3–4\,\mu \times 6–7\,\mu$. One of the modes of transmission in man may be by salivary contamination, or by droplets. Of great importance in obstetrics is the fact that infection can be passed congenitally from mother to foetus, in some animals through several generations. The disease may be acquired during intra-uterine life if the mother is infected during the pregnancy.

Illness is a rare accompaniment of this common infection, and the best known manifestation of acquired toxoplasmosis is lymphadenopathy, which may be accompanied by the presence of glandular-fever-like cells in the blood.

The disease affects women more than men, and the peak incidence is between 25 and 35 years.

It is thought that in all cases of congenital toxoplasmosis

the disease is generalized at the start, but that some lesions of the internal organs heal during intra-uterine life, so that at birth the signs and symptoms are mainly neurological. The incidence of lesions is as follows (Eichenwald, 1960).

	% "Neurological"	% "Generalized"
Choroido-retinitis	94	66
Convulsions	50	18
Intracranial calcification	50	4
Jaundice	29	80
Hydrocephalus	28	0
Splenomegaly, Hepatomegaly	21	80–90
Microcephalus	13	25
Rash	1	0
Pneumonitis	0	41

and the overall mortality in both groups about 12%.

Diagnosis

T. gondii may be isolated from ventricular or cerebrospinal fluid, blood, lymph node or other tissue. Mice or multimammate rats are inoculated by the intracerebral, intraperitoneal or subcutaneous routes, and left for 6–8 weeks; their sera are tested for antibodies, and finally, after killing, a saline emulsion of brain is examined for toxoplasma cysts. Fertile hen's eggs or tissue cultures may be inoculated, but these methods are less sensitive. The histological appearance of excised lymph nodes may suggest toxoplasmosis.

Serological tests include the cytoplasm-modifying (dye) test of Sabin and Feldman, complement fixation, haemagglutination and fluorescence inhibition. "Toxoplasmin" is used for *in vivo* tests of allergy. The interpretation of serological tests can be very difficult, as latent infection is so common. Demonstration of a rising titre indicates active infection; and where it is not possible to demonstrate a rise, a dye test titre of 1:1000 is probably reliable evidence of current infection.

Treatment

Pyrimethamine, alone, or in combination with sulphonamides is used in treatment. Prophylactic therapy has been advocated for women suspected of being infected with *T. gondii* during pregnancy, but should only be undertaken under expert supervision in view of possible teratogenic effects.

Listeriosis (Seeliger, 1961; Gray and Killinger, 1966)

This is an infectious disease with a wide variety of clinical symptoms. Its aetiological agent is a Gram-positive, coccoid to filamentous rod, *Listeria monoytogenes*, which shows tumbling motility best demonstrated at room temperature (20°C). It grows aerobically, but at 37°C primary growth from clinical specimens may be poor, becoming apparent only after 3–5 days' incubation: *L. monocytogenes* is unlikely to be cultured from routine specimens, unless a special search is made.

The organism is pathogenic to laboratory animals, especially the mouse and the rabbit.

Its localization in the genital tracts of many vertebrates, including man, and its diaplacental transmission to the foetus, underlie its importance in human obstetrics.

Maternal infections usually take the form of a mild "flu-like" generalized infection, without symptoms referable to the genital tract. Pyelitis of pregnancy may be caused by *Listeria*. Abortion, or stillbirth, may follow the acute febrile infection. The diagnosis during pregnancy is established by bacteriological and serological tests, including blood cultures. Agglutinin titres in excess of 1:320, or those showing a substantial rise in titre only are diagnostic, and a positive complement fixation test at a dilution of 1:10 is suggestive of present or recent infection. In a number of proven cases of listeriosis of the newborn, the mothers had previously suffered from one to several abortions, suggesting that genital listeriosis may cause repeated abortion.

Evidence is accumulating that listeriosis is an important cause of neonatal death and foetal damage. Figures from Leipzig, Germany showed that the perinatal death rate of 3,246 deliveries in hospital was 5·42 per cent with a fatality rate of 0·154 per cent due to proven listeriosis infections. Fatal infections in neonatal life are rarely recorded in the United Kingdom. The disease is a typical foetopathia, there being a few cases confirmed as occurring in the 4th month of pregnancy, and many more in the 5th and succeeding months. If infection occurs in the late stages of gestation, dead foetuses or living children are born either prematurely or at term. If born alive, the children show uncharacteristic symptoms, usually ascribed to some non-infectious cause. The cardinal symptoms are respiratory distress, and circulatory failure, diarrhoea, and, occasionally, a papular exanthem. If the child survives more than 3 days, purulent meningitis supervenes and determines the fatal outcome.

The organism is sensitive *in vitro* to a number of antibiotics, but the drugs of choice are those of the tetracycline group. Penicillin and erythromycin have also been used in combination.

Rubella in Pregnancy, Foetal and Neonatal Life
(McCarthy and Taylor–Robinson, 1967)

A serious epidemic of rubella (1,800,000 cases) in the United States in 1964 gave impetus to further studies on the virus of rubella and on the pathogenesis of congenital infections.

The nature of the virion is still uncertain, but the combination of large size, sensitivity to ether, and ribonucleic acid, suggests that it resembles the viruses of the measles group, or rabies.

Cytopathic effects (CPE) are produced in primary cultures of human amnion (PHA), in thyroid cells, and in cells of rabbit origin. When the virus fails to produce CPE, its presence may be detected by failure of the culture to respond to challenge with another cytopathic virus (virus interference).

Serological tests include virus neutralization, complement fixation and fluorescent antibody methods.

Early reports of congenital rubella emphasized defects of the heart, eye and ear, but the name "expanded rubella syndrome" has been given to a wide spectrum of abnormalities observed after the 1964 epidemic. Prospective studies up to 1960, on summing up, showed that after maternal rubella in the 1st four weeks of pregnancy 47 per cent of liveborn children were defective; after rubella in the 2nd four weeks, 22 per cent; and in the next 2 four weeks periods, 7 per cent and 6 per cent respectively. In addition to teratogenesis, rubella in the first two months of pregnancy is associated with up to 53 per cent foetal death, as well as many premature births.

In addition to the classical triad of deafness, cataract, and cardiac anomalies (such as patent ductus arteriosus and ventricular septal defect) affected babes may suffer brain damage, resulting in mental retardation, microcephaly or hydrocephaly; retarded intra-uterine development, thrombocytopaenic purpura, anaemia, hepatosplenomegaly, unusual bone lesions, meningo-encephalitis, pneumonitis, myocarditis and hepatitis.

The virus crosses the placental barrier, and after congenital infection has been isolated from virtually every tissue. It may persist in the foetus throughout pregnancy, and, after birth, affected infants may excrete virus for some months, occasionally for periods up to a year. Most, if not all, foetal damage is presumed to be the direct result of viral multiplication in the tissues.

Postnatal rubella is probably the result of infection *via* the respiratory tract. The virus has been recovered from the nose, throat, and urine, from 7 days before until 10 days after, the appearance of the rash.

It is clear that the current studies on the pathogenesis of rubella may alter our views on prophylaxis, as there is every hope of a satisfactory live vaccine. Hitherto, the prophylactic use of γ globulin was given moderately favourable assessment, but this was before serological methods were available for estimating its potency, and before virological techniques for confirming the diagnosis in babies with suspected rubella syndrome. The dose given is usually 15 ml. Exposure to, and contraction of, the disease before the age of childbearing has long been held to be prophylactic. Current work indicates that second, inapparent infections may conceivably occur and the matter is still *sub judice*.

Cytomegalic Inclusion Disease (Timbury, 1967)

The cytomegaloviruses are members of the herpes group of viruses, and there are two serological types. They grow in human fibroblast cell cultures, producing cytopathic effects, with characteristic "owl's eye" intranuclear inclusions, and they can be isolated from the urine and from throat swabs.

About 50 per cent of the adult population has complement fixing antibody to these viruses, without any symptom of disease. The organisms are examples of "opportunistic pathogens", that is, they cause disease only when the normal resistance of the host is lowered. Adult infections are thus usually concomitant to severe debilitating diseases, e.g. neoplasia. The infection may be disseminated, or localized to the lungs or gastro-intestinal tract. Recent reports have indicated a possible association of the viruses with glandular fever.

Neonatal Infection

The newborn has a low resistance to the infection, and may develop severe generalized infection *in utero* or after birth from mothers with symptomless infections in which virus is excreted in the urine, or in the saliva. Neonatal disease is uncommon, but by no means a rarity, and the virus is usually transmitted *via* the placenta. The affected infants have jaundice, hepatosplenomegaly, blood dyscrasias such as thrombocytopaenia and haemolytic anaemia; microcephaly may be present, and the surviving infant may be mentally retarded. These viruses may be the cause of some cases of cerebral palsy. Some have speculated that cytomegalic inclusion viruses may be common causes of neonatal hepatitis.

Pathology

Characteristic intranuclear inclusions (owl's eye) are seen in enlarged cells found mainly in the salivary glands, liver, kidneys and lungs.

REFERENCES

Beattie, C. P. (1967), "Toxoplasmosis," in *Recent Advances in Medical Microbiology*, edited by Waterson, A. P., pp. 318–351. London: J. and A. Churchill Ltd.

Butler, N. R. and Bonham, D. G. (1963), *First Report of the British Perinatal Mortality Survey*. Edinburgh and London: E. S. Livingstone.

Colebrook, Dora C. (1935), *The Source of Infection in Puerperal Fever due to Haemolytic Streptococci*. London: H.M.S.O.

Cowan, S. T. and Steel, K. J. (1965), *Manual for the Identification of Medical Bacteria*, p. 84. Cambridge University Press.

Eastman, N. J. and Hellman, !. M. (Editors), *Williams Obstetrics 1966*, 13th ed. p. 333. New York: Appleton–Century–Crofts.

Eichenwald, H. F. A. (1960), "A Study of Congenital Toxoplasmosis with Particular Emphasis on Clinical Manifestations, Sequelæ and Therapy" in *Human Toxoplasmosis*, edited by J. Siim, p. 41. Copenhagen: Munksgaard.

Ellis, M. (1963), "Human Antitetanus Serum in the Treatment of Tetanus," *Brit. med. J.*, **i**, 1123.

Gardner H. L. and Dukes C. D. (1955), "Haemophilus vaginalis vaginitis", *Amer. J. Obstet. Gynec.* **69**, 962–976

Glynn, B. S., Cain, A. R. R. and Gillespie, W. A. (1967), "Bacteriology of the Neonatal Respiratory Tract," *Postgrad. med. J. Suppl.*, **43**, 99.

Gordon, John E. (1965), *Control of Communicable Diseases in Man*, 10th ed. New York: The American Public Health Assoc.

Gray, M. L. and Killinger, A. H. (1966), "Listeria Monocytogenes and Listeric Infections," *Bact. Revs.*, **30**, 309.

Harrison, C. V. (1966), "Toxoplasmosis," in *Recent Advances in Pathology*, 8th ed., edited by Harrison, C. V., pp. 207–210. London: J. and A. Churchill Ltd.

Janeway, C. A. (1966), "The Immunological System of the Child," *Arch. Dis. Childh.*, **41**, 358.

Kass, E. H. (1956)," Asymptomatic Infections of the Urinary Tract," *Trans. Ass. Amer. Phys.*, **69**, 56.

McCarthy, K. and Taylor-Robinson, C. H. (1967), "Rubella," *Brit. med. Bull.*, **23**, 185.

MacLane, C. M. (1939), "Pyelitis of Pregnancy: A five year study," *Amer. J. Obstet. Gyn,ec.*, **38**, 117.

Major, R. H. (1954), *A, History of Medicine*. Oxford: Blackwell.

Marmion, B. P. (1967) "The Mycoplasmas," in *Recent Advances in Medical Microbiology* edited by Waterson, A. P., p. 198. London: J. and A. Churchill Ltd.

Martius, H. (1941), "Zum Enstehungsmechanismus der Schwangerschaft spyelitus," *Zbl. Gynäk*, **65**, 812.

M.R.C. Memorandum (1967), No. 23: "Nomenclature of fungi pathogenic to Man and animals. Names recommended for use in U.K." (3rd ed.). London: H.M.S.O.

Public Health Laboratory Service Survey (Report 1960), Lidwell, O. M. (1961), *J. Hyg. Camb.*, **59**, 259.

Quinn, E. L. and Kass, E. H. (1960), *Biology of Pyelonephritis*. London: J. and A. Churchill.

Registrar General's Reports, 1954–1964.

Schaffer, A. J. (1966), *Diseases of the Newborn*, 2nd ed., pp. 116–142, 269–276, 400, 552, 713–767. Philadelphia and London: W. B. Saunders Co.

Seeliger, H. P. R. (1961), *Listeriosis*. Basel and New York: S. Karger.

Timbury, Morag C. (1967), *Notes on Medical Virology*. London and Edinburgh: E. and S. Livingstone.

Williams, R. E. O., Blowers, R., Garrod, L. P. and Shooter, R. A. (1966), *Hospital Infection, Causes and Prevention*, 2nd ed., p. 30. London: Lloyd Luke Ltd.

Wilson, G. S. and Miles, A. A. (1964), *Topley and Wilson's Principles of Bacteriology and Immunology*, 5th ed. London: Edward Arnold Ltd.

Wilson Clyne, D. G. (1963), *A Textbook of Gynaecology and Obstetrics* p. 144, p. 512. London: Longmans Green and Co. Ltd.

Winner, H. I. and Hurley, Rosalinde (1964), *Candida albicans*. London: J. and A. Churchill Ltd.

Winner, H. I. and Hurley, Rosalinde (Editors) (1966), *Symposium on Candida Infections*. Edinburgh and London: E. and S. Livingstone Ltd., and Boston: Little Brown.

2. URINARY INFECTION IN OBSTETRICS AND GYNAECOLOGY

W. BRUMFITT AND A. P. CONDIE

INTRODUCTION

Infection of the urine is a problem in all countries of the world. "Pyelitis of pregnancy" was recognized before the bacteriological era (Rayer, 1841) and in a review Sims (1965) describes pyelonephritis as the most frequent and important medical complication of pregnancy. "Cystitis" is a common disease of women of child-bearing age whilst after gynaecological surgery urinary infection is commonplace.

In 1956, Kass published carefully collected information on the importance of asymptomatic infection and stressed the need to recognize this condition since it was sometimes the precursor of severe symptomatic infections. The latter could be prevented by early detection and cure of the asymptomatic disease. Furthermore it has become apparent that chronic pyelonephritis is an important cause of renal failure and the relationship of all forms of urinary infection (including asymptomatic) to this condition requires consideration. The detection and treatment of urinary infection in obstetrics and gynaecology provides an excellent opportunity for the practice of preventive medicine whereas failure of recognition, and therefore treatment, may lead ultimately to chronic, irreversible disease.

The purpose of this chapter is to consider some important aspects of urinary infection in a general way and then to deal in more detail with those special aspects which relate to pregnant women and gynaecological patients.

BACTERIOLOGY

Common Pathogens of the Urinary Tract

Infections acquired outside hospital are due to *Esch. coli* in 90 per cent of patients and most of the remainder are due to either *Proteus mirabilis* or *Klebs. aerogenes*.

In contrast, infections acquired in hospital are due to a wider range of bacteria although *Esch. coli* is still found to be the most common cause. In addition to those organisms already mentioned *Strept. faecalis*, *Ps. aeruginosa* and other strains of *Proteus* (*rettgeri, morganii* and *vulgaris*) are found.

A major difference between domiciliary and hospital infections is that in the former the organisms are both sensitive to a wide range of antibiotics and have a predictable sensitivity pattern whereas infections acquired in hospital are much more likely to be resistant to antibiotics and the sensitivity pattern is unpredictable. Organisms isolated in a particular hospital are liable to be resistant to the antibiotics in most frequent use.

Serotyping of Esch. coli

By using specific antisera it is possible to categorize *Esch. coli* into 149 different O-types and since the antigenic structure is a stable property of bacteria it can be used as a definitive typing characteristic. Investigations using this method show that a small number of serotypes are responsible for the majority of domiciliary urinary infections. The common serotypes causing these infections are also those which most frequently inhabit the intestinal canal and it appears highly likely that the bowel is the reservoir of the bacteria responsible (Grüneberg, Leigh and Brumfitt, 1968).

Distinction between Relapse and Reinfection

An important application of serotyping urinary organisms is in differentiating between recurrence due to failure of treatment and reinfection by a new organism. Figure 1 summarizes some situations where failure of treatment has occurred. In general if significant numbers of two *different* organisms are isolated at intervals from a patient's urine then reinfection must have occurred, whereas if the same organism is isolated repeatedly, this is usually taken to indicate relapse. When an infection due to *Esch. coli* is followed by one due to *Proteus mirabilis* reinfection has obviously occurred but when *Esch. coli* reappears distinction can only be made by serotyping (Fig. 1). As will be seen later such distinction greatly influences the method of treatment. In practice reinfection is much more common than relapse but relapsing infection is usually more serious because it implies tissue involvement with or without abnormality of the urinary tract.

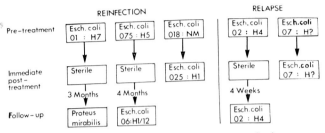

Fig. 1. Changes in urine culture after treatment of urinary infection. Note difference between reinfection and relapse.

HOST FACTORS ASSOCIATED WITH SUSCEPTIBILITY TO INFECTION

The normal urinary tract is sterile, except near the urethral orifice. Available evidence reviewed by Beeson (1955), points strongly to urinary infections starting from below and if the kidney is involved the bacteria have ascended up the ureter from the bladder. Infections transmitted via the blood stream are believed to be unusual.

Infection of the Lower Urinary Tract

Females are known to be more susceptible to urinary infection than males. Several reasons for this have been proposed, for example the proximity of the urethral orifice to the rectum and the moist environment around it favours bacterial growth. Furthermore, the urethra is only 5 cm. in length and the first 4 cm. are colonized by bacteria. It is susceptible to trauma during sexual intercourse and it is liable to be involved by infections of the vagina. Recently Stamey *et al.* (1968) have made the interesting observation that in the male, prostatic fluid is powerfully bactericidal but that no equivalent substance is produced by the female periurethral glands. Thus the female lacks the disinfectant barrier present in the male and this too may be a factor in determining the greater susceptibility to infection. Pasteur used urine as a culture medium and the bacteria which are found in urinary infection all grow well in it. Organisms such as *N. gonorrhoeae*, which do not cause urinary infection cannot multiply in the urine. However, even if bacteria which can multiply in the urine enter the healthy bladder in large numbers, infection is by no means certain to follow. Two mechanisms appear to be important in preventing the establishment of infection. First the "wash out" of bacteria resulting from complete bladder emptying (Cox and Hinman, 1961) is of great importance. As a result of complete emptying only a thin film of urine coating the bladder wall remains and hence the bacteria themselves come into contact with the mucosa. The second defence mechanism is the ability of the mucosa to eliminate bacteria in contact with its surface (Vivaldi, Munoz, Cotran and Kass, 1965). Consequently any process which alters normal micturition so that bladder emptying is incomplete leads to bacterial multiplication in the residual pool of urine thus allowing infection to become established and to persist.

Spread of Infection from the Bladder to the Renal Pelvis

The vesico-ureteric valves prevent bladder urine from ascending into the ureters during micturition. However, sometimes these valves become incompetent and urine is able to reflux. Vesico-ureteric reflux can be demonstrated by the micturating cystogram (Hodson and Edwards, 1960) and by this means reflux of infected urine has been shown to occur in patients with lower urinary tract infection. Such reflux may be due to oedema around the valves which makes them incompetent. However, it is also known that women with infection confined to the bladder early in pregnancy may later develop acute pyelonephritis although no inflammation of the lower urinary tract has occurred. The route of upward spread in these patients has not been established.

Infection of the Renal Tissues

The wedge-shaped distribution of infection in the kidney in man and experimental animals suggests that the most likely route of invasion is from the collecting tubules in the medulla and then outwards through corresponding nephrons (Beeson, 1967). The renal medulla is more susceptible than the cortex to infection by *Esch. coli* and several factors may be responsible. Normal immune mechanisms may be impaired by hypertonic conditions found in the medulla so that both complement activity and phagocytosis are inhibited. Complement may also be inactivated by ammonia, the concentration of which increases towards the distal end of the renal tubule (Beeson and Rowley, 1959). The relatively low rate of blood flow in the inner medulla has also been blamed. Finally the hypertonic conditions in the medulla may allow survival of bacterial variants as spheroplasts or L-forms, whereas in an isotonic environment the bacteria would have been killed. These various factors may work independently or together to increase the susceptibility of the kidney to bacterial invasion.

DIAGNOSIS OF URINARY TRACT INFECTION

In many patients a diagnosis of urinary infection is still being made on an evaluation of symptoms alone and treatment is instituted without bacteriological confirmation of infection. This practice results in much unnecessary treatment being given because several studies have shown that a substantial number of patients, especially female, complain of symptoms suggestive of urinary infection in the absence of organisms in the urine. In a survey of such patients in general practice in New Zealand, Gallagher *et al.* (1965) found that only 59 per cent of 130 unselected patients with symptoms of an acute lower urinary infection had infected urine. Similarly Mond *et al.* (1965) in a general practice study in London observed that in only 45 per cent of their patients with symptoms suggestive of urinary tract infection was the infection confirmed bacteriologically. However, half of these patients with symptoms but no bacteriuria had excess excretion of white blood cells suggesting that these patients had urethritis rather than infection within the bladder.

It is thus obvious that symptoms such as dysuria, frequency or nocturia must not be used alone to diagnose urinary infection which must be confirmed by accurate bacteriological examination of the urine. In a study of bacteriuria in pregnancy we found that symptoms such as frequency, nocturia and urgency were complained of just as often by non-bacteriuric control patients as by those with confirmed bacteriuria (Condie et al., 1968). Surprisingly even loin pain and tenderness on palpation in the absence of fever did not correlate well with finding of infected urine although the presence of these signs along with fever or rigors was almost always associated with infected urine and therefore pointed to acute pyelonephritis.

Great caution must be exercised in the interpretation of symptoms suggestive of urinary infection in the light of these observations. Placing the label "urinary tract infection" on a patient is a serious step nowadays because it is likely to lead to a chain of investigations including pyelography causing unnecessary inconvenience and discomfort to the patient.

A further important disadvantage of relying on symptoms to diagnose infections of the urinary tract is that many of these infections, confirmed bacteriologically, remain asymptomatic even in some cases where there is involvement of renal tissues. Inadequate treatment is particularly liable to convert symptomatic infections to asymptomatic ones.

Collection of Specimens

Bacteriological examination of a carefully collected uncontaminated specimen of urine is the *sole* method of diagnosing infection of the urinary tract. Collection of an uncontaminated urine specimen from a female patient is not easy but with care a minimally contaminated specimen can be collected at normal micturition. The need for catheterizing with its attendant risk of introducing infection (Beeson, 1958; Brumfitt, Davies and Rosser, 1961) can usually be avoided for the collection of routine specimens.

Scrupulous attention to technique in the collection of specimens of urine from female patients is essential for accurate diagnosis. Actual techniques have varied especially in the method of pre-collection cleansing of urethral meatus and vulva. Turner (1961) in comparing the degree of contamination of 200 specimens collected from patients whose vulvae were washed by a nurse, with midstream specimens from 200 different unprepared patients, concluded that cleaning of the vulva before collection of urine specimens from antenatal patients was not worthwhile. However, Kass (1968) noted that in his clinic there was approximately 20 per cent of excess contamination in the unprepared patient over that encountered following thorough washing.

We have found that without washing an unacceptable degree of contamination followed, while using a simple washing procedure with a single swab after labial separation contamination was reduced to a minimum and a confidence level for infection of 95 per cent was obtained when two consecutive specimens were positive. We must, therefore, subscribe to the view that swabbing is necessary and also that adequate instruction of the patient is vital. We originally used antiseptic solutions for vulval cleansing but since Roberts et al. (1967) have pointed out that such solutions might contaminate the urine and reduce the bacterial count sufficiently to mask the infection, we have been using either soap solution or sterile water with satisfactory results. The important point about any method employed is that its success in reducing the number of contaminated specimens to a minimum should be proved in sound bacteriological terms before it is routinely adopted. The patient must be carefully instructed in the correct technique of cleansing and collection and where possible be supervised by a trained nurse. She must be instructed to wash her hands and swab the introitus from before backwards while separating the labia with two fingers of one hand. She then squats over a toilet and passes urine into a sterile plastic container held in the other hand after letting the first part of the stream go directly into the toilet. The lid is placed on the container and the specimen is either cultured within the hour or is refrigerated at 4°C until culture is possible. Small numbers of bacteria in urine which is left at room temperature multiply to give a false positive result. In this respect co-operation of nursing staff in hospitals is by no means always perfect and the custom of the specimen of urine being collected by the night staff at 7 a.m. and being left on a bench in a warm place awaiting the laboratory opening at 9 a.m. is still all too prevalent! Collection of these specimens must be co-ordinated with laboratory collection times or refrigerated at once if this is not practicable.

In the great majority of patients infection can be diagnosed or excluded by examination of well taken urine specimens. In a few cases, however, the results of culture are persistently equivocal despite repeated examination of specimens. In such cases, or where there is persistent contamination, the problem may be solved by direct sampling of the urine by suprapubic aspiration. This procedure has been found to be safe in the non-pregnant woman (Stamey, Govan and Palmer, 1965) and in a large series of pregnant women also (Beard et al., 1965; Eykyn and McFadyen, 1968). The use of a urethral catheter is a less satisfactory alternative in cases of persistent contamination because of the danger of introducing infection (Brumfitt, Davies and Rosser, 1961). A further source of error may be that a true infection may have a falsely lowered bacterial count due to excessive hydration and frequency of micturition (Cox and Hinman, 1961). However, this would only occur with exceptional overhydration and frequency (O'Grady and Cattell, 1966).

Quantitative Bacteriological Methods

Marple in 1941 reported the need for quantitative colony counts for the accurate diagnosis of urinary infections but stressed the need for catheter specimens. The idea did not then gain general acceptance, however, and the simpler qualitative methods continued to be used. It was not until Kass (1956) published systematic analyses of bacterial counts that criteria were scientifically established which would allow differentiation to be made between true infection of the urine and contamination in ordinary voided specimens. Since then the need for catheter specimens has been obviated and large scale screening programmes have been made practicable, thereby allowing some clarification of our understanding of the prevalence and importance of urinary infections in whole populations. Kass found that patients with bacterial counts of over 100,000 organisms per ml. of urine usually had a similar level in subsequent specimens and the organisms were known urinary pathogens (usually Gram negative rods). Lower bacterial counts were usually associated with urethral commensals or mixed organisms suggestive of contamination and examination of a second specimen usually gave a negative result. Thus the term "significant bacteriuria" implies that bacteria are actually multiplying in the bladder urine and therefore that true infection is present. Under these circumstances the bacterial population will ordinarily exceed 100,000 per ml. of urine. However, bacteria may have entered the urine as contaminants from the container used for collection, from vaginal and faecal contamination, from the peri-urethral area and from the urethra itself. Urethral contaminants in urine rarely exceed 1,000 bacteria per ml., and other forms of contamination can be avoided by proper preparation of the patient and either prompt processing of the specimen or storage at 4°C.

100,000 organisms per ml. is widely accepted as the criterion of infection and should be used not only in research but for ordinary routine diagnosis. A number of published works on urinary infection are invalidated because infection was not defined in terms of quantitative bacteriology.

Description of the techniques for counting bacteria in the urine are beyond the scope of this chapter but the methods available have been reviewed (Brumfitt, 1968). Precise bacterial counts are necessary as a standard against which simpler tests can be compared and for the investigation of equivocal results but simpler methods are now available for the investigation of larger groups, such as pregnant women. The method which we find both suitable and economical merely involves dipping a sterilized absorbent filter paper strip of standard size into the urine and laying a measured area of the paper on to a well dried MacConkey plate. The test can be performed rapidly, 6 to 8 urine samples can be examined in duplicate on one culture plate and the results read very quickly (Fig. 2). Other methods consist of dipping a slide coated with culture medium into the urine or sampling the urine with a platinum loop of standard size. Quantitative estimation of white cells in the urine has also been recommended as a method of detecting urinary infection but the limit between normality and abnormality is not accurately defined. Difficulties arise in distinguishing between leucocytes and renal tubular cells and also because white cells are unstable in alkaline urine. Significant infection of

the urine is not always accompanied by an increased white cell excretion and this is particularly well demonstrated in bacteriuria of pregnancy. On the other hand there are a number of lesions of the urinary tract not of infective origin which are associated with inflammation and cause an abnormally high urinary white cell count. Thus estimation of white cell excretion is not only less accurate than counting bacteria but also less specific.

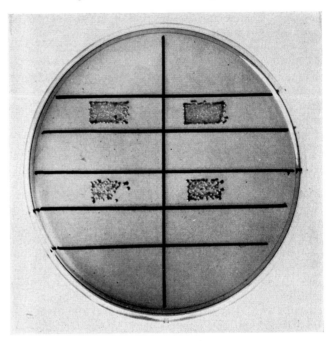

Fig. 2. Results obtained on 6 urines by the filter paper technique. Duplicate impressions have been made from each specimen, and the plates incubated overnight. The results are: urines 2 and 4 infected (more than 24 colonies on the inoculated area) and urines 1, 3, 5 and 6 uninfected.

LOCALIZATION OF INFECTION IN THE URINARY TRACT

Infection of the urine can be diagnosed by quantitative bacteriology but having reached this position it is important to know whether the renal tissues are involved. Evidence is accumulating to show that bacterial invasion of the kidney need not be accompanied by the classical features of acute pyelonephritis and indeed that urinary symptoms may be entirely lacking, so that the patient is suffering from "asymptomatic pyelonephritis". A major advance in the management of urinary infection will occur when it is possible to diagnose this condition of asymptomatic pyelonephritis in the individual patient.

Fairley, Bond and Adey (1966) studied a group of pregnant women by ureteric catheterization and found that about 40 per cent had bacteria in the renal pelvic urine suggesting renal invasion by bacteria. However such a procedure cannot be applied to routine use. More recently Fairley, Bond and Brown (1967) described an ingenious technique whereby ureteric urine can be sampled without passing ureteric catheters. The technique involves first catheterization of the bladder and collection of a specimen of bladder urine on which bacterial counts are carried out. Neomycin is then instilled to sterilize the bladder contents and after an interval the neomycin is removed by washing with sterile water. Subsequent urine specimens are collected through the urethral catheter at 10 minute intervals. This urine has therefore come straight from the ureters and bacterial counts from it represent those of urine in the renal pelvis. Valuable though it is, this test is time consuming and must be carried out in hospital. Treatment of the infection should be commenced as soon as the results of the test are known.

Two simple indirect methods can be used to detect asymptomatic pyelonephritis. The first depends upon the finding that when infection involves the renal parenchyma, specific antibodies against the infecting organism can be detected in the patient's serum. On the other hand, such antibodies are not found in significant titre when infection is confined to the lower urinary tract (Brumfitt and Percival, 1963; Winberg et al., 1963; Percival, Brumfitt and de Louvois, 1964). The second method of detecting renal involvement is to estimate renal concentrating ability (Winberg, 1959). Kaitz (1961) showed that defective concentration was present in 9 of 20 women with asymptomatic bacteriuria. We have recently confirmed that a proportion of pregnant women with asymptomatic bacteriuria have defective urine concentrating ability but that control non-bacteriuric pregnant women have no such defect. Furthermore, patients with defective concentration usually have a raised antibody titre against the infecting organism (Reeves and Brumfitt, 1968). It was also found that infections in these patients tended to be more resistant to treatment. We are at present investigating whether these patients with raised antibody titres and defective urine concentration are more likely to develop acute pyelonephritis or other complications.

Other methods of detecting asymptomatic pyelonephritis include detection of urinary enzymes and certain specific low molecular weight proteins. It is hoped that these methods will reflect kidney destruction and tubular damage respectively, and they are being evaluated at the present time.

BACTERIURIA IN PREGNANCY

This subject has been intensively studied over the past decade and the vast literature that has accumulated has recently been examined in some excellent reviews (Savage, Hajj and Kass, 1967; Whalley, 1967; Beard and Roberts, 1968).

Importance of Antenatal Screening

It has been known for many years that pregnant women were liable to have a large number of bacteria in their urine in the absence of symptoms (Dodds, 1931). Later Kass (1956, 1960) clearly demonstrated that acute pyelonephritis of pregnancy was particularly liable to develop in this group of bacteriuric women but that it seldom developed in non-bacteriuric pregnant women. He also demonstrated that treatment could substantially reduce the development of this serious complication and this has been confirmed by several subsequent studies. (Kass,

1959; Turner, 1961; Little, 1966; Kincaid-Smith and Bullen, 1965 and Condie et al., 1968). A relationship between untreated bacteriuria and other complications of pregnancy, including premature delivery, has also been suggested (Kass, 1960; Savage et al., 1967), but this is more controversial.

Nevertheless the possibility of preventing an attack of acute pyelonephritis and the hope of arresting the progress of a chronic disease at an early asymptomatic stage has led to greater appreciation of the importance of screening all antenatal patients for significant bacteriuria. However, this important type of preventive medicine is still neglected by the majority of antenatal clinics in this country despite reports of its economic practicability even in a busy clinic of a large general hospital (Williams et al., 1965b). It is suggested that screening all new antenatal patients for the presence of significant urinary infection should be as routine a part of antenatal care as screening for syphilis, anaemia, diabetes and rhesus immunization.

Prevalence of Bacteriuria in Pregnancy

The exact prevalence of bacteriuria during pregnancy is difficult to state because published reports show great variation. Most, however, fall into the range of between 5·0 and 6·5 per cent and studies showing higher percentages often include organisms which suggest contaminated specimens. It should be noted that there are strong indications that patients from lower socio-economic groups have a higher prevalence of bacteriuria during pregnancy (Henderson et al., 1962; Turck et al., 1962) and other workers have claimed a rise in prevalence with age and parity.

Acquisition of Bacteriuria

Bacteriuria has been studied in so much detail during pregnancy that there is a risk of concluding that this infection is often acquired during pregnancy. In fact there is evidence to suggest that pregnancy, with modern antenatal care, may be an incidental reason for detecting a chronic condition which was often present long before the pregnancy. For example, Sleigh et al. (1964) found that 8 per cent of a group of 397 nulliparous married women attending an infertility clinic in Edinburgh had bacteriuria compared with 6·6 per cent of 1,684 pregnant women from the same area. In Jamaica, Kass et al. (1965) found that 4 per cent of adult women had bacteriuria while Stuart et al. (1965) found the prevalence among pregnant women there to be 3·5 per cent. In Wales (Sussman et al., 1969) 3,578 non-pregnant women were screened for bacteriuria and this was found in two consecutive cultures in 126 (3·5%). A similar prevalence was found by Freedman et al., (1965) in Japan.

This evidence suggests that a small but definite proportion of adult women have significant bacteriuria (possibly related to marriage and intercourse) but that pregnancy itself need not cause any increase in the prevalence of bacteriuria except possibly for the associated increased need for catheterization of the bladder (Brumfitt, Davies and Rosser, 1961).

Few would now dispute the relationship of asymptomatic bacteriuria during early pregnancy and the subsequent development of acute symptomatic urinary tract infection. In his earlier studies Kass (1956, 1957 and 1960) reported that 40 per cent of patients found to have bacteriuria in early pregnancy developed acute pyelonephritis later in the pregnancy but that the acute complication did not occur in those women whose urine was sterile early in pregnancy. Different authors report a very wide range for the incidence of acute pyelonephritis following untreated bacteriuria in early pregnancy ranging from 14–63 per cent compared with 0–14 per cent among women whose urine was uninfected early in pregnancy (Whalley, 1967). These differences are partly due to strictness of the criteria used for the diagnosis of acute pyelonephritis, some using this label when only frequency and slight dysuria were complained of, symptoms which are often present even in patients whose urine is persistently sterile. In a recent report Savage, Hajj and Kass (1967), using very strict criteria for the diagnosis of pyelonephritis, found that this developed in 26 out of 108 patients with untreated bacteriuria compared with only 1·4 per cent of a random sample of non-bacteriurics. In our own study (Condie *et al.*, 1968) 23·3 per cent of a group of 86 untreated pregnant bacteriuric patients developed definite symptoms of acute pyelonephritis compared with 2 per cent of 150 non-bacteriuric controls.

The relationship between asymptomatic bacteriuria in pregnancy and chronic progressive pyelonephritis is less clear, since few prospective long term studies on patients with urinary infections are available. In some pregnant women bacteriuria is almost certainly a benign condition causing no obvious complications during the pregnancy and being easily eradicated by chemotherapy, often only after a single course of treatment. In others the urine cannot be kept persistently clear of bacteria even after several courses of different chemotherapeutic agents. Some of this latter group are probably at a stage of a disease where progressive renal damage may proceed to chronic renal failure.

Effect of Bacteriuria on Pregnancy

There is no doubt that many women who have bacteriuria detected in the first trimester will go through the pregnancy with no complications and deliver a normal baby of normal size at term. However, it has frequently been observed that such women seem to be more prone to certain complications than are patients whose urine is sterile throughout pregnancy. A direct association between bacteriuria and these complications is, however, by no means universally accepted and the possibility of preventing these complications by eradication of the bacteriuria is even more controversial.

Prematurity. An association between acute pyelonephritis and premature delivery is well known (Dodds, 1932). The finding in 1960 by Kass that 24 per cent of a group of women with asymptomatic bacteriuria delivered babies weighing less than 2,500 g. but that after eradication of the infection the incidence fell to 10 per cent, a level similar to his non-bacteriuric patients, led initially to hopes that

here was a method of substantially lowering the prematurity rate. Unfortunately further work has not always clearly demonstrated this association, and even where it has, the effect on the prematurity rate of treating the bacteriuria has not often been shown to be worthwhile. Some studies support the relationship (Le Blanc and McGanity, 1964; Kincaid-Smith and Bullen, 1965; Stuart, Cummins and Chin, 1965; Brumfitt, Grüneberg and Leigh, 1966; Condie *et al.*, 1968 and Grüneberg, Leigh and Brumfitt, 1969) while others do not (Bryant *et al.*, 1964; Sleigh *et al.*, 1964; Henderson and Reinke, 1965 and Little, 1966).

There are several reasons why studies of this question should produce such variable and often inconclusive results. First, the differing approaches to the problem, such as comparing bacteriuric patients receiving treatment with those given placebo or comparing bacteriuric women with matched non-bacteriuric controls or with the general population regardless of their urinary findings. In these studies also the criteria have varied for defining significant bacteriuria and in methods for its detection. Some do not specify that the bacteriuria must be persistent during pregnancy; in some in fact bacteriuria was only found at the time of delivery. Many authors treat bacteriurics as a homogeneous group, whereas it is probable that only certain bacteriuric women have a tendency to deliver prematurely, such as those with underlying chronic renal disease (Kincaid-Smith and Bullen, 1965) or those whose infection did not readily respond to chemotherapy some of whom were found to have serious renal abnormalities (Brumfitt, Grüneberg and Leigh, 1966). A further difficulty is to be able to take into account the effect of many other factors known to influence foetal size such as pre-eclamptic toxaemia, socio-economic factors, smoking, multiple pregnancy, uterine abnormalities, etc. Twin pregnancies for example must be excluded as demonstrated by Savage, Hajj and Kass (1967), who found a prematurity rate of 23·6 per cent in a group of untreated bacteriurics compared to 13·5 per cent in a random sample of the pregnant population. When they excluded multiple pregnancies, however, this difference was no longer statistically significant. It may be more difficult to show a relationship between bacteriuria and prematurity in more affluent populations (Wilson, Hewitt and Monzon, 1966) because the mean birth weight of babies (Gruenwald *et al.*, 1967) and the prevalence of bacteriuria (Turck *et al.*, 1962) are both linked to socio-economic factors.

Inaccuracies may also be due to considering prematurity by simple weight definition alone without separately considering the prematurely delivered babies from those who were "small for dates" at delivery. A better approach might be to study the mean birth weights in bacteriuric and non-bacteriuric groups instead of just the very low birth weights.

In our own study (Condie *et al.*, 1968) preliminary results showed a significant difference in prematurity rates between bacteriurics (23 premature out of 180 total births) and the controls (9 premature out of 180 total births). The mean birth weights for the bacteriurics (6 pounds 13·5 ozs.) and the controls (7 pounds 3·3 ozs.) were also significantly different although less so. Despite these lower birth weights the gestation length at delivery was slightly longer for bacteriurics than for the controls in contrast to the findings of Savage, Hajj and Kass (1967).

The greatest single problem in trying to demonstrate a possible association between bacteriuria and prematurity is that the incidence of both these conditions is relatively low and so very large numbers of pregnant women must be screened in order to obtain statistically significant results. Beard and Roberts (1968) noted the difference in prematurity rates between bacteriurics and non-bacteriurics from 11 major studies and they calculated that 6,000 patients would have to be screened for a 95 per cent probability that this difference was significant and for a 99 per cent probability over 13,000 patients would be required. A carefully designed study of this magnitude has yet to be reported.

Pre-eclamptic toxaemia. A significant increase in hypertension among pregnant women with bacteriuria has been reported (Stuart, Cummins and Chin, 1965 and Kincaid-Smith and Bullen, 1965) but others (Low *et al.*, 1964; and Little, 1966) have failed to show such a relationship. One of the problems is the different criteria used in various studies to define pre-eclamptic toxaemia and difficulties in standardizing blood pressure recording in large numbers of patients.

Anaemia. Few worthwhile studies of pregnancy anaemia in relation to bacteriuria have been reported and most workers have found no good evidence to support an association (Kaitz and Hodder, 1961; Savage *et al.*, 1967 and Little, 1966). An association between bacteriuria and low serum folate levels was reported by Martin *et al.* (1967), but their criteria for diagnosing significant bacteriuria were inadequate.

Thus while several well known complications of pregnancy seem to be more common in women who have bacteriuria early in pregnancy, the association is obviously not a strong one and may not even be a direct one. In this field many important questions remain unanswered and await very large scale studies for their solution.

Treatment of Bacteriuria During Pregnancy

Prevention of complications such as acute symptomatic pyelonephritis during pregnancy depends on the ability to eradicate bacteriuria completely and so there is great need to devise an effective treatment for this condition.

Two questions need to be answered: the best chemotherapeutic agents to use and how long treatment should be continued.

Kass (1960) found a high relapse rate when he treated bacteriuric women with short courses of therapy and he, therefore, advised that treatment be given continuously throughout pregnancy. As was pointed out by Williams and Leigh (1966) determination of the minimum inhibitory concentration (MIC) of sulphonamides against the infecting organism is more accurate than the disc test in predicting the result of treatment. In those patients whose bacteriuria is not easily eradicated by a short course of chemotherapy it is important to realize that renal tissue involvement or underlying renal abnormality may be present (Brumfitt,

Grüneberg and Leigh, 1966; Leigh, Grüneberg and Brumfitt, 1968) and that these patients especially need long-term follow-up and radiological investigation. The use of continuous therapy throughout pregnancy may prevent this selection process of those women most at risk and may also mask a renal focus of infection. In any case, the use of continuous maintenance therapy in these patients has proved no better than short term therapy.

It must be stressed that treatment which is adequate for eradicating asymptomatic bacteriuria in the majority of patients (i.e. a short course of oral therapy) may not suffice in an attack of acute pyelonephritis where a higher initial blood level may be desired. When the patient is sufficiently ill to be admitted to hospital parenteral therapy should be given at first. If the infection was acquired outside hospital it is likely to be sensitive to ampicillin which should be given at a dose of 500 mg. 6-hourly by the intramuscular route. When the temperature has fallen oral therapy can be substituted. Details of treatment of more complicated situations such as infections due to resistant organisms and bacteraemic shock are described in a review (Brumfitt and Reeves, 1969).

Chemotherapeutic Agents Suitable for Bacteriuria in Pregnancy

About 75 per cent of women with bacteriuria in pregnancy respond to sulphonamide therapy and this cure rate is similar to that obtained using a variety of chemotherapeutic agents. Further the majority of organisms are sensitive to the blood and urine levels obtained by the usual therapeutic doses, the drugs are cheap and toxic effects are few. Results with the long-acting sulphonamides are similar and these have the advantage over sulphadimidine that the patient has fewer tablets to take and is less likely to forget to complete the course. Stevens–Johnson syndrome has been reported following the use of long-acting sulphonamides (Beveridge *et al.*, 1964) but the association may be fortuitous (British Medical Journal, 1964). Sulphonamides are usually not used during the last few weeks of pregnancy because they are said to reduce the binding capacity of the plasma for bilirubin (Odell, 1959 and Dunn, 1964). However, it was thought by Adamsons and Joelsson (1966) that it is unlikely that dangerous levels of unconjugated bilirubin are ever reached in the foetus because of the ability of the placenta to transfer it quickly into the maternal circulation.

Ampicillin is an effective drug against the strains of *Esch. coli* commonly found in urinary infections but the results of primary treatment are similar to those obtained with sulphonamides. When patients whose bacteriuria had failed to respond to sulphonamides were treated with ampicillin, however, 60 per cent of them were cured (Brumfitt, Leigh, Percival and Williams, 1964) and it is, therefore, a useful drug for the treatment of these patients. Nitrofurantoin is also useful in both primary and secondary treatment. Some women experience nausea following its use and for this reason we like to restrict the dose to 100 mg. twice daily for the treatment of primary infections. These doses should be given last thing at night and after breakfast.

Tetracycline is effective in the treatment of bacteriuria but its use is not recommended because it is said to produce discolouration of the primary dentition (Davies, Little and Aherne, 1962) and high tone deafness has been reported in children born to mothers who were treated with streptomycin for tuberculosis during pregnancy, although it is less likely that a short course would cause this damage.

In any case failure of primary treatment of bacteriuria in pregnancy is often associated with renal tissue involvement (as shown by a raised serum antibody titre against the infecting organism) or radiological abnormalities (Leigh, Grüneberg and Brumfitt, 1968) and in these women the infection is often not eradicated even though several courses of different antibiotics are given.

LONG TERM PROGNOSIS OF BACTERIURIA IN PREGNANCY

The long term outlook for these patients who were known to have bacteriuria during pregnancy has not yet been clarified. While it is known that in children, unchecked urinary infection can progress within a decade to chronic pyelonephritis and renal failure, the risk to these adult women is less clear. It is certain that in some of them the infection is benign and easily cured but in others it is not and tends to persist or recur. In a prospective study Leigh, Grüneberg and Brumfitt (1968) studied a group of 157 women for 2 to 4 years after having bacteriuria during pregnancy. All of these patients had been treated, the bacteriuria eradicated and they had remained free of infection at 6 weeks post partum. At long term follow-up, however, 43 (27 per cent) were again found to have bacteriuria. This recurrent infection was found to be more than twice as frequent in those who had required more than one course of chemotherapy to eradicate the initial bacteriuria. Furthermore, radiologically demonstrable urinary tract abnormalities were found to be more common and more severe in the group who had been difficult to cure during pregnancy. It is tempting to surmise that this group will contain women likely to progress towards chronic pyelonephritis and renal failure and that close follow-up and prolonged treatment might prevent this. There is, however, no long term prospective study which is able to prove this and some authorities have questioned whether such patients develop renal lesions of sufficient severity to cause renal failure in later years (Stamey, personal communication).

Until these points have been clarified, we think that women who have had bacteriuria during pregnancy, and especially those who proved difficult or impossible to cure, should have further specimens of urine examined at 6 weeks post partum and again at 3 and 6 months, then probably yearly. An intravenous pyelogram should be carried out not less than 3 months post-partum when the physiological changes in the urinary tract due to pregnancy should have reverted to normal. Future follow-up should be planned according to the results of these preliminary investigations.

URINARY INFECTION IN THE PUERPERIUM

Infection of the urinary tract found during the puerperium may be a continuation of pregnancy bacteriuria in which case the factors involved are as already discussed in detail. Infections which are acquired de novo in the puerperium may be due to the use of a catheter during or after labour to relieve retention of urine caused by the atony of the bladder which is not uncommon after delivery.

Brumfitt, Davies and Rosser (1961) examined 320 women known to have sterile urine before delivery and studied mid-stream specimens of urine during the puerperal stay in hospital. Of 105 patients who were not catheterized 4·7 per cent developed infected urine, while out of 110 who were catheterized once for specimen collection 9·1 per cent developed infection. In contrast, where catheterization was necessary on clinical grounds in 105 patients 24 (22·8 per cent) developed infected urine and in 32 of these where the indication was retention of urine, 13 (40·6 per cent) became infected. The majority of these patients were asymptomatic and the infections tended to resolve spontaneously when the bladder function returned to normal or to be easily cured by a single course of chemotherapy. None of these women were found to have relapse of infection when urine was examined at the post natal clinic. This contrasts with the findings on follow-up of patients who had bacteriuria during pregnancy where relapse was not uncommon.

Unless women are screened for bacteriuria during pregnancy it cannot be known whether an infection discovered in the puerperium is a continuation of a preexisting bacteriuria or a new infection with, therefore, a different prognosis. All these patients need a further urine culture at 6 weeks post partum.

The collection of specimens for culture during the puerperium may present difficulty due to the flow of lochia from the vagina. In the light of the above evidence catheterization to obtain a specimen is unjustified and in practice an uncontaminated voided specimen can be collected if the lochial discharge is temporarily held back by placing a pledget of sterile cotton wool into the introitus before cleansing the urethral orifice and vulva in the usual manner.

URINARY INFECTIONS IN GYNAECOLOGY

Acute Infections

Apart from the post-operative situation urinary infection in the non-pregnant woman has not received such concentrated study as that associated with pregnancy. This is partly because acute symptomatic infections of the lower urinary tract are usually seen and treated in general practice and respond well to treatment. For example, a seven-day course of sulphonamide results in a 90 per cent cure rate.

The symptoms of dysuria and frequency are not always associated with infection of the urine and Mond *et al.* (1965) found that only about half of the female patients seen in general practice with such symptoms had significant bacteriuria. Further investigation showed that 47 per cent of the uninfected patients had an excess of white cells in the urine suggesting that urethritis, without infection of the urine, was the cause of the symptoms.

Some patients suffer recurrent attacks of frequency and dysuria which they find distressing. Study of the organisms in these recurrent cases usually shows different strains, proving that they are true recurrences and not persistence of the original infection. The history will sometimes reveal a precipitating cause, such as coitus, in which case recurrences can often be avoided by the patient taking a single dose of nitrofurantoin (100 mg.) just before or after intercourse. Where no precipitating cause can be identified and persistent attacks occur it is wise to carry out a full investigation, including pyelography and urethrocystoscopy, the latter to exclude polypi or bladder diverticula.

Acute urinary infection is easily treated by a 7 to 10 day course of sulphonamide and a 90 per cent cure rate can be expected, but a six week follow-up at which the urine is examined to confirm eradication of the infection is necessary. For recurrent infections the organism should first be eradicated and then long term prophylactic therapy given. Nitrofurantoin or sulphonamide once or twice daily are suitable for this purpose and should be continued for at least 6 months.

Although symptomatic lower urinary tract infections occasionally progress to acute pyelonephritis or are found to be associated with renal abnormalities they appear to be much more benign in these respects than asymptomatic bacteriuria of pregnancy.

Post-operative Infections

As indicated earlier in the chapter post-operative infections of the urinary tract in gynaecological patients are due to a wide range of organisms which show varying degrees of antibiotic resistance. Infections due to highly antibiotic resistant strains create an even more difficult problem when they cause septicaemia or bacteraemic shock and the urinary tract is known to be the most common source of such infections.

After major vaginal surgery urinary infection is common and this has usually been blamed on the widespread use of the urethral catheter in these cases—especially where the technique has been faulty. After repair of prolapse catheterization is necessary in about half the patients (Donald et al., 1962) and Paterson, Barr and MacDonald (1960) reported that 71 per cent of patients had infected urine post-operatively and a further 21 per cent developed it at a later stage. Gillespie et al. (1960) found that the incidence post-operatively in patients with indwelling catheters and open drainage was 98 per cent.

It is widely believed that once bladder function returns to normal after operation these infections tend to clear spontaneously but, nevertheless, at a 5 to 6 year follow-up of 47 patients after prolapse repairs Simmons and Baker (1963) found infection in 31·9 per cent. They found no single aetiological factor other than operation and catheterization in association with these urinary infections. Such

infections do not seem to cause serious renal damage because Cattell et al. (1963) in a follow-up of 88 of 102 patients previously reported by Durham et al. (1954) could find no evidence of progressive renal damage. Considering the importance of post-operative infection in gynaecology it is surprising how few prospective studies are available using proper bacteriological techniques. From the published literature it is difficult to come to a firm conclusion about its long-term importance.

In contrast a great deal of good work has been done on the aetiology and prophylaxis of post-operative gynaecological urinary infections. Prevention of these urinary infections can be attempted in three ways: prophylactic chemotherapy, local bladder antiseptics and special arrangements for bladder drainage.

Linton and Gillespie (1962) pointed out the probable sources of infection in these cases. Insertion of the catheter may introduce organisms from the catheter itself or, more likely, from the patient's urethra or introitus. When an indwelling catheter is used infection may enter after its insertion either by rising air bubbles in the case of open drainage or in the film of mucopus between the catheter and the urethral wall when the catheter moves in the urethra along with the patient's movements. They found that with intermittent catheterization infection was markedly reduced by disinfection of the urethra with chlorhexidine jelly before inserting the catheter or instilling 1/5,000 chlorhexidine aqueous solution into the bladder after catheterization. With indwelling catheters the infection rate was reduced from 85 per cent to 10 per cent by draining the catheter into a closed sterile vessel containing disinfectant and preventing movement of the catheter up and down in the urethra by anchoring it in place with a small pad of plastic foam moistened with chlorhexidine cream through which a Foley catheter was threaded, the plastic pad lying against the urethral orifice while the bag of the catheter was inflated in the bladder.

Prophylactic chemotherapy has been tried with apparent improvement (Hawkins, 1962 and Williams et al., 1962) but such therapy can only be regarded as an adjunct to the other prophylactic measures already described. In fact many workers reserve chemotherapy for established infections.

Urinary Infections in Gynaecological Out-patients

Information on the prevalence of bacteriuria in women referred to gynaecological out-patients is very limited. However, in a recent study of 1506 women attending for the first time 82 (5·4 per cent) were found to have significant bacteriuria on two successive occasions. Esch. coli accounted for 83 per cent of infections. Of special interest was the higher incidence in patients with carcinoma (20 per cent), fibroids (11 per cent), prolapse (10·5 per cent) and infertility (10 per cent). Radiological examination was carried out on 46 patients and 19 showed abnormalities (Williams et al., 1969). This data again emphasizes the potentially dangerous associations of asymptomatic bacteriuria.

THE RELATIONSHIP BETWEEN BACTERIURIA IN PREGNANCY AND CHRONIC PYELONEPHRITIS

There has recently been much debate about how often chronic pyelonephritis is the cause of renal failure. Numerous pathologists have tried to demonstrate the frequency of chronic pyelonephritis at autopsy and very divergent views have emerged. The value of these studies is limited by the variation in technique of the examination and lack of uniform histological criteria for diagnosis. Furthermore, in many cases proper evidence for the presence or absence of infection during life is not available and information about renal function is lacking. Because of these difficulties and the similarity of the histological changes found in pyelonephritis to those found in other renal disease, arguments based upon autopsy studies seem futile.

Several studies have shown a relationship between bacteriuria during pregnancy and the subsequent demonstration of X-ray abnormalities (Whalley, Martin and Peters, 1965; Kincaid-Smith and Bullen, 1965; Brumfitt, Leigh and Grüneberg, 1966; Leigh, Grüneberg and Brumfitt, 1968 and Gower et al., 1968). However, the possibility that both bacteriuria and renal damage were present before pregnancy cannot be refuted at present. In female children with urinary infection prospective studies have shown that progressive scarring and calyceal changes occur (Hodson, 1959; Smellie et al., 1964 and Smellie, 1967). One third of women who had bacteriuria during pregnancy were subsequently shown to have organic urinary tract disease which might represent disease initiated in childhood (Leigh, Grüneberg and Brumfitt, 1968). However, the answer to this question will only be solved by long-term and large scale prospective follow-up studies. Meanwhile it is difficult to see how bacteria multiplying in an already damaged kidney can fail to produce further damage, and it seems, therefore, imperative to detect and give long-term care to such patients.

REFERENCES

Adamsons, K. and Joelsson, J. (1966), Amer. J. Obstet. Gynec., 96, 437.
Beard, R. W., McCoy, D. R., Newton, J. R. and Clayton, S. G. (1965), Lancet, 2, 610.
Beard, R. W. and Roberts, A. P. (1968), Brit. med. Bull., 24, 44.
Beeson, P. B. (1955), Yale J. Biol. Med., 28, 81.
Beeson, P. B. (1958), Amer. J. Med., 24, 1.
Beeson, P. B. (1967), in Renal Disease, p. 382, ed. Black, D. A. K., Blackwell.
Beeson, P. B. and Rowley, D. (1959), J. exp. Med., 110, 685.
Beveridge, J., Harris, M., Wise, G. and Steven, S. L. (1964), Lancet, 2, 593.
British Medical Journal (1964), Leading Article 2, 1410.
Brumfitt, W. (1968), Recent Advances in Clinical Pathology, 5, 19. Churchill.
Brumfitt, W., Davies, B. I. and Rosser, E. ap. I. (1961), Lancet, 2, 1059.
Brumfitt, W., Grüneberg, R. N. and Leigh, D. A. (1966), Symposium on Pyelonephritis, p. 20. Edinburgh: Livingstone.
Brumfitt, W., Leigh, D. A., Percival, A. and Williams, J. D. (1964), Postgrad. med. J. Suppl., p. 55.

Brumfitt, W. and Percival, A. (1963), "Proc. 2nd International Congress of Nephrology," eds. Vostal, J. and Richet, G., Excerpta med. (Amst.), p. 260.
Brumfitt, W. and Reeves, D. S., (1969) J. infect. Dis., 120, 61.
Bryant, R. E., Windom, R. E., Vineyard, J. P. and Sanford, J. P. (1964), J. Lab. clin. Med. 63, 224.
Cattell, W. R., Curwen, M. P., Shooter, R. A. and Williams, D. K. (1963), Brit. med. J., 1, 923.
Condie, A. P., Williams, J. D., Reeves, D. S. and Brumfitt, W. (1968), in Urinary Tract Infection, p. 148, eds. O'Grady, F. and Brumfitt, W. Oxford U. P.
Cox, C. E. and Hinman, F. (1961), J. Amer. med. Ass., 178, 919.
Davies, P. A., Little, K. and Aherne, W. (1962), Lancet, 1, 743.
Dodds, G. (1931), J. Obstet. Gynaec. Brit. Emp., 38, 773.
Dodds, G. (1932), J. Obstet. Gynaec. Brit. Emp., 39, 46.
Donald, I., Barr, W. and McGarry, J. A. (1962), J. Obstet. Gynæc. Brit. Cwlth., 69, 837.
Dunn, P. M. (1964), J. Obstet. Gynaec. Brit. Cwlth., 71, 128.
Durham, M. P., Shooter, R. A. and Curwen, M. P. (1954), Brit. med. J., 2, 1008.
Eykyn, S. J. and McFadyen, I. R. (1968), in Urinary Tract Infection, p. 141, eds. O'Grady, F. and Brumfitt, W. Oxford U. P.
Fairley, K. F., Bond, A. G. and Adey, F. D. (1966), Lancet, 1, 939.
Fairley, K. F., Bond, A. G., Brown, R. B. and Habersberger, P. (1967), Lancet, 2, 427.
Freedman, L. R., Phair, J. P., Seki, M., Hamilton, H. B., Nefger, M. D. and Hirata, M. (1965), Yale J. Biol. Med., 37, 262.
Gallagher, D. J. A., Montgomerie, J. Z. and North, K. D. K. (1965), Brit. med. J., 1, 622.
Gillespie, W. A., Linton, K. B., Miller, A. and Slade, N. (1960), J. clin. Path., 13, 187.
Gower, P. E., Haswell, B., Sidaway, M. E. and de Wardener, H. E. (1968), Lancet, 1, 990.
Gruenwald, P., Funakawa, H., Mitani, S., Nishimura, T. and Takeuchi, S. (1967), Lancet, 1, 1026.
Grüneberg, R. N., Leigh, D. A. and Brumfitt, W. (1968), Urinary Tract Infection, p. 68, eds. O'Grady, F. and Brumfitt, W. Oxford U. P.
Grüneberg, R. N., Leigh, D. A. and Brumfitt, W. (1965), Lancet, 2, 1.
Hawkins, D. F. (1962), J. Obstet. Gynaec. Brit. Cwlth., 69, 585.
Henderson, M., Entwistle, G., and Tayback, M. (1962), Amer. J. publ. Hlth., 52, 1887.
Henderson, M. and Reinke, W. A. (1965), in Progress in Pyelonephritis, p. 27, ed. E. H. Kass. Philadelphia: F. A. Davis Co.
Hodson, C. J. (1959), Proc. roy. Soc. Med., 52, 669.
Hodson, C. J. and Edwards, D. (1960), Clin. Radiol., 11, 219.
Kaitz, A. L. (1961), J. clin. Invest., 40, 1331.
Kaitz, A. L. and Hodder, E. W. (1961), New Engl. J. Med., 265, 667.
Kass, E. H. (1956), Trans. Ass. Amer. Physns., 69, 56.
Kass, E. H. (1957), Arch. intern. Med., 100, 709.
Kass, E. H. (1959), Trans. Ass. Amer. Physns., 72, 257.
Kass, E. H. (1960), Arch. intern. Med., 105, 194.
Kass, E. H. (1968), Ann. Rev. Med., 19, 440.
Kass, E. H., Savage, W. and Santamarina, B. A. G. (1965), in Progress in Pyelonephritis, p. 3, ed. Kass, E. H. Philadelphia: F. A. Davis Co.
Kincaid-Smith, P. and Bullen, M. (1965), Lancet, 1, 395.
Le Blanc, A. L. and McGanity, W. J. (1964), Texas Rep. Biol. Med., 22, 336.
Leigh, D. A., Grüneberg, R. N. and Brumfitt, W. (1968), Lancet, 1, 603.
Linton, K. B. and Gillespie, W. A. (1962), J. Obstet. Gynaec. Brit. Cwlth., 69, 845.
Little, P. J. (1966), Lancet, 2, 925.
Little, P. J. and de Wardener, H. E. (1966), Lancet, 2, 1277.
Low, J. A., Johnson, E. E., McBride, R. L. and Tuffnell, P. G. (1964), Amer. J. Obstet. Gynec., 90, 897.
Marple, C. (1941), Ann. int. Med., 14, 2220.
Martin, J. D., Davis, R. E. and Stenhouse, N. (1967), J. Obstet. Gynaec. Brit. Cwlth., 74, 697.
Mond, N. C., Percival, A., Williams, J. D. and Brumfitt, W. (1965), Lancet, 1, 514.
Odell, G. B. (1959), J. Pediat., 55, 268.
O'Grady, F. and Cattell, W. R. (1966), Brit. J. Urol., 38, 149.

Paterson, M. L., Barr, W. and Macdonald, S. (1960), *J. Obstet. Gynaec. Brit. Emp.*, **67**, 394.

Percival, A., Brumfitt, W. and de Louvois, J. (1964), *Lancet*, **2**, 1027.

Rayer, P. (1841), Traité des Maladies des Reins et des Alterations de la Secretion Urinaire. Paris 1841.

Reeves, D. S. and Brumfitt, W. (1968), in *Urinary Tract Infection*, p. 53, eds. O'Grady, F. and Brumfitt, W. Oxford U. P.

Roberts, A. P., Robinson, R. E. and Beard, R. W. (1967), *Brit. med. J.*, **1**, 400.

Savage, W. E., Hajj, S. N., and Kass, E. H. (1967), *Medicine*, **46**, 385.

Simmons, S. C. and Baker, H. R. W. (1963), *J. Obstet. Gynaec. Brit. Cwlth.*, **70**, 968.

Sims, E. A. H. (1965), *Ann. Rev. Med.*, **16**, 221.

Sleigh, J. D., Robertson, J. G. and Isdale, M. H. (1964), *J. Obstet. Gynaec. Brit. Cwlth.*, **71**, 74.

Smellie, J. M. (1967), *J. roy. Coll. Physns.*, **1**, 189.

Smellie, J. M., Hodson, C. J., Edwards, D., Normand, I. C. S. (1964), *Brit. med. J.*, **2**, 1222.

Stamey, T. A., Govan, D. E. and Palmer, J. M. (1965), *Medicine*, **44**, 1.

Stamey, T. A., Fair, W. R., Timothy, M. M. and Chung, H. K. (1968), *Nature*, **218**, 444.

Stuart, K. L., Cummins, G. T. M. and Chin, W. A. (1965), *Brit. med. J.*, **1**, 554.

Sussman, M., Asscher, A. W., Waters, W. E., Evans, J. A. S., Campbell, H., Evans, K. T. and Williams, J. E. (1969), *Brit. med. J.*, **1**, 799.

Turck, M., Goffe, B. S. and Petersdorf, R. G. (1962), *New Engl. J. Med.*, **266**, 857.

Turner, G. (1961), *Lancet*, **2**, 1062.

Vivaldi, E., Muñoz, J., Cotran, R. and Kass, E. H. (1965), in *Progress in Pyelonephritis*, p. 531, ed. Kass, E. H. Philadelphia: F. A. Davis Co.

Whalley, P. (1967), *Amer. J. Obstet. Gynec.*, **97**, 723.

Whalley, P., Martin, F., and Peters, P. J. (1965), *J. Amer. med. Ass.*, **193**, 878.

Williams, D. K., Garrod, L. P., and Waterworth, P. M. (1962), *J. Obstet. Gynaec. Brit. Cwlth.*, **69**, 403.

Williams, J. D., Brumfitt, W., Leigh, D. A. and Percival, A. (1965a), *Lancet*, **1**, 831.

Williams, J. D., Leigh, D. A., Rosser, E. ap. I. and Brumfitt, W. (1965b), *J. Obstet. Gynaec. Brit. Cwlth.*, **72**, 327.

Williams, J. D. and Leigh, D. A. (1966), *Brit. J. clin. Pract.*, **20**, 177.

Williams, J. D., Thomlinson, J. L., Cole, J. G. L. and Cope, E. (1969), *Brit. med. J.*, **1**, 29.

Wilson, M. G., Hewitt, W. L., Monzon, O. T. (1966), *New Engl. J. Med.*, **274**, 1115.

Winberg, J. (1959), *Acta Paediat.*, **48**, 577.

Winberg, J., Anderson, H. J., Hanson, L. A. and Lincoln, K. (1963), *Brit. med. J.*, **2**, 524.

1. CYTOTOXIC DRUGS

T. A. CONNORS and M. E. WHISSON

Cancer could be adequately controlled by surgery and irradiation in most instances if it remained localized and did not invade surrounding tissue or metastasize. Successful treatment of widely disseminated cancer will depend on the discovery of agents which are selectively cytotoxic to tumour cells and which can be administered systemically. The drugs used at present are unfortunately by no means perfect anti-cancer agents. The majority of them act on a common pathway, the genetic apparatus of the cell. Since there is evidence that this apparatus is the same for both cancer cells and normal cells, it is difficult at first sight to see how the present agents ever act in a selective manner. In fact the selectivity usually obtained is slight and many types of cancer do not respond well to treatment. Other classes of tumour do respond to varying degrees but the selectivity is directed towards dividing cells rather than tumour cells since where tumour regression is observed it is usually associated with toxicity to certain host tissues also rapidly dividing, such as bone marrow. Not surprisingly the best results of cancer chemotherapy are obtained in the treatment of rapidly growing cancers such as choriocarcinoma, where there is a 70 per cent possibility of cure, lymphomas and leukaemias. It must however be stressed that rapidly growing tumours will not necessarily be sensitive to the present day agents. Experience in the laboratory shows that very great differences in sensitivity to drugs occur even amongst tumours which are identical in growth rate and similar in histopathology. Table 1 shows the effect of chemotherapeutic agents on the growth of two transplanted plasma cell tumours which grow in the C-mouse. In animals bearing either tumour one drug (CB 40–645) has an LD_{50} of 370 mg./kg. However the dose required to eradicate the PC6 plasma cell tumour is only 2·7 mg./kg. while the much higher dose of 340 mg./kg. is required to have the same effect against the PC5 plasma cell tumour. This Table illustrates that a tumour has an inherent sensitivity or resistance to each particular drug. Unfortunately this difference in sensitivity occurs not only between different types of cancer but also amongst members of any one tumour class similar in histology and other features. Although, for instance, there is a good chance of curing patients with choriocarcinoma with certain drugs, some of these tumours are quite refractory to treatment although one would find it impossible to distinguish them from tumours undergoing complete regression.

While the aim for the future must be the discovery of anti-tumour agents which act by other pathways than the present agents and may be truly selective in their anti-tumour effects, even at present some of the chemicals we already have can, under certain conditions, be highly selective. Such selectivity may arise as a result of the tumour metabolizing the administered agent in a unique manner so that it becomes more toxic, or conversely the normal sensitive tissues of the host may deactivate the cytotoxic drug. Host reactions may also be exercised against neoplastic cells in the post-treatment phase, during which time depleted normal tissues have a chance to recover. Following damage to all growing cells, the final result will then be selective elimination of the tumour cells.

The route of administration and also dosage regimen can greatly influence the response obtained. The accessibility of the tumour cells may also be an important factor, just as it is in the response of abscesses to anti-bacterial chemotherapy (Goldacre and Whisson, 1966). Tumour cells may survive for some time in totally ischaemic and apparently necrotic zones of tumours (Goldacre and Sylvén, 1959, 1962), and probably drugs reach these zones in only ineffective concentrations. Where it can be shown by intravascular dyes or other means that the centre of a growing tumour is ischaemic, then a much greater success may be expected when chemotherapy is combined with a careful enucleation of the tumour (Martin and Fugmann, 1960; Humphreys, Mantel and Goldin, 1966). Quite apart from the possibility of cells surviving anaerobically in the ischaemic zone, tumour size alone may determine the ultimate outcome of chemotherapy. In extensive studies using a murine leukaemia Skipper and colleagues (Skipper, Schabel and Wilcox, 1964; Skipper, Schabel, Wilcox, Laster, Trader and Thompson, 1965) have shown that drugs act like gunshot amongst a large flock of birds, always leaving a fixed percentage of survivors. Thus if a drug kills 99 per cent of the cells of the tumour the residue from a 200 g. mass (10^{11} cells) will be 2 g. (10^9 cells), which is usually much more than any immune response can handle. In fact mice cured chemotherapeutically of transplanted tumours, a method of immunization which in our hands gives stronger immunity than any other, can never reject more than 10^7 cells on reinoculation of the tumour. The immunological rejection of spontaneous tumour is no doubt much less efficient and it is quite obvious that early treatment is as important for success with chemotherapy as with radiation or surgery. Perhaps because chemotherapy is still often given with the intention of palliation rather than cure it is frequently given late in the disease, i.e. after the failure of surgery or irradiation.

SCREENING TESTS

Many different types of screening test for the detection of anti-tumour agents are used, and this fact alone is

TABLE 1

WIDELY VARYING RESPONSE OF TWO PLASMA CELL TUMOURS TO FOUR CLOSELY RELATED ALKYLATING AGENTS. THE TWO TUMOURS, ADJ-PC5 AND ADJ-PC6A HAVE IDENTICAL GROWTH RATES AND VERY SIMILAR HISTOPATHOLOGY, BUT THE ADJ-PC6A IS GENERALLY MUCH MORE SENSITIVE TO ALKYLATING AGENTS. THE REASONS FOR THIS DIFFERENCE IN SENSITIVITY ARE NOT KNOWN

COMPOUNDS CB40–645 AND CB40–678 (WARD, BLENKINSOP AND CO. NOS. 7007, AND 4247) ARE STRUCTURALLY RELATED TO VITAMIN K, WHEREAS CB1072 AND CB1074 ARE BELIEVED TO BE ACTIVATED IN TISSUES BY β-GLUCURONIDASE

Compound	LD_{50}	Response of ADJ–PC5		Response of ADJ–PC6A	
		90% Inhibitory Dose	Therapeutic Index	90% Inhibitory Dose	Therapeutic Index
CB40–645	370 mg./kg.	340 mg./kg.	1·1	2·7 mg./kg.	137
CB40–678	11·8 mg./kg.	1·4 mg./kg.	8	1·4 mg./kg.	8
CB1074	115 mg/.kg.	19 mg./kg.	6	1·5 mg./kg.	77
CB1072	22 mg./kg.	8·3 mg./kg.	2·7	0·2 mg./kg.	111

evidence of the inadequacy of any particular test to reliably select good anti-tumour agents (Connors and Roe, 1964). Most of the drugs at present in use in cancer chemotherapy have been selected because they were active against transplanted animal tumours. Figure 1 shows the result of such a test where animals bearing a tumour were treated with various dose levels of a drug. Then a number of days later the weights of the tumours in treated groups were compared with the weights of the tumours of a control group. The test is also designed to give an

LD_{50} for the drug so that a therapeutic index may be obtained for each compound. Experience with screens such as this has revealed that each type of transplanted tumour is highly individual in its response to drugs and for no tumour can we predict with any certainty drugs likely to be useful in the clinic in the treatment of any one type of cancer. Testing in the clinic is still largely empirical and many more controlled clinical trials are required before it will be possible to obtain optimal use even of the drugs presently available.

QUANTITATIVE TUMOUR INHIBITION AND TOXICITY TEST

TUMOUR .Adj.-pc5.............

CB. .40-433.............. Name .. .6.-.MERCAPTOPURINE.......................................

Solvent .. .Oil................. No. of injections ....1...... Route of Administration ... .I.P,....................

Date of implant ..4..6..66...... Date of 1st injection ....14..6..66.......... Date killed ..24..6..66...............

.........LD$_{50}$. 225 mg/Kg   ID$_{90}$ 150 mg/Kg   Therapeutic Index 1.5..................................

	CONTROL Untreated	...40...mg/Kg	...80..mg/Kg	..160.. mg/Kg	..320...mg/Kg	......mg/Kg	......mg/Kg
Tumour weights gms.	4.6 3.4 2.3 5.4	5.3 4.2 4.0	2.0 2.0 2.8	0.8 0.0 0.0	+ (Day 6) + (Day 6) + (Day 7)		
Mean tumour weight as per cent of control	115%	58%	7%	$^3/_3$ DEAD			
Per cent inhibition	STIM.	42%	93%				
Average body weight change gms.	-1.2	+0.4	+0.6	-3.4			

FIG. 1. Example of a screening test showing a positive result with 6-mercaptopurine against the Adj-pc5 plasma cell tumour growing in Balb/c-mice. The dose range spans the toxic and minimal effective levels, so that both toxicity (LD$_{50}$) and carcinostatic dose (ID$_{90}$ or 90% inhibitory dose) are measured in the one experiment. Tumour stimulation is frequently seen with carcinostatic agents at dose levels just below the minimal inhibitory level.

Alkylating Agents

Although many chemicals now used in the clinic were detected by their activity against animal tumours, the decision to test them against these experimental systems was often taken because they possessed some toxic effects which suggested they might be selective cytotoxic agents. Such was the case with the alkylating agents. The earliest members of this heterogeneous group of chemicals to show anti-tumour activity were the aliphatic nitrogen mustards. Studies firstly on sulphur mustard and then on the aliphatic nitrogen mustards were extensive during the years of the second World War because of their potential use as chemical warfare agents. Extensive toxicological studies showed that these agents were selectively affecting rapidly dividing cells—one of the major toxic manifestations being lymphopenia. The idea prevalent at the time that all cancers were rapidly growing led to the use of these compounds as anti-tumour agents firstly in the laboratory, where they were shown to inhibit a number of animal tumours, and subsequently in the clinic, where good remissions were obtained in Hodgkin's disease (Gilman and Philips, 1946). Since 1946 in excess of 3,000 alkylating agents have been synthesized and tested for anti-tumour activity (Bratzel, Ross, Goodridge, Huntress, Flather and Johnson, 1963).

Mechanism of Alkylation

An alkylation may be considered to be the replacement of the hydrogen atom of an organic molecule by an alkyl (R.CH$_2$–) group as shown in the following formula:

$$R.CH_2X + HR' \rightarrow R.CH_2R' + HX$$

Alkylating   Organic   Alkylated
Agent   Molecule   Molecule

The alkylating radical RCH$_2$– may be a compound one, (i.e. it may contain many different types of chemical grouping) the only requirement being that the carbon atom through which the attachment to the molecule R' is made is a fully saturated one (Ross, 1962). Alkylation can also be extended to include the addition of an alkyl group to a tertiary amine to form a quaternary ammonium compound or reaction with negatively charged ions (phosphate, carboxyl and hydroxyl) to form esters and ethers as shown in the following reactions:

$$R.CH_2X + {}^-OR' = RCH_2OR' + X^- \qquad (1)$$

Alkylating   Ionized
Agent   Hydroxyl

$$R.CH_2X + {}^-OOCR' = R.CH_2OOCR' + X^- \qquad (2)$$

Ionized
Carboxylic
Acid

Basically all the alkylating agents can be considered to react by the formation of an intermediate positively charged ion—the carbonium ion:

$$R.NH.CH_2CH_2Cl \rightarrow R.NH.CH_2CH_2{}^+$$

Nitrogen   Carbonium
Mustard   Ion

This positively charged ion will be extremely reactive to molecules which contain negatively charged centres. Many molecules in the cell contain such negatively charged centres and the alkylating agents will be particularly reactive towards ionized thiols as may be found in amino-acids, enzymes and structural proteins, towards ionized acidic groups found in nucleic acids and proteins and towards uncharged amino groups occuring in amino-acids and proteins. It is obvious that when an alkylating agent is administered, provided it penetrates the cell, an enormous variety of chemical reactions can take place in all types of cell. Much of the compound will probably hydrolyse harmlessly (by reaction with intracellular water) but many proteins, nucleic acids and other important cell constituents will be alkylated.

At first sight it would seem difficult to sort out whether one particular type of alkylation leads to cell death or whether cytotoxicity is the result of alkylations of many different sites. Studies using physiological dose levels of alkylating agents where the dose of agent was restricted to the minimum dose which could cause death, revealed that DNA synthesis was particularly affected by alkylating agents. The work of Lawley and Brookes (1965) showed that the N^7 atom of the guanine in DNA was very susceptible to alkylation.

Alkylating agents require to be at least difunctional (i.e. they must have two alkylating groups) before they show any selective anti-tumour effect and this eventually led to the supposition that the alkylating agents killed cells by reacting with two adjacent guanine molecules in the DNA helix. Once DNA had been cross-linked in this way its replication was interfered with and the death of the cell resulted. Cross linked DNA products have in fact been isolated after reaction with DNA and this theory explains why only small dose levels of alkylating agents are required to kill cells, since it requires only of the order of one cross-link per 10^5 nucleotides to deactivate a whole molecule of DNA. This theory also conveniently explains why rapidly dividing tissues, with a large number of cells synthesizing DNA at any one time, are particularly

sensitive to the action of the alkylating agents. Non-dividing cells such as the parenchymal cells of the liver may be alkylated to the same extent but in this case since they are not synthesizing DNA there is no evidence of toxicity. Even if they are stimulated to divide *after a suitable interval*, e.g. by partial hepatectomy, there is still no obvious toxicity. This is apparently because the cells are able to repair alkylated DNA. When the interval between alkylation and the onset of DNA synthesis is short the cell is lethally injured (Roberts, Brent and Crathorn, 1968). Differences in sensitivity of tissues growing at equal rates and the development of resistance to alkylating agents may in part be explained by the differential capacity of the tissues to repair alkylated DNA. In addition both normal and neoplastic tissues contain cells which are in a prolonged resting phase. In this state they are not susceptible to alkylating agents and can probably repair alkylated DNA. Such cells can enter a growth phase if their growing neighbours are killed by alkylating agents (Bruce, 1966). A speculative approach to cancer chemotherapy may be to induce cancers to undergo rapid division and then, when they are in the susceptible state, to treat them with alkylating agents.

Monofunctional Alkylating Agents

Whilst it is a general requirement that the alkylating agents must be at least difunctional to be tumour inhibitory, there is now a new class of active monofunctional agents which form an important exception. The simplest of these (I) is a more effective inhibitor of the Walker carcinoma than the difunctional agent (II) or the trifunctional derivative (III).

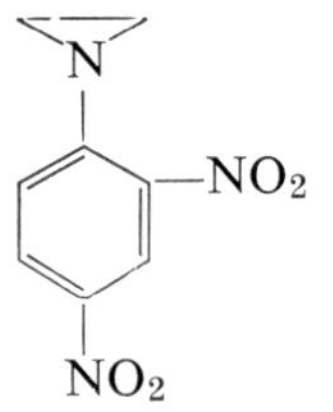

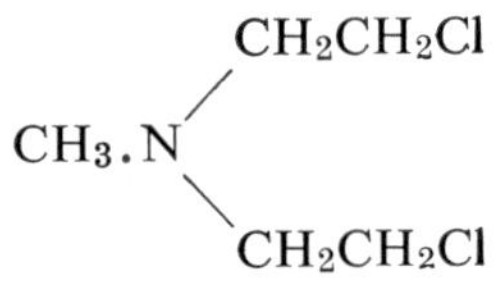

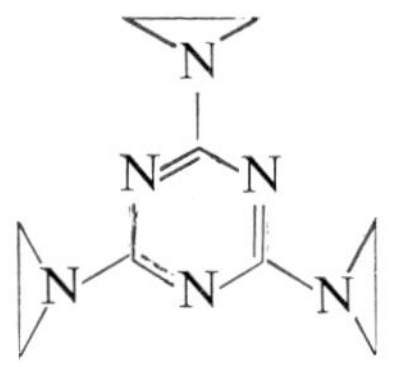

At the time of writing it is considered likely that compound (I) and its more recently developed derivatives may have a completely different mode of action from the polyfunctional agents.

Aromatic Nitrogen Mustards. The aromatic nitrogen mustards have perhaps provided the most important alkylating agents in clinical use. The first derivative to be synthesized, aniline mustard (IV) achieved limited clinical trial in 1948, and since that time numerous derivatives have been synthesized. The earliest derivatives

$$M = -N(CH_2CH_2Cl)_2$$

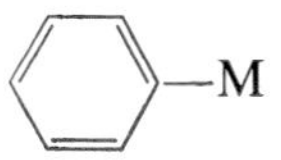

(IV) 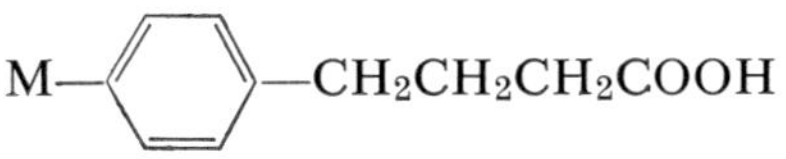   (V)

represented the attempts of the chemist to change the physical properties of the molecule and one of the most successful was the fatty acid chlorambucil (V), which is used at the present day for the treatment of ovarian carcinoma (Masterson and Nelson, 1965). The idea of using the dichloroethyl arms ($-N(CH_2CH_2Cl)_2$) as the cytotoxic groups and a natural molecule to carry this "warhead", (Bergel, 1961) into the cell, led to the design of many nitrogen mustards incorporating so called natural structures. Perhaps the most successful examples of this approach are melphalan (VI), degranol (VII; R = $-NH.CH_2CH_2Cl$) and dibromomannitol (VII; R = Br).

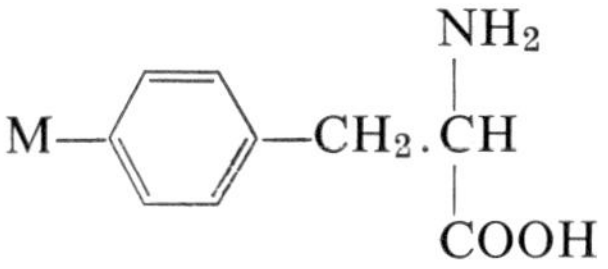

(VI)

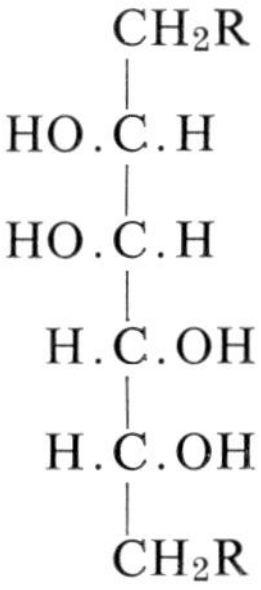

(VII)

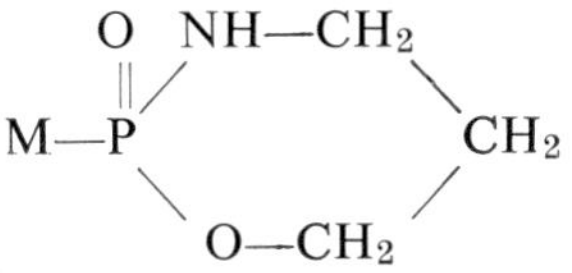

(VIII)

These agents and a related mannitol derivative, mannitol myleran (VII; R = $-OSO_2CH_3$) find widespread application in the treatment of cancer, and are useful in the treatment of carcinoma of the ovary and cervix. Mannitol myleran in particular has induced useful remissions in ovarian carcinoma (Černý, Šándor, Winkler, Ujházy, Uhrínová, Petrek, Siracky and Halko, 1965). Of all the alkylating agents, endoxana (VIII) Cyclophosphamide (Cytoxan in the U.S.A.), shows the widest range of anti-cancer activity in the clinic. It is for instance employed

for the treatment of carcinoma of the endometrium once treatment with progestogens has failed. This compound was designed in an attempt to prepare a "latently active" derivative. Latently active alkylating agents are chemicals which due to their structure are chemically rather inert. However metabolic reactions are known to take place in the body which could convert these compounds into chemically very reactive (and therefore highly cytotoxic) derivatives. The general hope with this approach is that tumours will be more efficient in this lethal synthesis than normal tissues (Ross, 1962). Endoxan is in itself chemically unreactive but it was prepared in the hope that it would be acted on by tumour phosphamidase enzymes to release an active alkylating agent. Endoxan has indeed a good effect on a variety of experimental tumours but its active metabolite or its method of activation are as yet unknown.

Other Alkylating Agents

Once it was established that the nitrogen mustards were inhibiting tumours because of their alkylating properties a number of other types of chemical alkylating agents were tested for their anti-tumour effects. Animal screening tests revealed that members of the epoxides (e.g. IX), sulphonoxyalkanes (e.g. X) and ethyleneimines (e.g. XI) could also inhibit the growth of some animal tumours.

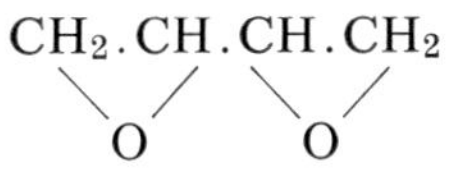

(IX)

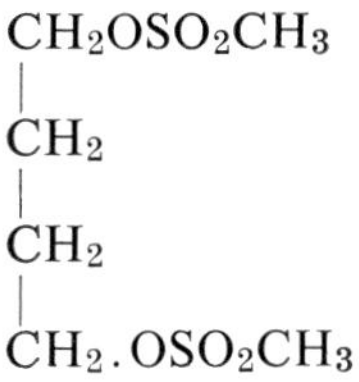

(X)

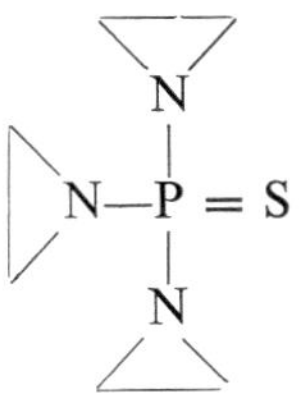

(XI)

These agents act in basically the same way as the nitrogen mustards and have provided a number of derivatives of clinical use the most notable being myleran (X) which finds particular use in the treatment of chronic granulocytic leukaemia. Thio-Tepa (XI) has been used in the treatment of ovarian carcinoma and carcinoma of the breast and TEM (III) for ovarian carcinoma.

On the whole the alkylating agents have not proved outstanding in the treatment of gynaecological cancers and one expects no more than 30–40 per cent objective remission rate of the more sensitive tumours (e.g. uterine and ovarian carcinoma) even where optimal dosage schedules are employed.

Attempts to improve Selectivity

During the past decade as the drawbacks of the alkylating agents have been realized so attempts have been made to improve their selectivity. The case of endoxan has already been mentioned, and selectivity achieved by structural modification of the injected derivative probably also accounts for the effect of aniline mustard (IV) on experimental plasma cell tumours (Whisson and Connors, 1965). It was observed that a plasma cell tumour which was quite resistant to the action of most alkylating agents

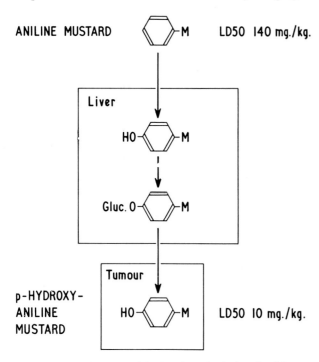

FIG. 2. Aniline mustard is thought to be hydroxylated in the liver to form the para-hydroxy derivative. It is postulated that in the liver this is immediately conjugated to the glucuronide which, being extremely water soluble, is relatively non-toxic. Tumours which have very high glucuronidase levels reconvert the glucuronide to the highly toxic para-hydroxyaniline mustard and so are selectively inhibited.

underwent complete regression, even when well established, after administration of a small dose of aniline mustard. Studies of related structures led to the development of a hypothesis that aniline mustard was metabolized according to the scheme shown in Figure 2. Aniline mustard is converted in the liver into a hydroxylated derivative which is much more toxic than aniline mustard itself. However the toxic effects of this derivative are not seen since it is immediately converted also in the liver to its glucuronide which is probably quite non-toxic. If the plasma cell tumour had an extremely high glucuronidase level it would reconvert the glucuronide to the highly toxic hydroxy-derivative inside the tumour. The finding that this plasma cell tumour had in fact an extremely high

glucuronidase level added support for this mechanism of action (Connors and Whisson, 1966) and shows how under certain conditions a considerable degree of selectivity may be obtained with the alkylating agents. In order to design more selective latent derivatives it is obvious that a fuller knowledge must be obtained of the metabolic pathways of tumours and their enzyme content etc. Once differences are found between the tumour and sensitive host tissues, the chemist may design alkylating agents which are selectively activated by a tumour. However it must be borne in mind that not only are there many different types of tumour based on pathological and morphological classifications but even tumours similar by these criteria may nevertheless differ widely in their biochemistry. It is obvious then that if an alkylating agent is designed to be activated by a particular enzyme then the tumour must have an abundance of this enzyme compared to the host tissues sensitive to alkylating agents. If such an alkylating agent is to be used rationally it must be determined beforehand whether the tumour has a high level of the relevant enzyme. Since tumours are so individual in their biochemical make-up then the means must be available to biopsy each tumour to detect whether it has a high level of the enzyme and is therefore liable to be particularly sensitive to the drug. Aniline mustard or preferably its O-glucuronide might be rationally used against tumours shown to have a very high β-glucuronidase level.

It appears to be a common feature of many tumours both animal and human that they are slightly more acid than normal tissues (Eden, Haines and Kahler, 1955; Meyer, Kammerling, Amtam, Koller and Hoffman, 1948). Theoretically the difference can be exploited by alkylating agents in a number of ways. It can be used to allow certain basic alkylating agents to concentrate in tumour cells (Reid, 1964) or other types of alkylating agent to be activated. This difference in pH can be accentuated by glucose and has certainly improved the efficacy of the alkylating agent TEM experimentally (Connors, Mitchley, Rosenoer and Ross, 1964).

Recently it has been found that many nitrogen mustards bind to serum proteins in such a way as to protect them from hydrolysis (Wade, Whisson and Szekerke, 1967). The serum proteins can therefore act as carriers of these alkylating agents and may confer selectivity by virtue of the greater permeability of the capillaries of tumour tissue. Fibrinogen is rapidly trapped as fibrin in experimental tumours (Isliker, Cerottini, Jaton and Magnetat, 1964) and alkylating agents bound to fibrinogen might show a great gain in selectivity by being deposited in the region of the tumour.

By attempts such as these the alkylating agents are being made more selective in their toxicity. As more is understood about the biochemistry of different tumours so there is a better chance of employing the above drugs in a more rational way.

Antimetabolites

Any compound that interferes with the utilization of a body metabolite by virtue of its close similarity in chemical structure may be defined as an anti-metabolite. In practice the only anti-metabolites employed with advantage in cancer chemotherapy are derivatives structurally similar to purines, pyrimidines and folic acid. These derivatives interfere at one stage or another with the biosynthesis of nucleic acids. Not surprisingly then, these derivatives have many similar effects to alkylating agents and they show selective toxicity to rapidly proliferating cells rather than cancer cells. As with the alkylating agents best responses in the clinic are usually with the fast growing lymphomas and leukaemias. Perhaps the most impressive results of cancer chemotherapy are obtained in the treatment of choriocarcinoma. Treatment with the anti-folic acid methotrexate (XII)

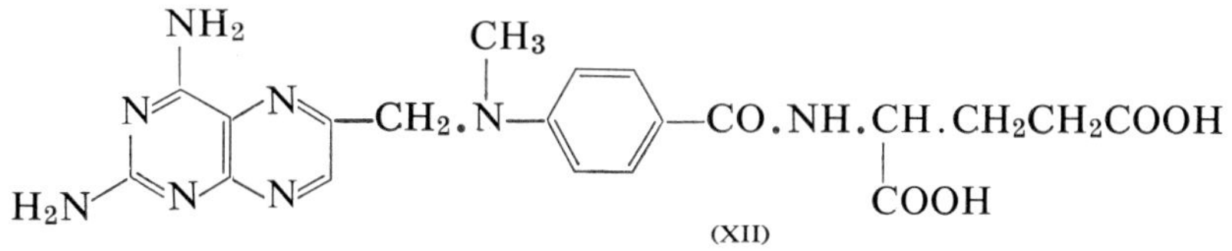

Many more potential folic acid antagonists have been synthesized over the years but none have displaced methotrexate in the clinic.

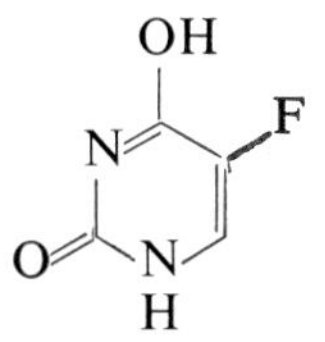

6-mercaptopurine (XIII) was one of the first anti-purines synthesized and like methotrexate is still extensively used in cancer chemotherapy mainly against acute leukaemia in children but also against choriocarcinoma. This compound is converted *in vivo* to its ribotide which is the active form of the drug. The drug acts by interfering with nucleic acid synthesis. A number of different pathways may be involved in this inhibition of DNA synthesis—for instance 6MP interferes with the formation of adenylic and guanylic acids from inosinic acid. Many

or with the anti-purine 6-mercaptopurine (XIII)

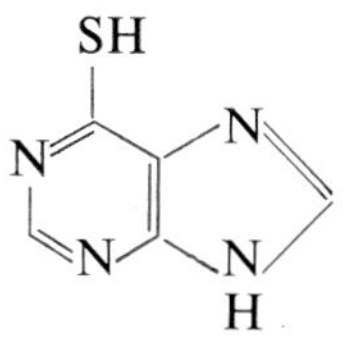

can lead to cures in as high as 70–80 per cent of cases. Methotrexate is also used in the treatment of sarcoma of the uterus when good but short term responses are seen in about one-third of patients treated. 5-fluorouracil (XIV) and its ribotide are also useful in the treatment of carcinoma of the breast (late postmenopause), ovary, and uterine body. 30–40 per cent objective remissions may be expected under optimum conditions but these are usually only short term effects.

Folic acid is involved in a large number of biochemical pathways (Stock, 1966). Its role after reduction to tetrahydrofolic acid is to transfer groups containing single carbon atoms to molecules as they are being built up into various important cell constituents (e.g. nucleotides). Methotrexate and its earlier known analogue aminopterin combine with the enzymes (folic or dihydrofolic reductase) that reduce folic acid to the active form responsible for the so-called "one carbon" transport. The folic acid antagonists can kill cells by interfering with a variety of cell functions. It is likely that the most important cytotoxic action of these derivatives is to prevent the synthesis of DNA by inhibiting the methylation of deoxyuridylic acid to thymidylic acid:

derivatives of 6MP have been synthesized and some, such as the 5-butyl glycine ethyl ester (Butoglycin) are claimed to have advantages over the parent drug (Semonský, Černý and Jelínek, 1967). 5-fluorouracil (XIV) is structurally so similar to uracil that it substitutes for it in many metabolic reactions. This compound can again interfere with cell metabolism in a number of different ways. It is incorporated for instance in the place of uracil into RNA and can block the assembly of ribosomes from ribosomal RNA (Sells and Crudup, 1966). It appears that fluorouracil, after conversion to 5-fluorodeoxyuridylic acid, causes its main toxicity by preventing the formation of thymidylic acid from uridylic acid.

As with the alkylating agents resistance may develop to any one of these agents. Resistance may arise in a number of ways. In the case of methotrexate some cells have been shown to have a greatly increased level of folic reductase but others show a restricted permeability to the drug. Cells resistant to 6-mercaptopurine have usually lost the enzymes required to convert the drug into the active ribotide. Cells resistant to 5-fluorouracil may be impermeable to the drug or fail to convert it to the ribotide. In other cases the structure of thymidylate synthetase, the enzyme which converts uridylic acid to thymidylic acid, is said to be altered.

Natural Products

Many products of natural origin have been screened for potential anti-tumour action. The most important of these now in clinical use are the actinomycins and the vinca alkaloids, members of which are highly effective in the treatment of choriocarcinoma. The actinomycins are a series of closely related peptides produced by certain streptomyces. Each actinomycin consists of two peptide lactone rings linked by a phenoxazine chromophore group. They differ from one another only in the amino-acid content of the peptide chains. Actinomycin D has proved particularly successful in the treatment of Wilm's tumour in combination with X-rays. The actinomycins combine with DNA but their action is not to inhibit DNA synthesis

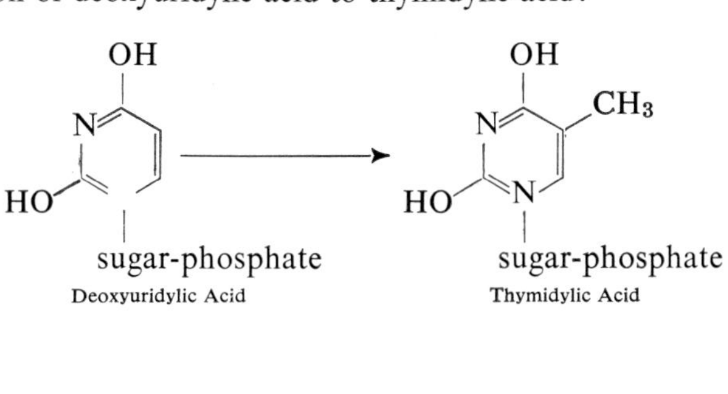

Deoxyuridylic Acid   Thymidylic Acid

but to prevent DNA dependent RNA synthesis. Presumably the chemical attaches to DNA in such a way as to interfere with the action of RNA polymerase. As an end result these derivatives inhibit protein and RNA synthesis.

Vincristine and vincaleukoblastine are two of the vinca alkaloids which are used clinically. These compounds are thought to inhibit the utilization of certain amino-acids, particularly glutamine, by interfering with the formation of the amino-acid—S–RNA complex.

Mitomycin C isolated from streptomyces is an antibiotic which appears to act by alkylation of DNA after enzymatic reduction *in vivo* (Iyer and Szybalski, 1964).

Amongst other antibiotics which have been shown to have anti-tumour activity are the glutamine antagonists azaserine and DON, puromycin which affects protein synthesis, and mithramycin which is used in the treatment of cancer of the testis.

Miscellaneous Agents

New types of agent are continually being discovered as a result of their activity against animal tumours. The most important recent discovery has been the finding that asparaginase can cause complete regression of certain animal tumours. It is now recognized that asparagine is an essential amino-acid for certain tumours. This in fact makes it the ideal chemotherapeutic agent for such tumours since asparagine is not an essential amino-acid for normal tissues and highly purified asparaginase should have none of the side effects usually associated with anti-tumour agents. Preliminary clinical results have shown that where tumours can be shown to be asparagine requiring they regress on treatment with asparaginase.

Cytosine arabinoside which specifically affects cells during DNA synthesis, natulan used in the treatment of Hodgkin's disease, methylgloxal bis (guanylhydrazone), and hydroxyurea are all examples of new classes of derivative which may eventually prove to be very effective against particular types of cancer.

DOSAGE SCHEDULE

Anti-cancer drugs are frequently given in prolonged continuous courses following the tradition developed for anti-bacterial chemotherapy. There is evidence however that this may not be the optimal schedule for many drugs and tumours. In acute leukaemia, for instance, methotrexate was much more effective in maintaining remissions when given intramuscularly twice weekly than when given orally daily (Zubrod, Schepartz, Leiter, Endicott, Carrese and Baker, 1966).

Many drugs are most effective at a particular point in the cell cycle. The alkylating agents for example are most toxic to cells in the early post mitotic phase (the G_1 period) and in the early stage of DNA synthesis (Roberts, Brent and Crathorn, 1968). Cytosine arabinoside acts on cells during the DNA synthetic phase only, and Skipper and others (Skipper, Schabel and Wilcox, 1967) have studied in detail the effect of different dosage schedules of this drug on the L1210 leukaemia. They showed that if the drug level was kept high in the animal by perfusion or frequent administration throughout two doubling times of the tumour, followed by a similar course of treatment after a host recovery period of 6 more doubling times, then they could achieve a 100 per cent tumour cell kill. This contrasted with other dosage schedules where a 100 per cent cell kill was never obtained and therefore only an extension of survival time was obtained and not a cure. In translating this result to the clinic one meets major difficulties. The doubling time of human tumours is very variable and may be of the order of months. There is also the probability that there is extensive cell death and many cells may be out of cycle in a resting (G_0 phase). Further research is required on the cell kinetics of human tumours before rational and highly effective dosage schedules can be organized such as that for cytosine arabinoside against the mouse L1210. Following Skipper's work and assuming a cycle time of three days for human cancer cells, an optimum schedule for S-phase active drugs (e.g. anti-metabolites and alkylating agents) would be an intensive course for one week followed by a period of three weeks for recovery from toxicity and then followed by another week of therapy. This sequence would be continued for a time dependent on the percentage cell kill occuring during each course. Treatment is often stopped too soon and our modern understanding of cell kinetics should soon permit us to predict the number of courses of partially effective drugs required for complete cure. However, until better drugs are found the number of courses of treatment required for 100 per cent kill of the cancer cells may well be more than the patient can tolerate. In addition, the kinetic studies indicate that only when the first course of therapy results in better than a 90 per cent tumour cell kill is chemotherapeutic cure a possibility.

Route of Administration

The efficacy of cancer drugs can be influenced not only by the dosage regimen chosen but also by the route of administration. Cobb (1966) has shown, for instance, that two alkylating agents may have the same anti-tumour effects when administered intrarterially close to the tumour but one of them loses all its activity if it is given by the intraperitoneal route. Many alkylating agents are very unstable in water and must be administered soon after solution or dissolved in non-polar solvents such as ethanol. The instability of certain nitrogen mustards in water has been used to design agents for special use in localized infusion studies (Davis and Ross, 1965). Sulphur mustards have been prepared which have half lives of only a matter of seconds. By injection close to the site of the tumour the active alkylating agent may be expected to reach the tumour in a high concentration but any drug escaping into the systemic circulation would be expected to hydrolyse before reaching sensitive sites such as the bone marrow. Topical application may also be useful in certain cases, and for this purpose an excellent solvent would seem to be dimethyl sulphoxide (Leake, 1967).

In conclusion the present status of chemotherapy is

that the majority of drugs at present available are more selective towards rapidly dividing cells rather than cancer cells. The most sensitive human tumours are those which are fairly rapidly growing—the lymphomas, especially Burkitt's lymphoma, acute leukaemia and choriocarcinoma. With many other clinical tumours the slight regressions or temporary hold-ups of tumour growth observed produce little benefit in terms of survival time and are probably not due to any selective cancerostatic action of the drug. Rather, such effects are secondarily induced in the tumour by toxic effects on the patient. On the other hand with relatively rare tumours such as Burkitt's lymphoma true selectivity does exist. It is perhaps too much to say that for every tumour there is a selective drug if only one had the means of knowing which one. However, there is no doubt that if all the known drugs could be considered for every human tumour very many more examples of dramatic remission due to chemotherapy would be in the literature. Future research perhaps will concentrate not only on improving the efficiency of the drugs we already have, by studying optimal dosage schedules etc., but by developing sensitivity tests which will enable one to determine in advance whether the tumour is likely to be highly sensitive to a particular drug. Some progress has already been made in testing drugs on short term cultures of biopsy specimens of human tumours. However, a lot more must be known about the metabolism of anti-tumour agents and about the biochemistry of individual tumours before one can begin to use anti-cancer agents rationally. New types of cancer chemotherapeutic agents may arise by chance, as for instance the discovery of asparaginase, where a particular chemical is shown to cause regression of an animal tumour. Further studies by the experimentalists may reveal the features of a tumour that make it sensitive to the drug. The last stage in the process will be to detect human tumours with these same features which should also be sensitive to the drug. The drug can then be administered knowing that the chances of tumour regression are high.

REFERENCES

Bergel, F. (1961), "New Developments in Carcinochemotherapy," *Brit. med. J.*, **2**, 399.

Bratzel, R. P., Ross, R. B., Goodridge, T. H., Huntress, W. T., Flather, M. T. and Johnson, D. E. (1963), "A Survey of Alkylating Agents, *Cancer Chemotherapy Reports*, **26**, 1.

Bruce, W. R. (1966), "The Action of Chemotherapeutic Agents at the Cellular Level and the Effects of these Agents on Hematopoietic and Lymphomatous Tissue," Proceedings of the 7th Canadian Cancer Conference, Honey Harbour, June 1966.

Černý, V., Šándor, L., Winkler, A., Ujházy, V., Uhrínová, M., Petrek, C., Siracký, J. and Halko, J. (1965), "Mannitol-busulphan in Advanced Ovary Carcinoma," *Neoplasma*, **13**, 181.

Cobb, L. M. (1966), "The Influence of the Route of Administration of Nitrogen Mustard and Melphalan upon their Anti-tumour Activity in the Rat, *International Journal of Cancer*, **1**, 329.

Connors, T. A. and Roe, F. J. C. (1964), *Evaluation of Drug Activities: Pharmacometrics* (D. R. Laurence and A. L. Bacharach) Vol. 2, p. 827. New York: Academic Press.

Connors, T. A. and Whisson, M. E. (1966), "Cure of Mice Bearing Advanced Plasma Cell Tumours with Aniline Mustard: The relationship between glucuronidase activity and tumour sensitivity." *Nature, London*, **210**, 866.

Connors, T. A., Mitchley, B. C. V., Rosenoer, V. M. and Ross, W. C. J. (1964), "The Effect of Glucose Pretreatment on the Carcinostatic and Toxic Activities of Some Alkylating Agents, *Biochem. Pharm.*, **13**, 395.

Davis, W. and Ross, W. C. J. (1965), "A Highly Reactive Sulfur Mustard Gas Derivative for Localized Infusion Studies," *J. med. Chem.*, **8**, 757.

Eden, M., Haines, B. and Kahler, M. (1955), "The pH Rat Tumours Measured in Vitro," *J. nat. Cancer Inst.*, **16**, 541.

Gilman, A. and Philips, F. S. (1946), "The Biological Actions and Therapeutic Applications of the β-chlorethyl Amines and Sulfides," *Science*, **103**, 409.

Goldacre, R. J. and Sylvén, B. (1959), "A Rapid Method for Studying Tumour Blood Supply using Systemic Dyes," *Nature, Lond.*, **184**, 63.

Goldacre, R. J. and Sylvén, B. (1962), "On the Access of Blood-borne Dyes to Various Tumour Regions," *Brit. J. Cancer*, **26**, 306.

Goldacre, R. J. and Whisson, M. E. (1966), "The Biology of Large Solid Tumours Regressing with Nitrogen Mustard Treatment: A study of the mouse plasma cell tumour ADJ–PC–5 and the Walker carcinosarcoma 256," *Brit. J. Cancer*, **20**, 801.

Humphreys, S. R., Mantel, N. and Goldin, A. (1966), "Chemotherapy and Surgery of Spontaneous Tumours of Mice," *Europ. J. Cancer*, **2**, 1.

Isliker, H., Cerottini, J. C., Jaton, J. C. and Magnentat, G. (1964), in *Chemotherapy of Cancer* (ed. Plattner, P.) p. 278. Amsterdam: Elsevier.

Iyer, V. N. and Szybalski (1964), "Mitomycins and Porfiromycin: Chemical mechanism of activation and cross-linking of DNA," *Science*, **145**, 55.

Lawley, P. D. and Brookes, P. (1965), "Molecular Mechanism of the Cytotoxic Action of Difunctional Alkylating Agents and of Resistance to this Action," *Nature*, **206**, 480.

Leake, Chauncey D. (Ed.) (1967), "Biological Actions of Dimethyl Sulphoxide," *Annals of the New York Academy of Science*, **141**, 1.

Martin, D. S. and Fugmann, R. A. (1960), "Clinical Implications of the Interrelationship of Tumour Size and Chemotherapeutic Response," *Ann. Surg.*, **151**, 97.

Masterson, J. G. and Nelson, J. M. (1965), "The Role of Chemotherapy in the Treatment of Gynecologic Malignancy," *Amer. J. of Obstet. Gynec.*, **93**, 1102.

Meyer, K., Kammerling, E., Amtam, L., Koller, M. and Hoffman, S. (1948), "pH Studies of Malignant Tissue in Human Beings," *Cancer Res.*, **8**, 513.

Reid, J. M. (1964), "The Synthesis and Properties of some Potential Cytotoxic Agents." Thesis submitted for the degree of Doctor of Philosophy, University of London, 1964.

Roberts, J. J., Brent, T. P. and Crathorn, A. R. (1968), "The Mechanism of the Cytotoxic Action of Alkylating Agents on Mammalian Cells: Inactivation of the DNA template and its repair," in *Symposium on Interaction of Drugs and Sub-cellular Components in Animal Cells*. London: J. & A. Churchill Ltd.

Ross, W. C. J. (1962), *Biological Alkylating Agents*. London: Butterworths.

Sells, B. H. and Crudup, K. (1966), "Ribosome Production during recovery from Puromycin Treatment: Influence of 5-fluorouracil," *Biochim. biophysic. Acta*, **123**, 253.

Semonský, M., Černý, A. and Jelínek, V. (1967), "Antineoplastisch wirksame N-[(6-Purinylthio)Valeryl]-Aminosäuren," 5th International Congress of Chemotherapy, Vienna, 1967.

Skipper, H. E., Schabel, F. M. Jr., Wilcox, W. S. (1967), "Experimental Evaluation of Potential Anti-cancer Agents XXI: Scheduling of arabinosylcytosine to take advantage of its S-phase specificity against leukaemia cells," *Cancer Chemotherapy Reports*, **51**, 125.

Skipper, H. E., Schabel, F. M. Jr., Wilcox, W. S. (1964), "Experimental Evaluation of Potential Anti-cancer Agents XIII: On the criteria and kinetics associated with curability of experimental leukaemia." *Cancer Chemotherapy Reports*, **35**, 1.

Skipper, H. E., Schabel, F. M. Jr., Wilcox, W. S., Laster, W. R. Jr., Trader, M. W. and Thompson, S. A. (1965), "Experimental Evaluation of Potential Anti-cancer Agents XVIII: Effects of therapy on viability and rate of proliferation of leukemic cells in various anatomic sites," *Cancer Chemotherapy Reports*, **47**, 41.

Stock, J. A. (1966), in "The Chemotherapy of Neoplasia" (Vol. 4 of *Experimental Chemotherapy*). R. J. Schnitzer and F. Hawkins (eds.). New York and London: Academic Press.

Wade, Roy, Whisson, M. E. and Szekerke, M. (1967), "Some Serum Protein Nitrogen Mustard Complexes with High Chemotherapeutic Selectivity," *Nature Lond.*, **215**, 1303.

Whisson, M. E. and Connors, T. A. (1965), "Cure of Mice Bearing Advanced Plasma Cell Tumours with Aniline Mustard," *Nature, Lond.*, **206**, 689.

Zubrod, C. G., Schepartz, S., Leiter, J., Endicott, K. M., Carrese, L. M. and Baker, C. G. (1966), "The Chemotherapy Program of the National Cancer Institute: History, analysis, and plans," *Cancer Chemotherapy Reports*, **50**, 479 and 536.

2. THE EFFECTS OF TERATOGENIC DRUGS

H. TUCHMANN-DUPLESSIS

Since 1956 it has been known that drugs can act in a teratogenic way against the foetus. It was then first recognized that sex steroids used in the treatment of threatened abortion could masculinize female foetuses. The full potential danger of drugs however was not realized at that time because it was generally considered that the placental barrier completely protected the growing embryo.

The thalidomide catastrophe resulted in recognition of the possibility of impairing the normal development of a human embryo by giving a drug in therapeutic dosage to the mother even when it did not harm the mother.

Recently experimental screening methods have been devised which aim to determine whether a drug is likely or not to have adverse effects on the growing embryo. A W.H.O. Study Group have published the result of their discussion on the prognostic value and limitations of drug testing before clinical use. We will therefore here, only consider the conditions under which teratological action takes place and the drugs which produce abortions, congenital malformations or functional anomalies which may be discovered only after birth during the stage of adaptation to extra-uterine life.

Teratological Principles

The general principles of teratogenesis are basically not different from those underlying harmful effects in adults.

Teratogenic action however, is more complex because antenatally one is dealing with two biological systems—the developing embryo and the mother's body.

Whether or not congenital malformation occurs depends upon various factors—the developmental stage of the embryo, its genetic constitution, the physiological or pathological state of the mother and the specificity of the agent used. It is only when all these conditions coexist that a teratogenic agent will be able to produce a malformation.

(a) Embryonic Conditions

A drug can act directly on the embryo or indirectly through a metabolite which has been formed in the mother's body.

The results therefore depend not only on the nature and the dose of the agent used for the mother's condition, but also to a large extent on the exact stage of development of the embryo. The critical period in human beings for the embryo lies between the 13th and 60th days after conception. It is possible for foetal abnormalities to be produced later (Fig. 1). The morphological type of malformation usually depends on the embryonic stage in which the drug is administered.

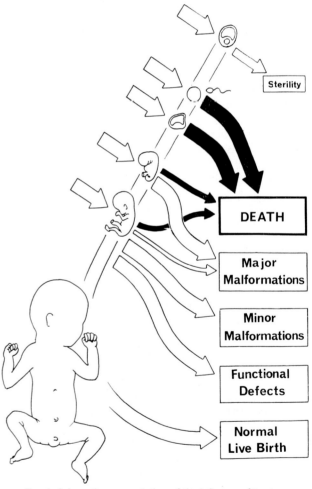

FIG. 1. Schematic representation of the influence of teratogenic factors on gametogenesis and various stages of embryonic and foetal development. During the preimplantation period strong teratogenic agents kill the embryo. During embryogenesis from day 13 to 60 teratogenic agents are embryotoxic or produce major congenital malformations. During the following foetal period minor morphological and functional malformations can be produced.

Each and every organ has a critical period in which its development can be deranged. A few of the various teratogenic agents that exist can however show a "preferential" effect on specific organs. The three best known teratogens effecting humans—radiation, rubella and thalidomide—although they may act at the same period against the embryo, do induce different types of abnormalities (Fig. 2).

rat. Thalidomide which produces obvious malformations of the rabbit is apparently safe for the rat.

Clinical observations in humans have shown comparable information about the variations in susceptibility to teratogens. For instance, among women who took thalidomide at the critical stage of pregnancy, less than 25 per cent gave birth to deformed babies, the remainder apparently escaping any ill-effect from the drug.

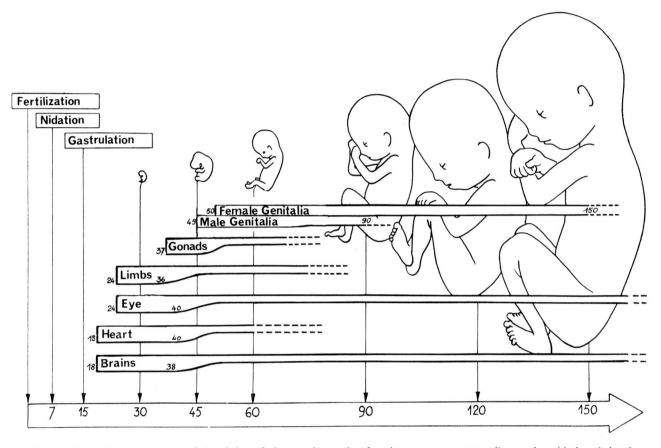

FIG. 2. Schematic representation of the timing of the morphogenesis of various organs, corresponding to the critical periods of teratogenic susceptibility. I am greatly indebted to my collaborator Doctor P. Haegel who prepared this diagram and Fig. 1.

Mental retardation, abnormalities of the central nervous system and malformations of the eye predominate after X-ray therapy; there is impairment of somatic growth, cataract, malformations of the heart and deafness commonly following rubella infection; while the thalidomide abnormalities are characterized by skeletal malformation, associated with normal growth and well-developed intelligence.

(b) Genetic Susceptibility

The way an embryo reacts to external agents depends upon its genetic constitution. This can vary not only between different species of animals but also within a definite species changing from strain to strain and even sometimes between individuals of the same strain. Cortisone which is a potent teratogenic agent in the rabbit and in the mouse does not produce any malformations in the

(c) Maternal Conditions

Not only does the developmental stage and the genetic constitution of the embryo matter but the action of the drug must depend also on the physiological and pathological condition of the mother.

Among physiological factors, age, diet, local uterine conditions, hormonal balance and environmental conditions play the largest role. Experimental and clinical data show that the risks of malformation and perinatal mortality are higher in very young mothers than in those of average age and still higher in the much older age groups.

As far as the diet is concerned specific deficiencies of nutrients, especially vitamins, minerals and essential amino-acids are more dangerous than general undernutrition. In the human population furthermore, the physiological status of the mother depends not only upon her intake of food but also on her social habits, climate and variations according to season. The larger number of malformations in lower social groups is generally ascribed to malnutrition, alcoholism and chronic diseases (but see Gopalan. Sec. V, Chap. 4).

A pathological condition, particularly one such as a chronic metabolic disease or toxaemia, hypertension, obesity and diabetes may bring about favourable conditions for the causation of congenital malformations.

Diabetes especially deserves attention because in diabetic and pre-diabetic mothers abortions, foetal mortality and congenital malformations are far more frequent than in the population as a whole.

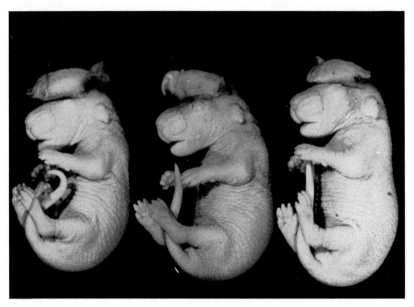

FIG. 3. Anencephaly in mouse foetuses treated with T.W.R. 1339.

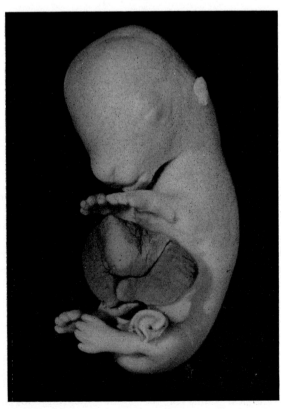

FIG. 4. Coelosomia in a rabbit foetus treated with T.W.R. 1339.

The figures given in the literature are variable. According to Miller *et al.*, (1944) and Barns (1949–50) the foetal mortality in diabetic women is 3 times higher than in the general population. In a study made in our department based on 150 diabetic women Turpin (1967) found that the perinatal mortality was 24 per cent as compared to 3 per cent in non diabetic women.

The figures are also variable concerning the frequency of congenital malformations.

In a group of 1742 children born from diabetic mothers Sindram (1955) found 4·9 per cent congenital malformations. White (1952) 12 per cent. Oakley (1953) also estimates that the state of anomalies is 6 higher in the offspring of diabetic women than in the general population. Turpin (1967) finds only a 3 fold increase of anomalies in diabetic mothers.

Even though we cannot explain the increased incidence of congenital malformation in children of mothers with metabolic diseases there can be no doubt that these conditions do favour the teratogenic action of those drugs that can act in this way. To give an instance, we can cite the influence of impaired maternal metabolism receiving Triton W.R. 1339. This compound which produces hyperlipaemia and hypercholesterolaemia in rodents happens to be embryotoxic and teratogenic in the rat, the mouse and the rabbit (Tuchmann-Duplessis and Mercier-Parot, 1964) (Fig. 3 and 4).

Teratogenic Agents

There are a great number of drugs in a variety of chemical groups capable of producing congenital malformations in mammals including the human. Until we can work out the classification of teratogenic drugs on a physiological or a pharmacological basis, which we cannot yet, we must perforce consider them here in an arbitrarily selected order.

Vitamins

Experimental data on the influence of vitamins in animals demonstrate that vitamin deficiencies are the worst of the dietary deficiencies as they lead to inhibition of growth in utero, they kill the embryo or they sometimes produce malformations.

Vitamin Deficiencies. The first example of congenital malformation produced exogenously was the teratogenic action of vitamin A deficiency in the pig, discovered by Hale in 1933. For the past twenty years it has been established that deficiency of Vitamin A can produce a large variety of congenital malformations in other species as well including the rat, the mouse and the rabbit.

In spite of a mass of experimental work it is still open to question whether deficiency of Vitamin A can be teratogenic in man. Sarma (1959) reported microcephaly in association with microphthalmia in a child born to an Indian woman who had Vitamin A deficiency. This single case report may or may not be significant.

Other vitamin deficiencies, E, B2, and pantothenic acid can also produce abnormalities of the central nervous system, and of the eye and skeleton in rats. But there is no evidence of a similar reaction in human beings.

The only vitamin deficiency which is known to be teratogenic in man is folic acid deficiency which can be produced by deficient diet or by folic acid antagonists—aminopterine and x methyl folic acid. Clinical cases have been observed after the administration of aminopterine and we will go further into this problem in the section devoted to the effects of anti-tumour drugs.

Deficiencies of other vitamins such as ascorbic acid, biotine, pyrodoxine thiamine and vitamin K do not seem to be teratogenic.

Excess of Vitamins. High doses of vitamin A (40 to 50 thousand i.u. per day) interfere with intra-uterine development and produce from 30 to 90 per cent of gross malformations in the rat (Cohlan, 1953; Giroud et al., 1954). Giroud also had rats with malformations on doses of 500 i.u. Vitamin A per day.

It has been claimed that large doses of Vitamin D taken during pregnancy could cause hypercalcaemia with hardening of the bones of the vault and base of the skull. No malformations have occurred.

It has been claimed that a synthetic compound menadione with properties similar to those of Vitamin K can cause ill effects on the foetus. Given in large doses in the second half of pregnancy menadione can lead to neonatal jaundice. This condition does not occur after the administration of non-synthetic Vitamin K.

Hormones

Several hormones are teratogenic for animals. The masculinizing effect of certain sex hormones has been well established in man.

Androgenic Steroids

The use of testosterone or its analogues in human beings in pregnancy, or in rodents, can lead to masculinization of female foetuses.

In girls the masculinization of the urogenital sinus takes the form of hypertrophy of the clitoris and atrophy of the labia. If the drug has been given before the 12th week of pregnancy complete fusion of the labia may occur.

The masculinizing effect of compounds related to testosterone was first shown in the rabbit by Courrier and Jost (1942) after they had administered ethinyl-testosterone. Later when synthetic steroids with a 17 hydroxy group were used therapeutically they were shown to have similar effects on the foetus to those of methyltestosterone. After Wilkins had reported the first case (1960) a further hundred cases or more of masculinization of female foetuses associated with the use of 17 α ethinyl testosterone and 17 α ethinyl 19 nortestosterone have been described to date.

Several groups have investigated the influence on gonads and on pre-natal development of steroids because they are frequently used as oral contraceptives. Ten years of clinical experience has shown conclusively that contraceptive steroids do not cause any mutations, nor produce any congenital malformations. The risk of masculinization of the female foetus is so small that it can for all practical purposes be ignored.

Yet, although contraceptive steroids do not alter matters morphologically, their action in causing possible upsets in the pituitary-hypothalamic system cannot be completely brushed aside. In rodents the hypothalamus and the higher centres of the nervous system are specific sexually. For this reason hormones that act during the critical stages of histogenesis of the brain are potentially capable at least of impairing sexual behaviour and modifying the gonadotrophic activity of the pituitary. Monkeys that have been masculinized in utero by giving progestogens to their mothers show permanent changes in sexual behaviour.

Corticosteroids

Cortisone produces cleft palates and a number of cardiac abnormalities in mice and rabbits. Hydrocortisone and ACTH has similar effects in mice. The incidence of malformations varies according to the dose of cortisone and the strain of the animal that is being studied. The rat and monkey are resistant to the teratogenic action of corticoids. In the rat however, high doses of cortisone bring about an inhibition of prenatal development, and atrophy of the adrenal cortex and the newborn are very fragile. Most of them die from cachexia or inter-current infections (Mercier-Parot, 1957).

We are still assessing the susceptibility of the human foetus to cortisone. Several cases of cleft palate have been observed in infants born to mothers that have been with cortisone during the pregnancy. Popert (1962) who analysed several hundred cases he found in the literature, discovered that one per cent of children exposed to cortisone in utero had cleft palates. This incidence is slightly higher than in a random sample and Popert therefore considers cortisone to be a weak teratogen in humans.

Taking into account however the fact that cortisone is only administered to women who have some pathological condition one must be diffident in making any definite statement co-relating the cleft palates that have been observed with the cortisone therapy. Although the risk of giving cortisone seems to be slight since this is still uncertain, it is wiser to administer this hormone to pregnant women only if the medical condition really justifies taking the risk.

Sudden withdrawal of corticosteroids at birth when infants have been born to mothers on high doses of this hormone during the latter part of the pregnancy may result in serious damage in the week or so after birth. In those few cases reported haemorrhage, atrophy and necrosis of the adrenal cortex have been found.

Thyroid Function

The human thyroid starts functioning towards the end of the first trimester of pregnancy. The gland develops mainly under the influence of foetal thyroid stimulating hormone. For this reason agents that can act on the release of TSH or the secretion of thyroxine can inhibit the foetal thyroid.

Large doses of thyroxine injected into the pregnant rat can cause retardation of thyroid development. It is not likely however that such an inhibition of the thyroid could occur in human beings because the placental permeability to thyroxine is minimal. Propylthiouracil however, crosses the placenta rapidly and so interferes with the thyroxin synthesis of the foetal thyroid and can produce foetal thyroid abnormalities and especially goitre formation.

Prenatal hypothyroidism can also be blamed for some abnormalities of the development of the central nervous system and may be responsible for mental deficiency in the offspring.

As may be recalled administration of iodine and iodines to the mother during pregnancy can produce goitres in the offspring. In some cases the enlargement of a thyroid may produce obstruction in the trachea with resulting serious respiratory distress, rarely leading to death by asphyxia.

Radiopaque compounds as well as radioactive iodine given in early pregnancy can lead to congenital hypothyroidism and so affect the outcome of the pregnancy.

In the rat when large doses of thyroxine were administered 20 per cent of the offspring had cataracts (Giroud et al., 1954). (See also Sec. X, Chap. 5.)

Pituitary Hormones

Growth hormone has no specific action on the developing embryo. Until recently foetal gigantism was attributed to excessive amounts of somatotropic hormones acting on protein and carbohydrate metabolism in the mother.

Personal observations (1955) have shown that STH neither stimulates nor has teratogenic action on the offspring.

STH by exerting a non-specific toxic effect can cause retardation of growth in the foetus of the rat (Fig. 5). Human Gonadotrophins which often produce multiple and premature ovulation can lead to multiple pregnancies and they have been incriminated as causing foetal deformities. Although a large number of infants have been

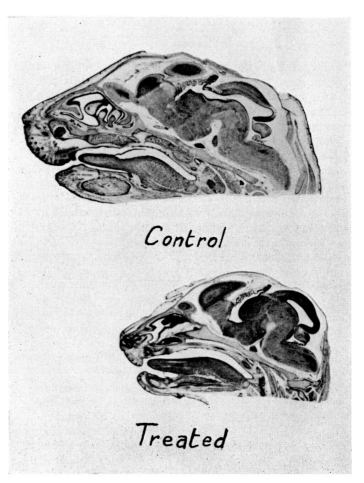

FIG. 5. Section of the head of rat foetuses treated by S.T.H. The growth inhibition is due to a non-specific toxic effect.

born, including a successful quintuplet pregnancy, as reported by Higgins et al., (1966) we can make no definite statement as to the potential danger of human pituitary gonadotrophins.

The influence on the other two pituitary hormones ACTH and TSH has already been mentioned when discussing corticoids and thyroid function.

Insulin and Hypoglycaemic Agents

The hypoglycaemic hormone produced by the pancreas is probably not teratogenic although isolated cases of malformations have been reported in the mouse and in the rabbit. Studies in the Rhesus monkey using labelled insulin show that insulin is rapidly transferred from the mother to the embryo. The placenta permeability however must be limited since the concentration for a labelled hormone in the umbilical venous blood is only a fraction of that present in the maternal circulation. Most of the results obtained in animals, as in human beings, indicate that administration of insulin to pregnant mothers does not harm the embryo.

Oral Hypoglycaemic Drugs

Several hypoglycaemic sulfonamides—carbutamide, tolbutamide and a dimethylbiguanide are teratogenic in rodents. Table 1. In most cases the abnormalities are

TABLE 1

TABLE DEMONSTRATING THE MEAN OF THE RESULTS OBTAINED AFTER INFLUENCE OF VARIOUS HYPOGLYCAEMIC AGENTS TO PREGNANT RATS

Treatment	Percentage aborted	Average number of foetuses	Percentage of abnormalities*
Control	2	9·4	0
Carbutamide	38	4·4	23
2259 RP	33	9	0
Tolbutamide	36	8	2
Chlorpropamide	10	6·8	0
Dibiguanide	17	7·5	0·5

* Account has only been taken of serious abnormalities recognizable macroscopically.

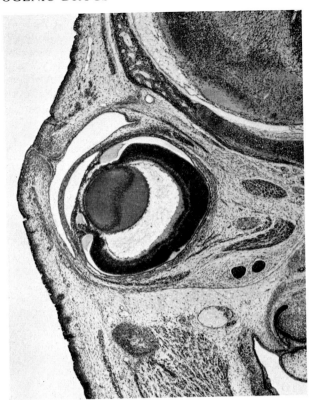

FIG. 7. Section of the eye of a carbutamide treated foetus. Atrophy of the optic nerve, some fibres are directed to the cornea (gray spot on the upper right).

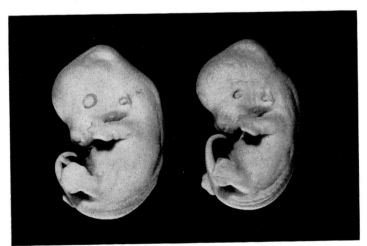

FIG. 6. Rat foetuses. On the left the control, on the right a carbutamide treated foetus with microphtalmia.

observed in the eye and the central nervous system; yet skeletal abnormalities, cleft palate and even shortening of the maxilla can be produced (Tuchmann-Duplessis and Mercier-Parot, 1963).

The teratogenic action does not seem to be related to the chemical structure of the compound nor to its specific pharmacological properties (Figs. 6, 7 and 8).

In human beings, abortions and the production of malformations have been attributed to the use of hypoglycaemic

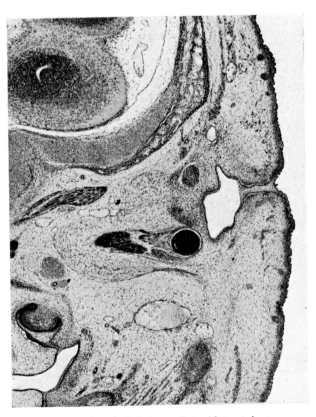

FIG. 8. Microphtalmia in a carbutamide treated rat.

agents. No definite conclusions however can be drawn since the available clinical data indicates that normal and abnormal children can be born to mothers who have received copious amounts in early pregnancy. Until there is more information on the subject oral hypoglycaemic agents should be considered to be less safe than insulin and therefore should be avoided in therapeutic treatment of pregnant women.

Hyperglycaemic Agents

Repeatedly, experiments on alloxan diabetes have shown malformations in mice. Glucagon is teratogenic in the rat. Administering 300–600 gammas of glucagon by injection we were able to observe various eye malformations ranging from glaucoma to microphthalmia, (Fig. 9). Other hyperglycaemic agents such as galactose 2 desoxyglucose and fluroacetate are also teratogenic in the rat (De Meyer, (1961).

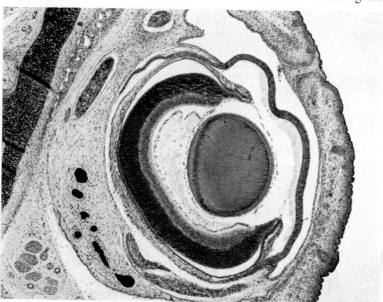

FIG. 9. Glaucoma in a glucagon treated rat. The cornea is very broad, and wrinkled.

TABLE 2

CHEMICAL STRUCTURE OF THREE GLUTARIMIDES. ONLY THALIDOMIDE IS TERATOGENIC

Thalidomide (α-phtalimido-glutarimide)

Doridene (α-phenyl-α-ethyl-glutarimide)

Aturbane
(Chlorhydrate of α-phenyl-α-[β'diethylamino-ethyl]-glutarimide)

TWR 1339

The frequent association of diabetes and upsets in lipid metabolism have led us to examine the action of a surface agent—Triton WR 1339—which causes hyperlipaemia and a significant rise in total body cholesterol. Large doses of TWR 1339 cause a high percentage of abortions and 15–20 per cent of gross malformations in rodents. These results suggest that the various fertility troubles observed in diabetics may be related not only to the condition of hyperglycaemia but also to other metabolic disorders (Tuchmann-Duplessis and Mercier-Parot, 1964). A hypocholesteraemic agent, Triparenol (Mer 29) produces multiple malformations of the central nervous system in rats and mice (Roux *et al.*, 1961).

Tranquilizers

Several have been incriminated as causing human malformations following clinical and experimental demonstration of the teratogenic action of thalidomide.

Glutaramides

We investigated two chemically related compounds of thalidomide, α phenyl and α ethylglutarimide (Doriden) and α phenyl beta diethyl amino ethyl glutarimide (Aturban) which had become suspect. No malformations could be observed even using very high doses, including those toxic to the mother. (Tuchmann-Duplessis and Mercier-Parot, 1964). This is an example that demonstrates how chemical structure, pharmacological properties and teratogenic action are all independent of one another. (Table 2.)

Phenothiazines

A large number of phenothiazines have been used for long periods in pregnancy to relieve tension and nausea. Although in a few isolated cases slight teratogenic action of chlorpromazine and prochlorpromazine have been reported in the rat there has been no proof of any toxic effect on a human foetus whether the drug has been taken for a short time or for several months. Careful observations made using Librium shows that this tranquilizing drug is not teratogenic.

Imipramine given in large doses in the rabbit has been found to be teratogenic. Clinical claims about this antidepressant as well as about Haloperidol which is a very active buturophenone, have not been confirmed.

Large doses of Haloperidol can delay implantation in the rat and in the mouse. In our experience this action is due to a modification of the gonadotropic activity of the maternal pituitary leading to excessive releases of luteotrophic hormone.

Reserpine which is used in hypertension and in psychiatric disorders may affect the foetus. A syndrome characterized by lethargy, bradycardia, hypothermia and nasal congestion has been described. A similar syndrome due to depletion of the catecholamine stores could be produced in guinea pigs. No abnormalities however were observed.

Serotonin (5-hydroxytryptamine) which interferes with reserpine metabolism when administered to mice in early pregnancy can cause resorption and malformations. In the second half of pregnancy 5-hydroxytryptamine rapidly leads to foetal death. Robson et al., (1965) attribute the harmful action of serotonin to impairment of the functional activity of the placenta.

Modification of serotonin metabolism and especially a high level of serotonin production is considered to be one of the causes of habitual abortion in human beings (Sadowsky et al., 1963).

Lysergic Acid Diethylamide (LSD)

Recent investigations have shown that LSD can impair prenatal development. In the rat foetal resorption, inhibition of growth and stillbirth can occur. In the mouse a few cerebral malformations have also been observed.

Chromosome alterations and chromatid breaks have been observed in white blood cells in patients treated with LSD. Similar alterations have been confirmed in vitro when LSD has been added to cell cultures. Chromatid breaks have been observed in two infants whose mothers took LSD during pregnancy.

Zellweger et al., (1967) reported an abnormal child born to a nineteen year old mother who took LSD on the 25th, 45th and the 98th day after her last menstrual cycle. Chromatid breaks were found in the mother as well as the deformed child.

This single reported case does not enable us to draw any definite conclusion as to the possible teratogenic action of LSD since several mothers have given birth to normal children after having been treated with LSD.

Ganglion Blocking Agent

When hexamethonium bromide has been used in toxaemia pregnancy occasional cases of paralytic ileus of the newborn have followed. Although hexamethonium crosses the placenta rapidly and reaches the foetal circulation in a concentration of 50 per cent of that present in the maternal blood, it is still uncertain as to what extent such a complication is directly related to this drug.

Hypnotics

Oxybarbiturates and thiobarbiturates are not teratogenic. Since the placental transfer is rapid the concentration of barbiturates to foetal blood is approximately 70 per cent that in the maternal circulation. High doses may depress foetal activity without producing real damage.

Phenmetrazine

This drug widely used in the treatment of obesity has been incriminated as causing several cases of diaphragmatic hernia and also malformations of the limbs. Since many infants have been born to mothers treated during pregnancy with phenmetrazine without any abnormalities the clinical evidence does seem to be not very convincing. Our experience with rodents, rats, mice and rabbits using phenmetrazine have not shown teratogenic effects (unpublished data). Investigations performed by Cahen et al., (1964) using another anorexic agent—2-diethyl amino-propiophenone failed to reveal teratogenic effects.

Analgesics

In most animals and in human beings salicylates cross the placenta rapidly and are found in the umbilical cord blood. High doses of acid salicylic acid (aspirin) can cause foetal resorption and congenital malformations in rodents. The widespread use of salicylates however in human beings suggests that even large doses taken during pregnancy are not dangerous to the human foetus. Where patients have glucose-6-phosphatase dehydrogenase deficiency however, overdoses might theoretically be considered to cause abnormalities.

Other analgesics such as morphine, meperidine, scopolamine, chloral hydrate, which all cross the placenta are not teratogenic. Administered in the last months of pregnancy however, morphine does have a definite depressant action on the foetus. In the foetal rabbit large doses of morphine can interfere with cardio-vascular function.

In mothers addicted to morphine the foetus can develop a syndrome of physiological dependence on morphine. In such rare cases a withdrawal syndrome from morphine has been observed in the new born.

Antihistamines and Antinauseant drugs

The frequent use of these drugs in early pregnancy is the explanation why several of them, meclezine, cyclizine, trifluorazine, have been incriminated as causing foetal abnormalities. In rodents, large doses of cyclizine, chlorcyclizine and meclezine have been shown to produce a large variety of abnormalities of the eye, the central nervous system and of the face and the palate, (Tuchmann-Duplessis and Mercier-Parot, 1963; King, 1963; Narrod and King, 1965). Although several extensive epidemiological studies have been made by various teams in the U.S.A., in Australia, in Sweden and in the United Kingdom, it is still not possible to draw any definite conclusion as to the influence these drugs have. No proof of teratragenic action has been definitely established in man, (James, 1963; David, 1963; Mellin, 1963; McBride, 1963; Yerushalmy, 1965; Sadusk, 1965).

Alkaloids

Cafeine and nicotine as well as reserpine and morphine which have already been mentioned have been incriminated as having harmful effects on the growing embryo. In the mouse, cafeine can impair the evolution of pregnancy and cause a few malformations (Nishimura, 1964). Epidemiological studies on the influence of smoking have definitely shown that nicotine has a deleterious effect. In women who smoke 20 or more cigarettes per day the prematurity rate is twice as high as in mothers who do not smoke. According to Lowe, (1959); Frazier et al., (1961); Herriot et al., (1962) infants of smoking mothers are not only premature but they also weigh less at any given stage of gestation.

It has been suggested that chronic hypoxia of the smoking mother might be the cause of the lower foetal weight (Haddon et al., 1961).

Anticoagulants

The administration of dicoumarin derivatives has been reported as causing different types of foetal haemorrhage resulting in a few cases in foetal or neonatal death. Although bihydroxycoumarin is nearly completely bound to plasma proteins, coumarin and its analogues cross the placenta and have a stronger anticoagulant effect on the foetus than on the mother.

The harmful effect of bihydroxycoumarin may also be due to the enzymic immaturity of foetal liver. There is a deficient detoxication mechanism which is brought about by conjugation with glururonic acid. That is why even minute quantities of free bihydroxycoumarin are able to interfere with prothrombin synthesis in the liver.

The influence of treatment with coumarin in early pregnancy is still uncertain. Three personal observations of cases in which coumarin was administered before conception and during the first two months of pregnancy have resulted in deliveries of normal babies.

Heparin, which does not cross the placenta in quantities of biological significance, has apparently no harmful effect on the foetus.

Antitumour Drugs

A large number of antitumour drugs have been investigated. The majority of them have harmful effects on the embryo, since they are embryotoxic and frequently also teratogenic.

Antitumour drugs can be divided into three groups according to the mechanism of their action: alkylating agents, antimitotics, and antimetabolites. Since it is not possible to make a short survey of the data accumulated on this subject only the most important results will be given.

Among the alkylating agents which act on cell metabolism as do radiations, nitrogen mustard, cyclophosphamide, triethylenemalamine, chlorambucil and busulfan or myleran are the most teratogenic in rodents. Three of these compounds, cyclophosphamide, chlorambucil and busulfan have been incriminated as causing malformations in humans.

The antimitotic drugs, colchicine, desacetylmethyl-cochicine, podophyline and urethane are in the main embryotoxic. Urethane and podophyline can also produce some malformations. There is some suspicion, not confirmed, that podophyline can produce malformations in human beings.

The worst substances for teratogenic effect are found in the group of antimetabolites. It is our experience that actinomycin D, 6-chloropurine, 6-mercaptopurine, azathioprine or imuran and the folic acid antagonists, aminopterin and x-methyl folic acid have had the most teratogenic

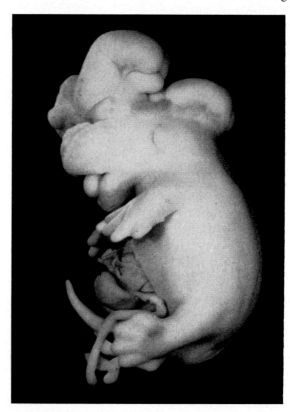

FIG. 10. Anencephaly and coelosomia in a mouse foetus treated with x-methyl folic acid.

action in rodents and in the cat. (Figs. 10 and 11.) They can produce a large variety of malformations of the central nervous system, the eye, the viscera and in the skeleton.

In the rabbit imuran and mercaptopurine can bring about malformations of the limbs similar to those observed in infants born to mothers treated with thalidomide. (Figs. 12, 13, 14, 15.) Aminopterin is also teratogenic for human beings, as demonstrated by Thiersch (1952).

The greater the difference in general toxicity and embryo toxicity is for most of the antitumour drugs, the greater is the teratogenic action.

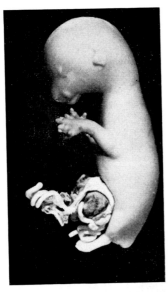

FIG. 11. Coelosomia and shortening of the inferior part of the body in a cat foetus treated with x-methyl folic acid.

Antibiotics

Most antibiotics such as penicillin, streptomycin, dehydrostreptomycin, tetracycline, oxytetracycline, and oxymethyl penicillin traverse the placental barrier rapidly and appear in high levels in the embryo and in the amniotic fluid.

Penicillin which has been used extensively in pregnancy appears to be quite harmless for the embryo.

Streptomycin administered to a mother can be detected within a few minutes in the foetus. Its well known toxity for the nervous system, which is even more pronounced in

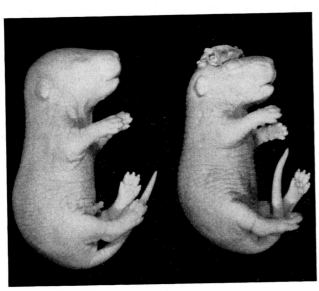

FIG. 12. Anencephaly in a mouse foetus treated with 6-mercaptopurine. On the left a normal foetus.

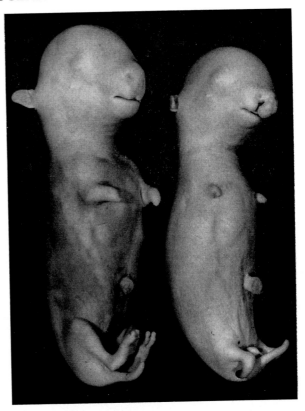

FIG. 13. Severe leg deformities and hare lip in rabbit foetuses treated with 6-mercaptopurine.

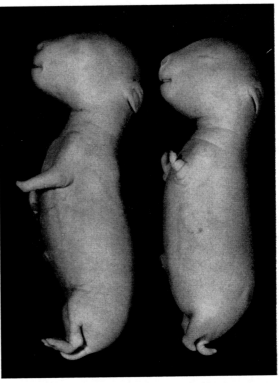

FIG. 14. Severe leg malformation in rabbit foetuses treated with azathioprine.

young animals than in adults, has given rise to the suspicion that streptomycin will cause lesions of the vestibule in the young foetus. A few cases of neonatal deafness have been reported in the children of mothers treated with streptomycin for tuberculosis. The incidence however of this abnormality is so low that one can still not be certain as to the teratogenic effect of streptomycin.

Tetracycline has been cited as the cause of human skeletal malformation. In our personal experience with rats using doses 60 to 100 times higher than the clinical doses, we have not observed any malformations. The antibiotic promptly crosses the placenta and it can be detected in the skeleton and in the teeth even one month after birth.

sulphathiazole, and sulphamerazine can produce congenital malformations in rats. Only one of these compounds, sulphasoxazole (Gantrisin) has been shown to be embryopathic in humans.

Sulphonamides may bring about an increase in the frequency of the incidence of kernicterus, since they cause penetration of unconjugated bilirubin into the central nervous tissues. Similar adverse effects have not been shown to occur in the foetus.

The statement has often been made that drugs that are dangerous to the new born infant should be considered as potentially harmful to the foetus when they are given to the mother. Exceptions to this rule must however be found because many drugs, as for instance chloramphenicol

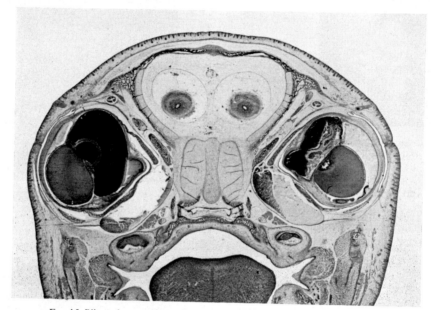

FIG. 15. Bilateral eye malformations in a rabbit foetus treated with azathioprine.

The clinical claims as to the teratogenicity of tetracycline have not yet been confirmed, although it is well established that hypoplasia and yellow or brown discolouration of the primary teeth can occur in infants whose mothers have been treated with tetracyclines. It is possible that temporary retardation of neonatal growth may be due to deposition of tetracyline in the skeleton.

Chloramphenicol, which is very toxic to premature new born children in whom it produces the "gray syndrome" does not seem to have any harmful effect on the foetus when administered to the mother during pregnancy.

Novobiocin interferes with the metabolism of bilirubin and increases the likelihood of neonatal jaundice in the new born. In rats this antibiotic also inhibits enzymatic processes in the liver and reduces the activity of glururonyl transferase.

Sulphonamides

Most sulphonamides reach the same blood concentration in the foetus as in the maternal circulation within one or two hours. Long acting compounds such as sulphapyridine, sulphasoxazole, sulphacetamide, sulphadiazine,

which are toxic to infants never reach dangerous foetal levels when administered to the mother.

Antiprotozoals

Quinine, which has been used more than any other drug against malaria has also been used as an abortifacient and has often been considered to be dangerous to the foetus. In rodents high doses of quinine can cause cochlear damage. In human beings it has been claimed that abortions, a few cases of deafness and some eye malformations have occurred after quinine therapy during pregnancy. The rarity of congenital deafness however can be attributed to this drug in spite of its widespread use and the absence of any correlation between the frequency of damage to the inner ear and endemic malarial areas makes it still doubtful as to whether this drug has any teratogenic action.

If quinine is used to induced labour, thrombocytopenia may occur in the mother and the new born. Quinine brings about thrombocytopenia by combining platelets and giving them the properties of a weak antigen. Neonatal thrombocytopenia therefore results from the transplacental passage of both antibody and quinine. It is appropriate to state that other drugs, as for example thiazides such as **chlorothiazide,** may produce thrombocytopenia by direct action on megacaryocytes.

The newer antimalarial drugs such as **pentaquine** and **primaquine** are not potentially dangerous for the foetus. Where the foetus however has a metabolic disorder of the erythrocyte formation, intravascular haemolysis and methaemaglobinemia may occur.

Chloroquine, which is a compound related to quinine and used in malaria, in collagen diseases and in lupus erythematosis has been incriminated as the cause of several cases of cochlear and vestibular defects, and of mental retardation. Since it is known that chloroquine administered to adults may lead to reversible toxic effects on the nerves, it is not possible to rule out embryotoxic effects.

Atrican, which is a trichomonacidal substance, has no harmful effects on the embryo. In our experience this amino nitro thiazole has not produced resorption nor malformations in the rat, the mouse or the rabbit. High doses may be toxic to the mother animal but no teratogenic effect has been reported in humans.

Another trichomonacidal drug, **metronidazole,** which is supposed to interfere with the purine metabolism, was at one time thought to be dangerous for the foetus. So far no clinical material has supported this contention.

Smallpox vaccinia may be mentioned as a substance that has been thought to cause human malformations. The precise effect of smallpox vaccination on the foetus has still not been properly established. Tondury (1963) reported an abortion occurring on the 83rd day after the last period when revaccination had been carried out 52 days after the period. The foetus showed generalized vaccinial necrosis of the skin. The presence of the vaccine virus could be demonstrated.

Green *et al.,* (1966) reported two cases of foetal vaccinia leading to spontaneous deliveries of stillborn foetuses. Vaccina virus was isolated from the placenta and from the foetal liver.

When Bourke *et al.,* (1964) carried out a prospective study on 112 pregnant women receiving smallpox vaccination they were not able to demonstrate any harmful foetal effects.

CONCLUSIONS

From experimental and clinical material it is possible to conclude that drugs which may be harmless for the mother may be harmful for the foetus and may cause congenital malformations.

Some of the differences in toxicity of drugs in the foetus as compared with the adult must be due to underdevelopment of the foetal metabolising enzyme systems of the liver as well as to the functional immaturity of the foetal kidney.

The increased foetal susceptibility to drugs is often related to the absence of enzymic systems to synthesize and conjugate glucuronides.

Although a large number of drugs have been shown to be teratogenic in animals a similar action in humans has only been proven in a few cases in specially favourable circumstances. Such a correlation could be shown for thalidomide, androgens and androgen-like steroids, coumarin derivatives and antitumour agents such as myleran, aminopterin, chlorambucil and cyclophosphamide. Other drugs however must be suspect and among these are thiouracil, iodine, antinauseants, oral hypoglycaemic agents, and long acting sulphonamides.

Since teratogenic action is irreversible, a decision to prescribe a drug should only be taken after an evaluation has been made of its potential danger to the embryo as compared with the risk of depriving the mother of its beneficial effects. The potential teratogenic danger of certain drugs however should not in its turn lead to therapeutic nihilism and thus deprive women throughout half their lives of the beneficial action of new drugs.

All photographs except figure 10 are from experiments of H. Tuchmann-Duplessis and L. Mercier-Parot.

Fig. 10 is from experiments of H. Tuchmann-Duplessis, Lefebvres-Boisselot and Mercier-Parot.

FURTHER READING

In the bibliography references indicated by one star are general reviews, those indicated by two stars are books.

*Adamsons, K. and Joelsson, I. (1966), "The Effects of Pharmacologic Agents upon the Fetus and Newborn," *Amer. J. Obstet. Gynec.,* **96**, 3, 437.

*Baker, J. B. E. (1960), "The Effect of Drugs on the Foetus," *Pharmacol. Rev.,* **12**, 1, 37.

Barns, H. H. F., Lindan, O., Morgans, M. E., Reid, E. and Swyer, G. I. M. (1950), "Foetal Mortality in Pregnant Rats Treated with Anterior Pituitary Extract and in Alloxan Diabetic Rats," *Lancet,* **1**, 841.

Barns, H. H. F. and Morgans, M. E. (1949), "Pregnancy Complicated by Diabetes Mellitus," *Brit. med. J.,* **1**, 51.

Bourke, G. J. and Whitty, R. J. (1964), "Smallpox Vaccination in Pregnancy: a Prospective Study," *Brit. med. J.,* 5397–1544.

*Burns, J. J. and Conney, A. H. (1964), "Therapeutic Implications of Drug Metabolism," *Seminars in Hematology,* **1**, 4, 375.

Cahal, D. A. (1965), "Drug Embryopathies, Preventive Measures: The British Point of View," *Symp. on Embryopathic Act. of Drugs.* London: J. and A. Churchill, 279.

*Cahen, R. L. (1964), "Evaluation of the Teratogenicity of Drugs," *Clin. Pharmacol. Therapeutics,* **5**, 4, 480.

*Cahen, R. L. (1966), "Experimental and Clinical Chemoteratogenesis," *Advances in Pharmacology,* **4**, 263.

**Ciba Foundation Symposium on Congenital Malformations* (1960). London: J. and A. Churchill.

Cohlan, S. Q. (1953), "Excessive Intake of Vitamin A as a Cause of Congenital Anomalies in the Rat," *Science,* **117**, 535.

Courrier, R. and Jost, A. (1942), "Intersexualité foetale provoquée par la pregneninolone au cours de la grossesse," *C.R. Soc. Biol.,* **136**, 395.

David A. and Goodspeed, A. H. (1963), "Ancoloxin and Fetal Abnormalities," *Brit. med. J.,* **1**, 121.

Degenhardt, K. H. (1965), "Probleme der Humangenetik," *Med. Welt,* **50**, 2784.

Degenhardt, K. H. (1966), "Entwicklungsentgleisung Spezieller Organanlagen," *Naturw. Rdsch.,* **19**, 1, 13.

De Meyer, R. and De Plaen, J. (1964), "An Approach to the Biochemical Study of Teratogenic Substances on Isolated Rat Embryo," *Life Sciences,* **3**, 709.

*Fave, A. (1964), "Les embryopathies provoquées chez les Mammifères," *Thérapie,* **1**, 1.

Frazier, T. M., Davis, G. H., Goldstein, H. and Goldberg, I. D. (1961), "Cigarette Smoking and Prematurity: a Prospective Study," *Amer. J. Obstet. Gynec.*, **81**, 988.

Giroud, A. and Martinet, M. (1954), "Influence de la souche de rats sur l'apparition des cataractes thyroxiniennes," *Arch. Franç. Pediat.*, **11**, 168.

*Giroud, A. and Tuchmann-Duplessis, H. (1962), "Malformations congenitales: Rôle des facteurs exogènes," *Pathologie et Biologie*, **10**, 1, 119.

Giroud, A. (1963), "Vitamine A et tératogenèse," *Teratogenesis*. Schwabe and Co. Edit., 440.

Green, D. M., Reid, S. M. and Rhandy, K. (1966), "Generalised Vaccinia in the Human Fœtus," *Lancet*, **1**, 7450, 1296.

Haddon, W. Jr., Nesbitt, R. E. and Garcia, R. (1961), "Smoking and Pregnancy: Carbon Monoxide in Blood during Gestation and at Term," *Obstet. Gynec.*, **18**, 262.

Herriot, A., Billewicz, W. Z. and Hytten, F. E. (1962), "Cigarette Smoking in Pregnancy," *Lancet*, **1**, 771.

Higgins, G. C. and Ibbertson, H. K. (1966), "A Successful Quintuplet Pregnancy following Treatment with Human Pituitary Gonadotrophin," *Lancet*, **1**, 114.

James, J. R. (1963), "Ancoloxin and Foetal Abnormalities," *Brit. med. J.*, **1**, 59.

King, C. T. G. (1963), "Teratogenic Effects of Meclizine Hydrochloride on the Rat," *Science*, **141**, 353.

Koller, Th. and Erb, H. (1964), "Medikamentöse Pathogenese fetaler Missbildungen," *Acta Genet. Basel.* Basel: S. Karger.

Lowe, C. R. (1959), "Effect of Mothers' Smoking Habits on Birth Weight of Their Children," *Brit. med. J.*, **2**, 673.

McBride, W. (1963), "Cyclizine and Congenital Abnormalities," *Brit. med. J.*, **1**, 1157.

Mellin, G. W. and Katzenstein, M. (1963), "Meclozine and Fetal Abnormalities," *Lancet*, **1**, 222.

Mercier-Parot, L. (1957), "Influence de la cortisone et de l'hormone corticotrope sur la gestation et le développement post-natal du rat," *Biol. méd.*, **96**, 6.

Miller, H. C., Hurwitz, D. and Kuder, K. (1944), "Fetal and Neonatal Mortality in Pregnancy Complicated by Diabetes Mellitus," *J. Amer. med. Ass.*, **124**, 271.

Murakami, U. (1966), "Teratogenesis of Craniofacial Malformations in Animals," *Arch. Environmental Health*, **13**, 695.

Narrod, S. A., Wilk, A. L. and King, C. T. G. (1965), "Metabolism of Meclizine in the Rat," *J. Pharmacol. Exp. Ther.*, **147**, 380.

**Nishimura, H. (1964), *Chemistry and Prevention of Congenital Anomalies*. Springfield: Charles C. Thomas, 111.

Oakley, W. (1953), "Prognosis in Diabetic Pregnancy," *Brit. med. J.*, **50**, 1453.

Popert, A. J. (1962), "Pregnancy and Adrenocortical Hormones," *Brit. med. J.*, **1**, 967.

Robson, J. M., Poulson, E. and Sullivan, F. M. (1965), "Pharmacological Principles of Teratogenesis," *Symp. Embryopathic Act. of Drugs*. London: J. and A. Churchill, 21.

Roux, Ch. and Dupuis, R. (1961), "Action tératogène du Triparanol," *C.R. Soc. Biol.*, **155**, 12, 2255.

Sadowsky, A., Pfeifer, G., Sadowsky, E., Tsur, C. and Sulman, F. G. (1963), "Serotonin Metabolism in Habitual Abortion," *Obstet. Gynec.*, **22**, 6, 778.

Sarma, V. (1959), "Marternal Vitamin A Deficiency and Fetal Microcephaly and Anopthalmia," *Obstet. Gynec. N.Y.*, **13**, 299.

Sindram, I. S. (1955), *Zwangerschap en suikerziekte*. Amsterdam: H. J. Paris, 313.

**Stoll, R. and Maraud, R. (1965), "Introduction à l'étude des malformations," *Monographies de Physiologie Causale*. Paris: Gauthier-Villars.

*Sutherland, J. M. and Light, I. J. (1965), "The Effect of Drugs upon the Developing Fetus," *Pediatric Clin. of North America*, **12**, 3, 781.

**Symp. on Embryopathic Activity of Drugs* (1965). London: J. and A. Churchill.

**Teratogenesis* (1963). Basel: Schwabe & Co.

Thiersch, J. B. (1952), "Therapeutic Abortions with a Folic Acid Antagonist, 4 Aminopteroylglutamic Acid (4 amino P G A, administered by the oral route)," *Amer. J. Obstet. Gynec.*, **63**, 1298.

Töndury, G. (1963), "Über den Infektionsweg und die Pathogenese von Virusschädigungen beim menschlichen Keimling," *Teratogenesis*. Schwabe & Co., 379.

Tuchmann-Duplessis, H. and Mercier-Parot, L. (1963), "Action du chlorhydrate de cyclizine sur la gestation et le développement embryonnaire du rat, de la souris et du lapin," *C.R. Acad. Sci.*, **256**, 3359.

Tuchmann-Duplessis, H. and Mercier-Parot, L. (1963), "Repercussions des neuroleptiques et des antitumoraux sur le développement prénatal," *Teratogenesis*. Schwabe & Co., 490.

*Tuchmann-Duplessis, H. (1964), "Aperçu sur la tératogenèse expérimentale," *Rev. Roum. Embr. Cyt.*, **1**, 1, 1.

*Tuchmann-Duplessis, H. and Merceir-Parot, L. (1964), "Influence des facteurs externes sur la production des malformations congénitales," *Arch. Biol. (Liège)*, **75**, suppl. 1099.

Tuchmann-Duplessis, H. and Mercier-Parot, L. (1964), "Avortements et malformations sous l'effet d'un agent provoquant une hyperlipémie et une hypercholestérolémie," *Bull. Acad. nat. Méd.*, **148**, 19–20, 392.

*Tuchmann-Duplessis, H. (1965), "Design and Interpretation of Teratogenic Tests," *Biological Council Symp. on Embryopathic Activity of Drugs*. London: J. and A. Churchill, 56.

Turpin, A. L. (1967), *A propos de 150 cas de grossesses diabétiques*. Thèse Faculté de Médecine Paris, Cafedith Edit. Paris.

White, P. (1952), "Diabetes Complicating Pregnancy," in Joslin, E. P., Root, H. F., White, P. and Marble, A., *Treatment of Diabetes Mellitus*, 9th edition, 676. Philadelphia: Lea and Febiger.

WHO Scientific Group (1967), "Principles for the Testing of Drugs for Teratogenicity," *Wld. Hlth. org. tech. Rep. Ser.*, 364.

Wilkins, L. (1960), "Masculinization of Female Fetus Due to Use of Orally given Progestins," *J. Amer. med. Ass.*, **172**, 1028.

Wilson, J. G. (1964), "Experimental Teratology," *Amer. J. Obstet. Gynec.*, **90**, 7, 1181.

Wilson, J. G. (1964), "Teratogenic Interaction of Chemical Agents in the Rat," *J. Pharmacol.*, **144**, 3, 429.

**Wilson, J. G. and Warkany, J., (1965), *Teratology: Principles and Techniques*. Chicago: Univ. of Chicago Press.

Woollam, D. H. M. (1967), *Advances in Teratology*. Logos Press, Academic Press, 1 and 2.

Yerushalmy, J. and Milkovich, L. (1965), "The Evaluation of the Teratogenic Effect of Meclizine in Man," *Amer. J. Obstet. Gynec.*, **93**, 553.

Zellweger, H., McDonald, J. S. and Abbo, G. (1967), "Is Lysergic Acid Diethylamide a Teratogen?" *Lancet*, **2**, 7525, 1066.

3. THE USE OF ERGOT IN OBSTETRICS

J. CHASSAR MOIR

Ergot has long been the drug of choice for the control of postpartum haemorrhage. This reputation is based on its speedy action in bringing about a pronounced and sustained uterine spasm, together with its freedom from undesirable side effects even when administered in comparatively large dosage. Although some qualifications are necessary in view of recent knowledge these claims are still substantially true and, despite the availability of other oxytocic drugs, ergot continues to hold a high place in obstetric practice.

History

The history of ergot is of interest and has some meaning even in present day work. Old writings and woodcuts, and frescoes in certain old churches, all testify to the existence of a peculiar illness that appeared from time to time in South Germany and France. This disease was characterized by an intense burning in the fingers and toes, and on occasions the symptoms progressed to gangrene of the extremities. Because St. Antony and his followers provided help for the victims, the disease came to be known as St. Antony's Fire. In the course of time certain peculiarities were recognized, and it became obvious that this disease, unlike smallpox, the "Black Death", and other epidemics that ravaged Europe in the Middle Ages, was not truly infectious but was a form of poisoning caused by the eating of bread made from diseased corn. Rye was then the main crop, and in damp seasons the rye-heads were often heavily contaminated with "black spurs" which, as we now know, are the ears of the corn distorted and discloured by the growth of a specific fungus. Thus it was that ergot (the "argot"—a spike of dead wood of the early writers) first became known for its poisonous properties. How, and when, the substance came to be used in medicine is unknown, but there is documentary evidence that by the 16th century the "black spurs" were used by certain midwives "to expedite lingering labour". For this purpose the diseased grains were sought in local granaries, were powdered and doused with boiling water; and in the infusion so prepared a seemingly miraculous power was found which could make weak pains strong and strong pains so powerful that delivery of the baby could be accomplished in an incredibly short time. The introduction of ergot into official medicine was long delayed, but when its use was described by Dr. John Stearns of New York State in 1808, great interest was aroused and, as can be seen from the medical journals of the time, it became the "wonder drug" of the time and the object of endless praise. But, as has so often happened in medical history, enthusiasm outstripped judgment; the dangers were not appreciated; many a woman died from a ruptured uterus, and many a foetus was lost because of the "violent and almost incessant action which it induces" (Dr. Stearns' words). By the end of the century these dangers came to be realized; and medical opinion, already wavering, was now sharply turned against the use of ergot in labour. This can be seen by the words of a would-be wit who, writing to the editor of a medical journal, proposed that the *pulvis ad partum* should be renamed the *pulvis ad mortem*.

Thus was the knowledge of ergot and its properties slowly and painfully acquired. The drug has long since ceased to be used before the birth of the child because—all too easily—a spasm is provoked, and this is so even with a dilute intravenous "drip". But, by the same token, the drug is ideal for the prevention or arrest of haemorrhage caused by abnormal uterine relaxation after the birth of the baby.

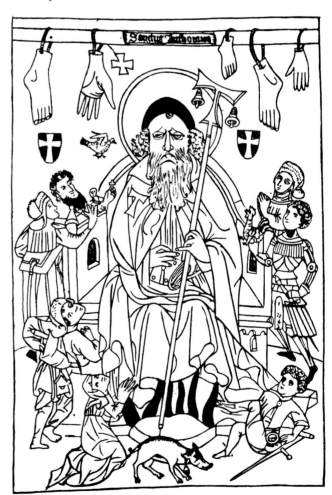

FIG. 1. A representation of Saint Antony surrounded by maimed suppliants. From the rail above hang relics left by the sufferers of gangrenous ergotism.

Pharmacology

Perhaps no crude drug in the Pharmacopoeia has been subjected to so much analytical investigation as has ergot. This is not the place to go into the complicated but fascinating story of the elucidation of its many and varied chemical principles. Suffice it to say that a round score of alkaloids have now been isolated. Some are dextrarotatory and without oxytocic action; an equal number are laevo-rotatory and do possess this action. First to be isolated were the large-moleculed alkaloids such as ergotamine (Femergin and Gynergin). These have a very slow but sustained action, and, incidentally, are the ones most likely to cause gangrene if the administration is long continued. Much later, the small-moleculed ergometrine was obtained which has the remarkably rapid "John Stearns" effect even when administered by mouth. The presence of this hitherto unidentified principle was established in 1932 (Moir, 1932). Three years later, and after observing the effect—or lack of effect—of innumerable chemical fractions on the behaviour of the uterus in puerperal women, the new alkaloid was isolated which reproduced in every respect the traditional clinical action. The proposed name was *ergometrine*, and this was generally accepted throughout Europe, although in the U.S.A. the term *ergonovine* (Ergotrate) is still preferred. An interesting variant is the semi-synthetic methyl-ergometrine, marketed by the Sandoz Company under the name of Methergin, which faithfully reproduces the clinical effects of ergometrine.

Present-day Use of Ergot

The spasm-producing properties of ergometrine make it the drug of choice for prevention or arrest of postpartum haemorrhage caused by uterine relaxation. For *prevention* the drug can be given by the mouth, either in the form of a crude extract (although this has been dropped from the British Pharmacopoeia) or as 0.5 to 1.0 mg. of the alkaloid dissolved in a small quantity of water. The effect becomes apparent within 5 to 7 minutes, or slightly more if the patient has a full stomach. Given by intramuscular injection it acts more rapidly, and by intravenous injection of 0.25 to 0.5 mg. a response is seen in as short a time as 45 to 60 seconds. The sustained uterine spasm which is at first induced changes after 10 to 15 minutes to regular, strong contractions which continue with decreasing force for a further 30 to 40 minutes.

As explained, one of the chief reasons for ergometrine's reputation in the *treatment* of postpartum haemorrhage, is its rapidity of action. When this is important, the intravenous injection of 0.25 mg. is the method of choice. (Oxytocin can also be used in this circumstance, but should never be injected intravenously, even after the delivery of the foetus, save in the minute dosage of 1, or at the most, and with great caution, 2 International Units; preferably, however, oxytocin should be given as a dilute "oxytocin drip". Oxytocin also has the disadvantage of a shorter duration of action.)

Sometimes, however, an intravenous injection may be inconvenient because of lack of assistance or other reason, and an intramuscular injection may then be necessary. Here, the rapidity of action is less conspicuous, and the patient may lose much blood in the six or seven minutes that elapse before the ergometrine takes effect. One way of hastening its action is to mix it with hyaluronidase which acts as a "dispersant". This, however, has the disadvantage that valuable time may be lost in making the necessary solution, and the cost is high.

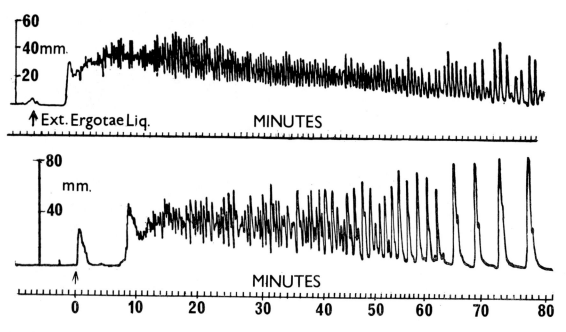

FIG. 2. *Top:* The tracing which first showed the presence of an unidentified active principle in crude ergot. *Bottom:* The first tracing to be made with the purified alkaloid, later to be named *ergometrine*.

Over many years I have occasionally used another method which may seem dangerous but which, in fact, is simple and safe if used in properly selected cases. This is to inject ergometrine (0·5 mg.) directly into the uterine corpus via the abdominal wall. The method is simple. Assuming that the bladder is empty and that the uterus can be easily palpated through the abdominal wall—and the method is suitable only for such cases—the fundus is manipulated forwards and the overlying skin painted with an antiseptic solution. The syringe needle is then boldly thrust into the uterine substance and the ergometrine solution injected. This method has a slight advantage over the usual form of intramuscular injection, for a contraction starts at the point of injection and slowly spreads over the rest of the uterus; meantime, the drug is also absorbed into general circulation and redistributed to the uterine muscle as a whole. If this method is used before the expulsion of the placenta there is an added advantage that the upper pole (fundus) of the uterus contracts before the lower pole, thus reducing the possibility of an incarceration of the placenta.

Yet another way of obtaining a quick response to an intramuscular injection is to use a mixture of ergometrine and oxytocin; such a solution is marketed under the proprietary name of Syntometrine. With it, a uterine response can be expected after 2½ to 3 minutes. This preparation is, however, not suitable for intravenous injection because of the large dose of oxytocin which it contains and, in my opinion, has no clear advantage over the straightforward *intravenous* injection of 0·25 mg. of ergometrine as described in an earlier paragraph.

It is sometimes recommended that ergometrine administration should be repeated within 10 or 20 minutes. There is however no clear purpose achieved by so doing and, with the possibility of over-dosage, the practice may be harmful.

In the past, when uterine sepsis was a greater hazard than it is today, sub-involution of the uterus was a much discussed topic, and the term itself came to be invested with a sinister meaning. Ergot was then commonly administered in the belief that it would hasten involution and secure what in loose hospital parlance was termed "a nice tight uterus". There was, however, no theoretical basis for the contention that ergot would hasten normal involution, nor did carefully controlled measurement give any support to this widely held belief (Russell and Moir, 1943).

The Use of Ergot before the Birth of the Placenta

One of the major changes in obstetrical technique in recent years has been the free use of oxytocic drugs before the birth of the placenta, and there is no doubt that a carefully timed intravenous injection of ergometrine enables the obstetrician to expel the placenta almost immediately after the birth of the child thus virtually eliminating the third stage of labour. The advantage is the greatly reduced incidence of postpartum haemorrhage (ten-fold according to some writers); the disadvantage is the increased incidence of a retained placenta.

If this technique is used certain points must be observed. The foetal presentation must be cephalic and the injection must be timed to coincide with the birth of the anterior shoulder. This ensures that the drug is given after all mechanical hindrance to the easy birth of the child is at an end; also, that the lower pole of the uterus is held open by the body of the foetus, so providing a free passage for the birth of the placenta which will be delivered within the next one, or two, minutes. With the foetus born, the obstetrician places his hand over the uterus and, with the first sign of the powerful contraction induced by the ergometrine, he expels the placenta by the method of his choice.

Although this technique has very great advantages, two dangers must be clearly stated. The method is permissible only if the possibility of a twin pregnancy can be excluded. Should an error be made in this respect, the spasm induced by the ergot may cause the death of the retained foetus. In this connection I can recall a tragic case. A woman believed to have twins was given an intravenous injection of ergometrine after the birth of the second foetus. She was then found to have triplets; the third foetus, when extracted, was dead.

Another troublesome but less dangerous event is the incarceration of the placenta by a muscular spasm of the thick lower edge of the upper uterine segment (not of the cervix itself as is often incorrectly stated). This complication is usually the result of the obstetrician failing to express (or to extract) the placenta at the optimum time. Fortunately, the circumstance is not dangerous because the contracted uterus does not bleed, and urgent treatment is not required. However, it is reasonable to make a gentle vaginal examination because the placenta will sometimes be found to be half extruded into the vagina, whence it can be easily hooked out by the finger, helped by gentle traction on the cord. If however the placenta is not felt, it is best to allow time—about 30 minutes—for the ergometrine effect to diminish. If, after this interval, the placenta still remains incarcerated an anaesthetic should be administered and a manual extraction performed, remembering that the fingers must first be inserted through the constricting muscle ring and the latter gently stretched before the placenta can be grasped and extracted.

During Caesarean section most surgeons employ an oxytocic agent to check haemorrhage during and after the extraction of the placenta. For this purpose ergometrine is ideal; it can be given intravenously by the anaesthetist, or by direct injection into the uterine fundus by the operator.

Action of Ergometrine on the Non-pregnant and Early-pregnant Uterus

Although ergometrine is conspicuously successful in bringing about a spasm in the uterus at term, it has comparatively little effect on the intact uterus of early pregnancy. Only if the uterus is already active (i.e. aborting) does the drug exert any useful action, and even then it is probably less efficient in conventional dosage than is oxytocin.

In the non-pregnant uterus the action of ergometrine is

also comparatively slight, although experimental recordings show that the contractions during menstruation are increased in force and frequency. Ergometrine is, however, not a drug that can be expected to check menorrhagia.

Ergometrine as a Cause of Hypertension

The final question to be considered is the possibility of danger caused by the occasional sudden rise of blood pressure that may occur after the injection of ergometrine.

The very full pharmacological testing to which ergometrine was subjected before being released to the medical profession, gave no indication of hypertension after administration in any reasonable dosage, nor did the clinical use of the drug in its early days—which was most carefully controlled—give any evidence of such an action. It therefore came as a surprise to find that in recent years isolated instances of sudden dangerous hypertension to 200 mm/Hg. systolic or over, combined with intense headache, have been recorded.

Before going further let us first consider the changes in blood pressure that normally occur after the birth of the baby. There is surprisingly little documentary evidence on this subject, but small-scale observations made by myself and my assistants go to show that after the birth of the placenta the blood pressure often rises by 5 or even 10 mm/Hg. Now, it is a well recognised fact that if the placenta is long retained, the patient's blood pressure may fall to a low level even in the absence of significant bloodloss. One can well suppose, therefore, that the clinical improvement following the successful removal of the placenta is often associated with a rise of systolic blood pressure of well over ten mm/Hg. The observations made by Baillie (1963) who recorded an elevation of blood pressure during Caesarean section when ergometrine was injected to help in the delivery of the placenta, can mostly —if not wholly—be explained by these facts, although it is difficult to account for his finding that toxaemic patients show a greater rise than others.

The very marked hypertension referred to in the paragraph before last is, however, of a very different order.

Most conspicuous, perhaps, is the report by Ringrose (1962) of a woman who, after the intravenous injection of ergometrine, developed a hypertension of 190/120 mm/Hg. and eventually died: at post-mortem examination extensive haemorrhages were found in both cerebral hemispheres. It would be tempting to dismiss such an extraordinary occurrence as an example of some pathological condition unassociated with ergometrine sensitivity; but to do so would be unjustifiable until fuller information is gathered of the frequency of hypertension after the injection of ergometrine; and such evidence is still awaited. In a small series of personally observed cases no significant change has been seen in the blood-pressure after the injection of ergometrine, but I have knowledge of at least two cases, supervized by colleagues, who have witnessed a dangerous elevation of blood pressure after the injection. The possibility that women who develop a hypertension are already under the influence of other drugs whose action is potentiated by the ergometrine, must be considered; but so far there is no convincing evidence in support of this theory.

As with all clinical problems, a balanced judgment must be maintained. Assuming that the intravenous or intramuscular injection of ergometrine does sometimes cause a dangerous hypertension, this can only occur on very rare occasions—perhaps once in many hundred instances; and against this possibility must be weighed the undoubted benefit conferred on the patient by the prevention of dangerous postpartum haemorrhage. From these considerations one fact clearly emerges. Ergometrine should not be given in unnecessarily large doses nor should its administration be recklessly repeated.

REFERENCES

Baillie, T. W. (1963), *Brit. med. J.*, **1**, 585.
Dudley, H. W. and Moir, J. C. (1935), *Brit. med. J.*, **1**, 520.
Moir, J. C. (1932), *Brit. med. J.*, **1**, 1119.
Moir, J. C. (1955), *Canad. med. Assoc. J.*, **72**, 727.
Ringrose, C. A. D. (1962), **87**, 712.
Russell, S. and Moir, J. C. (1943), *J. Obstet. Gynaec. Brit. Emp.*, **50**, 94.

1. THE GENETICS OF CONGENITAL MALFORMATIONS

CEDRIC CARTER

Malformations present at birth have a varied aetiology. A minority appear due to purely environmental factors such as foetal infection or teratogenic drugs, a minority are due almost entirely to genetic factors such as chromosome anomalies or mutant genes of large effect; most, however, of the types of malformation with a relatively high incidence are probably due to a complex interaction of genetic predisposition and environmental triggers.

The purely environmental causes of malformation, infection by rubella in the first trimester of pregnancy, thalidomide intoxication in the first trimester, and the effects of large doses of radiation, are valuable in showing the importance of timing in causing malformation. Their contribution to the total load of malformation, except perhaps in the case of epidemic years of rubella, or the peak year of the thalidomide disaster in Germany, is small. (See Sec. XII, Chap. 2.)

MALFORMATIONS DUE TO CHROMOSOME ANOMALY

(a) Non-disjunction

Abnormalities of chromosome behaviour in germ cell formation are common. In particular chromosome non-disjunction (the failure of members of a chromosome pair to separate at cell division) during the formation of ovum or sperm, is common. The effect is the production of an ovum or sperm with one missing, or one extra, chromosome. If such a gamete takes part in zygote formation, the zygote in turn will have one missing chromosome (monosomy for that chromosome), or one extra chromosome (trisomy for that chromosome).

For example, non-disjunction of the sex chromosome pair at the first or second stages of meiosis may lead to zygotes with monosomy for a single X-chromosome, usually called the XO genotype, or trisomy for the sex chromosomes in the form of XXX or XXY genotypes. Similarly non-disjunction, at the second meiotic division, of the Y chromosome may produce the XYY genotype. Most zygotes with the XO genotype abort, and this genotype is one of the most common found in early spontaneous abortions. Those XO foetuses that reach term, about 3 in 10,000 female births, have some or all of the congenital malformations characteristic of Turner's syndrome. There is probably no foetal loss with the trisomies of the sex chromosomes, and a little over 1 in 1,000 females have the XXX genotype and about 2 per 1,000 of males the XXY genotype; but neither of these have any striking incidence of structural congenital malformations. Simple nuclear sexing by buccal smear is an effective screening procedure to detect XXX and XXY genotypes, but will not detect XYY individuals. No estimate is yet available of the population incidence of the XYY genotype.

No complete monosomies of the autosomes (the chromosomes other than the sex chromosome) are viable. Most trisomies of the autosomes are also non-viable and abort, but about 2 in 1,000 of foetuses which reach term have a trisomy of one of the two smallest, 21 or 22 (G group), chromosomes and have Down's syndrome (mongolism)*. Appreciably fewer, perhaps 3 in 10,000 have trisomy of a large acrocentric chromosome of the 16–18 or E group (in most instances it is 18 that is involved), and a similar number trisomy of the 13–15 (D group), in most instances it is 15 that is involved. As with G trisomy, D and E trisomic genotypes are characterized by a specific syndrome of malformations, Patau and Edward's syndrome respectively.

A striking feature of the trisomic genotypes is that they occur with increasing frequency as maternal age increases. For example, trisomy 21 is present in about 1 in 2.000 births to mothers under the age of 25, but in about 10 in 1,000 births to mothers over the age of 40 years. The reason for this maternal age effect has not yet been found. It is understandable that autosomal trisomies will produce syndromes. Hundreds of genes are present in triplicate and the organisms' metabolism, therefore, will be disturbed in many different ways.

(b) Structural Change

In addition to syndromes of multiple malformations due to abnormalities of the total number of chromosomes, such syndromes may also occur due to the absence of part of a chromosome or the presence of extra chromosome material following structural alteration of one or more chromosomes.

The origin of structural anomalies is breakage of one or more chromosomes, followed by the loss of chromosome material, or by anomalous rejoining of raw ends. The latter may involve exchange of material between chromosomes. The exchange will initially, in most instances, be balanced, there being neither gain nor loss, but only re-arrangement of chromosome material and so no clinical effects are produced. When, however, an individual with such a balanced interchange forms germ cells a proportion of these will have an unbalanced chromosome complement with either extra or missing chromosome material. The best known example is an

---

* There has been much discussion as to whether trisomy 21 or 22 is responsible for Down's syndrome. It may well be that trisomy of either member of the G group of chromosomes will cause the syndrome.

interchange between a D and G chromosome, to give a chromosome with most of the material of both the D and G chromosomes. Assuming segregation is primarily for the larger, D, chromosome such an individual may form germ cells:

(a) with normal D and G chromosomes, giving a normal zygote;

(b) with a normal D and no G chromosome, giving a zygote which is not viable;

(c) with the D/G translocated chromosome, giving a zygote which develops into a clinically normal individual but with the same genotype as the parent;

(d) with the D/G and a G chromosome which since, an extra G chromosome is present, gives a zygote which develops into a child with Down's syndrome. The risks in practice are not yet accurately established, but a woman carrying a D/G translocation appears to have about a 1 in 5 chance, where the pregnancy goes to term, of having a child with Down's syndrome.

(c) The Load of Chromosomal Anomalies

There is now evidence that 25 per cent of early abortions are associated with chromosome anomalies. Since about 16 per cent of recognizable pregnancies terminate in an abortion, it follows that about four per cent of zygotes have a chromosome anomaly. About 3 in 4 of such zygotes must abort leaving about 1 child in 100 at term with a chromosome anomaly. Two of the commonest anomalies found in abortuses are triploidy (the presence of 3 of each chromosome, 69 in all), and the XO genotype. Probably about 50 per cent of G trisomy foetuses abort.

Most of the abortions associated with chromosome anomalies are due to fresh mutations (usually nondisjunction) and it is only rarely that repeated abortions can be attributed to a balanced chromosome interchange in one or other parent.

MALFORMATIONS DUE TO MUTANT GENES

(a) The Nature of Gene Mutation

Gene mutations, unlike chromosome mutations, are not visible under the microscope. There is good reason to believe that often the mutation may involve only the substitution of one single base for another of the 100 or more triplets of bases which constitute the operationally specific part of a structural gene. Each triplet of bases in a structural gene codes one amino-acid in the peptide whose production is controlled by the structural gene. Two or more peptides then combine to form a biologically active protein, often an enzyme. The most likely effect of the base change in a structural gene is to substitute one amino-acid for another in the peptide. The effect of a gene mutation is, then, essentially a single specific chemical change. The most typical conditions due to mutant genes are the haemoglobinopathies and inborn errors of metabolism such as phenylketonuria, amaurotic family idiocy, and galactosaemia. Understandably, however, mutant genes, no doubt by similar mechanisms, may also produce anomalies which may be classed as malformations. If the protein product of the gene is required for structural development a mutation in that gene will cause malformation.

Gene mutations are individually much rarer than chromosome mutations, and so specific conditions due to mutant genes tend, if at all serious, to be rare. There are, however, a great many genes that may mutate and it is estimated that about 1 live-born child in 100 is affected by a condition due to a mutant gene; most of these conditions, however, do not involve congenital malformation. No doubt some early abortions are due to gene mutations which in either the heterozygous or homozygous state are incompatible with life, but there is no direct evidence for this as yet.

(b) Dominant, Recessive and X-linked Conditions

When a gene mutation first occurs in a germ cell, the zygote will nearly always receive a normal gene on the corresponding chromosome coming from the other germ cell. The zygote is then said to be heterozygous for the mutant gene. If this heterozygous state causes clinical abnormality, the condition so caused is called a *dominant* condition. Many mutant genes, however, particularly those causing enzyme defect, cause no clinical abnormality in heterozygotes. The production of enzyme may be halved, but this causes no disturbance unless the enzyme system is placed under unusual stress. The first recipient of such a gene will be a clinically unaffected heterozygote. Clinical abnormality occurs only when zygotes are formed homozygous for the mutant gene because both parents happen to be heterozygous for that mutant gene. The likelihood of such similarity in parents is increased if they are blood relatives, for example first cousins. Since there is no selection against heterozygotes, recessive mutant genes build up in the population to relatively high frequencies. Most individuals are heterozygous for one or more such genes.

Mutant genes on the X-chromosome have the special feature that, since males have only one X-chromosome, a boy or man will be clinically affected if this X-chromosome carries the mutant gene. A woman, however, may be heterozygous for the gene and in many instances such heterozygotes will be clinically little affected.

Some examples of straightforward dominant congenital malformations are: classical achondroplasia, mandibulofacial dysostosis, acrocephalo-syndactyly (Apert's syndrome), cleidoncranial dysostosis, many instances of polydactyly, syndactyly and brachydactyly, polycystic kidneys (of the type which usually does not cause renal failure till adult life), subvalvular aortic stenosis, cleft lip and/or cleft palate with mucous pits of the lower lip, aniridia, and several types of congenital cataract.

Straight-forward recessive congenital malformations include: most forms of congenital deafness, the majority of instances of very severe microcephaly, infantile polycystic kidneys with cysts in the liver, Morquio's type of osteochrondrodystrophy and Hurler's syndrome (both essentially inborn errors of mucopolysaccharide metabolism), female pseudohermaphroditism due to congenital adrenal hypoplasia (essentially an inborn error of steroid metabolism), Ellis-van-Creveld syndrome, the severe form of epidermolysis bullosa dystrophica and ichthyosis congenita.

Straight-forward X-linked congenital malformations include: one form of congenital hydrocephalus due to aqueduct stenosis, one form of anhidrotic congenital ectodermal dysplasia, Albright's hereditary osteo-dystrophy, megalocornea, one form of microphthalmia, and male pseudohermaphroditism due to the testicular feminization syndrome.

More Complex Determination of Common Malformations

Of the conditions simply genetically determined des-cribed above, only Down's syndrome may be considered a common malformation in the sense of having an in-cidence of 1 or more in 1,000 total births. The other common malformations in people of North-West European stock are the major malformations of the neural tube, that is spina bifida cystica and anencephaly, cardiac malformations (if these are considered as a whole), cleft lip with or without cleft palate, talipes equinovarus, con-genital dislocation of the hip and infantile pyloric stenosis. It may be argued whether the latter two conditions are truly congenital malformations, but it is conventional to include them. Most other populations show appreciably lower incidences of neural tube malformations, though relatively high incidences are also found in Alexandria and Bombay. Cleft lip (±cleft palate) is relatively common in Mongolian populations, particularly Japan and Malaya. African populations show a relatively high incidence of ulnar polydactyly, but otherwise have a rather low malformation rate.

The best evidence that both genetic and environmental factors are concerned in the aetiology of these common malformations comes from twin studies. For example, a large scale twin study from Southern Germany showed that only about 25 per cent of the monozygotic twins of patients with talipes equinovarus were similarly affected, so that intra-uterine environmental factors must be important, but that an even smaller proportion of like-sexed dizygotic twins were also affected, so that genetic factors must also be important in the aetiology of the condition. The same situation applies for congenital dislocation of the hip, pyloric stenosis and cleft lip (±cleft palate). There is for all these conditions a mono-zygotic twin concordance of well below 50 per cent, but a like-sex dizygotic twin concordance of 5 per cent or less. No satisfactory twin studies for neural tube or cardiac malformations are yet available, but the monozygotic twin concordance is probably less than 25 per cent for these conditions.

Large scale family studies support the hypothesis that these common malformations are due to a complex genetic-environmental interaction and further indicate that the genetic predisposition is probably polygenic. The family pattern is best established for uncomplicated cleft lip (±cleft palate). This malformation is genetically and embryologically distinct from midline cleft palate without cleft lip. Family studies in Denmark, in Utah in the United States, and London have shown a consistent

pattern. In the general population the incidence in these areas is about 1 in 1,000 total births. In first degree rela-tives, sibs or children, the incidence is about 4 per cent, that is 40 times the population incidence. In second degree relatives, aunts and uncles or nephews and nieces, the incidence is about 7 per thousand, that is 7 times the population incidence, and in third degree relatives about 2·5 per thousand, that is only $2\frac{1}{2}$ times the population incidence.

This pattern cannot be attributed to single mutant gene effects and is far too regular to be due wholly to the similarities of environment that one finds within families. It can, however, be readily explained if one assumes that the malformation is caused by extreme deviation of an underlying, continuously variable character, analogous say to stature or intelligence. Polygenic determination of such a character will tend to give such normally distri-buted variation. If it is assumed that those beyond a threshold are at risk of developing the malformation, then it is possible to estimate how many relatives of the patients will also be beyond the threshold and so at risk. This is illustrated for first (e.g. sibs and children of patients) and third (e.g. first cousins) degree relatives in Figure 1.

Where the mean value on the underlying variable of those affected differs from the population mean by x units, the mean of first degree relatives will differ by $x/2$ units (since on average they share half their genes in common with the patients), of second degree relatives by $x/4$, and third degree relatives by $x/8$ units. The hypothesis will give family patterns close to those actually observed for cleft lip (±cleft palate).

With increasing incidence of malformation, on this hypothesis the absolute risk to relatives will increase, but the risk relative to the general population incidence will fall. Similarly, if the malformation has a higher incidence in one sex than the other, then one would expect with this mechanism of inheritance that the relative risks will be highest in the sex in which the general population incidence is lower. This is well seen with infantile pyloric stenosis.

Some absolute and relative risks in common congenital malformations are shown in Table 1. The effect of the male sex preponderance in pyloric stenosis is shown in this table, as is the tendency for the factor, by which the incidence in relatives is greater than that in the general population, to fall as the population incidence increases.

The next stage in the understanding of the aetiology of the common malformations will come from the discovery of the mechanisms by which the genetic predispositions act and the nature of the environmental triggers also required before the genetic predisposition leads to mal-formation. At present only in the case of congenital dislocation of the hip do we have some knowledge of these factors. Here a genetically determined joint laxity (especially in males) and a genetically determined shallow acetabulum form part at least of the genetic predisposition. The intra-uterine malposition of flexed hips, extended knees and extroverted feet, which is often associated with breech lie in primiparae, is one element and perhaps the

MODEL FOR POLYGENIC INHERITANCE OF HARELIP ($\pm$ C. P.)

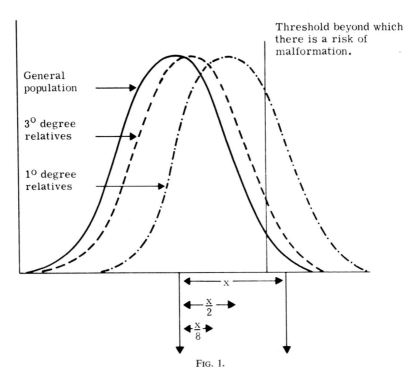

Fig. 1.

most important of the environmental component in the aetiology.

GENETIC COUNSELLING IN RELATION TO CONGENITAL MALFORMATIONS

Genetic counselling in relation to congenital malformations is useful not only in answering parents' questions on the risk of recurrence in later pregnancies, but also in alerting the medical profession to early diagnosis of malformations which are not externally visible, for example aganglionic megacolon or pyloric stenosis.

(a) Chromosome Anomalies

The great majority of syndromes due to chromosome anomalies arise as a result of fresh mutations in parents who are themselves chromosomally normal. Here the risk of recurrence is low. The risk is also low where a child is affected as a result of a freshly occurring structural chromosomal anomaly and both parents have normal chromosomes. Relatively high risks of recurrence may exist when one or other parent has a balanced chromosome interchange, and also where one or other parent is a mosaic with mostly normal cells but some trisomic cells.

It is not practicable, with present facilities, to carry out chromosome examinations on lymphocyte and fibroblast culture of all parents who have had a chromosomally abnormal child. Where a mother under 30 years of age has a child with a trisomy syndrome, such as Down's syndrome, it is desirable to examine the chromosomes on a lymphocyte culture of the child. If trisomy is present the parents may be given a low risk of recurrence.

TABLE 1

INCIDENCE IN RELATIVES OF PATIENTS WITH COMMON MALFORMATIONS COMPARED WITH THE POPULATION INCIDENCE

	Cleft lip (±cleft palate[1])	Congenital disolocation of hip females only[1]	Pyloric stenosis: females only[1]	Pyloric stenosis: males only[1]	Spina bifida[2]
Population incidence	1/1,000	2/1,000	1/1,000	5/1,000	4/1,000
MZ twins	×300	×300	Not known	Not known	Not known
1st degree relatives (sibs and children)	×35	×35	×100	×10	×10
2nd degree relatives (aunts, uncles, nephews and nieces)	×7	×3	Not known	×5	Not known
3rd degree relatives (first cousins)	×2½	×2	×3	×1½	×2

[1] Data or references in Carter, C. O. (1965). In "Progress in Medical Genetics." (Ed. Steinberg and Bearn). Vol. IV., Chapter 3.
[2] Carter, C. O., Laurence, K. M. and David, P. (1968). J. Med. Gen. **5**, 81.

Mosaicism of normal and G trisomy cells in one or other parent is not excluded, but will seldom be present. If the child is found to have a structural chromosomal anomaly, for example a D/G interchange, in a child with Down's syndrome, the chromosomes of both parents should be examined on lymphocyte culture. If these are found normal, again a low risk of recurrence may be given. If a chromosome interchange is found in one or other parent then the risk appropriate to the specific interchange should be given. Where parents are willing to chance another preganancy it is now possible to determine whether a chromosome anomaly is or is not present early in the pregnancy from a culture of amniotic cells and to offer the parents a termination if Down's syndrome will develop. Where a child has died before his or her chromosomes have been examined, both parents should be investigated.

(b) Conditions Due to Mutant Genes of Large Effect

Genetic counselling for conditions due to mutant genes of large effect depends on recognizing the condition and knowing its established pattern or patterns of inheritance, together with an appreciation of the pattern of inheritance indicated by individual family trees. With straight-forward dominant conditions, the rule is that there is a 1 in 2 risk to the offspring of affected individuals and little risk to the offspring of unaffected members of the family. Where a child with such a dominant condition is born to unaffected parents it has very probably been affected as a result of a fresh mutation and the risk of recurrence in further children of the two parents is low. Gonadal mosaicism, whereby a portion of one gonad of a clinically normal parent contains the mutant gene, is a mechanism by which there could be an increased risk to further children, but in practice this seems to be a rare phenomenon.

With recessive conditions, assuming, as will usually be the case, that both parents are normal (though after the first affected child, known to be heterozygous carriers of the mutant gene concerned), the risk of recurrence in later children of the two parents is 1 in 4. In contrast, there is little risk of the condition appearing in the offspring of the patient, if he or she survives, provided that he or she does not marry a heterozygote (or homozygote) for the mutant gene concerned. This will be unlikely unless the patient marries a near blood relative. A marriage between two homozygotes for the same mutant gene, when all offspring will be affected, has occurred with congenital deafness, where there is a tendency for intermarriage of patients. However, since a number of different mutant genes may cause recessive congenital deafness, in most instances of such intermarriages the offspring will be unaffected. The risk to the offspring of the unaffected sibs, of patients with recessive conditions, is low, again provided that these sibs do not marry a blood relative. Where parents with a 1 in 4 risk are prepared to take the chance it is already possible to visualize instances, for example with Hurler's syndrome, where it will be possible in the future to decide, from amniotic fluid cells, whether the embryo is or is not affected.

With X-linked conditions, determined by mutant genes on the X-chromosome much depends on recognizing whether the mother or sister of an affected boy is or is not a heterozygous carrier. If any other male in the family is affected it may be assumed that the mother of an affected boy is a carrier. The risk to any further sons of being affected is then 1 in 2 and the risk of any daughter being a carrier like the mother is 1 in 2. If no other male in the family is affected, there is a possibility, though probably less than a half chance, that the boy is affected as a result of a fresh mutation and later children are not at risk. Tests for the heterozygote state may be available.

(c) Conditions Due to more Complex Genetic Predisposition

With malformations such as cleft lip or spina bifida cystica it is not possible to base estimates of risks on theoretical considerations. It is, however, possible to give empirical estimates of risks based on large scale family studies. It is important to remember, however, that these empirical estimates are valid for the population studied and not necessarily for other populations. In the case of spina bifida cystica the recurrence risk of spina bifida cystica or anencephaly is of the order of 6 per cent in south-east Wales, an area with a high population incidence. It may well be less in south-east England and less still in some low incidence areas such as Japan. With polygenic inheritance it is to be expected that the risk in relatives compared to the population incidence will be higher where the malformation is rare, but the absolute risk will be lower. It is also noteworthy that whereas with, say, a recessive condition the risk of recurrence in a subsequent pregnancy is 1 in 4, whether the parents have already had one, two or even three affected children, with polygenic inheritance the recurrence risk is likely to increase according to the number of previously affected children. With recessive inheritance all parents at risk have the same risk; with polygenic inheritance and a threshold some parents will have an appreciably higher risk of having children beyond the threshold than other parents, and such "high risk" parents will be found especially among those who already have had two affected children.

It must be remembered that common malformations may also occur as part of syndromes which are due to chromosome anomalies or to mutant genes of large effect and have the recurrence risks considered in sections (a) and (b). For example, cleft lip and palate is part of the D trisomy syndrome, and also of the dominant Van de Woude's syndrome.

Some approximate empirical recurrence risks for common uncomplicated congenital malformations appropriate for Britain are given below:

Spina bifida and anencephaly	1 in 20 risk of spina bifida cystica or anencephaly after one affected child. This arises to about 1 in 10 if mother has already had two affected children.

Congenital malformations of the heart	1 in 50 risk of the same or similar type of heart malformation. Probably raised if parents have already had two children with similar malformations.
Cleft lip (±cleft palate)	1 in 30 risk for sibs or children of patients. Raised to 1 in 10 if one or other parent is affected and perhaps also 1 in 10 if parents have already had two affected children.
Pyloric stenosis	If index patient is male—1 in 20 for sons and brothers and 1 in 40 for daughters or sisters. If index patient is female—1 in 5 for sons and brothers and 1 in 10 for daughters and sisters.
Congenital dislocation of the hip	If index patient is female—1 in 100 for sons and brothers, and 1 in 15 for daughters and sisters. Somewhat higher risk where the index patient is male.
Talipes equinovarus	1 in 50 for brothers and sisters.
Aganglionic megacolon (Hirschsprung's disease)	Where the index patient has a short segment affected—1 in 20 for brothers, 1 in 100 for sisters. Where the index patient has a long segment affected—1 in 10 for sibs of either sex.

Overall it will be seen that these extra recurrence risks are not high when seen in the perspective that about 1 child in 50 will have some at least moderately serious malformation. The recurrence risks are for the same variety of malformation, there is no general increased risk of malformation. It is also noteworthy that where a couple have had children with two unrelated malformations the recurrence risks should be given independently for each malformation.

Specialist genetic clinics are gradually being established in university medical centres as staff trained both in medicine and genetics become available, from which practitioners may seek help in cases of difficulty or where special tests are likely to be helpful.

Prevention in the Future

The majority of children with chromosome anomalies are affected as a result of a fresh instance of non-disjunction. Probably little can be done to prevent non-disjunction apart from encouraging births at younger maternal age, and it is difficult to visualize any effective therapy for conditions such as Down's syndrome. The most promising future line of prevention, once appropriate technical methods of amniocentesis and culture of amniotic cells are refined would appear to be the early screening of the embryo for chromosome anomalies and the offer to the parents of a termination of the pregnancy when this does not occur naturally.

For conditions due to mutant genes, since there is but a single biochemical lesion, replacement or other therapy may well be possible in the future. Genetic counselling will reduce the incidence of such conditions, particularly as it becomes increasingly possible to detect the heterozygous carrier of recessive and X-linked conditions. Increasingly too it will become possible, by biochemical examination in amniotic cell culture, to screen early embryos for conditions due to mutant genes of large effect.

With conditions due to the interaction of complex genetic predisposition and intra-uterine environmental factors, prevention will come, once the detailed mechanisms are known, from the recognition of embryos genetically at risk (at first perhaps because the parents have already had one child with the malformation) and their protection from the additional intra-uterine environmental triggers.

BIBLIOGRAPHY

General

Fraser Roberts, J. A. (1967), *Introduction to Medical Genetics.* 4th Edition. Oxford University Press.
Carter, C. O. (1962), *Human Heredity.* Penguin Books (1967 reprint).
Norman, A. P. (Ed.) (1965), *Congenital Abnormalities in Infancy.* Blackwell.
Stevenson, A. C., Johnston, H. A., Stewart, M. I. P. and Golding, D. R. (1966), Suppl. to Vol. 34 of the Bulletin of the World Health Organization. *WHO*, Geneva.

Chromosome Anomalies

Hamerton, J. L. (Ed.) (1962), *Chromosomes in Medicine.* Heinemann.
Bartalos, M. and Baramki, T. A. (1967), *Medical Cytogenetics.* The Williams and Wilkins Co., Baltimore.

Conditions Due to Single Genes

McKusick, V. (1968), *Mendelian Inheritance in Man.* 2nd Edition. The Johns Hopkins Press.

Common Conditions with Complex Inheritance

Carter, C. O. (1965), "The Inheritance of Common Congenital Malformations." In *Progress in Medical Genetics* (Ed. Steinberg and Bearn), Vol. IV.

2. THE RELATION OF NATIONAL AND GEOGRAPHIC VARIATIONS TO MATERNAL AND CHILD HEALTH

ROMA N. CHAMBERLAIN

One of the great achievements of medicine in the twentieth century has been the world wide improvement in maternal and child health. This improvement has been brought about by many factors, among the most important being the introduction of chemotherapy and antibiotics and the advances of knowledge in the care of the mother and child during pregnancy and childbirth. However, such dramatic effects could not have been achieved had it not been for the parallel improvements which were occurring in social conditions, especially in nutrition and housing.

The standard of maternal and child care varies very considerably from one country to another, and as knowledge increases and the techniques of medical care become more intricate so the gap between the under-developed countries, some hardly touched by modern civilization, and the advanced countries with their highly sophisticated medical services may well tend to widen rather than diminish.

In order to compare the results between countries it is necessary to have a fairly uniform pattern for the collection of statistics. Ideally one would like to compare morbidity rates but in the few countries which collect such figures, they are nearly all based on hospital statistics and are unlikely to be comparable. Maternal and infant mortality rates are at the present time the only figures available for assessing the variations on an international basis. There are several criteria which must be fulfilled if false assumptions are not to be made. These were described in the 1966 Annual Report of the Chief Medical Officer of the Ministry of Health, England and Wales (1967). The countries must be able to estimate their populations fairly accurately and therefore to have had a census in the recent past. Each must have a reliable system of registration of births and deaths and use an agreed definition for live and still births with a uniform classification of causes of death. In the following tables only those countries which have had a census within the last ten years and coded by the Statistical Office of the United Nations as having at least a 95 per cent registration of vital events have been included.

International statistics for maternal and infant mortality rates are based on live births so that the definitions of both viability of the foetus and of live birth can effect the results. Not all countries in the tables use the W.H.O. definition for live and stillbirth[1]. The effect of this on the infant

figures will be discussed later but as the number of maternal deaths is small compared with the number of births, it is probably not of great importance when considering maternal mortality rates.

In the countries with small populations and consequently few maternal deaths the results are likely to be affected by chance. Table 1 shows the maternal mortality rates for the years 1962–64 for selected countries. It shows the variation which can occur from year to year. The standard error is given with the maternal mortality rates for the year 1963 in Table 2 to give an estimate of the variation due to chance.

Whether a death is assigned to causes directly due to pregnancy and to childbirth or to associated causes is likely to effect the mortality rates, particularly where the number of deaths is small. In some countries, for example Scotland, a specific question may be asked on the death certificate as to whether the patient had been pregnant or not, while in others it is left to the certifying doctor to decide whether he considers the pregnancy is relevant to the cause of death. The possible effect of this on the statistical results can best be illustrated by the example of pulmonary embolism. If deaths which occur after puerperal phlebitis and thrombosis are included, pulmonary embolism is the fourth highest cause of maternal death in England and Wales. Here a detailed confidential enquiry has been carried out on every maternal death since 1952. At first there were very few reports of deaths due to pulmonary embolism occurring during early pregnancy, nearly all the deaths reported occurring after childbirth. Since the first report for 1952–54, however, the

---

[1] "Live birth is the complete expulsion or extraction from its mother of a product of conception, irrespective of the duration of pregnancy, which, after such separation, breathes or shows any evidence of life, such as beating of the heart, pulsation of the umbilical cord, or definite movement of the voluntary muscles, whether or not the umbilical cord has been cut or the placenta is attached; each product of such a birth is considered live born."

"Foetal death is death prior to the complete expulsion or extraction from its mother of a product of conception, irrespective of the duration of pregnancy; the death is indicated by the fact that after such separation the foetus does not breathe or show any other evidence of life, such as beating of the heart, pulsation of the umbilical cord, or the definite movement of voluntary muscle."

Foetal deaths are usually divided into four groups as follows:—

Group 1. Less than 20 completed weeks of gestation, described as "early foetal deaths".

Group 2. 20 completed weeks of gestation but less than 28, described as "intermediate foetal deaths".

Group 3. 28 completed weeks of gestation and over, described as "late foetal deaths".

Group 4. Gestation period not classifiable in Groups 1, 2, or 3. Late foetal deaths correspond to stillbirths in many countries.

TABLE 1

MATERNAL MORTALITY RATES PER 100,000 LIVE BIRTHS IN VARIOUS
COUNTRIES FOR THE YEARS 1962 TO 1964

Country	Year		
	1962	1963	1964
Australia	35·9	27·2	32·7
Austria	69·0	60·0	48·6
Belgium	32·9	30·8	—
Bulgaria	73·8	71·1	46·6
Canada	40·7	35·4	30·2
Czechoslovakia	46·9	36·0	—
Denmark	20·6	25·5	15·6
Finland	51·6	49·8	42·3
France	42·8	38·2	32·5
Germany, West	87·1	82·8	69·4
Hungary	76·9	67·3	53·0
Iceland	42·6	20·8	63·3
Ireland	43·7	34·8	46·9
Israel	40·7	49·6	16·3
Italy	97·7	88·2	—
Japan	112·0	102·5	97·8
Netherlands	33·4	32·8	33·1
New Zealand	29·2	40·2	32·2
Norway	20·9	20·5	23·0
Poland	37·4	36·1	48·9
Portugal	116·7	87·7	84·3
Rumania	106·6	85·1	—
Spain	53·5	59·8	—
Sweden	13·0	26·6	19·6
Switzerland	56·6	34·5	—
U.K.: England and Wales	35·6	28·5	25·9
Northern Ireland	30·7	41·9	17·5
Scotland	40·3	38·0	23·0
U.S.A.	35·2	35·8	33·1
Yugoslavia	159·8	137·3	—

numbers have been rising. This rise may not necessarily be due to an increase in the number of deaths from this cause. The results of the enquiry have aroused interest in the association of pulmonary embolism with early pregnancy, so that 15 years ago a doctor may not have recorded the fact that the patient was pregnant on the death certificate and the death would not have been assigned to maternal causes. Now that the importance of the association has been appreciated, it is much more likely that he will record the pregnancy and the death will be correctly assigned.

Another pitfall when comparing international statistics is the difficulty which sometimes occurs in assigning a death to a single cause. If, for example, a patient suffering from toxaemia of pregnancy has an antepartum haemorrhage, is delivered by Caeserean Section and on the seventh day after birth has a fatal pulmonary embolism, it will depend on the way in which the certificate is completed as to which cause the death is assigned.

All these points have to be borne in mind when considering the results from a wide range of countries.

Table 2 shows the Maternal Mortality rates per 100,000 live births according to certain causes for the year 1963. A few countries included in Table 1 have had to be omitted as the figures for the causes were not available for the year

1963. The statistical criteria already mentioned, which are necessary to ensure a reasonable comparability, mean that the tables only include those countries which have reached a high state of development in the collection of their statistics. There is a wide range in the results achieved. Japan has a mortality rate five times that of Norway. In Japan the rates for sepsis are low but there is an outstandingly high number of deaths from toxaemia. In the majority of countries and particularly those where the number of deaths is small, the rates are liable to vary according to chance. In Denmark, for instance, in 1963 there were four deaths from toxaemia, one death from haemorrhage and one from sepsis.

While international mortality statistics are a guide to the results which are being achieved in different countries, they are of little value in the study of the racial and epidemiological patterns of disease. Hospital in-patient statistics are equally of little help. From time to time special studies are made in an endeavour to elucidate some of the racial differences. The difficulties of collecting comparable morbidity statistics were highlighted at the Conference of the International Society of Geographical Pathology held in London in 1960 when the incidence of eclampsia and pre-eclampsia was reviewed by delegates from many countries. Doll and Hanington (1961) reported on a special study sponsored by the Society on the incidence of these diseases. The study was carried out independently in a number of centres throughout the world but despite careful central planning and control, it was impossible to reach any but the most tentative conclusions. It was found that the percentage of women in whom the systolic blood pressure rose to 145 mm. Hg or above was greatest in Ireland, Scotland and England and the lowest in Nigeria and Japan. Doll and Hanington postulated that generally the response of the cardiovascular system to pregnancy varied from one country to another and that the response had no obvious relation to diet and in particular its protein content. The high death rate in Japan was referred to by Baird (1961) in his summing up of the Conference, when he reported that the Japanese delegates considered this to be due to the poor antenatal care in the rural districts of Japan. Takaki, Magari, and Yuasi (1961) while referring to the better care in the towns considered that diet and particularly an increasing protein intake had an adverse effect.

It is interesting to note the findings of Barron and Vessey (1966) who carried out a study of the obstetric behaviour of immigrant groups. It was confined to births occurring in the Lambeth Hospital during 1958–60 and therefore a selected group but they found that pre-eclampsia was only one-third as common among the West Indian women as among the British which was similar to the findings of Doll and Hanington. The West Indian patients also had a shorter second stage of labour, a lower forceps rate and a higher incidence of intact perineum after delivery than the Irish or the British. The many factors which may account for this are discussed in the original paper.

Table 3 shows the regional distribution for maternal mortality in England and Wales according to the major causes for the years 1961–64. The total maternal mortality

TABLE 2

MATERNAL MORTALITY RATES PER 100,000 LIVE BIRTHS ACCORDING TO CERTAIN
CAUSES IN VARIOUS COUNTRIES FOR THE YEAR 1963

Country	Maternal sepsis	Toxaemia of pregnancy and puerperium	Haemor-rhage of pregnancy and childbirth	Abortion without sepsis or toxaemia	Abortion with sepsis	Total	
						Rate	Standard error
Australia	3·8	4·2	4·2	2·5	3·0	27·2	3·4
Austria	11·1	8·2	8·9	2·2	5·2	60·0	6·8
Belgium	2·5	3·8	3·1	4·4	1·9	30·8	4·4
Bulgaria	6·1	15·1	20·4	8·3	8·3	71·1	7·3
Canada	4·1	6·0	6·7	0·9	4·5	35·4	2·8
Czechoslovakia	4·2	3·0	3·0	2·5	2·5	36·0	3·9
Denmark	1·2	4·9	1·2	1·2	4·9	25·5	5·6
Finland	3·6	9·7	10·9	7·3	3·6	49·8	7·8
France	2·6	5·4	4·9	4·1	2·0	38·2	2·1
Germany, West	11·5	15·4	13·9	4·6	5·3	82·8	2·8
Hungary	5·3	15·9	9·8	3·8	15·9	67·3	7·1
Israel	8·6	6·5	6·5	4·3	Nil	49·6	10·4
Italy	7·7	25·5	16·7	1·8	3·1	88·2	3·0
Japan	3·9	39·9	24·8	4·2	1·1	102·5	2·0
Netherlands	6·4	4·4	6·0	2·0	0·4	32·8	3·6
New Zealand	7·7	15·5	9·3	Nil	1·5	40·2	7·9
Norway	Nil	6·3	4·7	Nil	Nil	20·5	5·7
Poland	4·5	6·5	10·5	1·4	2·2	36·1	2·5
Portugal	10·8	13·7	29·7	4·2	8·0	87·7	6·4
Rumania	5·1	9·2	23·1	2·4	27·8	85·1	5·4
Sweden	Nil	12·4	1·8	3·5	Nil	26·6	4·9
Switzerland	2·7	4·5	5·5	2·7	2·7	34·5	5·6
U.K.: England and Wales	3·3	5·7	4·4	1·6	3·7	28·5	1·8
Northern Ireland	15·0	3·0	6·0	Nil	Nil	41·9	9·6
Scotland	11·7	5·8	5·8	Nil	2·9	39·0	6·1
U.S.A.	4·0	7·1	6·1	1·6	4·9	35·8	0·9

TABLE 3

MATERNAL DEATH RATES PER 100,000 TOTAL BIRTHS FOR CERTAIN CAUSES BY STANDARD
REGIONS, 1961–1964, ENGLAND AND WALES, AND URBAN AND RURAL AGGREGATES

Region	Maternal sepsis*	Toxaemia of preg-nancy and childbirth	Abortion	Other causes	Total pregnancy and childbirth	
					Total	Excluding abortion
England and Wales	4·0	5·5	6·1	14·8	30·3	24·2
Northern	3·2	6·5	6·1	13·0	28·8	22·7
East and West Ridings	3·6	6·8	4·8	12·9	28·1	23·2
North Western	6·1	5·3	5·5	14·6	31·6	26·1
North Midland	2·9	6·8	4·7	13·3	27·7	23·0
Midland	4·5	6·1	8·0	14·4	33·0	25·0
Eastern	2·8	2·8	3·5	19·5	28·6	25·1
London and South Eastern	2·9	4·6	9·7	17·7	34·9	25·3
Southern	4·5	2·7	3·1	9·8	20·1	17·0
South Western	4·6	7·9	0·4†	10·0	22·8	22·4
Wales	4·8	6·9	7·9	16·4	36·0	28·1
Urban and rural aggregates						
Conurbations	3·5	5·0	9·0	17·2	34·6	25·6
Outside conurbations						
Urban areas						
Population: 100,000+	4·2	5·7	6·0	12·2	28·1	22·1
50,000–100,000	3·9	7·1	3·6	13·9	28·5	24·9
less than 50,000	5·0	6·7	4·5	15·6	31·8	27·3
Rural districts	3·6	4·2	3·8	11·6	23·2	19·4

* Not including abortions.   † One death only.

rates were highest in the Welsh, Midland, and London and the South Eastern Regions. The high rate in the South East was due, however, to the effect of Greater London, the rate including abortions being 39 per 100,000 total births in Greater London and 22·8 in the remainder of the South Eastern Region, or if abortions are not included the difference was 26·9 for Greater London and 20·3 for the rest of the Region. The pattern for individual diseases varied slightly, thus the rates for sepsis were high in the North Western Region but low in London and the South East; for toxaemia they were high in the South West, Wales and the North but low in the South and East; and for abortion they were high in London and the South Eastern Region and Wales and low in the South. The high rate for abortion in the South East was due to the effect of Greater London where the death rate was 12·1 per 100,000 total births compared with the rest of the South East where it was 2·5.

In the same table the mortality rates have been analysed according to the density of population. The highest mortality rates were found in small towns with populations of less than 50,000, except in the case of abortion when the rates in conurbations were double those of the smaller towns and urban areas. The individual conurbations usually had higher rates than their surrounding regions but there were two exceptions: in the Northern Region, Tyneside had a rate of about half that of the remainder of

the Region, and in the North Western Region, where there are two conurbations, Merseyside was below and South East Lancashire was above the rate for the rest of the Region.

It is generally agreed that now a maternal death is so rare an event in childbirth, perinatal and infant mortality rates are of greater significance than maternal mortality rates in assessing the standards of care, even though the lack of uniformity in the collection of data has a greater effect than on the maternal statistics. Countries vary in the extent to which they comply with the W.H.O. definitions of live and stillbirth. Some countries such as England and Wales have no definition for a live birth and differ slightly from the W.H.O. definition of a stillbirth. In others the differences are much greater. Thus a baby may not be considered to be born alive unless it is still living at the time of the registration of the birth, for example, in France within three days or in Spain within 24 hours; or a child under a certain weight, length, or gestation period may not be recorded as a live birth, or for that matter as a birth at all, unless it lives for more than 24 hours. In a few countries any child over 26 weeks gestation is considered viable, as compared with the more usual 28 weeks; while in Japan some of their statistics relate to foetal deaths with a gestational age of four months and over.

Table 4 shows the mortality rates for late foetal deaths and for infants dying aged 0–6 days, 0–27 days and under

TABLE 4

MORTALITY RATES FOR LATE FOETAL AND INFANT DEATHS PER 1000 LIVE BIRTHS

Country	Late foetal deaths	Infant mortality				
		0–6 days	0–27 days		Under 1 year	
	1964*	1963	1964	1965	1964	1965
Australia	(12·6)	12·8	13·6	13·2	19·1	18·5
Austria	12·6	—	20·2	21·2	29·2	27·9
Belgium	15·1	15·1	16·6	—	25·3	24·0
Bulgaria	10·0	—	15·0	13·8	32·9	30·8
Canada	12·2	16·1	17·3	—	24·7	—
Czechoslovakia	8·6	10·3	13·1	—	21·4	25·3
Denmark	(11·5)	13·1	14·3	—	18·7	18·7
Finland	9·8	12·3	13·7	13·6	17·0	17·6
France	15·8	9·6	15·9	15·4	23·3	22·1
Germany, West	12·8	17·8	18·9	18·4	25·3	23·9
Hungary	11·7	22·5	26·7	27·5	40·0	38·8
Ireland	—	14·1	18·2	17·2	26·7	25·2
Israel	13·8	12·0	15·8	15·6	28·2	27·4
Italy	21·0	17·9	21·9	—	35·5	35·6
Japan	(27·0)	9·2	20·4	18·5	12·4	11·7
Netherlands	13·6	10·4	11·6	11·4	14·8	14·4
New Zealand	13·0	11·4	12·4	12·1	19·1	19·5
Norway	(12·7)	10·1	11·8	—	16·4	—
Poland	11·3	14·1	21·7	—	47·7	41·5
Portugal	26·8	15·8	26·0	25·4	69·0	64·9
Rumania	15·2	—	15·0	13·7	48·6	44·1
Sweden	11·3	11·0	11·7	10·6	14·2	13·3
Switzerland	11·3	14·2	14·3	—	19·0	17·8
U.K.: England and Wales	16·6	12·3	13·8	13·0	19·9	19·0
Northern Ireland	19·8	16·6	18·3	17·7	26·3	25·0
Scotland	18·1	14·6	16·4	15·9	24·0	23·1
U.S.A.	12·8	16·4	17·9	17·7	24·8	24·7

* Figures in brackets are for 1963.

TABLE 5

INFANT (I.E. UNDER ONE YEAR OF AGE) MORTALITY RATES PER 1000
LIVE BIRTHS FOR CERTAIN CAUSES (I.S.D. "B" LIST) FOR THE YEARS
1963 AND 1964

Country	Congenital malformations (B.41)		Birth injuries, P.N. asphyxia, and atelectasis (B.42)	
	1963	1964	1963	1964
Australia	3·75	3·71	4·53	4·68
Austria	3·90	4·36	5·79	5·71
Belgium	5·00	4·52	3·25	3·40
Bulgaria	3·22	2·51	5·11	4·86
Canada	4·44	4·35	5·58	5·37
Czechoslovakia	4·56	4·33	6·83	7·24
Denmark	4·09	4·04	7·16	6·68
Finland	3·70	3·16	6·94	6·49
France*	3·68	3·63	3·39	3·35
Germany, West	4·30	4·11	5·63	5·45
Hungary	6·51	6·32	11·06	11·49
Iceland	3·54	3·34	3·96	5·22
Ireland	7·29	7·15	4·32	5·14
Israel	4·66	4·74	5·11	5·43
Italy	3·53	3·40	6·75	6·20
Japan	2·00	1·96	1·72	1·78
Netherlands	4·01	3·80	4·01	3·91
New Zealand	4·02	2·91	4·53	4·68
Norway	3·03	3·17	4·20	4·53
Poland	4·47	4·71	5·24	5·56
Portugal	2·31	2·63	4·18	4·78
Rumania	3·14	—	4·74	—
Sweden	3·44	3·11	5·05	4·85
Switzerland	4·10	4·32	6·66	4·75
U.K.: England and Wales	4·20	4·15	5·22	5·23
Northern Ireland	6·46	6·17	6·76	6·37
Scotland	5·24	4·94	7·11	7·61
U.S.A.	3·56	3·53	6·56	6·27
Yugoslavia	1·45	1·59	4·65	4·49

* Excluding children born alive but dead before registration of birth, in France within 3 days.

one year. It is of particular interest to see that the high fœtal and infant mortality rates do not follow the same geographical distribution as the maternal mortality rates. Thus Japan has an infant rate death rate near the average of the countries selected despite its high maternal mortality rate.

Table 5 shows the infant mortality rates according to certain causes from the International classification "B" List. It shows the variations which occur between the different countries, although some of this is undoubtedly due to varying practices in the assignment of the death to a single cause.

Table 6 shows the causes of late foetal deaths for the countries with available statistics. It is interesting to note that 37 per cent of the foetal deaths in Japan were due to maternal causes, mainly toxaemia of pregnancy. Their results cannot be compared with other countries because they use a widely different definition of stillbirth. Hereditary factors are likely to play a greater part in infant than in maternal mortality as many forms of congenital malformations are known to be genetic in origin. Babies with congenital abnormalities often die from asphyxia or infection and the death may be assigned to these causes. However, foetal and infant death rates from congenital malformations are higher in the U.K. and Ireland than in other countries.

The geographical and racial distributions of congenital malformations is a subject which has aroused interest over many years. Only a proportion are manifest at birth and many do not become diagnosable until much later. In order to make an accurate assessment of the incidence of any disease it is necessary to relate it to a known population. For this reason most of the studies are related to incidence at birth and to congenital malformations which are fairly common and easily recognisable. Lamy and Frézal (1961) speaking at the first International Conference

TABLE 6

LATE FOETAL MORTALITY PER 1000 LIVE BIRTHS BY CAUSE, AVERAGE ANNUAL RATES FOR THREE LATEST AVAILABLE YEARS (1961–63)

Country	Diseases of pregnancy and childbirth	Difficulties of labour	Placental and cord conditions	Congenital malformations	Diseases of foetus	All causes
Belgium	0·49	0·48	2·55	1·36	8·75	14·55
Canada	0·99	0·77	4·57	1·66	3·66	12·34
Denmark	0·64	1·23	4·34	1·27	4·14	12·08
Finland	1·50	0·50	4·20	1·76	4·75	13·42
Germany, West	0·60	1·20	2·52	0·88	7·05	13·13
Hungary	0·47	0·40	2·06	1·51	7·50	12·39
Israel	1·58	0·72	3·65	1·15	6·15	13·76
Japan*	31·93	5·14	5·82	0·82	29·37	98·20
Netherlands	2·36	1·23	3·83	1·59	4·25	14·81
New Zealand†	2·28	0·62	4·44	1·85	3·18	13·17
Rumania (1963 only)	3·40	1·74	3·29	1·82	7·23	15·60
Switzerland	1·59	0·70	3·07	1·02	4·93	11·84
U.K.: England and Wales	3·18	1·39	5·11	3·47	4·12	18·44
Northern Ireland	4·60	1·19	4·64	4·67	5·58	21·81
Scotland	4·41	1·36	4·32	4·95	4·05	20·33

* These figures include only those attended by a physician. The figures also appear to include deaths which occur from the fourth or following months of gestation.

† Before 1962 excluding Maoris.

on Congenital Malformations reviewed the studies which had been made on the incidence and the following information was taken from their paper which also gives the details of the studies referred to, by whom they were conducted and the references.

Anencephaly is a condition most easily studied and one known to vary with both race and geographical location. It has a higher incidence among Caucasians than Negroes; it is commoner among Sikhs than other Indians; it has a low incidence among Hakka Chinese; there is a decreasing

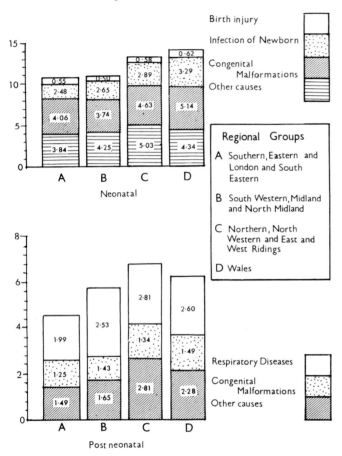

FIG. 1. Neonatal and post-neonatal death rates per 1000 live births by regional groups. This diagram has been adapted from an illustration appearing in Regional and Social Factors in Infant Mortality. Spicer and Lipworth published by H.M.S.O. from whom permission to reproduce was obtained.

frequency from Northern Ireland and Scotland to Southern England where the rate is higher than Continental Europe; and there are regional variations in France. A positive correlation exists between the incidence of anencephaly and that of spina bifida and meningoceles; however, spina bifida is much more frequent than anencephaly in Switzerland and Sweden, whereas, in Japan it is three times less common. Of the other malformations recognisable at birth, anophthalmia-micro-ophthalmia is significantly higher among Japanese than Caucasians; polydactalia is commoner among Negroes than among members of the Mongolian races and even more than among Caucasians;

hare lip and cleft palate varies little among Caucasian populations but is higher among members of the Mongolian races and lower among Negroes. Lamy and Frézal summed up by saying that there is only very fragmentary data available on the incidence of congenital malformations.

In England and Wales, regional differences in perinatal and infant mortality have been recognised for many years and a considerable amount of work has been carried out analysing the factors affecting the distribution. In 1955, Heady, Morris, Daly and Stevens published a series of papers on "social and biological factors in infant mortality". In the third paper of the series (Daly, Heady and Morris, 1955), they found that these regional variations were due to causes other than differences in respect to age and parity distribution. The stillbirth rates were highest in Wales and lowest in the Southern part of England. The neonatal death rates were also highest in Wales but lowest in the Eastern region. Since then various further studies have been made. Heady and Heasman (1959) and Spicer and Lipworth (1966) continued the 1955 survey confirming the findings. Diagram 1 and Table 7 are taken from the book by Spicer and Lipworth.

This latest survey was carried out on babies born in 1964. When comparing the death rates in the four areas, regional differences for age and parity and social class were standardised by applying to the known numbers in each social class, age and parity group in each of the four areas, the corresponding rates for England and Wales as a whole. This gave the number of deaths for each region which would have been expected if their rates had been the same as the whole country. The ratio of the observed number to this expected number, expressed as a percentage, allows comparison by region unaffected by other factors. The results are shown in Table 7 below.

TABLE 7

STILLBIRTH AND INFANT DEATHS IN ENGLAND AND WALES. STANDARDISED MORTALITY RATIOS FOR STILLBIRTHS AND INFANT DEATHS BY REGIONS

Regional Groups*	Stillbirths	Neonatal	Post-neonatal
A	87	94	86
B	104	94	97
C	110	110	118
D	116	114	108

* For key to Regional Groups see Fig. 1.

Babies born in the South and Eastern parts of England were at an advantage as far as stillbirths and infant deaths were concerned, while the experience of those born in Wales and Northern England was far less favourable. The same regional patterns have remained despite all the changes which have occurred in medical care.

In England and Wales the only national morbidity statistics available are those based on hospital admissions but unfortunately they are of limited value as the regional morbidity ratios are affected by the varying hospital confinement rates. In common with a number of other countries, there is in England and Wales a scheme for the notification of all congenital malformations observed at birth. The scheme is voluntary and has been in operation since 1964. Its primary purpose is not to provide incidences of congenital malformations but to act as a monitoring system to ensure that any future tragedy similar to that which occurred with thalidomide could be detected much earlier. It does give some information on the incidence of some of the abnormalities which are easily recognisable at birth. About 16 per cent of the total live and still-births are notified as having a congenital malformation. Some of the conditions are very slight, on the other hand the figures for conditions which cannot be immediately recognised, e.g., congenital heart disease, are inaccurate and the extent of notification variable. However, defects of the central nervous system and hare lip and cleft palate show a distribution which confirms the findings in individual studies.

Table 8 shows the incidence by region for 1965. As it can be seen malformations of the central nervous system are commoner in Wales and in the North West of England and lowest in the South East of England. On the other hand there is practically no variation in the regional

hard to disentangle as poor medical care often accompanies undernutrition and bad housing. In those countries with high standards, both medical and social, the biological factors have an increasing influence so that contraception and the extent to which abortion is induced for medical or social reasons will effect the results. Finally in the background are the racial differences, and very little is known about these, for even in congenital malformations which are probably the best documented the knowledge is admitted to be fragmentary.

Professor Sir Dugald Baird summed it up when he said at the International Society of the Geographical Pathology conference;

"Epidemiological research depends upon the accurate and systematic observation and recording of clearly definable facts in a known population or a representative sample of it. Unfortunately in many under developed countries even mortality statistics are not often available so that it is impossible to discover much about the incidence of disease. Even in a highly developed country like Britain, regional comparisons are usually impossible because of the inadequacy of morbidity statistics."

TABLE 8

CERTAIN CONGENITAL MALFORMATIONS BY STANDARD REGIONS,* ENGLAND AND WALES, 1965, PER 10,000 TOTAL BIRTHS

Region	All defects of C.N.S.	Anencephalus	Encephalocele	Hydrocephalus spina bifida	Cleft lip and cleft palate
North	54·72	18·74	1·33	27·69	14·43
Yorkshire and Humberside	44·81	14·63	0·69	25·34	12·10
North West	60·20	22·24	1·29	30·70	12·89
East Midland	49·48	18·15	1·45	26·35	13·82
West Midland	50·99	15·69	1·45	28·18	12·28
East Anglia	41·00	11·93	1·12	20·87	12·67
South East	36·51	10·96	1·11	19·18	13·30
South West	44·69	14·54	1·86	22·73	12·68
Wales I (South)	69·89	24·46	2·04	38·15	14·85
Wales II (North)	43·64	14·81	1·56	22·60	14·81

* The Standard Regions were modified in 1965, so that they do not correspond with those in Table 3, Fig. 1, or Table 7.

pattern for cleft lip and palate which is in line with the finding that there is an even distribution among Caucasian populations.

This chapter has discussed a few of the many facets in the regional and geographical pattern of maternal and child health. This pattern as we have seen can be affected by four factors:

1. Medical standards.
2. Social standards in the widest sense.
3. Biological factors in the population structure, e.g. the age and parity of the mother.
4. Racial differences.

For most of the world population the medical and social standards are the important factors and are reflected in the maternal and infant mortality rates. The two factors are

ACKNOWLEDGEMENTS

I wish to thank Dr. Hill and the staff at the General Register Office for their help and particularly for preparing the figures for Table 3. Diagram 1 and Table 7 are reproduced from the General Register Office study on Medical and Population Subjects No. 19, Regional and Social factors in Infant Mortality with permission of the Controller of H.M. Stationery Office.

REFERENCES

Annual Report of the Chief Medical Officer of the Ministry of Health, London, (1967): *On the State of the Public Health*, 1966. H.M.S.O., London.

Baird, D. (1961), "General Summary." *Pathologie et Microbiologie (Basel)*, **24**, 557–560.

Barron, S. L. and Vessey, M. P. (1966), "Immigration—A New Social Factor in Obstetrics." *Brit. med. J.*, **1**, 1189–1194.

Daly, C., Heady, J. A. and Morris, J. N. (1955), "Social and Biological Factors in Infant Mortality III." *Lancet*, **i**, 445.

Doll, R. and Hanington, E. (1961), "International Survey of Eclampsia and Preeclampsia, 1958–59: Epidemiological Aspects," *Pathologie et Microbiologie (Basel)*, **24**, 531–541.

Epidemiological and Vital Statistics Report, (1966), **19**, 257–334.

Epidemiological and Vital Statistics Report (1966), **19**, 380–381.

Epidemiological and Vital Statistics Report, (1967), **20**, 437–486.

Heady, J. A. and Heasman, M. A. (1959), *Social and Biological Factors in Infant Mortality. Gen. Reg. Office. Studies on Medical and Population Subjects*, No. 15. H.M.S.O. London.

Lamy, M. and Frezal, J. (1961), *The Frequency of Congenital Mal formations. First International Conference on Congenital Malformations*, 1960. Philadelphia and Montreal: J. B. Lippincott and Company.

Spicer, C. C. and Lipworth, L. (1966), *Regional and Social Factors in Infant Mortality. Gen. Reg. Office. Studies on Medical and Population Subjects No. 19.* H.M.S.O. London.

Takaki, F., Magari, M. and Shu Yuasi (1961), *Pathologie et Microbiologie (Basel)*, **24**, 459–473.

World Health Statistical Annual, 1963. Volume 1. (1966). Geneva: W.H.O.

3. COMPUTERS

L. C. PAYNE

The principles of computers embrace far wider areas of application than simply calculation and accounting. Properly understood and applied they have a profound and continuing part to play in improving the effectiveness of medical procedures. This will not be accomplished however until doctors generally acquire proficiency in a computer language, so that they can translate their specialized knowledge and experience into a suitable form to enlist computer-assistance. This job cannot be handed over entirely to computer scientists and technicians. Doctors must lead.

In order not to misunderstand the role of computers it is necessary to recognize that computing power, like electric power, is entirely undifferentiated until it is applied. To apply electric power some apparatus must be designed which enables the electric power to be used to some purpose. The apparatus may be well-designed, badly designed or indifferently designed, depending on the designers' collective knowledge of both electricity and the application to which it is to be put, as well as their resourcefulness in conceiving an effective arrangement for the purpose. If electric power is misapplied we do not blame the electric generator, but rather the designers of the electronic or electric apparatus. Nor can we or do we expect electrical engineers to be able to design all the devices which can usefully use electricity, ranging from kettles to kapnographs, colorimeters to cardiographs, and so on. Even less could we have asked Michael Faraday, genius though he was, to even guess at the many uses to which electricity would be put. Yet we have all, obstetricians and gynaecologists included, come to depend very much on both electrical and electronic apparatus in one form or another.

So it is with computers. The computer is a *machine*, no more and no less, for performing *any specified data-procedure*. Being a machine both data and the data-procedure must be suitably codified by expressing them in a *computer language*. A data-procedure written in the form of a computer language is called a *programme*. When both data and programme are inserted into a computer, the computer simply causes the procedure to operate on the data step by step. *This is all a computer does*, and obstetricians and gynaecologists may, like many others, be forgiven if they do not readily see in this simple truth profound implications greatly exceeding those that emanated from the first twitch of electrical energy on a galvonometer. Let me attempt to explain.

Obviously if the data supplied to a computer is numerical and the data-procedure is an arithmetical one, then the *action* arising when the computer applies the arithmetic data-procedure to the numerical data is *calculation*. But what if the data is the English and Russian vocabularies and the data-procedure embodies the rules of syntax in these languages? Clearly the *action* arising when the computer applies this procedure to this data is *translation*. Similarly if the data is the musical notes and the procedure embodies the canons of composition in some form, then the computers *action* resulting from applying this procedure to this data will be to *compose* a tune. If the data is that supplied by instruments on an oil-refining process and the procedure embodies the rules by which adjustments are to be made, then the computers *action* will *control* the process. If the data is that elicited from a patient by a clinician during a clinical examination and the procedure embodies a way in which this can be compared with a listed set of differentiating syndromes, prognoses and therapies, then the computers *action* in applying this procedure to this data will be to *produce a differential diagnosis* with corresponding prognoses and therapies. And so on. Almost every intelligent action can be looked at in this way: there are almost as many data-procedures as there are thought processes.

Until now of course there has been no incentive to examine our actions critically in this way, the computer being the first machine in history (apart from elementary calculators, counters and sorting machines) which can process data (in the broadest sense of the word) flexibly and incredibly quickly. We take it for granted that muscle plus machine is in very many situations far more effective than muscle alone, without it offending human vanity in any way. But when it comes to assessment, decision and judgment—the province of intelligence—where information must be selected and weighed before action is taken, we have had to rely hitherto *necessarily* and *exclusively* on mind alone, and the very suggestion that mind plus machine can in very many situations be far more effective than mind alone is upsetting—to some at least!

As a versatile data-engine the role of the computer in medicine is as wide as the many different ways in which data is or could be used. This includes the great variety of uses of medical record data in the management of health and sickness in patients, in epidemiology and social medicine, and so on; it includes the vast and growing field of laboratory measurements and analysis whether for routine or research purposes; it includes diagnosis, therapy and prognosis; it includes the bio-medical sciences which depend heavily on mathematical and statistical analysis; it includes patient monitoring in which data proliferates from continuous recording; it includes paramedical activities such as dietetics, radiation treatment planning, nursing administration, hospital planning, catering, supplies, finance, and so on. The opportunities for implementing, refining and extending many procedures in almost every department of the health, medical and welfare services, are legion, and as awareness of these opportunities become more widespread, the tempo of practical application is gaining momentum, and steadily but inevitably precipitating a major involvement of medicine with technology.

Although computers, being machines, have no capacity for thought, they can certainly implement the thinking (or lack of it) embodied in the procedures specified to them. Their *actions* therefore can and do exhibit intelligence (or lack of it) to the extent that intelligent procedures can be explicitly prescribed, or programmed as it is called. Computers can therefore be programmed to examine and classify electrocardiographs, and considerable success in this has already been achieved; they can be programmed to detect cardiac arrythmias, or say changes in myocardial contractility, from data connected directly to them from patients; they can be programmed to detect acidosis or hypoxia in foetuses from data collected directly from the mother by means of electrodes (similar to those used in the foetal electrocardiograph) comfortably situated in a fabric belt worn round the abdomen; they can be programmed to store extensive and updated information on differentiating syndromes, prognoses and therapies; they can be programmed to retrieve disease conditions from such "libraries" whose differentiating syndromes are measurably similar to observed symptoms, signs, and so on, thus producing a differential diagnosis in response to a telephone call; they can also be programmed to print out further tests and signs which should be sought for to clarify the diagnostic situation, and they can be programmed to print out relevant treatments; they can be programmed to calculate radiation dosage distributions for the radiotherapeutic treatment of cancer patients; they can be programmed to produce schedules of duties for nurses; they can be programmed to store and scan medical records *not* simply to produce *statistics* but to *reveal significant changes* in cross-infection, drug utilization, morbidity, phocomelia, durations of stay, length of waiting lists, and so on. In fact there is no limit to what they can be programmed to do once medical people have

learned to provide the data in suitable form, rather than in the present form, which virtually relegates it to medical records libraries for perpetuity!

What computers can do in terms of quality is entirely determined by the procedures prescribed for them. Computing power (like electric power) is undifferentiated and useless until a programme is prepared; the programme may be well-designed, badly designed or indifferently designed, depending on the designers' collective knowledge of both computers and the application to which they are being applied, as well as their resourcefulness in conceiving an effective procedure. If the computing power is misapplied the computer cannot be blamed, it lies at the door of the designers of the programme. Nor can we expect computer scientists to be able to design all the programmes determining the uses to which computing power can be put. Only an obstetrician can define a useful obstetric procedure, but only an obstetrician with computer programming competence can define a useful obstetric procedure and programme it for practical implementation by computer.

The barrier therefore is not technology or even finance (computer time can be hired very cheaply) but *education*. Computers are *not* calculators; in fact these days the thing computers do least is compute! Calculation merely happens to be one special class of data-procedure that computers can perform and it is reasonable therefore that mathematicians and accountants should use computers for their work. The more fundamental fact to bear in mind however about computers is that they can operate (through data-procedures) on *any* kind of objective data; these versatile machines have liberated us from mathematics and what we need to do now is to liberate computers from mathematicians. Only suitably trained doctors can decide how computers can best be used in medicine, and only suitably trained obstetricians and gynaecologists can decide how computers can best be used in assisting them in their professional activities.

Of necessity, this paper can only stimulate obstetricians and gyncaeologists to take steps to instruct themselves. Understandably an obstetrician or gynaecologist may aver that he does not in fact have much data, and that he is primarily concerned with the patient. This attitude however is taking far too narrow a view of data. The really valuable role of the computer (once it is properly understood and applied) is not in producing figures, but in improving medical *management*. All managers, whether of patients, hospitals or factories, are endeavouring to control a changing and developing situation, but they can only respond to those changes in a situation of which they are aware, and only respond with that set of actions of which their limited knowledge allows. They will not respond to those changes of which they are unaware, and moreover will not do so with all the confidence of not even knowing that they do not know. Such, for example, was the confidence with which thalidomide was being administered to expectant mothers with such tragic effects for so long. There is certainly no room for complacency because as Sir Derek Dunlop has pointed out (*British Medical Journal*, 21.8.65), "It has been estimated that from 10 to 15 per cent of patients in our general hospitals are suffering to a greater or lesser extent from our efforts to treat them". With computers the possibility exists of devising data-procedures which will enable (to a far greater extent than exists or could exist without computers), physicians, surgeons and administrators to know what is happening and not what has happened. This will apply to the more timely awareness of cardiac arrythmias and of foetal distress as to what is going on in a hospital; it will enable us to control, evaluate and compare, the effectiveness of medical activity, as it will enable us to screen, monitor and manage the health of the whole community far better than we can at the present time.

THE TECHNOLOGY

A more detailed description of how such procedures can be developed and organized cannot be given without reference to the nature of computer systems. The heart of every computer system is its store in which both the active programme and active data on which it is operating are contained (see figure); reference data, such as medical

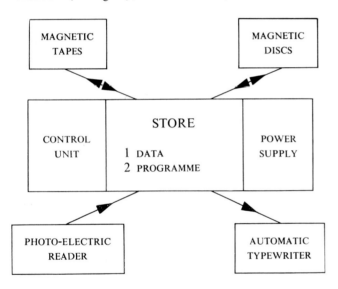

records, is filed either on magnetic tapes or magnetic discs which provide large capacity file storage. This data can be transferred to and from the active store as required. New data and programmes are commonly inserted into the active store via a photo-electric reader which accepts data in the form of either punched paper tape or punched cards. Results are commonly printed out directly onto an automatic typewriter.

To get data into a computer therefore requires it to be converted into punched form. This is achieved by having the data typed on a keyboard with a punched attachment; every time a key is pressed it causes a coded row of holes to appear on a continuous piece of paper tape, or as a coded column of holes on a punched card (usually with a capacity of 80 columns and measuring about 7 inches by 4 inches). Anything that can be typed therefore (such as a medical record) can be inserted into a computer. Graphical data, such as that provided by an electrocardiograph, a blood pressure recorder, a biochemical autoanalyser,

and so on, can also be turned into punched paper tape form by means of a small device, called an analogue-to-digital converter, attached to the instrument producing the graphical data. This device simply samples the height of the curve at regular intervals and represents each height as a coded row of holes on the paper tape. Graphs in punched paper tape form can thus be inserted into the computer store for inspection and analysis by a suitable programme. Pictures also, such as radiographs or micro-photographs of cervical smears, can similarly be turned into punched paper tape form: each point on the picture is scanned (television-like so that a million points can be scanned in a second!) and each point is assigned a number corresponding to its contrast level, which is then coded as a row of holes on paper tape. It may be of interest to mention that an attempt to develop a programme which will cytologically examine cervical smears is presently being sponsored by the Medical Research Council.

Getting the data prepared however is only one aspect; the other is to design the programme. The need for the programme is due to the fact that a computer is *only intrinsically capable of the most elementary operations* (such as add, compare, subtract, and so on) which typically it performs at around a million times a second. This feature coupled with the fact (by no means obvious) that *any explicit data-procedure can be broken down into a sequence of these elementary operations* (doing this is called programming), enables a computer to carry out any data-procedure which has been analysed in this way. Each of the elementary operations is given a simple code, and if a data-procedure is analysed into such elementary operations and each assigned its particular code, the data-procedure is said to be programmed in *machine language. A computer can only carry out a data-procedure which is in this form.*

The trouble about machine languages however is that they are (*a*) *special* to each type of computer so that re-programming is required for each type of computer, and (*b*) so *detailed* that they require a considerable amount of tedious programming effort and therefore expense. Not surprisingly therefore programming techniques have developed a much more efficacious method in the form of what are called *high-level languages*. These languages are an attempt (*a*) to provide a stylized language much closer to everyday language, and therefore more easily learned, and (*b*) to provide a language which can be accepted by *any* computer. Economy is thus affected in the time taken to write the programme, and also in the fact that a programme developed for one type of computer can be used on any other type of computer.

Considerable progress has been made in devising these "universal" languages of which the most widely used are FORTRAN and ALGOL (others are COBOL and PL1), but one must add at once that although these languages attempt to be universal they all have a long way to go in achieving this goal. Much remains to be done and much is being done, but it is likely to be a continuing task for many years to come. The problem is that a computer language such as ALGOL, developed principally for calculations (*ALGe*braic *O*riented *L*anguage) is by no means well suited to many aspects of medical data processing.

Programmes written in a high-level language cannot be performed directly by a computer: they have first to be translated into machine language. To transcribe one stylized language, such as ALGOL, into another stylized language such as machine language, is itself a data-procedure, and thus can be performed by a computer if a suitable programme is devised. Such a programme, and a monumental piece of programming it is too (usually provided by the computer manufacturer), is called a *compiler*. A computer with an ALGOL compiler will accept any data-procedure written in ALGOL and transcribe it automatically into machine language and thus carry it out. Similarly a computer with a FORTRAN compiler will accept any data-procedure written in FORTRAN, and so on. Ultimately of course one would like a compiler which would accept any procedure written in the English, German, French, American, and other languages, but since there are almost as many versions of these languages as there are individuals who speak them, then we shall probably have to settle for something less than the ultimate. It should be pointed out however that some ambitious compilers have already been written with an extensive vocabulary not only of words but phrases, and at the experimental level limited man-machine "conversations" have already taken place. These may not merit the description of conversation, but they show real promise of helping the computer user in (a) designing his programme (b) correcting his programme, and (c) obtaining answers to enquiries from data-banks of reference data stored inside the computer.

The astonishing increase in the speed of computers (it has grown from 1,000 operations per second 20 years ago to 1,000,000 operations per second today) is fast opening up a further capability in the form of the *computer utility*. Evidently a user typing in data and questions, and requiring answers at the rate of about 10 times per second, is not fully employing a computer capable of 1,000,000 operations per second. Thus in each second the computer can divide its time between hundreds of users (it could, for example, perform 1,000 operations for each of 1,000 users every second) and appear to each user to be offering him an exclusive service! This is the concept of *time-sharing*. To the extent that different users will require the use of different programmes then the computer must be capable of operating first one programme and then another according to some scheme of priorities. Complex though this certainly is, it is in fact just another data-procedure which can with effort be programmed, thus enabling the computer to provide a *"multi-programming"* service, as it is called.

What of the next 20 years? It will certainly see the computer permeating every aspect of our society. Mind plus computer in many contexts will be superior to mind alone, so wherever mind is used we can confidently expect some extension of its capability by using computer power. Computer literacy, that is fluency in a computer language, will be as widespread as the ability to drive. Computer literacy will enable doctors, biochemists, pharmacists,

radiologists, and so on, to formulate *their* specialized procedures in a way that can enlist the assistance of computer power. To do this they will have in their offices a data-terminal which they will be able to connect to computer centres by dialling; the location of the computer centres may be near or far. The data-terminal may take the form of a key-board (typewriter-like) for both communicating and receiving information, but it may be augmented with a cathode ray tube (television-like) with a "light-pen" for sending/receiving graphical information or for instantly receiving a complete medical record, radiograph, and so on. Much of the information resting in filing cabinets (often inaccessibly because of the time it takes to sort through it) will be stored in a data-bank so that it can be selectively and quickly retrieved by the computer at the press of a button. Operational systems (not experimental systems) are already installed and working incorporating all these features, so none of these developments is predicated on further technological progress. Further technological progress could lead to successful voice communications with computers, limited perhaps to a specialized vocabulary of phrases, but by no means limited in its utility.

The large time-shared central computer system described, with its data-banks of reference data serving a wide community of users, can now be augmented by another kind of computer facility. In recent years an entirely new technique, "micro-miniaturization", has enabled quite versatile computers to be built which are no bigger than a text-book. These are ideal for attaching "on-line", i.e. directly, to laboratory instruments, or to patient monitoring equipment during operative, recovery or intensive care phases to detect and evaluate changes in patients conditions and so to summon medical attention in response to changes of which they would otherwise be unaware. There is no doubt whatsoever that in time *computers will come between the patient and the doctor*, but only in the way that spectacles and the stethoscope do, namely to aid the human senses in being more fully aware of situations they are trying to manage. Remember we are talking of 24-hour quantitative surveillance with powers of selection, analysis, recording and communication—is it any wonder that anthropomorphisms get associated with such systems? None of this however will "take-over" the doctors function or any way diminish the decisions to be taken. On the contrary more decisions will be required because there will be more information, useful and relevant at that, given good design, to decide upon. Only ignorance simplifies decisions!

Equally with diagnosis. All that computers are going to do (properly used) is to enable up-to-date knowledge on disease and treatment to be systematically and, one hopes, professionally organized into an automatic library facility (A.L.F.—see Reference 1) accessible by telephone. In a matter of seconds, in response to a telephone call, information on as many as 30,000 disease profiles could be scanned to retrieve only what is relevant in a particular situation. The clinician will still have to decide but he will have more relevant information to decide from. Diagnosis will still be an art, but it will be a more refined art, requiring astute judgements to be made on more information than at present, and as Sir Ronald Fisher once said, "the errors arising from too much information are hardly likely to exceed those arising from too little".

When it comes to maintaining health rather than treating sickness, when it comes to evaluating one kind of therapy compared with another, when it comes to identifying high-risk profiles correlated with a pre-symptomatic disposition towards a particular disease, when it comes to epidemiology, when it comes to a far more critical appreciation of what medicine is doing, and to thinking how it can widen its scope to prevent sickness, that is towards health management rather than sickness management, then the computer is indispensable because it is the only hope of being able to achieve these things economically and intellectually (the variety is too great for unaided cerebral units along to cope with). It is hoped that enough has been said of computer techniques for this potential capability to be apparent, and for obstetricians and gynaecologists to begin to train and organize themselves to harness the benefits in their fields of activity.

FURTHER READING

"Introduction to Medical Automation," Pitman Medical Publishing Company, 1966. L. C. Payne.

4. STATISTICAL METHODS IN MEDICINE

C. C. SPICER

INTRODUCTION

It has been said that many clinicians regard statistics in the same way that some people regard ghosts. They do not believe in them but they are frightened of them. This point of view seems to have arisen from a misunderstanding of the aims and methods of statistics and is as unfortunate as an attitude of superstitious respect or outright rejection. In a chapter of this length it is not possible to treat the technical methods of statistics in detail. One can only attempt to explain some of the principles underlying the application of these methods and to show that for some purposes they are an important tool of medical research.

The basic reason for the existence of a body of statistical method is the need to be able to make reliable inferences from inherently variable observations. Virtually all observations on the real world are subject to some variation and it is a task of the experimental scientist, as a rule, to reduce this variation to a minimum in relation to the effects he is trying to study. The use of pure chemicals, clean glassware, genetically uniform strains of laboratory animals and standardized laboratory conditions are all examples of the precautions a scientist has to take in order to preserve the sensitivity and repeatability of his experiments. However, even in the best of experiments there usually remains a hard core of variability which may nevertheless be ignored because it is so small in relation to the main results. For example, the growth curves of rats with and without a vitamin in their diet may be quite erratic in both cases but differ so enormously that the erratic variations do not affect the main conclusions of the experiment.

The success of the laboratory scientist in controlling unwanted variation has obscured the fact that valid results may be obtained from variable material, and that in many biological situations variability is an inherent factor. It is for example impossible to visualize a human population without a certain degree of variation in its major properties. For some purposes it may be desirable to confine one's observations to relatively homogeneous sub-groups but this might correspondingly reduce the applicability of the findings. In any case the biologist and, particularly, the clinician has often to take his material as he finds it and make the best of it that he can, and it is here that the statistician can often make a useful contribution in providing a rational approach to the treatment of variability.

In many peoples minds the suspicion lurks that statistics are an attempt to make bad data into good by mathematical ingenuity. In fact, the approach of the statistician is to isolate the uncontrollable variations and measure them, and to consider the magnitude of any effect being studied in relation to its measured variability. His answer is often in the form of an assessment of "statistical significance". This is an estimate of the probability of the truth of the hypothesis that is being tested and is derived by the statistician from some mathematical model of the test situation. Consider, for example, two treatments being compared on 100 patients each. If on one treatment 90 patients are improved and on the other only 10, most people would agree that, for some reason, one treatment is very probably better than the other. If 47 patients are improved on one and 53 on the other it is likely that there is little or no difference in the effectiveness of the treatments.

The statistician attempts to give a numerical value to this probability of a real difference between the treatments so that experiments in which more doubtful results (e.g. 61 and 55) have been obtained can have an objective measure assigned to the probability of a true difference. The statistical judgment is expressed by saying that if there is no real difference between the treatments then the observed difference would have occurred in some given proportion of similar trials. If for example 90 per cent of trials of two equally effective treatments would have given a difference as large as or larger than that observed then it is probable that no real treatment difference exists. In order to calculate a numerical probability measure the statistician has to construct a mathematical version of the situation and his judgments cannot be valid unless this model is appropriate. It need not be exact any more than the ideal triangles of the geometer need correspond exactly to the real triangles of the surveyor, but it must be reasonably close.

Two points about significance tests, which are often misunderstood need special emphasis. First, there has arisen, through well justified experience, a convention that a result which has only a 5 per cent or 20 to 1 chance or less of having occurred, is "significant" and is said to be "significant at the 5 per cent level". This is purely a convention and has no absolute justification *except* experience. Other levels of significance can be used if the experimenter feels they are more appropriate.

Secondly a "non-significant" result, as usually quoted, according to the above rule, does not necessarily imply that no treatment difference (for example) exists, but that the observations as they stand are compatible with a range of possible differences, one of which is zero. If the control of error is poor or the number of subjects is small the experiment may be compatible also with quite large and practically useful differences. The existence of these can only be confirmed by improving the conduct and design of the experiment or increasing the number of observations, or both, the current results having returned a verdict of "Not Proven".

The idea on which the statistical approach is based and which the statistician uses as a basis for his calculations is that of a distribution. It is meaningless to speak of the "height" of a human population. There is a variety of heights which a human being may have ranging from the unusually short, through a more normal group, to the unusually tall. There is in fact a "distribution" of heights and to give anything like a true picture of the population it is necessary to accompany a statement of the "normal" average, or most usual height by some account of the scatter about the normal. If the curve of the distribution can be given an adequate mathematical expression then all its properties can be summed up in the form of a few, perhaps 2 or 3, numerical constants from which can be calculated for example the fraction of the population with heights between certain limits, or less than a given value. It is one of the most important findings of applied statistics that a comparatively small number of mathematical forms can, for all practical purposes, describe most of the types of variability that are encountered. Given these mathematical expressions it is possible to make an exact approach to the choice of descriptive constants and the derivation of tests of significance.

The applications of statistical method fall broadly into the two categories of description and analysis but there is also a body of experience on statistical inference and experiment arising from practical applications which requires special consideration, and I shall discuss the subject under these three heads.

DESCRIPTIVE STATISTICS

The characterization of a statistical distribution demands, as stated above, at least two measurements, one of which gives some idea of the most typical value of the distribution and the other of the scatter around this typical value. Other properties of the distribution may require specification but they are not usually of great interest to the non-statistician and will not be touched on in this article.

The most widely used, and in many ways the best, "typical measure" is the ordinary *arithmetic mean*. It is easy to compute, readily understood, and has some very desirable properties as a basis for statistical analysis. The disadvantages of the arithmetic arise mainly when the underlying distribution is asymmetrical. If it is symmetrical or nearly so, the mean will be very close to the most frequently observed value and is then a good typical measure. But if the distribution is very asymmetrical and particularly if it has one or two "rogue" outliers a long way from the main body of observations, the mean may

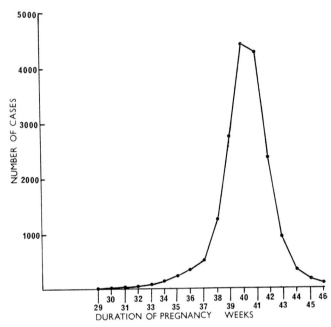

FIG. 1. Duration of pregnancy for 17,708 male births in multiparae (After Timonen, *et al.* Researches performed by the National Board of Health in Finland, No. 5. Helsinki, 1969). The curve is noticeably "skew" with a sharp cut-off at 46 weeks and a long tail extending back to the early weeks of pregnancy.

not be a very typical measure. Very asymmetrical distributions are not uncommon in medicine. The distribution of duration of pregnancy for example has a long "tail" extending back to 4–8 weeks and a comparatively sharp fall off after the 40th week. In this case the arithmetic mean is biassed to short durations and is well away from the most usual duration. If one was concerned with the date of foetal death the situation would be even worse since most deaths probably take place near conception or near delivery and the average date would fall somewhere in between, in a highly untypical position.

To remedy some of these deficiencies various other measures may be used, the most obvious being the *mode* or most frequent value, and the *median*: a value such that

50 per cent of the observations fall above it and 50 per cent below.

The mode has obvious uses when the most common value is overwhelmingly predominant. For example no one would attach much importance to the average number of leaves on a clover plant when the modal value of three is so characteristic.

The median has not such obvious advantages but clearly gives a good idea of the central value of a distribution. Neither of these measures are affected by the presence of a few extreme observations but the median may be affected by asymmetry of the distribution in much the same way as the mean. Neither is so straightforward to calculate as the mean, and neither is satisfactory from the mathematical point of view as a basis for tests of significance.

From the point of view of the non-statistician a graph of the distribution is an indispensable adjunct to the use of any of these measures.

The scatter of a distribution is again capable of description in many ways. The range from the highest to the lowest observation, for example, is a simple index of total spread. Another possibility is the sum of the deviations of each observation from the average, all taken as having a positive sign. Many others have also been proposed such as the range on either side of the mean outside which a given fraction of the observations lie. However, the most generally useful measure has been found to be the *standard deviation*. This is calculated by taking the deviations of the observations from the mean, squaring them, and taking the average of the summed squares. The square root of this average is the standard deviation.[1]

It is difficult to explain in simple terms the reasons for the superiority of the standard deviation over the other measures of scatter. A useful property is that squaring the deviations gets rid of the awkward differences of sign. Higher even powers such as the fourth would also do this but they are much more trouble to calculate and, compared with the simple square, greatly over-emphasize relatively unimportant outlying observations, and random fluctuations. These and other advantages of the square of the standard deviation have proved so valuable in mathematical analysis that it forms the basis of many statistical procedures and has been given the dignity of a special name: the *variance*. (Professor Greenwood once said that this was also a definition of the attitude of one statistician towards another) and it will often be encountered in this form in statistical publications. It is probably sufficient for the non-statistician to regard the variance and standard deviation as the only important measure of scatter.

There remains one other class of descriptive statistics which must be mentioned but cannot be adequately explained in the space available. These are the measures of *association*. They arise from the lack of absolute correspondence between variations of one quantity and that of another when we consider this combined distribution. For example tall men in general tend to have tall wives and short men short wives but the relation is rather a loose one. This is in contrast with many problems in the more exact sciences: for example the increase in length of an iron bar can be very closely predicted from a known increase in temperature.

Probably the most important index to be remembered as a measure of association is the correlation coefficient which is a kind of analogue of the standard deviation in which squaring the deviations is replaced by multiplying and averaging the deviations from their respective means of corresponding variables, e.g. deviation of husbands height from the mean husbands height multiplied by the deviation of his wife's height from wives mean height.[2] For further information the reader must be referred to the literature. Here it is only possible to say that the correlation coefficient is standardized so that it always lies between $+1$ and -1. The former indicates "perfect" association in which increase of one variable accompanies an exactly proportional increase in the other; the latter an inverse but still perfect relationship. Zero indicates no relationship. Intermediate values show varying degrees of association. The situation can be understood more clearly from Figure 2 than from attempts at verbal explanation.

There are many snags and limitations about the use of the correlation coefficient (usually given the symbol "r") and it is mentioned here mainly for completeness as readers may meet it in the literature. An unstandardized form which does not lie between $+1$ and -1 is known as the *Covariance* on the analogy with the variance, discussed above.

ANALYTICAL STATISTICS

It is clearly not possible to give a detailed account of analytical statistics here. It seems worthwhile, however, to discuss briefly an example which may give some idea of the nature of the analytical approach.

Suppose we are testing the response of patients to a drug in comparison to a control group who have had no treatment or a placebo. The results might be set out in a 2×2 table as follows:

	Improved	*Non-improved*	*Total*
Treated Patients	11	3	14
Controls	8	8	16
Totals	19	11	30

---

[1] Mathematically the variance is defined as

$$\text{Variance} = \frac{S(x_i - \bar{x})^2}{n - 1}$$

where S denotes summation, $(x_i - \bar{x})$ is the deviation of the ith observation from the mean $(\bar{x})$, and n is the number of observations. The standard deviation is the square root of the variance.

[2] The mathematical definition of the correlation is

$$r = \frac{S(x_i - \bar{x})(y_i - \bar{y})}{\sqrt{S(x_i - \bar{x})^2 S(y_i - \bar{y})^2}}$$

where $(x_i - \bar{x})$ and $(y_i - \bar{y})$ are deviations of corresponding values of x and y about their means $(\bar{x}, \bar{y})$.

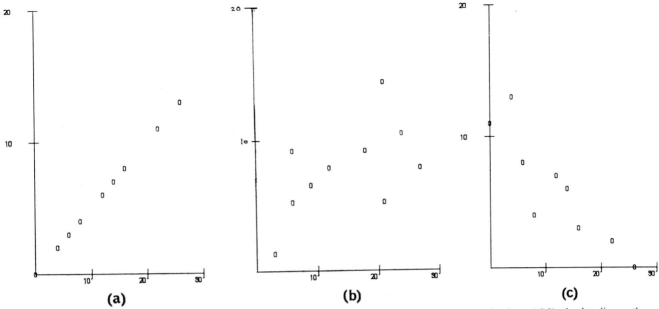

FIG. 2. This figure illustrates the nature of the correlation coefficient. Diagram (a) shows perfect correlation (r = +1·0): the data lie exactly on a straight line. Diagram (b) shows a loose positive correlation (r = +0·56). Diagram (c) shows an example of negative correlation (r = −0·89).

On the face of it the treated patients have done better, but we would not expect the proportions improved in the two groups to be identical even if the treatment was useless and what is required is some test which will tell us how likely the observed results would be if there was really no treatment effect at all. The mathematician can provide such a test given the assumption that there is no effect and that the patients form a homogeneous group unaffected by whether they were chosen to be controls or treated.

What the mathematician does, in effect, is to say: given 14 treated and 16 controls out of which 19 responded and 11 did not, let us vary the entries in the body of the table, in all possible ways, while preserving the marginal totals (14, 16, 19 and 11). Some of these ways will show an advantage for the treated patients and some will not, but if the treatments are equally effective large apparent improvements or non-improvements in the two treatment groups will be rare. Tables can then be calculated which specify the rarity of the observed result in numerical terms, on the assumption that there is no real difference between the treatments, the true proportion improved being the same for each and approximated by the overall totals as about 19:11.

In the present case the mathematical model is simple and reasonable (though its validity is not universal and others have been proposed). In more complicated cases the models are correspondingly more elaborate and the assumptions necessary to make them mathematically tractable may be rather suspect. Only experience and detailed mathematical analysis can bring to light the virtues and limitations of a statistical technique.[3]

[3] Generally speaking results of this kind which compare frequency of response to different treatments are examined by a statistical procedure known as the χ^2 test. This measures the deviations of the observations from the values they would be expected to take on the basis of some hypothesis: e.g. that there is no treatment effect.

Fortunately most of the tests in common use appear to be remarkably "robust" (to use G. E. P. Box's term) and their practical application is comparatively unaffected by the approximations and assumptions on which they are based. Only practical experience ultimately justifies the use of statistical methods, and it should be emphasized that the demonstration of their robustness rests as much on the fact that they have not apparently led anyone seriously astray in practice as on mathematical theory.

STATISTICAL INFERENCE AND EXPERIMENT

We have so far discussed mainly the theoretical background of statistical techniques. Their application in a medical context has led to some important general principles and has also emphasised the difficulties that arise from the nature of medical practice.

A good deal of the usefulness of statistics arises from the fact that the behaviour of populations or aggregates is often much more predictable than that of the individuals that compose them. This is in many ways alien to the attitude of the doctor who prefers to regard each patient as an individual to be treated on his merits as a particular

The χ^2 test is not confined to simple two-way tables but can be used to compare, for example, a number of treatments to which subjects may respond in several ways such as "no response", "improved", "much improved", "cured".

Formally, χ^2 is defined as:

$$\chi^2 = S\left[\frac{(\text{Observed} - \text{Expected})^2}{\text{Expected}}\right]$$

where S denotes summation over all categories of the table, "Observed" is the actual number of observations in a category and "Expected" is the number calculated on some hypothesis as expected to be there.

problem. The mechanical application of a statistically derived rule on the grounds that it works out for the best in a majority of cases is distasteful and may account for some of the resistance to statistical methods in the medical profession. However, in the last twenty years or so the statistically controlled trial has shown itself such a valuable tool that a discussion of its basic principles is essential in any account of medical statistics however brief.

The underlying ideas of the clinical trial are essentially simple and consist mainly of eliminating, so far as possible, the effects of bias and preconception in the observers and the patients and providing a valid test of statistical significance for the results. The first of these is not intrinsically a statistical question but statisticians probably have more experience of it than most scientists as the commonest misuse of statistics is to select from a population the cases which support a hypothesis and quietly discard the rest. The practice is, of course, by no means confined to medicine and may, in some circumstances lead to correct inferences. For example, Sir Ronald Fisher once produced evidence that the experimental results which Mendel published were almost certainly selected to demonstrate most conclusively the correctness of his hypothesis. Such a process may be justifiable in the case of a Mendel but is highly dangerous for the ordinary mortal. In medicine the pressure for a solution, that is an effective treatment, is so great that the temptation to seize on an interesting new idea ahead of the evidence has to be resisted with particular firmness.

The principle that is adopted in planning a clinical trial is therefore to define the population under study and its varieties and subdivisions as clearly as possible *before* the experiment and then ensure by some objective randomizing process that the experimental population is as alike as possible to the control in all relevant, or supposedly relevant, subdivisions. As a simple example the comparison between two treatments might be made by choosing pairs of patients alike in such thing as age, sex, place of residence and social class and then deciding which treatment each gets by tossing a coin. More elaborate experiments require more elaborate random selection procedures and extensive tables now exist of random numbers and permutations of numbers for this purpose.

A further precaution which has been found almost essential wherever it can be applied is to conceal the nature of the treatment from both the doctor and the patient. This is clearly impossible in all experiments for example those in surgical treatment or with dangerous drugs where the physician must be ready to deal with side effects, but should be applied wherever possible. I would add that it is also wise in many cases to extend it to the statistician during his analysis if there is any danger of subjective elements creeping into it.

Some of these principles have been recognized fairly explicitly for over 50 years and in occasional instances for much longer; for example Fibiger conducted a trial of diphtheria antitoxin in 1898 which would have satisfied modern criteria and even earlier examples can be cited. More recently it was pointed out by Sir Ronald Fisher that, besides its value in eliminating subjective bias, randomisation is the essential mathematical basis for providing valid tests of significance by which to assess the results.

The main criticisms of clinical trials arise more from the difficulties of medical experiment as a whole than from any logical flaw in their structure. Many of the ethical objections that arise would apply equally or more strongly to less rigorous alternatives. The use of randomization procedures may appear to introduce the atmosphere of the gambling saloon into medicine but is really a reflection of the fact that medical experiment, like gambling, is often of an essentially statistical nature and the choice confronting the physician is not between a statistical and a non-statistical approach but between the use of good and bad statistics.

The clinical trial in its classical form has been objected to on the grounds that it requires the experiment to be carried to its bitter end even if it becomes obvious at an early stage that one or more of the treatments is manifestly superior or harmful. Such impressions should always be regarded with suspicion but may well be justified. Statistical theory has provided a partial answer to this problem, in some cases, in the form of what are called *Sequential Trials*. These allow the trial to be discontinued at the earliest moment at which a judgment can be objectively formed. They also have the advantage that the analysis and arithmetic can be done in graphical form without elaborate calculation. A simple example of such a trial is the comparison of two treatments which are administered at random to pairs of patients matched for their relevant characteristics. If both treatments fail or both succeed the results are ignored, but if one fails and the other succeeds the successful treatment is given a score which is added cumulatively during the trial. This cumulative score can be plotted graphically on paper on which are drawn boundary lines provided by the statistician. The positions of these boundary lines are determined by the size of treatment difference it is practicable to detect and the risks which can be accepted of the consequences of a wrong decision. When the cumulative score crosses one of the boundaries the corresponding treatment is taken as the better and the experiment is terminated.

The main disadvantages of this type of trial are that it may give a very poor estimate of how good the better treatment is, and that appropriate designs exist for only a rather simple and limited variety of experiments. In addition some designs permit the unlikely but possible occurrence of very long drawn out experiments as the sample size is not fixed in advance. This can be avoided by the use of fixed sample size designs at the expense of sometimes coming to a "don't know" decision—which may, of course, be an entirely reasonable conclusion. In view of their limitations it is not advisable for the non-statistician to use sequential methods uncritically and without advice from a statistician, but in appropriate circumstances they can be a very valuable and economical type of experiment.

The clinical trial is a rigorous and well founded statistical tool, but it can only be used in circumstances where the experimenter has fairly full control over the patient, and his environment. It is, however, an essential part of medical research to evaluate the aetiological factors of disease and, except in very special cases where volunteers can be used, it is not possible to use techniques such as random allotment, that have been successful in clinical trials. Most aetiological studies must be done retrospectively and in nearly all of them the control group has to be selected on grounds that are plausible rather than rigorous. The result of this is that the grounds for inference are much more uncertain than in the clinical trial, and the statistical techniques less firmly based.

An outstanding example of the difficulties that arise in this field is provided by the intense controversy that has been aroused by studies on the aetiology of lung cancer. In obstetrics a similar example is provided by the influence of the mother's smoking habits on the birth weight of her child. It has been shown that the children of mothers who smoke during pregnancy tend to have lower birth weights than those of non-smoking mothers. Statistical theory is of use here in demonstrating that the differences in birth weight are most unlikely to have arisen by chance. It cannot however give any information as to whether the differences are necessarily due to associated differences in the smoking habits of the mothers. Only the medical and biological worker viewing the evidence as a whole can decide whether it is satisfactory to him or not. In the present example it is clear that the non-smoker may be a very different person from the heavy smoker, and even the smoker who could give up different from the one who cannot. Unless the controls are a reliable counterpart to the affected cases no amount of statistical significance testing alone can demonstrate *causal* associations.

In gynaecology very complex problems of the same kind have arisen in attempts to determine the aetiology of carcinoma of the cervix. By comparing patients with cervical carcinoma with control cases various factors such as fertility, marital status, age at first sexual intercourse, social class, and religious denomination have been shown to differ between cases and controls. Some of the factors are themselves related to one another in a complex manner. Once again the controls cannot be regarded in the same way as those in a properly randomized experiment, and it must be realized that this situation, where strictly controlled experiments cannot be carried out on human beings, is intrinsic in much medical research and will be repeatedly encountered in the future. It should be clearly recognized that the limitations are not so much those of statistical method as of clinical experimentation.

REFERENCES

The number of elementary textbooks on statistical methods is legion and it would be invidious to pick out any particular one. As an introductory text, however, Sir Austin Bradford Hill's "Principles of Medical Statistics" remains unchallenged for the medical worker. Sir Ronald Fisher's works, though fundamental, are largely unintelligible to the medical reader, but Chapters 1–3 of "The Design of Experiments" will repay serious study. The other books cited below have been chosen as being useful and relatively non-technical introductory texts.

Armitage, P. (1960), "Sequential Analysis." Oxford: Blackwell Scientific Publications.

Cox, D. R. (1967), "The Planning of Experiments." New York: John Wiley and Son, (Paperback).

Finney, D. J. (1955), "Experimental Design and its Statistical Basis." Chicago: Chicago University Press.

Fisher, Sir Ronald A. (1966), "The Design of Experiments." Edinburgh: Oliver and Boyd, (Paperback).

Hill, Sir Austin Bradford (1966), "Principles of Medical Statistics." *The Lancet*, London.

Witts, L. J. (Ed.) (1959), "Medical Surveys and Clinical Trials." London: Oxford University Press.

5. ULTRASONICS

C. N. SMYTH

Introduction

The principal application of ultrasound is to diagnosis, and the pulse-echo Sonar, or Radar like, range finding technique is used for the delineation of structures while the continuous-wave Doppler principle is used for foetal heart-rate observation and blood-flow measurement. Ultrasound is used at high intensity for cleaning instruments and occasionally for sterilization.

Therapeutic applications are rarely encountered in the gynaecological patient and would be ill advised in the pregnant patient. Some methods from other branches of medicine are included here to illustrate the possibilities.

In several countries the use of ultrasonic agitation to augment radiotherapy in the treatment of malignant disease is receiving research attention.

The pulse-echo diagnostic method with cathode-ray tube visualization and photographic recording has three main forms of use. (In more elaborate equipments storage tubes or "memotron" cathode-ray tubes are used so that the final image can be seen in its entirety before it is photographed.)

1. "A" scan in which the sound beam is fixed in direction and the returning echoes are displayed against time (=distance) in a graph with echo amplitude as ordinate (Fig. 1).

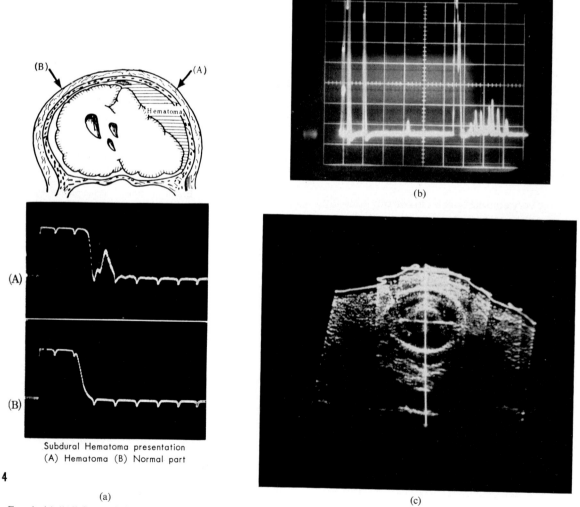

Subdural Hematoma presentation
(A) Hematoma (B) Normal part

(a)

(b)

(c)

FIG. 1. (a) "A" Scans. Subdural haematoma (*courtesy of Japan Radio Co. Ltd.*). (b) Fetal cephalometry (*courtesy of Mr. E. I. Kohorn*). A, Scan only; P, proximal echo from foetal head; D, distal echo from foetal head; M, midline echo; U, echo from posterior wall of uterus. (c) Transverse suprapubic scan of foetal head showing mid-line echo pattern. Measurement of the biparietal diameter is taken at right angles to the mid-lines (*courtesy of Professor Ian Donald, University of Glasgow*).

2. "B" scan in which again the beam direction is fixed but the echoes are displayed as light intensity modulation of the cathode-ray tube screen. Time is abcissa and the ordinate is a slow time scale so that successive observations in a rapid time sequence are displayed one beneath the other. In this way the excursion of moving structures can be measured (Fig. 2). A new name for this is T.P. mode (time position).

injection of air or contrast medium is necessary to delineate tissue planes, and pictures (Sonograms) can be made by doctors or clinicians with very little training and interpreted with practice. The equipments are costly, as costly as X-ray installations, but are now commercially available in several countries, Donald (1958–67), Holmes (1954), Kossoff (1964), Siemens (1969), Kretz (1969).

The resolution of fine structure obtainable by ultra-

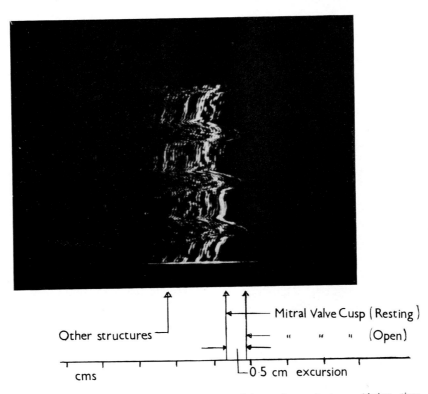

FIG. 2. "B" Scan. Movements of mitral valve and deeper heart structures. Abcissa, time base proportional to depth. (Time scale—15 microseconds/cm). Ordinate, time base 1 cm/second. Pulse repetition frequency—300/second (*courtesy of Mr. R. J. Blackwell*).

3. "C" or compound B scanning uses light intensity modulation but the position and direction of the abcissa moves on the surface of the cathode-ray tube in sympathy with the position and direction of the examining probe. This method builds up a plan of the structures producing echoes (Fig. 3). There are variations of the method depending on whether the beam moves in orthogonal co-ordinates only or rocks as well in order to obtain normal incidence with as many underlying structures as possible.

In some equipments the sound emitting probe makes direct contact with the body surface while in others a tank, or bag of water, is interposed to improve automation and delay multiple echoes beyond the picture range (Fig. 10).

Clinical Considerations

Ultrasonics by the pulse-echo, Sonar, method is now being widely applied to diagnosis especially for obstetrics and gynaecological tumours. The method is to soft tissues what X-rays are to hard tissues and bone. With Sonar no

sonics is very much inferior to that obtainable from X-rays. Theoretically the resolution is 1,000 times worse because ultrasonic waves have a wavelength of 0·1 to 1·0 mm. depending on the frequency used. The resolution available in radiology is measured in ångström units and seldom necessary for diagnosis, so in fact the apparent limitation in Sonar is not so consequential.

In practice with water immersion of the subject as practised in Australia, Robinson (1967), and America, Thompson (1967) the 2 MHz resolution is of the order of 2·5 mm. and by contact scanning of the order of 4·0 mm. These figures are worse than the wavelength limitation for the reasons given in the technical section, Kossoff (1964).

Diagnosis depends on the following information provided by several Sonograms; in difficult problems as many as 9 pictures may be required from each patient.

1. The shape and size of tissue boundaries.
2. Distortion of organs, e.g.: Bladder or Uterus.
3. The sonic transparency of the contents of organs or cysts or growths.

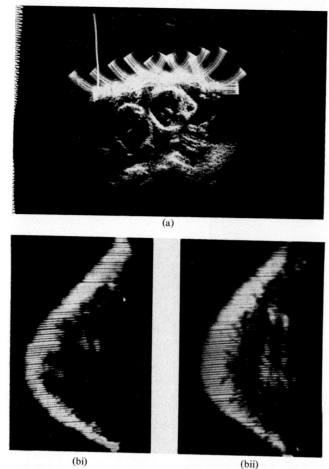

(a)

(bi)   (bii)

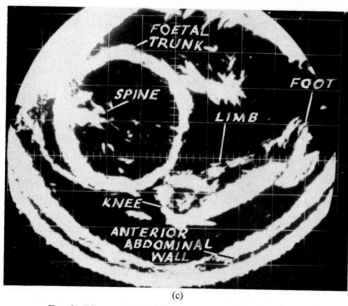

(c)

FIG. 3. "Compound or 'C'" Scan. (a) Transverse section through twins at head level. $2\frac{1}{2}$ MHz—(*courtesy of Mr. E. I. Kohorn.* (b) Fibroadenoma of breast—(*courtesy of Japan Radio Co. Ltd.*). (i) normal, (ii) tumour. (c) Foetal Section—(*courtesy of Commonwealth Acoustic Laboratories, Sydney, D. E. Robinson*). (a) Was obtained by contact scanning with olive oil as the coupling liquid film. (b) and (c) were obtained by the water immersion method in which the water bath is separated from the patient by a "rho-c" rubber membrane.

4. The variation of "transparency" (Trans-sonicity) at different frequencies of ultrasound.

5. The degree of insonation necessary to make echoes from within the uterus or a cyst visible.

6. Pulsation or respiratory movement of echoes.

For example, the uterus might be seen to be larger than normal and to have a cavity filled with trans-sonic liquid when examined at 1·5 MHz. When examined at higher gain there might be the suspicion of a small foetus and the suggestion of hydramnios. On repeating the examination at 2·5 MHz and high gain, the cavity is seen to be filled with small flecks. At this frequency and low gain the organ appears relatively opaque and the deep parieties cannot be visualized. The correct diagnosis is hydatidiform mole (Fig. 4).

Fibroids are transsonic at 1 MHz and relatively opaque at 5 MHz. Cancellous bone is very opaque to ultrasound above 1 MHz.

To make many diagnoses the exactness of the dimensions of the picture are not important and low resolution is acceptable. For measurements of head size, week-by-week foetal growth, or baby weight from the area of multiple sections, or to recognize spina bifida or other gross congenital abnormalities, the highest definition is desirable.

There are techniques of scanning deep in the body by passing small probes into the organs through blood vessels. The adult heart can be scanned through the femoral vein. The uterus and foetus can be examined through the cervix and probes can readily be passed into the bladder. These techniques overcome the difficulty of surface reflections and multiple echoes in the sub-cutaneous layers which obscure certain investigations, Kimoto (1964), Pell (1964).

PRINCIPAL APPLICATIONS

A. Gynaecological and Obstetric

Non Pregnant Uterus: Fibroids and differentiation from carcinoma and ovarian cysts. (Donald, 1966)

Early Pregnancy: Pregnancy, multiple pregnancy, mole. Incomplete abortion 6 weeks gestation onwards. Results speculative before 7 weeks. (MacVicar, 1963)

Late Pregnancy: Cross-sections of trunk and head for foetal size. Determination of head orientation and axis for biparietal head size and growth rate measurements. Gross congenital deformities. Spaldings sign in intrauterine death. (Willocks, 1964, Thompson, 1965)

Labour: Head size, orientation and disproportion. (Robinson, 1967)

Placenta: Site from 10 weeks to term, placental size from multiple sections. (Kohorn, 1968)

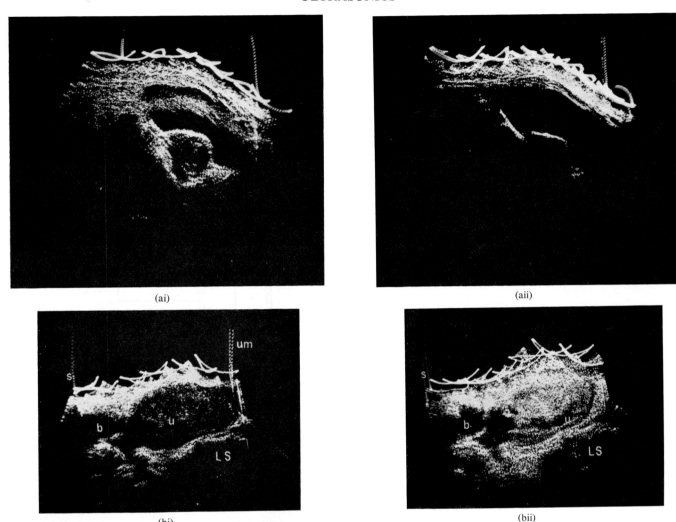

(ai)

(aii)

(bi)

(bii)

FIG. 4. "Compound Scans". (a) Fibroid at 2·5 MHz (i) and 5·0 MHz (ii) inspection frequencies and comparable apparatus sensitivity. Longitudinal section through full bladder. Dotted line marks symphysis pubis. (*courtesy of Professor Ian Donald, University of Glasgow*). (b) Hydatidiform mole at 2·5 MHz and two gain or sensitivity adjustments. (i) —35 db. (ii) —20 db. S, symphysis pubis; um, umbilicus; b, full bladder; u, uterus; LS, longitudinal section (*courtesy of Mr. E. I. Kohorn and Mr. R. J. Blackwell*).

Foetus:	Recognition of falx, orbits, foramen magnum. Foetal death is only recognizable by loss of pulsating echo from foetal heart. (This is easier to recognize by the Doppler effect instrument, vide page 698 Electronics) than by the pulse-echo technique. (Robinson, 1967)
Neonate:	Detection of head injury, subdural haemorrhage by "A" scope or Compound scanning recognition of mid-line shift. (Gordon, 1964)
Maturity:	Increasing opacity of foetal skull bone.

B. Non Obstetric or Gynaecological

Liver:	Growths, cysts, sclerosis. (Donald, 1966. Wells, 1967.)

Heart:	Tumours and carcinomata (McCarthy, 1967. Wells, 1968.) Dimensions and valve movements. (Hertz, 1964 and 1965, Edler, 1965.)
Head:	Tumours, traumatic damage. (Grossman, 1965.)
Breast:	Tumours and carcinomata. (Wells, 1968.)

Other Diagnostic Techniques

The pulse-echo method by "A" or by "Compound" scanning can be supplemented by "B" scanning for visualizing the extent of movement of heart-walls or valves. The method is to display "A" scan traces of the moving tissue boundaries repetitively below one another so that the moving boundaries form a time graph as shown in Fig. 2, Edler (1965).

With collimated probes the transmission of ultrasound through the body in a chosen direction can be recorded

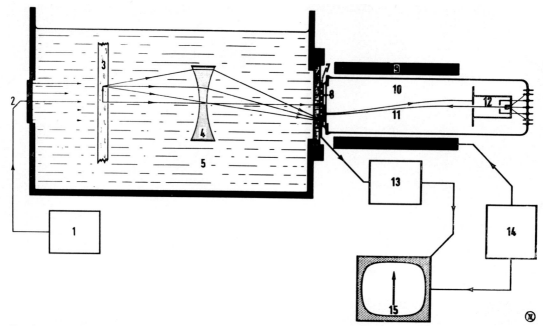

FIG. 5. Ultrasound image camera. (1) 4 MHz oscillator; (2) ultra-sound transmitter; (3) material under inspection; (4) acoustic lens; (5) water; (6) oil contained by metallized plastic film; (7) signal plate; (8) quartz plate; (9) deflection and focus coils; (10) ultrasound camera tube; (11) electron beam; (12) electron gun; (13) video-frequency amplifier; (14) deflection generator; (15) image of defect in material. (*Reproduced by permission of the Editor of the Proceedings of the Institution of Electrical Engineers*).

and the absorption or scattering measured at select frequencies. The method has been used to observe temperature differences in the brain, and to study the nature of tumours. There is a possible application to the detection of intracranial haemorrhage in the newborn (Fig. 1).

Sound-fields can be registered as pictures by several techniques, for example photographic development is accelerated by agitating the developer and uniformly exposed light sensitive plates (in contact with jelly-base developer) will develop in relation to ultrasonic insonation. The method is however insensitive and requires several milliwatts of power per cm.², Rust (1949). A more sensitive method is to make a television camera with a piezo-electric end-plate in place of the usual photo-electric face-plate, Fig. 5. Ultrasound at 4 MHz has a wavelength in water of 0·025 cm. and such short waves can be focussed by plastic lenses if source, object and lens are immersed in water, or another suitable medium, to match the body, Tarnoczy (1965). Fig. 6 is an example of this technique, Sokolov (1949), Smyth (1963), Jacobs (1965), Turner (1965). The method is very sensitive, about 10^{-7} watts/cm.², and provides the best resolution possible, namely that comparable with one wavelength. Pictures can be made in 0·02 sec. Unfortunately the camera tubes are small and a single picture is at present limited to about 4 sq. cms. of body surface.

Ultrasonic holograms, Gabor (1948 and 1966) can be made by visualizing or scanning the ultrasound field from two interfering ultra-sound beams, one of which has passed through the body, Gregus (1966), Halstead (1968).*

* Also, (Fishlock, 1966); (Mueller, 1966); (Preston, 1967); (Metherell 1967).

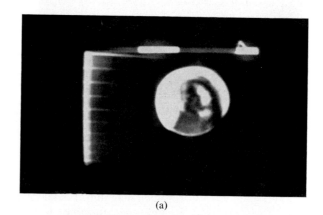

(a)

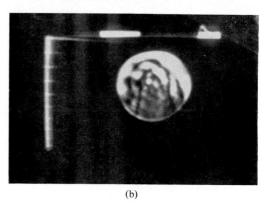

(b)

FIG. 6. Ultrasonic-camera picture of tip of thumb *continuous wave technique*. (*a*) reflection; (*b*) transmission. (*Reproduced by permission of the Editor of the Proceedings of the Institution of Electrical Engineers*).

The ultra-sound camera makes this process practicable and may provide a "3D" view of internal organs. At present the technique is limited to research projects.

With the advent of colour television displays, the ultrasonic properties of tissues at different frequencies or at different velocities can be reproduced as a colour picture. Jacobs has described a view of the hand in which the blood vessels are white and scintillating while the stationary tissues have a fixed colour, Jacobs (1967).

Blood-flow in accessible vessels has been measured by pulse delay measurements up-stream and down-stream, or by the Doppler frequency shift method, Franklin (1966). Where the vessel can only be inspected from a distance the velocity profile can be determined from the Doppler frequency shift spectrum and changes in flow recorded. The measurement of absolute flow in remote vessels

requires a knowledge of the vessel diameter, of its angle to the inspecting ultrasonic beam and of the viscosity of the blood in the particular patient. At best the answer is approximate, Stone (1967).

Therapeutic Applications and Safety

In surgery intense ultrasound (20–250 watts/cm.²) has been used to control Meniére's Disease, Bullen (1963), and to relieve Parkinsonian tremor and ablate neoplasms, Lele (1962).

Research presently in progress in several countries is showing that for certain types of malignant cell ultrasonic agitation can assist the destruction of the tissue by radio-therapy, Woeber (1965).

Ultrasonic cleaning is used in many hospitals for cleaning instruments, Crawford (1963). It has also been

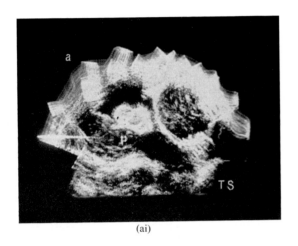

(ai)

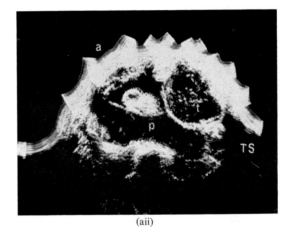

(aii)

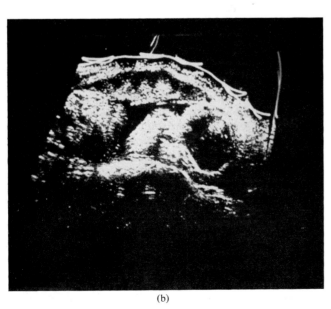

(b)

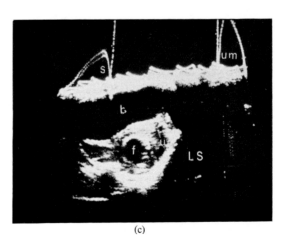

(c)

FIG. 7. (a) Placentography (i) and (ii). Transverse scan of abdomen 2 cm above the umbilicus demonstrating the placenta (p) which is clearer at low gain. (ii.) a, anterior abdominal wall; t, transverse scan of foetal trunk (*courtesy of Mr. E. I. Kohorn and Mr. R. J. Blackwell*). (b) Placentography. Upper anterior placenta. Vertical marks on skin surface indicate position of umbilicus and top of symphysis pubis. Longitudinal scan in mid-line. (*Reproduced by courtesy of Professor Ian Donald, University of Glasgow*). (c) 9 week foetus demonstrating conceptus (f) in uterus (u). Longitudinal scan. s, symphysis; um, umbilicus; b, full bladder; (*by courtesy of Mr. E. I. Kohorn and Mr. R. J. Blackwell*).

TABLE 1

CHARACTERISTICS OF ULTRASONIC VIBRATIONS IN WATER

Intensity	Frequency	Amplitude of Vibration	Acceleration	Velocity
1 watt/cm.^{2} = 10^4 w./m.^{2}	30·0 MHz	4·0 . 10^{-4} Microns or 4 Angstrom Units	1·6 Million "G"	
1 watt/cm.^{2} = 10^4 w./m.^{2}	5·0 MHz	24·0 . 10^{-10} Metres	0·26 Million "G"	
1 watt/cm.^{2} = 10^4 w./m.^{2}	2·5 MHz	48·0 . 10^{-10} Metres	0·13 Million "G"	81 mm./sec.
1 watt/cm.^{2} = 10^4 w./m.^{2}	1·0 MHz	120·0 . 10^{-10} Metres	0·052 Million "G"	
10 milliwatts/cm.^{2} = 100 w./m.^{2}	30·0 MHz	0·4 . 10^{-10} Metres	0·16 Million "G"	
10 milliwatts/cm.^{2} = 100 w./m.^{2}	5·0 MHz	2·4 . 10^{-10} Metres = Diameter of Hydrogen atom	0·026 Million "G"	8·1 mm./sec.
10 milliwatts/cm.^{2} = 100 w./m.^{2}	2·5 MHz	4·8 . 10^{-10} Metres	13,000 "G"	
10 milliwatts/cm.^{2} = 100 w./m.^{2}	1·0 MHz	12·0 . 10^{-10} Metres	5200 "G"	

used to sterilize fluids, particularly milk, but it is an expensive and uncertain method and may not break up viruses or spores.

Ultrasound is used in physical medicine for the treatment of arthritic conditions and for softening post-operative keloid and fibrous tissue in Dupuytren's contracture. These indications point to applications in gynaecological surgery, or for the relief of dysmenorrhoea, Summer (1963).

Its use for dissolving stones has been reported, Knight (1963), but investigation of its value in accelerating the dissolution of thrombi is negative. Low intensity ultrasound has been shown experimentally to promote healing (Dyson *et al.*, 1968).

Ultrasound acts by producing focused heat and by producing extreme accelerations, up to 1,000,000 G!, which lead to cavitation. Cavitation arises at high sound intensities when the accelerations produce negative intramolecular pressures and release gases from solution. When the minute bubbles formed collapse again intense shock waves are set up which have a disrupting effect on weak bonds, loosen dirt and break up bacteria, Antony (1963), Table 1.

Table 1 tabulates the particle displacements, velocities and accelerations for water molecules vibrating at ultrasonic frequencies. It may give the impression that considerable disruptive forces are present, but this is not in fact the case. The accelerations and peak velocities are transient and exist only for millionths of a second and are negligible in comparison with thermal motions. The thermal energy of a particle at temperature T is $\frac{1}{2} KT$ where K is Boltzman's constant (1·38 × 10^{-23} joule/°C). For a hydrogen atom this is 1,550 metres/sec. and for the heavier water molecule, 364 metres/sec. If one water molecule collides and reverses direction in a millionth of a second, the acceleration would be 1·2.10^9 times gravity. Against this the figures of Table 1 are negligible.

The kinetic energy of the particle movements, $\frac{1}{2} mV^2$, can be taken as a measure of the power for destruction and is often measured in electron volts, (i.e. the energy to transfer one electron through a potential change of one volt). Thermal energies necessary to achieve changes in

molecular arrangements are of the order of one electron volt. Thermal energies at room temperature are about 1/40th of an electron volt. Ultrasonic energies at 1 watt per cm.^{2} in the frequencies quoted in Table 1 are from 10^{-9} to 10^{-8} electron volts.

Sound and ultrasound exert a static force on surfaces against which they are reflected. The force varies with the reflection coefficient and is maximal at 100 per cent reflection where the pressure is given by the formula:

Force,* (Newtons/metre^2) = 2. Sound intensity (watts/cm.^{2}) ÷ velocity of propagation (metres/sec.).

This pressure can lead to the migration of particles distributed in liquid suspension and may lead to streaming and migration of intracellular bodies with some disruption of cell function. Such movements could occur at low powers where the ordered effect of coherent ultrasonic vibrations act in one direction and are more effective than the larger random forces due to thermal agitation. The subject has been studied by Hughes (1965).

Ultrasound increases the absorption of unguents, promotes growth, Gordon (1965), (at least in vegetables), softens mucus and other polymers, prevents barnacles adhering to ships and has a thousand other effects. These qualities are mentioned not for their direct relevance but because a knowledge of general effects may stimulate new lines of enquiry. It may also increase healing rates (Dyson *et al.*, 1968).

The intensity of insonation involved in diagnostic techniques is very low compared with the intensities necessary to produce the therapeutic effects.

The effects of ultrasound are not cumulative as radiation doses are, because with ultrasound we are dealing with a transient state of matter which disappears on the cessation of insonation. With radiation each particle is of high energy and the danger arises from the increasing probability of a direct hit or mutation as the total life dose increases.

Various workers have studied the biological effects of ultrasound and no teratogenic effects have been reported

* See next chapter, Electronics and Clinical Measurements, for reference to SI units.

under 10 watts/cm.², (Acoustic Society, Reference 3), Murray Smyth (1965), Hughes (1965), Knight (1968), Lele (1962) and Garg (1967).

The intensities of ultrasound used in diagnosis are of the order of 30 milliwatts/cm.² in the Doppler method, and in the pulse-echo method, 1 watt/cm.² peak or 1 mW/cm.² mean values. There are no reported cases of suspected damage to patients or the early foetus, although pioneers of the subject have been at pains to notice any untoward effects.

Methods of measuring ultrasonic intensities have been described by Mikhailov (1964), Brown (1967) and Stephens (1966).

Technical Considerations

Ultrasonic waves are sound-waves but of supra-audible frequency. They are organized movement or vibrations of matter at atomic dimensions and are propagated by a disturbance of the intra-atomic electric forces which link molecules in solids and liquids and operate in gases when near collisions occur. The qualities of a material to transmit ultrasound depend on density and elasticity.

In gases and liquids only compressional waves are propagated, but in solids and gels the particle displacement may be across the direction of wave propagation and give rise to two types of wave with different velocities and directions with respect to the source.

Ripple waves can be propagated at the interfaces and surfaces of a solid or liquid and these again have a velocity which is slow and peculiar to the material, Stephens (1966).

Medical diagnostic applications are limited to the use of compressional waves which in saline at body temperature have a velocity of 1,500 metres/sec. Where the waves enter solid matter other forms of wave motion may be excited and give rise to echoes of a confusing nature. These adverse effects are particularly noticeable when the wave enters the material obliquely and for this reason the tissues are examined orthogonally in most applications.

TABLE 2

RELATION BETWEEN FREQUENCY AND WAVELENGTH FOR SALINE, ULTRASOUND VELOCITY 1500 METRES/SECOND
(velocity = frequency × wavelength)

Frequency	Wavelength	
0·5 MHz	3·0 mm.	
1·0	1·5	
2·5	0·6	
5·0	0·3	
10·0	0·15	
30·0	0·05	
300·0	5 microns	1 micron = 10^{-6} metre
3000·0	0·5 microns = wavelength of visible light	

For compressional waves the relation between wavelength and frequency is shown in Table 2. At millimetre wavelengths the sound waves are diffracted at discontinuities, and where there is a change of material. They are reflected from plane surfaces as light waves would be. Waves are scattered by irregularities of structure which are large compared with a wavelength, but small surface changes such as cellular structure are too small and provide a specular mirror-like surface. Cells have little effect up to 5 MHz but at frequencies above this the sound is scattered and lost to an increasing extent. The clear fluid of the eye enables frequencies of up to 20 MHz to be used, Baum (1968). The lung on the other hand is opaque to frequencies above 1 MHz, because of the air content.

The sound waves in the front of a flat transmitter vary in intensity for some distance in a rhythmical pattern due to the interfering effects of waves from different parts of the crystal surface. This zone, called the Fresnel zone or "near field", extends until there is less than half a wavelength path difference between a point on the axis and any part of the crystal; beyond this distance the field is graded but ripple free (Fig. 8) Table 3 gives the dimensions for different crystal diameters and wavelengths, Kossoff (1964). The effect is reduced for short pulses due to the presence of many odd harmonics.

Attempts to explore the echo capabilities of the body with such a probe in the near field region is therefore beset with limitations, Hodgkinson (1966), and as the probe is moved one reflecting point may appear as a line or succession of dots. If the probe is not flat but focused by a converging lens in front of the crystal, or by using a hollow ground crystal, the field can be concentrated to a point at one particular range. (The range can be varied by the use of variable power, liquid-filled, plastic lenses under variable pressure.)

Between the crystal and the reflecting layer in the body and between different parallel layers in the tissue planes, multiple echoes may be formed and these return to be received in an indistinguishable and inextricable mixture. With such difficulties it is remarkable that ultrasonics aids visualization at all, but it does. The definition can be improved if separate transducers are used for transmitting and receiving with a small area of overlap as drawn in Fig. 9. This is sometimes called the "split beam" method and was used in radar to give angular discrimination. The timing of echoes is a measure of the distance of a reflecting surface below the probe, or would be if the sound had the same velocity in all tissues, if the beam went in a straight line and was not refracted to a bent path, and if the force of application did not disturb the resting position of the internal parts.

Movement of the parts can be overcome by the use of a water-filled balloon to separate the patient from the probe. The method also reduces multiple echoes by delaying the second echo off the picture. Water immersion techniques add to the picture definition but increase the inconvenience of the method for the patient. The water bath may only contact the patient through a thin "ρc" rubber membrane.

Contact probes are easier and speedier to use and are the method currently in use in hospitals in the U.K.

Scanning procedures are a matter of experience combined with a knowledge of the characteristics of a particular machine. The probes must be well coupled to the surface with oil or jelly to maintain an air free space, and the maximum angulation to the surface for clear echoes, determined by experiment and the speed of scanning and the ratio of angulations to lateral displacement adjusted

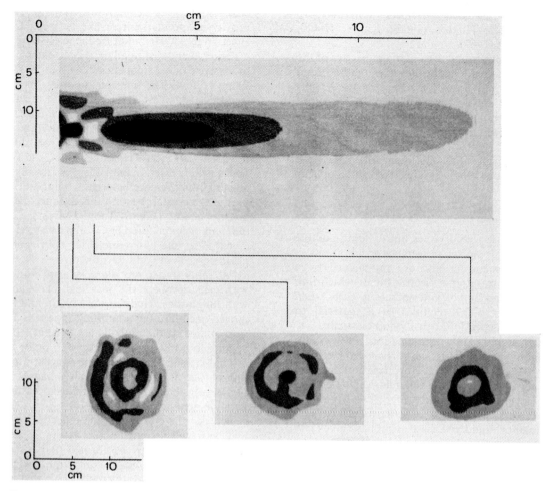

Fig. 8. Longitudinal section and 3 cross sections of "Iso-sonogram" of ultrasonic probe, pulse operation at 1 MHz (*courtesy of W. L. Hodgkinson, U.K. Atomic Energy Authority, Didcot, Berkshire, England*).

TABLE 3

The Far or Uniform field extends beyond $3\cdot14\ a^2/L$ where L is the wavelength and a the radius of a plane circular transmitter. The angle of the probe given defines the angle from the axis for half power, 3 db. attenuation, in the far field region.

Probe Diameter	1 MHz.		2 MHz.		5 MHz.	
	Distance	*Angle*	*Distance*	*Angle*	*Distance*	*Angle*
3 mm.	4·7 mm.	11°33′	9·4 mm.	5°45′	23·00 mm.	2°18′
5 mm.	13·0 mm.	6°54′	26·0 mm.	3°27′	65·00 mm.	1°23′
10 mm.	54·0 mm.	3°27′	104·0 mm.	1°44′	270·00 mm.	0°44′
15 mm.	117·0 mm.	2°18′	335·0 mm.	1°9′	580·00 mm.	0°28′
25 mm.	327·0 mm.	1°23′	654·0 mm.	0°44′	1·63 m.	0°17′

to suit the depths of the structure being investigated. The maximum pulse repetition rate is about 1,000 scans per second (each echo-train occupies about a millisecond). The placenta requires long sweeps across the surface with little angular change. The foetal head on the other hand reflects waves of normal incidence and the probe angulation must repeatedly sweep through normal incidence as the lateral or longitudinal traverse is made (Fig. 7).

The "swept gain" control which is provided to increase sensitivity for echoes of greater range and so to overcome the attenuation of deep echoes, has to be adjusted for the best results with certain types of dense tumour or unusually trans-sonic cysts.

For foetal growth measurements the bi-parietal diameter is most accurately measured by "A" scan techniques with an independent precision double-pulse timing unit to mark and identify the scalp echoes and measure the distance between them. Even with this refinement the results are only correct on 70 per cent of patients unless the foetus is first examined by compound scanning to elicit the correct orientations for the biparietal measurement.

When a sound wave impinges on an interface between two materials, some of the sound is transmitted through and some is reflected back. The proportion reflected

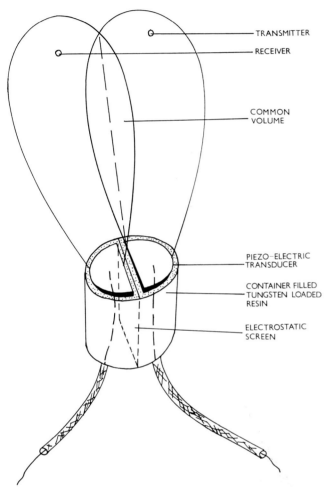

FIG. 9. Principle of the split beam highly directional probe.

depends on the changes in density and elasticity encountered. The reflection constant is given by the formula $(r - 1)^2/(r + 1)^2$ where r is the ratio of the acoustic impedances of the two materials (Table 4). Acoustic impedance is the product of the acoustic velocity and the density of the material. Velocity is proportional to the square root of the elasticity divided by density. Some typical values are tabulated in Table 1. To make good acoustic coupling to the body, transducers must be coupled by a liquid medium to exclude an air interface and double reflection losses. Olive oil, or K-Y jelly or water are suitable materials.

Ultrasonic waves are usually engendered by piezo-electric materials such as quartz or by synthetic ceramics such as barium titinate or lead-zirconium titinate. When these materials are electrically polarized there is a change

of dimensions in the direction of the applied voltage of the order of 1 part in 10^{10} per volt/cm. The effect is magnified by mechanical resonance in the thickness of the transducer because transducer materials are exceptionally hard and the power generated is only poorly radiated into water or body fluids. Because of this difficulty to transfer energy to other materials, piezoelectric transducers tend to "ring" or resonate for some time after they are pulsed. (In contact with water they lose about 7 per cent of their energy each cycle of vibration). Damping of the vibration can be aided by loading the reverse side with an absorbing material of matched acoustic impedance such as can be made by centrifuging tungsten high density powder into epoxy resin as it polymerizes. By this technique transducers can be made that will transmit 1 microsecond duration pulses into the body.

Receivers, or microphones for ultrasound employ the same materials and construction as transmitters. Often the same probe serves both purposes. They work because application of force to piezo-electric materials generates an electric charge by disturbing the balance of ionic charges in the crystal lattice. The magnitude of the transduced voltage is about 10^{-6} volt/dyne/cm.^{2}, or 10^{-5} volt/newton/ m.^{2}. 1 watt of ultrasound/cm.^{2} in water is equal to 135 dynes pressure/cm.^{2}, or 13·5 newtons/m.^{2}.

The forces that hold solids and liquids together are largely electrical in nature and of the order of 10^8 volts/cm. It is not surprising therefore that distortions of certain

TABLE 4

ACOUSTIC PROPERTIES OF MATERIALS

Material	Density gm./ml.*	Sound Velocity metres/sec.	Impedance Kgm./metre^2	Reflection Against Saline %
Water	1.00	1440	$1·44 \times 10^6$	2
Sea Water	1·03	1456	1·50	0
Castor Oil	0·95	1490	1·45	1·6
ρC rubber	—	1040	1·52	0·32
Carbon Tetra-chloride	1·6	920	1·47	1·0
Mercury	13·6	1400	19·0	85
Methyl alcohol	0·80	1100	0·88	26
Limb tissues mixed	1·02–1·06	1500	1·60	3·0
Muscle	1·07	1600	1·68	3·5
Bone	1·9	—	—	—
Brain Liver Spleen Blood	1·04– 1·06	1500– 1600	1·55– 1·65	1·0– 5·0
Fish	1·06	1790	1·9	11·7
Polythene	1·1	2000	2·2	18·9
Polystyrene	1·06	2300	2·45	24
Perspex	1·2	2600	3·1	34·7
Aluminium	2·7	6300	17·0	83
Quartz	2·7	5800	15·6	81
Steel	7·7	5850	45·0	93·5
Air	—	341	—	100

* To convert to kilograms/metre^3, multiply by 1000.

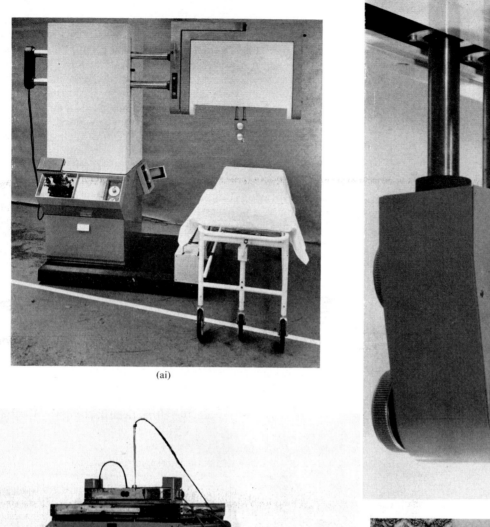

(ai)

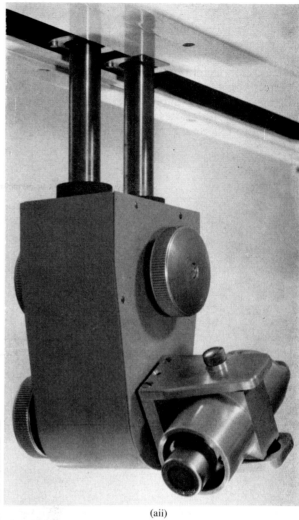

(aii)

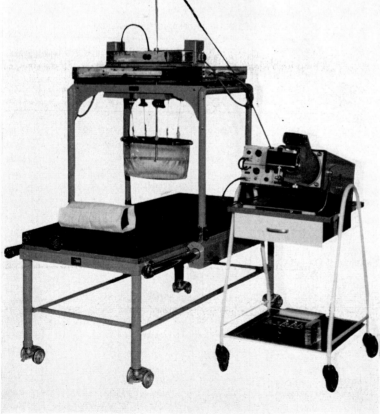

(b)

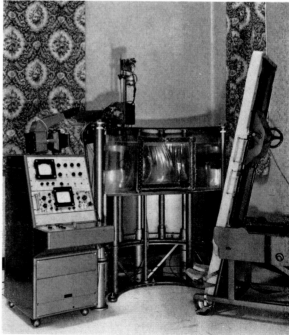

(c)

Fig. 10. Ultrasonic pulse-echo sonographs: (a) Nuclear Enterprises contact scanning Diasonograph. (i) Complete equipment, (ii) Rocking probe. (b) Japan Radio Co. Equipment. (c) Commonwealth Acoustic Laboratories Equipment.

crystals can produce changes in surface charge and that applied voltages can produce in some assymetrical insulating materials a change in dimensions. Light waves and electro-magnetic waves produce weak electric fields and their interactions with matter are slight although known effects. More recently it has been noted that laser light can produce intense electric fields of the order of 10^7 volts per cm. and pulsed laser light will set up ultrasonic vibrations in transparent media, Stephens (1966). The effect has been thought to be detrimental in ophthalmic lazer surgery.

Sensitivity and Resolution

Table 5 gives the sound field intensities for the images at aperture F1 for spherical objects of different sizes. The sizes are given in water wavelengths so that the table is applicable to different frequencies.

TABLE 5

BACK SCATTERED ENERGY FROM SMALL SPHERES,
Rayleigh Formula

Ratio scattered energy to incident energy in aperture F1	Diameter of Object in Wavelengths
2.10^{-4}	5
10^{-5}	0·8
10^{-10}	0·05

The limiting sensitivity of receivers working with microsecond pulses is of the order of 10^{-11} watts/cm.^{2}. Assuming that the "F" number of the probe (ratio of diameter to distance from object) is 1/20 for a deep echo then the energy received is $1/20^2$ or 1/400 of the figure given in the table. To this must be added the transmitting inefficiency which by the reciprocity theorem also equals 1/400. For each direction the path attenuation factor to allow for absorption and scattering may be 1/10, making 1/100 altogether. The energy loss is therefore $16·10^6$.

If the pulse peak input is limited to 1 watt per cm.^{2} to avoid cavitation then the diffraction loss must not exceed 10^5 times. This corresponds to a hard object of 1 wavelength diameter.

These figures illustrate that the method has more than adequate sensitivity for the resolution capabilities of directional probes, which is of the order of 10 wavelengths.

Image camera techniques are less sensitive, about 10^{-7} watts/cm.^{2}, 10^{-3} watts/m.^{2}, and may only penetrate through 10 cms. of tissue but the resolution is as high as the wavelength will allow, that is about $\frac{1}{2}$ mm. at 4 MHz.

In these considerations it is assumed that the electrical circuits, which transduce the probe movements and the angulation of the sound beam in the body to a picture on the cathode-ray tube, function perfectly and do not introduce distortions. In practice mal-adjustments of the time-base and sine-cosine potentiometer circuits can very easily destroy definition and the equipments need to be checked and calibrated frequently on dummy objects of known configuration. Practical methods for adjustment and calibration are given by Fleming (1968), in an article that also illustrates errors in foetal head shape and size introduced by circuit errors.

All pictures made by Professor Ian Donald, University of Glasgow, Mr. E. I. Kohorn and Mr. R. J. Blackwell, University College Hospital, London were obtained on Nuclear Enterprises Diasonographs.

The pictures provided by Mr. E. I. Kohorn, M.Chir., F.R.C.S., M.R.C.O.G., and Mr. R. J. Blackwell, were made in the Department of Obstetrics and Gynaecology, University College Hospital, London.

REFERENCES

Because of the relative novelty of this technique in clinical diagnostic work many clinicians will wish to become acquainted with the research background which continues and which has preceded acceptance of the method as routine hospital procedure, and for this reason the subject has been given extensive references with titles, some of which have been abbreviated for convenience.

Those marked in the list with an asterisk are of a general explanatory nature and included for general reading.

Antony, O. A. (1963), "Ultrasonic Cleaning," *Ultrasonics*, **1**, 194–198.
Baum, G. (1968), "Ophthalmic Ultrasonography," *Ultrasonics*, **6**, 43–47.
*Brown, B. and Gordon, D. (1967), *Ultrasonic Techniques in Biology and Medicine*. Iliffe.
Bullen, M. A., Wells, P. N. T., Freundlich, H. A. and Angell, J. G. (1963), "Treatment of Meniére's Disease," *Ultrasonics*, **1**, 2–8.
Crawford, A. E. (1963), "Ultrasonic Cleaning," *Ultrasonics*, **1**, 65.
*Donald, I., MacVicar, J. and Brown, T. G. (1958), *Lancet*, i, 1188.
*Donald, I. (1961), "Tissue Interfaces by Ultrasonic Echo-sounding," *Brit. J. Radiol.*, **34**, 539–546.
Donald, I. (1965), "Diagnostic uses in Obstetrics and Gynaecology," *J. Obstet. Gynaec. (Brit. Comm.)*, **72**, 907–917.
Donald, I. (1966), "Sonar Examination of the Abdomen," *Ultrasonics*, **4**, 119–124.
Donald, I. and Abdulla, U. (1967), "Further Advances in Ultrasonic Diagnosis," *Ultrasonics*, **5**, 8–12.
Donald, I. (1967), "Sonar . . . in Obstetrics and Gynaecology," *Advances in Obstetrics and Gynaecology*, Vol. 1, Baltimore: W. & W.
Dyson, M., Pond, J. B., Joseph, J. and Warwick, R. (1968), "Stimulation of Tissue Regeneration," *Clin. Sci.*, **35**, 273–285.
Edler, I. (1965), "Mitral Valve Function by Ultrasound Echo-method," *Diagnostic Ultrasound*, pp. 198–228. New York: Plenum Press.
Fleming, J. E. E. and Hall, A. J. (1968), "Scanning Calibration and Effects of Mal-adjustment," *Ultrasonics*, **6**, 160–166.
Fishlock, D. (1966), "Sound in 3-D," *New Scientist*, 8th December, p. 562 (Holograms).
Franklin, D. L., Watson, N. W., Pierson, K. E. and van Citters, R. L. (1966), "Doppler Flowmeter," *Amer. J. Med. Elect.*, **5**, 24–28.
Garg, A. G. and Taylor, A. R. (1967), "Effect of Pulsed Ultrasound on the Brain," *Ultrasonics*, **5**, 208–212.
*Gordon, A. G. (1963), "Ultrasound in Agriculture," *Ultrasonics*, **1**, 70–77.
*Gordon, G. (1964), *Ultrasonics as a Diagnostic and Surgical Tool*, Livingstone.
Gabor, D. (1948), "A New Microscopic Principle," *Nature*, **161**, 777. (Also *Electronics and Power*, July 1966, pp. 230–234.)
Gregus, P. (1966), "Pictures by Sound," *Perspective*, **14**, 287–302.
Gregus, P. (1964), "Ultrasonic Propagation in the Eye," *Ultrasonics*, **2**, 134–136.
Grossman, C. C. (1965), "Acoustic Phenomena in the Detection of Brain Tumours," *Ultrasonics*, **3**, 22–24.
Halstead, J. (1968), "Ultrasound Holography," *Ultrasonics*, **6**, 79–87.
Hertz, C. H. (1964), "Heart Investigations," *Med. Electron. Biol. Engn.*, **2**, 39–45.
Hertz, C. H. (1965), "The Continuous Registration of the Movement of Heart Structure . . .," *Ultrasonic Energy*, University of Illinois Press, ed. by Eliz. Kelly, pp. 294–302.
Hodgkinson, W. L. (1966), *Ultrasonics*, **4**, 138–142.

*Holmes, J. H., Howry, D. H., Posakony, G. I. and Cushman, C. R. (1954), *Trans. Amer. Clin. and Climatolog. Assn.*, **66**, 208.

Hughes, D. E. (1965), "Biological Implications of the Action of Weak Ultrasound," *Ultrasonic Energy*, University of Illinois Press, ed. by Eliz. Kelly, pp. 9–22.

Jacobs, J. E. (1965), "Applications of Ultrasound Image Converters in Biology," *Biomechanics*, ed. by Kenedi, Pergamon Press.

Jacobs, J. E. (1967), "Colour Display, Ultrasound Image Converters," Vancouver Conf. Bio-Medical Engn. Centre, Northwestern Univ. Ohio.

Kimoto, S., Omoto, R., Tsunemoto, M., Muroi, T., Atsumi, K. and Uchida, P. (1964), "Ultrasonic Intravenous Probes," *Ultrasonics*, **2**, 82–86.

Knight, P. R. and Newell, J. A. (1963), "Ultrasonics in Cholelithiasis," *Lancet*, **i**, 1023.

Knight, J. J. (1968), "Effects of Airbourne Ultrasound on Man," *Ultrasonics*, **6**, 39–42.

Kohorn, E. I., Suter, P. E. N., Rees, J. M. and Blackwell, R. J. (1968), "Ultrasonic Compound . . . in O. and G," *Brit. Med. J.*, **1**, 112–113.

*Kossoff, G., Robinson, D. E., Liu, C. N. and Garrett, W. J. (1964), "Design Criteria for Ultrasonic Visualization," *Ultrasonics*, **2**, 29–38.

Kretz (1969), Kretztechnik A4871 Zipf, Germany, "Ultrasonic Diagnosis".

Lele, P. P. (1962), "Lesions with Ultrasound," *J. Physiol.*, **160**, 494–512.

MacVicar, J. and Donald, I. (1963), "Early Pregnancy," *J. Ostet. Gynaec. (Brit. Comm.)*, **70**, 387–395.

McCarthy, C. F., Read, A. E. A., Ross, F. G. M. and Wells, P. N. T. (1967), "Scanning of the Liver," *Quart. J. Med.*, **36**, 517–524.

Metherell, A. F., El-Sum, H. M. A., Dreher, J. J. and Larmore, L. (1967), "Image Reconstruction from Sampled Acoustical Holograms," *Applied Physics Letters*, **10**, No. 10, pp. 277–278.

Metherell, A. F. and El-Sum, H. M. A. (1967), "Simulated Reference . . . Acoustical Hologram," *Applied Physics Letters*, **11**, No. 1, pp. 20–22.

Mikhailov, I. G. (1964), "Methods of Measuring the Absolute Intensity of Ultrasonic Waves in Liquids and Solids," *Ultrasonics*, **2**, 129–133.

Mueller, R. K. and Sheridon, N. K. (1966), "Sound Holograms and Optical Reconstruction," *Applied Physics Letters*, **9**, No. 9, pp. 328–329.

Pell, R. L. (1964), "Clinical Investigations," *Ultrasonics*, **2**, 87–89.

Preston, K., Jr. and Kreuzer, J. L. (1967), "Ultrasonic Imaging . . . Holographic Technique," *Applied Physics Letters*, **10**, No. 5, pp. 150–152.

Robinson, D. E., Kossoff, G. and Garrett, W. J. (1966), "Artefacts in Ultrasonic Visualization," *Ultrasonics*, **4**, 186–194.

Robinson, D. E., Garrett, W. J. and Kossoff, G. (1967), "Ultrasonic Echoscopy in Clinical Obstetrics and Gynaecology," C.A.L. Report 40, Commonwealth Acoustic Laboratories, Sydney, Australia.

Rust, H. (1949), "Chemical Reactions for Acoustic Pictures," *Naturwissenschaften*, **36**, 374.

Siemens (1969), *Biomedical Engineering*, **4**, 36–37.

Smyth, C. N., Poynton, F. Y. and Sayers, J. F., *Proc. I.E.E.*, **110**, 16–28. Also (1963) *J.I.E.E.*, **9**, 4030E, and "Ultrasound Image Camera," *Ultrasonics* (1966), **4**, 15–20.

Smyth, C. N. (1967), "Ultrasound in Clinical Practice," *Ultrasonics*, **6**, 59.

Smyth, M. G., Jnr. (1965), "Animal Toxicity Studies with Ultrasound . . .," *Proc. of 1st Int. Conf. Pittsburg. Diagnostic Ultrasound*, p. 296.

Sokolov, S., Ya. (1949), "The Ultrasonic Microscope," *Doklady Akad. Nauk., S.S.S.R.*, **64**, p. 333.

*Stephens, R. W. B. and Bates, A. E. (1966), *Acoustics and Vibrational Physics*, p. 600. London: Arnold.

Stone, H. L., Stegall, H. F., Bishop, V. S. and Laenger, C. (1967), "Intravascular Doppler Effect Probe for Flow Measurement," *7th Int. Conf. Med. Biol. Eng.*, p. 215. Stockholm: Almquist and Wicksell.

Summer, W. and Patrick, K. M. (1963), *Ultrasonic Therapy*, Elsevier, Holland.

Tarnoczy, T. (1965), "Sound Focusing Lenses and Wave Guides," *Ultrasonics*, **3**, 115–127.

Thompson, H. E., Holmes, J. H., Gottesfeld, K. R. and Taylor, E. S. (1965), "Fetal Growth," *Amer. J. Obstet. Gynec.*, **92**, 44–50.

Thompson, H. E., Holmes, J. H., Gottesfeld, K. R. and Taylor, E. S. (1967), "Obstetric and Gynecological Uses . . .," *99*, 672–682.

Turner, W. R. (1965), "Ultrasonic Imaging," *Ultrasonics*, **3**, 182–187.

Wells, P. N. T. and Evans, K. T. (1968), "Examination of Human Breast," *Ultrasonics*, **6**, 220–228.

Willocks, J., Donald, I., Duggan, T. C. and Day, N. J. (1964), "Foetal Growth," *J. Obstet. Gynaec. (Brit. Comm.)*, **71**, 11.

Woeber, K. (1965), "Ultrasound in the Treatment of Cancer," *Ultrasonic Energy*, **9**, 137, ed. by Eliz. Kelly, Univ. of Illinois Press.

*1. "Ultrasonics in Medicine, Diagnosis and Surgery," April 1967. Special Review Issue, *Ultrasonics*, **6**, pp. 59–125.

*2. "Diagnostic Ultrasound," (1965), *Proc. of the Int. Conf. at Pittsburg*. New York, U.S.A.: Plenum Press.

*3. "The Human Effects of Ultrasonic Radiation," (1967), *British Acoustical Society*—Symposium, Physics Dept., Imperial College, London, S.W.7. Ed. by Dr. Stephens.

*4. "Ultrasonic Energy," *Biological Investigations and Medical Applications*, ed. by Eliz. Kelly, University of Illinois Press, 1965.

*5. "Electronics Review," (1966), *Electronics*, **39**, 24, pp. 37–38.

6. ELECTRONICS AND CLINICAL MEASUREMENTS

C. N. SMYTH

Introduction

Electronic kymographs with transducers to detect and record temperatures, pressures, forces, heart rates, blood flow, perspiration, rates of growth and biological potentials of the electrocardiogram or encephalogram make a physiological laboratory of the labour ward. Knowledge is increased and norms are established, pathological situations are recognized early and information or data is collected against which defects appearing in childhood may be correlated. Chemical auto-analysers and blood cell estimators and automatic cancer screening by flying spot microscope and computer add to the specialized armamentarium of the Obstetric and Gynaecology Department.

The data collects in the absence of the clinician. With little additional nursing and technical staff, diagnoses become simpler and more exact.

Ultrasonic diagnosis is discussed in chapter 5.

Two people need to be converted to such methodology, the clinician and the patient. The latter presents no difficulty. Accurate and simple explanations and samples of the record for scrap books suffice, providing the techniques are applied with charm and without discomfort.

With contraction gauges fixed to the abdomen an oxytocin infusion can be set up and adjusted to a satisfactory rate to give regular contractions within 30 minutes. Without such help and relying on clinical impressions half-a-day may go by achieving the same end with the same degree of safety.

Most instruments need some supervision and this in itself establishes a closer relationship between the nurses or technicians and the patient, with many indirect benefits from casual observation and increased confidence.

The clinician needs training and experience to convince himself of the safety of methods, and the improvement which results.

Few clinicians who have followed foetal distress with every heart beat of the foetus clearly visible and analysed, for conduction defects and wave shape changes, will hasten unduly to a Caesarean section if normal delivery in reasonable time is practicable, and the effects of oxygen therapy, repositioning of the mother and other actions can be observed as they occur.

The instant confirmation of foetal life and consciousness by ultrasonic cardiology, the equally rapid diagnosis of a mole or of pregnancy completes conviction.

There remains the final problem of expense and extra nursing or technical assistance. What is a foetal life worth*, what is the cost of mental retardation, or of a chorion epitheloma recognised later than necessary?

* In the United Kingdom, in a 1,000 patient per annum hospital, the continuous cost would be about £4 a patient or £400 a life saved! This sum includes amortization of the capital expenditure.

The possibility for improvement in obstetric care and the reduction of paediatric and adult morbidity are substantial, while present clinical practice leaves little room for complacency.

Electronics has a connotation synonomous with the recording of physiological data for diagnosis or the control of treatment. It is with this limited aspect that this chapter is concerned. In a larger context electronic instruments are familiar in many obstetric and gynaecological departments as illustrated in Table 1.

Equipments require expert design, construction, maintenance and use. Bedside measurements require no less careful preparation but can often be used by clinical staff, nurses, or ward technicians. The care of the equipment is usually the responsibility in England of Chartered Engineers, or in some instances, Hospital Physicists, and in the U.S.A. of electronics technicians. Particular caution is required with mains operated devices in case unwanted earth currents endanger the patient or staff. The use of multiple equipments and equipments simultaneously with diathermy are particular hazards.

The clinician needs to understand the physical effects which are transduced and the clinical implications of the results and also to appreciate the causes of error in each type of observation.

Except for the recording of biological potentials, electronics makes the intermediate step between the physical effect it is desired to observe and the indicated or graphed result. Electrical systems bring flexibility for remote use, and sensitivity and accuracy that exceeds human ability.

A system for measurement or control comprises the *transducer* to turn the physical effect to be observed, say a movement, into an electrical voltage change, *bridge circuits* to arrange a null balance of the effect so that only increments and not the standing electrical output are amplified in most applications. Direct current or alternating current *amplifiers* to suit the type of transducer, wired or telemetered *pathways* to the polygraph or data logging or visual *display* required for the particular application. Data *processing circuits* to record average, peak, integrated or rate of change from the logged data. Mains or battery *power supplies* to operate the various equipments.

The electronic circuit comprises *passive elements* through which current flows; these are resistance, capacitance and inductance; and *active elements*, valves and transistors which switch in larger amounts of power from the energy supplies, that is from batteries or electronic oscillators or the mains supply. The circuit resistance regulates the current flow but the rate of change of current and the discrimination or selectivity of the circuits to respond to particular frequencies are controlled by the inductance and capacitance. Inductance comprises coils of wire usually

TABLE 1

DEPARTMENTAL ELECTRONIC EQUIPMENTS AND METHODS

1. *X-ray*

Diagnostic and Therapy
Dose control gear
Arteriography rapid injection rams

2. *Diathermy*

Surgery and Therapy
Dose meters
Temperature measurement

3. *Special Techniques*

Thermography
Laser surgery
Cryo-surgery

4. *Pressure and Flow Monitoring*

Regional perfusions
Control of Labour

5. *Cardiology*

Electrocardiograph
Phonocardiograph
Ultrasonic movement detection

6. *Laboratory* (Chemical, Endocrine, Haematology, Serology, Cytology, Immunology.)

Autoanalysers
Chromotography
Electronic weighing
Cell counters
Cell size estimators

7. *Computers*

Note keeping
Laboratory records
Dispensary records
Data processing:
    Averaging, Statistics, Recall, Search facilities.
Bibliographies

8. *Special purpose computers*

Elimination of "noise", transient averaging
Cardiology, digitized results
Foetal cardiology
Foetal Encephalography
Foetal stimulus response averaging

9. *Radio-isotope metabolism and localization study*

Scalers
Counters
Rate meters
Scintillation counters
Scanning for placental site (e.g. technetium 99m.)

10. *Ultrasonics*

Diagnostic, body scanning
Head, mid-line displacement, for
birth distortions
Rates of growth
Cardiology

11. *Miscellaneous*

Autotypists, Photostat machines, Closed Circuit Television, Tape Recorders

enhanced by a magnetizable core. Capacitance comprises closely spaced conductors of large area separated by air or by an insulating material. No steady or direct or average current can flow through a capacitance, but a to-and-fro current can alternate in it. Inductance slows down the rate of current change, capacitance tends to increase it. At high frequencies the energy stored in inductance or capacitance may not be able to return to the circuit in the time of a current alternation; it is lost as

TABLE 2

PRINCIPLE COMPONENTS USED IN CLINICAL ELECTRONIC MEASUREMENTS

Transducers to turn the following parameters into electrical currents:

Movement, Force, Pressure	by Inductance, Capacitance or Resistance changes. Piezo-electric effect
Position, Growth	Ultrasonics (echo)
Temperature	by Temperature coefficient of Resistance or Capacitance or the Thermo-electric effect. (Thermo-junctions)
Light and Colour	Photo-electric and photo-conductive cells
Sound	Microphones, Carbon resistance, Variable inductance Variable capacitance, Piezo-electric
Humidity	Fibre length, salt conductivity
Drop rate counters	Electrolyte conductivity, photoelectric.
Flow rates	Electromagnetic induction Ultrasonics, Anemometers and thermostroms
Hydrogen ions, Kations pCO$_2$, pO$_2$	Glass and polarographic electrodes Colorimeters

Amplifying and data processing circuits

Bridge circuits and Calibrating circuits
Direct and Alternating current amplifiers
Direct to Alternating current converters and rectifiers
Frequency modulators, transmitters and telemetering receivers
Averaging, Integrating, Peak registering, Differentiating (Rate of Change), Rate circuits
Stimulators, counters, timing circuits, pulse generating circuits
Analogue computers
Transient averaging computers
Analogue to digital converters
Digital computers

Data Display Devices

Indicating meters, pointer or digital (numerical)
Oscillographs, transient and Memotron storage tubes
Chart recording polygraphs. Photographic, Ultraviolet, Ink, Ink jet, Hot Stylus, Teledeltos, Xerographic, Carbon paper
Numerical printers
Automatic typewriters

Miscellaneous Devices

Demand operated infusion pumps
Stimulators, timing circuits, pacemakers (for cardiac resuscitation or sphincter control)
Mains energising and battery recharging circuits for the above equipments

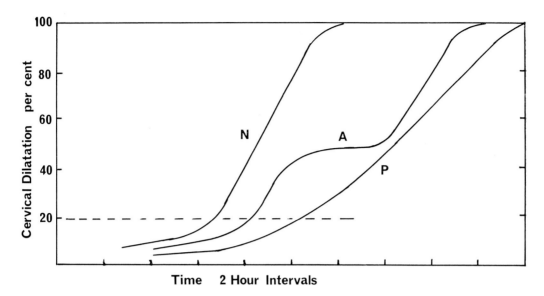

FIG. 1. Cervical dilatation curves or "cervimetry" illustrative of normal labour (N), arrested labour (A), and prolonged and difficult labour (P).

radiated wireless waves and can be received by another circuit at a distance, (Barwick, 1967, Smyth and Wolff, 1960).

In most countries special frequencies are set aside for medical telemetering. In the United Kingdom 102·2–102·4 MHz is allocated but low power devices for telemetering from the body with a range of less than 1½ metres may be of any frequency between 300 KHz and 30 MHz. For very short ranges signals can be telemetered by direct magnetic coupling between the fields of one inductance and another. The method does not radiate at low frequencies, about ½MHz, and is safe at low powers. It is used for implanted telemetering systems. Licences are necessary for each type. (GPO. 1968).

There are three ways in which transducers are commonly used; to produce or change a direct current, to change the magnitude of an alternating current, or to change the frequency of oscillation of an electronic source. The first two methods are generally used with wired pathways. The frequency modulation system is particularly valuable with telemetered systems since the strength of the received signal is not important, only the frequency of oscillation has to be counted to elicit the transmitted information. With biological telemetering multiple receivers or rotating aerials are necessary if the signal is not to be lost at certain orientations of the transmitter when it is free to move within the patient.

Other electronic elements used in transducers are photoelectric and photoconductive cells, thermo-electric couples, one way current flow barriers called rectifiers or diodes, and a variety of resistive, capacative, or inductive materials which are temperature dependent and can be used for temperature measurement.

Table II gives a number of transducer principles and lists the circuits and display devices that may be used with them.

By way of example the following techniques are illustrated, and their clinical significance discussed:

1. The Recording of Cervical Dilatation.
2. Intra-uterine pressure measurements.
3. Head-to-cervix force measurements.
4. The Electrohysterograph.
5. Foetal Cardiology.
6. Foetal and Neonatal Tests.
7. pH, pCO_2 and Oxygen tension measurements.
8. Polygraphs and Data Display methods.

THE RECORDING OF CERVICAL DILATATION

Graphs of cervical dilatation as a function of time vary in shape to accord with types of labour. The slowness of starting dilatation and the rate of dilatation in mid-labour and the slowing of the rate towards full dilatation are characteristics associated in different degree with different categories of patients.

Graphing the rate of dilatation from hourly examinations is the profitable procedure, noting at the same time the frequency and strength of contractions. Friedman (1967) gives average examples and limits for these curves. (Fig. 1). A most common abnormality is a cessation of dilatation associated with an adverse presentation.

Various instruments have been devised for measuring the rate of cervical dilatation, but they are not comfortable for long periods of use. Friedman and Von Micsky (1963), Fig. 2. Halliday (1952) and Smyth (1954) are examples. Clinical observation and digital examination as frequently as necessary serve as the best guides to progress in most labours. The problem with cervical measuring devices is the mode of attachment to the cervix. Even though the gauge offers no constraint to dilatation or retraction, the point of first attachment to the rim does not remain "the rim" as dilatation proceeds. Pain and distortion are introduced if the tissues are held by the attachments for too long and not left free to slide over the internal tissue planes. Figure 2 is excellent in the labour patient, and the Smyth gauge or balloons have been used in the post-partum, non-pregnant and early abortion patient to study the cervical response to drugs (Schild, 1951).

Intra-uterine pressures

If a cavity is divided into two parts by a *flat* elastic diaphagm or by a lax diaphragm the hydrostatic pressure in the two parts must be equal, Figure 3(a). This theorem applies whether one is considering the cellular, vascular or gross dimensions of an organ and is very pertinent to the development of uterine pressures and to pressure differ-ences which may occur between the placental sinuses and the amniotic fluid and parts of the foetal circulation.

Pressures in a large liquid filled space are not the same everywhere. Pressure increases with depth by the weight of the ambient liquid above, just as atmospheric pressure varies with altitude. In the uterus the pressure difference between the fundus and cervix is about 20 mm. Hg. for the ambulant patient at term; for the recumbent patient it is about 15 mm. Hg. When contractions occur the *increase* in pressure is the same everywhere.

The pressures in the tissues and cavity of a viscus at any horizontal level are determined by the turgidity of the blood vessels in the walls until or unless the tissue is ischae-mic. The predominant thin walled vessels are the capil-laries and venules. They buffer any pressure change the muscular fibres may initiate. If sphincters act on the arteries or veins to obliterate flow, the pressure developed will depend on erectile or other haemodynamic factors. Only when flow is arrested can the myometrium of itself contract the surface area of the uterus and, after a spherical or limiting shape is produced, raise the pressure inside. A fall in intra-uterine pressure which sometimes precedes contractions marks these flow change and shape change effects.

The pressure on the outside surface of the uterus is that of the peritoneal space. The pressure on the inside wall of the uterus is higher as a result of the integrated strain of the myometrium and fibrous tissue which hold together the contents and the vascular flow through the walls. If the walls are thick then the pressure drops gradually through the wall thickness and at any layer the pressure is divided inversely as the ratio of the wall tensions, deep and super-ficial to the point of measurement. Figure 3(c).

In the empty thick walled uterus an open ended catheter or a microballoon could (if the cervix made a tight seal round the catheter) be subject to very high pressures. The successive layers of muscle would act to integrate a high central pressure; the inner layers would have no blood flow as the pressure exceeded arterial blood pressure. The highest pressures recorded reach 500 mm. Hg. Hendricks (1964). In general terms the multiplication of pressure which can appear as a viscus empties is the natural log-arithm of the ratio of the inside to outside diameters. Figure 4. For a ratio of 50 times this would be 3·9 times.

Liquids are very incompressible. If a uterus of 5 litres was of fixed shape the addition of one cubic millimetre of blood would raise the pressure to about 500 mm. Hg.! If the shape were that of a Rugby football and the surface area remained constant, the addition of 25 ml. blood would change the shape to spherical. After this any further increase of pressure with volume would depend on the myometrial resistance to stretch. Unless the myometrial stretch reflex over-compensates this volume change uterine contractions are in fact uterine expansions.

These basic considerations point to certain conclusions of value when measuring pressures in the amniotic cavity by the various methods available.

Firstly

When catheters are used, the tambour to which they are connected must be at the same level as the site at which the measurement is required and must be calibrated for zero pressure at this site, or a correction for the changed level added to all measurements. The only exception is when the catheters are air filled and work with air filled balloons.

Secondly

When the catheter is terminated in a balloon the balloon must not be full or the rubber under tension, otherwise the intra-balloon pressure will be greater than the site pressure, neither must the balloon empty completely into the tambour at maximum pressure or the reverse will be the case. As long as the balloon is flaccid there can be no error.

Thirdly

When open ended catheters are used, the pressure read-ings will be correct providing there is sufficient tissue fluid to distend the tambour. With cardiac manometers the volume displacement required for 100 mm. Hg. pressure will be of the order of 10^{-5} ml. The catheters need side holes if the tip is not protected against contact with the viscus wall. If the catheter is $\frac{1}{2}$ mm. diameter a closing force of 1 gramme will produce an artefact pressure of 400 mm. Hg., and if the catheter is bent the pressure artefact may be further increased.

When fine catheters are used the accidental presence of air bubbles slows the response time and where they occur near a change in diameter, i.e. coupling to taps or needles, surface tension effects will introduce errors that may be as large as + or − 12 mm. Hg.

Fourthly

Intramural pressure measurements should allow for the fall in pressure which occurs through the wall thickness.

Fifthly

There is not likely to be a pressure difference between the placental tissue and the amniotic fluid space because the separating membrane is lax: at least until there is free drainage of fluid. When a pressure difference does occur there is a movement of foetal blood to the low pressure side with a resulting bradycardia, a common occurence in late labour.

Finally

If, through the abdominal wall, the uterine wall can be flattened without it making contact with the foetus; then because there is no pressure gradient across a flat surface, the force to flatten is a measure of the pressure within. This is the principle of the guard-ring electromanometer or tocodynamometer. Figure 5 Smyth (1957)(1966). The body wall becomes its own tambour. This instrument measures the force of application in the centre area only. The large plate allows the area of contact to vary as the pressure changes and allows one belt tension to suffice for a wide range of pressures. The gauge must be applied so that it is nearly in whole contact with the patient between contractions and in contact over more than the central area at the height of a contraction. Too much pressure will sink it on to the foetus, and give artificially high pressure readings. When the uterus is "dry" the device no longer measures pressures, although it will still indicate contractions. The device is useful for observing the induction of labour and controlling oxytocin infusions. Smyth (1958).

External manometers which indent the uterus, or follow curvature changes, are subject to errors from local muscle tensions.

Figure 6 shows a relationship between cervical dilatation rates and contraction rates for different rates of uterine effort on the Montevideo scale. The product of the "intensity" of the contractions (in mm. Hg.) multiplied by their frequency (contractions per 10 min.) is expressed in mm. Hg. per 10 min. or Montevideo Units. The "intensity" is defined as the rise in amniotic pressure produced by the contraction. The intensity is therefore the pressure increase above the tonus or base line, and since this base line is not constant but fluctuates a few millimetres, changes of pressure are not included unless they rise at least 5 mms. above the immediate level of the contraction pattern. Caldeyro-Barcia (1961). The Montevideo scale confuses frequency and amplitude but the graph emphasizes that there is an optimum contraction frequency for the shortest labour (unless incipient foetal-distress demands slower progress) this is 22 contractions per hour irrespective of their strength. Faster rates decrease the strength, slower rates allow the cervix to regress in dilatation. Figure 6. The observation has a relation to the control of oxytocin infusions by pressure measurements. Lindgren (1964) gives the pressures necessary to initiate labour.

In this section all pressures have been quoted in mm. Hg. or torrs. With the introduction of the SI, MKS system of units, the torr is no longer recommended although it will doubtless be used for blood pressure measurements for a long time. The correct measurement of pressure will become the Newton per square metre (N/m²). A Newton is 10^5 dynes, (equal to a weight of a little over 100 gms.). The full implications are given in the pamphlet from the Royal Society (1968). (1 mm. Hg. (1 torr.) is equal to 133·322 Nm⁻²). (See Metrication, p. vi.)

Head-to-Cervix Force Measurements

Small flattened balloons or specially designed strain gauges, (Smyth 1954, Lindgren 1955), are used to measure

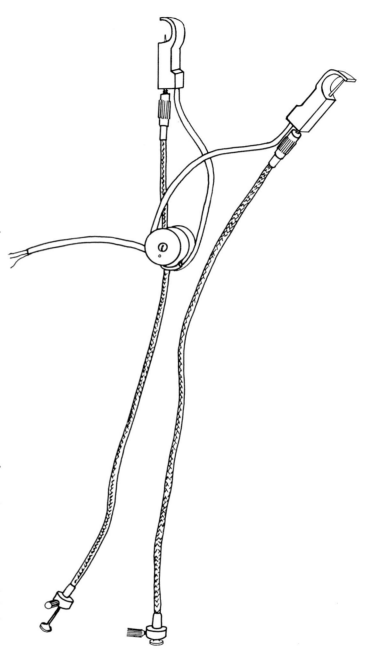

FIG. 2(a).

FIG. 2(a) and 2(b). Friedman-von Micsky cervigraph. There is a resistance transducer at the hinge. It can be pinned to the cervix for short intervals without discomfort while the efficiacy of the contractions is ascertained as illustrated in 2(b).

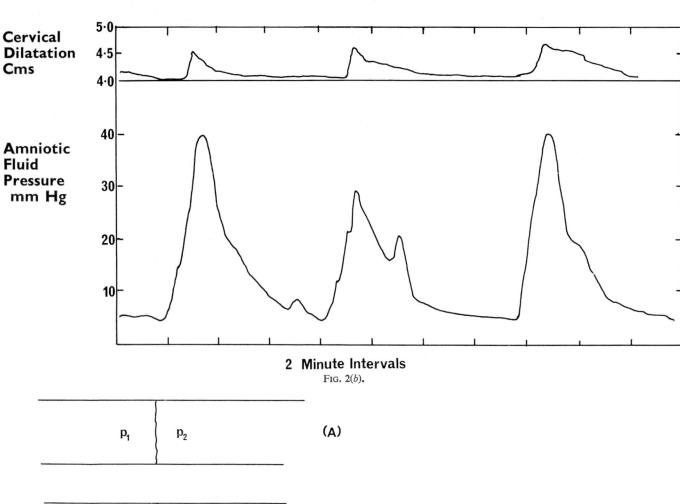

Cervical Dilatation Cms

5·0
4·5
4·0

Amniotic Fluid Pressure mm Hg

40
30
20
10

2 Minute Intervals

FIG. 2(*b*).

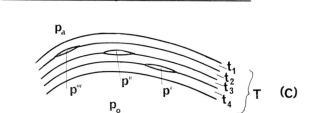

p_1 p_2 **(A)**

R
p_1 T p_2 **(B)**

p_a
t_1
t_2
t_3
t_4
p''' p'' p' T **(C)**
p_o

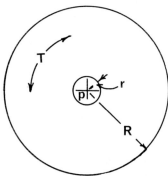

T r p R

FIG. 3. Principles of pressure distribution and measurement. At (A) a lax diaphragm, or an elastic diaphragm only remains flat when there is no pressure difference between opposite sides. $p_1 = p_2$. At (B), p_1 exceeds p_2 and the diaphragm comes under tension T gms per cm of width and assumes a spherical shape. $T = R(p_1 - p_2)$ where R is the radius of curvature. For a cylindrical shell the tension would be doubled as it acts only in one direction. In (C) is shown part of the thick wall of a viscus such as the uterus. It is idealized as 4 concentric shells with tensions $t_1 - t_4$ making a total tension of T. P's denote pressures in the spaces shown. The intra-mural cavities are infinitely thin so as not to distort the wall geometry. Each shell contributes to the pressure within and nothing to the pressure without. The pressure at p is therefore:

$$\frac{p_0 - (p_0 - p_a)}{T} \cdot (t_4 + t_3)$$

and similarly for other sites. Where the pressure is the result of tensions in two directions having different curvatures, the proportions must be separately assessed and added arithmetically.

FIG. 4. In a thick walled organ such as the postpartum uterus, with a very small cavity, high pressures could be developed as a result of the accumulated muscular work on the small central space. If the organ is assumed to develop a uniform tension throughout and to be composed of concentric spherical shells from radius r to R, then the internal pressure would be given by the expression: $p = T \log_e R/r$, where e is the base of natural logarithms. T is the tension per cm².

the force between the presenting part and the dilating cervix in labour. The results are particularly helpful toward the rational treatment of long labours with complications or those being studied experimentally. If labour is not progressing to completion in a patient with ruptured membranes, who has had 100 good natural or oxytocin produced contractions, these measurements may point to a need for reassessment of proportions, to another search for obstruction, or for the need to relax an undeveloped lower segment. The position for balloons or gauges is indicated in Figure 7, and typical recording in a normal patient is shown in Figure 8.

The forces near the crown of the head should be several times greater than amniotic fluid pressure and rise and fall with the fluid pressure, (Lindgren and Smyth, 1961).

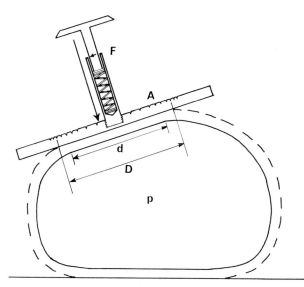

FIG. 5a. The uterus is flattened to a circle of diameter "d" by the application of a flat plate under force F to the abdominal wall. The surface contact area of diameter "D" and area "A" can be read on the transparent plate by the area calibration circles inscribed on it. If p is the pressure in the uterus at the level of the plate then $F = A \cdot p$ very nearly in the thin patient, but there is an error because $D \neq d$, and some force is required to flex the skin at the edges of contact.

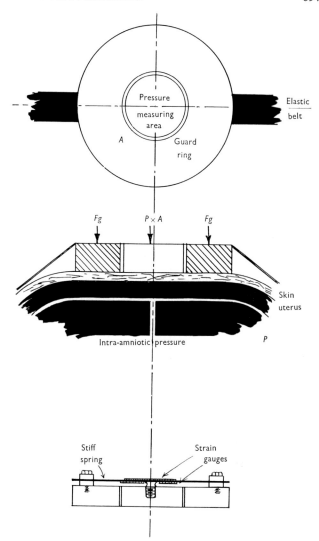

FIG. 5b. The guard-ring electromanometer shown overcomes the errors of the instrument shown in 5a by measuring P.A. only, the force on the central disc, and disregarding the force applied to the co-planar guard-ring Fg. The two are joined together by a stiff spring to which resistance strain gauges are attached. The device turns the body wall into a tambour and makes an absolute reading of pressure within from outside. The instrument is calibrated by applying a weight to A with the instrument inverted.

Flattening of the curves at the higher pressures shows that progressive labour is under way.

The integrated retaining force exerted axially by the cervix must equal the downward force of the fluid pressure on the section of head exposed to the hydrostatic pressure. Where the forces on the cervix are low, some other force preventing delivery must be sought. We know of no recorded cases of failure of the cervix to dilate when the forces upon it are normally large: except for the traumatically scarred cervix.

The graphs of Figure 8 illustrate the effect of rupturing the membranes in increasing the force at the larger diameters and reducing the forces nearer the occiput. This redistribution increases head moulding and expedites delivery. Most moulding occurs in the first stage and

tends to regress in the second stage. The value of membranes in protecting the head of the premature child from excessive moulding is emphasised by these studies.

The Electrohysterograph

Electrohysterography is the recording of slowly varying potentials from the abdominal surface in sympathy with labour contractions. (They are said not to be present in Braxton Hicks contractions.). The subject is controversial in that the origin of the potentials is obscure and they may be a sweating or vascular response to pain. Workers who have studied the subject by intrauterine methods and intramyometrial electrodes have discovered fast action potentials contributing to the spread of the contraction wave. The

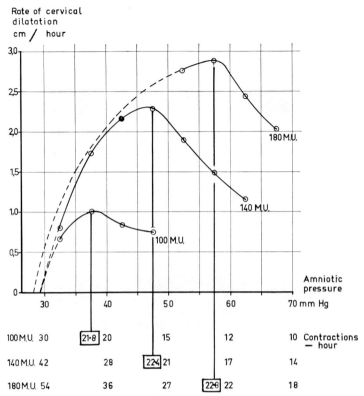

100 M.U.	30	21·8	20	15	12	10 Contractions — hour
140 M.U.	42		28	22·4	21	17	14
180 M.U.	54		36	27	22·6	22	18

Fig. 6. Average rates of cervical dilatation in mid-labour as a function of the contraction pressures for 3 groups of patients, those with weak uterine action, 100 Montevideo units, average action 140 MU and strong action 180 MU. It is seen that for all classes the optimum frequency of contractions is nearly constant and equal to 22 contractions per hour.

reader who wishes to work in this field should consult Dill and Maiden (1948), Steer and Hirsch (1950) and Halliday and Heyns (1952), and Larks (1960).

Jung (1958), Sureau (1955) and Kao (1959) have published recordings from animal and human subjects with intra-uterine electrodes.

Foetal Cardiology

Foetal electrocardiography has been practised for 60 years and foetal phonocardiography for the same order of time. Valuable as these techniques can be for the differential diagnosis in fœtal distress and for the early diagnosis of viable pregnancy or multiple pregnancy, they are subject to artefacts and require trained technicians to work them satisfactorily. With intra-uterine electrodes, Smyth (1953), or the Hon (1963) scalp electrode, artefacts can be avoided, but the sterile intra-uterine procedures reserves the technique for labour ward emergencies. The advent of ultrasonic Doppler principle heart-beat monitors, free of artefacts and simple to apply at any time after 11 weeks gestation, has made the former methods obsolete except for wave-form analysis. The Doppler instruments have been shown to be free of teratogenic effects in animals. They work at 35 mW. cm^{-2}., at which sound level adverse effects are not to be expected (Smyth, M., 1966).

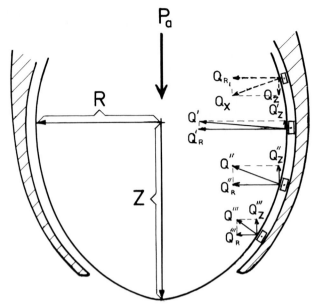

Fig. 7. Illustrates the section of a fetal head of semi-axes R and Z cms. The amniotic fluid pressure is Pa gms/cm^2. The head-to-cervix forces at the positions shown are normal to the head surface and of magnitudes Q', Q'', Q''' and Q_x gms per cm^2. Each has components parallel to R and Z. The sum of the Z components of the pressures at all levels and circumferences add up to the pressure Pa times the area of fluid contact with the head. Q_x acts in opposition to Q'', Q' contributes little to the Z component of retaining force. The R components constitute the moulding forces on the head and tend to elongate it in the Z direction.

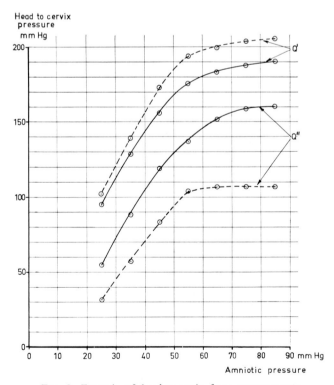

Fig. 8. Example of head-to-cervix force measurements made with gauges positioned as shown in Figure 7. The forces were measured per unit area and are therefore expressed as "pressures". Full lines—membranes intact, dotted lines—after rupture of membranes.

The artefacts which affect foetal cardiology have been maternal and foetal movements, maternal biological potentials from other tissues, room noise, static and mains electrical interference. In mid-pregnancy foetal electro-cardiography is for some patients prevented by excess vernix caseosa rendering the foetal skin non-conducting.

The Doppler instruments are immune to noise and slow foetal movements and to electrical interference and readily provide heart-rate recordings. The probes can be light and rest on the abdomen without the need for a constraining belt.

For the differential diagnosis of foetal distress, the electro-cardiographic recording of extrasystoles and con-duction defects in the R wave remains useful. Certain types of congenital heart lesions are also shown by the electro-cardiogram. With computer techniques the "p" and "t" waves can be demonstrated from recordings made with abdominal electrodes, (van Bemmel, 1966).

The phonocardiograph (Palmrich, 1951–53) elucidates the systolic and diastolic times separately. In physio-logical bradycardia, due to transient occlusion of the cord or other cause, only the diastolic time is affected and the

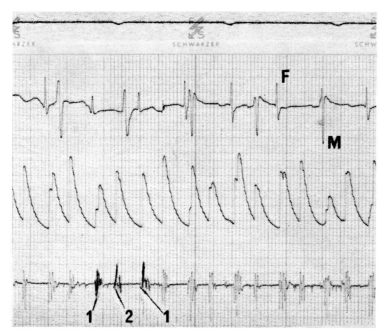

Fig. 9. Example of foetal electrocardiogram from abdominal electrodes (F). The maternal escape potentials are of equal amplitude (M). The lowest line is the phonocardiograph transduced by a moving iron telephone earpiece mounted in a cellular rubber shield and air spaced from the abdominal wall. The centre line is the rectified, smoothed and amplified phonocardiogram prepared for rate measurement. The top line marks seconds.

The Doppler principle is to transmit a 2 MHz ultrasonic sound wave toward the foetal heart from a piezo-electric crystal, and to receive on an adjacent crystal the reflected sound. The returning sound will be of the same frequency unless the reflector is moving when there will be a frequency change proportional to reflector velocity. The beat note formed between the ingoing and outgoing ultrasound falls in the audible range for reflector movements above 6 cms/second. Except in elaborate equipments, there is no discrimination between receding and advancing reflecting surfaces and there are two sounds for each heart beat. The similarity with normal heart sounds makes counting easy. These instruments also note the flow of blood in the cord and larger maternal arteries, and have been used to outline the anteriorly placed placenta and to detect placenta praevia vaginally.

With these devices the foetal heart rate can be followed throughout labour contractions, and types one and two bradycardia differentiated, (Caldeyro–Barcia, 1960, Hon, 1964).

rhythm remains regular. When anoxia or metabolic acidosis is excessive there are changes in systolic time and rhythm.

Equipments for electrocardiography and phonocardio-graphy have been reviewed, (Smyth, 1958b).

Figure 9 shows foetal ECG, and PCG recordings simul-taneously.

Figure 10 shows Doppler principle records made from a commercial instrument, (SK, 1967).

Foetal and Neo-natal Tests

The increasing interest of the obstetrician in the quality as well as the quantity of "his product" has led to the introduction of stimulus response tests which can be conducted on the foetus or neonate, (Bench, 1967, Smyth, 1965).

The value of such tests has not yet been well established, for the necessary correlation with adult behaviour must take many years. Prechtl (1967) has published significant surveys correlating obstetric disorders with impaired physical and mental performance.

Tests are designed to glean as much information as practicable of the obscure foetus, and to study the neo-nate through reactions which involve a minimum of learning.

Andersen (1963), Clark and Polgar (1960), and Severing-haus (1960) and Flenley (1967).

pH measurements are made directly in reference to a neutral or calomel half-cell with a capillary glass electrode in which the blood can be measured and later removed

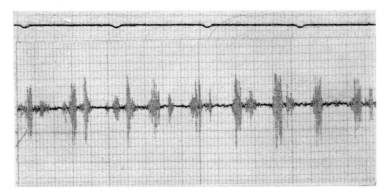

Fig. 10. Foetal heart movements from an early case of pregnancy, recorded from the "Doptone" instrument. 2 MHz ultrasonic waves directed to the foetus through the abdominal wall and a full bladder are reflected from the moving heart walls to given the beat-note recorded here. The instrument can be used from 10 weeks gestation and is not affected by extraneous noises, electrical interference or slow foetal-patient movements. The upper line marks seconds.

In this way it has been hoped to test the structural integrity of the neo-nate rather than its acceptance of social instruction.

Methods employed (in addition to routine neurological, cardiological, respiratory and other function tests) are to surprise the small patient by sounds or light (adding touch, taste and other factors for the neonate) and to record the response through changes in heart rate (breathing and sweating also in the neonate).

Transducers used in this work are the ultrasonic doppler effect or the electrocardiograph for heart rates, skin conductivity for sweating, and thermo-junctions to time respiration. Body movements are recorded from cot movements transduced by air displacement anemometers or piezo-electric accelerometers.

A typical neonatal record is shown in Figure 11.

The normal foetus is conscious of extraneous sounds and shows a transient tachycardia and movements when surprised by loud sounds (70 db. in the uterus, 90 db. at the abdominal surface), even when the mother is unaware of the stimulation, Murphy (1962) and Smyth, Bench (1967). The foetus habituates to repetitions of the stimulus. It has been found that foetuses that do not respond are at risk. The test is readily performed by tapping a stethoscope briskly for a few seconds while listening to the heart; it may come to be recognized as an early warning of foetal distress, or as an indication for foetal blood sampling in labour.

The average effect for different initial heart rates is illustrated in Figure 12.

pH, pCO_2 and Oxygen tension measurements

The rapid measurement of blood gas tensions and base excess values in microsamples of foetal blood (less than 0·1 ml.) obtained by the Saling technique (1965) has become a ward method through the work of Astrup and Siggaard-

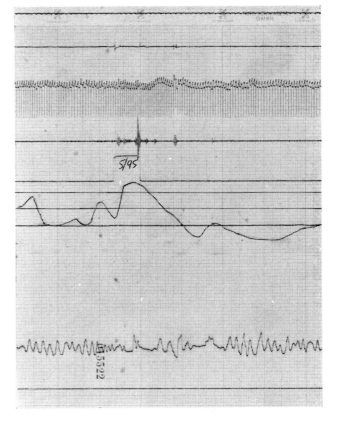

Fig. 11. Typical neonatal response to sound stimulation. The stimuli are pre-recorded on a tape recorder so that the same random sequence of notes and stimulus durations can be played to each child at the same acoustic intensity. Note the "startle" at the onset of stimulation followed by the changed respiration pattern and heart-rate rise and fall. 1st line, seconds; 2nd line, cost movement; 3rd line, e.c.g. (electrocardiogram); 4th line, vocalization or cry; 5th line, stimulus marker (5 seconds at 95 db); 6th line, heart rate; 7th line, respiration.

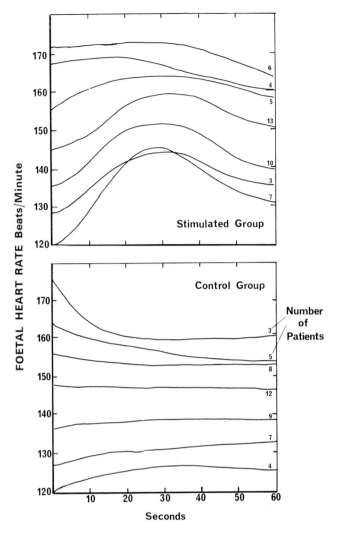

FIG. 12. The foetal heart-rate fluctuates continuously within 5 beats per minute of the average rate. The rate changes last from only a few seconds to a minute or so. Over these small changes there are short period rate changes related to foetal activity and other unknown factors. When the normal foetus is stimulated by sounds there is a reaction shown by an increase in heart rate lasting for about a minute. The magnitude of the reaction varies, on average, with the initial heart-rate. The heart-rate changes for stimulated and unstimulated foetuses are shown. The test was repeated a large number of times on each patient and the results averaged by computer. The smoothed curves above show the difference acoustic stimulation makes to the heart-rate regression toward normal values when stimulation begins at different initial heart-rates.

for further tests. pH measurements are usually made on two fractions of the sample for each assay as there is a systematic difference between the first two uses of an electrode after it has been cleaned, amounting to as much as 0·01 unit pH.

Measurements of pCO_2 and base excess or deficit are determined through pH measurements made on blood under standard conditions while blood pH is measured on the sample as collected anaerobically.

The pH electrode is a specific acceptor of hydrogen ions. With special glasses electrodes can be made to accept sodium or potassium or other ions selectively (Hinke, 1961).

pCO_2 is measured in the Severinghaus electrode, by determining the extent to which the blood can modify the pH of an adjacent layer of bicarbonate solution. A pH electrode is covered with absorbent cellophane, or silk, soaked in weak bicarbonate solution and then covered overall by a gas porous layer of Teflon foil. The outer layer is covered with the blood to be examined at controlled temperature. CO_2 perfuses to change the bicarbonate pH according to the Hesselbach equation. The electrode is calibrated against CO_2 and O_2 gas mixtures.

Another method of measuring blood pCO_2 is to equilibrate the microsamples of blood with known CO_2 tensions (say 4 and 8 per cent CO_2 mixtures, 28·4 and 56·8 mm. Hg.) at 37°C and 100 per cent humidity and to measure their pH. The pCO_2 of the original blood can then be found by interpolation. According to Astrup there is a correction factor proportional to the degree of deoxygenation of the blood, but it is common practice to disregard this correction. Beard (1967) states that the uncorrected figures are in the best agreement with the Severinghaus method.

pO_2 is measured by equilibrating small samples of saline or bicarbonate with the micro blood sample and measuring the oxygen tensions in these liquids by polarography or by means of a fuel cell.

In the Clark electrode the principle of polarography is employed between a 25 micron diameter platinum electrode and an electrolytically purified silver annulus. The microsample of saline (or KCl, or a mixture according to taste, the device has to be calibrated) joins these two electrodes and is covered by Teflon foil. The electrode at 37°C is brought into contact with the anaerobic sample of blood for a minute and then a potential of 0·6 volt is applied between the electrodes. The current which flows after a chosen time, circa 10^{-8} amp., say 20 seconds, is taken as the reading appropriate to the calibration. In the absence of oxygen in the solution the current speedily falls to zero as hydrogen covers the platinum electrode. If oxygen is present the platinum catalyses a reaction with the hydrogen and the formation of water allows the electrode to conduct again.

With the dimensions specified a partial equilibration is effected proportional to oxygen tension. The method is reliable in the concentrations found in foetal or adult blood and is more discriminating than comparative colourimetry with red and infra-red light which is an alternative method (Stott, 1953).

The fuel cell method uses oxidation of lead in alkaline solutions. The equilibrated bicarbonate is continuously or intermittently passed to a minute silver-lead cell and the total current which flows between the electrodes is a measure of the oxygen consumed. Each oxygen atom gives off 2 electrons. 1 ampere second is $6·3 \times 10^{18}$ electrons. The current is large and amplifiers are not necessary (Hunt, 1964, Mackereth, 1964, Briggs, 1964, Smyth, 1968).

Polygraphs and Data Display methods

The choice of apparatus will depend much on the staff available, but where technical assistance is limited and recordings are in demand at all hours of the day and night, equipment which has only to be switched on and have the appropriate transducers attached to the patient has much to commend it. From this particular viewpoint, polygraphs that use ink or hot stylus and need adjusting if the paper speed is varied should be avoided. Those that write with carbon paper or on ultraviolet sensitive paper, or that record by xerography, are to be preferred; with these the writing constants are independent of ambient temperature and ink blockages. It is an advantage if alarms are provided to indicate the end of paper supplies and other failures, as the machines must work for long periods without attention. The length of obstetric data records makes cost considerations important and polygraphs that employ ordinary plain paper for the record save much expense.

Magnetic tape data recorders are economical and assist data transfer where records will be used for computer storage and analysis. They should have frequency modulated channels for slowly varying parameters like uterine action. Separate tapes for fast cardiac studies and slow uterine measurements are an advantage. Time recognition marks should be added automatically to all paper and magnetic tape records.

Certain parameters such as heart rate, uterine work and peak pressures can be measured on digital voltmeters and displayed near the patient. The readings can be typed automatically or printed numerically at regular intervals to provide a tabulated record of labour.

In the choice of equipment, attention should be given to the stability of zero and amplitude calibration over periods of several hours, to a short initial warming up period before the calibration becomes stable, and to independence from ambient temperature variations. For cardiology the frequency response needs to be higher than for the equivalent adult records. Foetal ECG records must show changes at 200 Hz. if conduction defects arising in early foetal distress are to be seen.

The increasing use of computers in hospital records must eventually influence the design of electronic monitors, and for this reason new installation can benefit from the advice of systems engineers associated with the local or regional computer centre.

References

The following references extend the text which, because of the extent of the subject, is very abbreviated. They are chosen either for their originality or for the value they have as reviews of sections of the subject, and for their extensive bibliographies. The text books listed at the end make profitable general reading in the applications and principles of medical instrumentation.

REFERENCES

Barwick, R. E., Fullagar, P. J. (1967), *Proc. Ecol. Soc. Aust.*, **2**, 27–49.

Beard, R.W. (1967), Queen Charlotte's Hospital, London. Lecture Course, "Foetal Sampling."

van Bemmel, J. H., van der Weidde, H. (1966), I.E.E.E. trans. *Biomed. Eng. BME*, **13**, 175.

Bench, R. J., and Smyth, C. N. (1967), *Digest, 7th Int. Conf. Med. and Biol. Engineering*. Almquist and Wiksell, 26, Gamla Brogatan, Stockholm. p. 244.

Briggs, R., Viney, M. (1964), *J. Sci. Instrum.*, **41**, 78.

Caldeyro-Barcia, R. (1960), *Pediatria* (Spanish), **29**, 91.

Caldeyro-Barcia, R. (1961), *Oxytocin*, Oxford: Pergamon Press.

Dill, L. V., and Maiden, R. M. (1948), *Amer. J. Obstet. Gynaec.*, **56**, 213.

Flenley, D. C., Millar, J. S., and Rees, H. A. (1967), *Brit. med. J.*, 349.

Friedman, E. A. (1967), Text. "Labor." New York: Meredith Pub. Co. (Butterworths, U.K.)

Friedman, E. A., and von Micsky (1963), *Amer. J. Obstet. Gynaec.*, **87**, 789.

GPO (1968), *Med. and Biol. Telemetry Devices*, W.6802, London: H. M. Stationery Office.

Halliday, E. C., and Heyns, O. S. (1952), *J. Obstet. Gynaec. Brit. Emp.*, **59**, 309–322.

Halliday, E. C., Jacobs, G., van Wyk and Heyns, O. S. (1958), *J. Obstet. Gynaec. Brit. Emp.*, **65**, 409–413.

Hendricks, C. H. (1964), *J. Obstet. Gynaec. Brit. Comm.*, **71**, 712.

Hinke, J. A. M. (1961), *J. Physiol.*, **156**, 314–335.

Hon, E. H. (1963), *Amer. J. Obstet. Gynaec.*, **86**, 772–784.

Hon, E. H. (1964), *Med. Electron. Biol. Eng.*, **2**, 71–76.

Hunt, T. K. (1964), *Lancet*, **ii**, 1370.

Jung, H. (1958), *Forschr. Geburtsh. Gynäk.*, **7**, 4–14.

Kao, C. Y. (1959) *Amer. J. Physiol.*, 196.

Larks, S. D. (1960), Text. (pub. Charles C. Thomas, Springfield, Illinois.)

Lindgren, C. L. (1955), *Acta obstet. gynec. scand.*, **38**, 211.

Lindgren, C. L. (1964), *Bibl. Gynaec. Fasc.*, **42**, 125–140.

Lindgren, C. L., and Smyth, C. N. (1961), *J. Obstet. Gynaec. Brit. Comm.*, **68**, 901.

Mackereth, F. J. H. (1964), *J. Sci. Instrum.*, **41**, 38.

Murphy, K., and Smyth, C. N. (1962), *Lancet*, **i**, 972.

Palmrich, A. H. (1951), *Zbl. Gynäk.*, **73**, 1699.

Palmrich, A. H. (1952), *Gynaecologa*, (*Basel*, **133**, 29, and **134**, 117.

Palmrich, A. H. (1953), *Z. Geburtsh. Gynäk.*, **138**, 304–307.

Polgar, G., Forster, R. E. (1960), *J. appl. Physiol.*, **15**, 706.

Prechtl, H. F. R. (1967), *Brit. med. J.*, **4**, 763–767.

Royal Society (1968), *Metrication in Scientific Journals*, Pamphlet from Royal Society, London, S.W.1.

Saling, E. (1965), *J. Int. Fed. Gynec. Obstet.*, **3**, 101.

Severinghaus, J. W. (1960), *Anaesthesiology*, **21**, 717; also Text, Churchill, London (1959).

Schild, H. O., Fitzpatrick, R. J., and Nixon, W. C. W. (1951), *Lancet*, **i**, 250.

Siggaard-Andersen, O. (1963), *Acid-base status of the blood*, Monograph, Munksgaard, Copenhagen; also *Scand. J. clin. Lab. Sci.*, **15**, Suppl. 69–76.

SK (1967), Smith, Kline Instrument Co., Welwyn Garden City, Herts. England.

Smyth, C. N. (1953), *Lancet*, **i**, 1124.

Smyth, C. N. (1954), *Comptes-Rendus du Congress Int. Gynae. Obstet.* (S. A. George, Geneva), p. 1030.

Smyth, C. N. (1957), *J. Obstet. Gynaec. Brit. Emp.*, **64**, 59, see also *Lancet* (1966), **i**, 1152.

Smyth, C. N. (1958), *Lancet*, **i**, 237.

Smyth, C. N., and Farrow, J. L. (1958b), *Brit. med. J.*, **2**, 1005.

Smyth, C. N., and Wolff, H. S. (1960), *Lancet*, **ii**, 412.

Smyth, C. N. (1965), *J. Obstet. Gynaec. Brit. Comm.*, **72**, 6.

Smyth, C. N. (1966), *Med. Electronics and Biol. Engin.*, **5**, 69–73.

Smyth, C. N., and Bench, R. J. (1967), *Digest of 7th Int. Conf. Med. and Biol. Eng.* Almquist and Wiksell, 26, Gamla Brogatan, Stockholm. p. 244.

Smyth, Murray G., Jnr. (1966), *Diagnostic Ultrasound*, Proc. of the 1st International Conference, Pittsburg, 1965, p. 296. (Publishers, Plenum Press, New York.)

Steer, C. M., Hirsch, H. J. (1960), *Amer. J. Obstet. Gynaec.*, **59**, 25.

Stott, F. D. (1953), *J. Sci. Instrum.*, **30**, 120.

Sureau, C. (1955), *Etude de L'Activite Electrique de L'Uterus* .... Paris: R. Foulon.

Texts for General Reading

Electrophysiological Technique, by C. J. Dickinson (1950), Offices of Electronic Engineering, 28, Essex Street, Strand, London.

Principles of Electronics, by L. T. Agger (1956), Macmillan and Co. Ltd., (New York: St. Martin's Press).

Electronics for Biological Research, by P. E. K. Donaldson, (1958), Butterworth's, London.

Physical Laws and Effects, by C. Frank Hix Jnr. and Robert P. Alley (1958), Chapman and Hall Ltd., London. (John Wiley and Sons, Inc., New York.)

Fetal Electrocardiography, by S. D. Larks (1961), Charles C. Thomas, Springfield, Illinois, U.S.A.

Fetal Electrocardiography and Electro-encephalography, by R. L. Bernstine (1961), Charles C. Thomas, Springfield, Illinois, U.S.A.

An Introduction to Medical Automation, by L. C. Payne (1966), Pitman Medical Publishing Co. Ltd., London.

Engineering in the Practice of Medicine, by Bernard L. Segal and David G. Kilpatrick (1967), The Williams and Wilkins Company, Baltimore.

7. IRRADIATION

B. WINDEYER

The use of ionizing radiations in medicine started immediately after the discovery of X-rays by Roentgen in 1895. The diagnostic uses of these new rays were soon apparent. Before many months had passed, it was also found that the rays had a profound biological effect causing erythema of the skin and the regression of some superficial malignant tumours.

There has been, in the seventy four years since Roentgen's discovery, continuous progress in the development of techniques and in the interpretation of X-ray findings so that, at the present time, diagnostic radiology has become a discipline of the first importance in medicine. It is now possible with modern techniques and sometimes, with the use of appropriate contrast media, to examine and obtain invaluable information about almost every organ and tissue in the body, normal and pathological.

As a therapeutic agent, X-rays were used in the first few years in attempts to treat a wide variety of conditions: acute and chronic infections, asthma, skin eruptions of every kind as well as benign and malignant tumours. Apparatus was crude and unreliable. Output of radiation was inconstant both as regards quality and quantity and many difficulties had to be overcome to obtain any constancy in therapeutic effect.

Experience was gained by trial and error and after some years of experience it gradually became apparent that X-ray treatment had real value in the treatment of various forms of malignant disease and in the management of skin dermatoses. Depilation could be produced and the function of various organs could be altered, for example, ovarian function could be suppressed with the production of a menopause.

The discovery of radium by Marie Curie brought another agent into therapeutic use. It was expensive and difficult to obtain but the profound biological effect of radium was immediately appreciated. It also had to be used empirically and gradually experience was built up. Radium had the advantage that it could be used by application to the surface, by implantation directly into the tissues so that heavy dosage could be delivered locally to a tumour, or by insertion into the normal body cavities. Cancer of the cervix uteri was a condition which appeared to be suitable for treatment in this way.

The use of radium was mainly in the hands of the gynaecologists who found it useful for the treatment of uterine cancer and of some surgeons who used it for a wide variety of forms of malignant disease.

X-rays and radium therefore developed along rather different lines as therapeutic agents and were scarcely considered as alternative or complementary forms of treatment except by the dermatologists who made use of both.

Radiation Damage and the Development of Radiation Protection.

Among the reports of some successes and of failure from treatment, there began to appear descriptions of cases where severe local inflammatory reactions had occurred, sometimes followed after heavy dosage by deed ulceration which was painful and showed little tendency to heal. There was also an accumulation of evidence that radiologists who exposed their hands to the beam and received repeated small doses were suffering from an intractable dermatitis which after the lapse of some ten or more years developed into skin cancer. Similar damage was noted on the hands of radium workers and some radiologists were reported to have died from unexplained anaemia. All these reports gave rise to considerable alarm and in 1921 the British X-ray and Radium Protection Committee was formed. Others followed and in 1928 the International Commission on Radiological Protection was formed by the International Radiological Congress. The study of radiological protection thus began nearly 50 years ago to protect the medical radiological workers and it has become of increasing importance to a much wider section of the population with the more widespread use of ionising radiations, not only for medical purposes but also in almost every activity of modern life.

The realization that not only local damage to exposed portions of the body and general damage to the body as a whole can occur but also that quite small doses to the gonads can cause genetic damage is of great importance in the development of the use of ionizing radiations and nowhere is it more important than in irradiation techniques in gynaecology and obstetrics.

There are now Recommendations of the International Commission translated into national Regulations and Codes of Practice which, if scrupulously observed, ensure that the benefits of the use of ionizing radiations can be obtained without undue risk.

Dose Measurement and Dose Distribution.

The next major step forward in the use of ionizing radiations was the determination of accurate methods of dosage measurement and of accurate knowledge of the distribution of radiation in the tissues.

The purely empirical approach to radiation treatment was replaced by standardized techniques, well documented and based on accurate observation, and follow-up of patients. Outstanding leadership was given by two clinics, the Radiumhemmet in Stockholm under the direction of Gösta Forsell and the Fondation Curie in Paris under the direction of Claude Regaud. Among their achievements was the development of techniques for the radium treatment of cancer of the cervix. The Heyman technique and the Paris technique have stood the test of time and for some forty years have been used either in their original or some modified form in many clinics throughout the world.

There was not, however, any satisfactory unit of dosage and it was not possible to make any real correlation of the dose given by X-rays and that given by radium and this became a matter of increasing importance, particularly in the treatment of uterine cancer where, in more advanced cases, both local radium application and X-rays from the surface had to be employed. The introduction of the *roentgen* both for X-rays and radium as a unit of dose based on the degree of ionization caused by the radiation, and later the *rad* as a unit of absorbed dose, made it possible to determine accurately the dose distribution in the tissues from various techniques. By definition a roentgen is the quantity of X- or gamma-radiation such that the associated corpuscular emission per 0·001293 grammes of air produces, in air, ions carrying one electro-static unit of quantity of electricity of either sign. A rad, the radiological unit of absorbed dose is 100 ergs per gramme.

Radiotherapy as a Separate Discipline

At about the same time in the 1930's there came to fruition a movement to combine the therapeutic uses of X-rays and of radium in the hands of the same clinician and the discipline of radiotherapy became established. General radiology became replaced by separate disciplines of diagnostic radiology and radiotherapy and the radiotherapists gradually took over the use of radium from the surgeons and in many instances from the gynaecologists. It was generally appreciated in the new discipline that the planning of treatments, the measurement of dose and dose distribution and such matters as the protection of patients and of operating personnel demanded the collaboration of those with specialized knowledge of physics. The practice of radiotherapy has therefore become a matter of teamwork with clinically trained physicists as essential members of the team.

Development of Apparatus

The next landmark of major importance in radiotherapy was the development of apparatus.

Although there had been continual improvements in the output, the reliability and the clinical convenience, the main type of X-ray apparatus in use up to 1939 was limited to the 200 to 250 kilovolt range. The quality of radiation did not afford a sufficiently high percentage depth dose to enable the adequate irradiation of deeply situated tumours without extensive and sometimes excessive irradiation of superficial and surrounding organs and tissues. There were some machines working at peak voltages of one million or more but generally they were in the nature of laboratory or experimental models and not thoroughly reliable and convenient for clinical use.

The vast increase in knowledge of electronics and the progress of electrical engineering between 1939 and 1945 immediately made available a new range of apparatus for routine clinical use. Reliable X-ray machines of constant and very high output, designed and engineered for accurate clinical application with great flexibility of movement, are now readily available working at peak voltages in the range of one to ten million volts and more. This quality of radiation is commonly known as supervoltage radiation as distinct from orthovoltage, the 200 to 250 kilovolt range, and it has particular advantage in the treatment of many forms of malignant disease.

1. Investigation of dose distribution showed that radiation produced by the 200 to 250 kilovolt range of apparatus has an increased specific absorption in bone as compared with soft tissue. This means that with radiation of this quality there is an increased dose in bone and a greater danger of bone necrosis and also that a tumour underlying bone, as may be the case in some growths in the pelvis, is shielded and may receive inadequate dosage. With supervoltage there is no such specific absorption in bone and therefore less risk of bone necrosis and greater certainty of adequate dose in the planning of treatment.

2. The percentage depth dose is adequate to enable the irradiation of deep seated tumours to a desired dose with relatively simple field arrangements.

3. There is little side scatter of radiation and therefore the beam is sharper and there is less radiation of surrounding tissues.

4. The maximum dose from each field is some millimetres below the skin and intense skin reactions do not occur though care must be taken to avoid subcutaneous damage with fibrosis, as different individuals react differently to radiation.

5. The integral or total body dose is reduced and there is therefore less likelihood of radiation sickness.

At the same time as the developments in electronics and high voltage engineering and also due to the stimulus of military requirements, there was a tremendous advance in knowledge of radioactivity. It became possible to produce radioactive isotopes of all elements and many of them could be produced in quantity in nuclear reactors. Each such radioactive substance has its own characteristics in regard to the type of radiation emitted and the time period of its decay. Some of them, in particular radioactive cobalt and radioactive caesium, emit gamma rays i.e. highly energetic X-rays, and have been found to be efficient substitutes for radium for therapeutic purposes. They can be obtained in quantity and are much less expensive than radium. Radioactive cobalt with a half life of 5·3 years can be obtained with high intensity of radiation from a reactor and is used with sources up to 5000 to 10,000 curies in heavily protected apparatus which emits a beam of radiation (a curie is the quantity of radon in radioactive equilibrium with 1 gramme of radium, the quantity which decays at the rate of $3·7 \times 10^{10}$ disintegrations per second). The quality of the beam of gamma radiation from cobalt is such that it is equivalent to the beam of radiation produced by an X-ray machine working at about three million volts.

Radioactive caesium is a decay product from nuclear reactors with a half life of 30 years. It cannot be obtained with the same high intensity of radiation and the quality of its gamma emmission is comparable to the beam of X-ray apparatus working at peak voltages of 700 kilovolts.

This quality is such that there is no specific selective absorption in bone and, though inferior in some respects to radioactive cobalt, a caesium unit with a source of 2000 curies provides efficient apparatus with the main advantages of supervoltage X-ray therapy.

These two radioactive substances (Co-60 and Cs-137) and some others provide convenient and sufficiently long-lived sealed sources to be used as substitutes for radium for either interstitial or intracavitary applications. Radioactive gold (Au-198) with a half life of 2·67 days is a convenient substitute for radon seeds for permanent implants.

In addition to these relatively long-lived artificially produced radioactive substances which are used as substitutes for radium in sealed sources, there are many others—and the number of such substances and the form and purpose for which they are used is continuously increasing—which are used as unsealed radioactive substances for diagnostic and research purposes. They are invaluable tools, whose use has opened up completely new prospects and new methods of medical and biological research. Some few of them, such as radioactive isotopes of iodine and phosphorus, are also used for therapeutic purposes.

Significant advances in radiotherapy are unlikely to come from further accumulation of knowledge about dose measurement and distribution, and only marginal benefit will probably come from further elaboration of apparatus. The greatest hope for further significant improvement is in obtaining greater knowledge of the biological action of radiation and at the present time this is the most important field of endeavour. Further knowledge of the biological action of radiation both in its qualitative and quantitative aspects is also important in radiation protection. The measures of protection which have been adopted both nationally and internationally have undoubtedly reduced the hazards so that they compare favourably with any of the risks of normal civilized life. It is, however, a matter of considerable importance in a far wider field than medical irradiation, now that ionizing radiations are used extensively in industrial processes and many aspects of research.

Greater knowledge may further reduce some hazards and may make possible the more extensive use of these radiations without excessive costs in protective measures.

RADIOBIOLOGY

Knowledge of the biological action of radiations has been accumulating since radiations were first used.

The gross biological effects of radiation on tissues are now well documented. However the exact mechanism of their action at a subcellular and molecular level is still a matter for experiment. At the doses used in radiotherapy, it is likely that an effect on specific sensitive or vital targets within the cell is necessary, rather than a general denaturing effect on cytoplasm. The radiation produces ionization and free radicals within the aqueous media of the cell. These may then react with components of cell structure. It is thought that the principal lethal effect on cells is an alteration in the desoxy-ribonucleic acid (DNA)

of the chromosome apparatus. Some of this may be repaired by intracellular recovery processes, with subsequent normal viability of the cell and reproductive integrity. However, with increasing magnitudes of dose fewer of the irradiated cells will be capable of recovery and subsequent continued division. This effect, with varying degrees of magnitude, is observed in both normal and malignant tissues. The radiosensitivity of the dividing normal cells of a tissue may well be of the same order as that of the tumour arising within it. However the normal tissue maintains a homeostatic control for the replacement of damaged tissue and is able to respond with increased proliferation and replacement. This response is absent in the malignant tumour. Provided that a suitable combination of total dose and number of component fractions is selected, it is then possible to achieve tumour destruction without irreparably damaging the normal stroma. Less than complete killing of the tumour cells may result from an inadequate dose, an incompletely covered tumour volume or reduced radiosensitivity of certain cells within the tumour. The most significant factor in the latter component is areas of hypoxia due to a poor blood supply. Current trials involving the use of hyperbaric oxygen during radiation therapy are designed to reduce such radioresistant hypoxic cells to as small a proportion of the total number as possible.

All the principles of the treatment of malignant disease are based on the knowledge that, though ionizing radiations have a damaging or a destructive effect on all living tissue according to the size of the dose delivered, there is a selective effect and that some organs, some tissues and some cells are more sensitive than others. It was realized in the early years that the haemopoietic tissues were particularly radiosensitive, that the function of the ovary and the testis could be grossly damaged and that certain malignant tumours were more radiosensitive than the normal tissues in which they were growing. It has been known for many years that irradiation of the eye is hazardous and that cataract formation is likely to occur. It is not yet accurately known what is the primary lesion in a cell which is caused by radiation and knowledge is deficient about all the processes involved in the elimination of a tumour treated by radiation. Controlled investigations with the use of neutrons as a means of radiation are being undertaken because it has been shown that the effect of neutrons is relatively independent of the oxygenation of the cell.

There are many other aspects which need elucidation, such as the effects of fractionation of dose, the influence of the vasculature of the tumour and the tumour bed, and the possible influence of immunological processes on the elimination of irradiated tumours.

It would appear that radiotherapy, having passed through various stages of empiricism, realization of hazards and protection, accuracy in dosage, professional and scientific organization, and development of apparatus, is now in the stage where continued improvement is likely to come from a greater knowledge of radiobiology and the application of this knowledge by radiotherapists with a high standard of clinical knowledge and experience.

THERAPEUTIC USES OF IONIZING RADIATIONS

It is convenient to consider the therapeutic uses of ionizing radiations in Obstetrics and Gynaecology in the two categories of (1) a variety of non malignant conditions and (2) malignant conditions.

(1) Non Malignant Conditions

The knowledge that irradiation by X-rays or radium could induce an artificial menopause led to the treatment of some non malignant conditions by methods of irradiation as an alternative to surgical operation.

In those patients who are coming to the end of reproductive life, aged 40 and over, the dose necessary to produce an artificial menopause is a small one of less than 500 rads to the ovaries. This is because the ovarian follicles remaining in the ovary are all in some stage of maturation and become more radiosensitive in the process of maturation. In the case of young women, say in the 20 to 30 decade, there is a high proportion of immature follicles which are much more radioresistant. In these younger women, the dose required to produce a definitive menopause is considerably higher though a temporary menopause is caused by the lower dose, due to the destruction of those follicles which are undergoing maturation. Surgical advances and the introduction of the whole science of gynaecological endocrinology has altered the picture in the management of many non malignant conditions previously treated by radiotherapy. Many patients used to be treated for irregular bleeding at and around the menopause by the production of a definitive menopause by irradiation and some patients in much younger age groups were treated for severe and intractable menorrhagia by the production of a temporary menopause as an alternative to hysterectomy.

A Committee on Radiological Hazards to Patients set up by the Ministry of Health in England stated in its report in 1960 that the induction of a temporary menopause by means of irradiation of the ovaries or attempts in infertile women to stimulate the ovaries by direct irradiation cannot be justified.

There is evidence that the induction of a menopause by the intrauterine insertion of radium for such conditions may be associated with an increased incidence of cancer of the body of the uterus some ten to twenty or more years later (Dickson, 1969). This additional factor has been an important one in determining the present general policy that there are other better and safer methods than irradiation for the treatment of these non malignant conditions.

The destruction of ovarian function by irradiation is, however, sometimes indicated in the treatment of cancer of the breast. There is unequivocal evidence of hormonal dependance in a proportion of cases of cancer of the breast, and regression of skeletal metastases after surgical removal of the ovaries was demonstrated by Beatson in 1896. Ovarian ablation has become a standard procedure in the treatment of many patients with advanced cancer of the breast. Despite the psychological trauma involved, it may be indicated in the treatment of young women with rapidly growing tumours of poor prognosis and for those in the age group around the menopause there are frequent indications. It is of value also sometimes in older women, even ten years after menstruation has ceased.

Surgical removal of the ovaries is the quickest and surest procedure but there are some patients for whom there are contra indications or who refuse surgery and irradiation of the ovaries is an alternative. Although menstruation may be permanently stopped in the case of a woman over 40 years of age by a dose of less than 500 rads to the ovaries, this does not ensure destruction of oestrogenic activity from the ovaries and it is necessary to give higher dosage. A total dose of 2000 rads to each ovary by supervoltage radiation, spread out over a period of three weeks in six or more fractions, does appear to be adequate and can be delivered with only minimal reaction during the course of radiotherapy to the breast tumour.

2. Malignant Disease

Cervix Uteri

The successful treatment of cases of cancer of the cervix by radium insertion was among the first notable achievements of radiotherapy. Techniques became standardized at the Radiumhemmet in Stockholm and at the Fondation Curie in Paris and these two techniques gradually spread throughout the world. They differed in the types of applicator which were used and particularly in the time over which the treatment was given. The Stockholm technique was an interrupted one in which the total dose was given over three weeks in three applications of approximately 24 hours each and the Paris technique was a continuous application over 5 to 7 days with daily removal and replacement of the apparatus. The amounts of radium used were different but the same order of total dose was reached. Both techniques consisted essentially of the introduction of a linear source into the uterine cavity extending from the external os to the fundus and the packing of sources in the lateral fornices of the vagina as far laterally as possible and a further vaginal source below the cervix. Various modifications to these techniques were made, but essentially their principles have been the same and they have persisted as the method of radium treatment of cancer of the cervix for upwards of 50 years.

The dosage at first was empirical and was assessed in terms of milligramme hours or in millicuries destroyed, a function of the strength of the source and the time in which the application was made. The Manchester Clinic in its modification introduced a dosage system which assessed the dose delivered to the tissues at two main points of interest within the pelvis, and further knowledge of dose distribution has enabled accurate calculation to be made of the dose at various other points so that excessive radiation can be avoided at points of vulnerability such as the rectal wall.

The results of radiotherapy in cancer of the cervix throughout the world, the overwhelming majority carried out by intracavitary application of radium or some radioactive nucleide used as a substitute, have been collected and reported annually by an international committee based on Radiumhemmet. An internationally agreed classification of the stages of advancement determined on the basis of clinical examination was drawn up originally under the aegis of the League of Nations and with some subsequent modification is used, with strict criteria for statistical presentation, to give a basis for comparing the results of different clinics.

At the same time that radiotherapy was being developed, the techniques of radical surgical removal were also undergoing rapid development and there has been for many years a considerable division of opinion about the relative advantages and disadvantages of each method of treatment. It was agreed that radiotherapy was the only rational method of treatment for those cases where the growth was fixed and complete surgical ablation could not be performed and it was shown that in addition to palliation some proportion of these cases had prolonged and lasting cure. The argument centred on the earlier case which could be removed by Wertheim's hysterectomy or similar radical surgery. It was shown that the local lesion could be healed in a high proportion of early cases by radium treatment but it was also shown that the best techniques of radium treatment to the cervix would not destroy metastases in lymph nodes at the side wall of the pelvis. Techniques were then devised for supplementary irradiation by X-rays to the parametria and pelvic walls. The combined dose, delivered by the intracavitary radium which falls off rapidly with increasing distance from the cervix and by X-rays directed to the parametria, could be assessed with reasonable accuracy but it was difficult to give unassailable proof that such techniques really destroyed the lymph node metastases.

The argument for radical surgery was that it is not possible to determine, on clinical examination, whether lymph nodes are involved at the pelvic wall or not, that they could be removed efficiently by radical dissection, and that there was no proof that if metastases were present they could be destroyed by radiation.

There have been continued improvements in techniques both in radiotherapy and in surgery and the results of both methods have improved, in terms of long term survival and in reduction of morbidity, and the two opposing points of view have come much closer together.

The use of supervoltage radiation with its increased percentage depth dose and abolition of specific selective absorption in bone has meant that adequate dosage can be delivered to the parametria and pelvic walls with certainty and without excessive reaction to superficial tissues. Accurate techniques, making used of shaped metal filters which modify the dose distribution within the individual radiation beams, have been developed. Using wedge shaped filters, it is possible to build up the dose received at the pelvic wall with a lesser dosage to the already heavily irradiated central portions, which have been the site of the radium treatment. Using this combination technique, an appropriate uniform dosage throughout the pelvic structures can be obtained. There is also now adequate and unequivocal evidence that pelvic lymph node metastases can be destroyed by supervoltage radiation.

Accuracy of dose distribution and dose measurement do not, however, determine the complete elimination and permanent healing of either the primary lesion or the lymph node metastases in all cases. There are variations in the biological response of squamous cell carcinoma of the cervix to radiation and some do not heal completely and some recur after an interval of months or years.

There are now a number of collaborative studies in which initial radiotherapy is followed by radical surgery so that the advantages of both could be obtained and the results in terms of long-term survival and of subsequent morbidity may be of great interest and importance.

It is now possible, with supervoltage radiotherapy, to deliver homogeneous dosage to the whole of the pelvis with a relatively simple technique in women of medium size with three ports of entry, one anterior and two posterolateral or, in large women, with four ports of entry, two anterolateral and two posterolateral. Such techniques have been used in more advanced cases of carcinoma of the cervix in an attempt to cure extensive pelvic disease by external irradiation alone. It appeared that there would be a theoretical advantage in that adequate dosage could be given in this way to all the tissues involved without over-irradiation of superficial tissues and without the complication of the varying dose from intracavitary radium.

It could not be expected that a high proportion of long term cures would result because advanced pelvic growth must mean a likelihood of extra pelvic and more distant metastases. There have been some patients completely healed and without any sign of disease for periods of eight and nine years but there has also been a relatively high proportion of patients who developed local recurrence at the site of the original growth in the cervix. It is in accord with radiobiological studies in general that a larger mass of tumour tissue may be more difficult to destroy by radiation. This is due to several factors, in part being the reduced probability of being able to destroy a larger number of cells with a dose of radiation which is fixed by the tolerance of normal surrounding tissue. In addition there is the likelihood of a larger number of poorly oxygenated cells being present within large tumour masses. There may in the future be alterations in technique leading from further radiobiological knowledge which will alter the problem but at present the practical procedure is to increase the dose in the region of the cervix by the addition of intracavitary radium application.

The problem is not, however, the same as that posed in the earlier years with orthovoltage X-rays, when external irradiation was a supplementary treatment to the main radium application, which was designed to spread the field irradiated as far as possible out to the pelvic walls. It is now possible and advisable to give the required extra dose to the site of the original growth by a more simple technique, consisting of a single applicator with a line source of radium, or of Cobalt-60 as a substitute, extending from below the cervix up to the fundus of the uterus.

The greater knowledge that has been gained about radiation hazards and protection of personnel has brought a realization that the standard intracavitary radium techniques make the greatest single contribution to the dose received by the staff of a radiotherapy department and certainly to the nursing staff of the wards. In order to lessen this dose, modifications in technique have been devised to permit "after loading" of the radium sources. With the patient anaesthetized, suitably shaped applicators not yet loaded with radium are placed in the cavity of the uterus and in the vaginal fornices. They are sufficiently long to project beyond the introitus where they are held rigid by a harness. Subsequently the radium can be quickly inserted into the applicators and later removed with a minimum of exposure. A further development of after loading techniques has been the design of the Cathetron. This apparatus consists of a well protected lead safe in which is housed nine sources of Cobalt-60. By remote control from outside the room the Co-60 sources can be pushed forward with an accuracy of a few millimetres down a flexible catheter which can be attached to a metal catheter already inserted into the uterus or vagina. Three sources and three catheters at one time can be used so that the traditional distribution of radium can be followed if required or a single line source can be used. Each source can be up to four to five curies so that the dose given by the older radium techniques over 24 hours can, if required, be delivered in fifteen minutes.

Such apparatus obviously makes a great contribution to the protection problem and can reduce the dose to personnel to negligible quantities. It also gives the opportunity for flexibility of technique, particularly as regards fractionation of the total dose. There are, however, new questions raised as to possible differences in tissue response and possible dangers from the much greater intensity of radiation.

Corpus Uteri

The usual type of adenocarcinoma of the body of the uterus is sensitive to radiation and if adequate dosage is given it can be made to disappear. When the tumour is operable surgical extirpation is the usual method of choice often after preliminary intracavitary radium therapy. There are patients with inoperable growths and others who because of age or general condition might be deemed unsuitable for operation and who are treated by radiation and a multiplicity of techniques has been used. They vary from a modification of the techniques used for cancer of the cervix with rather heavier dosage in the uterus and less in the vagina, to the use of a spring loop loaded with a number of cobalt sources, the insertion of a line source in the uterus from cervix to fundus with extra sources placed in each cornu of the uterus and filling the whole uterine cavity with multiple beads of Co-60. There is a greater tendency to use external radiation with super-voltage and the same principles apply as in cancer of the cervix, in that additional intracavitary radiation must be given to increase the dose at the site of the maximum tumour. With increasing safety of operation there are fewer patients who are unsuitable for surgery on account of age or general condition and these radiotherapy techniques are mainly confined to the advanced and inoperable cases.

It has been observed with some frequency that recurrence may occur in the vault of the vagina or lower down the vagina or at the introitus after hysterectomy for cancer of the body of the uterus, even though the operation may be a radical one.

Preoperative irradiation by the insertion of radium applicators in the uterus and the vaginal fornices is given in order to reduce the risk of such recurrence.

Preoperative radiation is preferable to postoperative local radiation as, in addition to the delay necessary to allow healing, it is not possible to obtain an adequate distribution of radiation by placing applicators in the vaginal vault. It is the same difficulty of adequate placement of applicators and the consequent limitation of dosage to one side of the growth that makes intracavitary radium treatment of stump carcinoma of the cervix a difficult and unsatisfactory technique. In all such cases the intracavitary radium should be considered as a supplement to planned external radiation of supervoltage quality.

Carcinoma of the Vagina

The majority of cases of carcinoma involving the vaginal walls are initially carcinoma of the cervix which is in an advanced stage of the disease and has spread across one or more of the fornices to invade the vaginal wall. Primary carcinoma of the vagina is relatively rare but the radiotherapist is not uncommonly faced with isolated vaginal recurrence from primary tumours of the body of the uterus, of the ovary and of the cervix after radical hysterectomy.

In the case of advanced carcinoma of the cervix with vaginal involvement the problems are essentially those of treatment of carcinoma of the cervix but it is necessary to include the vagina down to the introitus in the volume of tissue irradiated. This is done by appropriate extension of the fields of external irradiation and by supplementary intracavitary application also extending down to the introitus.

Primary cancer of the vagina, if sufficiently localized, and isolated metastases may be treated satisfactorily by interstitial implantation with needles of radium or Cobalt-60 of appropriate length or by the implantation of radioactive tantalum (Ta, 182, half life 111 days) or iridium wire (Ir-192, half life 74 days), perhaps with a supplementary dose from a central vaginal applicator. In all cases the total dose must be carefully planned and the position of the radioactive sources inserted must be measured after they have been checked by radiography using standard technique.

Carcinoma of the Vulva

Malignant growths of the labia do not usually respond well to radiotherapy, and radical vulvectomy, where this is possible, is a preferable procedure. Even with advanced growths extensive destruction of the whole vulval tissues by diathermy coagulation is usually to be preferred but there is a useful place for radiotherapy in growths around the urethra. They respond well to interstitial implantation of radium needles. A homogeneous dose can be planned and delivered by needles implanted parallel to a catheter in the urethra with a further plane of needles at right angles to this under the mucosa of the vulva.

External irradiation is usually reserved for the palliation of the most advanced tumours.

Cancer of the Ovary

In the great majority of instances, cancer of the ovary comes for irradiation after an initial laparotomy and the problems of radiotherapy vary greatly according to the findings of the initial operation. When the tumour is a localized one, either unilateral or bilateral, it may be considered that the disease has been completely removed by surgery but there are many disappointments seen after what has been apparently a most satisfactory clearance and there does seem to be value in giving postoperative treatment to the whole pelvis by supervoltage radiation as a routine.

Certainly such treatment is indicated if there is doubt about complete removal and in those cases where there is a suspicion of the spilling of malignant cells if a cystic tumour has ruptured during removal. There does appear to be an improvement in the rate of five year survival when post operative irradiation has been given but it is difficult to evaluate individual cases. Patients with observed peritoneal metastases studded over the pelvis have had prolonged survival and apparent cure but it is known that such metastases may regress after laparotomy and removal of the primary tumour without any radiation.

It has been advocated that in cases with operable cancer of the ovary, it is preferable to remove the ovaries but to leave the uterus so that it can be used as a site for intracavitary radium application. The whole problem of external irradiation of the pelvis has been greatly changed by the development of apparatus and the introduction of supervoltage radiation and it would appear to be preferable to make a complete clearance of uterus and ovaries.

Unfortunately many patients are seen with much more advanced disease. Palliation and occasional apparently complete disappearance of a fixed and inoperable tumour can by achieved by external irradiation of the pelvis. Some of them have marked ascites and this may disappear with the response of the primary tumour. When, however, the disease is more widespread throughout the peritoneal cavity and no longer localized in the pelvis the achievement of radiotherapy is much more limited and problematical. There are undoubtedly some cases where multiple tumours studded over the peritoneum do regress but generally radiotherapy to the abdomen above the pelvis is rarely beneficial except to cause regression of an individual mass which may be giving pain.

Heavy radiation of the upper abdomen is also hazardous in that damage may be caused to the kidneys or to bowel, particularly if a loop of intestine is bound down and immobile in association with a mass of growth.

Ascites may sometimes be reduced by the intraperitoneal instillation of radioactive gold or yttrium in colloidal solution but it is doubtful if this is superior for intra-peritoneal therapy to such cytotoxic substances as nitrogen mustard or thiotepa. Intraperitoneal instillations are most useful in cases where there are multiple seedling deposits and are rarely of benefit when large masses of growth can be palpated.

The response to radiotherapy of cancer of the ovary depends on the nature of the primary lesion. In general, papillary adenocarcinoma is moderately radiosensitive but the rarer pseudomucinous growths, usually of slower evolution, are not likely to have any rapid or marked response. Of the rarer tumours dysgerminomas usually have a higher degree of radiosensitivity and radiotherapy has an important role in their treatment.

Inguinal Lymph Nodes

For many years it has been taught that metastases in inguinal lymph nodes were resistant to radiotherapy and that it had little place in their treatment. Experience has shown that the harder qualities of radiation are effective in destroying inguinal lymph node metastases. This has been demonstrated in patients with inoperable metastases and the evidence is unequivocal as the metastases have been demonstrated by biopsy. It has been considered that surgical block dissection of operable inguinal metastases was the most appropriate treatment. Block dissection has not been free from morbidity or from recurrence and there appears a gradual tendency for more stringent selection of early cases for submission to the procedure. It is now reasonable to consider the use of radiation as a preoperative measure or as an alternative to surgery.

DIAGNOSTIC RADIOLOGY

Diagnostic radiology has made outstanding advances in elucidating the problems of every discipline in medicine and in obstetrics and gynaecology it has many a vital role to play.

There are the general examinations necessary and practical for many disciplines in medicine, such as chest radiography, the determination of abnormalities in bone structure, the function of the alimentary tracts and other abdominal organs, and the presence or absence of metastases in bone and soft tissue. Arteriography, venography and lymphography have brought new possibilities for the diagnosis of abdominal and pelvic disease.

Specific to the problems of obstetrics and gynaecology are the examinations of pelvimetry, placentography and utero-salpingography which have become essential methods of investigation and are now used universally.

Such investigations do, however, raise particular problems with regard to the hazards of ionizing radiations. It has been recognized for many years that the ovary is particularly radiosensitive and more recently that the foetus can be damaged by quite small doses of radiation. Although it is radiosensitive at all stages, it has been determined that the foetus is particularly liable to damage during the early weeks of pregnancy in the period of organogenesis and even before the pregnancy is clinically diagnosed. The International Commission on Radiological Protection has made specific recommendations on this subject and the following is an extract from the Commission's report:—

Exposure of Women of Reproductive Capacity

The recommendation permitting dose accumulation at rates up to 3 rems* in a quarter should not apply in circumstances involving abdominal exposure of women of reproductive capacity. Such women should be occupationally employed only under conditions where the dose to the abdomen is limited to 1·3 rems in a quarter, corresponding to 5 rems per year delivered at an even rate. Under these conditions, the dose to an embryo during the critical first two months of organogenesis would normally be less than 1 rem, a dose which the Commission considers to be acceptable. By definition a rem is the quantity of any ionizing radiation such that the energy imparted to a biological system per gramme of living matter by the ionizing particles present in the focus of interest, has the same biological effectiveness as 1 rad of from 200 to 250 KV X-rays* (Roentgen Equivalent Main).

Exposure of Pregnant Women

It is likely that a pregnancy of more than two months duration would be recognized by the woman herself or by her physician. While many of the critical stages of embryogenesis are now past, recent evidence indicates that even after the second month the foetus is still especially radiosensitive. In particular, the possible induction of leukaemia and other malignant conditions must be considered. Recent studies in children indicate that exposure of the foetus in utero to doses of a few rads of X-rays can increase the incidence of malignant disease within the subsequent decade. Furthermore, investigation has shown that exposure of foetuses to doses of a few rads of X-rays can give rise to detectable somatic mutations, resulting in the condition of pigment mosaicism, although this condition does not appear to be hazardous.

In the report of the Committee on Radiological Hazards to Patients set up by the Ministry of Health in England the following is an extract relevant to obstetrics and gynaecology:—

Obstetrics

While diagnostic radiology in obstetrics has undoubtedly contributed to the saving of lives of many mothers and babies, in general all radiological examinations should be kept to a minimum during pregnancy. In particular, radiological examinations of the urinary and alimentary tracts should whenever possible be avoided during pregnancy. Those of the sacro-iliac joints and lumbar spine should whenever possible be deferred until after confinement.

The time when radiation is most likely to cause foetal damage is during the first few weeks. Therefore hysterosalpingography for the diagnosis of early pregnancy is quite unjustified, and even straight X-ray examination should be employed only in exceptional circumstances. Radiological examination for the estimation of foetal maturity should be undertaken only when there is clear need. Multiple pregnancy or breech presentation may properly be established by X-ray examination when the clinical diagnosis is in any doubt. Other malpresentations and suspected foetal abnormality fully justify X-ray examination, as does suspicion of placenta praevia when accurate clinical diagnosis is not immediately feasible.

Pregnant women should be submitted to pelvimetry only after thorough clinical examination by an experienced obstetrician. The full radiological examination is necessary for only a small proportion of primigravidae and a very few multigravidae, but once decided upon the examination should be thorough. Of the four radiographic projections in common use—erect lateral, antero-posterior, subpubic arch and outlet, and supero-inferior or inlet—the last named presents by far the highest dosage to both maternal ovaries and foetal gonads and should be omitted whenever possible.

AVERAGE GONAD DOSES IN MILLIROENTGENS PER EXPOSURE TO FOETAL GONADS AND MATERNAL OVARIES IN PELVIMETRY.

Projection	Dose to	
	Maternal Ovary	Foetal Gonads.
1. Antero-posterior	460	630
2. Lateral	577	535
3. Sub-pubic arch and pelvic outlet	670	140
4. Supero-inferior, pelvic inlet or Thom's	992	2242

In view of the relative magnitude of the maternal and foetal gonad doses delivered in obstetric X-ray procedures, especially pelvimetry, most careful radiographic technique and expert supervision is always desirable. In particular the beam size should be restricted to the smallest dimensions practicable in every instance.

At the present time routine chest X-ray examination may be expected to reveal one active and hitherto unsuspected case of pulmonary tuberculosis for every 500 pregnant women X-rayed and is therefore on this basis worthwhile. To reduce to the minimum the already small genetic hazard involved, full sized films should be used with full precautions and then preferably not after the twenty-fourth week of pregnancy.

In general medical and surgical practice, the possibility of pregnancy should be considered and inquiry made concerning the recent menstrual history of any woman of child-bearing age before any abdominal radiological investigations or the use of radioactive isotopes are instituted.

Gynaecology

Hysterosalpingography is a procedure that demands special co-operation between clinician and radiologist to restrict the number of films and the amount of fluoroscopy. The Panel considers that image intensification should be employed in this procedure whenever feasible. To reduce the exposure in fluoroscopy, full dark adaptation should be achieved before it is performed. Hysterosalpingography should not be carried out after the presumed day of ovulation.

In urinary stress incontinence clinical diagnostic methods are efficacious and cysto-urethrography is required only in quite exceptional circumstances.

In the last few years new methods of investigation have been evolved such as scanning of the body by sensitive counters which will determine the localization of radioactive isotopes absorbed into particular tissues or organs. It is possible to obtain accurate localization of metastases in bone after administration of Ca-47 or Fluorine-18. The site of metastases may be determined by scanning in this way frequently even before they can be visualized by X-ray diagnostic techniques. Techniques have also been devised for placentography by scanning after the administration of radioactive technetium or radioactive indium. It is possible to obtain placental localization by point to point measurement of the site of uptake of the radioactive nucleide with a dose which will deliver as little as 10 millirads to the foetus and with a scanning technique which produces a picture equally informative as that produced by arteriography and X-rays, the dose to the foetus being no more than 20 millirads. This dose of 20 millirads is more than ten times less than that given to the foetus by the X-ray technique if only two films are taken.

It is to be hoped that placental scanning will be adopted for this reason in preference to the alternative techniques of diagnostic radiology and that constant vigilance will always be observed to reduce unnecessary radiological exposure.

REFERENCES

Radiological Hazards to Patients, Second Report of the Committee, Ministry of Health, HMSO, 1960, **35**, 116.

Dickson, R. J. *The Late Results of Radium Treatment for Benign Uterine Haemorrhage*, 1969, Br. J. Radiol., **42**, 582.

Beatson, G. T. 1896, 'On the Treatment of Inoperable Cases of Carcinoma of the Mamma: Suggestions for a new method of Treatment with illustrative cases', *Lancet* 2, 104–107, 162–165.

8. ISOTOPES AND THEIR USE IN RELATION TO OBSTETRICS AND GYNAECOLOGY

HAYAMI FUJIMORI

I. A Concept of Radioactive Isotopes

Matter is composed of molecules, a molecule is composed of atoms, and an atom is constituted chiefly of a central nucleus. The diameter of the nucleus is approximately 10^{-13} cm, while the diameter of the atom as a whole is about 10^{-8} cm.

If we compare an atom with an apple, a molecule consisting of atoms would be the size of the Earth. Around the nucleus rotate small particles called electrons. If the nucleus represents the sun and the electrons the encircling planets, the combination may be thought of as a miniature solar system.

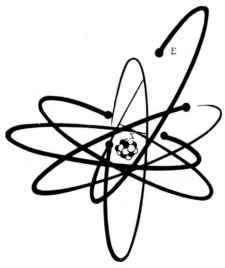

FIG. 1. E: electrons, N: nucleus.

There are two major particles within the nucleus, i.e. the proton and the neutron. The proton has a positive electrical charge and has a mass of 1.7×10^{-24} gram, while the neutron has no electrical charge and is approximately the same mass as the proton. The electron has a negative electrical charge equal in magnitude to that of a proton, and is 1/1840 of the mass of a proton or neutron. Therefore, the mass of the atom is about the same as the total mass of protons and neutrons in the nucleus, because of the low mass of the electrons. An atomic number (Z) is given to each atom according to the number of its protons, and this is the same as the atomic number assigned to the element in the chemical periodic table. The total number of protons and neutrons in the nucleus is termed the mass number.

Based on the precise scientific research of physicists and chemists, it has been confirmed that the chemical characteristics of individual atoms do not depend upon the number of neutrons but upon the number of protons in the nucleus.

All atoms of a given element, therefore, are not necessarily of the same mass. For example, hydrogen exists as one of three types of atoms. The most common type has a single proton in the nucleus and one electron in an orbital ring. The second type of hydrogen atom has a neutron in the nucleus in addition to the proton (Fig. 2). Consequently its mass is twice that of the most common type of hydrogen atom. The third type of hydrogen atom has two neutrons and one proton in the nucleus, and it weighs three times as much as the most common type of hydrogen atom.

There are six forms of the oxygen atom. The most

common form of oxygen has eight neutrons and eight protons in the nucleus, and consequently eight electrons in an orbital ring. The rarer type of oxygen atom has ten neutrons and eight protons in the nucleus (Fig. 3).

The rarer oxygen atoms have the same number of protons and electrons, and therefore the same atomic number, and so they behave chemically in the same way as their more common brothers. They are termed "isotopes".

One hundred and three kinds of atoms, from Hydrogen to Lawrencium have been discovered up to the present.

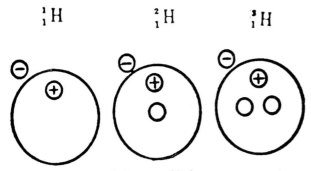

FIG. 2. Isotopes of hydrogen.

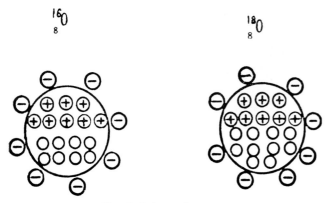

FIG. 3. Isotopes of oxygen.

The physical behavior of the isotopes of an element differs according to the number of particles in the nucleus.

The nucleus of some isotopes is unstable, so that the atom disintegrates to form another atom, emitting during the process some type of radiation.

Three types of radiation were described as *alpha* (α), *beta* (β) and *gamma* (γ) by Rutherford. Additional types of radiation were later discovered.

Alpha radiation consists of alpha particles, which are a combination of two protons and two neutrons. The alpha particle is the same as the nucleus of a helium atom ($_2^4$He).

Beta radiation consists of beta particles. The beta particle is an electron.

Gamma radiation is a kind of electromagnetic wave like x-rays, but generally with a shorter wave length than x-rays.

Among the isotopes, those producing radiation are called "radioactive isotopes (RI)". RI behave chemically in the same way as their stable brothers, but they disinte-

grate to other atoms of different mass while emitting radiation.

For example:

Radium ($_{88}^{226}$Ra) decays to Radon ($_{86}^{222}$Rn), and emits an alpha particle i.e., $_{88}^{226}$Ra $\rightarrow$ $_{86}^{222}$Rn $+$ $_2^4$He.

Radon decays further to Radium A ($_{84}^{218}$Po) and Radium A decays to Radium B ($_{82}^{214}$Pb). By successive disintegrations Radium finally decays in this way to Lead.

In addition to the natural radioactive isotopes such as Radium, many kinds of radioactive isotopes have been produced artificially by physicists, among whom Curie-Joliot, Lawrence, Livingston, Kerst, and McMillan are most famous. Such isotopes are called "artificial radioactive isotopes".

Each radioactive isotope decays at a rate specific for that particular isotope. The time required for 50 per cent of a radioisotope to decay is called the "half-life".

The disintegration scheme of each radioactive isotope is also specific for that particular isotope.

Radioactive isotopes are used in the diagnosis of various diseases, as tracers in the study of organ function, and in the treatment of malignant diseases and also non-malignant diseases, e.g. Thyrotoxicosis. The pattern of radioactive decay type of radiation and the half-life of the individual radioactive isotope are important considerations in selecting the radioisotope to be used.

II. Measurement of Radioactivity

The unit of radioactivity is the curie. It is defined in terms of the number of atoms of the given isotope disintegrating in one second.

1 curie (Ci) = 3.7×10^{10} disintegrations per second

1 millicurie (mCi) = 3.7×10^7 disintegrations per second

1 microcurie (μCi) = 3.7×10^4 disintegrations per second

Special instruments have been designed for the accurate measurement of radioactivity.

III. Special Precautions for the Use of Radioactive Isotopes in the Obstetrical and Gynecological Fields

The application of radioactive isotopes in medical practice has increased markedly in the past ten years Special attention, however, should be paid to techniques for the proper use of radioactive isotopes in the obstetrical and gynecological fields because radioactive isotopes incorporated into the body may have a harmful influence not only on the female genital organs, but in pregnancy, also upon the fetus.

Even with doses hitherto considered safe for diagnosis radioactive pharmaceutical agents may exert a harmful influence upon women when they are pregnant, because then the organs are less resistant and more sensitive to many factors as compared with their resistance and sensitivity in the non-pregnant state.

It is therefore important to take precautions such as selecting the correct radioactive pharmaceutical agent and administering it in the correct dose to cause the minimum amount of harm. We also have to consider the ability of some radioactive pharmaceutical substances to cross the placenta and thus affect the fetus.

I would like to quote the findings from an interesting paper by Weis who used sodium chloride ^{22}Na for a study. Weis reported that the half clearance time of sodium chloride ^{22}Na from the uterus was doubled whenever the pregnancy was complicated by toxaemia, bleeding, infection or by a twin pregnancy.

When discussing this paper Holly commented as follows: Recent studies at Johns Hopkins University as reported by the National Academy of Science suggests 25r as the safe total maximum irradiation for patients up to the age of 30.

IV. Diagnostic Use of Radioactive Isotopes

(1) Method of Detection of Uterine Cancer using ^{32}P

Radioactive phosphorus (^{32}P) emits only beta particles as it decays to stable sulfur. Its half-life is 14·3 days; the peak energy of its beta particle is 1·7 mev., with an average energy of 0·7 mev.; the maximum range of tissue penetration is about 8 mm., and the average range is approximately 2 mm.

All tissues of the body contain phosphorus. Phosphorus introduced into the blood stream in the form of a readily diffusible phosphate ion will be incorporated in all tissues of the body, and especially those tissues which utilize phosphorus in their metabolic processes. The rapidly

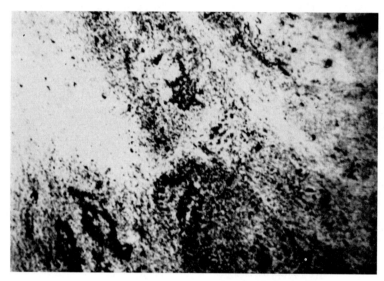

Fig. 4. Microradioautograph of cancerous tissues of the uterus.

Kety estimated that the exposure for the fetus in utero was 2·5r when 5μCi of ^{24}Na was given. ^{24}Na is an isotope with a shorter half life than ^{22}Na. Holly asked Dr. Bruns whether an estimate of total irradiation had been made for ^{22}Na, especially in patients who had been the subject of a serial study.

^{24}Na or ^{131}I has been used diagnostically for locating the placenta, but ^{99m}Tc or ^{113m}In which has far less radiation effect upon the fetus is now being used as a tracer (see p 717).[1] ^{131}I is widely used in order to evaluate thyroid function as well as to measure the quantity of circulating thyroid hormone. It should however be remembered that ^{131}I administered to a pregnant woman passes through the placenta and may effect the fetus by its accumulation in the thryoid tissue (see Chapter by Tuchmann-Duplessis Sec. XII, Chap. 2. In 1959 a new *in vitro* test for thyroid function was developed by Hamolsky *et al*. Using this test no radioactive pharmaceutical agents were administered to pregnant women and therefore the harmful effect to the fetus was avoided (see p. 717).

growing malignant tumor tissue takes up this element in significantly greater amount than normal tissue, so this element can be used for the detection of uterine cancer. Many methods are described in medical literature (e.g. by Schubert, by Müller, by Tabuchi, and by Iwai). These methods, however, all have certain disadvantages. A method devised by the author Fujimori in 1958 is considered to be more rational in principle and simpler in technique.

It was confirmed by the author that, after ^{32}P administration, a greater number of black spots could be seen micro-radioautographically in malignant cells than in other cells.

The radioactivity of the four phosphorus fractions of these cancerous tissues was measured with a Geiger-Müller counter, i.e. the radioactivity of acid-soluble phosphorus, the RNA phosphorus, the DNA phosphorus and phospholipid. According to the results obtained, the acid-soluble phosphorus fraction showed the highest specific radioactivity. Many researchers believe that acid-soluble phosphorus is more abundant in malignant than in normal cells.

---

[1] The physical half life of ^{22}Na is 2·6 years, of ^{24}Na is 15 hours.

From these findings it is believed that ^{32}P administered as a tracer is concentrated in cancerous tissues in significantly greater amounts than in other tissues, and therefore that malignant changes in the cervix can be shown by increased radioactivity.

In the past, a solution of ^{32}P was injected intravenously or intramuscularly and had to pass into the general circulation before reaching the uterus. Relatively large doses were necessary in order to get a measurable concentration in the malignant tissue.

The author administered the ^{32}P (in the form of sodium acid phosphate in 20 ml. of 20% glucose solution), 1 to 5 microcuries per kg. of body weight into the femoral artery, simultaneously occluding it distally (Fig. 5 and 6). This

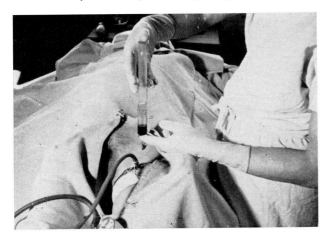

FIG. 5. Administration of ^{32}P into the femoral artery, simultaneously occluding it distally.

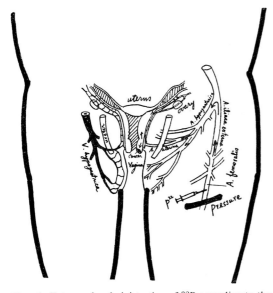

FIG. 6. Retrograde administration of ^{32}P according to the method mentioned in Fig. 5.

procedure forced retrograde passage of the tracer solution into the uterine arterial circulation without passing through the rest of the body, bringing a much higher concentration of ^{32}P to the lesion with a lower total dosage, than with intravenous injection.

In 19 patients with proved cervical cancer (including 6 cases of carcinoma in situ) and 14 with benign erosion or no lesion of the cervix, radio-phosphorus was administered as above. At two, four, twelve and twenty-four hours after injection biopsy specimens were taken, dried and ashed, and their radioactivity was measured with a Geiger-Müller counter. Simultaneously blood was drawn and the radioactivity of the dry-ashed serum samples was measured. Expressed in counts per minute per gram of tissue or serum, the radioactivity of the cervical biopsy specimens was expressed as a percentage of the radioactivity of the serum.

Fourteen of the 19 cases (or 73%) with proved malignancy gave a value of more than 120% of the serum value, while of the 14 cases without malignancy (one a glandular erosion and the other a mucous polyp), only 2 cases (or 14%) gave a value over 120%. It is of great interest that four of the six cases of carcinoma in situ (the so-called Stage 0) gave a value higher than the demarcation level of 120%. In any case, these results show that a significantly higher percentage of malignant lesions gave a radioactivity value of over 120% of that of serum in comparison with nonmalignant lesions of the cervix.

The radioactivity of lymph nodes with and without histologically demonstrable cancerous metastases was measured four to six hours after the administration of ^{32}P when the radical removal of uterine cancer was performed, and was compared with that of simultaneously drawn sera. It was also of interest that in metastatic malignancy there was a statistically significant difference between the radioactivity of involved and uninvolved lymph nodes.

Clinical application of this method was performed as follows: A needle-type Geiger counter (probe counter) of 0·8-cm diameter and 18·5 cm length was found to be useful for measuring radioactivity of the external and internal surfaces of the cervix after the intra-arterial injection of ^{32}P. A cervix with malignant lesions showed a radioactivity two to four times higher than those without such lesions.

The diagnostic accuracy of various methods of detecting cancer of the cervix was compared with that of the final histological diagnosis (Table 1).

TABLE 1

Histological Diagnosis	Malignant		Non-malignant (erosion)	
Colposcopy	79/82	96·5%	204/205	99·0%
^{32}P	69/79	90·7%	109/113	97·0%
Gross examination	184/224	82·1%	277/300	90·3%
Smear	72/82	87·0%	118/126	94·0%

The diagnostic accuracy of this method of detecting cancer of the cervix was 90·7% in 79 cases with proven cancer and 97·0% in 113 cases without cancer.

It is also possible to detect local and distant metastases of choriocarcinomas using ^{32}P.

A patient with malignant chorionepithelioma with metastases to the vaginal wall and with neurological signs and abnormal brain-wave patterns indicating metastases in the right parietal lobe of the brain, was given ^{32}P intramuscularly. The needle counter inserted into the vagina near the metastases gave significantly higher counts than other normal parts of the body. Furthermore, the counts over the right parietal lobe were higher than over the left parietal lobe.

(2) Method of Determining the Patency of the Fallopian Tubes using Radioactive Isotopes

A method of determining the patency of the Fallopian tubes using radioactive isotopes was introduced by Stabile and Leborgne in 1956. This method consists of the measurement of radioactivity excreted into the vagina through the Fallopian tubes, the uterine cavity and the cervical canal, after radioactive gold colloid (^{198}Au) has been injected into the abdominal cavity.

In 1956 Fujimori published another method using radioactive phosphorus ^{32}P to determine the patency of the Fallopian tubes and called this method "radio-intubation".

Radio-intubation is based on the fact that the patency of the Fallopian tubes can be judged from the appearance of radioactivity in the urine measured every five minutes, after 5 ml. of sterile saline solution containing 1μCi/ml of ^{24}Na or ^{32}P has been introduced into the uterine cavity (Fig. 7–10). Experimental results obtained are shown in Figure 10.

When the Fallopian tubes on both sides are functioning and patent, the radioactivity in the urine begins to rise within only five minutes from the introduction of the solution into the uterine cavity, and the peak is reached in about thirty minutes. This is due to the fact that the solution flows out into the abdominal cavity through the Fallopian tubes, is absorbed into the general circulation through the peritoneum and is then excreted in the urine.

When the Fallopian tubes on both sides are occluded, radioactivity in the urine shows less increase with a lower peak about thirty minutes after the introduction of the solution.

When the tube on one side is occluded or the tubes on both sides are in a spastic condition, the peak of the curve is reached in about thirty minutes, but the curve is not as steep or as high as the curve for patent Fallopian tubes on both sides, but it is steeper and higher than the curve for occluded Fallopian tubes on both sides (Fig. 11).

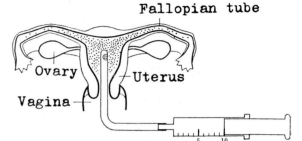

FIG. 7. "Radio intubation".

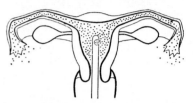

FIG. 8. A case with patent fallopian tubes on both sides.

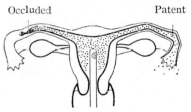

FIG. 9. A case with patent fallopian tube on one side.

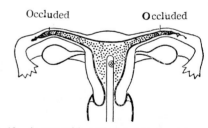

FIG. 10. A case with occluded fallopian tubes on both sides.

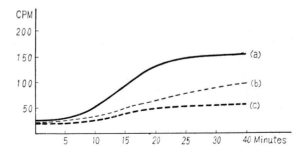

(a) CPM in the urine of a case with patent fallopian tubes on both sides.
(b) CPM in the urine of a case with a occluded fallopian tube on one side.
(c) CPM in the urine of a case with occluded fallopian tubes on both sides.

FIG. 11. Three kinds of CPM curves indicating the patency of the fallopian tubes.

The author believes the radiation effects of the radioactive isotopes as used here are negligible because of the small dose administered. Even with very much greater dosage no harmful effect upon Drosophila was found experimentally.

There was good correlation between this method and gross findings at laparotomy in 89% of the cases.

It can be said that this method is simple and is rapid for diagnosing patency of the Fallopian tubes. It however, has the disadvantage that there is no kymographic record and no X ray photograph such as are obtained with conventional Rubin testing or hysterosalpingography.

(3) Method of Estimating Thyroid Function using ^{131}I

^{131}I is used widely to evaluate thyroid function as well as to measure circulating thyroid hormone. It should, however, be remembered that ^{131}I administered to the pregnant woman passes through the placenta and may produce some untoward effect upon the fetus.

Hamolsky et al. developed in 1959 an in vitro test for thyroid function based upon their fundamental study in 1957 on the uptake of liothyronine by red blood cells as a method of estimating thyroid function.

Mitchell was the first to modify the test by using an anion exchange resin in place of red blood cells. However, the characteristics of granular resins vary from day to day. To simplify the Triomet-131 (liothyronine^{131}I) uptake test, Abbott Laboratories developed an exclusive Triosorb resin sponge (polyurethane resin-embedded sponge) which acts as a replacement for red blood cells in the blood cell uptake test.

The resin-sponge offers several advantages over red blood cells:—increases the accuracy of handling in the laboratory, reduces the time required, and obviates the use of red blood cells, thus increasing the safety and simplicity of the in vitro uptake test.

Clinical results on Japanese women obtained by the Triosorb test in the author's department are as follows:

1. The mean value of the Triosorb test using resin-sponge (RSU), was 29.5 ± 1.9% at the high-temperature phase of basal body temperature and 28.1 ± 1.2% at the low-temperature phase of basal body temperature in healthy adult women.

2. The mean value of RSU in pregnant women at two months was 27.1 ± 1.75% and at seven months 20.3 ± 1.8%.

3. The value of RSU five days post partum was 21.5 ± 0.8%, that is, much lower than normal. It returned, however, to the normal value at one month post partum.

4. The mean value of RSU in women complaining of sterility (184 cases) was 30.0 ± 0.6%.

5. The mean value of RSU in pregnant women with threatened abortion (17 cases) revealed 28.4 ± 1.5%. Therefore, if the value of RSU in pregnant women shows continuous increase in repeated tests, this could indicate threatened abortion, except in the presence of hyperthyroidism.

(4) Scintigram

(a) Scintiscanning for determining the location of the placenta. ^{131}I-labelled and ^{132}I-labelled human serum albumin (HSA), (Weinberg et al., 1957; Hibbard, 1961); ^{24}Na chloride (Browne and Veall, 1950); ^{51}Cr-labelled red cells (Paul et al 1963) and ^{51}Cr-labelled HSA (Johnson et al., 1964) have been used for placental scanning. Recently however, ^{99m}Tc (McAfee et al., 1964) and ^{113m}In (Stern et al., 1967) are most widely used.

^{99m}Tc can be obtained as the daughter nuclide of ^{99}Mo (half life 2.5 days). The physical half-life is 6 hours. β emission is absent and 140-KeV γ ray is emitted.

^{113m}In can be obtained as the daughter nucleide of the long lived parent ^{113}Sn (half-life 118 days) in a nuclide generator. The physical half-life is 1.7 hours, the β emission is absent and 390-Kev γ ray is emitted.

Because of the characteristics mentioned above of both these pharmaceutical products maternal and fetal exposure with either is theoretically lower than with any of the others mentioned, namely ^{131}I, ^{132}I, ^{24}Na, ^{51}Cr.

The maternal and fetal exposure has been estimated in practice by some authors as follows:

Normal Placenta

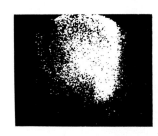 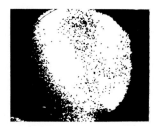

anterior left lateral

Patient N.M. 8M
Prognosis Nomal Delivery

Fig. 12. Scinticamera. ^{113m}In Cl$_3$ 3mCi (Illustration reproduced by permission of Dr. H. Kakeki.)

Placenta Praevia

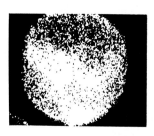 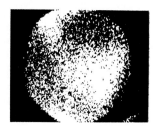

anterior right lateral

Patient O.T. 8M
Prognosis Cesarean Section

Fig. 13. Scinticamera. ^{113m}In Cl$_3$ Ci. (Illustration reproduced by permission of Dr. H. Kakeki.)

Weinberg *et al* (1963) estimated the exposure at 85 millirad in maternal blood, 41·8 millirad in the maternal ovary, 230 millirad in the maternal thyroid gland, 5·4 millirad in the fetus with a higher concentration of 26 millirad in the fetal thyroid gland, after placental scanning using 5μCi of ^{131}I-HSA.

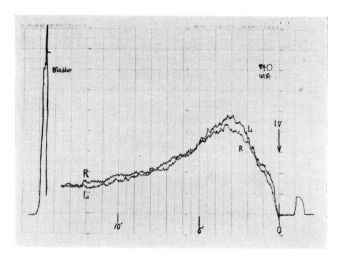

FIG. 14. Renogram revealing normal function on both sides. (Illustration reproduced by permission of Dr. Y. Mitani and Dr. R. Shukuwa.)

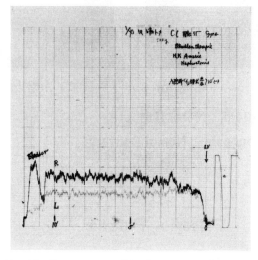

FIG. 15. Renogram revealing the presence of extensive damage to kidney function on both sides. (Illustration reproduced by permission of Dr. Y. Mitani and Dr. R. Shukuwa).

Y. Anno (1968) estimated the exposure at 7·2 millirad in the maternal ovary, 4·8 millirad in the fetus. On the other hand J. McAfee (1964) estimated the concentration in the fetal thyroid gland at 10–35 millirad.

Anno (1968) estimated the exposure at 8·9 millirad in the maternal ovary and 11·3 millirad in the fetus after placental scanning using 1000 Ci of [113m]InFe (OH)3Y had been carried out.

It can be seen that in placental scanning using [113m]In little or no activity is localized in the region of the bladder from excretion of the radio-pharmaceuticals. This results

in an important advantage for [113m]In transferrin over [99m]TcHSA. If the excretion in the bladder had been of a high level confusion would arise with a low-lying placenta as it does in placental scanning using [99m]TcHSA (Kakeki).

(b) Radioactive Isotope Renogram (RIRG). The procedure is as follows: 5 ml. of physiological saline solution or distilled water containing 20–30μCi of ^{131}I-Hippuran is injected intravenously and the concentration of gamma-emitting isotope passing through the kidney tissue is recorded at the lumbar surface over the kidney using a scintillation detector and collimator designed for RIRG.

Figure 14 shows renograms of the kidneys with normal function on both sides.

Figure 15 shows renograms of a patient 49 years of age with cancer of the cervix in stage IV. The renogram reveals the presence of extensive damage to kidney function on both sides due to the advanced uterine cancer.

V. Therapeutic Use of Radioactive Isotopes in the Gynecological Field

Radioactive isotopes recently used for the therapy of gynecologic malignant tumors are: [226]Ra, ^{60}Co, [198]Au, ^{32}P, [157]Cs.

(1) [60]Co

[226]Ra was used widely up to ten years ago, following the discovery of this element by the Curies. However, as one of the big contributions made in the use of atomic energy in the medical field, the discovery of the biological action of ^{60}Co has caused this radioisotope to take a prominent place in therapy.

Radioactive cobalt, ^{60}Co, a product deliberately irradiated in a reactor, has a half-life of 5·3 years. It decays to [60]Ni by emitting a beta particle of 0·31 mev and gamma radiations of 1·17 and 1·33 mev.

The advantages of ^{60}Co over radium in therapeutic use are its flexibility in the form of its application, i.e. needles, solution, suspension, plaster-like form, pearl-like particles, non-flaking corrosion-resistant alloy, and its low cost. However, the short half-life of 5·3 years is a serious disadvantage.

(a) Local irradiation. Small needles of ^{60}Co are inserted into malignant tissue in the cervical canal in place of small sources of [226]Ra.

(b) Split method of Barnes. Twelve or more long ^{60}Co needles are inserted into the parametrial and cervical tissues. This method is effective in advanced uterine cancer. It is, however, not widely used because of extensive side effects.

(c) Application of ^{60}Co solution. A rubber bag is inserted into the urinary bladder, and ^{60}Co solution is instilled into the rubber bag for the treatment of cancer of the bladder and surrounding tissues.

The use of isotope solution in the bladder had a run for a short time, but is not now seriously considered except, perhaps, for some cases of multiple papillomatoma. There has been a great deal of fibrosis of the bladder caused by this technique (Sir Brian Windeyer).

(d) Application of small ^{60}Co rods in a nylon tube. Small rods of ^{60}Co are put into a nylon tube until it is filled to the desired length. At surgical intervention in uterine cancer, the tube is threaded into the tissues close to lymph node metastases, which are irradiated locally by the ^{60}Co string.

The suture is removed after several days, when adequate local irradiation has been received.

(e) Plastic Radio-Cobalt preparation—the so-called Plastobalt Macro method of Becker and Scheer. (Figs. 16

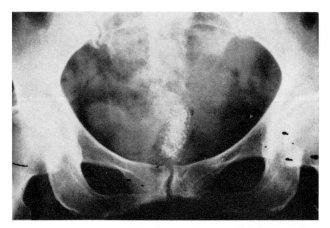

FIG. 16. Plastobalt Macro inserted into the vagina.

and 17.) Plastic chicle gum is impregnated with many small ^{60}Co particles, 0·2 mm. in diameter and with 40μCi radioactivity in each particle.

This preparation is called "Plastobalt Macro" supplied by Buchler A. G. Plastobalt Macro is suitable for use in local irradiation of a cancerous region with an uneven

bladder or rectum. This procedure is very effective for the treatment of inoperable cancer (Fig. 18).

(g) Cobalt teletherapy. One of advantages of cobalt teletherapy is the cheapness of this source. The source costs less than $10,000 and yet it provides the radiation equivalent of $25 million worth of radium.

Another advantage of cobalt teletherapy is that radiation from this source offers better skin tolerance, less absorption in bone, more accurate tumor dosage and better depth dosage than that from conventional X-ray machines. Therefore, radioresistant carcinomas of the cervix and advanced ovarian cancer may be treated effectively by cobalt teletherapy.

(2) Radioactive Cesium ^{137}Cs

Radioactive cesium, ^{137}Cs, is a fission product which has a half-life of 37 years.

^{137}Cs decays to ^{137}Ba by emitting beta particles of 0·5 meV and 1·20 meV, and gamma radiation of 0662 meV from ^{137}Ba.

^{137}Cs has a lower energy than ^{60}Co, but longer half-life than the latter. This source, therefore, appears to be the most economical and desirable isotope for teletherapy.

However, the radiational output from the same volume of a source of ^{137}Cs is less than that of a source of ^{60}Co. The sphere of irradiation therefore is limited.

(3) Radioactive Gold ^{198}Au

Radioactive gold, ^{198}Au, has a half-life of 2·69 days. It decays to mercury, ^{198}Hg, with two beta emissions of 0·29 (1%) and 0·97 (99%) meV and three gamma emissions

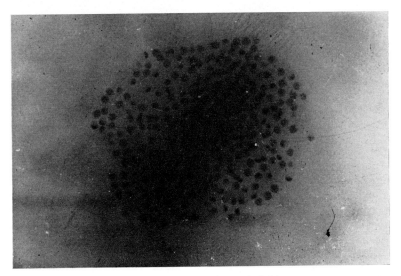

FIG. 17. X-ray picture of plastobalt Macro.

surface, for example, a cauliflower-like or crater-like surface.

(f) ^{60}Co pearl method devised by Jones and Kepp and Czech, Becker and Scheer. Many pieces of ^{60}Co pearls each 0·6 mm. in diameter respectively are joined in a long chain on a thread, and the chain is inserted into the uterine cavity, the cervical canal, vaginal canal, urinary

of 0·411 (100%), 0·68 (1%) and 1·09 (0·2%) meV. The relatively low energy beta particles have a short range of a maximum of 3·8 mm. in tissue or water with an average energy of 0·32 meV, and an average path of less than 1 mm.

^{198}Au is used clinically in the form of a sterile colloidal solution for the treatment of ovarian cancer and carcinomatous peritonitis and pleurisy by intracavitary infusion.

A colloidal solution of ^{198}Au with particle sizes in the range of 0·003 to 0·007 micron to 0·1 to 0·2 micron is most widely used for interstitial, intratumoral and intracavitary injection.

The initial maximum dose into an abdominal cavity with a cancerous effusion is 150 mCi as recommended by Abbott Laboratories, with subsequent infusion as required at monthly intervals. In some cases, however, nausea, vomiting, weakness, malaise, paralytic ileus and diarrhoea are observed as characteristic systematic side effects of ^{198}Au infusion.

In the author's experience, a ^{198}Au dose of 150 mCi is too much for the Japanese female patient. A dose of

studies on the mechanism of ^{198}Au as a cancerocidal agent *in vivo* and *in vitro*, it may be said that radio-gold particles penetrate into cancer tissue and into normal tissue. When colloidal radio-gold ^{198}Au is injected intraperitoneally, a large part of it is fixed to the serous lining, thus reducing effusion from the peritoneum, and is fixed to the surface of the cell membrane, thus helping to destroy the cancer cell. A small quantity is picked up by the lymphatic system and the blood stream, and is then deposited in the spleen and liver or excreted in the faeces and urine.

Carcinocidal effects of colloidal radio-gold ^{198}Au are not intensive. There is a little superficial injury to the tumor surface, causing a certain superficial fibrosis and

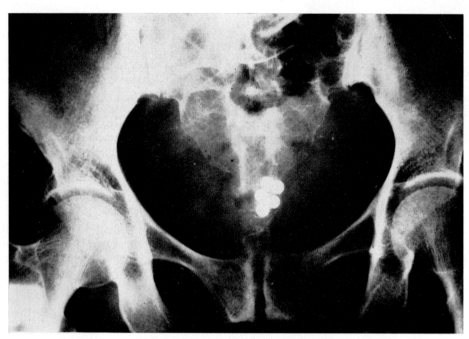

FIG. 18. Five pieces of ^{60}Co pearls inserted into the uterine cavity.

50 mCi of ^{198}Au per month for intra-abdominal cavitary infusion is used, and it has been found safe and effective for the Japanese female patient.

Intratumoral and interstitial injection of ^{198}Au for uterine cancer. Intratumoral injection of colloidal gold ^{198}Au results in many millions of point sources emitting beta rays diffusely throughout the injected volume of tissue. Considerable effect can be obtained in the cancerous tissue with relatively little damage to the surrounding normal tissue because the tissue penetration of beta radiation from the colloidal radio-gold is relatively short. A further advantage of colloidal radio-gold ^{198}Au is that concentration of this substance in regional lymph nodes by reticuloendothelial phagocytosis has been observed after its intraparametrial injection. The author, however, cannot yet confirm the therapeutic significance of the concentration of colloidal radio-gold in the regional lymph nodes for the treatment or prophylaxis of lymph node metastases.

Mechanism of colloidal gold ^{198}Au as a cancerocidal agent. Based on the experimental results of the author in

some capillary injury along with the inhibitory influence on the production of malignant ascites. Following the above-mentioned influence of ^{198}Au on malignant lesions, the patient feels much better subjectively and has increased appetite, so that life may be prolonged. No complete cure, however, is expected from the administration of colloidal radio-gold ^{198}Au alone.

(4) Radioactive Phosphorus ^{32}P

In the obstetrical and gynecological fields, no radioactive phosphorus is used routinely for therapeutical purposes. In the author's clinic, it has been confirmed experimentally that ^{32}P has a mild carcinocidal effect, and in the U.S.A. has been found helpful in the control of ascites.

REFERENCES

Abbott Laboratories (1960), "Trimet™ (Radio-L-Triiodothyronine) for use in an in Vitro test in the Diagnosis of Thyroid Disease," *Radio-Pharmaceuticals by Abbott.*
Abbott Laboratories (1965), "Triosorb™ Abbott's T-3 Diagnostic KIT," *Abbott Radio-pharmaceuticals March* 1965.

Barnes, A. C., Morton, J. L. and Callendine, G. W., Jr. (1950), "Use of Radioactive Cobalt in the Treatment of Carcinoma of the Cervix," *Amer. J. Obstet. Gynec.*, **60**, 1112.

Becker, J. und Scheer, K. E. (1956), "Die radioaktiven Isotopen in der Geburtshilfe und Gynäkologie," *Fortschtschritte der Geburtshilfe und Gynäkologie III.* Basel: S. Krager AGG.

Czech, H., Kepp, R. K., and Wolthaus, G. (1950), "Ergebnisse der Behandlung der bösartigen Genitaltumoren an der Universitäts-Frauenklinik Göttigen in der Jahren 1937–44," *Strahlentherapie*, **82**, 321.

Czech, H. (1951), "Die intrauterine Radiumbestrahlung des Gebärmutterkörperkarzinom an der Universitäts-Frauenklinik Göttingen," *Strahlentherapie*, **84**, 524.

Fujimori, H. (1955), "Radioactive Isotopes in Obstetrical and Gynecological Fields" (published in Japanese), Igakushoin Ltd., Tokyo, Japan.

Fujimori, H. (1958), "Some New Applications of Radioactive Isotopes in the Obstetrical and Gynecological Fields," *J. Jap. Obstet. Gynec. Soc.*, **5**, 227.

Fujimori, H. und Kawai, I. (1961), "Diagnostische Untersuchungen des Uteruskarzinom mit Radioisotopen," *Zbl. für Gynäk.*, **83**, 5.

Fujimori, H. and Noda, S. (1965), "Diagnosis of Metastases of Choriocarcinomas using Radioactive Isotope ^{32}P." Read at the 3rd Asiatic Congress of Obstetrics and Gynecology, 11–13 January, 1965.

Fujimori, H., Yamada, F., Morimura, M., Yonekawa, W., Toyama, T. and Kawabata, O. (1966), "Application of Triosorb Test in the Fields of Obstetrics and Gynecology," *Jap. J. Nucl. Med.*, **3**. Proceedings of 5th Annual Meeting of the Japanese Society of Nuclear Medicine, 29, 30 August, 1965, Kyoto.

Hamolsky, M. W., Stein, M. and Freedberg, A. S. (1957), "The Thyroid Hormone-Plasmo Protein Complex in Man. LI. A New in Vitro Method for Study of 'Uptake' of Labelled Hormonal Components by Human Erythrocytes," *J. Clin. Endocr.*, **17**, 33.

Hayashi, M., Koizumi, H. and Kimura, K. (1958), "A method for Diagnosis of the Patency of the Fallopian tubes using ^{198}Au," (published in Japanese), *Sanka to Fujinka*, **25**, 947.

Iwai, M. and Fukuda, T. (1964), "Diagnosis of Uterine Cancer using ^{32}P" (published in Japanese), *Kaku Igaku*, **1**, 32.

Jones, D. E., cited by Schwiegk S. 681.

Kakeki, H. (1966), "Scintigram using ^{99m}Tc," read at the 6th Annual Meeting of the Japanese Society of Nuclear Medicine, Tokyo.

Mitani, Y., Seki, T., Soo, C., and Sawa, T. (1964), "Some Observations on Renogram of Outpatients with Carcinoma of the Uterine Cervix after Discharge as a Screening Renal Function Test," *Jap. Nucl. Med.*, **3**, 72.

Mitani, Y., Shukuwa, R., Seki, T., Soo, C., and Sawa, T. (1966), "On Renograms of the Urinary Tract Changes of Gynecological Diseases Except for Carcinoma of the Uterine Cervix," *Jap. Nucl. Med.*, **5**, 58.

Mitchell, M. L., Handen, A. B. and O'Rourde, M. E. (1960), "The In-vitro Resin Sponge Uptake of Triodothyronine-^{131}I from Serum in Thyroid Disease and in Pregnancy," *J. Clin. Endocr*, **20**, 1474.

Müller, J. H. (1953), "Tumordiagnostik, Künstliche Radioaktive Isotope in Physiologie Diagnostik und Therapie redigiert von H. Schwiegk," Berlin, Göttingen, Heidelberg: Springer-Verlag, S.584.

Schubert, G. (1955), "Die Radioisotope in Diagnostik und Therapie," *Arch. Gynäk.*, **186**, 337.

Schwiegk, H. (1955), "Künstliche Isotope in Physiologie Diagnostik und Therapie redigiert von H. Schwiegk," Berlin, Göttingen, Heidelberg: Springer-Verlag.

Stabile, A., Leborgne, F. (1956), "Emploi des radioisotopes (Au 198) pour l'étude de la perméabilité tubaire isopéristaltique," *Gynéc. prat.*, **7(5)**, 259.

Stabile, A. and Leborgne, F. E. (1956), "Emprego de radio-isotopos (Au 198) no estudo da permeabilidate tubária isoperistáltica," *An. brasil. Ginec.*, **42**, 1.

Tabuchi, A. (1958), *The 10th Annual Meeting of Japanese Society of Obstetrics and Gynecology*, **10**, 1164.

Tubis, M. (1964), "A Review of Original Radioisotope Research Projects. Lecture presented under the sponsorship of the Japanese Society of Nuclear Medicine and the Japanese Radioisotope Association, April, 1964."

Weis, E. B. Jr., Bruns, P. D. and Stewart Taylor, F. (1958), *Amer. J. Obstet. Gynec.*, **76**, 340.

METRICATION

Since some of our contributors have started to use the International System of units in writing their chapters, we have thought it wise to incorporate, with permission, the major part of the pamphlet *Metrication in Scientific Journals*, published by The Royal Society of London, 1968.

THE EDITORS

SI (which is the abbreviation in many languages for Système International d'Unités) is an extension and refinement of the traditional metric system. It embodies features which make it logically superior to any other system as well as practically more convenient: it is rational, coherent and comprehensive.

It is fortunate that now that the time has come to discard completely the time-honoured native units (which are not without their advantages), there is to hand a fully developed International System to take their place. Over the years much thought has been given to extending and improving the metric system until finally in 1960 the Conférence Générale des Poids et Mesures, the body responsible for maintaining standards of measurements (of which the U.K. is an active participant), formally approved SI. Already nearly thirty countries have decided to make it the only legally accepted system and it is destined to become the universal currency of science and commerce.

The main features of SI are as follows:

1. There are six basic units (see below), the metre and kilogramme taking the place of the centimetre and gramme of the old metric system.
2. The unit of force, the newton (kg m s^{-2}), is independent of the Earth's gravitation, and the often confusing introduction, in some branches of science and technology, of g into equations is no longer necessary.
3. The unit of energy in all forms is the joule (newton × metre), and of power the joule per second (watt); thus the variously defined calories, together with the kilowatt hour, the B.t.u. and the horsepower are all superseded.
4. 'Electrostatic' and 'electromagnetic' units are replaced by SI electrical units.
5. Multiples of units are normally to be restricted to steps of a thousand and similarly fractions to steps of a thousandth.

Lists are appended of the basic SI units, of some derived SI units, of compatible units, and also examples of units which run counter to SI, the use of which is accordingly to be actively discouraged. Also listed are the names and symbols of the prefixes representing numerical factors: these are both convenient in obviating the need to write large numbers of zeros or in some instances high powers of 10, and also helpful in establishing familiarity with the numerical framework of modern science. It will be noted that the recommended prefixes are limited to $10^{\pm 3n}$.

BASIC SI UNITS

Physical Quantity	Name of Unit	Symbol for Unit
Length	metre	m
Mass	kilogramme	kg
Time	second	s
Electric current	ampere	A
Thermodynamic temperature	degree Kelvin	°K
Luminous intensity	candela	cd

Symbols for units do not take a plural form.

SUPPLEMENTARY UNITS

Physical Quantity	Name of Unit	Symbol for Unit
Plane angle	radian	rad
Solid angle	steradian	sr

These units are dimensionless.

DERIVED SI UNITS WITH SPECIAL NAMES

Physical Quantity	Name of Unit	Symbol for Unit	Definition of Unit
Energy	joule	J	kg m^2 s^{-2}
Force	newton	N	kg m s^{-2} = J m^{-1}
Power	watt	W	kg m^2 s^{-3} = J s^{-1}
Electric charge	coulomb	C	A s
Electric potential difference	volt	V	kg m^2 s^{-3} A^{-1} = J A^{-1} s^{-1}
Electric resistance	ohm	Ω	kg m^2 s^{-3} A^{-2} = V A^{-1}
Electric capacitance	farad	F	A^2 s^4 kg^{-1} m^{-2} = A s V^{-1}
Magnetic flux	weber	Wb	kg m^2 s^{-2} A^{-1} = V s
Inductance	henry	H	kg m^2 s^{-2} A^{-2} = V s A^{-1}
Magnetic flux density	tesla	T	kg s^{-2} A^{-1} = V s m^{-2}
Luminous flux	lumen	lm	cd sr
Illumination	lux	lx	cd sr m^{-2}
Frequency	hertz	Hz	cycle per second
Customary temperature, t	degree Celsius	°C	$t/°C = T/°K - 273.15$

FRACTIONS AND MULTIPLES

Fraction	Prefix	Symbol	Multiple	Prefix	Symbol
10^{-1}	deci	d	10	deka	da*
10^{-2}	centi	c	10^2	hecto	h*
10^{-3}	milli	m	10^3	kilo	k
10^{-6}	micro	μ	10^6	mega	M
10^{-9}	nano	n	10^9	giga	G
10^{-12}	pico	p	10^{12}	tera	T
10^{-15}	femto	f			
10^{-18}	atto	a			

* To be restricted to instances where there is a strongly felt need, such as may be experienced in the early days of metrication in favour of the centimetre as the unit of length in certain biological measurements.

Compound prefixes should not be used, e.g. 10^{-9} metre is represented by

$$1 \text{ nm, } not \text{ } 1 \text{ m}\mu\text{m}.$$

The attaching of a prefix to a unit in effect constitutes a new unit, e.g.

$$1 \text{ km}^2 = 1 \text{ (km)}^2 = 10^6\text{m}^2$$

$$not \text{ } 1 \text{ k(m}^2) = 10^3\text{m}^2.$$

Where possible any numerical prefix should appear in the numerator of an expression.

EXAMPLES OF OTHER DERIVED SI UNITS

Physical Quantity	SI Unit	Symbol for Unit
Area	square metre	m²
Volume	cubic metre	m³
Density	kilogramme per cubic metre	kg m⁻³
Velocity	metre per second	m s⁻¹
Angular velocity	radian per second	rad s⁻¹
Acceleration	metre per second squared	m s⁻²
Pressure	newton per square metre	N m⁻²
Kinematic viscosity diffusion coefficient	square metre per second	m² s⁻¹
Dynamic viscosity	newton second per square metre	N s m⁻²
Electric field strength	volt per metre	V m⁻¹
Magnetic field strength	ampere per metre	A m⁻¹
Luminance	candela per square metre	cd m⁻²

UNITS TO BE ALLOWED IN CONJUNCTION WITH SI

Physical Quantity	Name of Unit	Symbol for Unit	Definition of Unit
Length	parsec	pc	30·87 × 10¹⁵ m
Area	barn	b	10⁻²⁸ m²
	hectare	ha	10⁴ m²
Volume	litre	l	10⁻³ m³ = dm³
Pressure	bar	bar	10⁵ N m⁻²
Mass	tonne	t	10³ kg = Mg
Kinematic viscosity diffusion coefficient	stokes	St	10⁻⁴ m² s⁻¹
Dynamic viscosity	poise	P	10⁻¹ kg m⁻¹ s⁻¹
Magnetic flux density (magnetic induction)	gauss	G	10⁻⁴ T
Radioactivity	curie	Ci	37 × 10⁹ s⁻¹
Energy	electronvolt	eV	1·6021 × 10⁻¹⁹ J

Until such time as a new name may be adopted for the kilogramme as the basic unit of mass, the gramme will often be used, both as an elementary unit (to avoid the absurdity of mkg) and in association with numerical prefixes, e.g. μg.

EXAMPLES OF UNITS CONTRARY TO SI WITH THEIR EQUIVALENTS*

Physical Quantity	Unit	Equivalent
Length	ångström	10⁻¹⁰ m
	inch	0·0254 m
	foot	0·3048 m
	yard	0·9144 m
	mile	1·609 34 km
	nautical mile	1·853 18 km
Area	square inch	645·16 mm²
	square foot	0·092 903 m²
	square yard	0·836 127 m²
	square mile	2·589 99 km²
Volume	cubic inch	1·638 71 × 10⁻⁵ m³
	cubic foot	0·028 316 8 m³
	U.K. gallon	0·004 546 092 m³
Mass	pound	0·453 592 37 kg
	slug	14·593 9 kg
Density	pound/cubic inch	2·767 99 × 10⁴ kg m⁻³
	pound/cubic foot	16·0185 kg m⁻³
Force	dyne	10⁻⁵ N
	poundal	0·138 255 N
	pound-force	4·448 22 N
	kilogramme-force	9·806 65 N
Pressure	atmosphere	101·325 kN m⁻²
	torr	133·322 N m⁻²
	pound (f)/sq. in.	6894·76 N m⁻²
Energy	erg	10⁻⁷ J
	calorie (I.T.)	4·1868 J
	calorie (15°C)	4·1855 J
	calorie (thermochemical)	4·184 J
	B.t.u.	1055·06 J
	foot poundal	0·042 140 1 J
	foot pound (f)	1·355 82 J
Power	horse power	745·700 W
Temperature	degree Rankine	$\frac{5}{9}$ °K
	degree Fahrenheit	$t/°F = \frac{9}{5}T/°C + 32$

* Fuller lists are to be found in the National Physical Laboratory's *Changing to the metric system* (Anderton & Brigg). London: H.M.S.O. (1966).

INDEX